Gynecological Imaging

Jean Noel Buy
Michel Ghossain

Gynecological Imaging

A Reference Guide to Diagnosis

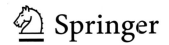 Springer

Jean Noel Buy

Service Radiologie
Hopital Hotel-Dieu
Paris
France

Michel Ghossain
Department of Radiology
Hotel Dieu de France
Beirut
Lebanon

ISBN 978-3-642-31011-9   ISBN 978-3-642-31012-6   (eBook)
DOI 10.1007/978-3-642-31012-6
Springer Heidelberg New York Dordrecht London

Library of Congress Control Number: 2013932135

Printed on acid-free paper

Springer is part of Springer Science+Business Media (www.springer.com)

To Ouria for all her advices, the quality of her work in the follow up of the files and in the archive of the bibliography, for her help in the elaboration and the accomplishment of this project.
To Amanda, my daughter, to Roxane.
To my Parents and all my Family.

Foreword

Gynecologic Imaging is a new book by Prof. Jean-Noel Buy which intergrades the fundamental science of gynecologic disease with the powerful abilities of modern digital imaging techniques. I have known Jean-Noel since he arrived in San Francisco in 1980 to study advanced digital imaging in my laboratory. Quick to recognize the potential of digital imaging in the understanding of abdominal and gynecologic disease, he was able to publish a number of original papers based upon his work in San Francisco. Returning to France he rapidly rose to the rank of Full Professor at the oldest and most famous hospital in Paris – The Hotel Dieu Hospital where much of the incredible material, found in *Gynecologic Imaging* was amassed. *Gynecologic Imaging* is the triumph of Dr. Buy's career and deserves to become a classic text which correlates gynecologic science with the modern imaging techniques of Computed Tomography, Ultrasonography, and Magnetic Resonance Imaging.

Jean-Noel Buy is eminently qualified to write this authoritative text. His career has been spent at a hospital with a special focus on gynecologic disease. The scope and depth of material available has enabled a truly unique and comprehensive text to be written. Approximately 1,000 pages in length the book is organized into 10 parts and 37 chapters. Multiple color drawings, tables, charts as well as macroscopic and microscopic findings are closely correlated with over 4,000 superb digital images. Readers will find the clarity and cohesiveness of a book, written almost exclusively by one author, refreshing. The radiologist, gynecologist, surgeon, medical student and all clinicians involved in the diagnosis and treatment of gynecologic disease will acquire a greater ability to understand, interpret and integrate the imaging findings in gynecologic disease and how to best use this knowledge in daily clinical practice.

Jean-Noel presented his idea to write a definitive text on gynecologic disease to me several years ago. I have enjoyed watching and at times discussing with Jean-Noel the book's progress. While it has taken time to complete, the wait has been worth it. I believe *Gynecologic Imaging* will rapidly find a place in the library of all who are or will be involved in the diagnosis and treatment of the wide spectrum of gynecologic abnormalities.

Seattle, Washington

Albert A. Moss, MD, FACR
Professor of Radiology
Chairman Emeritus
University of Washington School of Medicine

Acknowledgments

My heartfelt thanks and gratitude to:

1. Professor J. Ecoiffier and Professor D. Vadrot who allowed me to become a Professor of Radiology.
2. Professor Albert A. Moss (Full Professor in University of California in San Francisco) and later Chairman (in University of Washington in Seattle) who played an important role in my knowledge and capabilities which have enriched me, and played an essential role in my formation.

   Professor A. Margulis (Chairman in the University of San Francisco) who graciously accepted me for a visiting fellowship and who instructed me in UCSF.
3. Thanks to the gynecologists, surgeons and pathologists who enabled me to advance in the knowledge and way to deal with patients and to establish correlations between radiology and clinical, surgical and pathological findings. Thanks to Professor Pujade Eric, oncologist who created the Gineco group, where the most uncommon cases particularly of adnexal masses were discussed.

   Heartfelt thanks to Missis Ute Heilmann who accepted realization of this project, Claus-Dieter Bachem who showed deep concern in guiding me in the edition and giving me precious advices, Alwin Metter in the realization of pictures and drawings, Karthikeyan for all his appropriate questions for the revisions and Meike Stoeck for the numerous advantages in directing me.

Jean Noel Buy

Contents

3 Peritoneum

Contents

6   Broad Ligament

7   Complications of Adnexal Masses

8   Pelvic Inflammatory Disease (PID)

Contributors

Mourad Aissat, MD Surgical Department, Cochin Hospital, Paris, France

Jean Paul Akakpo, MD Radiology Department, La Pitie Salpetriere Hospital, Paris, France

Bruno Deval, MD Surgical Department, Geoffroy Saint Hilaire Clinic, Paris, France

Kamel Hassen, MD Radiology Department, Hotel Dieu Hospital, Paris, France

Denis Jacob, MD Gynecological Surgery, Paris, France

Danielle Hugol, MD Pahology Department, Hotel Dieu Hospital, Paris, France

Pascal Rousset, MD Radiology Department, Hotel Dieu Hospital, Paris, France

Catherine Sciot, MD Radiology Office (Private Practice), Rue Pierre Louys, Paris, France

Dominique Vadrot, MD Radiology Department, Hotel Dieu Hospital, Paris, France

General

Part 1

Embryology of the Urogenital System and Intersexual Disorders

1

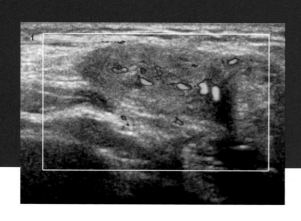

Contents

1.1   Embryology of the Urogenital System

The urogenital system develops from the intermediate mesenchyme derived from the dorsal body wall of the embryo (Fig. 1.1).

At the beginning of the third week, an opacity formed by a thickened linear band of epiblast—the primitive streak—appears caudally in the median plane of the dorsal aspect of the embryonic disc.

Shortly after the primitive streak appears, cells leave its deep surface and form mesenchyme, a tissue consisting of loosely arranged cells suspended in a gelatinous matrix. Mesenchymal cells are ameboid and actively phagocytic.

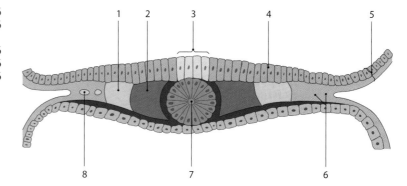

Fig. 1.1 *1* Intermediate mesenchyme (mesoderm), *2* paraxial mesoderm, *3* neural groove, *4* embryonic ectoderm, *5* amnion, *6* coelomic spaces, *7* notochord, *8* lateral mesoderm [Adapted from Moore [1]]

J.N. Buy, M. Ghossain, *Gynecological Imaging*,
DOI 10.1007/978-3-642-31012-6_1, © Springer-Verlag Berlin Heidelberg 2013

3

Mesenchyme forms the supporting tissues of the embryo, such as most of the connective tissues of the body and connective tissue framework of glands.

Some mesenchyme forms mesoblast (undifferentiated meso-derm) which forms the intraembryonic or embryonic mesoderm.

A longitudinal elevation of mesoderm, the urogenital ridge, forms on each side of the dorsal aorta. The part of the urogenital system giving rise to the urinary system is the nephrogenic cord; the part giving rise to the genital system is the gonadal ridge

1.1.1 Development of the Urinary System [1]

1.1.1.1 Kidneys and Ureters

Pronephroi

They are represented by a few clusters and tubular structures in the neck region

The pronephric ducts run into the cloaca.

The pronephroi soon degenerate; most of the length of the pro-nephric ducts persists and is used by the next set of kidneys.

Mesonephroi (Figs. 1.2 and 1.3)

They appear late in the fourth week caudal to the rudimentary pronephroi.

They consist of glomeruli and tubules. The mesonephric tubules open into bilateral mesonephric ducts, which were originally the pronephric ducts.

The mesonephric ducts open into the cloaca.

The mesonephric ducts degenerate toward the end of the first trimester.

Metanephroi (Fig. 1.4)

The primordial of permanent kidneys begins to develop early in the fifth week, from two different sources:
1. The metanephric diverticulum is an outgrowth from the meso-nephric duct near its intrance into the cloaca. The stalk of the diverticulum becomes the ureter and the cranial portion the col-lective system.
2. The metanephrogenic blastema is derived from the caudal part of the nephrogenic cord.

1.1.1.2 Urinary Bladder

The expanded terminal part of the hindgut, the cloaca, is an endo-derm-lined chamber that is in contact with the surface ectoderm at the cloacal membrane. The cloaca receives the allantois ventrally, which is a fingerlike diverticulum.

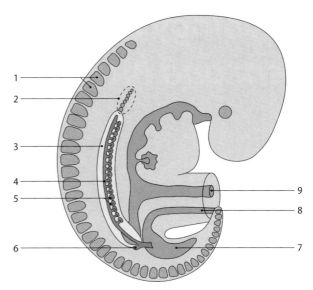

Fig. 1.2 *1* Somites, *2* pronephros, *3* nephrogenic cord, *4* mesonephric duct, *5* mesonephric tubules, *6* metanephric diverticulum, *7* cloaca, *8* allantois, *9* omphaloenteric duct [Adapted from Moore [1]]

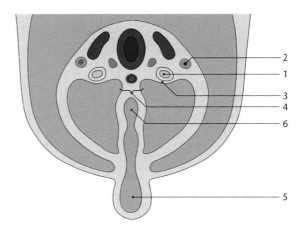

Fig. 1.3 *1* Nephrogenic cord, *2* nephrogenic duct, *3* urogenital ridge, *4* dorsal mesentery, *5* umbilical vesicle, *6* midgut [Adapted from Moore [1]]

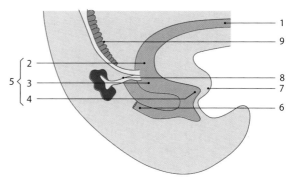

Fig. 1.4 *1* Allantois, *2* vesical part, *3* pelvic part, *4* phallic part, *5* urogenital sinus, *6* rectum, *7* genital tubercle, *8* metanephric diverticulum, *9* meso-nephros [Adapted from Moore [1]]

The cloaca is divided by a wedge of mesenchyme, the urorectal septum (Figs. 1.4 and 1.5), that develops between the allantois and the cloaca, in two parts:

The rectum and cranial part of the anal canal dorsally

The urogenital sinus ventrally

By the seventh week, the urorectal septum has fused with the cloacal membrane (Fig. 1.6), dividing it into a dorsal membrane and a larger ventral urogenital membrane. The area of fusion of the urorectal septum with the cloacal membrane is represented in the adult by the perineal body.

The urogenital system is divided in three parts:

A cranial vesical part that forms the bladder, but its trigone is derived from the caudal ends of the mesonephric ducts.

A middle pelvic part that becomes the entire urethra in females.

A caudal phallic part that grows toward the genital tubercule (primordium of the clitoris).

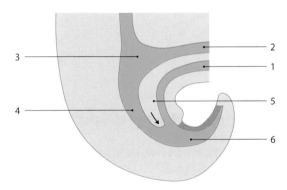

Fig. 1.5 *1* Allantois, *2* omphaloenteric duct, *3* midgut, *4* hindgut, *5* urorectal septum (with *arrow*), *6* cloaca [Adapted from Moore [1]]

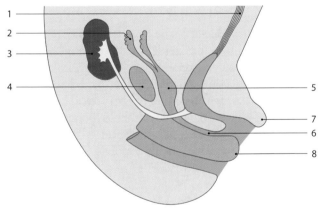

Fig. 1.6 *1* Urachus, *2* uterine tube, *3* kidney, *4* ovary, *5* uterus, *6* vagina, *7* clitoris, *8* urorectal septum [Adapted from Moore [1]]

1.1.1.3 Urethra

The entire urethra is derived from endoderm of the urogenital sinus.

1.1.2 Development of the Gonads

The gonads are derived from three sources:
1. Mesothelium (mesodermal epithelium) lining the posterior abdominal wall
2. Underlying mesenchyme (embryonic connective tissue)
3. Primordial germ cells

1.1.2.1 Indifferent Gonad

At the fifth week, a thickened area of mesothelium develops on the medial side of the mesonephros. Proliferation of this epithelium and the underlying mesenchyme produces a bulge on the medial side of the mesonephros—the gonadal ridge (Fig. 1.7). Fingerlike epithelial cords—the gonadal cords—soon grow into the underlying mesenchyme. The indifferent gonad consists of an external cortex and an internal medulla.

1.1.2.2 Primordial Germ Cells

These large spherical cells are visible early in the fourth week among the endodermal cells of the umbilical vesicle (yolk sac) near the origin of the allantois.

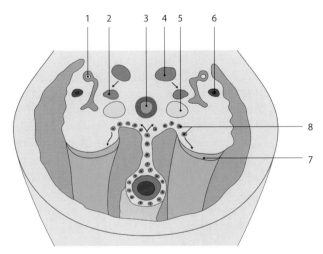

Fig. 1.7 *1* Mesonephric duct, *2* suprarenal medulla, *3* aorta, *4* sympathic ganglion, *5* suprarenal cortex, *6* paramesonephric duct, *7* gonadal ridge, *8* primordial germ cells [Adapted from Moore [1]]

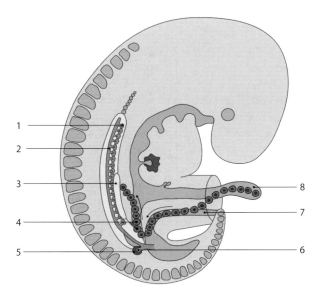

Fig. 1.8 *1* Mesonephros, *2* mesonephric duct, *3* primordium of gonad, *4* primordial germ cells, *5* metanephrogenic blastema, *6* metanephric diverticulum, *7* allantois, *8* umbilical vesicle (yolk sac) [Adapted from Moore [1]]

During folding of the embryo, the dorsal part of the umbilical vesicle is incorporated into the embryo.

As this occurs, the primordial germ cells migrate along the dorsal mesentery of the hindgut to the gonadal ridges (Fig. 1.8).

During the sixth week, the primordial germ cells enter the underlying mesenchyme and are incorporated in the gonadal cords.

1.1.2.3 Sex Determination

Development of the male phenotype requires a Y chromosome. The SRY gene for a testis-determining factor (TDF) has been localized in the sex-determining short arm region of the Y chromosome. It is the TDF regulated by the Y chromosome that determines testicular differentiation. Under the influence of this organizing factor, the gonadal cords differentiate into seminiferous cords.

Development of the female phenotype requires two X chromosomes. A number of genes and regions of the X chromosome have special roles in sex determination. Consequently, the type of sex chromosome complex established at fertilization determines the type of gonad that differentiates from the indifferent gonad. The type of gonad present then determines the type of sexual differentiation that occurs in genital ducts and external genitalia.

Testosterone, produced by the fetal testes, dihydrotestosterone (see Chap. 3), a metabolite of the testosterone, and the anti-Mullerian hormone (AMH) determine normal male sexual differentiation. Primary female sexual differentiation in the fetus does not depend on hormones; it occurs even if the ovaries are absent and apparently is not under hormonal influence.

1.1.2.4 Development of Testes

TDF induces the gonadal cords to condense and extend into the medulla of the indifferent gonad, where they branch and anastomose to form the rete testis.

The rete testis becomes continuous with 15–20 mesonephric ducts that become efferent ductules. These ductules are connected with the mesonephric duct, which becomes the duct of the epididymis.

1.1.2.5 Development of the Ovaries

Before birth, the ovary is not identifiable histologically until approximately the tenth week.

Gonadal cords do not become prominent, but they extend into the medulla and form a rudimentary rete ovarii.

Cortical cords extend from the surface epithelium of the developing ovary into the underlying mesenchyme during the early fetal period (Fig. 1.9). This epithelium is derived from the mesothelium.

As the cortical cords increase in size, primordial germ cells are incorporated into them.

At 16 weeks, these cords break up into isolated clusters of primordial follicles each of which consists of an oogonium, derived from a primordial germ cell, surrounded by a single layer of flattened follicular cells derived from the surface epithelium.

Although many oogonia degenerate before birth, the two million or so that remain enlarge to become primary oocytes before birth.

After birth, the surface epithelium of the ovary flattens to a single layer of cells continuous with the mesothelium of the peritoneum at the hilum of the ovary.

1.1.3 Development of Genital Tract [1]

1.1.3.1 Development of the Female Genital Ducts and Glands

1. During the fifth and sixth weeks, the genital system is in an indifferent state. Two pairs of genital ducts are present the mesonephric ducts (or Wolffian ducts) and paramesonephric ducts (or Muller ducts) (Fig. 1.7).
2. The paramesonephric ducts develop lateral to the gonads and to mesonephric ducts on each side from longitudinal invaginations of the mesothelium on the lateral aspects of the mesonephroi. The edges of these paramesonephric grooves approach each other and fuse to form the paramesonephric ducts. The funnel shaped cranial ends of these ducts open into the peritoneal cavity. Caudally, the paramesonephric ducts run parallel to the mesonephric ducts until they reach the future pelvic region of the embryo. Here, they cross ventral the mesonephric ducts, approach each other in the median plane, and fuse to form a Y-shaped uterovaginal primordium (Fig. 1.6).
3. This tubular structure projects in the dorsal wall of the *urogenital sinus*[1] (see definition later) and produces an elevation, the sinus tubercle, which defines the site of the future hymeneal membrane.
4. Contact of the uterovaginal primordium with the urogenital sinus induces the formation of paired endodermal outgrowths—the sinovaginal bulbs. They extend from the urogenital sinus to the caudal end of the uterovaginal primordium. The sinovaginal bulbs fuse to form a vaginal plate. Later, the central cells of this plate break down, forming the lumen of the vagina.

---

[1] At fifth week, a septum divides the cloaca into rectum and urogenital sinus that later on will give rise to bladder, urethra, and phallus.

Fig. 1.9 (**a**) (At the *top*) *1* Neural tube, *2* sympathetic ganglion, *3* aorta, *4* paramesonephric duct, *5* primordium of suprarenal medulla, *6* primordium of suprarenal cortex, *7* hindgut, *8* gonadal ridge, *9* indifferent gona, *10* primordial germ cells, *11* primary sex cord, *12* mesonephric duct, *13* aggregation of neural crest cells. (**b**) (*Below*) *14* Uterine tube, *15* surface epithelium, *16* primordial, ovarian follicle, *17* mesonephric duct and tubule, *18* degenerating rete ovarii [Adapted from Moore [1]]

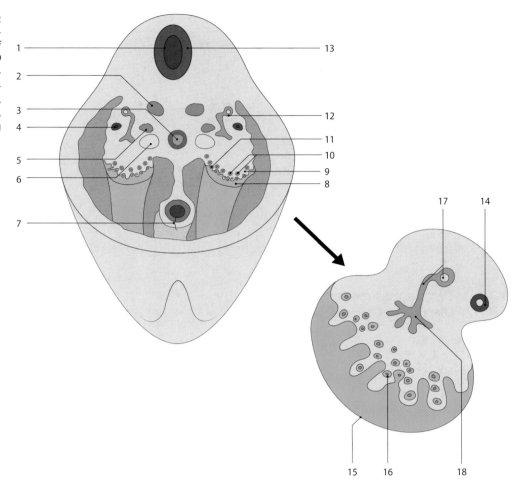

The epithelium of the vagina is derived from the peripheral cells of the vaginal plate.

Until fetal life, the lumen of the vagina is separated from the cavity of the urogenital sinus by a membrane—the hymen. The membrane is formed by invagination of the posterior wall of the urogenital sinus, resulting from expansion of the caudal end of the vagina. The hymen usually ruptures during the perinatal period.

The unfused portion of the ducts gives rise to the tubes. The uterovaginal primordium gives rise to the body and cervix of the uterus and superior part of the vagina.

The anatomical origin of tubes, uterus, and vagina is summarized in Table 1.1.

At tenth week, the Mullerian ducts are completely fused (entire septum gone).

Fusion of the paramesonephric ducts also brings together a peritoneal fold that forms the broad ligament and two peritoneal compartments the rectouterine pouch and the vesicouterine pouch. Along the sides of the uterus, between the layers of the broad ligament, the mesenchyme proliferates and differentiates into cellular

Table 1.1 Anatomical origin of tubes, uterus, and vagina

Muller ducts	
Unfused part	Tubes
Uterovaginal primordium(fused part)	Uterus body and cervix
	Upper vagina
Urogenital sinus:	Lower vagina

tissue the parametrium, which is composed of loose connective tissue and smooth muscle.

The histological origin of epithelium and connective tissue of tubes, uterus, and vagina is summarized in Table 1.2.

The urogenital sinus in which the vagina opens enlarges as the embryo growths, so that it becomes the vestibule of the adult external genitalia.

Consequently, the vestibule is lined, except for a variable portion anterior to the urethral orifice, by the endodermal epithelium of the urogenital sinus.

Table 1.2 Histological origin of epithelium and connective tissue of tubes, uterus, and vagina

Embryological origin	Type of tissue of tube, uterus, and vagina
1. Muller duct of mesodermal origin	
Mesothelium	Epithelial component of the tubes the uterus body, the cervix
Mesenchyme	Subepithelial stroma of the mucosa (tube, uterine corpus, endocervix, upper part of the vagina)
	Muscularis (tube, myometrium, upper vagina)
	Muscularis and fibrous stroma of the cervix
2. Urogenital sinus	
Mesenchyme	Muscularis of the lower part of the vagina
3. Peripheral cells of the vaginal plate	Epithelium of the vagina

Table 1.3 Mesonephric ducts, remnants, and location

Appendix vesiculosa	Cranial end of the mesonephric duct	Lateral to ovary
Epoophoron	Efferent ductules and duct of the epididymis	Mesovarium
Paroophoron	Rudimentary tubules	Mesosalpinx
Gartner's duct cyst	Ductus deferens and ejaculatory duct	Mesometrium Lateral wall of the uterus and vagina

1.1.3.2 Mesonephric Ducts Remnants

In female embryos, the mesonephric ducts regress because of the absence of testosterone, and only a few nonfuctional remnants persist (Table 1.3).

The mesonephric ducts, remnants, and their location are reported in Table 1.3.

1.1.3.3 Development of the Male Genital Ducts and Glands

In the presence of fetal testes:
- Sertoli cells begin to produce Müllerian-inhibiting substance (MIS), also called anti-Mullerian hormone (AMH), at 7 weeks. MIS causes the paramesonephric ducts to disappear by epithelial-mesenchymal transformation.
- Interstitial cells produce testosterone in the eighth week. Testosterone stimulates:
  (a) The mesonephric ducts which will give rise to the epididymis and the ductus efferens
  (b) Glands development:
    – Seminal glands (from lateral outgrowths of the caudal end of each mesonephric duct)
    – Prostate (from the prostatic part of the urethra)
    – Bulbourethral glands (from the spongy part of the urethra) The paramesonephric ducts remnants are reported in Table 1.4.

Table 1.4 Paramesonephric ducts, remnants, and location

Hydatid of Morgagni	Cranial end of the paramesonephric duct	Lateral to infundibulum

1.1.4 Development of External Genitalia and of the Inguinal Canals [1]

1.1.4.1 Common Development in Female and Male

Up to the seventh week, the external genitalia are similar in both sexes. Distinguishing sexual characteristics begin to appear during the ninth week, but the external genitalia are not fully differentiated until the 12th week.

In the fourth week, proliferating mesenchyme produces a *genital tubercle at the cranial end* of the cloacal membrane (Fig. 1.10).

Labioscrotal swellings and urogenital folds soon develop on each side of the cloacal membrane. The genital tubercle elongates to form a primordial phallus

When the urorectal septum fuses with the cloacal membrane at the end of the sixth week, it divides the cloacal membrane in a dorsal anal membrane and a ventral urogenital membrane (Fig. 1.11).

The urogenital membrane lies in the floor of a median cleft, the urethral groove, which is bound by the urogenital folds. The anal and urogenital membranes rupture a week later, forming the anus and urogenital orifices. The urethra and the vagina open in a common cavity, the vestibule.

1.1.4.2 Development of Male External Genitalia

Masculinization of the indifferent external genitalia is induced by testosterone produced by the interstitial cells of the fetal testes.

As the phallus enlarges and elongates to become the penis, the urethral folds form the lateral walls of the urethral groove on the ventral surface of the penis.

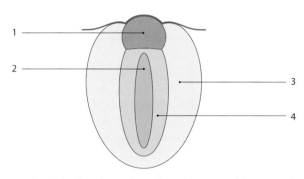

Fig. 1.10 *1* Genital tubercle, *2* cloacal membrane, *3* labioscrotal swelling, *4* urogenital fold [Adapted from Moore [1]]

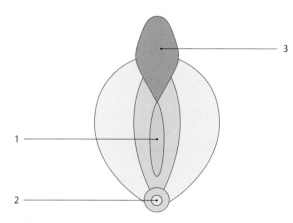

Fig. 1.11 *1* Urogenital membrane, *2* anal membrane, *3* primordial phallus [Adapted from Moore [1]]

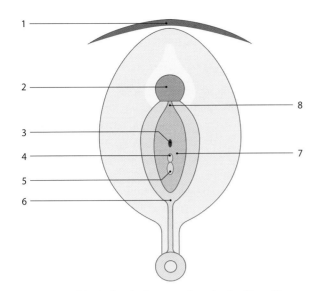

Fig. 1.12 *1* Mons pubis, *2* clitoris, *3* external urethral orifice, *4* hymen, *5* vaginal orifice, *6* posterior labial commissure, *7* vestibule of vagina, *8* anterior labial commissure [Adapted from Moore [1]]

1.1.4.3 Development of Female External Genitalia (Fig. 1.12)

(a) The primordial phallus gradually becomes the clitoris.
(b) The urogenital folds fuse posteriorly to form the frenulum of the labia minora or nymphes. The unfused parts form the labia minora.
(c) The labioscrotal folds fuse posteriorly to form the posterior labial commissure and anteriorly to form the anterior labial commissure and the mons pubis. The unfused parts form the labia majora.

1.1.4.4 Auxiliary Genital Glands

Buds grow from the urethra into the surrounding mesenchyme and form the bilateral mucus-secreting urethral glands and paraurethral glands. These glands correspond to the prostate in the male.

Outgrowths from the urogenital sinus form the greater vestibular glands in the lower third of the labia majora. These tubuloalveolar glands also secrete mucus and are homologous to the bulbourethral glands in male.

1.1.4.5 Development of the Inguinal Canals

(a) The gubernaculum. As the mesonephros degenerates, a ligament the gubernaculum develops on each side of the abdomen from the caudal pole of the gonad.
The gubernaculum passes obliquely through the developing anterior abdominal wall at the site of the future inguinal canal and attaches caudally to the internal surface of the labioscrotal swellings (future labia majora).

The gubernaculum is also attached to the uterus near the attachment of the uterine tube. The cranial part becomes the ovarian ligament, the caudal part the round ligament of the uterus.

(b) The processus vaginalis. The processus vaginalis is an evagination of peritoneum, develops ventral to the gubernaculum, and herniates through the abdominal wall along the path formed by the gubernaculum. The vaginal process carries along extensions of the layers of the abdominal wall with it, which forms the walls of the inguinal canal. This relatively small processus vaginalis obliterates and disappears before birth. A processus vaginalis that persists after birth is called a *canal of Nuck*.

1.1.5 The Adult Derivatives and Vestigial Remains of Embryonic Urogenital Structures

These are reported in Table 1.5 [1].

Table 1.5 Adult derivates and vestigial remains of embryonic urogenital structures

Male	Embryonic structure	Female
Testis	**Indifferent gonad**	Ovary
Seminiferous tubules	**Cortex**	Ovarian follicles
Rete testis	**Medulla**	Rete ovarii
Gubernaculum testis	**Gubernaculum**	Ovarian ligament
		Round ligament
Efferent ductules of testis	**Mesonephric tubules**	Epoophoron
Paradidymis		Paroophoron
Appendix of epididymis	**Mesonephric duct**	Appendix vesiculosa
Duct of the epididymis		Duct of the epoophoron
		Gartner duct
Ductus deferens		
Ureter, pelvis calices, collecting tubules	**Metanephric diverticulum**	Ureter, pelvis calices, collecting tubules
Appendix of testis	**Paramesonephric duct**	Hydatid (Morgagni) Tube
		Uterus
		Vagina (upper part)
Bladder	**Urogenital sinus**	Bladder
Urethra		Urethra
Prostatic utricle		Vagina (lower part)
Prostatic gland		Urethral and paraurethral glands
Bulbourethral glands		Greater vestibular glands
Seminal colliculus	**Sinus tubercle**	Hymen
Penis	**Phallus**	Clitoris
Ventral aspect of penis	**Urogenital folds**	Labia minora
Scrotum	**Labioscrotal swellings**	Labia majora

According to Ref. [1]

1.2 Intersexual Disorders [2]

1.2.1 Definition

Intersexuality implies a discrepancy between the morphology of the gonads (testes/ovaries) and the appearance of the external genitalia [2].

Intersexual conditions are classified according to the histologic appearance of the gonads [2].

1.2.2 Classification

Classification of these disorders is reported in Table 1.6.

Table 1.6 Classification of intersexual disorders

> **1. Disorders associated with a normal chromosome constitution**
>   **1. Female pseudohermaphrodism**
>   Fetal defect
>   **Androgenital syndrome**
>   21-alpha-hydrxoylase deficiency
>   11-beta-hydroxylase deficiency
>   Maternal influence
>   Maternal ingestion of progestins and androgens
>   Maternal virilizing tumor
>   **2. Male pseudohermaphrodism**
>   Gonadal defects
>   **Persistent Mullerian duct syndrome**
>   **End-organ defects**
>   Disordered androgen receptor binding
>   **Androgen insensitivity syndrome** (testicular feminization)
>   Disordered testosterone metabolism
>   5-alpha-reductase deficiency
> **2. Disorders associated with an abnormal chromosome constitution**
> **Sexual ambiguity infrequent**
>   Klinefelter syndrome
>   Turner syndrome
>   Pure gonadal dysgenesis
> **Sexual ambiguity frequent**
>   True hermaphrodism = ovarian and testicular tissue in the same or opposite gonads
>   Mixed gonadal dysgenesis = abnormal testis + contralateral streak gonad

1.2.3 Description of the Disorders

These disorders are classified in two main categories according to the fact there are associated with a normal or an abnormal chromosome constitution.

1.2.3.1 Disorders Associated with a Normal Chromosome Constitution

Female Pseudohermaphrodism

Female pseudohermaphrodism occurs as a result of excessive androgens in utero in an individual. The main findings are:

Karyotype XX.

Two ovaries.

Elevated level of androgens during embryogenesis, which usually results in phenotype male.

Tumors, if appearing, are always benign.

A Common Cause Is Congenital Adrenal Hyperplasia

The manifestations of the syndrome are summarized most easily through an understanding of the biosynthetic pathways of mineralocorticoid, glucocorticoid, and sex steroids (see Chap. 3)

This syndrome is related in 95 % of cases to a 21-hydroxylase deficiency (inherited as an autosomal recessive trait caused by an abnormal gene on chromosome 6) and in 5 % to a 11-beta-hydroxylase deficiency.

These enzymes convert pregnenolone and participate in the formation of aldosterone in the glomerulosa and of cortisol in the fasciculata. Absence of one of these enzymes deviates the conversion of the pregnenolone in delta-4-androstenedione, which can convert in testosterone or estrone.

The main findings are reported in Table 1.7.

Table 1.7 Congenital adrenal hyperplasia

> 1. 46 XX chromosome. Normal ovaries
> 2. Masculinization of the external genitalia (excessive production of androgens by the fetal suprarenal glands) causes varying degrees of:
>   Clitoral hypertrophy
>   Partial fusion of the labial majora
> 3. Persistent urogenital sinus

Male Pseudohermaphrodism

Definition: A heterogeneous group which are characterized by:

1. 46XY karyotype, chromatin-negative nuclei
2. Testes: inadequate production of testosterone and MIS by the fetal testes
3. External genitalia usually female or ambiguous (may be male) variable

The defect may be:

In the gonad leading to insufficiency of androgens, MIS, or both

In the end-organ defects in which developing tissues are unresponsive to androgens or MIS

A Common Cause Is Androgen Insensitivity Syndrome

A common cause is *androgen insensitivity syndrome* (Figs. 1.13 and 1.14). The familial disorder transmitted through the female.

The diagnosis may be suggested by the knowledge that in situ or maternal parent of the patient has the disorder, by the finding of a testis in an inguinal hernia sac in a prepubertal girl, by the failure of the menarche to occur at the time of puberty, or by the development of symptoms or signs caused by a gonadal tumor or an adnexal cyst.

Explanation of the syndrome:

1. *46 XY chromosome*: Testes. There are usually in the abdomen or the inguinal canals. On gross examination, the testes in the adult are typically slightly reduced in size. Discrete firm nodules (hamartomas or Sertoli cell tumors) commonly protrude from the sectioned surfaces. The Sertoli cell tumors may form larger masses. Occasionally nodules of seminoma are encountered.
2. Testes (epithelial cells or Sertoli cells) produce MIS that results in absence of tubes uterus and vagina.

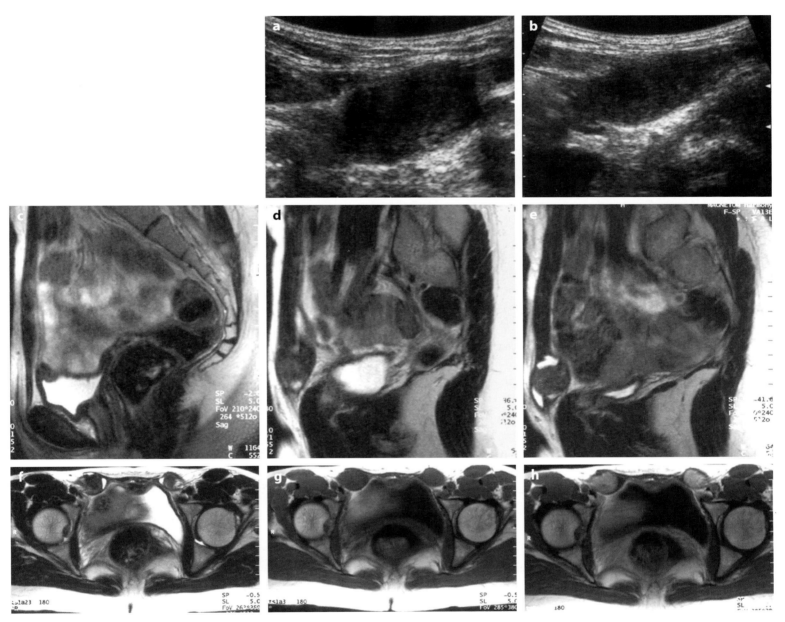

Fig. 1.13 Androgen insensitivity syndrome. A 31-year-old woman with primary amenorrhea, bilateral inguinal mass, and female phenotype (Karyotype XY). Testosterone 2.96 ng/ml, DHEA normal, prolactinemia 76.7 ng/ml (normal <25 ng/ml). TAS displays right (**a**) and left (**b**) testis in the inguinal region. MR T2 midline sagittal (**c**) shows absence of uterus; parasagittal (**d**) and left parasagittal (**e**) and axial T2 (**f**) display bilateral inguinal testis with tissular portion containing some small hyperintense structures at the periphery. Axial MR T1 (**g**) and after contrast (**h**): the tissular portion looks homogeneous and significantly enhances [Adapted from Moore [1]]

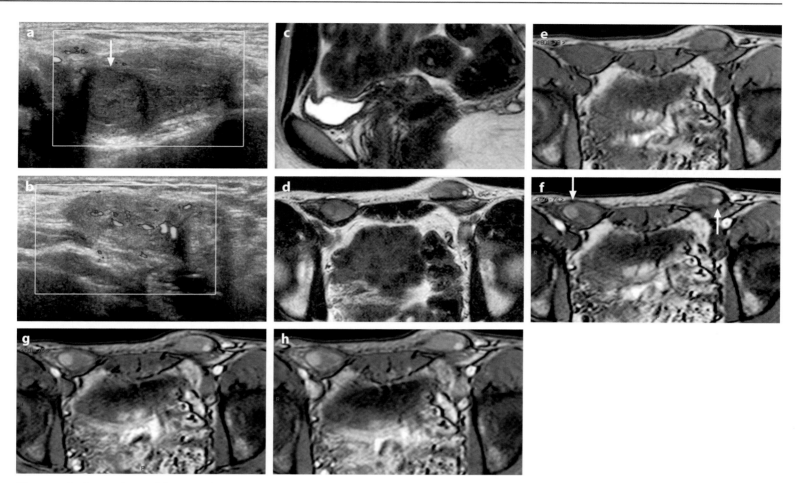

Fig. 1.14 Androgen insensitivity syndrome. Primary amenorrhea. Female phenotype. Karyotype XY. US (**a**, **b**) with a high-frequency superficial probe displays a bilateral testis in the inguinal regions. A slightly hypoechoic nodule is depicted in the right ovary (*arrow*). MR sagittal T2 (**c**) does not display a vagina. Axial T2 (**d**) depicts a right testes in the inguinal canal, containing a small nodule and a left testis at the level of the external orifice of the inguinal canal, containing small cysts. DMR without injection (**e**) and at the arterial phase (**f**) depicts in the right testis a nodule (*arrow*) with an early diffuse contrast uptake very suggestive of an endocrine tumor; a smaller nodule of the same type (*arrow*) is also present in the left testis. At the venous phase (**g**) and on the delayed (**h**) contrast uptake in the tumors slightly increases. Prospective diagnosis: bilateral endocrine tumors in the testes (Sertoli adenomas). This patient has not been yet operated [Adapted from Moore [1]]

3. Testes (interstitial cells or Leydig cells) produce androgens which normally induce masculinization of the indifferent external genitalia. In this syndrome, the failure of the end-organs to respond to androgens is thought to result from a deficiency of the cytosol receptor or the nuclear apparatus involved in the complex mechanism of androgen activity. This is the reason why the external genitalia are female, but the vagina usually ends in a blind pouch.

Findings of AIS are reported in table (Table 1.8).

Table 1.8 Findings of androgen insensitivity syndrome (AIS)

1. 46XY chromosome
2. Testis in the abdomen or in the inguinal canals
3. Aplasia of tubes, uterus, and vagina until the hymen due to secretion of Müllerian-inhibiting substance (MIS) also called anti-Mullerian hormone (AMH) secreted by the Sertoli cells of the testis
4. Normal external female genitalia (insensitivity to androgens secreted by the interstitial cells of the testis)
5. Most testes contain bilateral hamartomas (Sertoli cell adenomas) from 1 to 10 mm
Malignant tumors (mainly seminomas) or other malignant germ cell tumors may develop mainly after 25 years

Differential diagnosis: Mayer-Rokitansky-Kuster-Hauser syndrome (Fig. 1.15).

Main findings are reported in Table 1.9.

Table 1.9 Mayer-Rokitansky-Kuster-Hauser syndrome

Main features
– 46XX chromosome
– Normal ovaries
– Hypoplasia of the tubes, aplasia of uterus and vagina until the hymen
– Normal external female genitalia
Associated abnormalities
– Renal anomalies (40–50 % of cases)
– Associated skeletal or spinal anomalies in 10–12 % of cases
– Hearing loss in 10–25 % of cases

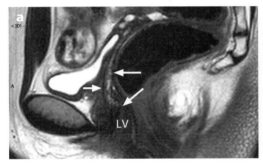
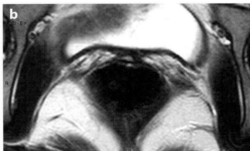
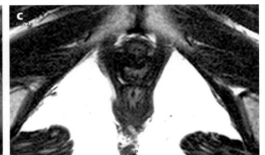
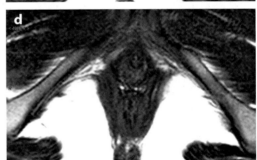

Fig. 1.15 Mayer-Rokitansky-Kuster-Hauser syndrome. Twenty-years-old woman with amenorrhea. (1) *Absence of vagina.* (**a**) MR Sagittal T2 on the midline displays absence of vagina almost until the introitus, with adipose tissue between two lines very likely representing the rectovaginal septum (*long horizontal arrow*) and the vesicovaginal septum (*short horizontal arrow*). The lower vagina (*LV*) is present with a cone shape and an apex (*oblique arrow*); the junction with remnant vagina is well depicted. (**b–d**) Axial T2 at three different levels: Through the middle part of the posterior wall of the bladder (**b**) allows to definitely confirm the absence of vagina until the introitus. At the level of the posterior and inferior part of the pubis (**c**) displays the a normal vestibular vagina. Through the inferior half of the urethra (**d**) depicts the fusion of the anterior wall of the inferior part of the vestibular vagina with the urethra. (2) *Tubal remnants.*

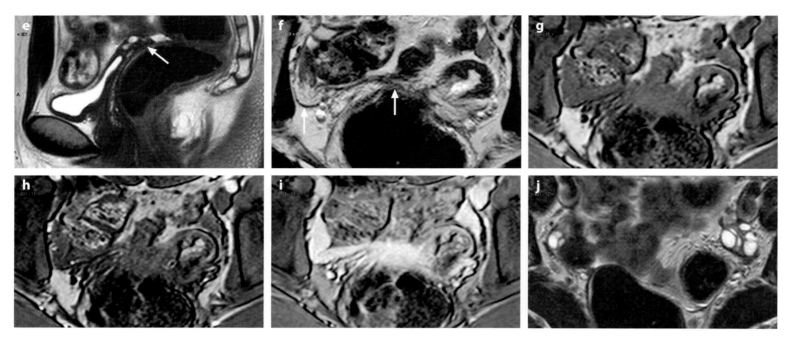

Fig. 1.15 (*continued*) (**e**, **f**) Sagittal T2 through the midline (**e**) displays between the upper part of the bladder and rectum low-intensity tissue (*arrow*). Axial T2 through this tissular mass (**f**) shows a central mass (*central arrow*) with irregular borders related to a remnant of the uterus and laterally two tubular structures with a hyperintense signal related to tubal remnants (*lateral arrow*). On DMR without injection (**g**) and at the arterial phase (**h**), tubal arterial vessels are visualized in the tubal remnants. On the delayed (**i**), a significant contrast uptake is visualized in the uterus and tubes remnants, with a characteristic fold appearance in the right tube at the venous phase. (3) *Normal ovaries* are visualized on axial T2 (**j**) [Adapted from Moore [1]]

The Persistent Mullerian Duct Syndrome

The Mullerian duct syndrome seems to be a heterogeneous group of disorders caused by different defects in the Mullerian-inhibiting system; mutations in the MIS gene are responsible for at least half of the cases. The remainder appeared to be caused by mutations in the receptor for the gene products.

The main findings are reported in Table 1.10.

Table 1.10 Main findings of the persistent Mullerian duct syndrome

Karyotype XY
Gonads: unilateral or bilateral cryptorchid testes
Wolffian duct structures
External genitalia normal or almost normal
Inguinal hernia in which prolapses an infantile uterus and fallopian tubes

1.2.3.2 Disorders Associated with an Abnormal Chromosome Constitution

Some of these disorders are characterized by a gonadal dysgenesis.

Definition of Gonadal Dysgenesis

Macroscopically, gonadal dysgenesis is characterized by a gonadal streak. The gonadal streak is an elongated structure with the gross appearance of an infantile ovary.

Microscopically, the ovary is composed almost exclusively of ovarian stroma, typically without ova at the time of puberty. Exceptionally, a few remain, and Graafian follicles and even corpora lutea may develop, usually within the first few postpubertal years.

Sexual Ambiguity Infrequent

Klinefelter Syndrome

The main findings are reported in Table 1.11.

Table 1.11 Klinefelter syndrome

Karyotype 47 XXY
Diagnose suspected at adolescence
Gynecomastia, obesity, or eunuchism
Small testes
Associated gonadal (seminomas, teratoma, embryonal cell carcinoma) and extragonadal neoplasms

Turner Syndrome

The main findings are reported in Table 1.12 (Fig. 1.16).

Table 1.12 Main findings of Turner syndrome

Karyotype 45X, less frequently mosaic 45X/46XX, and 46XX with isochrome X (duplication of one arm of the X with loss of the other arm)
Newborn: findings related to lymph stasis
Patients who reach adolescence undiagnosed present with primary amenorrhea
Bilateral streaks

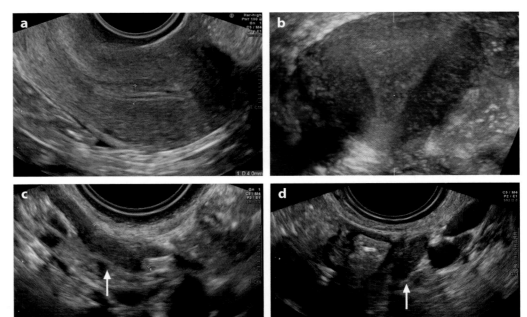

Fig. 1.16 Turner syndrome. Thirty-two-year-old woman, karyotype X0, hormonal treatment. EVS (**a**) and with 3D reformation (**b**) depict a uterus of normal size with a normal proportion between the body and the cervix, with a normal endometrial cavity. Transverse views of the right ovary (**c**) and of the left ovary (**d**) display bilateral small and flattened ovaries (*arrows*), without any secondary follicle, corresponding to bilateral streaks [Adapted from Moore [1]]

Pure Gonadal Dysgenesis (Some Forms)

The main findings are reported in Table 1.13.

Table 1.13 Pure gonadal dysgenesis

Karyotype 46XY (more common) or 46XX
Streak gonads generally
Internal genitalia include Mullerian structures (fallopian tubes and uterus)
Phenotypically normal or hypoplastic external genitalia

Sexual Ambiguity Frequent

Mixed Gonadal Dysgenesis

Main findings are reported in Table 1.14.

Table 1.14 Mixed gonadal dysgenesis

1. Chromatin-negative nuclei
2. Testis on one side (more or less normal structurally and functionally) and undifferentiated gonad on the other side
3. Internal genitalia female
4. External genitalia range from normal male through intermediate depending partly on the androgen output of the testis

True Hermaphrodism

Definition: well-formed ovarian and testicular tissue most commonly in the same gonad (ovotestis) or as two separate gonads

The main findings are reported in Table 1.15.

Table 1.15 Main findings of true hermaphrodism

1. Most frequent karyotypes are 46XX (60 %) mosaic (presence of two or more cell lines) (30 %). 46 XY (10 %)
2. Gonad: 　Nature: most frequent ovotestis 　　Second most common ovary on the left side 　　Uncommonly testis 　Location depends on the nature of the gonad: 　　Ovotestis In the inguinal canal or labioscrotal swelling 　　Increasing amount of ovarian tissue: ovarian fossa 　　Testis 63 % in scrotum 15 % inguinal 22 % ovarian fossa
3. Genital organ adjacent to the gonad depends on the nature of the gonad: 　Fallopian tube often adjacent to an ovary, or epididymis adjacent to a testis
4. Phenotype male 3/4 patients evaluated for gynecomastia 　Phenotype female 1/4 patients evaluated for amenorrhea or failure to develop secondary changes

The testicular tissue is typically more normal structurally and functionally than that of mixed gonadal dysgenesis, so that three-fourths of the patients are phenotypic males.

1.3 Congenital Abnormalities Related or Not to Intersexual Disorders

Embryology of these disorders may involve the ovaries, the different segments derivated from the mullerian ducts and from the urogenital sinus. These are reported in the following chapters.

1.3.1 Of the Ovary

They are described in chapter 6.

1.3.2 Of the Derivates of the Mullerian Duct (Tube, Uterus Body and Cervix)

They are described in chapter 19.

1.3.3 Of the Mullerian Duct and the Urogenital Sinus (Vagina)

They are described in chapters 19 and 30.

1.3.4 Of the Vulva

They are reported in chapter 35.

References

1. Moore KL, Persuad TVN (2008) The developing human. Clinically oriented embryology, 8th edn. Saunders, Philadelphia, pp 243–284
2. Robboy SJ, Bentley RC (2002) Embryology of the female genital tract and disorders of abnormal sexual development. In: Blaustein's pathology of the female genital tract, 5th edn. Springer, New York, pp 3–36

Anatomy and Radioanatomy of the Pelvis and the Perineum and Anatomical Locations of Pelvic and Perineal Masses

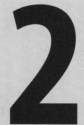

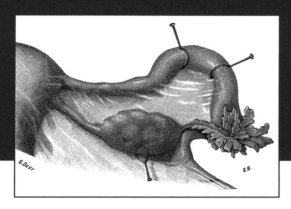

Contents

Diagnosis of the origin of a pelvic mass is one of the most common and difficult problems encountered in pelvic imaging.

Precise location of the mass is one of the fundamental steps in the radiological diagnosis of a pelvic mass. A precise knowledge of the anatomy of the pelvis (topographic and descriptive) with anatomical sections in the different planes (axial, coronal and sagittal) is essential to localize precisely a pelvic mass and eventually according to the nature of the mass (especially in case of malignant tumor) to precise its extension. Knowledge of the anatomy can only be understood with a precise knowledge of embryology of the genital organs, the genital tract and the external female genitalia [1] but also of the peritoneum, and the urinary tract (mainly the ureters and the bladder), and of the GI tract (small bowel and colon and rectosigmoid) which can be involved in different pathologic processes of the gynecological organs.

The topographic diagnosis is different according to the exclusively or mainly cystic nature of the mass, or its mixed, mainly solid or exclusively solid nature.

2.1 Anatomy and Radioanatomy of the Pelvis and the Perineum

2.1.1 Female Genital Tract Is Situated in the Pelvis and in the Perineum

2.1.1.1 The Pelvis Is Limited By

- Upward by the plane passing through the promontory of the sacrum, the arcuate line of the ilium, the iliopectineal line, and the posterior surface of the pubic crest.
- Laterally, the pelvic wall formed above the arcus tendineus (which is a thickening of the aponeurosis of the internal obtuatus) by the obturator internus above, and the levator ani below.
- Backward the piriformis covered by fascia over piriformis and the sacrum covered by the presacral fascia
- Downward the pelvic floor is formed by the levator ani covered by the fascia of the pelvic diaphragm;
- Levator ani and coccygeus form the pelvic diaphragm and delineate the lower limit of the true pelvis.

2.1.1.2 The Perineum Is Limited By

- Anteriorly, the pubic symphysis and its arcuate ligament
- Posteriorly, by the coccyx.
- Anterolaterally, the ischiopubic rami and the ischial tuberosities
- Posterolaterally, the sacrotuberous ligaments

J.N. Buy, M. Ghossain, *Gynecological Imaging*,
DOI 10.1007/978-3-642-31012-6_2, © Springer-Verlag Berlin Heidelberg 2013

- The deep limit of the perineum is the inferior surface of the pelvic diaphragm, its superficial limit the skin.
- An arbitrary limit joining the ischial tuberosities divides the perineum into an anterior urogenital triangle and a posterior anal triangle.

Female genital tract is composed of:
1. The ovary, which is only related by a thin mesovarium to the posterior part of the broad ligament and although entirely not covered by peritoneum, is considered as an intraperitoneal organ, because it lies in the peritoneal cavity.
2. Derivatives of the Muller duct, which give rise to the tubes, the body of the uterus, the cervix, and the upper vagina (see Chap. 1), which lie under the peritoneum of the bottom of the pelvic cavity, and therefore are subperitoneal.
3. The lower part of the vagina, which arises from the vaginal plate (see Chap. 1.1.3.1). During embryologic development this part will give rise to two portions:
   - An upper portion which migrates upward to fuse with the upper part of the vagina (which arises from the Muller duct). These two parts will form the subperitoneal segment of the vagina.
   - A lower portion under the hymeneal membrane which lies in the perineum and opens into the vestibule. This portion will form the perineal segment of the vagina.

These organs, intraperitoneal, subperitoneal, and perineal, present anatomical relationships with:
- The extraperitoneal space lateral to the parietal pelvic peritoneum
- The retroperitoneal space, mainly via lymphatic and nervous structures
  Moreover, in radiological practice:
- Masses of the female genital tract can be difficult:
  - To differentiate from extra female organs, GI tract, urinary tract, peritoneum, broad ligament, extraperitoneal, retroperitoneal nervous structures, and even in uncommon cases from parietal masses
  - To precisely locate as ovarian, tubal, uterine in origin, or in case of a double location contiguous or separated to precise the organ of origin

2.1.2   The Different Anatomical Spaces of the Female Genital Tract and Perineum

2.1.2.1 Definitions

Peritoneum [2]: a single layer of flattened mesothelial cells, lying on a layer of loose connective tissue

The mesothelium usually forms a continuous surface, but in some areas may be fenestrated; neighboring cells are joined by junctional complexes but probably permit the passage of macrophages.

The submesothelial connective tissue may contain macrophages, lymphocytes, and adipocytes (in some regions).

Mesothelial cells may transform into fibroblasts, which may play an important role in the formation of peritoneal adhesions after surgery or inflammation of the peritoneum.

Peritoneal cavity: a virtual space lying between the parietal peritoneum and the visceral peritoneum. It may contain physiologically a small amount of peritoneal fluid (<30 cc).

After ovulation, secondary to rupture of the dominant follicle, a little more of fluid is seen in the Douglas.

During menstruation, blood may escape from the uterine tubes into the pelvic peritoneal cavity.

Intraperitoneal organ: although not situated in the peritoneal cavity (between the two layers of peritoneum), an organ entirely (small bowel, appendix, cecum, sigmoid) or almost entirely covered with visceral peritoneum (like in the abdomen, liver, stomach, spleen).

Retroperitoneal organ: an organ situated behind the posterior parietal peritoneum.

Organ lying in the peritoneal cavity: an organ situated in the peritoneal cavity, almost entirely not covered by peritoneum like the ovary (but only connected to the posterior leaf of the broad ligament by the mesovarium).

Meso is composed of the apposition of twofolds of visceral peritoneum (except for the transverse mesocolon which has fourfolds, two from the foregut, two from the midgut).

Root of peritoneum is the area of reflection and attachment of the meso on the posterior parietal peritoneum.

Extraperitoneal tissue (transversalis fascia) separates the parietal peritoneum from the muscle layers of the abdominal wall.

2.1.2.2 The Different Anatomical Spaces

The Intraperitoneal Space

The intraperitoneal space containing the intraperitoneal segments of the GI tract, covered by visceral peritoneum:
1. Small bowel attached by the mesentery to the posterior parietal peritoneum along its root extending from the duodenojejunal junction to the ileocecal junction
2. Cecum usually suspended by a short mesentery and appendix with its short mesoappendix connecting it to the lower part of the ileal mesentery
3. Sigmoid with the mesosigmoid connected to the posterior parietal peritoneum by its two roots:

   The primary root from the inferior angle of the aorta bifurcation to the posterior junction of the rectosigmoid junction

   The secondary root from the origin of the primary one, descending obliquely along the primitive and external left iliac artery

The Subperitoneal Space

The Roof: The Broad Ligament (Figs. 2.1, 2.2, and 2.3)

Peritoneal Folds
1. Mesosalpinx (Fig. 2.4a–c)

   It covers the tube except the fimbriae of the tubal infundibulum which project from its free lateral end into the peritoneal cavity. It is attached laterally to the suspensory ligament of the ovary and medially to the ovarian ligament.

   It contains vascular anastomoses between the uterine and ovarian vessels, the epoophoron (Fig. 2.4d), the paroophoron, and the proximal part of the Gartner canal.

Fig. 2.1 Anterior view of the broad ligament.
1 Uterus, *2* cervix, *3* vagina, *4* left ovary, *5* utero-ovarian ligament, *6* tube with its infundibulum, *7* tubo-ovarian ligament, *8* Morgagni hydatid, *9* round ligament, *10* broad ligament with its anterior (*a*), middle (*b*), and posterior (*c*) wings; *11* posterior leaf of the broad ligament, and *12* infundibulopelvic ligament

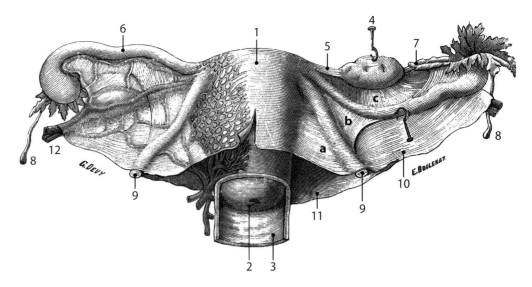

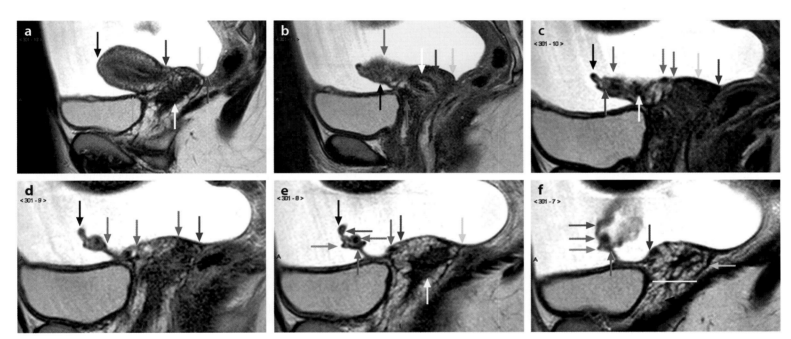

Fig. 2.2 Landmarks: Contiguous sagittal sections of the broad ligament from the midline (black landmark) to the left pelvic wall (purple landmark) (cervix in the middle sagittal plane, uterus body oriented to the right) (last figure with bars). (**a**) Section through the middle sagittal plane of the uterus body (black landmark). Uterus body (between *black arrow* and *blue arrow*), right paracervix (between *blue* and *yellow arrows*), right vaginal wall (*white arrow*), vesicouterine pouch (*pink arrow*), Douglas (*purple arrow*). (**b**) Section at the junction of the left lateral border of the uterus and the mesometrium (*red landmark*). Myometrium (*black arrow*), mesometrium (*gray arrow*), cervix inner stroma (*white arrow*), external stroma (*blue arrow*), vesicouterine septum (*red arrow*), posterior fornix of the vagina (*yellow arrow*). (**c**) Section through the inner mesometrium (*green landmark*). Mesosalpinx (between *black* and *gray arrows*) containing the medial branch of the tubal artery (*black arrow*), the tube (*purple arrow*). Mesometrium above the Mackenrodt's ligament (between *gray* and *red arrows*) containing vessels particularly the ascending segment of the uterine artery (*white arrow*). Uterine artery (*red arrow*) at the junction of Mackenrodt's ligament and mesometrium. Mackenrodt's ligament (between *red* and *green arrows*). External cervix lateral stroma (*yellow arrow*), posterior fornix of the vagina

(*blue arrow*). (**d**) Section through the inner Mackenrodt's ligament (purple landmark). Mesosalpinx (between *black* and *gray arrows*), mesometrium above the Mackenrodt's ligament (between *gray* and *red arrows*), Mackenrodt's ligament (between *red* and *green arrows*), posterior fornix of the vagina (*blue arrow*). (**e**) Section just lateral to the previous one (yellow landmark). Mesosalpinx (between *black* and *green arrow*), containing medial tubal artery (*purple arrow*), and uterine artery (*red arrow*), round ligament containing its artery (*brown arrow*), mesometrium above the Mackenrodt's ligament (between *green arrow* and *blue arrow*). Uterine artery in its latero uterine segment (*gray arrow*), Mackenrodt's ligament (between *blue* and *yellow arrows*), vagina lateral wall (*white arrow*). (**f**) Section at the level of the medial face of the ovary (brown landmark). Mesosalpinx with anastomoses between uterine and ovarian arteries (*red arrow*), tubal artery with a low signal (*purple arrow*) along the tube. Round ligament (*brown arrow*) containing its low signal artery. Mesometrium between the *green arrow* and the *blue arrow*. White line at the level of the lower part of the cervix. Mackenrodt's ligament between the *blue arrow* and the *yellow arrow*, above the white line. Below the white line, paravaginal subperitoneal tissue (*black arrow*)

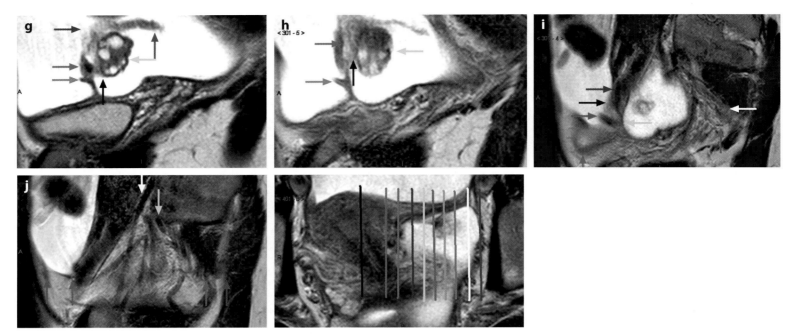

Fig. 2.2 (*continued*) (**g**) Section through the middle part of the ovary at the level of change in direction of the salpinx (orange landmark). Round ligament (*brown arrow*), mesosalpinx containing uterine artery (*red arrow*), mesovarium (*black arrow*), ovary (*yellow arrow*), tube with ampullary portion (*blue arrow*) and infundibulum (*purple arrow*). (**h**) Section through the mesovarium (gray landmark). Infundibulopelvic ligament contains ovarian artery (*red arrow*), mesovarium (*black arrow*), ovary lateral third (*yellow arrow*), round ligament (*brown arrow*). (**i**) Section through the junction of the lateral part of the broad ligament and the extraperitoneal space (white landmark). Medial part of the extraperitoneal space (*blue arrow*) containing the left external iliac vein. Anterior (*black arrow*) and posterior (*yellow arrow*) peritoneal leaves of the mesometrium close to their attachment to the extraperitoneal space. Round ligament at the beginning of its extraperitoneal segment (*green arrow*). Anterior and posterior subperitoneal spaces (between *red arrows*). Retroperitoneal space (*white arrow*). (**j**) Section through the extraperitoneal space (Bordeaux red landmark). Anterior subperitoneal space (between *green arrow* and anterior *red arrow*), extraperitoneal space (between *red arrows*), retroperitoneal space (between posterior *red arrow* and *purple arrow*), external iliac artery and vein (*white arrow*), arterial and venous branches of the hypogastric artery and vein (*yellow arrow*)

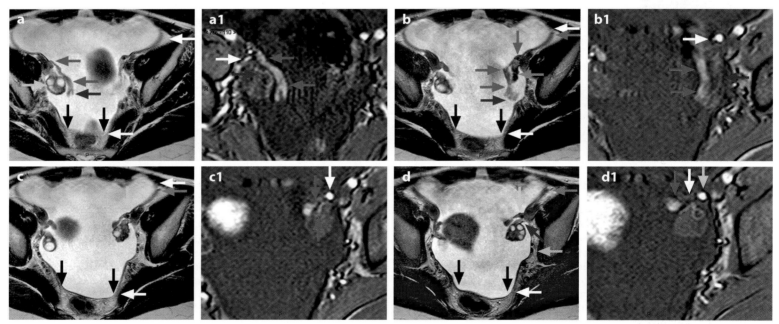

Fig. 2.3 Landmarks: Contiguous axial sections of the broad ligament from the top (black landmark) to the pelvic floor (lower purple landmark) using axial T2 and DMR (at the arterial phase) sequences at the same level (last figure with bars). (**a**) Section (axial T2), through the right adnexa (black landmark). Right ovary (*yellow arrow*), right tube ampulla (between *red arrows*), infundibulum (between the more distal *red arrow* and *blue arrow*). Extraperitoneal space (between *white arrows*), retroperitoneal space (between *black arrows*). (**a1**) Same section (DMR, arterial phase): right ovarian artery (*white arrow*) and intraovarian branches (*blue arrow*), tubal arteries (*red arrows*). (**b**) Section (axial T2) through the left adnexa (*red landmark*): infundibulo pelvic ligament containing the low signal intensity ovarian artery (*green arrow*), left superior ovarian cortex (*orange arrow*), left tube ampulla (between *red arrows*) infundibulum (between the more distal *red arrow* and *blue arrow*). Extraperitoneal space (between *white arrows*), retroperitoneal space (between *black arrows*). Round ligament (*brown arrow*). (**b1**) Same section (DMR, arterial phase): left ovarian artery (*white arrow*) and intraovarian branches (*blue arrow*), tubal arteries (*red arrows*). (**c**) Section (axial T2) through both adnexa (green landmark). Left infundibulopelvic ligament containing the ovarian artery (*yellow arrow*). Extraperitoneal space (between white arrows), retroperitoneal space (between *black arrows*). Round ligament (*brown arrow*). (**c1**) Section (DMR, arterial phase): left ovarian artery (*white arrow*) and intraovarian branches (*green arrow*), lateral tubal artery (*red arrow*). (**d**) Section (axial T2) (purple landmark) junction between the isthmus and the ampulla. Ovarian artery (*yellow arrow*) mesovarium with lateral leaf in continuity with the posterior leaf of the parietal pelvic peritoneum (*blue arrow*) uterine artery in its extraperitoneal segment (*pink arrow*). Retroperitoneal space (between the two *black arrows*), junction between the retroperitoneal space and the extraperitoneal space (*white arrow*), round ligament (*brown arrow*). (**d1**) Section (DMR, arterial phase): ovarian artery (*yellow arrow*) lateral tubal branch of the ovarian artery (*white arrow*) anastomosis between ovarian artery and tubal artery (*green arrow*), intraovarian arteries (*red arrow*)

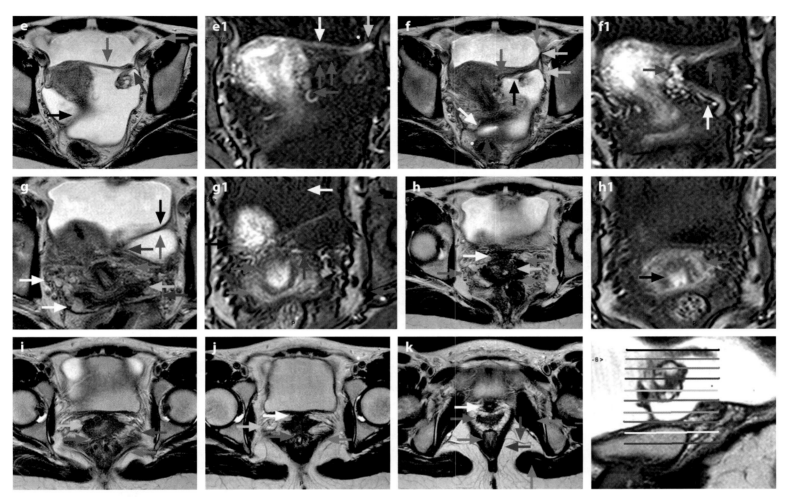

Fig. 2.3 (*continued*) (**e**) Section (axial T2) (yellow landmark). Round ligament at the beginning of its extra peritoneal location (*brown arrow*). Isthmic portion of the tube and mesosalpinx in its superior portion (*red arrow*), mesovarium (*blue arrow*), right uterosacral ligament (*black arrow*). (**e1**) Section (DMR, arterial phase). Uterine artery: ascending segment in the mesometrium along the lateral border of the uterus body (horizontal *red arrow*), uterine artery in the mesosalpinx (vertical *red arrows*), medial tubal branch (branch of division of the uterine artery in the superior portion of the mesosalpinx) (*white arrow*). Terminal portion of the uterine artery in the mesosalpinx (*yellow arrow*) anastomosing with the ovarian artery. (**f**) Section (axial T2) through the ovarian ligament (*brown landmark*). Ovarian ligament indicating the inferior part of the mesosalpinx (*black arrow*), uterine artery in the mesosalpinx (*red arrow*), round ligament in its proximal portion (*brown arrow*), anterior and posterior leaves of the broad ligament joining the lateral parietal peritoneum (*yellow arrows*), right uterosacral ligament (*white arrow*), Douglas (*purple arrow*). (**f1**) Section (DMR, arterial phase): uterine artery in its transverse segment (*white arrow*) at its ascending segment (*purple arrow*) in the mesosalpinx (*red arrow*), superior uterine vein lateral and below the transverse segment of the uterine artery (*blue arrow*), ureter crosses between uterine artery and vein, not visualized on this sequence. (**g**) Section (axial T2) (orange landmark), anterior (*black arrow*) and posterior (*red arrow*) leaves of the mesometrium clearly defined by fluid in the peritoneal cavity containing the low signal intensity of the round ligament, Mackenrodt's ligament (between *blue arrows*) with its paracervical portion (*green arrow*) and para-

vaginal portion lateral to the fornix (*yellow arrow*). On the right side lateral limit between Mackenrodt's ligament and the extraperitoneal space (*white arrows*). (**g1**) Section (DMR, arterial phase): fluid in the peritoneal cavity (*white arrow*); artery of the round ligament just behind *white arrow*. Transverse segment of the uterine artery (*blue arrow*), intrauterine arteries (*black arrow*), cervical arteries (*red arrow*), vaginal arteries (*green arrow*), arteries of the extraperitoneal space (between *purple arrows*). (**h**) Section (axial T2) (gray landmark) through the lower part of the Mackenrodt's ligament: uterovesical septum (*white arrow*), lateral fornix (*green arrow*), lower part of the cervix (*yellow arrow*), junction of the Mackenrodt's ligament and the extraperitoneal space (*red arrow*), rectovaginal septum (*orange arrow*). (**h1**) Section (DMR, arterial phase): cervical arteries (*black arrow*), vaginal arteries (*red arrow*). (**i**) Section (axial T2) (white landmark): uterovesical septum (*black arrow*), vaginal wall (*yellow arrow*), rectovaginal septum (*red arrow*), paravagina (*purple arrow*), iliococcygeus muscle (*green arrow*). (**j**) Section through the top of the rectovaginal septum (lower purple landmark), vesicovaginal septum (*white arrow*), paravagina (*yellow arrow*), rectovaginal septum (*red arrow*), iliococcygeus muscle (*brown arrow*). (**k**) Section through the lower part of the subperitoneal space just above the pelvic floor, urethra (*white arrow*), vagina (*red arrow*), lower part of the rectum (*green arrow*) just above the rectoanal junction, iliococcygeus muscle lower part (*blue arrow*) just above the puborectal muscle, obturator internus (*orange arrow*), gluteal maximus (*brown arrow*), posterior perineum:ischiorectal fossa (*gray arrow*)

2. Mesovarium (Fig. 2.4a–c)

It projects from the lower and lateral part of the posterior fold of the mesosalpinx to the hilum of the ovary. All the rest of the ovary is devoid of peritoneum.

It carries vessels and nerves to the ovary.

The ovarian ligament attaches the inferomedial extremity of the ovary to the lateral angle of the uterus posteroinferior to the uterine tube. The ovarian ligament is continuous with the medial border of the round ligament.

The upper pole of the ovary is connected to the posterior part of the infundibulum of the tube by the tubo-ovarian ligament.

3. Mesometrium or Parametrium of Virchow (3) (Figs. 2.4a, b and 2.5)

It is the largest part of the broad ligament.

(a) It is limited by:

Upward, the lower part of the mesosalpinx.

Downward, the subperitoneal tissue covering the pelvic floor.

Medially, the lateral border of the uterus and the vagina until the introitus.

Laterally, upward the suspensory or infundibulopelvic ligament, which is attached to the upper part of the lateral face of the ovary; below this ligament.

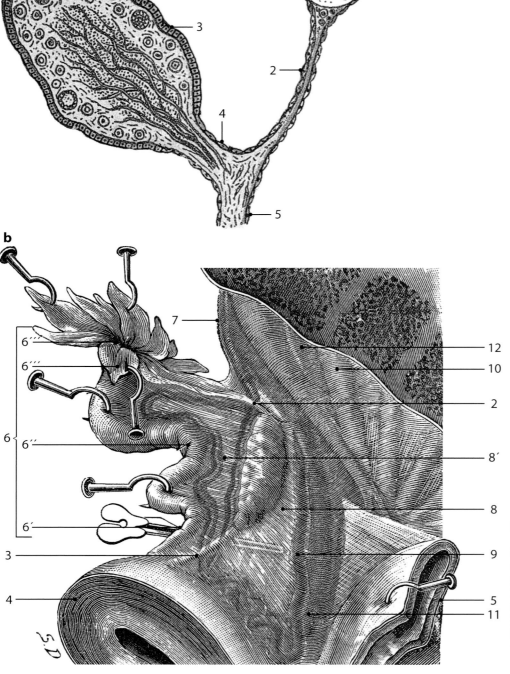

Fig. 2.4 (a) *1* tube, *2* mesosalpinx, *3* ovary, *4* mesovarium, *5* mesometrium. **(b)** *1* Ovary, *2* Tuboovarian ligament, *3* Ovarian ligament, *4* Uterus, *5* Rectum, *6* Tube with 6' isthmus, 6" ampulla, 6‴ infundibulum, *7* Suspensory or Infundibulopelvic ligament containing in its thickness the ovarian artery and vein and lymphatics, *8* Mesometrium, 8' Mesosalpinx, *9* Uterine artery, *10* Sacral plexus, *11* Ureter, *12* Internal iliac vein

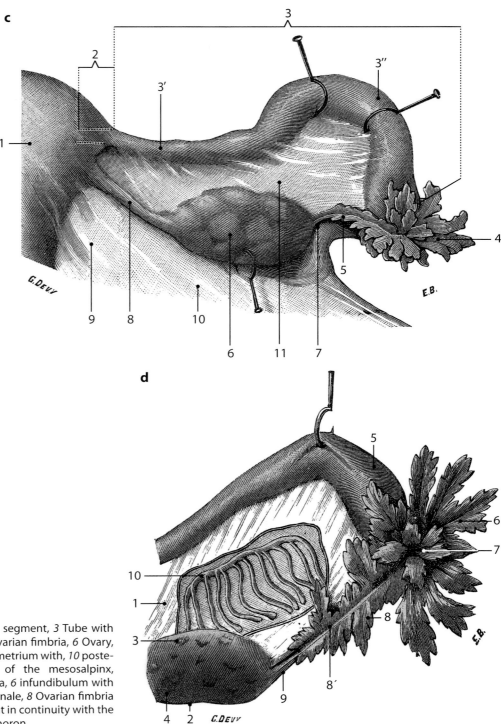

Fig. 2.4 (*continued*) (**c**) *1* Uterus, *2* Tube intramural segment, *3* Tube with *3'* Isthmic portion, *3"* Ampulla, *4* Infundibulum, *5* Ovarian fimbria, *6* Ovary, *7* Tuboovarian ligament, *8* Ovarian ligament, *9* Mesometrium with, *10* posterior leaf, *11* Mesosalpinx. (**d**) *1* Posterior leaf of the mesosalpinx, *2* Ovary with *3* De Graaf's follicles, *4* Scars, *5* Ampulla, *6* infundibulum with two concentric circles of fimbriae, *7* Ostium abdominale, *8* Ovarian fimbria with *8'* its longitudinal gutter, *9* Tuboovarian ligament in continuity with the longitudinal gutter of the ovarian fimbria, *10* Epoophoron

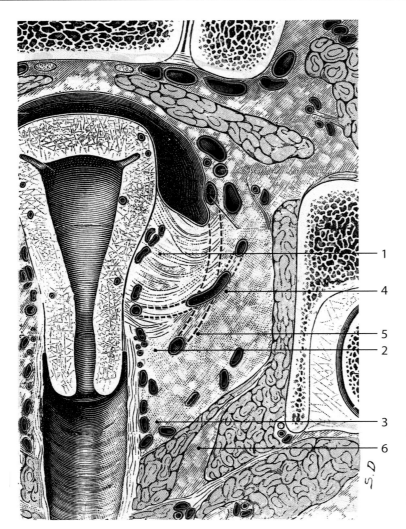

Fig. 2.5 Coronal section through the middle of the broad ligament.
1 Mesometrium, *2* paracervix, *3* paravagina, *4* uterine artery, *5* ureter, *6* levator ani

Forward the anterior peritoneal fold:
- Medially, descends on the anterior face of the uterus body until the isthmus, reflects onto the bladder forming the uterovesical fold
- Laterally, is heightened by the proximal part of the round ligament which inserts on the uterus just below the uterine tube

Backward, the posterior peritoneal fold descends over the posterior face of the uterus body, the upper cervix, the posterior fornix until the lower border of the posterior lip of the exocervix then reflects on to the front of the rectum to form the Douglas pouch.
(b) It contains:
Loose connective tissue and smooth muscle
The uterine artery
The ureter
1. Uterovesical fold at the level of the isthmus (Fig. 2.6) The continuum with the anterior parietal peritoneum raised by:
On the midline, the median umbilical ligament (obliteration of the lumen of the urachus, derivative of allantois) (see Chap. 1.1.1)
Laterally, the medial umbilical folds over the obliterated umbilical arteries

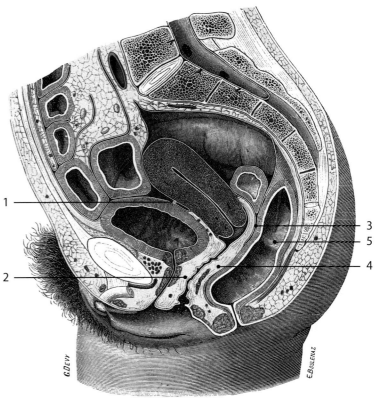

Fig. 2.6 Sagittal view through the middle part of the uterus.
1 Vesicovaginal cul de sac, *2* vesicovaginal septum, *3* Douglas pouch, *4* rectovaginal septum, *5* rectum

2. Douglas pouch:
The top is at the level of the torus (Fig. 2.6:1121 p 353).
The anterior leaf covers the posterior part of the cervix, than reflects over the posterior fornix.
The bottom is at the level of the inferior border of the posterior lip of the cervix.
The posterior leaf reflects over the anterior and lateral borders of the rectum until the rectosigmoid junction.
The lateral parts (called the ring of Waldeyer) are arciform heightened by the subperitoneal uterosacral ligaments.

Ligaments
1. *Round Ligament* (Fig. 2.1)
As the ovarian ligament with which it is continuous, the round ligament is issued from the gubernaculum of the embryo (see Chap. 1).
Near the uterus, it contains much smooth muscle, which progressively diminishes until the terminal part which is purely fibrous
  1. In the Mesometrium
    It starts from the uterus body just below and anterior to the lateral cornua.
    It passes diagonally down and laterally within the mesometrium.
  2. It crosses the obturator nerve and vessels, the obliterated umbilical artery.
    Just before the deep inguinal ring, it passes over the epigastric artery.
  3. It traverses the inguinal canal.
  4. It terminates on the mons pubis.

2. *Uterosacral Ligaments* (Fig. 2.7)

They arise from the posterior surface of the cervix on both sides of a little transverse protrusion the torus uterinus. The ligaments go backward around the lateral faces of the rectum and are attached to the front of the sacrum. They constitute the roof of the sacrorectovaginal septum. They contain fibrous tissue and smooth muscle.

3. *Ligaments of Mackenrodt* (Fig. 2.5)

It is limited by:

The superior part of the cervix with the transverse segment of the uterine artery immediately below

Inferiorly: the inferior border of the lateral fornix of the vagina

Medially: lateral wall of the uterine cervix, lateral fornix of the vagina

Laterally: is continuous externally with the fibrous tissue which surrounds the pelvic blood vessels of the pelvic wall.

Forward: the supravaginal part of the cervix is

Backward: the uterosacral ligaments

It contains:

The ureter crossing the inferior part of the transverse segment of the uterine artery, the uterine vein (superior and lateral branch as it passes below the ureter, above the vaginal artery)

Cervicovaginal artery, superficial and deep uterine veins

Lymphatics

4. *Pubocervical Ligament*

From the anterior part of the cervix and the upper vagina, diverge around the urethra attach to the posterior aspect of the pubic bones.

The Floor

The Levator Ani (See Figures Chap. 37)

Comprises two parts: a superolateral part, the iliococcygeus muscle; and an inferomedial part, consisting of the puborectalis and the pubovisceralis

1. A superolateral part: the iliococcygeus muscle

   (a) Origin: the ischiatic spine; the arcus tendineus, which is a thickening of the obturator fascia covering the medial and upper part the obturator internus muscle (a little lower than its superior border) extending from the ischiatic spine behind, running along the inferior border of the obturator canal, to the body of the pubis in front.

   The pubis body is 1 cm lateral to the pubic symphysis and 5 mm above its lower border

   (b) Direction: its general direction is inward and downward; its inferior and medial attachment is on the horizontal puborectalis.

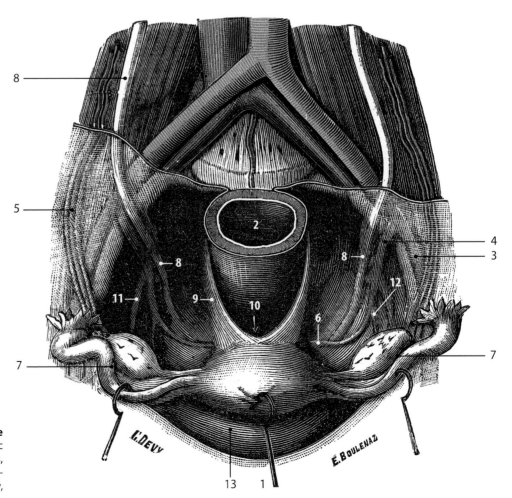

Fig. 2.7 Frontal view of the posterior part of the broad ligament. *1* Uterus, *2* rectum, *3* external iliac vessels, *4* internal iliac vessels, *5* utero-ovarian vessels, *6* uterine artery, *7* ovary and tube, *8* ureter, *9* uterosacral ligaments, *10* Douglas, *11* obturator artery, *12* vesicovaginal artery, *13* bladder

(c) End: The more anterior fibers intersect with those of the opposite side forming sort of a strap around the 3/4 posterior of the rectum.

The middle and posterior fibers end for some of them with the tip of the coccyx, but mainly with the anococcygeal raphe. This raphe is continuous with the fibroelastic anococcygeal ligament, which is applied and partly attached to its inferior surface.

2. An inferomedial part comprising the puborectalis and the puboviceralis

The puborectalis

(a) Origin: the posterior face of the body of the pubis just above the lower border, slightly lateral to the midline

(b) Direction: anteroposterior, almost horizontal slightly backward and downward, roughly 1 cm height; its upper portion is directly in contact with the lower border of the iliococcygeus

(c) End: a sling dorsal to the anorectal junction

The puboviceral comprises three different fascicles:

1. The pubovaginalis
   - Origin: the body of the pubis just above the lower border, medial to the puboperinealis
   - End: Posterolateral vaginal wall at the level of the mid-urethra

2. The puboperinealis
   - Origin: the body of the pubis, lateral to the previous one
   - End: perineal body

3. The puboanalis
   - Origin: the body of the pubis (higher than the previous ones) medial to the insertion of the iliococcygeus
   - Direction: slightly oblique backward and downward; immediately after its insertion, goes between the puborectalis and the puboperinealis, then follows the medial border of the puborectalis
   - End: the lateral border of the anal canal and the intersphincteric space

The ischiococcygeus muscle does not belong to the levator ani. It lies just in contact with the most posterosuperior portion of levator ani; it is a small muscle which extends from the ischiatic spine to the lateral margin of the coccyx and the fifth sacral segment along the sacrospinous ligament, closing the pelvic floor between the piriformis and the posterior part of the iliococcygeus.

The Piriformis

It mainly arises from the anterior face of the sacrum from the anterior parts of S2, S3, S4 by three digitations, which are attached to the bone between the pelvic sacral foramina, and to the grooves leading from foramina. The muscle passes out of the pelvis through the greater sciatic foramen. It inserts into the medial side of the upper border of the greater trochanter.

Obturator Internus

This muscle and the fascia over its upper inner surface form part of the anterolateral wall of the true pelvis. The lateral part of obturator internis is attached to the structures surrounding the obturator foramen, and to the medial part of the obturator membrane. This muscle is covered on its medial part by a thick fascial layer; this parietal pelvic fascia is well differentiated as the obturator fascia. This fascia arches below the obturator vessels and nerve, investing the obturator

canal, and is attached anteriorly to the back of the body of the pubis. A thickening of this fascia , the tendinous arch of the levator ani gives a firm attachment to the levator ani (see above).

The Content
From the front to the back

In Front, the Urinary Axis
In front, the urinary axis with the bladder (which arises from the urogenital sinus except the trigona which arises from the mesonephric ducts) and the upper half of the urethra (which arises from the urogenital sinus) (see Chap. 1).

Below the Bladder the Urethra
Female urethra is 4 cm length, 6 mm in diameter.
The urethra has:

1. Origin: internal urethral orifice, the middle of the symphysis pubis. It runs anteroinferiorly in front of the anterior vaginal wall, with a slight anterior curve from its origin to its end.

2. Mainly a subperitoneal segment: Above the inferior fascia of the pelvic diaphragm

   Anteriorly: in the normal female, the bladder neck (which is the internal urethral orifice) sits above the pelvic floor supported predominantly by the pubovesical ligaments (fibromuscular tissue extending from the bladder neck to the inferior aspects of the pubic body), the endopelvic fascia of the pelvic floor, and levator ani; these support the urethra at rest. With elevation of intra-abdominal pressure, the levators contract, increasing urethral closure pressure to maintain continence.

   This anatomical arrangement alters after parturition and with increasing age, such as the bladder neck lies beneath the pelvic floor particularly when the intra-abdominal pressure rises. The mechanism described above fails to maintain continence (stress incontinence as a result of urethral hypermotility).

   Posteriorly: the anterior vaginal wall

3. A short perineal segment

   In the deep perineal space: crosses medially the perineal membrane posteriorly to its anterior attachment to the pubourethral ligament of Henlé (transverse perineal ligament) and to the arcuate ligament (both of them forming the sus urethral lamina of Testut)

   In the superficial perineal space: runs between the anterior aspect of the bulbs of the vestibule immediately behind their anterior junction (the commissura bulborum)

4. End: urethral meatus

   In the vestibule of the vulva

   Anterior to the tubercle of the anterior wall of the vagina

   c. 2.5 cm behind the glans clitoridis

   Relationships:

   Backward: the anterior vaginal wall

   The wall consists of an outer muscle coat and an inner mucosa.

In the Middle, the Genital Axis
In the middle, the genital axis with the derivates of the Muller duct (see Chap. 1) tubes, uterus body, cervix , and vagina with two parts (one issued from the Muller duct and the other above the hymeneal membrane issued from the urogenital sinus).

In the Back, the GI Tract Axis

In the back, the GI tract axis with the rectum (which arises from the hindgut). In fact the rectum has two segments:

1. The intraperitoneal segment
2. The subperitoneal segment enclosed in perirectal fascia and separated from it by the mesorectum

The Vesicovaginal Septum

The vesicovaginal septum (Fig. 2.6) between posterior wall of the bladder and the anterior wall of the vagina.

The Rectovaginal Septum

The rectovaginal septum (Fig. 2.6) between the posterior wall of the vagina and the anterior perirectal fascia.

Laterally

Posteriorly, the sacrorectogenital fasciae (see Chap. 17)
The roof is formed by the uterosacral ligament. The floor is at the level of the levator ani
Anteriorly and laterally:

(a) The peritoneum forms:
   The median umbilical fold covering the urachus
   The medial lateral folds covering the obliterated umbilical arteries
(b) In front and below these folds is the subperitoneal space of Retzius defined as:
   The apex: the umbilicus
   The floor: the pelvic fascia covering the anterior part of levator ani immediately behind pubic symphysis
   Anteriorly: the fascia transversalis covering the inner part of the anterior abdominal wall
   Posteriorly: the peritoneum with the median and medial umbilical folds
   Laterally: a cellular sheet, which is a condensation of subperitoneal issue heightened by the umbilicovesical arteries called by Testut the umbilicovesical aponeurosis

Vascularization (Fig. 2.8)
The Extraperitoneal Space

This anatomical space is the compartment lateral to the lateral pelvic parietal peritoneum. Although it is not individualized in anatomic textbooks, it is isolated here because it is a particular space concerning the pathways of extension.

In front, it is limited by the pubis.
Backward, it is limited by the ischiatic spine.
It is in continuity with the subperitoneal and retroperitoneal spaces.
Medially it is limited by the lateral parietal peritoneum.
It contains from inside to outside:

1. The parietal pelvic ureter. It is adherent to the lateral part of the peritoneum. It lies close the uterine artery and behind it, behind the posterior leaf of the mesometrium, before entering the Mackenrodt ligament.
2. The hypogastric gain of Faraboeuf raised by the hypogastric branches of the hypogastric artery and veins. The hypogastric artery gives from the front to the back:
   (a) The vesical arteries
   (b) The uterine artery (usually with a common trunk with the umbilical artery at its origin) and its branches

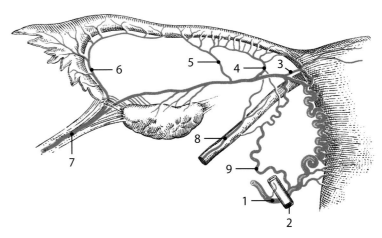

Fig. 2.8 *1* Uterine artery, *2* ureter, *3* artery of the fundus, *4* medial tubal artery, *5* middle tubal artery, *6* lateral tubal artery, *7* ovarian artery and suspensory ligament of the ovary, *8* artery of the round ligament, *9* anastomose between the uterine artery and its terminal portion (From EZES)

(c) The middle hemorrhoidal artery (which will give the inferior hemorrhoidal artery, also called the pudendal artery). Lymph nodes in a space limited by:
   1. In front, the posterior part of the iliac external vein; backward the pelvic parietal ureter; and outward the obturator nerve. In oncologic surgery, this space is the fundamental area of lymphadenectomy
   2. The nervous plane with the obturator nerve

The Retroperitoneal Space (Fig. 2.9)

From the back to the front:

1. *The sacrum*
2. *Immediately in front of the sacrum, parietal pelvic fascia*: a plane formed by the presacral fascia and immediately laterally in contact, the fascia over piriformis
   (a) *The presacral fascia*
      Its limits are as followed:
         Above, the promontory
         Below, the posterior part of the anorectal junction
         Laterally, the posterior part of the tendinous arches of the pelvic fascia(a thick white band extending from the lower part of the symphysis pubis to the inferior margin of the spine of the ischium).
         Behind the fascia: the presacral veins
         In front of the fascia: the right and left hypogastric nerves, coming from the superior hypogastric plexus
   (b) *Immediately laterally Fascia over piriformis*
      It is very thin and fuses with the periosteum in front of the sacrum at the margins of the anterior sacral foramina. It ensheathes *the sacral anterior primary rami which lies behind the fascia* (GRAY 1360) [2].
      The internal iliac vessels lie in front of the fascia over piriformis, and their branches draw out sheaths of the fascia and extraperitoneal tissue into the gluteal region.
3. *In front, the hindgut with the end of the sigmoid and the rectum*
   (a) From the promontory to the inferior part of the primary root of the mesosigmoid (usually S3), the sigmoid with its posterior meso and laterally the posterior parietal peritoneum.

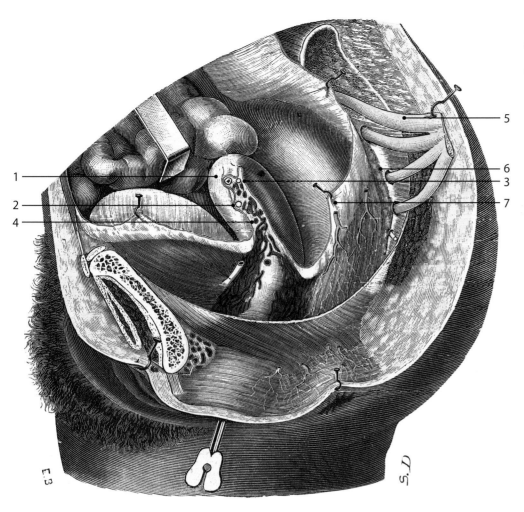

Fig. 2.9 Lateral view of the inner part of the broad ligament and of the retroperitoneal space. *1* Tube, *2* round ligament, *3* utero-ovarian ligament, *4* venous plexus, *5* sacral plexus, *6* fascia of piriformis, *7* posterior parietal peritoneum

(b) Below this level, the peritoneum covers the anterior part of the rectum until the bottom of the Douglas and ascends from this bottom posteriorly, according to an obliquely line until the inferior part of the primary root of the mesosigmoid, and from that part, continues with the posterior parietal pelvic fascia. At this level, the rectum is considered as intraperitoneal.

Laterally, it is in continuity with the posterior parietal peritoneum. Below this level, visceral fascia ensheathes the rectum until the anorectal junction. The rectum is subperitoneal with its visceral mesorectal fascia.

The Perineal Space (Figs. 2.10 and 2.11)

Perineal space is the anatomical compartment below the pelvic floor and is diamond shaped.

It is limited by:

- The deep limit: the inferior surface of the pelvic diaphragm (formed by levator ani and coccygeus) covered with the deep fascia lining the inferior surface of the levator ani, which is continuous at its lateral origin with the fascia over obturator internus below the attachment of levator. It lines the deep portion of the ischioanal fossa and its lateral walls
- The superficial limit: the skin which is continuous with that of the medial aspects of the thighs and the lower abdominal wall

- Anteriorly: pubic symphysis and arcuate ligament, the transverse ligament of Henle
- Posteriorly: coccyx
- Anterolaterally: isciopubic rami and the ischial tuberosities
- Posterolaterally: sacrotuberous ligaments

Perineum

Perineum is divided by a line joining the ischial tuberosities into an *anterior genital triangle and a posterior genital triangle.*

It contains:

1. The posterior anal triangle
2. The urogenital triangle from the deep part to the skin. This urogenital compartment contains:
   - The deep perineal space (deep limit: the inferior surface of the pelvic diaphragm)
   - The superficial perineal space (superficial limit: the superficial perineal fascia)
   - The vulva or pudendum or female external genitalia (the upper limit, the superficial perineal fascia; the lower limit, the skin)

In the middle of the line joining the ischial tuberosities is the *PERINEAL BODY*

It is a poorly defined aggregation of fibromuscular tissue located at the junction between the anal and urogenital triangles.

It is attached to many structures in both the deep and superficial urogenital spaces:

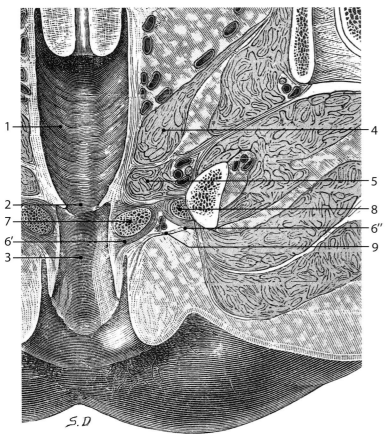

Fig. 2.10 Coronal section through the middle part of the vagina. *1* Subperitoneal vagina, *2* vaginal introitus, *3* vestibular vagina, *4* levator ani, *5* deep transverse muscle, *6′* bulbospongious muscle, *6″* ischiocavernous muscle, *7* bulb of vestibule, *8* crus of clitoris, *9* superficial aponeurosis of perineum (From Testut)

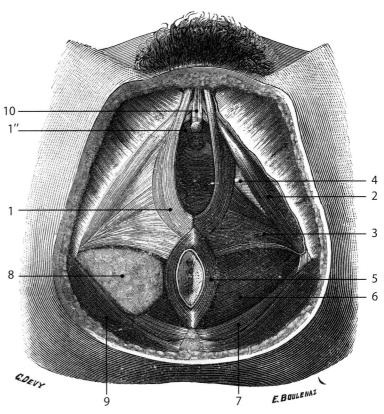

Fig. 2.11 Superficial perineal space. On the left side superficial fascia or Colles' fascia has been removed. *1* Bulbospongiosus muscle, *1′* internal fascicle, *1″* external fascicle, *2* ischiocavernous muscle, *3* superficial transverse perinei, *4* perineal membrane, *5* external anal sphincter, *6* evator ani, *7* ischiococcygeus muscle, *8* adipose tissue of the ischiorectal fossa, *9* gluteus maximus, *10* clitoris (From Testut)

- Posteriorly fibers from the middle part of the external anal sphincter and the conjoint longitudinal coat
- Superiorly the rectovaginal septum including fibers from levator ani (puborectalis and pubovaginalis)
- Anteriorly the deep transverse perinei, the superficial transverse perinei, the bulbospongious
- The perineal body is continuous with the perineal membrane and the superficial perineal fascia.

Anal Triangle [2, 3] (Fig. 2.10)

It is limited by:

(a) Superficially: superficial fascia continuous with the superficial fascia of the perineum, thighs and buttocks.
(b) Deeply: deep fascia lines the inferior surface of the levator ani and is continuous at its lateral origin with the fascia over the obturator internus below the attachment of levator. It lines the deep portion of the ischioanal fossa and its lateral walls.

It contains

(a) Ischioanal fossa limited by:
- Laterally:
- Anterolaterally, the deep fascia over obturator internus deeply, and ischial tuberosities more superficially
- Posterolaterally, the lower border of gluteus maximus and the sacrotuberous ligament

- Anteriorly:
- Superficially the posterior aspect of the urogenital triangle. Deep to this there is no fascial boundary between the fossa and the tissues deep to the perineal membrane as far anteriorly as the posterior surface of the pubis below the attachment of levator ani.

(b) Anal canal
The anal canal has a mucosa, a submucosa, an internal anal sphincter, and an external anal sphincter separated by a longitudinal layer.

1. Internal anal sphincter: It is a well defined ring of obliquely oriented smooth muscle fibers continuous with the circular muscle of the rectum, terminating at the junction of the superficial and subcutaneous components of the external sphincter.

2. External anal sphincter: It is an oval-shaped complex of striated muscle fibers.
- The uppermost fibers blend with the lowest fibers of the puborectalis; anteriorly some of these upper fibers decussate into the superficial transverse perineal muscles; posteriorly some fibers are attached to the anococcygeal ligament.
- The majority of middle fibers surround the lower part of the internal sphincter; this portion is attached anteriorly to the perineal body, posteriorly to the anococcygeal ligament
- The lower fibers lie below the level of the internal anal sphincter and are separated from the lowest anal epithelium by submucosa

3. Longitudinal layer is situated between the internal and external sphincters.
   - It contains the conjoint longitudinal coat and the intersphincteric space with its connective tissue components
   - The conjoint longitudinal coat has two components: an upper muscular and a lower fibroelastic component
   - The muscular component is formed by the fusion of striated muscle fibers from puboanalis with smooth muscle from longitudinal muscle of the rectum.
   - The layer then becomes completely fibroelastic, and splits into septa. The most peripheral septa extend through the external sphincter into the ischioanal fossa; the most central septa pass through it

(c) Anococcygeal ligament

   It runs between middle portion of the external anal sphincter and the coccyx. The lowest portion of the presacral fascia lies above the deep part of the ligament and between the two lie the most posterior fibers of the raphe of the iliococcygeus

Urogenital Triangle

Urogenital triangle [2, 3] (Figs. 2.10 and 2.11): extends from the inferior surface of the pelvic diaphragm to the lower limit of the labia and mons pubis. It is divided into two parts by a strong perineal membrane: the *deep perineal space* and the *superficial perineal space*

Deep Perineal Space

(a) Is limited by
   - Deeply: the endopelvic fascia of the pelvic floor
   - Superficially: the perineal membrane
   - Medially: it leaves passage to the urethra and the vagina

(b) It contains from deeply to superficially:
   1. The endopelvic fascia of the pelvic floor
   2. The deep perineal space between the endopelvic fascia and the fascia over deep transverse perinei. It is filled with adipose tissue. It is the narrow continuation of the ischioanal fossa extending until the body of the pubis
   3. The fascia above deep transverse perinei (superior sheet of the middle aponeurosis from Testut)
   4. The transverse perinei
   5. The perineal membrane

Superficially: the perineal membrane (inferior fascia of the urogenital diaphragm)
This membrane is triangular, attached:
   - Laterally to the periosteum of the ischiopubic rami
   - The posterior border: is fused with the deep part of the perineal body and is continuous with the fascia over the deep transverse perinei. The upper sheet is continuous posteriorly with the lower part of the rectovaginal septum
   - Anteriorly at the apex: fascia over transverse perinei and the perineal membrane join to form very tight aponeurotic fibers, the transverse ligament of Henlé also called the pubourethral ligament. Its apex is attached the arcuate ligament of the pubis

It is divided almost in two halves by the vagina and urethra such that it forms a triangle on each side of these structures which join anteriorly the pubourethral ligament of Henlé (just behind the arcuate ligament) links the two sides anteriorly

(c) It contains: the deep transverse perinei superficial to the transvers perinei: the urethral sphincter mechanism the urethral sphincter mechanism consists of intrinsic striated and smooth muscle of the urethra and the pubourethralis component of the levator ani. It surrounds the middle and lower thirds of the urethra.
   - Under: compressor urethra, arises from ischiopubic rami of each side by a small tendon. Fibers pass anteriorly to meet with their controlateral counterparts in a flat band anterior to the urethra, below sphincter urethrae
   - Under: sphincter urethrovaginalis: arises from the perineal body pass on each side of the vagina and urethra to meet their controlateral counterparts in a flat band anterior to the urethra, below compressor urethra

(d) The perineal membrane is divided almost in two halves by the vagina and urethra crossed by:
   - On the midline: the urethra 2–3 cm behind the inferior border of the symphysis pubis, the vagina
   - Behind the pubis the pubourethral ligament, the deep dorsal vessels, and nerves of the clitoris
   - Anterior to the transverse perinei, the posterior labial vessels and nerves

Superficial Perineal Space [2, 3] (Table 2.1) (See Chap. 34)

(a) Is limited by:
   - Deeply: the perineal membrane the deep perineal fascia is attached to the ischiopubic rami and to the posterior margin of the perineal membrane and perineal body over the membranous layer. In front, it fuses with the suspensory ligament of the clitoris and the fasciae of external oblique and the rectus sheath.
   - Superficially: the superficial perineal fascia also called Colles' fascia is attached to:
     - Posteriorly: the fascia over the superficial transverse perinei and the posterior limit of the perineal membrane
     - Laterally: the margins of the ischiopubic rami and the ischial tuberosities. From here it runs more superficially to the skin of the urogenital triangle, lining the external genitalia and then in continuity with the fascia of Scarpa of the anterior abdominal wall.

(b) It contains:
   1. The deep perineal fascia is attached to the ischiopubic rami and to the posterior margin of the perineal membrane and perineal body over the membranous layer. In front, it fuses with the suspensory ligament of the clitoris and the fasciae of external oblique and the rectus sheath.
   2. Superficial transverse perinei: laterally is attached to the medial and anterior aspect of the ischial tuberosity, medially the perineal body

Table 2.1 Components of the vulva

Anatomical compartment		
Anatomical structures	**Vulva**	**Superficial perineal space**
1. Labial formations		
Mons pubis	Mons pubis	
Labia majora	Labia majora	
Labia minora	Labia minora	
2. Erectile organs		
Clitoris		
Corpora cavernosa		Corpora cavernosa
Corpus clitoridis	Corpus clitoridis (1/2 anterior)	Corpus clitoridis (1/2 posterior)
Glans	Glans	
Bulbs of the vestibule	Bulbs of the vestibule (anterior part: join to the posterior part of corpus clitoridis)	Bulbs of the vestibule (posterior and middle part)
3. Glands		
Greater vestibular glands	Greater vestibular glands (anterior part)	Greater vestibular glands (posterior and middle part)
Ducts	Ducts	
Skene's glands	Skene's glands	Skene's glands
Skene's ducts	Skene's ducts	Skene's ducts
4. Vestibule (between labia minora)		
Urethra	Urethral meatus (in vestibule)	Urethra (perineal portion)
Vagina	Vaginal orifice (in vestibule)	Vagina (part of perineal portion)
	Hymen	

2. In its middle part: Vestibule
   The vestibule contains vaginal orifice (Introitus) hymen vaginae
   External urethral orifice also called: External urethral meatus
3. Erectile organs: the clitoris and the bulbs of vestibule
   Clitoris: Posterior portion of the corpus clitoridis and its two corpora cavernosa covered superficially by ischiocavernous muscle lie in the superficial perineal space
   Anterior portion of corpus clitoridis and the glans belong to the pudendum
   Bulbs of vestibule (posterior portion) are covered superficially by bulbospongious muscles in the medial part of the superficial perineal space; the anterior portion of the bulbs are thin in the vestibule.
4. Glands
   The greater vestibular glands or Bartholin's glands are situated in the superficial perineal space; each opens into the vestibule by a duct of c. 2 cm in the groove between the hymen and a labium minus
   The Skene's glands are situated all along the subperitoneal and the perineal portions of the urethra. Small glands and minute recesses or lacunae open into the urethra. Near the lower end of the urethra, number of these glands group together and open into a duct, named the paraurethral duct. Each runs down into the submucous tissue of the urethra and ends in a small aperture on the lateral margin of the external urethral orifice.

3. Bulbospongiosus attaches to the perineal body; on each side is separate; covers the superficial part of the vestibular bulbs; and greater vestibular glands run anteriorly on each side of the vagina to attach to the corpora cavernosa clitoridis
4. Ischiocavernosus attaches on the ischiopubic ramus on both sides of the corpus clitoridis ends in an aponeurosis attached to the sides and under surface of the of the crus

(c) Between the medial parts of the bulbospongious muscles, cross:
   • The lower part of the urethra
   • The lower part of the vagina

Vulva or Pudendum or Female External Genitalia [3] *(Table 2.1) (See Chap. 34)*

Definition: Anatomical compartment of the perineum situated below the superficial perineal space of the anterior genital triangle limited by:
• Deeply: the superficial perineal fascia
• Superficially: the skin
• In fact this anatomical space contains two types of anatomical structures: structures which entirely belong to this space (labial formations, vestibule), structures which belong to the superficial perineal space (bulbs of the vestibule) or both (clitoris)

It contains:
   1. Labial formations: Mons pubis, labia majora, labia minora

2.2 Anatomical Locations of Pelvic Masses

2.2.1 Gynecologic Pelvic Masses

2.2.1.1 Ovary (Fig. 2.12)

Typical findings in favor of a location to the ovary are reported in Table 2.2.

2.2.1.2 Tube (Figs. 2.13 and 2.14)

Typical findings in favor of a location to the tube are reported in Table 2.3

2.2.1.3 Uterine Masses Distorting the Contour of the Uterus

1. *Mainly subserous leiomyoma (sessile or pedunculated)*
   Anatomy:
      Continuity with the uterus or visualization of the pedicle
      Differential diagnosis:
      1. Ovarian fibrothecoma
      2. Carcinoma of the ovary
   As far as vascularization of subserous leiomyoma, it is mainly furnished by the large marginal segment of the uterine artery and of ovarian tumors by the thin ovarian artery and the tubo-ovarian artery, vascular findings, and contrast uptake of these processes are quite different. Vascularization and contrast uptake are reported in Table 2.4 (Fig. 2.15 and 2.33).

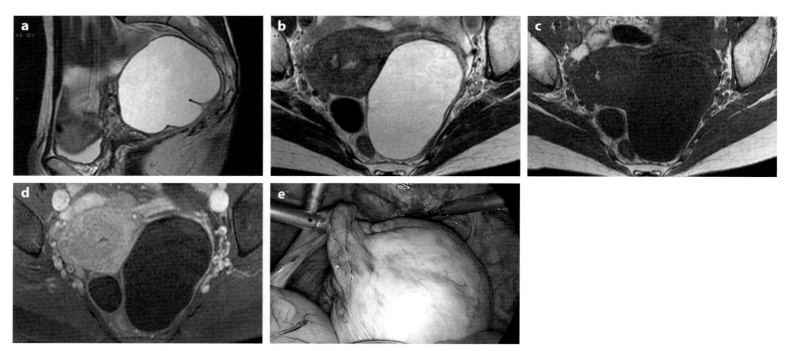

Fig. 2.12 Unilocular mucinous cystadenoma. Fifty-three-year-old woman. MR Sagittal T2 (**a**) and axial T2 (**b**) T2 display a unilocular cystic mass, with convoluted inferior border which discusses a possibility of hydrosalpinx. Visualization of the normal right ovary, while a normal left ovary independent of the mass is not visualized and the fact as the tumor is completely surrounded by a low intensity rim are in favor of an ovarian origin. On axial T1 (**c**) signal intensity is slightly superior to urine. On fat suppression after injection (**d**) a contrast uptake around the mass is in favor of an ovarian mass. Prospective diagnosis: ovarian cystic benign tumor. A hydrosalpinx is much more unlikely. Coelioscopy (**e**): confirms the mass is ovarian in origin. Microscopy: mucinous cystadenoma (cellular type not précised)

Table 2.2 Findings in favor of a location to the ovary

1. **Anatomy**
Usually in the ovarian fossa, limited in front by the external iliac vein, behind by the uterine artery and the pelvic ureter; may be in front, behind, inward, higher
Separated from the uterus (may be adherent)
Infundibular ligament and tubo-ovarian vessels arrive in the mass
2. **Shape and structure**
Round or oval
External cortex, hypoechogenic, low signal on T2 (related to high concentration of collagen)
When small or benign surrounded by ovarian parenchyma
After contrast (CT MR), a ring of contrast surrounds completely the mass
3. **Differential diagnosis**
(a) Cystic: hydrosalpinx, paraovarian cyst, inclusion peritoneal cyst, Tarlov cyst
(b) Solid masses
Benign: fibrothecoma versus subserous leiomyoma
Malignant: ovarian carcinoma versus leiomyoma

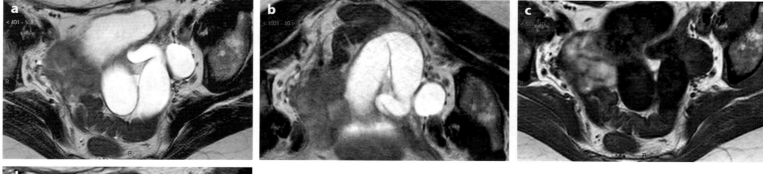
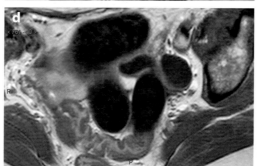

Fig. 2.13 Left hydrosalpinx. A 53-year-old woman. Interannexial total hysterectomy 10 years ago. Pelvic pain US examination demonstrates a left hydrosalpinx but is enable to know if it is unilateral or bilateral. MR axial T2 supine (**a**) displays a left tubular adnexal extra-ovarian collection typical for a hydrosalpinx. Axial T2 on prone position (**b**) demonstrates that the fluid is slightly moving in the tube; this sequence can be helpful in the differential of other cystic adnexal masses. Medial face of the left ovary lies against the isthmic ampullary junction; ovary contains a functional cyst (which has slightly increased in size 2 weeks after the US). Axial T1 without injection (**c**) shows the content of the dilated tube is a watery fluid; after injection (**d**), a slight contrast uptake is visualized in the wall of the hydrosalpinx

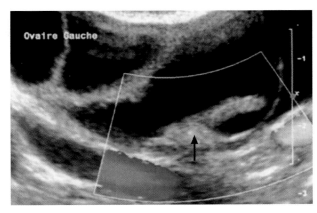

Fig. 2.14 Plica in a hydrosalpinx. In a tubular shape cystic adnexal mass related to an hydrosalpinx, localized tissular portion can simulate a papillary projection. When the digitiform shape and the oblique orientation are present like in this case, these morphologic findings are very helpful to distinguish it from a papillary projection in an ovarian cyst and to diagnose a plica (*arrow*). However, in some cases, the plicae can be smaller and round, impossible to distinguish from an endocystic papillary projection

Table 2.3 Findings in favor of a location to the tube

1. **Anatomy** Subperitoneal in the upper part of the broad ligament, except the infundibulum which is intraperitoneal. Ampulla and infundibulum medial to the ovary 2. **Shape and structure** Tubal shape with increasing diameter toward the periphery. Particular shape of the infundibulum Foldings of the outer wall, plicae of the inner wall with the possibility of the very suggestive cogwheel sign 3. **Differential diagnosis** (a) Cystic hydrosalpinx, paraovarian cyst, inclusion peritoneal cyst, Tarlov cyst (b) Solid benign and malignant most in a hydrosalpinx

2.2.2 Broad Ligament

2.2.2.1 Paratubal or Paraovaian Cysts (Fig. 2.16)

According to the embryologic origin, there are two types: paramesonephric and mesonephric cysts.

Table 2.4 Findings in favor of a location to the uterus

	Subserous leiomyoma	Ovarian fibrothecoma	Ovarian carcinoma
Artery (Doppler, DCT, DMR)	Peripheral, circular	Central	Central Tumoral thin and irregular
Contrast uptake (DCT, DMR)	High, mainly at the periphery	Low, on the delayed phase straight	High and heterogeneous

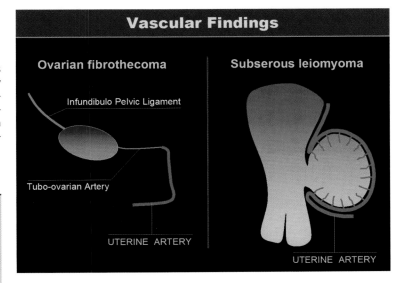

Fig. 2.15 Vascularization of ovarian fibrothecoma versus vascularization of subserous leiomyoma. Vascularization of a fibrothecoma is produced by the ovarian artery and the tubo-ovarian artery of the uterine artery which are of small caliber so that vascularization is poor and mainly central. On the opposite, vascularization of a subserous leiomyoma is produced by the marginal segment of the uterine artery and its branches (the arcuate arteries and the perforating arteries) with a characteristic peripheral vascularization more or less associated with a central vascularization

The main findings of paramesonephric cysts are reported in Table 2.5.

The main findings of mesonephric cysts are reported in Table 2.6.

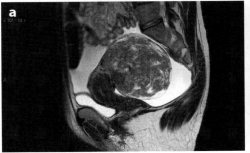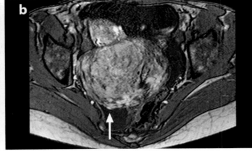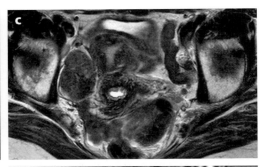

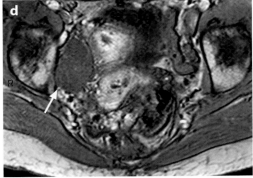

Fig. 2.16 Subserous leiomyoma versus ovarian fibroma. (1) Subserous leiomyoma. Sagittal T2 (**a**) displays a pediculated subserous leiomyoma. DMR axial at the arterial phase (**b**) depicts a rich peripheral vascularization (*arrow*) associated to a central vascularization, typical for a subserous leiomyoma. (2) Ovarian fibroma. On axial T2 (**c**), the right pelvic mass is in contact with the right border of the uterus body. Although location to the ovary is likely, DMR axial at the arterial phase (**d**) does not depict any peripheral vascularization at this phase (*arrow*) which is typical for ovarian fibroma. These vascular findings are very helpful to distinguish subserous leiomyoma from adnexal masses as in this case an ovarian fibroma

Table 2.5 Paramesonephric cysts (arise from Mullerian structures)

Definition
Lined by an epithelium which contains numerous ciliated cells. Some cysts may have papillary infoldings similar to endosalpingeal folds
The Hydatid of Morgagni is by far the most common
Definition
It is lined by ciliated and nonciliated cells and may have small epithelial
Findings
Dangling from one of the fimbriae
Ovoid or round
2–10 mm in diameter
Cystic: serous content

Table 2.6 Mesonephric cysts (arise from Wolffian structures)

Definition
Lined by an epithelium which contains only a few or no ciliated cells
May have a prominent muscular coat
Anatomy
2.1. Epoophoron, paroophoron (mesonephric tubules)
In the mesosalpinx
Easy to localize when clearly separated from the ovary; may be in contact with the ovary and in this case impossible to distinguish from an ovarian cyst arising in the ovarian cortex
2.2. Appendix vesiculosa, Gartner duct (mesonephric duct)
In the medial part of the mesometrium either lateral to the body of the uterus, more commonly in the paracervix or the paravagina
Shape and structure
Round or oval
Usually purely cystic, may contain papillary projection

2.2.2.2 Cystic and Solid Masses
(Fig. 2.17) **of the Mesometrium**

The main findings of cystic and solid masses of the mesometrium are reported in Table 2.7.

Table 2.7 Findings in favor of location to the mesometrium

Anatomy
Mass separated from the lateral border of the uterus, moving apart the anterior and posterior leaves of the broad ligament
Round ligament, more rarely uterosacral ligament pushed upward by the mass
Lateral extension until the pelvic wall
Inward displacement of the lateral wall of the bladder
Downward extension until the pubic symphysis
Mass effect on the pelvic ureter in its parametrial portion
Vascularization mainly by branches of the uterine and ovarian artery
Shape and structure
Mainly solid

2.2.3 Peritoneal Masses

2.2.3.1 Peritoneal Inclusion Cyst
(Figs. 2.18 and 2.19) (See Chap. 16)

Peritoneal pseudocyst occurs in different circumstances, all of them related to peritoneal adhesions: (1) after pelvic surgery, (2) after PID, (3) after endometriosis

Definition: It is defined histologically by an inner sheet of peritoneal flat cells of mesothelial type.

These cells usually secrete clear fluid responsible for the development of the cyst. But in some circumstances, different kinds of fluid may be encountered.

Findings in favor of peritoneal inclusion cysts are reported in Table 2.8.

2.2.3.2 Splenic Parenchyma

Splenosis

Definition: implantation of splenic tissue on the peritoneum after splenectomy

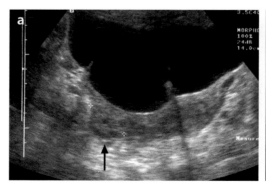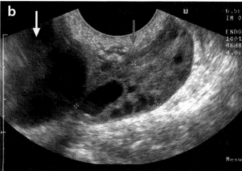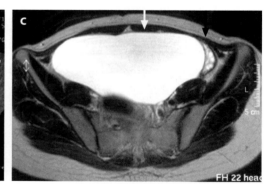

Fig. 2.17 Transverse TAS (**a**) displays a unilocular cystic mass with bosselated borders anterior to the uterus; a normal right ovary is depicted (*arrow*). Examination with the endovaginal probe in the lateral portion of left flank (**b**) depicts the left normal ovary (*red arrow*) pushed laterally by the cyst (*white arrow*). (**c**) MR axial T2 confirms the extra-ovarian location of the cyst (*white arrow*) in contact with the left normal ovary (*black arrow*). Coelioscopy: resection of the cyst. Microscopy: left paraovarian cyst

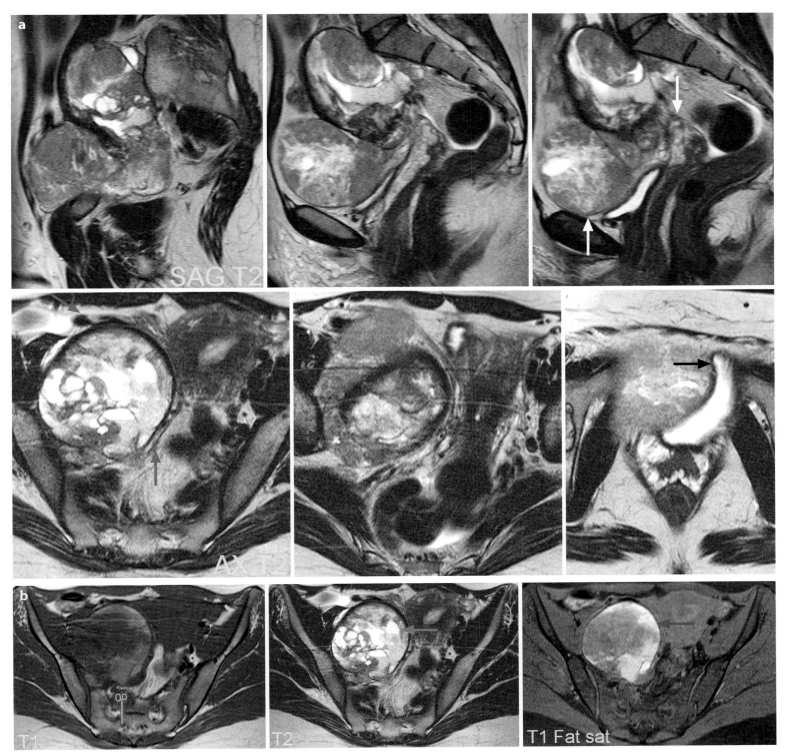

Fig. 2.18 High-grade synoviolosacoma of the broad ligament. (a): MR sagittal T2 (in three contiguousplanes) displays a well delineated mass moving apart the anterior and posterior leaves of the broad ligament (*white arrows*). On Axial T2 at three different levels, the mass (1) pushes inward and upward the round ligament (*anterior red arrow*) and backward the posterior leaf of the broad ligament (*posterior red arrows*), (2) extends laterally until the pelvic wall (*blue arrow*) (3) extends downward until the pubic symphysis pushing inward the lateral wall of the bladder (*black arrow*). **(b):** On axial T2, the mass contains solid tissue of intermediate signal with multiple cystic spaces (*green arrow*). On axial T1 (*pink arrow*) and on fat suppression (*purple arrow*), the solid portions contain hemorrhagic areas. Prospective diagnosis; tumor of the broad ligament. Cystic cavities and hemorrhagic changes suggest the possibility of a sarcoma. Definite diagnosis: high-grade synoviolosarcoma of the broad ligament

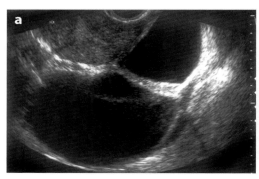 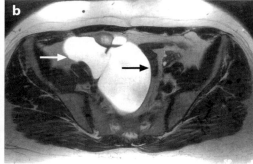

Fig. 2.19 High-grade synoviolosacoma of the broad ligament. (**a**): MR sagittal T2 (in three contiguousplanes) displays a well delineated mass moving apart the anterior and posterior leaves of the broad ligament (*white arrows*). On Axial T2 at three different levels, the mass (1) pushes inward and upward the round ligament (*anterior red arrow*) and backward the posterior leaf of the broad ligament (*posterior red arrow*), (2) extends laterally until the pelvic wall (*blue arrow*) (3) extends downward until the pubic symphysis pushing inward the lateral wall of the bladder (*black arrow*). (**b**): On axial T2, the mass contains solid tissue of intermediate signal with multiple cystic spaces (*green arrow*). On axial T1 (*pink arrow*) and on fat suppression (*purple arrows*), the solid portions contain hemorrhagic areas. Prospective diagnosis; tumor of the broad ligament. Cystic cavities and hemorrhagic changes suggest the possibility of a sarcoma. Definite diagnosis: high-grade synoviolosarcoma of the broad ligament

Table 2.8 Findings of mucocele

Anatomy: medial border of the cecum usually
Morphologic findings: elongated cystic mass
Differential diagnosis: hydrosalpinx

*Mucocele of the appendix may be associated with a mucinous ovarian tumor

Peritoneal nodules, ranging from punctuate to 7 cm in diameter, are scattered widely throughout the abdominal and less the peritoneal cavity (Fig. 2.20). Splenic tissue in the pelvis has the same echogenicity, density on CT, or signal on MR as the nodules situated in the left subphrenic space.

Pelvic Accessory Spleen

Exceptionally, pelvic accessory spleen can be present (Fig. 2.21).

2.2.4 Extraperitoneal Masses

Lymph node metastases of pelvic carcinoma is the major cause of masses in this space; a fundamental finding to differentiate them from intraperitoneal masses particularly ovarian masses is the peritoneum lying medial to these extraperitoneal masses (Fig. 2.22).

Cystic masses in this space are mainly related to lymphoceles.

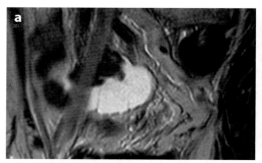 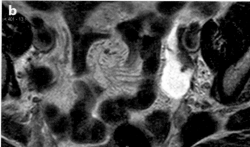 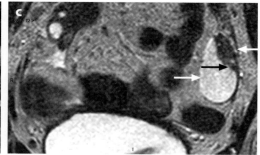
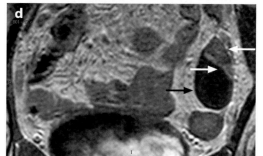

Fig. 2.20 Left peritoneal pseudocyst. Fifty-four-year-old woman. Total hysterectomy with conservation of the adnexae performed 3 years before. Left pelvic pain. Sagittal T2 (**a**) and axial T2 (**b**) display a unilocular cystic collection lying against the left lateral parietal pelvic peritoneum. Coronal T2 (**c**) depicts from outside to inside the normal ovary (*upper white arrow*), the distal portion of the ampulla of the tube and its infundibulum (*black arrow*) the peritoneal pseudocyst in contact with the medial face of the ovary with its thin medial wall (*lower white arrow*). Coronal T1 after injection (**d**) depicts contrast uptake in the ovary (*upper white arrow*) in the distal portion of the tube (*lower white arrow*), while the wall of the pseudocyst on its medial border looks very thin (*black arrow*)

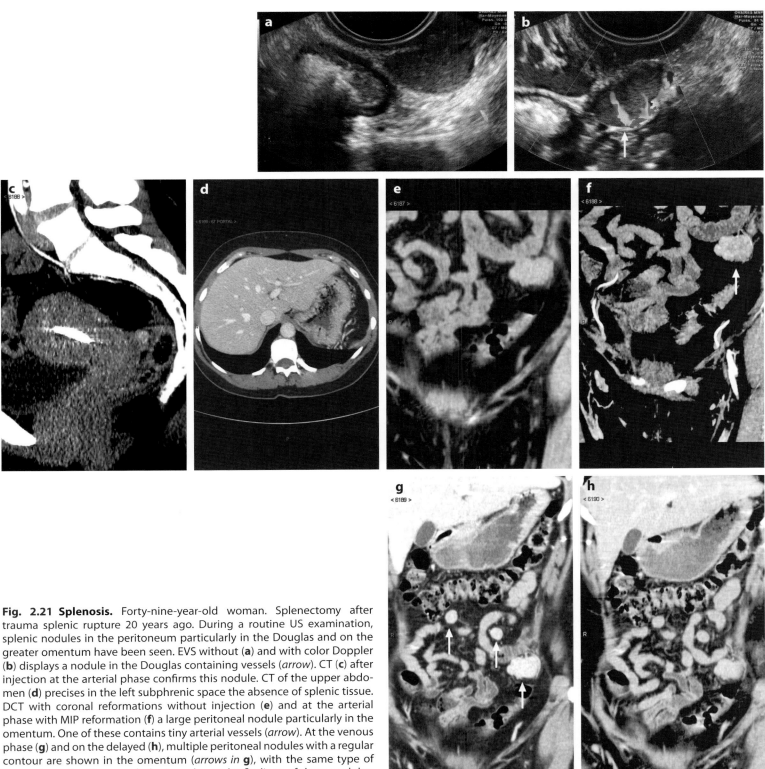

Fig. 2.21 Splenosis. Forty-nine-year-old woman. Splenectomy after trauma splenic rupture 20 years ago. During a routine US examination, splenic nodules in the peritoneum particularly in the Douglas and on the greater omentum have been seen. EVS without (**a**) and with color Doppler (**b**) displays a nodule in the Douglas containing vessels (*arrow*). CT (**c**) after injection at the arterial phase confirms this nodule. CT of the upper abdomen (**d**) precises in the left subphrenic space the absence of splenic tissue. DCT with coronal reformations without injection (**e**) and at the arterial phase with MIP reformation (**f**) a large peritoneal nodule particularly in the omentum. One of these contains tiny arterial vessels (*arrow*). At the venous phase (**g**) and on the delayed (**h**), multiple peritoneal nodules with a regular contour are shown in the omentum (*arrows in* **g**), with the same type of contrast uptake. The morphologic and vascular findings of these nodules, the previous splenectomy, are typical for splenosis

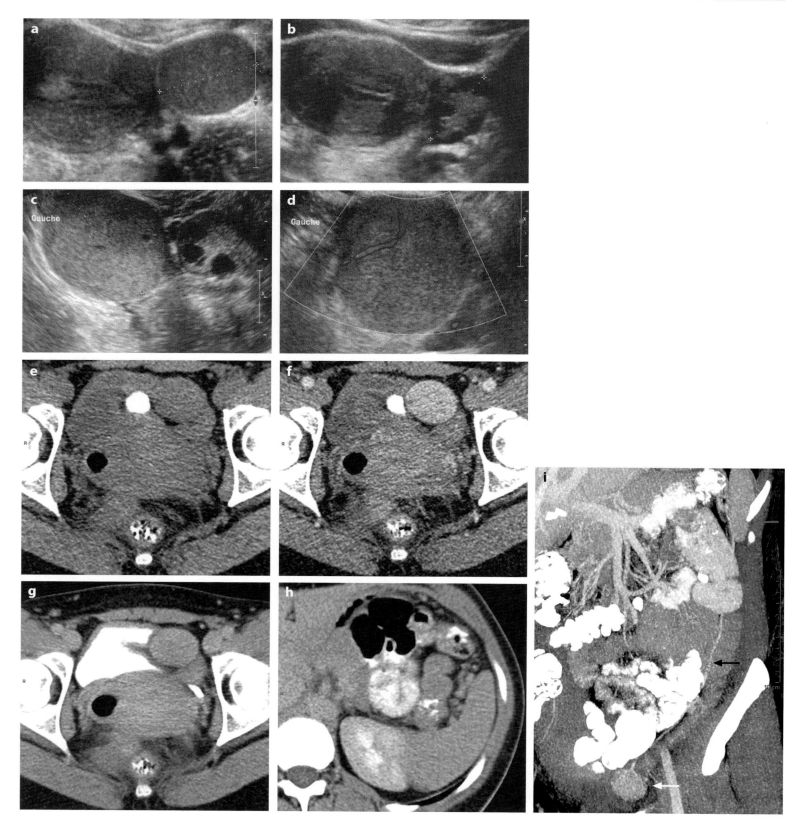

Fig. 2.22 Pelvic accessory spleen. EVS (**a–c**) displays a round echogenic homogeneous mass, separated from the uterus in (**a**) and from the ovary in (**b**, **c**), containing vessels on color Doppler (**d**). DCT without injection (**e**) and at the arterial phase (**f**) display a round mass with an early and homogeneous contrast uptake; on the delayed (**g**), contrast uptake is identical to the spleen (**h**). CT with oblique coronal reformation and MIP (**i**) depicts the accessory spleen (*white arrow*) related by a cord (*black arrow*) to the lower pole of the spleen (*red arrow*). Prospective diagnosis: pelvic accessory spleen. Coelioscopy confirmed the diagnosis

2.2.5 GI Tract Pelvic Masses

1. Sigmoid (Figs. 2.23 and 2.24)
2. Small bowel:
   Mobility of the mass
   Presence of air within the mass (Fig. 2.25)
3. Appendiceal Mucocele (Fig. 2.26)

Findings of mucocele are reported in Table 2.9.

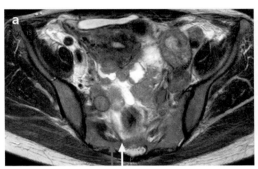
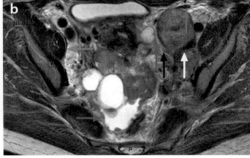
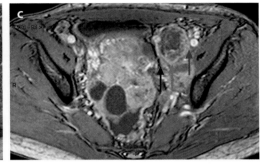

Fig. 2.23 Undifferentiated carcinoma of the ovary with lymph node metastases. MR axial T2. (**a**) (1) piriform fascia (*white arrow*), (2) anterior sacral ramus (*red arrow*). (**b**) (1) Lymph node metastases (*white arrow*), (2) extraperitoneal space (*black arrow*), (3) round ligament (*red arrow*) pushed forward by the lymph node, (4) left parietal pelvic peritoneum (*vertical green arrow*), (5) right parietal pelvic peritoneum (*horizontal green arrow*) lined by ascites, (6) parietal fascia (*brown arrow*). (**c**) MR axial, arterial phase displays in the left extraperitoneal space from inward to outwars: *1* peritoneum (*black arrow*), *2* a metastatic lymph node (*red arrow*) (an ovarian mass could not be in this location), *3* the extraperitoneal space lateral to the iliac vessels (*blue arrow*)

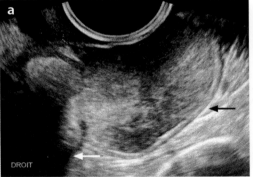
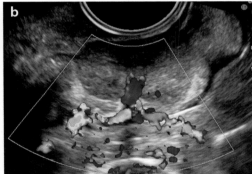
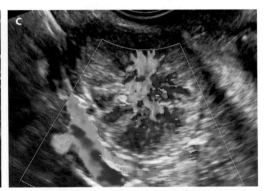

Fig. 2.24 Invasive adenocarcinoma of the sigmoid. A 82-year-old woman without THS right mass latero-uterine discovered during routine US examination. EVS (**a**) displays a right latero-uterine tissular mass (*black arrow*) with regular borders, communicating with the lumen of the sigmoid (*white arrow*). Right ovary is normal. On color Doppler (**b–d**), a vascular pedicle is depicted along the medial border of the bowel (**b**); the hypervascularization is central with a very particular radiated distribution (**c**). Prospective diagnosis: endoluminal sigmoid solid mass which particular vascularization suggesting the possibility of a villous tumor. Surgery: endoscopic resection of the polyp. Microscopy: adenocarcinoma p T1 N0 well differentiated developed at the surface of a tubulovillous adenoma

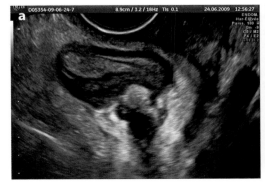
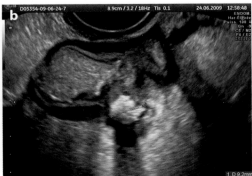

Fig. 2.25 Fifty-five-year-old woman; left pelvic pain CRP 108. EVS (**a**, **b**) display (1) a thickening if the sigmoid wall, (2) a diverticulum, and (3) an echogenic thickening of the mesosigmoid. These findings help to differentiate inflammation or an abscess of the sigmoid from a pelvic inflammatory disease with salpingitis

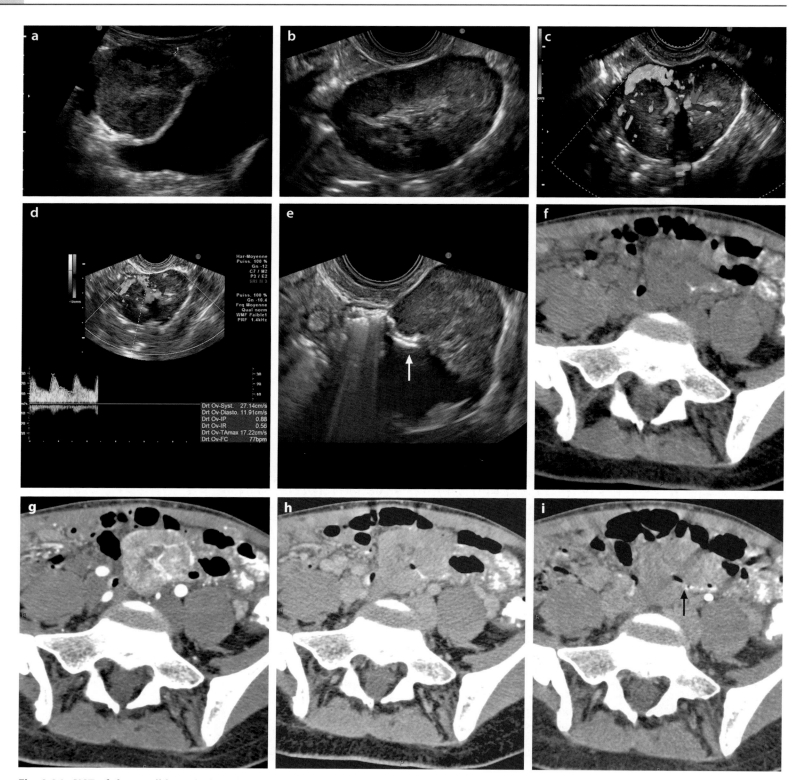

Fig. 2.26 GIST of the small bowel. Thirty-two-year-old woman. During a routine examination, a pelvic mass is discovered. TAS (**a**), a 4-cm mass in the left portion of the pelvis, close to the bladder is visualized; left kidney lies in the left lumbar fossa and is normal. EVS (**b**) (1) demonstrates that the mass is extra-ovarian, (2) better depicts the oval shape and the structure of the mass, particularly a central echogenic area. On color Doppler (**c**), a large pedicle and a high degree of central vascularization are displayed, with a high velocity on pulsed Doppler (**d**). On (**e**), gaz is entering into the mass (*arrow*). DCT without injection (**f**) displays that the mass is in front of the sacrum. At the arterial phase (**g**), a large vascular pedicle and rich peripheral and central vascularization are depicted. At the venous phase (**h**), an important washout is shown. On (**h**) and the delayed (**i**), presence of air and GI contrast uptake are going into the mass proving the mass is small bowel in origin (*arrow*). Surgery resection of the tumor with termino-terminal anastomosis. Pathology: GIST

Table 2.9 Surgical and radiologic findings of peritoneal inclusion cysts

Common
Size: usually between 4 and 10 cm
Mainly or exclusively cystic
Wall and septa thin and regular
Solid tissue can be present (related to inflammatory tissue)
Usually not round, conforming to surrounding structures
Lying against the peritoneum
Most commonly multilocular, may be unilocular
Adhesions to surrounding structures vey common (bladder, sigmoid)
Uncommon
May resemble simple free peritoneal fluid
Small papillae present (exceptionally)
Differential diagnosis
1. Mainly hydrosalpinx (which can be associated)
2. More rarely cystic ovarian mass or paraovarian cyst

2.2.6 Urinary Pelvic Masses

Pelvic kidney is the main differential (Fig. 2.27)

2.2.7 Neurogenic Masses

2.2.7.1 Tarlov Cyst

Tarlov cyst (Fig. 2.28 and 2.32) may be confused with an ovarian cyst on US.

On MR, the posterior location and the communication with a sacral foramen are typical for this type of cyst.

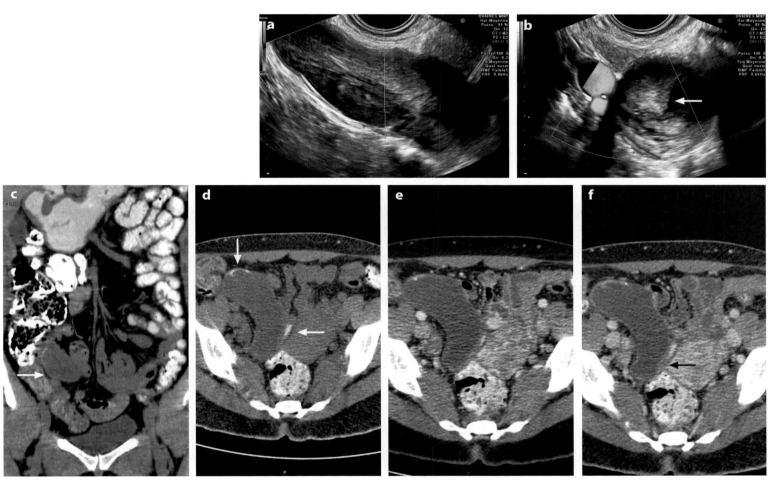

Fig. 2.27 Borderline mucinous tumor of the appendix. Forty-five-year-old woman. Right pelvic pain and sensation of a mass in the right iliac fossa. EVS longitudinal (**a**) and transverse (**b**) display an echogenic tubular mass in the right iliac fossa, with a regular vessel in the wall, containing an echogenic material without color flow (*arrow*). Location of the mass close to the cecum and the tubular shape suggest an appendicular origin. CT without injection and with coronal reformation (**c**) clearly displays the mass is appendicular (*arrow*). The transverse view without injection (**d**) depicts calcification in the wall (*arrow*). On DCT at the arterial phase (**e**) and at the venous phase (**f**) below a calcification, a slight contrast uptake is visualized in a localized thickening of the wall (*arrow*)

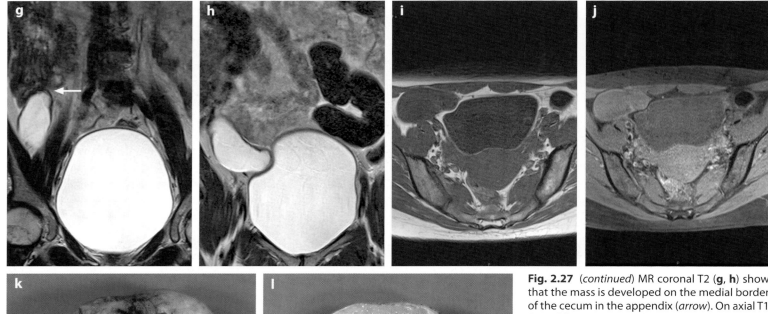

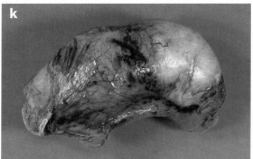

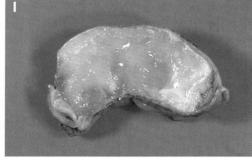

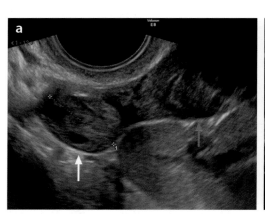

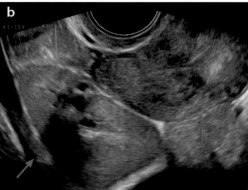

Fig. 2.27 (*continued*) MR coronal T2 (**g**, **h**) show that the mass is developed on the medial border of the cecum in the appendix (*arrow*). On axial T1 (**i**) and fat suppression (**j**), content of the appendix is about the same signal as pelvic muscles and does not correspond to clear fluid. (**k**) Macroscopic specimen. (**l**) Longitudinal section of the appendix: content is mucoid; a focal slight thickening of the wall is displayed. Microscopy: mucinous cystadenoma with a little focus of borderline tumor

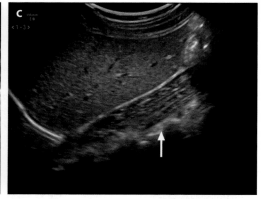

Fig. 2.28 Right pelvic kidney. EVS (**a**) right pelvic mass (*red arrow*) separated from normal right ovary (*white arrow*). EVS (**b**) right pelvic mass with a kidney shape in the pelvis (*red arrow*), separated from the uterus (*green arrow*). TAS (**c**) of the right lumbar fossa (*arrow*) does nor displays any kidney

2.2.7.2 Cystic Neurinoma (Fig. 2.29)

1. Morphologic and vascular findings
   Shape: round
   Solid patterns: highly vascularized, may be cystic
2. Topography: back to the presacral fascia

2.2.8 Perineal Masses

Cystic (diverticula of the urethra (Fig. 2.31), vaginal cysts, cysts of the greater vestibular glands) can be easily located in the perineum (see Chap. 35).

Location and extension of solid masses of the perineum are clearly depicted on MR (see Chap. 36).

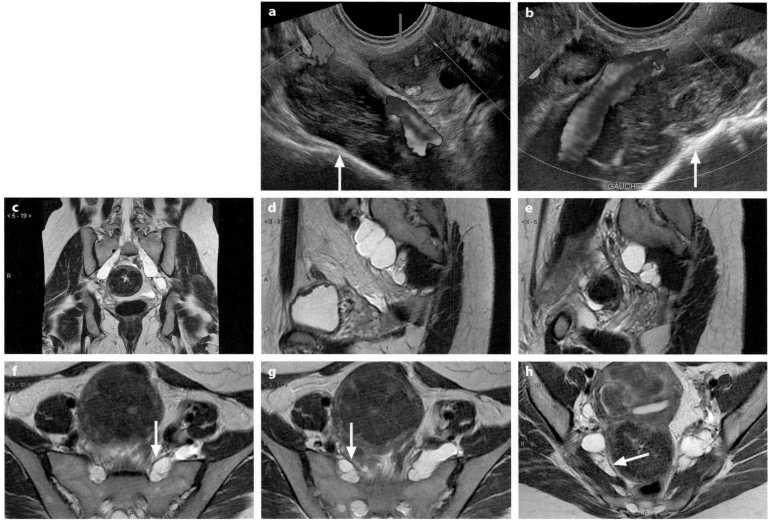

Fig. 2.29 Bilateral Tarlov's cysts. EVS displays behind external iliac pedicles, on the right (**a**) and the left sides (**b**) extra-ovarian low echogenic ovoid cystic masses (*white arrows*). Normal right ovary (*green arrow in* **a**) and left ovary (*green arrow in* **b**) are displayed medial to the external iliac vessels. MR coronal T2 (**c**), right parasagittal T2 (**d**), and left parasagittal T2 (**e**) show that these oblong collections are coming out from the sacral foramina and are typical for Tarlov's cysts. On axial T2 (**f–h**), the fascia over piriformis (*white arrows in* **f**, **g**, **h**), which is situated in front of the sacral plexus, is pushed forward by the collections. This anatomical landmark allows to localize these structures which are nervous in origin

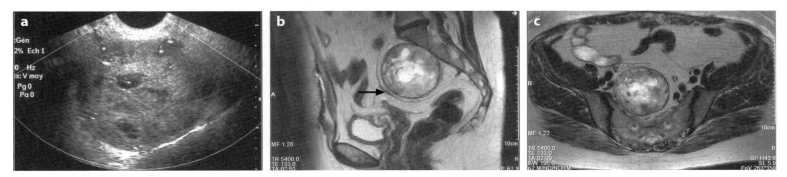

Fig. 2.30 US (**a**) mixed echogenic mass considered as a uterine leiomyoma. MR sagittal T2 (**b**) and axial T2 (**c**) display the presacral fascia pushed forward by the mass (*arrow in* **b**) proving its neurogenic origin. Pathology: neurinoma

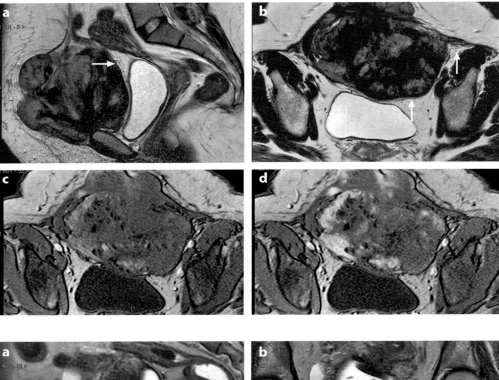

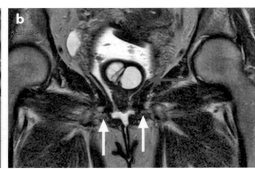

Fig. 2.31 Desmoid tumor of the anterior abdominal wall. MR sagittal (**a**) and axial T2 (**b**) display a parietal mass arising in the anterior abdominal wall extending anteriorly in the subcutaneous tissue and posteriorly pushing backward the fascia transversalis (*arrows*) and the anterior subperitoneal space particularly the anterior of the bladder. On DMR at the arterial phase (**c**), arterial vessels are mainly located at the periphery of the tumor, and at the venous phase (**d**), a significant contrast uptake in the same location was visualize. Resection of the mass was performed. Pathology: desmoid tumor

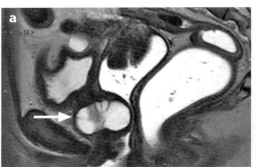

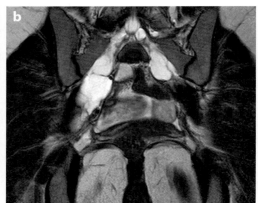

Fig. 2.32 Urethral diverticulum. MR sagittal T2 (**a**) displays a collection (*white arrow*) around the urethra, very suggestive of a diverticulum, which seems to be situated in the upper half of the urethra and therefore in the subperitoneal space. On coronal T2 (**b**) the collection (*red arrow*) is situated above the deep transverse perinei muscle (*white arrows*), definitely allowing to precise its subperitoneal location

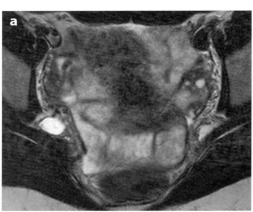

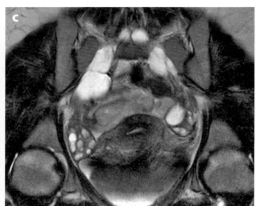

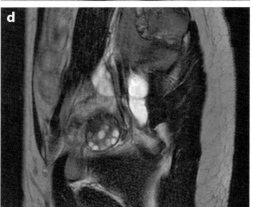

Fig. 2.33 Tarlov' cysts. MR AXIAL T2 (**a**) displays two normal ovaries. Coronal T2 (**b**) and Coronal oblique T2 (**c**) depict bilateral extraovarian collections coming from the sacral foramen on both sides related to Tarlov cysts. Right parasagittal T2 (**d**) depicts the communication of the cyst with the foramen

2.2.9 Parietal Masses

As far as anatomy of the abdominal wall, of the fascia transversalis and parietal peritoneum is clearly depicted, MR gives precise pre-surgical informations about the topography and pelvic extension of these masses (Fig. 2.30).

References

1. Moore KL, Persuad TVN (2008) The developing human. Clinically oriented embryology, 8th edn. Saunders, Philadelphia, pp 243–284
2. Stranding S (2005) Gray's, anatomy. The anatomical basis of clinical practice, 39th edn. Elsevier Churchill Livingstone, New York, Chap. 69: pp 1127–1138; Chap.102: pp 1321–1326; Chap.104: pp 1331–1338; Chap. 106: pp1353–1354; Chap. 107: pp 1355–1371
3. Testut L (1931) Appareil urogenital, Peritoine. In: Latarget A. Traité d'anatomie humaine. 8th edn revue par, G Doin et Cie Editeurs, Paris, pp 1–595

Ovarian and Adrenal Hormonal Synthesis

3

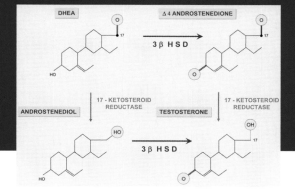

Contents

Why This Chapter in This Textbook?

Because without a basic knowledge of biochemistry of ovarian and adrenal synthesis of androgens and synthesis of estrogens by the ovary and peripheral organs particularly adipose tissue especially in obese patients, it is impossible to understand the role and the mechanism of action of these hormones in:

1. The sex differentiation (Chap. 1) and consequently the anatomy of female genital tract (Chap. 2)
2. The role of these hormones in the histology of the ovary (Chap. 5) and of the female genital tract particularly in the histology of the endometrium (Chap. 21)
3. In the causes of hyperandrogenism and hyperestrogenism
   (a) The causes of hyperandrogenism in:
      Adrenogenital syndrome (Chap. 1)
      Functional disorders (Chap. 7)
      Ovarian infertility (Chap. 8)
      Sex cord cell tumors (Chap. 11)
      Tumors of the ovary with functioning stroma (Chap. 13)
      Hyperandrogenism of ovarian and adrenal origin (Chap. 14)
   (b) The causes of hyperestrogenism
      Sex cord cell tumors (Chap. 11)
      Tumors of the ovary with functioning stroma (Chap. 13)
4. The role of these hormones in the benign and malignant disorders of the female genital tract (mainly Chaps. 22, 24, and 25)
5. Understanding of hormonal treatment in women during the reproductive age and after menopause
   The hormonal synthesis in the ovary and in the cortex of the adrenal gland is reported in the figure biochemistry (Fig. 3.1).

J.N. Buy, M. Ghossain, *Gynecological Imaging*,
DOI 10.1007/978-3-642-31012-6_3, © Springer-Verlag Berlin Heidelberg 2013

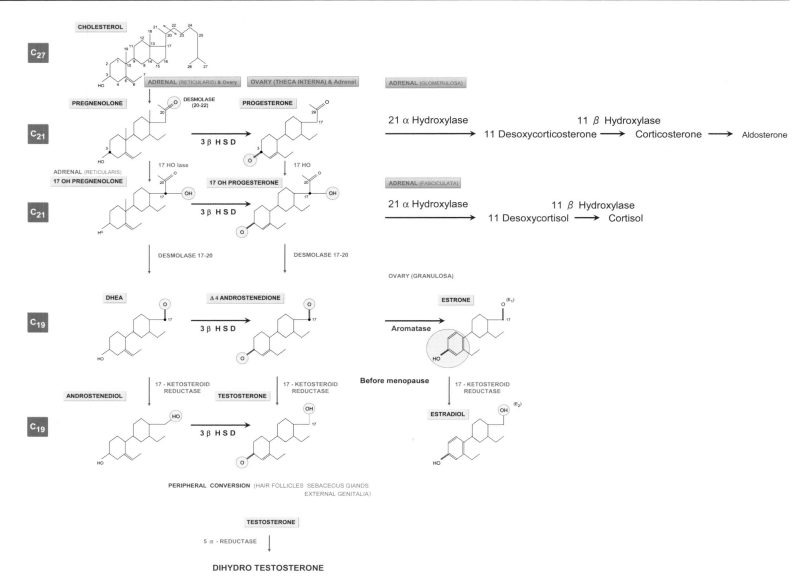

Fig. 3.1 Biochemistry. Major pathways of hormonal synthesis in the ovary, in the suprarenal cortex of the ladrenal gland and in the peripheral tissues. 3 β HSD: 3 β hydroxysteroid deshydrogenase, DHEA = Dehydroepiandrosterone

3.1   Ovarian Hormonal Synthesis (Fig. 3.1)

3.1.1   During the Reproductive Age Years

3.1.1.1 From Day 1 to 14

From Day 1 to 7

From day 1 to 7, development of approximately ten antral follicles from 2 to 6 mm in diameter happens in each ovary. Secretion of estrogen is low.

At day 7, a dominant follicle in one of the ovaries about 10 mm in diameter is clearly individualized.

From Day 8 to 14

Under the stimulation of FSH, this dominant follicle grows of 2.5 mm each day and will reach a size of 23 mm at day 14. This dominant follicle will synthesize 90 % of the secretion of estrogen.

The internal theca receives the cholesterol brought by the vessels. Under the influence of LH, the internal theca synthesizes delta-4-androstenedione. The lateral chain of the cholesterol is first broken by a desmolase which converts the cholesterol into pregnenolone. Then, two different pathways of biosynthesis are possible in the ovary and in the adrenal.

In the ovary, the preferential pathway is the conversion of pregnenolone into progesterone then into androstenedione.

In the reticularis of the adrenal, the preferential pathway is the conversion of pregnenolone into 17-OH-pregnenolone and then to DHEA. This last metabolite in turn can be converted into delta-4-androstenedione, or in androstenediol, and both of them in testosterone. In the peripheral tissues (hair follicles, adipose tissue), testosterone can be converted in dihydrotestosterone which is responsible of pilosity.

At each level of this last pathway, the enzyme 3-beta-hydroxydeshydrogenase can convert the metabolites in their equivalents in the other pathway.

In the internal theca of the ovarian follicle, under the influence of the FSH (its secretion steadily increases after day 7), the androstenedione passes into the granulosa where it is converted in estrone. This estrone through a dehydrogenation is converted in estradiol.

Twenty-four to forty-eight hour before ovulation, the high secretion of estrogen initiates a peak of LH. This LH peak is responsible for the rupture of the dominant follicle.

3.1.1.2 From Day 14 to 28

From Day 14 to 21

The ruptured de Graaf follicle transforms in corpus luteum. Vessels that ended in the internal theca before rupture invade the granulosa. Granulosa cells and internal theca cells transform in luteal and paraluteal cells, respectively. These cells will secrete a large amount of progesterone with a peak at day 21.

From Day 21 to 28

In the absence of pregnancy, secretion of progesterone decreases progressively.

Twenty-four to forty-eight hour before menstruation, the fall of progesterone induces a contraction of the myometrial and basal arteries at the base of the endometrium and induces an infarction of the endometrium with a slash of the spongious and the compact layers with a preservation of the basal layer.

3.1.2 After Menopause

The follicles are atretic. The stroma contains interstitial cells which secrete androgens mainly testosterone but also androstenedione.

Secretion of estrogens is very low. However, androgens can be converted in estrogens by an aromatase in the peripheral tissues mainly adipose tissue.

3.2 Adrenal Gland Hormonal Synthesis (Fig. 3.1)

The adrenal gland comprises the peripheral cortical adrenal gland and the central medullary gland. The cortical adrenal gland contains three different layers: (1) a peripheral outer layer the glomerulosa which secretes aldosterone, (2) a middle layer the fascicularis which secretes corticosteroid hormones, and (3) an inner layer the reticularis which secretes androgens. Whereas the zona glomerulosa is primarily regulated by the angiotensin II, both the zona fasciculata and the zona reticularis are regulated by the ACTH.

In the zona reticularis, the major pathway of androstenedione synthesis is through DHEA; hydroxyprogesterone, however, can also be an important precursor for androstenedione when precursor is produced in excess, as in 21-hydroxylase deficiency.

In the zona glomerulosa, progesterone is converted by a 21-α-hydroxylase in 11-desoxycortisone, then in corticosterone and then in aldosterone.

In the zona fasciculata, the 17-hydroxyprogesterone is converted by a 21-α-hydroxylase in deoxycortisol and then in cortisol.

This explains why in case of a congenital deficit in 21-α-hydroxylase, there is an excess of production of androgens leading to a hyperplasia of the adrenal glands (see Chap. 1).

Methods of Examination and Methods of Analysis of a Pelvic Mass or Process

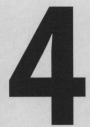

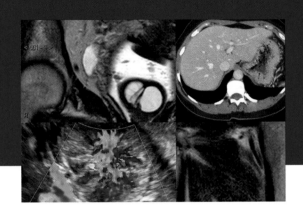

Contents

4.1 Bases of Diagnosis

Diagnosis of the nature of a pelvic mass is suggested on clinical, radiologic and biological findings.

4.1.1 Clinical Findings

Family genetic inheritance
Previous treatments:
    Medical treatment
    Surgical and pathologic reports
    Radiotherapy chemotherapy antioncogenic molecules
Clinical findings
Day of the menstrual cycle
Hormonal treatment

4.1.2 Radiologic Findings

Comparison with previous radiologic documents
Ultrasound, CT scan, MR, PET scan data

4.1.3 Biological Findings

Plasmatic tumoral markers:
    CA125, CA19-9, and ACE, particularly in case of suspicion of ovarian surface epithelial stromal tumors
    LDH, beta-HCG, and alpha-fetoprotein in case of suspicion of malignant germ cell tumors
    Inhibin in case of suspicion of a granulosa tumor
    SCC in case of suspicion of epidermoid carcinoma of the cervix, the vagina, and the vulva
    LDH in case of suspicion of uterine leiomyosarcoma

J.N. Buy, M. Ghossain, *Gynecological Imaging*,
DOI 10.1007/978-3-642-31012-6_4, © Springer-Verlag Berlin Heidelberg 2013

In case of suspicion of ovarian metastases, CA 19-9 in case of GI tract carcinoma, CA 15-3 in case of breast carcinoma
These markers are not only fundamental in the diagnosis of nature of a tumor, but also in the follow-up of a woman operated from a pelvic malignant process.
Findings of an inflammatory process (CRP, white cell count number, sedimentation rate)
Hormonal checkup:
Estrogens, progesterone, and androgens mainly for functional lesions and endocrine tumors
LH and FSH in case of suspicion of ovarian deficiency, or perimenopause, or suspicion of polycystic ovarian disease

4.2 Methods of Examination

4.2.1 US

1. Transabdominal ultrasound.
2. Endovaginal ultrasound.
3. Color Doppler: no contrast is used.

4.2.2 MR

4.2.2.1 Usual Protocol

1. Systematically is performed:
   Sagittal and axial T2 sequences (using recently 2-mm sections).
   Axial T1 and axial T1 fat suppression.
   Coronal T2 is performed particularly when the topography of the mass (ovarian, uterine, tubal, or other) is not clearly depicted on the previous sequences.
2. Two diffusion sequences are sometimes performed in the axial plane using a b0 and a b1000.
3. In most cases and particularly when a non purely cystic mass is displayed, DMR is performed in the axial plane using multisection sequences as follows:
   Noncontrast sequence:
   At the arterial phase 20–30 s after injection
   At the venous phase 50–60 s after injection
   Followed by four other sequences until 3 min

Curves of contrast uptake are evaluated in one or two areas of the lesion, and are compared preferentially to the curve of contrast uptake in the iliac external artery which is a constant landmark instead of choosing different references (inner or outer myometrium, pelvic muscle).
A delayed sagittal sequence is performed in some cases.

4.2.2.2 Particular Indications

1. Diagnosis and evaluation of endometriosis (sagittal and axial thin 2-mm sections are performed on T2 particularly to evaluate the uterosacral ligaments)
2. Evaluation of prolapse
   After preparation of the colon before the examination and voiding of the bladder immediately before examination in order to obtain a good straining.
   T2 sequences in the three different planes are performed.
   At least two sequences during straining.

4.2.3 CT

The day before the examination, the patient absorbs oral contrast in order to opacify the colon the day of examination.
The day of examination, the patient absorbs oral contrast 20 min before the examination in order to opacify the small bowel.

4.2.3.1 Usual Protocol

Four different sequences are performed:
Abdominopelvic CT without injection.
Abdominopelvic CT at the arterial phase (25 s after injection of 100 cc of IV contrast at a rate of 4 ml/s). This sequence associated with MIP reformation studies the type of arterial vascularization of the lesions.
Abdominopelvic CT or thoracoabdominopelvic CT (in case of suspicion of malignant disease) 60 s after injection. This sequence studies the type of contrast enhancement of the lesions and is fundamental to evaluate extension.
Abdominopelvic CT 4 min after injection in order to evaluate the degree of contrast enhancement on the delayed and to depict the topography of the ureters, which is essential for the surgeon in the preoperative checkup.

4.2.3.2 In Case of Suspicion of Involvement of the Rectum or the Large Bowel

Enema coupled with CT realized in prone position can be performed in a second time to rule out or confirm extension to the GI tract and to precise the degree of extension.

4.3 Methods of Analysis

Whatever the imaging modality performed, diagnosis of a gynecologic process is based on the following four different data.

4.3.1 Location of the Mass

Based on a clear comprehension of embryology and anatomy (see Chaps. 1 and 2).

4.3.2 Morphologic Findings

Based on the knowledge of the macroscopic and microscopic findings which are essential to suggest a specific type of process or even of a diagnosis. They are the common trunk of the findings displayed on the different imaging modalities with different expressions according to the radiation beam performed (US, X-ray, electromagnetic).

4.3.3 Vascular Findings

Which depend on:

1. The type of vascularization of the organ and of the tissue concerned in this organ (e.g., the ovarian artery is not as wide as the uterine artery).
2. The pathologic process involved, i.e., benign neoplasm or malignant invasive or noninvasive atypical proliferative, endocrine tumor, and inflammatory process.

4.3.4 Extension

Loco regional or metastatic, through direct continuity or via arteries, veins or lymphatics.

These different reasons outline the necessity to perform:

1. A reproductible protocol of examination based on different sequences each of one needing to be performed in the goal to look for a specific information.
2. A clear method of analysis of results on each of these sequences with a clear definition of each of the findings suggestive of a type of process and of their specific value isolated or gathered.

At the end of the analysis of one type or another of imaging modalities, with association of clinical findings, and eventually biological findings, three main different situations can be encountered:

1. The diagnosis of benignity or malignancy can be ascertained. Even a specific type of diagnosis can be suggested.
2. In other cases, only a differential diagnosis can be suggested. According to the findings of the US examination, one type or another type of imaging modality must be performed, which will or will not resolve the problem.
3. A lesion is detected, without being able to characterize the type of process.

Ovary

Part 2

Embryology, Anatomy, and Histology

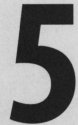

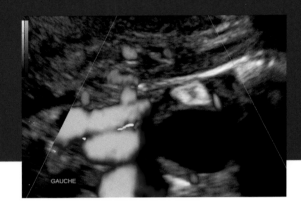

Contents

5.1 Embryology [1]

See Chap. 1

5.2 Anatomy [2, 3]

5.2.1 Description

The ovary lies in the peritoneal cavity behind the broad ligament linked to the junction of the mesometrium and the mesosalpinx by a thin double leaf of peritoneum the mesovarium (Fig. 5.1).

During reproductive age, the normal ovary is oval in shape, measures about 3 cm length, and has a cross-sectional surface <6 cm^2 and a volume <8 cm^3. Its surface is smooth in young women.

After menopause, size decreases gradually and becomes more flattened usually with a slightly nodular surface.

The ovary has two lateral and medial faces, superior and inferior poles, and anterior and posterior borders.

The lateral face contacts a depression of the parietal peritoneum, the ovarian fossa. On the extraperitoneal side, this fossa is limited in front by the posterior border of the external iliac vein and at the back by the uterine artery and the companion pelvic ureter (Fig. 5.2).

The medial face is in relationship with the infundibulum of the tube.

The superior pole is in relation with the fimbriae.

The inferior pole points downward toward the pelvic floor.

The anterior border faces the mesovarium.

The posterior border is free.

J.N. Buy, M. Ghossain, *Gynecological Imaging*,
DOI 10.1007/978-3-642-31012-6_5, © Springer-Verlag Berlin Heidelberg 2013

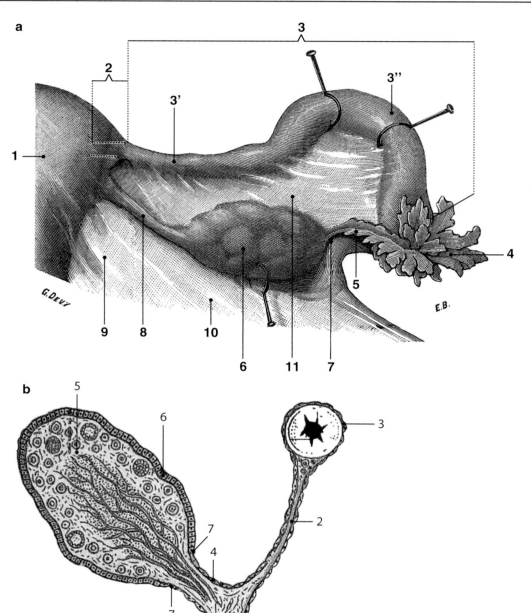

a

Fig. 5.1 (a) **Posterior view of the left adnexa (The infundibulo pelvic ligament is drawn downward).** *1* uterus, *2* tube: Intramural segment (1 cm in length), *3* tube: *3'* Isthmic segment (2 cm in length) and *3''* ampullary portion (6 cm in length), *4* Fimbriae, *5* Fimbria ovarica (Ovarian Fimbria), *6* Ovary, *7* Infundibulopelvic ligament (attachment), *8* Ovarian ligament, *9* Broad ligament: Mesometrium, *10* Broad ligament: External part, *11* Broad ligament: Mesosalpinx. (b) Lateral view of the left adnexa. *1* Broad ligament: Mesometrium, *2* Broad ligament: Mesosalpinx, *3* Tube, *4* Broad ligament: Mesovarium containing blood vessels to the ovarian hilum, *5* Ovary: Stroma, *6* Ovary: Surface Epithelium, *7* Ovary: Hilus (From Testut [3])

b

5.2.2 Peritoneal Attachments (Fig. 5.1)

1. Infundibulopelvic ligament: It is a peritoneal fold that is attached to the upper part of the lateral surface of the ovary. It contains the ovarian vessels and nerves. It passes superiorly over the external iliac vessels and genitofemoral nerve and passes between the posterior parietal peritoneum and the lumbar portion of the ureter. On the right side, the ligament is attached to a fold of peritoneum posterior and inferior to the caecum and the appendix. On the left side, the ligament is higher than on the right and is lateral to the junction of the descending and sigmoid colon.

2. Ovarian Ligament

   Embryology: Definition of the gubernaculum: As the mesonephros degenerates, a ligament the gubernaculum develops on each side of the abdomen from the caudal pole of the gonad. The gubernaculum passes obliquely through the developing anterior abdominal wall at the site of the future inguinal canal and attaches caudally to the internal surface of labioscrotal swellings. It will give rise to the ovarian ligament and to the round ligament of the uterus.

   Anatomy: The ovarian ligament attaches the inferomedial extremity of the ovary to the lateral angle of the uterus posteroinferior to the uterine tube. It lies in the posterior leaf of the broad ligament.

   The ovarian ligament is continuous with the medial border of the round ligament.

3. Mesovarium

   The mesovarium attaches the anterior border of the ovary to the back of the broad ligament. It carries blood vessels and nerves to the ovarian hilum.

   The uterine tube arches over the ovary and ascends in front of the anterior border of the ovary, then curves over its tubal end and passes down on its medial surface.

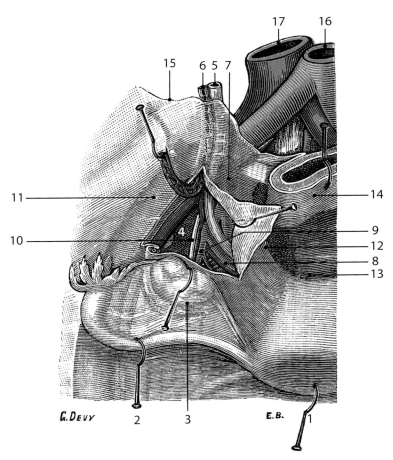

Fig. 5.2 *1* uterus, *2* tube, *3* ovary, *4* ovarian fossa, *5* ureter, *6* ovarian artery, *7* internal iliac artery, *8* uterine artery, *9* obturator artery, *10* obturator nerve, *11* external iliac artery, *12* parietal peritoneum, *13* douglas, *14* rectum, *15* parietal peritoneum, *16* aorta, *17* inferior vena cava

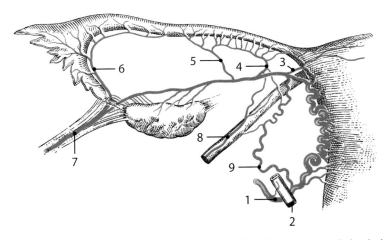

Fig. 5.3 *1* uterine artery, *2* ureter, *3* artery of the fundus, *4* medial tubal artery, *5* middle tubal artery, *6* lateral tubal artery, *7* ovarian artery and suspensory ligament of the ovary, *8* artery of the round ligament, *9* anastomose between the uterine artery and its terminal portion

5.2.3 Vascular Supply and Lymphatic Drainage

5.2.3.1 Arteries (Fig. 5.3)

1. The Ovarian Artery

   It descends behind the peritoneum crosses in front the lumbar ureter, crosses in front and medially the external iliac pedicle, and passes behind the external iliac vein. Here the artery turns

medially in the ovarian suspensory ligament, continues in the mesosalpinx, and passes back in the mesovarium.

2. The tuboovarian branch of the uterine artery originates at the end of the uterine artery (close to the origin of the tube) where the artery bifurcates in the artery of the fundus of the uterus and the tuboovarian artery. This artery lies in the mesosalpinx and anastomoses with the ovarian artery (sometimes forming a plexus) before entering the mesovarium or enters separately into the mesovarium.

5.2.3.2 Veins

The ovarian veins emerge from the ovary as a plexus in the mesovarium and the suspensory ligament. Two veins issue from the plexus which merge further in a single vein. The right one enters the VCI and the left one the left renal vein.

5.2.3.3 Lymphatic Drainage

Lymphatic drainage is via three main routes:
- Lomboaortic following the ovarian artery to pre- and lateral aortic nodes below the origin of the renal arteries
- Iliac nodes situated behind the external iliac artery, in front of the uterine artery
- More rarely, inguinal nodes

5.3 Histology [4]

5.3.1 The Ovary in Adulthood

5.3.1.1 Surface Epithelium (Figs. 5.4 and 5.5)

It consists of a simple layer of modified mesothelial cells. The cells vary from flat to cuboidal to columnar, and several types may be seen in different areas in the same ovary. The surface cells are separated from the underlying stroma by a distinct basement membrane.

Epithelial inclusion glands and their cystic counterparts arise from cortical invaginations of the surface epithelium and have lost their connection with the surface. They measure usually from 2 to 5 mm. An epithelium-lined cyst greater than 1 cm is designated a cystadenoma.

Histochemical studies have demonstrated glycogen, as well as acid and neutral mucopolysaccharides within surface epithelial cells. Unlike extraovarian mesothelial cells, surface epithelial cells have 17-beta-hydroxysteroid-deshydrogenase activity.

Surface epithelial cells are immunoreactive:
- For cytokeratin, Ber-EP, desmoplakin, vimentin, and TGF-alpha
- For receptors of estrogen, progesterone, and epidermal growth factor

Several antigens associated with ovarian tumors of surface epithelial origin have been demonstrated including CA 125, CA19-9, and MH99.

5.3.1.2 Stroma (Figs. 5.4 and 5.5)

The stroma starts beneath the basal membrane and occupies the majority of the ovary, surrounding follicles and their derivates

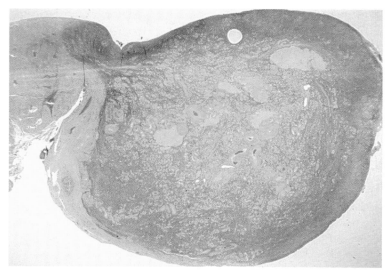

Fig. 5.4 Low magnified showing view the entire ovary. Cortical stroma that appears with a *purple color* is much more dense in the cortex than in the medulla. The outer cortex contains an antral follicle (at the *top*). On the left lies the hilum of the ovary

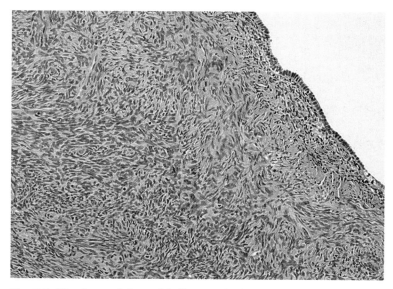

Fig. 5.5 Histology of the epithelium and adjacent stroma. Surface epithelium has a single layer of cuboidal or cylindric cells and in some areas has a double layer. Stroma is made of fusiform cells with a storiform pattern. In the outer cortex, there is an area of fibrosis (*pink* portion contrasting with *purple* adjacent stroma), which is quite common with increasing age

(corpus luteum and corpus albicans). The boundary between cortical and medullar stroma is arbitrary.

The stroma is composed of spindle-shaped cells and a network of reticulin and collagen fibers. Other types of cells may be present.

Spindle-Shaped Cells

The spindle-shaped stromal cells, which have scanty cytoplasm and resemble fibroblasts, are typically arranged in whorls or a storiform pattern.

The stromal cells are immunoreactive for vimentin, actin, and desmin as well as for estrogen progesterone and testosterone receptors.

Reticulin and Collagen Network

A dense reticulin network with a variable amount of collagen that is most abundant in the superficial cortex.

A variety of other cells may be found in the ovarian stroma:
1. Luteinized stromal cells
2. Enzymatic active stromal cells (EASC)
3. Decidual cells
4. Endometrial stroma-type cells
5. Smooth muscle cells
6. Fat cells
7. Stromal Leydig cells
8. Rare cells from the APUD system

MR Pattern (Fig. 5.6)

On T2, the outer cortex just beneath the surface epithelium appears as a low-intensity regular band because of the high concentration of collagen.

The stroma appears with an intermediate signal.

5.3.1.3 Follicles

Before Birth

1. Primordial germ cell.
2. *Oogonia* proliferate by mitosis.
3. *The primary oocyte (46,XX) and the primordial follicle.*

Oogonia enlarge to form primary oocytes: They contain 46XX chromosomes and double the quantity of DNA. Primary oocytes begin the first meiotic division. Connective tissue cells surround them and form a single layer of flattened follicular epithelial cells, constituting primordial follicles.

After Puberty

Folliculogenesis refers to the continuous process occurring throughout reproductive life whereby cohorts of primordial follicles undergo maturation during each menstrual cycle.
1. *The Primary Oocyte (46,XX) and the Primary Follicle* (Fig. 5.7)
    The primary oocyte (46,XX) becomes surrounded by a covering of amorphous glycoprotein material, the zona pellucida.
    The follicular epithelial cells become cuboidal or columnar, forming a primary follicle.
2. *The Secondary Follicle or Preantral Follicle*
    The follicular (granulosa) cells proliferate forming three to five concentric layers around the oocyte. As they increase in size, they migrate into the deeper cortex and medulla.
    The internal theca is made of epithelioid cells with an abundant reticulin network and vessels.
    The external theca merges gradually with the ovarian stroma.
3. *The Tertiary or Antral Follicle* (Fig. 5.8)
    Simultaneously the surrounding ovarian stromal cells become specialized into several layers of theca interna cells and an outer poorly defined layer of theca externa cells.
    Secretion of mucopolysaccharide-rich fluid by the granulosa cells results in their separation by fluid-filled clefts. The latter coalesce to form a single large cavity or antrum lined by several layers of granulosa cells.

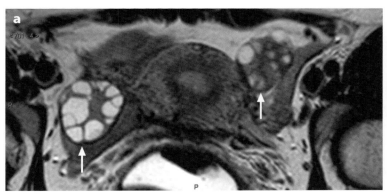
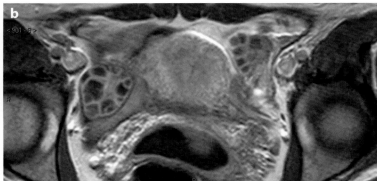

Fig. 5.6 Normal ovaries at day 5. Twenty-three-year-old woman. MR performed because of dysmenorrhea; MR axial T2 (**a**) displays normal ovaries. The outer cortex (*arrows*) appears as a regular low-intensity band related to an important quantity of collagen. The stroma is of intermediate signal.

More than ten antral follicles from 2 to 9 mm in diameter are present in the cortex. On T1 after injection (**b**), there is a slight contrast uptake in the outer cortex. Contrast uptake is more pronounced in the cortex, surrounding the follicles than in the medulla

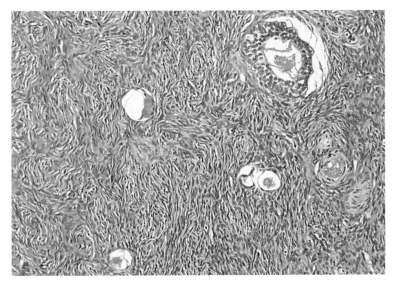
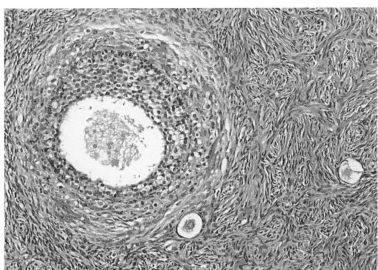

Fig. 5.7 The primary follicle (upper left corner) is surrounded by amorphous glycoprotein material, the zona pellucida. Several layers of follicular cells, cuboidal or columnar, are now present

Fig. 5.8 There is now a single large cavity or antrum lined by several layers of granulosa cells. The surrounding ovarian stromal cells are now differentiated into several layers of theca interna cells and an outer poorly defined layer of theca externa cells. Vessels are seen in the theca interna

On EVS, antral follicles as small as 2 mm can be detected. By cycle days 5–7, a varying number of antral follicles of 2–6 mm in diameter can be seen in both ovaries.

On MR, these follicles appear with a high signal intensity within the ovarian cortex (Fig. 5.6).

4. *The Mature or de Graaf Follicle*

   (a) As the follicle enlarges because of continued fluid secretion into the antrum, the oocyte reaches its definite size and an eccentric position at one pole of the follicle. At this point, the granulosa cells proliferate to form the cumulus oophorus (that contains the oocyte and protrudes into the antrum).

   (b) The primary oocyte (46,XX) increases in size and shortly before ovulation completes the first meiotic division (the chromosome number is reduced from diploid to haploid) to give rise to the secondary oocyte (23,X) and the first polar body. The secondary oocyte receives almost all the cytoplasm, and the first polar body receives very little; the polar body is a small, nonfunctional cell that soon degenerates.

Hormone Synthesis (see Chap. 3)

1. Estradiol (E2). Synthesis of estradiol starts in the internal thecal cell where androgen, mainly androstenedione, is synthesized under the stimulation by LH. Then under the action of aromatase, androstenedione is converted in estrone in the granulosa cells, which then is converted in estradiol (E2). Secretion of E2 is mainly produced in the mature follicle between day 7 and the ovulation; only a small amount of estradiol is secreted by the antral follicles.

2. Inhibin. A glycoprotein is synthesized by the granulose cells. Although inhibin is mainly under the control of LH, it reduces by negative feedback FSH secretion.

3. AMH. It is secreted by the granulosa cells of primary follicles and antral follicles. It is highest in preantral and antral follicles <4 mm diameter.

   On EVS, at day 7, this mature follicle, which at that time is called the dominant follicle, measures 10 mm in diameter. Then it grows usually 2 mm a day until ovulation, reaching a diameter of

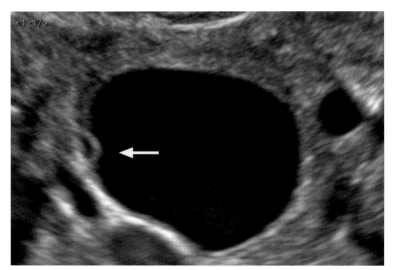

Fig. 5.9 Graafian follicle day 13. Follicle of 24 mm with a cumulus oophorus (*arrow*)

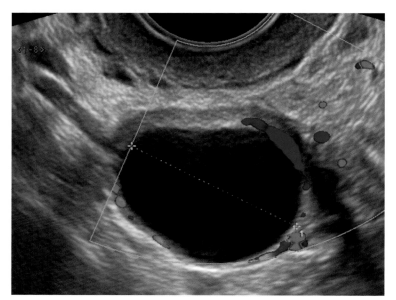

Fig. 5.10 Mature follicle at day 13. Peripheral vascularization is visible in the wall of the mature follicle, indicating an impending ovulation

20–25 mm by the time of ovulation. The cumulus oophorus becomes visible at the end of this first part of the cycle and usually indicates imminence of the ovulation (Fig. 5.9). On color Doppler, thin regular vessel can be displayed in the wall (Fig. 5.10).

On MR on T2, the dominant follicle appears with a thin regular wall and with a high signal intensity. On DMR at the arterial phase, a peripheral vascularization can be depicted (Fig. 5.11). Some days before ovulation, a cumulus oophorus can be seen (Fig. 5.12).

5. *Rupture of the Follicle*
   (a) After ovulation the secondary oocyte begins the second meiotic division (each chromosome divides in each half or chromatid) but progresses only to metaphase, when division is arrested.

(b) If sperm penetrates the secondary oocyte, the second meiotic division is completed: Each chromatid is drawn to a different pole. Most cytoplasm is retained by one cell, the fertilized oocyte. The other cell, the second polar body, soon degenerates. As soon as the second polar is extruded, maturation of the oocyte is complete.

On EVS, the Graafian follicle decreases in size and becomes flattened, and fluid is visualized in the peritoneal cavity (Fig. 5.13). Exceptionally, ovulation can be depicted during the examination.

Corpus Luteum of Menstruation (CLM)

After ovulation on the 14th day of a typical 28-day menstrual cycle and in the absence of fertilization, the collapsed ovulatory follicle becomes the corpus luteum of menstruation. It is a round structure of 2 cm with a festooned contour and a center filled with a focally hemorrhagic coagulum.

Histology

1. The luteinized granulosa cells are 30–35-μm polygonal cells with abundant eosinophilic cytoplasm that contains numerous small lipid droplets, a spherical nucleus with one or two large nuclei, typical of steroidogenic cells.
2. The theca interna forms an irregular outer layer of several cells in thickness and ensheathes the vascular septa that extend into the center of the structure.
   When the septa are cut in cross section, triangular-shaped wedges of theca cells appear in the sulci of the convoluted, thick granulosa lutein layer. The luteinized theca cells are half the size of the luteinized granulosa cells; the nucleus is round or oval with a single nucleolus. The cytoplasm contains lipid droplets that are usually larger than those in the granulosa.
3. During maturation of the CLM, capillaries from the theca interna penetrate the granulosa layer and reach the central cavity. Fibroblasts that accompany the vessels form an increasingly dense reticulum within the granulosa layer and the inner fibrous layer that lines the central cavity.

Hormone Synthesis

The CLM mainly synthesizes progesterone (P) but also synthesizes estrone (E1), estradiol (E2), and androgens, mainly androstenedione.

After ovulation LH, FSH, and E2 fall, but the LH concentration is sufficient to maintain the CLM, producing a mid-luteal peak of P and E2.

If fertilization does not occur, the increased levels of P and estrogen result in the fall of FSH and LH to basal levels via a negative feedback mechanism, with a marked decline in P and E2 synthesis after the 22th day of the cycle.

These changes are accompanied by involution of the CLM and beginning of the menstruation.

On EVS, the corpus luteum of menstruation measures a little less than the pre-ruptured Graafian follicle; its mean diameter is 2 cm. A characteristic peripheral vascularization is visualized in its wall (Fig. 5.14); at that time, capillaries from the internal theca penetrate in the granulosa layer.

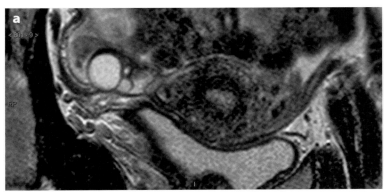

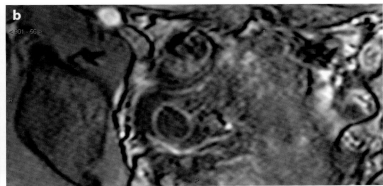

Fig. 5.11 Dominant follicle at day 12. MR coronal T2 (**a**) displays in the right ovary a follicle of 19 mm in diameter. Axial DMR performed at the arterial phase (**b**) depicts a characteristic rim of contrast uptake in the wall of the follicle

On MR (Fig. 5.15), on axial T2, the corpus luteum appears with a peripheral portion of an intermediate signal and a central portion more or less cystic;

On DMR at the arterial phase, a typical high contrast uptake in the peripheral portion is related with the endocrine type of vascularization with a rich network of capillaries.

Corpus Luteum of Pregnancy (CLP)

Following fertilization, placental HCG stimulates P production by the granulosa-luteal cells. P concentration within the postovulatory corpus luteum increases sixfold, whereas the E2 level drops to 10% of that within the preovulatory follicle.

HCG alone cannot maintain P secretion by the CLP. P secretion by the CLP begins to decrease by the end of the second month of gestation as the production of P is largely assumed by the placenta.

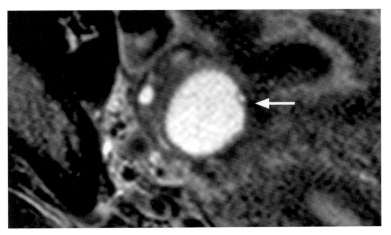

Fig. 5.12 Graafian follicle at day 13. MR axial T2 depicts a follicle of 23 mm containing a cumulus oophorus (*arrow*)

Corpus Albicans

The degenerating CLM converts in a corpus albicans. It is well circumscribed with convoluted borders and is composed almost entirely of densely collagen fibers with some fibroblasts. Occasionally, corpus albicans is focally calcified or cystic. Most are resorbed and replaced by ovarian stroma; they may persist in the ovarian medulla of postmenopausal women.

On EVS, its size is small (<5 mm) with a peripheral echogenic wall, with a hypoechogenic center (Fig. 5.16).

Atretic Follicles

Of the original 400,000 primordial follicles present at birth, 400 mature to ovulation; the remaining 99.9% undergo atresia. They contain high concentrations of androstenedione.

5.3.1.4 Hilus Cells

Histology

Ovarian hilus cells (hilar Leydig cells) are morphologically identical to testicular hilus cells except for having a female chromatin pattern.

They are more numerous during pregnancy, in parous women, with increasing age after menopause, and with increasing degrees of ovarian stromal proliferation and stromal luteinization.

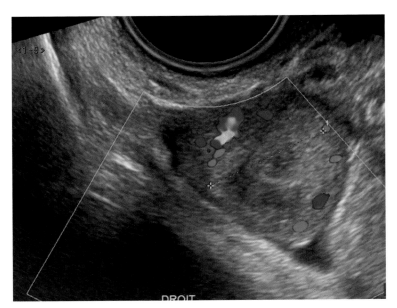

Fig. 5.13 Ovulation. The Graafian follicle has just ruptured. It has decreased in size and is flattened. Some follicular fluid is visualized in the ovarian fossa

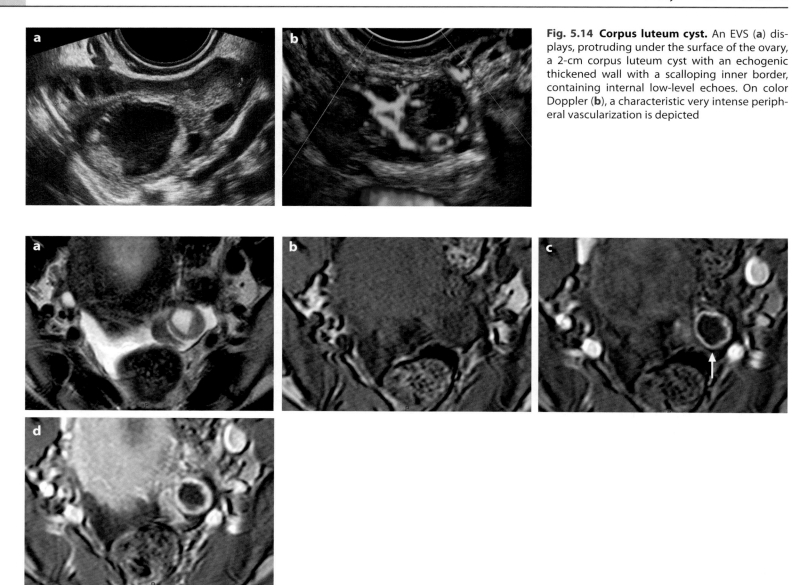

Fig. 5.14 Corpus luteum cyst. An EVS (**a**) displays, protruding under the surface of the ovary, a 2-cm corpus luteum cyst with an echogenic thickened wall with a scalloping inner border, containing internal low-level echoes. On color Doppler (**b**), a characteristic very intense peripheral vascularization is depicted

Fig. 5.15 Corpus luteum of menstruation. MR performed at day 21 of the menstrual cycle. MR axial T2 (**a**). In the left ovary, the corpus luteum has two components, a peripheral solid portion of intermediate signal and a central cystic portion of high signal intensity. On DMR without injection (**b**) and at the arterial phase (**c**) do not display vessels but an intense contrast uptake in the solid peripheral part (*arrow*), which expresses the predominant capillary type of this tissue related to its endocrine function. At the venous phase (**d**), a slight contrast diffusion is visualized

They are found in the ovarian hilus and the adjacent mesovarium. They characteristically ensheathe, or less commonly lie within non-medullary nerves, and frequently are juxtaposed to large venous or lymphatic sinusoids.

They can also lie within the ovarian stroma away from the hilus (stromal Leydig cells).

The cells are 12–25 μm in diameter, round or oval. They contain abundant eosinophilic cytoplasm, a spherical vesicular nucleus with one or two prominent nucleoli.

Hilus cells contain:

1. Specific crystals of Reinke, which are homogeneous eosinophilic non-refractile rod-shaped structures 10–35 μm long. They are better displayed with Masson's trichrome and iron-hematoxylin methods which stain them magenta and black, respectively. Spherical or ellipsoidal eosinophilic hyaline structures that represent very likely precursors of crystals can be identified often in greater number.

2. Peripheral eosinophilic granules, peripheral lipid vacuoles, and golden-brown lipochrome pigment. Normal Leydig cells are immunoreactive for inhibin and relaxin-like factor. Typically admixed with the hilus cells are delicate collagen fibrils and fibroblasts intermediate in appearance between the two cell types.

Hormone Synthesis

Hilus cells produce androstenedione in an amount higher than that secreted by ovarian stroma.

5.3.1.5 Rete Ovarii

It is a mesonephric remnant situated in ovarian hilum. It is composed a network of anastomosing, branching tubules with intraluminal

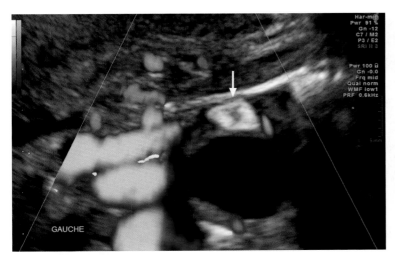

Fig. 5.16 Corpus albicans. EVS depicts in the cortex a typical corpus albicans (*arrow*) with a peripheral echogenic rim and a hypoechogenic center

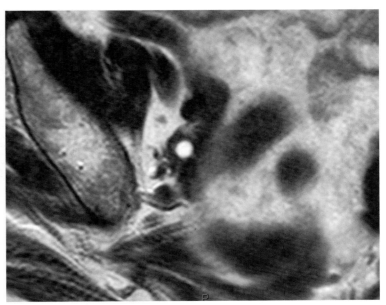

Fig. 5.18 Inclusion cyst. Eighty-year-old woman. MR axial T2 displays in the right ovary a 4-mm high signal intensity cyst related to an inclusion cyst

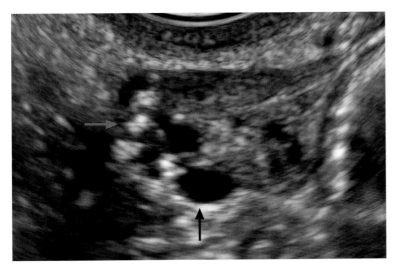

Fig. 5.17 Inclusion cysts and corpora albicantia. Menopausal woman. EVS routine examination. EVS depicts in the peripheral cortex inclusion cysts (*black arrow*) and calcified corpora albicantia (*red arrow*)

polypoid projections lined by an epithelium that varies from flat to cuboidal to columnar.

5.3.2   The Ovary in Menopause

5.3.2.1   Macroscopy

Most menopausal ovaries have a shrunken, gyriform, external appearance. The sectioned surface is usually predominantly solid, with occasional cysts several millimeters in the cortex. Small scars of corpora albicantia are present in the medulla.

5.3.2.2   Microscopy

Surface Epithelium

With advancing age, epithelial inclusion cysts are common .They can be multiple and scattered singly or in small clusters throughout

the superficial cortex; less commonly they extend into the deeper cortical or medullary stroma.

On EVS, inclusion cysts are commonly visualized (Fig. 5.17).

On MR, these inclusion cysts have a thin wall and measure less than 1 cm (Fig. 5.18).

Follicles

The characteristic feature of the postmenopausal ovary is the absence of primordial follicles and consequently of maturing follicle, corpora lutea, and atretic follicle.

Occasionally primordial follicles may persist for several years, accounting for sporadic ovulation and follicle cyst formation accompanied by postmenopausal bleeding. After this period, the only follicle-like structures encountered are unresorbed corpora fibrosa and corpora albicantia.

Stroma

The ovarian stroma has a wide variety of appearances. At one extreme of the spectrum, there is a stromal atrophy manifested by a thin cortex and minimal amounts of medullary stroma. The stroma is less cellular with an increase of intercellular collagen.

At the other extreme of the spectrum, there is marked proliferation of the stroma warranting the designation of stromal hyperplasia. Most women exhibit variable degrees of nodular or diffuse proliferation of cortical and medullary stromal cells.

Other changes include occasional luteinized stromal cells, broad irregular areas of cortical fibrosis or fibromatous nodules, cortical granulomas, and surface papillary stromal proliferations.

On EVS (Fig. 5.19), size of the ovary is reduced. Shape is not as oval and can be significantly flattened. Follicles are absent. Cortex can be very thin or irregularly thickened due to fibrosis. On color Doppler, vascularization is scanty or even absent.

On MR, on T2 the stroma appears with a low signal intensity, without any follicle (Fig. 5.20).

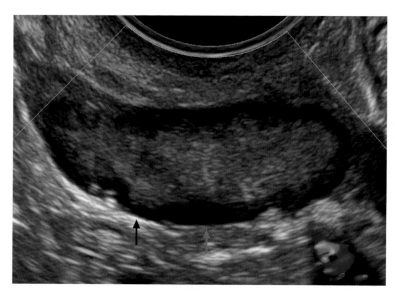

Fig. 5.19 Normal ovary of a menopause woman. Seventy-year-old woman. Routine examination. On EVS with color Doppler, the ovary measures 2.5 cm length, 1 cm width. The hypoechoic outer cortex is thin (*black arrow*) in some areas while in other areas there, it looks thickened (*red arrow*), very likely related to fibrosis. No follicle is present. Corpora albicantia are seen. No vessel in the stroma is displayed

5.3.2.3 Hormonal Synthesis

With cessation of follicular activity at the time of menopause, the ovarian stroma becomes together with the adrenal glands the major source of androgens. Testosterone and androstenedione are the major androgens secreted by the ovarian stroma.

Estrone is derived predominantly from the peripheral aromatization of androstenedione that occurs mainly in adipose tissue.

References

1. Moore KL, Persaud TVN, Torchia MG (2008) The developing human. Clinically oriented embryology, 8th edn. Saunders, Philadelphia, pp 243–284
2. Standring S (2005) Gray, anatomy. The anatomical basis of clinical practice, 39th edn. Elsevier Churchill Livingstone, London, pp 1331–1338, Chap 104
3. Testut L (1931) Appareil urogenital, peritoine. In: Latarget A Traité d'anatomie humaine. 8th edn. revue par. G Doin et Cie Editeurs, Paris, pp 1–595
4. Clement PB (2002) Anatomy and histology of the ovary. In: Blaustein's pathology of the female genital tract. Springer, New York, pp 649–673, Chap 15

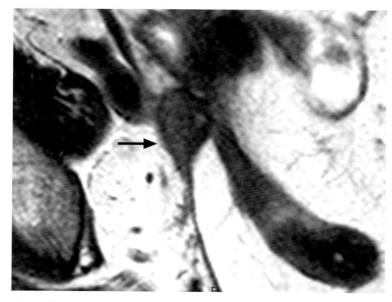

Fig. 5.20 Postmenopausal ovary. Fifty-seven-year-old woman without hormonal treatment. MR axial T2 depicts a normal 2-cm right ovary. The stroma at that age has an homogeneous low signal intensity with a thin outer cortex (*arrow*)

Congenital Lesions

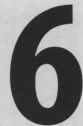

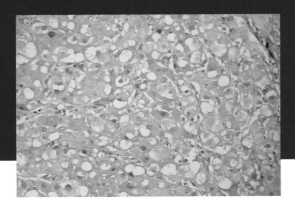

Contents

6.1 Absent Ovary [1]

In phenotypic females, absence of both ovaries usually is associated with an abnormal karyotype and a syndrome of gonadal dysgenesis. In such cases, bilateral streak gonads, or a unilateral streak gonad and a contralateral intra-abdominal testis are usually found.

Rarely, one ovary may be absent in an otherwise normal woman, usually representing an incidental finding at operation (Fig. 6.1). The differential diagnosis includes (1) ectopic ovary, which may lie at the level of the liver, close to the kidney, within the omentum, or within an inguinal hernia, and (2) adnexal torsion with atrophy or autoamputation.

6.2 Lobulated, Accessory, and Supernumerary Ovary [1]

1. *Lobulated Ovary*
   Definition: divided by one or several fissures into two or more lobes
2. *Accessory Ovary*
   Definition: normal ovarian tissue located in the vicinity of a normal ovary, with which it has a direct or ligamentous attachment
3. *Supernumerary Ovary*
   Definition: a similar structure usually, separated from the ovary, less than 1 cm in size, which may be located in the pelvis, the omentum, and the mesentery or can be retroperitoneal

J.N. Buy, M. Ghossain, *Gynecological Imaging*,
DOI 10.1007/978-3-642-31012-6_6, © Springer-Verlag Berlin Heidelberg 2013

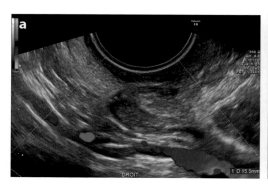
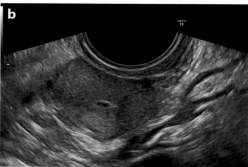

Fig. 6.1 Left absent ovary. Thirty-year-old woman; infertility. Absence of previous surgery. EVS (**a**) normal right ovary. EVS (**b**) in the left part of the pelvis, absence of the left ovary. Coelioscopy confirmed the diagnosis

6.3   Adrenal Cortical Rests [1]

Accessory adrenal cortical tissue is frequently observed within the wall of the fallopian tube and the broad ligament; it is exceptionally encountered in the ovary.

The adrenal rests are typically encapsulated nodules several milliliters in size.

Adrenal cortical tissue in these sites may be explained by the close proximity of the anlage of the adrenal cortex and the gonadal ridge during embryological development.

Ovarian adrenal cortical rests may be the origin of steroid cell tumors of the ovary that resemble to adrenal cortical tissue in both their histologic and endocrine manifestations. Such cases have been reported after resection of adrenal glands involved by congenital adrenal hyperplasia (Figs. 6.2 and 6.3).

6.4   Uterus-Like Ovarian Mass [2]

Definition: an ovary containing a central cavity lined by endometrial tissue and a thick wall of smooth muscle [2]

6.5   Splenic-Gonadal Fusion [1]

Definition: It results from fusion of the anlage of both organs during embryonic development.

A cordlike structure connecting the spleen to the left ovary or surrounding structures may be seen [1].

A case of discontinuous splenic-gonadal fusion has been reported [3].

In newborn female infants, splenic-gonadal fusion associated to undescended ovaries has been reported [4].

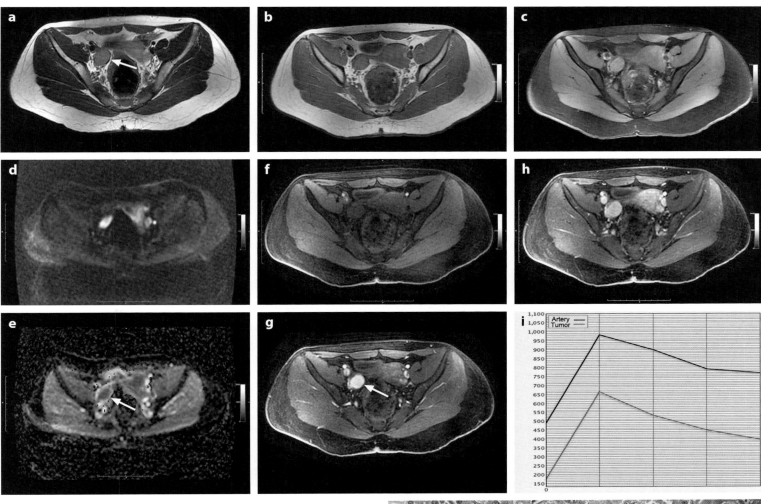

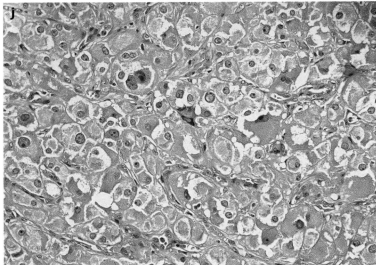

Fig. 6.2 Ovarian adrenal rest artery. Seventeen-year-old girl with known congenital adrenal hyperplasia operated of bilateral surrenalectomy at the age of 13. Due to the new development of hyperandrogenism findings and the appearance on US of a right ovarian mass, a MRI was performed. (**a**) Axial T2W image discloses a 35 × 25-mm right ovarian mass (*arrow*) of intermediate intensity between muscle and fat. (**b–c**) Axial T1W (**b**) and T1W-FS (**c**) images show the same level of the mass to have a low intensity slightly higher than that of muscle and normal ovarian parenchyma. (**d–e**) DWI at b1000 (**d**) and corresponding ADC map (**e**) show the mass (*arrow*) to have high signal intensity on DWI and an ADC value of 1.1×10^{-3} mm^2/s (mean of ADC at b500 and b1000). (**f–i**) DMR before (**f**), 25 s (**g**), and 70 s (**h**) after injection and corresponding time-intensity curves (**i**) show the mass to be homogeneously hyperintense with peak intensity at the arterial phase (*arrow* in **g**) and subsequent washout, typical of endocrine tissue. No obvious lesion was detected in the left ovary on MRI. Right ovariectomy was performed by coelioscopy and the left ovary was macroscopically normal. (**j**) At microscopy, the right ovarian tumor showed steroid cell with a microscopic appearance similar to that of the hyperplasia of the previously removed adrenal glands. These findings were confirmed by immunohistochemistry

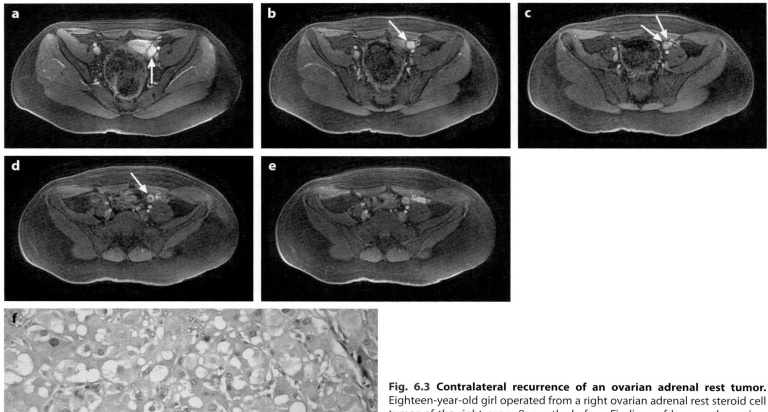

Fig. 6.3 Contralateral recurrence of an ovarian adrenal rest tumor. Eighteen-year-old girl operated from a right ovarian adrenal rest steroid cell tumor of the right ovary 8 months before. Findings of hyperandrogenism appeared again. Axial DMR5 (**a**) at the arterial phase shows a 17×13-mm ovarian mass situated in the left ovary (*arrow*) between the uterus and the left external iliac vessels. It has the same characteristics that of the previous removed right ovarian mass with peak intensity at the arterial phase. Axial DMR at the arterial phase (**b–d**) at adjacent higher levels show another similar lesion on **b** (*arrow*), two other on **c** (*arrows*), and another one with ring enhancement on **d** (*arrow*). This last lesion shows also center enhancement at the late phases (**e**). There is probably another smaller one lateral to it, seen on the arterial phase on (**d**). At laparotomy, the left ovary was indurate, and there were several nodules along the left lombo-ovarian ligament. All were removed and showed lesion with histologic appearance (**f**) comparable to the right ovarian mass

References

1. Clement PB (2002) Nonneoplastic lesions of the ovary. In: Kurman RJ (ed) Blaustein's pathology of the female genital tract. Springer, New-York, pp 675–727
2. Pai SA, Desai SB, Borges AM (1998) Uterus-like masses of the ovary associated with breast cancer and raised serum Ca 125. Am J Surg Pathol 22:333–337
3. Meneses MF, Ostrwski ML (1989) Female splenic-gonadal fusion of the discontinuous type. Hum Pathol 20:486–488
4. Putschar WCJ, Manion WC (1956) Splenic-gonadal fusion. Am J Pathol 32:15–33

Functional Lesions of the Ovary

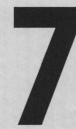

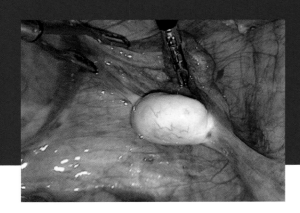

Contents

7.1 Introduction

Functional lesions of the ovary are by far the most common abnormalities encountered in the pathology of the ovary.

These lesions mainly involve the follicle (essentially during the reproductive age), less frequently the stroma cells (essentially after menopause), both as in the PCOD (in young women), or more rarely the Leydig cells (reproductive age group or menopause). During pregnancy, while the corpus luteum cyst is the most common functional lesion, very uncommon multifollicular ovaries (hyperreactio luteinalis) or solid nodules likely arising from stromal cells (pregnancy luteoma) can develop.

In clinical practice, these abnormalities can in many situations mimic tumoral lesions, mainly benign. Misinterpretation of their diagnosis can lead to unnecessary surgery and even more to inappropriate resections particularly in young women, which compromise the fertility, may be complicated with adhesions, or can lead to early menopause.

7.2 Functional Lesions in Nonpregnant Women During the Reproductive Age Group

There are a wide range of functional lesions in this age group. They vary from the single simple cyst to the more complex polycystic ovarian syndrome. For practical purposes, we divided this section in macrofollicular lesions (≥10 mm) and microfollicular lesions (<10 mm). Uncommon lesions involve the stroma.

Macrofollicular Lesions

These lesions result from excessive growth of one or several follicles with or without transformation in corpus luteum.

J.N. Buy, M. Ghossain, *Gynecological Imaging*,
DOI 10.1007/978-3-642-31012-6_7, © Springer-Verlag Berlin Heidelberg 2013

The most common and well defined is the unique follicle which can be non-luteinized (follicle cyst) or luteinized (corpus luteum cyst). The latter usually appears after rupture of the follicle but also has been described in some rare examples of luteinized unruptured follicle syndrome (LUF syndrome). These cysts may be complicated by hemorrhage.

Besides the common unilocular form, more complex patterns may be encountered in ultrasound representing bilocular or adjacent cysts.

Further more, multiple cysts superior to 10 mm in one or both ovaries led to the definition of the macrofollicular ovaries that could be divided in several sub-entities.

Microfollicular Lesions
They are dominated by the polycystic ovarian syndrome (PCOS) but can be encountered in women with no clinical or hormonal disturbance.

7.2.1 Follicle and Corpus Luteum Solitary Cysts

Definition
Follicle and corpus luteum are, respectively, termed follicle cyst and corpus luteum cyst when >3 cm [1].

Microscopically, follicle cysts are lined by an inner layer of granulosa cells and an outer layer of theca interna cells. The cells in either layer may be luteinized. Vascularization is weak and limited to the theca layer.

Corpus luteum cysts exhibit a convoluted lining composed of large luteinized granulosa cells and smaller luteinized theca interna cells with prominent outermost layer of connective tissue. Its wall is thicker. Vascularization is prominent at the periphery, essentially in the theca layer [1].

Content of follicle cysts and corpus luteum cysts varies from a serous or serosanguineous fluid to clotted blood, their hemorrhagic forms [1].

7.2.1.1 Non-Hemorrhagic Follicle Cysts

Common macroscopic and radiologic findings are summarized in Table 7.1 [1].

Ultrasound

The Cyst
Typically these cysts are unilocular, anechoic with a thin or non-visualized wall and without any papillary projection (Fig. 7.1). They usually measure from 3 to 8 cm in diameter. Larger cysts may occur rarely [1].

By definition a follicle cyst is >3 cm; otherwise, it is called follicle [1]. However, a follicle less than 3 cm that persists over one or more cycles can be assimilated to a small follicle cyst, but the denomination of persistent macrofollicle is more appropriate.

Table 7.1 Common macroscopic and radiologic findings of non-hemorrhagic follicle cysts

Size: between 3 and 8 cm
Round
Unilateral
Thin wall
Serous content
Unique
Unilocular
Absence of papillary projection

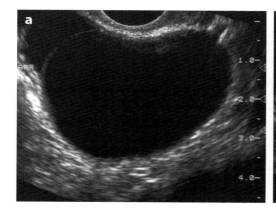
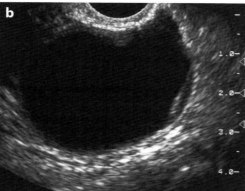

Fig. 7.1 Functional cyst with clear fluid. A 43-year-old women with left pelvic pain. (**a**) Endovaginal US displays a right unilocular anechoic cyst measuring 4.5 cm with a thin regular wall. An adjacent follicle is seen at the periphery. (**b**) Another view depicts an echogenic line near the inner wall of the cyst very likely related to a detachment of the granulosa. Coelioscopy with cystectomy was performed. Pathology revealed a functional follicular cyst

Its intraovarian location can be definitely diagnosed when the mass is encased in the ovarian parenchyma and/or surrounded by follicles which are pushed toward the periphery of the cyst.

In corpus luteum cyst, the wall is thicker. In color Doppler, vascularization in the wall is usually demonstrated.

Differential Diagnosis on US

The solitary follicle cyst should be distinguished from other purely ovarian and extraovarian cystic masses (Table 7.2).

When the ovarian origin is definite, the cyst cannot be differentiated from other purely cystic ovarian masses (Table 7.2) (Figs. 7.1, 7.2, 7.3, and 7.4). Follow-up is necessary to make the differential diagnosis.

When the ovarian origin is not sure, extraovarian unilocular cystic masses must be discussed:

1. Hydrosalpinx is the most common differential diagnosis. In the typical form of hydrosalpinx, tubular shape, plicae, mucosal folds when present allow to make the differential (Fig. 7.5). However, in some cases, only the ampullary portion of the salpinx may be dilated and simulates a unilocular cyst.
2. A paraovarian cyst can only be distinguished when it is clearly separated from the ipsilateral normal ovary (Fig. 7.6).
3. Peritoneal pseudocyst is rarely unilocular. Previous surgery or PID is usually suggestive.
4. When the location is posterior in the pelvis, a meningocele must always be kept in mind.

Whatever the type of mass, purely cystic masses on US are almost always benign. Most cases of follicle cyst and corpus luteum cysts regress spontaneously within 2 months, and this process can be accelerated by administration of a combined estrogen-progestogen preparation.

Table 7.2 Differential diagnosis of purely unilocular ovarian cystic masses on US, MR, and/or CT

Epithelial ovarian tumors
1. Serous cystadenoma
2. Mucinous cystadenoma (occasional)
Extraovarian unilocular cystic masses
1. Hydrosalpinx
2. Paraovarian cyst
3. Peritoneal pseudocyst
4. Uncommon: meningocele, bladder diverticulum
Ovarian non-epithelial unilocular cystic masses
Exceptional
1. Mature cystic teratoma (pediatric age)
2. Granulosa cell tumor (juvenile and adult type)

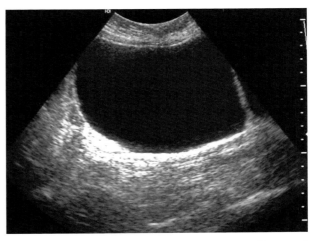

Fig. 7.2 Unilocular serous cystadenoma without papillary projection. Ultrasound shows an anechoic cyst without any papillary projection indistinguishable from a functional cyst. Only persistence on follow-up allowed suspicion of a neoplastic lesion. Histology confirmed the diagnosis of a serous cystadenoma

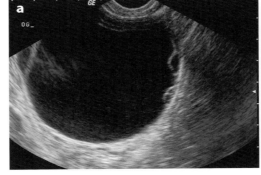

Fig. 7.3 Mucinous cystadenoma in a 40-year-old woman. (a) Transvaginal ultrasound shows a 7.4-cm cyst with anechoic fluid and thin wall. On the *left*, there is a loculation or an adjacent follicle. On the *right*, small loculations can be misinterpreted as granulosa detachments (compare to Fig. 7.1). (b) Another view of the left loculations. Follow-up showed persistence of the cyst. Coelioscopy and cystectomy were performed. Pathology: mucinous cystadenoma

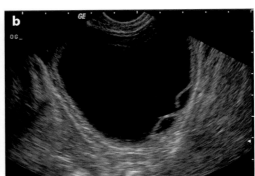
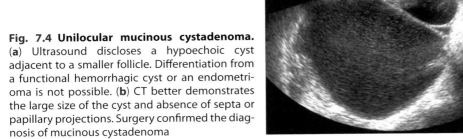
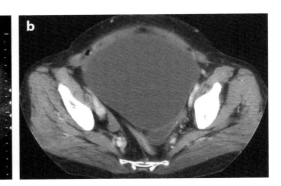

Fig. 7.4 Unilocular mucinous cystadenoma. (a) Ultrasound discloses a hypoechoic cyst adjacent to a smaller follicle. Differentiation from a functional hemorrhagic cyst or an endometrioma is not possible. (b) CT better demonstrates the large size of the cyst and absence of septa or papillary projections. Surgery confirmed the diagnosis of mucinous cystadenoma

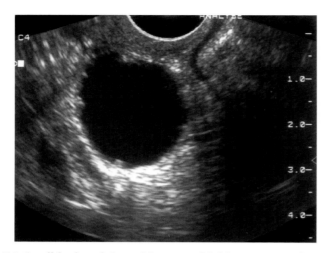

Fig. 7.5 Small hydrosalpinx with mucosal folds. Transvaginal sonography displays a small unilocular 2.5-cm cystic lesion with small intraluminal projections very suggestive of mucosal folds in a hydrosalpinx. Coelioscopy and pathology confirmed the diagnosis of hydrosalpinx

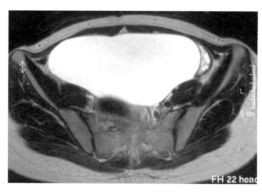

Fig. 7.6 Large paraovarian cyst laminating a normal left ovary. Axial T2W MR image discloses a large paraovarian cyst coming in close contact with the left ovary and laminating it. Distinction from an ovarian cyst is not possible, although one should expect the ovary to be more laminated with such a large cyst. Functional cyst can be as large as this one, although this is infrequent. Coelioscopy and pathology confirmed a left paraovarian simple cyst

MR and CT

Occasionally follicle cyst can be visualized on MR or CT.

On MR, performed without contrast, their signal is close to urine on T1- and T2-weighted images (Fig. 7.7). The wall is usually not visible on T1 where its signal is usually isointense relative to ovarian stroma, but usually visible on T2 where its signal is hypointense relative to ovarian stroma; after contrast, the wall shows in most cases greater enhancement than ovarian stroma [2].

On CT, their density is close to water density. After contrast injection, enhancement of the laminated normal ovarian parenchyma can be seen.

7.2.1.2 Follicle Hemorrhagic Cysts (FHC)

Macroscopic and Radiologic Findings

They are summarized in Table 7.3.

Table 7.3 Macroscopic and radiologic findings of hemorrhagic follicle cysts

Common
Size: 5–6 cm
Unilocular
Round
Unilateral
Unique
Thick wall
Uncommon
Bilateral
Multiple in the same ovary

Ultrasound

Cystic Content

Blood is known to have a variable sonographic appearance mostly related to the temporal sequence of clot formation and lysis. Classically fresh blood is anechoic, progressing subacutely to a mixed echogenicity and finally becoming anechoic. Therefore, it is not surprising that FHC have such variable features (Fig. 7.8). Some typical patterns are very suggestive of FHC [3–6]:

1. Diffuse echogenic pattern which seems to consist of a blood clot and often includes a small echo-free area (Figs. 7.8h and 7.9).

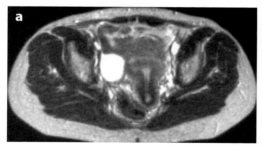
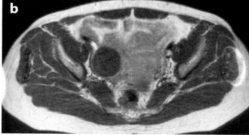

Fig. 7.7 Functional cyst with clear fluid. (**a**) MR, axial view, T2-weighted image. The content of the cyst has signal intensity close to urine. (**b**) MR, axial view, T1-weighted image with contrast injection. Regular cyst with a low signal intensity close to urine is displayed in the right ovary laminating the normal parenchyma

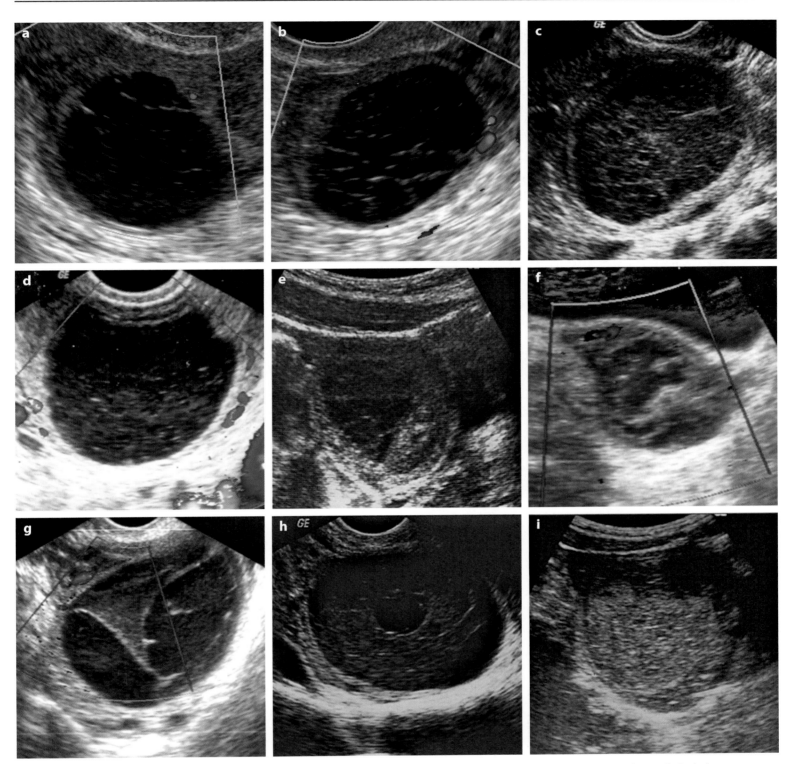

Fig. 7.8 Some but not all patterns of FHC: (**a**) scarce fibrin strands at the limit of visibility, (**b**) classical fine fishnet appearance, (**c**) coarse fishnet appearance looking like a sponge, (**d**) ill-defined fluid-debris level, (**e**) eccentric clot with associated slightly perceptible fishnet or reticular pattern, (**f**) irregular retractile clot, (**g**) stellate well-demarcated clot, (**h**) anechoic area inside diffuse echogenic content, (**i**) hyperechoic relatively homogeneous pattern. Although not always shown here, color or power Doppler was always performed to exclude vascularization inside the echoic content of the cysts. In all cases, follow-up or surgery confirmed the diagnosis

2. Whirled pattern of clotted blood or a mixed pattern with a clearly demarcated echogenic part (Fig. 7.10).
3. Multiple fine interdigitating "septations" giving a fishnet appearance (Fig. 7.11). These echogenic lines correspond to fibrin or other products of blood.
4. In other cases, some echogenic patterns are more heterogeneous, but containing in at least an area of the cyst one of the patterns described above (Fig. 7.12).

Some other patterns are not as characteristic:
1. Layering is uncommon. It is not specific [7, 8] (Fig. 7.13); this level can be seen in endometrioma and in dermoid cyst.
2. The pattern can be diffusely echogenic and heterogeneous (Fig. 7.14).
3. The cyst can be completely anechoic (with hemorrhage in the wall).

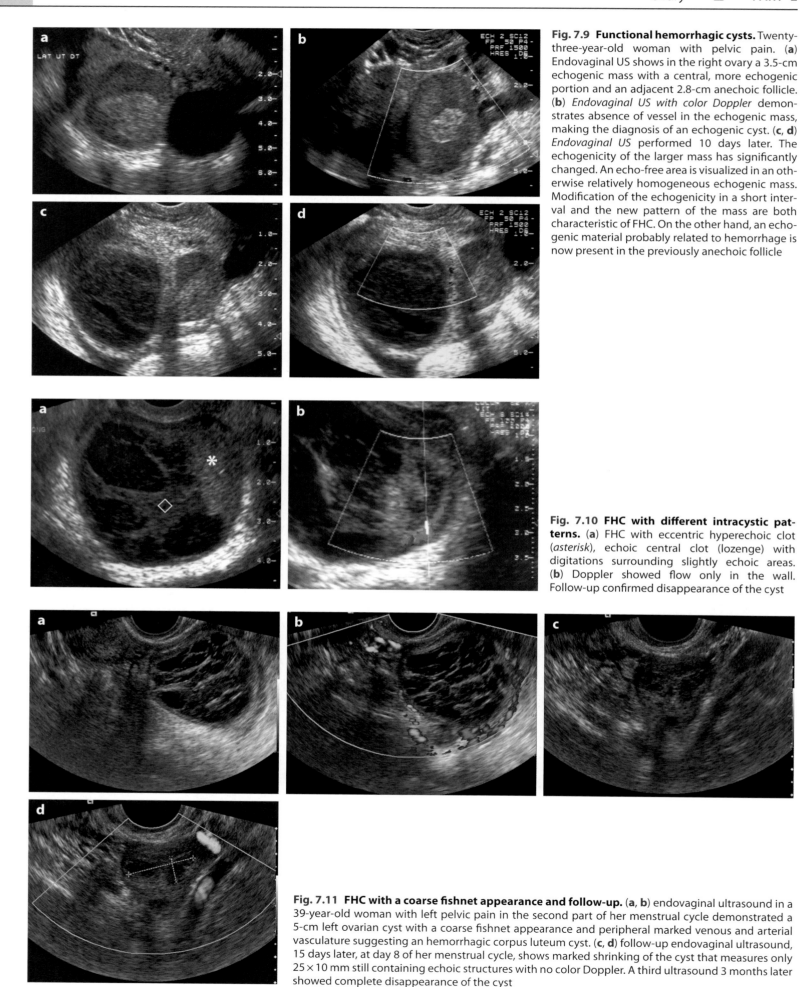

Fig. 7.9 Functional hemorrhagic cysts. Twenty-three-year-old woman with pelvic pain. (**a**) Endovaginal US shows in the right ovary a 3.5-cm echogenic mass with a central, more echogenic portion and an adjacent 2.8-cm anechoic follicle. (**b**) *Endovaginal US with color Doppler* demonstrates absence of vessel in the echogenic mass, making the diagnosis of an echogenic cyst. (**c, d**) *Endovaginal US* performed 10 days later. The echogenicity of the larger mass has significantly changed. An echo-free area is visualized in an otherwise relatively homogeneous echogenic mass. Modification of the echogenicity in a short interval and the new pattern of the mass are both characteristic of FHC. On the other hand, an echogenic material probably related to hemorrhage is now present in the previously anechoic follicle

Fig. 7.10 FHC with different intracystic patterns. (**a**) FHC with eccentric hyperechoic clot (*asterisk*), echoic central clot (*lozenge*) with digitations surrounding slightly echoic areas. (**b**) Doppler showed flow only in the wall. Follow-up confirmed disappearance of the cyst

Fig. 7.11 FHC with a coarse fishnet appearance and follow-up. (**a, b**) endovaginal ultrasound in a 39-year-old woman with left pelvic pain in the second part of her menstrual cycle demonstrated a 5-cm left ovarian cyst with a coarse fishnet appearance and peripheral marked venous and arterial vasculature suggesting an hemorrhagic corpus luteum cyst. (**c, d**) follow-up endovaginal ultrasound, 15 days later, at day 8 of her menstrual cycle, shows marked shrinking of the cyst that measures only 25 × 10 mm still containing echoic structures with no color Doppler. A third ultrasound 3 months later showed complete disappearance of the cyst

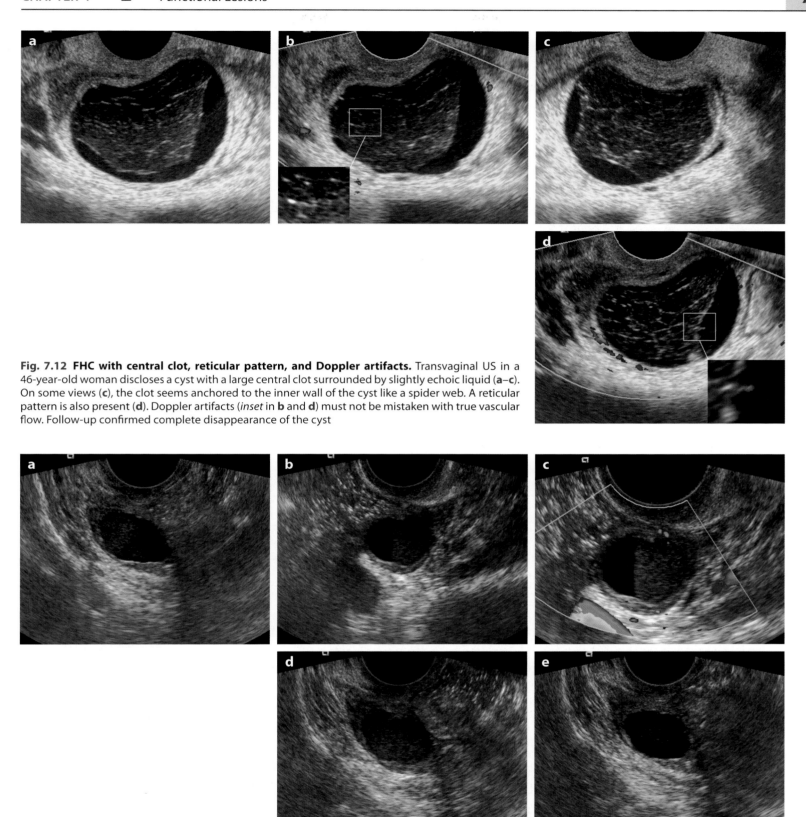

Fig. 7.12 FHC with central clot, reticular pattern, and Doppler artifacts. Transvaginal US in a 46-year-old woman discloses a cyst with a large central clot surrounded by slightly echoic liquid (**a–c**). On some views (**c**), the clot seems anchored to the inner wall of the cyst like a spider web. A reticular pattern is also present (**d**). Doppler artifacts (*inset* in **b** and **d**) must not be mistaken with true vascular flow. Follow-up confirmed complete disappearance of the cyst

Fig. 7.13 Corpus luteum with hemorrhagic cystic content and fluid level. (**a**) Oblique transvaginal US view in a woman in the second part of her cycle discloses a right ovarian 2.5 × 1.5-cm cystic structure with mixed echoic and anechoic content. (**b**) Strict sagittal view demonstrates the presence of a sharp fluid level. (**c**) Color Doppler shows vascular peripheral rim highly suggesting a cystic hemorrhagic corpus luteum. (**d**) Coronal view through the dependent part shows only echoic content. (**e**) Coronal view through the nondependent part shows only anechoic content. Follow-up confirmed disappearance of the cyst

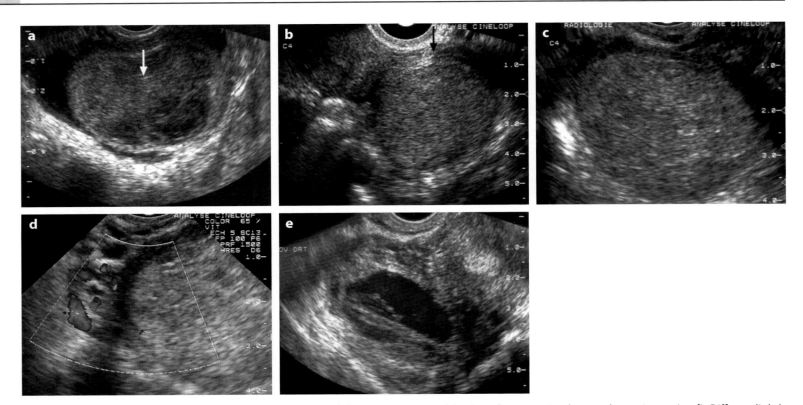

Fig. 7.14 FHC with atypical intracystic patterns. (**a**) FHC with heterogeneous intracystic pattern that can simulate a dermoid cyst. Note the linear echoic strands mimicking hair in dermoid cyst (*arrow*). (**b**) Homogeneously diffuse echoic pattern with slight more echoic eccentric area (*black arrow*), a combination that can simulate endometrioma. (**c**, **d**) Diffuse slightly hyperechoic and slightly heterogeneous avascular pattern that can suggest either endometrioma or dermoid cyst. (**e**) Fibrin digitations that can be confused with true septae in a multilocular cyst but avascular on Doppler

Wall

A thickened wall of 2–3 mm is usually present.
Acoustic enhancement is common.

Normal Ovarian Parenchyma

A normal ovarian parenchyma pushed toward the periphery is frequently observed.

Doppler

The main interest of color Doppler particularly when the form is not characteristic is to demonstrate the absence of vessel in the mass, which highly suggests its cystic nature [9]. Regular vessels can be visualized in the wall of the cyst.

Bilaterality and Multiplicity

Bilaterality and multiplicity in the same ovary are very uncommon.

Ultrasound findings of FHC are summarized in Table 7.4, and as endometrioma can have a close presentation, findings of endometriomas are reported in the same table.

Table 7.4 Ultrasound findings of endometriomas and functional hemorrhagic cysts

	Endometrioma	Functional hemorrhagic cyst
Size	<8 cm	<8 cm
Shape	Not round with protrusion	Round
Bilateral	1/2 to 1/3 of cases	Exceptional
Multiple cysts in the same ovary	Possible	Exceptional
Location	Ovarian fossa Displaced inward and backward	Ovarian fossa
Internal echo pattern	Ground glass pattern	Fishnet pattern Whirled pattern Heterogenous pattern
Clots	Echogenic foci Peripheral Round or curvilinear	Large hyperechoic central portion
Wall	Thick	Thick
Layering	Possible	Possible
Acoustic enhancement	Very common	Very common
Follow-up ultrasound	No modification in size and echo pattern	Modification in size and echo pattern
Normal parenchyma pushed toward the periphery	Common finding	Common finding
Adhesions	Possible	Absence

Table 7.5 Differential diagnosis of FHC

(a) Endometriosis
(b) Other cystic echogenic masses
   ■ Mature cystic teratoma
   ■ Tubo-ovarian abscess
   ■ Cystic epithelial tumor complicated with hemorrhage
(c) Tissular echogenic masses
   ■ Echogenic epithelial tumor with endocystic vegetation
   ■ Ovarian fibroma

Differential

The main differential diagnoses are listed in Table 7.5.
1. Differential diagnosis with endometriosis is detailed in Table 7.4.
2. Cystic mature teratoma typically has different morphological characteristics. However, in some cases, the echogenic pattern does not allow to make the differential so that MR or CT is necessary to make a specific diagnosis (Fig. 7.14).
3. More uncommonly, solid echogenic masses must be differentiated. Indeed, in some cases, vascularization can be difficult or impossible to demonstrate in a tissular mass as an ovarian fibroma or in a small vegetation resembling a clot in a cystic epithelial tumor (Fig. 7.15).

Resolution on follow-up ultrasound is a key finding for the diagnosis.

In all cases and particularly when the pattern of the cyst is not characteristic, two findings displayed on follow-up are characteristic for FHC [5] (Figs. 7.9 and 7.14):
– Decrease in size or even complete disappearance of the cyst usually after the next period
– Changing of the ultrasound pattern is depicted within 10 days
   Association: FHC can be associated in the same ovary with one or more endometriomas.
   Rupture (see Chap. 32)

MR [29]

Most commonly, the content of the cyst in FHC is hypointense on T1 (without and with fat suppression) contrary to endometrioma (Fig. 7.16). On T2 it is homogeneous or often heterogenous (Fig. 7.17).

Uncommonly, the cyst can have intermediate signal intensity on T1 that increases after fat suppression with heterogeneous signal on T2 (Fig. 7.18).

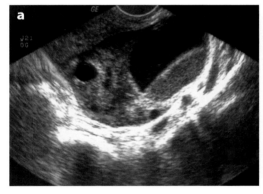
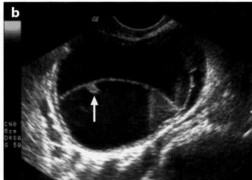

Fig. 7.15 Pseudovegetation in an FHC. Multiple hemorrhagic functional cysts in a 33-year-old woman under Clomid for ovarian stimulation: (**a**) Endovaginal oblique view shows a partly anechoic and partly echoic cyst. (**b**) Strict endovaginal sagittal view is necessary to well disclose the levels in the cysts. The small echoic structure against the wall of one of the cysts (*arrow*) is not vegetation but a small clot. All lesions disappeared on follow-up ultrasound

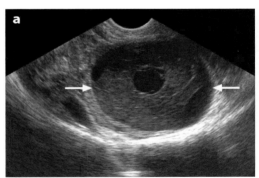
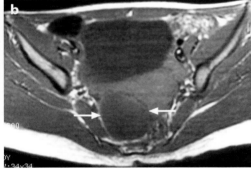
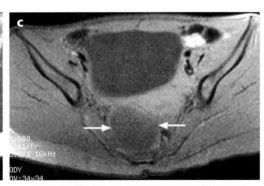
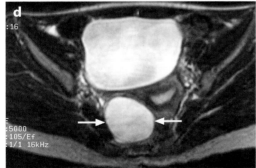

Fig. 7.16 FHC with a typical pattern on US and comparable to a simple cyst on MR. (**a**) Transvaginal US in a 26-year-old woman with pelvic pain in the second part of her menstrual cycle shows a 5.5-cm right ovarian cyst (*arrows*) with a typical pattern of FHC. (**b–d**) MR examination performed after 1.5 h demonstrates a homogeneous cyst (*arrows*), hypointense (i.e., with a signal intensity less than or equal to that of muscle) on T1-weighted images without (**b**) and with fat suppression (**c**); on T2-weighted images (**d**), the overall signal of the cyst was hyperintense, i.e., comparable to that of urine. A follow-up US examination after 12 days showed the disappearance of the cyst (Figures from Author's personal publication: Kanso et al. [29])

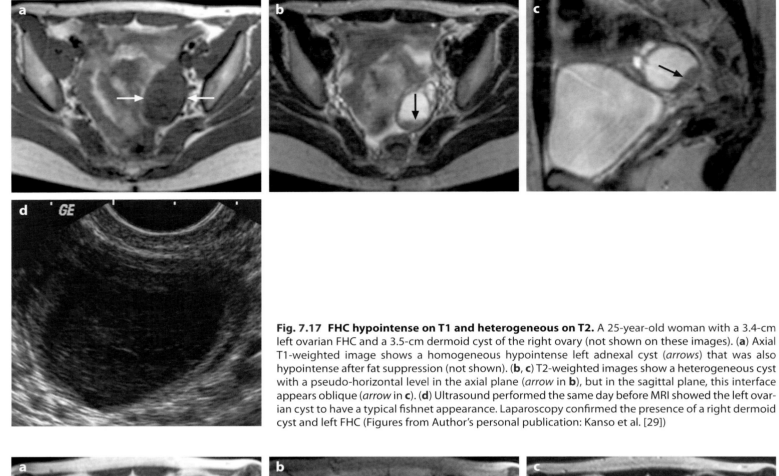

Fig. 7.17 FHC hypointense on T1 and heterogeneous on T2. A 25-year-old woman with a 3.4-cm left ovarian FHC and a 3.5-cm dermoid cyst of the right ovary (not shown on these images). (**a**) Axial T1-weighted image shows a homogeneous hypointense left adnexal cyst (*arrows*) that was also hypointense after fat suppression (not shown). (**b, c**) T2-weighted images show a heterogeneous cyst with a pseudo-horizontal level in the axial plane (*arrow* in **b**), but in the sagittal plane, this interface appears oblique (*arrow* in **c**). (**d**) Ultrasound performed the same day before MRI showed the left ovarian cyst to have a typical fishnet appearance. Laparoscopy confirmed the presence of a right dermoid cyst and left FHC (Figures from Author's personal publication: Kanso et al. [29])

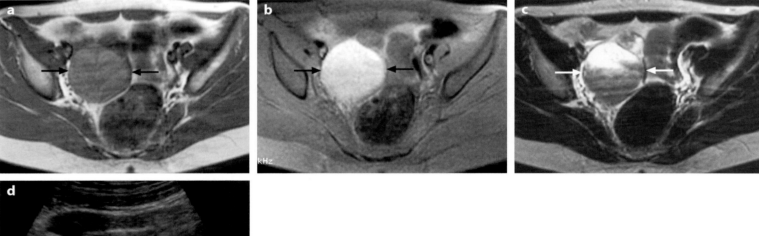

Fig. 7.18 FHC with intermediate signal intensity on T1 and high signal intensity on T1-weighted images with fat suppression. Axial MR images of a 6-cm surgically proven right FHC in a 16-year-old patient. (**a**) T1-weighted image shows a cyst (*arrows*) of intermediate signal intensity, slightly higher than that of muscle. (**b**) On T1-weighted image with fat suppression, the cyst (*arrows*) is relatively homogeneous and appears hyperintense. (**c**) T2-weighted image shows a heterogeneous cyst (*arrows*) with hyperintense and hypointense areas. (**d**) Ultrasound performed within 24 h shows an echoic pattern with some anechoic small areas (Figures from Author's personal publication: Kanso et al. [29])

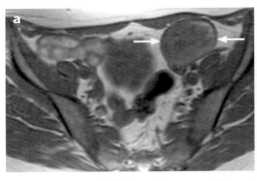
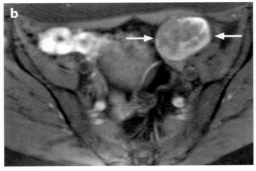
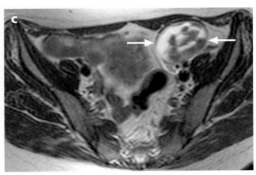

Fig. 7.19 FHC partially hyperintense on T1-weighted images. A 51-year-old patient with a 5.3-cm left FHC discovered incidentally on a pelvic MR performed for uterine adenomyosis. (**a, b**) T1-weighted image (**a**) shows a cyst (*arrows*) that is mainly hypointense, with small peripheral hyperintense components more evident after fat suppression (**b**). (**c**) On T2-weighted image, the cyst (*arrows*) appears very heterogeneous. The cyst disappeared spontaneously on follow-up examination (Figures from Author's personal publication: Kanso et al. [29])

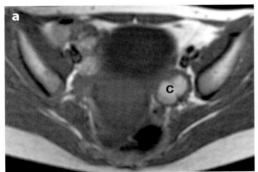
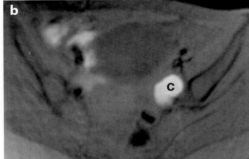
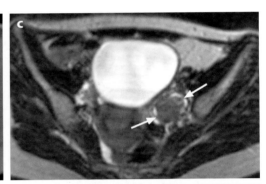
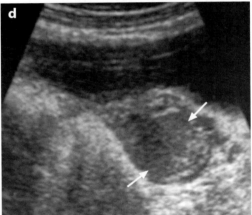

Fig. 7.20 FHC mimicking endometrioma. Axial MR images in a 26-year-old patient with a known left ovarian cyst persistent since 6 months. (**a, b**) T1-weighted images without (**a**) and with fat suppression (**b**) show an almost entirely hyperintense 3.2-cm left ovarian cyst (letter *c*) with internal notches. (**c**) On T2-weighted image, the cyst (*arrows*) exhibits low signal intensity. (**d**) Concomitant US shows a cyst (*arrows*) with echoic and hyperechoic content suggesting endometriosis. The MR and US imaging diagnosis was, incorrectly, an endometrial cyst. The patient, having refused any surgical or medical treatment, had an US examination 6 months later showing a decrease of the cyst size to 8 mm and its complete disappearance after another 6 months, hence confirming its functional nature (Figures from Author's personal publication: Kanso et al. [29])

Partial hyperintensity can be seen on T1 fat suppression (Fig. 7.19).

Exceptionally it can looks like an endometrioma (Fig. 7.20).

MR findings are summarized in Table 7.6.

Uncommonly, a particular pattern resembling a subacute hematoma designated as the "ring sign" has been reported [10].

- The peripheral portion has high signal intensity (close to fat) on T1 and T2.
- The central portion has a low intensity on T1 and intermediate signal intensity on T2.

This pattern has never been observed in endometriosis [10].

Table 7.6 Signal intensity of FHC and endometriomas on MR

T1	T1-FS	T2	FHC	Endometrioma
Low	Low	High (homogenous or heterogenous)	Most common	–
		Low	–	Rare
Intermediate	High	High (homogenous or heterogenous)	Uncommon	Uncommon
		Low	–	Uncommon
High	High	<Adipose tissue (homogenous or heterogenous)	Exceptional	Most common
		≥Urine (homogenous or heterogenous)	–	Less common

CT Scan

CT has no indication in the diagnosis of FHC except in case of rupture.

Without Contrast

Density of the mass is usually >20 HU (Fig. 7.21). Rarely the density of the cystic content is very high (85 HU). A fluid-fluid level may be visualized (Fig. 7.21). Hyperdense areas corresponding to clots can be demonstrated. These hyperdense areas are however different from the hyperdense focal clots seen in endometriomas which are more focal, denser and which can mimic calcifications [11]. However, in the majority of cases, differentiation from endometrioma is not possible.

After Contrast

IV contrast injection is mandatory when color Doppler does not definitely differentiate FHC from a solid mass (Fig. 7.22).

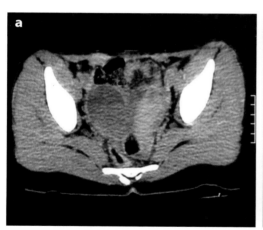
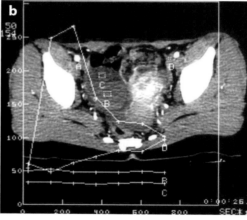

Fig. 7.21 FHC with fluid level documented by CT and time intensity curves. (a) CT with injection at the late phase shows a 6-cm right ovarian cyst with a density content superior to water, and fluid level. (b) Non-incremental dynamic MR at the level of cyst shows that the dependent part (*curve B*) has a density of 50 HU and a *flat curve* (from 0 to 12 min), proving absence of contrast uptake. The nondependent part (*curve C*) has a density of 30 HU and also a flat curve. The curves of the external iliac artery (*curve A*) and vein (*curve D*) are also displayed for comparison. The image displayed in b is at the arterial phase; note that the wall of the cyst is better displayed at the late phase

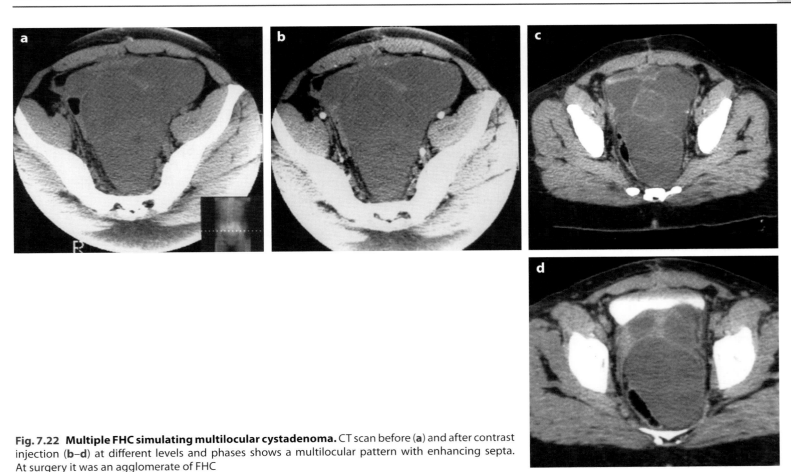

Fig. 7.22 Multiple FHC simulating multilocular cystadenoma. CT scan before (**a**) and after contrast injection (**b–d**) at different levels and phases shows a multilocular pattern with enhancing septa. At surgery it was an agglomerate of FHC

7.2.2 Multiple Follicular Cysts

7.2.2.1 Macrofollicular Ovaries

Several large follicles >10 mm, sometimes exceeding 3 cm, can be found in normal women, with undefined hormonal disorders, in some specific conditions such as macrofollicular dystrophy syndrome, in stimulated ovaries with or without hyperstimulation syndrome, in tamoxifen therapy, and in conditions associated to peritoneal inclusion cysts.

Macroscopy

– Size of the ovary >5 cm
– Multifollicular some >1 cm and up to 3 cm
– Uni- or bilateral

Imaging Findings

Two patterns can be observed:
1. The large follicles are clearly separated by normal ovarian stroma; the diagnosis of multifollicular ovaries is suggested (Fig. 7.23).

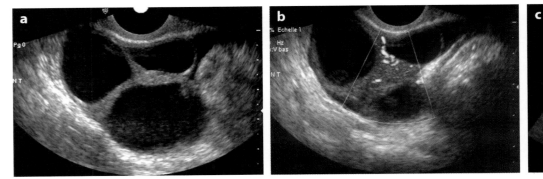
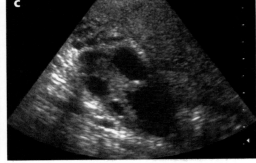

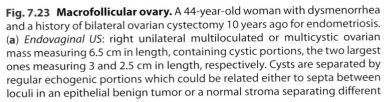

Fig. 7.23 Macrofollicular ovary. A 44-year-old woman with dysmenorrhea and a history of bilateral ovarian cystectomy 10 years ago for endometriosis. (**a**) *Endovaginal US*: right unilateral multiloculated or multicystic ovarian mass measuring 6.5 cm in length, containing cystic portions, the two largest ones measuring 3 and 2.5 cm in length, respectively. Cysts are separated by regular echogenic portions which could be related either to septa between loculi in an epithelial benign tumor or a normal stroma separating different follicle cysts. (**b**) *Endovaginal US with color Doppler* depicts vessels in the central echogenic portion which definitely confirms its tissular character without being able to precise the nature of this tissue. (**c**) Estroprogestin is administered and a *second US* is performed 5 weeks later. The cysts have significantly decreased in size, confirming the functional character of these lesions

Table 7.7 Differential diagnosis of benign multilocular cystic masses

Ovarian tumors
Mainly serous and mucinous cystadenoma
Uncommonly, granulosa cell tumor
Extraovarian cystic masses
Peritoneal inclusion cyst
Hydro- and pyosalpinx

2. The follicles are adjacent from one to the others; it is impossible to make differential diagnosis:
   (a) Between multifollicular and benign multilocular ovarian cystic masses (Table 7.7)
   (b) With multiloculated extraovarian cystic masses, particularly with hydrosalpinx (Fig. 7.24) and peritoneal inclusion cyst (Fig. 7.25)

Differential Diagnosis

Etiologies

(a) *Macrofollicular dystrophy syndrome* belongs to the group of dysovulation syndromes that are different from anovulation syndromes by the presence of a corpus luteum cyst after the peak of LH. This dysovulation is usually associated to hypofertility.

Duration of the cycle is longer (from 35 to 45 days). The first phase of the cycle is longer because of delayed ovulation; the luteal phase is shorter with a decrease in progesterone.

Clinically there is an intermittent painful ovarian hypertrophy, uni- or bilateral, associated with a premenarchal and premenstrual predominance. It is almost always associated with dysmenorrhea related to absence or delayed ovulation, and other symptoms with a premenstrual predominance such as pollakiuria, cystalgia, colitis, and mastodynias.

(b) *Ovarian stimulation and hyperstimulation syndrome*
The diagnosis is easy in the appropriate clinical context, i.e., ovarian stimulation. In case of excessive response to stimulation, a hyperstimulation syndrome can appear characterized by very large ovaries, ascites, and clinical disorders necessitating in some cases intensive care unit admission. The US ovarian pattern is close to that of hyperreactio luteinalis that is developed in the pregnant woman section. Torsion may be another complication.

(c) *Tamoxifen-related disorders*
In the follow-up of patients under tamoxifen therapy, effect on the endometrium is the main concern. However, it is a classical finding to observe multiple macrofollicles or follicle cysts in one or both ovaries that change in size, number, and position from one follow-up to another.

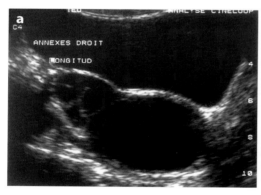 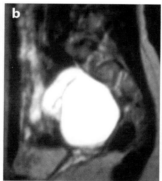 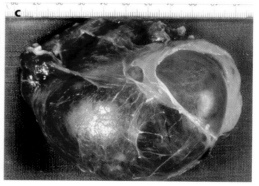

Fig. 7.24 Multiloculated hydrosalpinx. (**a–c**) Ultrasound (**a**), T2W MRI (**b**), and surgical specimen (**c**) of a right multiloculated hydrosalpinx. Communication between different loculi best seen on MRI is the best finding to suggest hydrosalpinx in this case (From Ref. [33]), with permission)

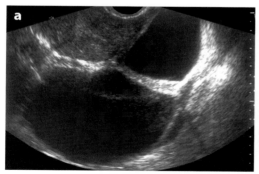 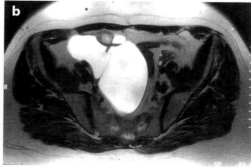

Fig. 7.25 Multilocular peritoneal inclusion cyst. (**a**) On US a multilocular cyst is seen close to the uterus. Differentiation between an ovarian cyst, a hydrosalpinx, and a peritoneal inclusion cyst is difficult. (**b**) On T2W MR image, the cyst is seen molding on adjacent organs, suggesting a peritoneal inclusion cyst (Fig. 7.26)

(d) *A particular form is associated to peritoneal inclusion cyst (PIC)*: Peritoneal inclusion cyst, after surgery (particularly non-laparoscopic) and after infections or endometriosis, usually surrounds the ovaries, favoring the development of macrofollicles and follicle cysts. These ovarian macrofollicles and cysts may be difficult to differentiate from loculations in the PIC.

Follow-Up: Except the peritoneal inclusion cysts, disappearance of these macrofollicles after suppression of the causal effect (tamoxifen or stimulation therapy) or after progestin therapy in macrofollicular dystrophy syndrome can be helpful to rule out an ovarian tumor (Fig. 7.23).

7.2.2.2 Microfollicular Ovaries: Polycystic Ovary Syndrome (PCOS)

Diagnosis of PCOS is based on an association of clinical, biological, and radiological findings.

In the typical form that in its most characteristic expression has been described by Stein-Leventhal, these different findings are associated, and the morphologic findings are particularly obvious.
However:

1. Some findings can be missing.
2. As it has been outlined by Pache et al. [12], there are minimal forms where anatomical changes of the ovary are so difficult to appreciate that US can display normal ovaries.
3. On the other hand,
   (a) Prepubertal girls, normal women, and young women with birth control pills can have morphologic abnormalities of the ovaries that can also resemble to PCOS.
   (b) Hyperandrogenism of adrenal origin produces anovulation and consequently may induce morphologic abnormalities of the ovaries that can mimic the morphology of PCOS.

Physiopathology [13]

1. Hypothalamus: There is an increase of the secretion of gonadotrophin-releasing hormone (GnRH) by the hypothalamic cells owing to an increase of the amplitude of LH secretion (in thin patients) or LH pulse frequency (in obese patients). This results in fluctuating raised level of LH.
2. Ovary: In the granulosa cells, there is an increase of IGFBP-2 and IGFBP-4 that decrease the action of IGF. This will lead to a decrease of the action of FSH on the granulosa cells.
   In the theca cells, there is an abnormal secretion of inhibin which is normally secreted by the granulosa cells. This will:
   (a) Decrease the secretion of FSH by the pituitary cells.
   (b) Increase the action of LH on the theca interna cells with a resulting increase of androgens. These androgens are not

converted in estradiol by the granulosa cells as it occurs normally because the aromatase is not activated by the FSH. They are released in the peripheral blood and converted mainly in the adipose tissue in estrone. The high level of estrone through endocrine action decreases the FSH secretion by the pituitary cells. The increased level of androgens also decreases the action of FSH on the granulosa cells.

3. There are an insulin resistance and hyperinsulinemia which occurs particularly in obese patients. This increase in insulin production decreases the IGFBP-1 secreted by the liver and increases the bioavailability of IGF1 in the plasma. Insulin and IGF1 will increase the action of LH on theca cells that stimulates the production of androgens.
4. In the adrenal glands, there is an increase of the androgen (DHA) secretion; 48 % of this androgen is extracted by the ovaries and converted into testosterone in the theca cells. The increased level of androgens also decreases the action of FSH on the granulosa cells. In PCOS, combined ovarian and adrenal hyperandrogenism is observed in 50 % of patients.

The results of these different and interacted mechanisms are an increase of the LH/FSH level ratio and moreover an increase of the LH/FSH bioactivity ratio with resulting hyperandrogenism and ovulatory dysfunction.

Pathology [1]

Gross Appearance (Fig. 7.26)

1. Typically bilateral, round and two to five times the normal size [1]
   Unilateral involvement is rare. Ovarian size can be normal in 28–40 % of cases. Shape can be oval.
2. Follicles
   Antral follicles increased twice with a mean number of 12.4, mainly ≤4 mm [14].
   Few or no stigmata of ovulation (i.e., corpus luteum or albicans), but corpus luteum has been described in as many as 30 % of otherwise typical cases of PCOS [1].
3. Stroma [14]
   Thickening of peripheral cortex about 50 % (fibrotic and hypocellular) and abruptly contrasted with sub-adjacent cortex.
   Tongues of similarly fibrotic stroma may extend into the deeper cortex.
   Within this zone, prominent venules and arterioles may be seen.

Microscopy

1. Atretic follicles have an inner lining composed of several layers of non-luteinized granulosa cells that may be focally exfoliated

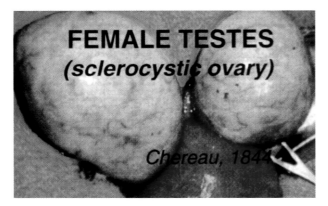

Fig. 7.26 Macroscopy of polycystic ovaries. Bilateral asymmetrical enlarged ovaries with glistening surface. Their size and shape oval on the right side and round on the left side explain the designation given by Chereau (1844) [30] as female testes

and an outer layer of theca interna cells which typically exhibit varying degrees of luteinization.

2. In the stroma, lutein cell nests are present in four of five cases [14]. So-called hyperthecosis, in which such nests are combined with marked stromal increase, is arguably a late stage of Stein-Leventhal morphology.

Clinical Findings

Related to ovulatory dysfunction: oligomenorrhea, amenorrhea, and sterility
Related to hyperandrogenism: hirsutism, acne, and seborrhea
    Acanthosis nigricans associated with insulin resistance
    Absence of findings of virilization
    According to morphotype, there are two forms:
– Obesity commonly associated with diabetes with insulin resistance
– Thin patients without diabetes

Biological Findings

1. LH increases, FSH normal or decreased, and LH/FSH increased.
2. Hyperandrogenism: increased delta-4-androstendione, normal testosterone.
3. Estrone is high due to peripheral conversion (particularly in obese patients) with a reversal of the estradiol-estrone ratio.
4. A hyperprolactinemia is commonly associated.

Ultrasound

The ultrasound findings are reported in Table 7.8.

Size

With transvaginal ultrasound, Pache et al. [12] found a mean ovarian volume of 9.8 cm^3 (approximate range 4–21 cm^3) in PCOS and 5.9 cm^3 (approximate range 2.5–8 cm^3) in normal subjects.

Table 7.8 Ultrasound findings in PCOS

1. Ovary
– Bilateral symmetrical or asymmetrical moderately enlarged and rounded ovaries
– Increased surface >6 cm^2 and increased echogenicity of ovarian stroma
– Numerous (≥12) and small (mean 4 mm) follicles with thick echogenic wall
– Absence of stigmata of ovulation (dominant follicle, corpus luteum)
2. Endometrial hyperplasia (obese)

Surface and Volume

The largest cross-sectional area of the ovary was considered increased when ≥6 cm^2 (Robert et al. [31]). Surface can be simply calculated (surface cm^2 = D_1 cm × D_2 cm × 0.8).
Volume is more difficult to calculate and has been considered as increased when >8 cm^3 [12]. Volume can be calculated using two orthogonal sections (volume cm^3 = D_1 cm × D_2 cm × D_3 cm × 0.5).

Roundness Index

According to Yeh et al., this index is designed by the ratio of the width over the length. Yeh et al. [15] found 25 % of ovaries in PCOS to be relatively round (i.e., roundness index >0.8) but bilaterally present in only 8.7 %. The occurrence of round ovaries in healthy individuals was 6 % in their series.

Asymmetry in Size (Fig. 7.27)

In Yeh et al. series, asymmetry (one is smaller than 50 % of the other) was found 20.9 % women with PCOS. Unilateral PCOS has been reported.

Stroma

The stroma is increased. The exact measurement of the surface of the stroma (excluding follicles) was shown to correlate with the total ovarian surface. Stroma could be considered enlarged when the largest cross-sectional area of the ovary was ≥6 cm^2 (Robert et al. [31]).

Echogenicity of the Stroma (Fig. 7.28)

The increased echogenicity of ovarian stroma as a marker of polycystic ovaries has been emphasized [12]. However, assessment of the echogenicity of ovarian stroma is subjective and not always present.

Follicles (Size and Number)

In Pache et al. series [12], median values of follicular size and number were, respectively, 3.8 mm and 9.8 in patients with PCOS compared with 5.1 mm and 5.0 in control subjects ($p < 0.001$).

The atretic follicles have a wall thicker than usual follicles with an increase of echogenicity.

Dominant follicle and corpora lutea are classically absent but have been occasionally reported (Goldzieher [32]).

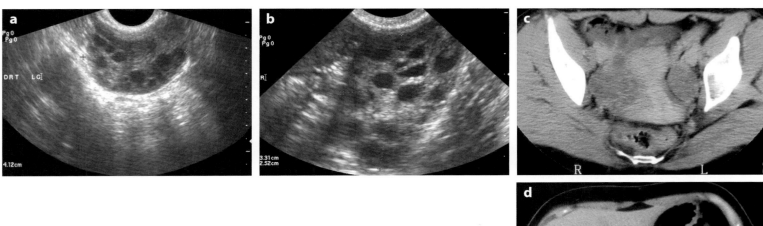

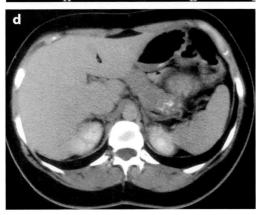

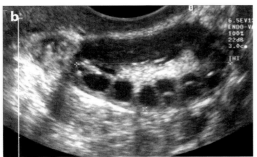

Fig. 7.27 Polycystic ovarian syndrome. A 28-year-old woman with hyperandrogenism, hirsutism, obesity, and oligomenorrhea. Testosterone and delta-4-androsténédione significantly increased. LH/FSH > 1. (**a**) Endovaginal US of the right ovary, longitudinal section: the ovary is increased in size (long axis: 4.1 cm). Its ovular shape is maintained. It contains more than ten follicles <10 mm. The stroma looks normal. (**b**) Endovaginal US of the left ovary, coronal section: the long axis of the ovary is 3.3 cm. Its shape is *round*. The roundness index is >0.7. It contains more than ten follicles <10 mm. The stroma looks increased, but its echogenicity is normal. (**c**) CT scan after injection displays bilateral polycystic ovaries slightly asymmetrical with a more rounded aspect on the right side. Analysis of the stroma is not as well visualized as on US. (**d**) CT scan of the adrenal glands is normal and rules out an adrenal origin. Selective samples in the adrenal and ovarian veins confirm the absence of a tumoral etiology

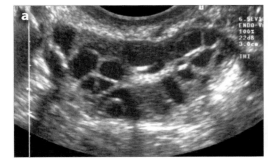

Fig. 7.28 Ultrasound of polycystic ovaries. (**a**, **b**) Two ultrasound views of polycystic ovaries show large ovaries with multiple small peripheral follicles and an echoic centrally located stroma

Uterus

In obese patients, manifestations are those of unopposed estrogenic stimulation, including menometrorrhagia, endometrial hyperplasia (Fig. 7.29), and exceptionally endometrial carcinoma [1].

Exceptionally endometrial carcinomas typically occur in obese patients under the age of 40. The tumors are almost always well-differentiated adenocarcinomas or adenoacanthoma with absent or only superficial myometrial invasion.

Doppler

Doppler has no interest in the diagnosis of PCOS. However, it has the interest to rule out an endocrine tumor. In some cases, it can detect a corpus luteum.

MR

When US has limitations in the correct visualization of the ovaries as in obese and virgin patients, MR can be performed. Findings are the same as on US. Abundant cellular stroma has been reported to show low signal intensity in all sequences [16].

CT Scan

CT has no indication in the diagnosis of PCOS. However, when the origin (adrenal or ovarian) of a hyperandrogenism on the basis of clinical and biological findings has not been established, CT has the importance to rule out a lesion of the adrenal glands.

If CT of the pelvis is performed for another reason, CT findings are the same as on the other imaging modalities.

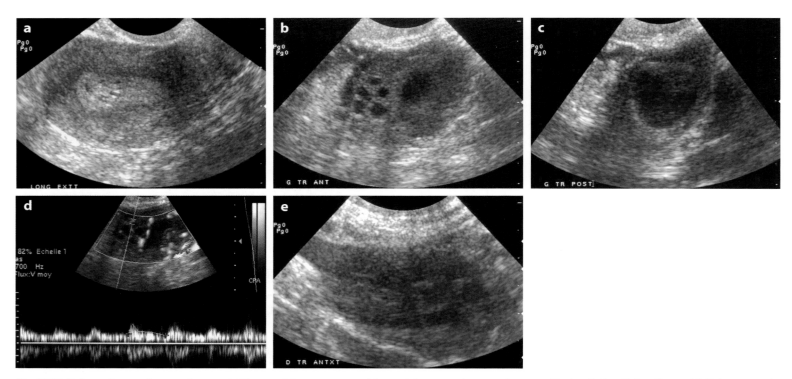

Fig. 7.29 Polycystic ovarian syndrome. A 25-year-old woman consulting for obesity, hirsutism, and amenorrhea. She was operated 9 months ago by coelioscopy for bilateral wedge resection of the ovaries. The pathologic diagnosis was Stein-Leventhal syndrome. She was treated with Clomid. (**a**) Thickening of the endometrium containing small echo-free cystic areas compatible with hyperplasia of the endometrium. (**b**) Endovaginal US of the left ovary: the ovary is normal is size (5.6 cm²). Small antral follicles are gathered in the medial part of the ovary. (**c**) A 1.7 dominant follicle is visualized in the posterolateral part of the left ovary. (**d**) Color Doppler displays vascularization in the ovary. (**e**) Endovaginal US of the right ovary displays an ovary normal in size which looks morphologically normal

7.2.3 Fibromatosis and Massive Edema

These two entities involve young women (13–39 years in fibromatosis and 9–32 in massive edema) with similar clinical manifestations and overlap in their histological features, explaining the reason why they are presented in this same chapter [17].

7.2.3.1 Fibromatosis

Definition

Fibromatosis is proliferation of spindle cells usually producing large amount of collagen like in an ovarian fibroma. But this proliferation is non-neoplastic, which means it is not circumscribed like in a benign ovarian tumor and that it surrounds follicular derivatives, contrary to an ovarian fibroma [17, 18].

The process varies from moderately cellular fascicles of spindle cells with a focal storiform pattern to relatively acellular bands of dense collagen [1].

Macroscopic and radiological findings are summarized in Table 7.9.

Clinical Findings

Menstrual abnormalities: irregularity, excessive bleeding, and amenorrhea.

Rarely hyperandrogenism: hirsutism and virilization [17].

Table 7.9 Macroscopic and radiological findings of fibromatosis

Unilateral (80 %)
Smooth or lobulated external surface
Topography:
– Usually: diffuse solid tissue containing small cysts
– Occasionally: localized or confined to the cortex
Foci of edema can be present
Torsion can be associated

Radiological Findings

(a) *Diffuse Pattern*

Radiologic findings are similar to those of ovarian fibroma, except that fibrous tissue surrounds the follicular derivatives, contrary to an ovarian fibroma [19]. Follicles up to 2.5 cm can be present [17].

On US the masses have an echogenicity close to myometrium with multiple areas of US attenuation. On color Doppler, few vessels are displayed.

On CT without contrast, density is slightly higher than that of myometrium. On MR, on T2 sequences, a diffuse area of hypointense stroma characteristic of fibrous tissue surrounding follicles allowed to suggest the diagnosis [19].

On the DCT and DMR, only slight contrast uptake is visualized on the delayed sequences, as it is usual in benign fibrous tissue proliferation [19].

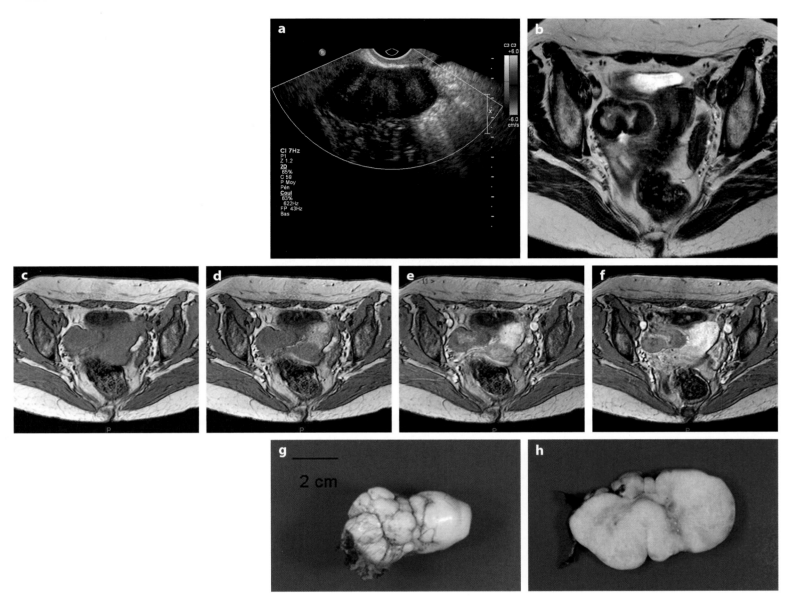

Fig. 7.30 Cortical fibromatosis. (**a**) EVS with color Doppler of the right ovary displays an oval mass containing multiple acoustic shadowing related to fibrous tissue. No vessel is depicted in the mass. These findings suggest an ovarian fibroma. (**b**) MR axial T2W depicts a convoluted surface and significant regular thickened cortex that are typical for cortical fibromatosis. (**c–f**) DMR without injection (**c**) and at the arterial phase (**d**) does not visualize any vessel. At the venous phase (**e**), slight contrast uptake is depicted in the thickened cortex, while contrast uptake is more intense in the medulla. Contrast uptake in the cortex slightly increases on the delayed phase (**f**). This type of contrast enhancement is typical for fibrous tissue and rules out a malignant ovarian tumor (**g, h**) Pathologic specimen displays a bosselated surface of the enlarged ovary (**g**). Longitudinal section (**h**) through the middle of the ovary confirms the thickened and regular outer cortex related to fibromatosis

(b) *Cortical Pattern*

In this form, the thickened cortex is typical for fibromatosis (Fig. 7.30).

(c) *Localized Pattern*

This form can mimic an ovarian fibroma on US. MR can help to make the differential diagnosis.

7.2.3.2 Massive Ovarian Edema

Definition

The enlarged ovary shows edematous hypocellular stroma surrounding follicles and their derivatives characteristically sparing the cortex.

The peripheral cortex most often thickened [17] is composed of dense collagen tissue.

Lutein cells may be seen.

Macroscopic and Radiologic Findings

They are summarized in Table 7.10.

Table 7.10 Macroscopic and radiologic findings of massive ovarian edema

Unilateral in 90 % of cases
Enlarged ovary
Hyperintensity on T2 images
Smooth surface
Focal fibromatosis is common
Torsion is observed in half of the cases

Clinical Findings

Three quarters of them present with abdominal pain, which may be acute and accompanied by abdominal swelling.

In the remaining patients, disorders of menstruation and hyperandrogenism can be seen.

Physiopathology

An explanation for massive edema is primary proliferation of the ovarian stroma with secondary torsion and edema (see also Chap. 32). On the other hand, massive edema may be simply fibromatosis with marked edema [17].

Few cases of lymphatic obstruction secondary to metastatic carcinoma within pelvic and para-aortic lymph nodes have been reported.

7.3 Functional Lesions in Postmenopausal (and in Perimenopausal) Women

7.3.1 Stromal Hyperplasia and Hyperthecosis

They are most commonly encountered in postmenopausal women.

(a) *Pathology*

Microscopy and Definition

Stromal hyperplasia (SH): The medulla and the cortex are replaced by a diffuse or nodular densely (closely packed) non-neoplastic proliferation of stromal cells; these cells are plumper than normal postmenopausal ovarian stromal cells [1].

Stromal Hyperthecosis (HT)

Luteinized stromal cells are scattered singly and in small nests or nodules throughout a hyperplastic ovarian stroma [18]. These luteinized cells synthesize androgens.

According to Nagamani [20], there are two types of HT:

Follicular derivates may lie within the hyperplastic stroma, but may be rare or absent in advanced cases. (type II of Nagamani).

In premenopausal women, sclerocystic changes similar to those seen in PCOS may also be present (type I of Nagamani).

Macroscopy (Fig. 7.31)

Both SH and HT are almost invariably bilateral.

The ovaries range from normal size to 7 cm in diameter, thus potentially mimicking an ovarian neoplasm.

They can be nodular or diffuse.

(b) *Stromal Hyperplasia*

SH may be found in women with disorders associated with androgenic or estrogenic manifestations including endometrial carcinoma and obesity [1].

To our knowledge, no imaging findings of stromal hyperplasia have been reported.

(c) *Stromal Hyperthecosis*

Clinical Findings

The clinical picture of HT evolves usually gradually.

Patients with hyperthecosis are usually obese and present a long-standing history of hirsutism. Hirsutism is more severe in patients with hyperthecosis compared to PCOS.

Signs of virilization: Clitoral enlargement and temporal balding can be present.

In premenopausal women, menstrual cycles are irregular and anovulatory.

Some patients with HT have the HAIR-AN syndrome: hyperandrogenism (HA), insulin resistance (IR), and acanthosis nigricans (AN).

Physiopathology

Circulating insulin level is higher than those in PCOS subjects. The effect of insulin on ovarian stroma cells may induce luteinization and convert them into steroidogenically active luteinized stroma cells.

A decrease in IGFBP-3 level has been observed in women with hyperthecosis of the ovary; this decrease may lead to an increase bioavailability of IGF-1. IGF-1 has stimulatory effect on androgen production by the ovarian stromal cells.

Biological Findings (Table 7.11)

1. LH is normal or low.
2. Hyperandrogenism:
   - The testosterone is markedly increased usually higher than in PCOS and may be in the tumor range (>200 ng/ml). Therefore, the possibility of a virilizing ovarian tumor should always be included in the differential diagnosis.
   - Androstenedione is less increased than testosterone.

Table 7.11 Biological findings of PCOS and hyperthecosis

PCOS	**Hyperthecosis**
LH increased; LH/FSH increased	LH normal
Androstenedione increased	Testosterone increased
Testosterone normal	Androstenedione less increased
Obese patient: estrogen increased	

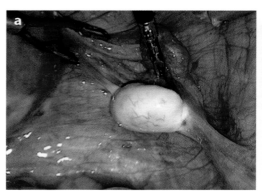 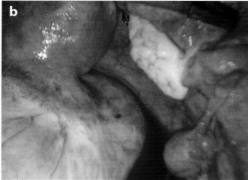

Fig. 7.31 Macroscopic patterns of hyperthecosis. (**a**) Coelioscopic view of a right ovary with hyperthecosis shows smooth but slightly bosselated surface. (**b**) Coelioscopic view of another right ovary with hyperthecosis shows marked nodular surface

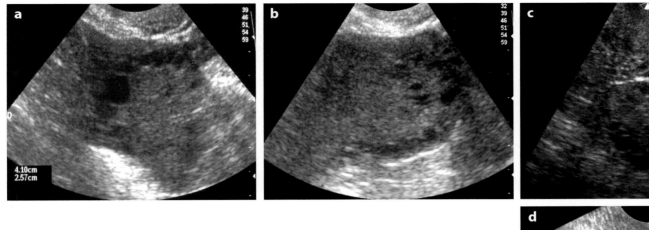

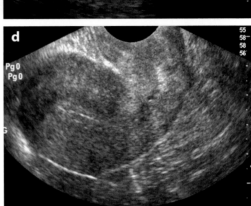

Fig. 7.32 Hyperthecosis. A 32-year-old woman with oligomenorrhea with Ferriman score of 42 and obesity (108 kg). Testosterone and delta-4-androstendione significantly increased. Suspicion of ovarian or adrenal tumor. (**a** and **b**) *Endovaginal US, longitudinal* (**a**) *and coronal* (**b**) *sections of the right ovary:* the right ovary is increased in size. It measures 4.1×2.6 cm (8.5 cm²). There is a significant increase of ovarian stroma associated with multiple antral follicles <10 mm. (**c**) *Endovaginal US of the left ovary:* the left ovary is of normal size measuring 2.7×2.2 cm (4.8 cm²). Its shape and its echogenicity are normal. (**d**) *Endovaginal US, longitudinal section of the uterus:* normal endometrium. *Venous samples* obtained by catheterism rule out an adrenal and ovarian tumoral etiology. The ovarian androgen was increased on both sides but was much higher on the right which seems to be correlated to the difference of size of the ovaries. *Surgery:* right adnexectomy. *Microscopy:* enlarged ovarian stroma with hyperthecosis

— Dihydrotestosterone is increased. It is mainly derived from peripheral conversion in normal women. Increased concentrations of dihydrotestosterone in ovarian vein of women with hyperthecosis indicate that the hyperthecotic ovaries possess 5-alpha-reductase activity. Increased secretion of DHT by the ovary could explain the severe hirsutism and virilization observed in these patients.

3. Estrogens: Estrone is increased because of increased peripheral conversion of androgen to estrogen. Estradiol is normal or low.

Imaging Findings

Ultrasound findings (Fig. 7.32) have been reported [21] and are summarized in Table 7.12.

The abnormalities are most commonly bilateral and symmetric. Hyperplasia of the stroma can be diffuse (Fig. 7.33) or pseudonodular (Fig. 7.34).

Shape can be oval or round (Fig. 7.35).

Table 7.12 Ultrasound findings in hyperthecosis

Usually bilateral and symmetrical
Ovaries increased in size
Round (suggestive) but can be oval
Hyperplasia of the stroma diffuse or nodular (suggestive)
Absence of follicle (after menopause) or some follicles at the periphery (before menopause)
No area of hypervascularization on color Doppler (useful to rule out an androgen-secreting tumor)

Echogenicity is most commonly isoechoic and homogeneous, more rarely pseudonodular (Fig. 7.34).

MR Findings (Fig. 7.36)

(d) *Differential Diagnosis*

These two functional disorders and fibromatosis must be distinguished from nonfunctional tumoral disorders as fibrothecoma (Table 7.13).

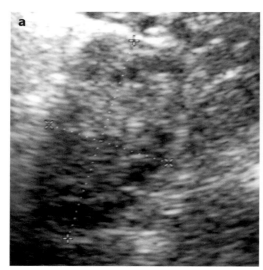

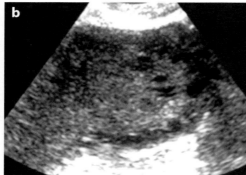

Fig. 7.33 Hyperthecosis in a 32-year-old woman considered as PCOS for a long time. During pregnancy findings of virilization. Testosterone: 2.3 ng/100 ml. On US stroma of both ovaries is significantly increased with few and small follicles at the periphery

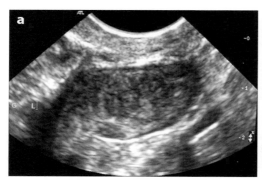

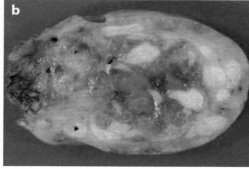

Fig. 7.34 Hyperthecosis with rapidly progressive virilization in a patient with menopause for 3 years. Testosterone level is 1.6 (2.5 times normal). (**a**) At ultrasound, the ovary is increased in size. Its shape is oval. Its pattern is pseudonodular. (**b**) Macroscopy specimen: multiple nodules are seen within the stroma (Figure from Author's personal publication: Rousset et al. [21])

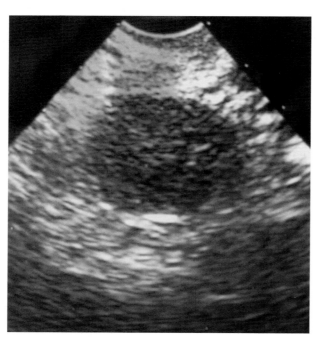

Fig. 7.35 Hyperthecosis with round shape. On ultrasound, a round shaped ovary is well disclosed in this patient with hyperthecosis (Figure from Author's personal publication: Rousset et al. [21])

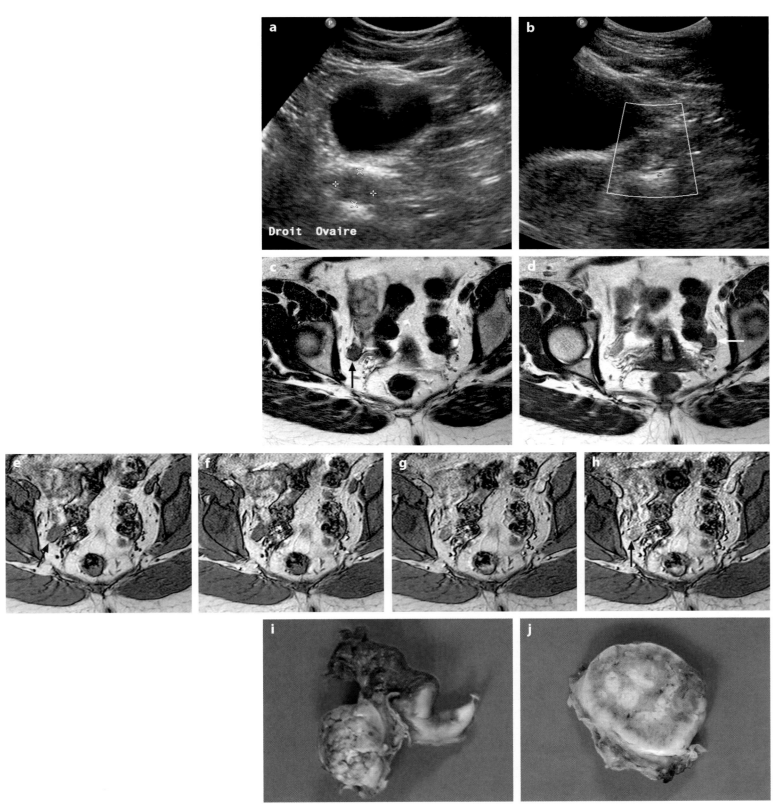

Fig. 7.36 Hyperthecosis in a 47-year-old diabetic woman with major hirsutism since 1 year (testosterone 1.3 ng/ml). (**a**, **b**) Ultrasound discloses two non-enlarged ovaries measuring 20 × 17 mm on the right (*cursors*) and 28 × 23 mm on the *left*. No significant follicle or vascular nodule is seen. (**c**, **d**) On T2WI the ovaries (*arrows*) are hypointense almost round shaped without follicles. (**e**, **h**) DMR before injection (**e**), at the arterial (**f**), portal (**g**), and late (**h**) phases, at the level of the right ovary (*arrow* in **e** and **h**) shows gradual uptake without hypervascular nodule suggestive of an endocrine mass. Similar findings were seen in the left ovary. (**i**, **j**) View of the surgical specimen. In (**i**) the right ovary is round shaped with small nodules on its surface. After section (**j**), stroma involved with hyperthecosis appears as a peripheral white layer and central white pseudonodules

Table 7.13 Stromal non-neoplastic and neoplastic disorders

	Age	Pathology	Luteinized cells	Follicles encompassed	Unilateral (U) Bilateral (B)	Hormonal changes
Non-neoplastic disorders						
Stromal hyperplasia	Postmenopausal menopausal	Multinodular or diffuse proliferation of densely packed stromal cells	No	No	B	No
Stromal hyperthecosis	Postmenopausal menopausal	Stromal hyperplasia and luteinized stromal cells	Yes	No	B	Yes
Fibromatosis	Mean 25 years	Non-neoplastic proliferation of spindle cells and abundant dense collagen	Yes (40 %)	Yes	U	Yes
Neoplastic disorders						
Fibroma	Mean 48 years	Neoplastic proliferation of spindle cells producing abundant dense collagen and varying degrees of intercellular edema	No	No	U	No

Table 7.14 Pathologic and radiologic findings of postmenopausal follicle cysts

– Small size (usually 0.2 up to 2.5 cm in diameter)
– Unilocular
– Uni- or bilateral (especially in perimenopausal patient)
– Unique or multiple (especially in perimenopausal patient)

7.3.2 Functional Cyst in Postmenopausal Women

Follicular cysts are commonly found in perimenopausal women, just after menopause and in patients with hormonal replacement. Disappearance of these cysts on follow-up examinations confirms their functional nature. If they persist, there very likely represent inclusion cysts or small cystadenomas.

Calcifications in the stroma are commonly associated.

Pathologic and radiologic findings are summarized in Table 7.14.

7.4 Pregnancy

7.4.1 Corpus Luteum Cyst
(Figs. 7.37, 7.38, and 7.39)

Corpus luteum of pregnancy has a thick convoluted wall and a central cystic cavity filled with fluid or a coagulum composed of fibrin and blood. The term "cyst" applies when the corpus luteum is >3 cm [1]. The term "hemorrhagic" could also be applied if one wants to emphasize on its hemorrhagic content but is often omitted because most corpora lutea have a hemorrhagic content.

When the cavity is large typically in the first trimester, the wall becomes stretched.

Obliteration of the cavity usually begins by the fifth month of gestation and is typically completed by term [1].

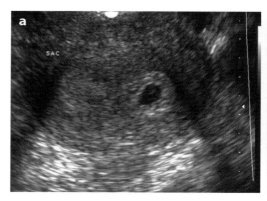 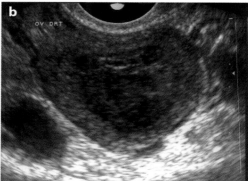 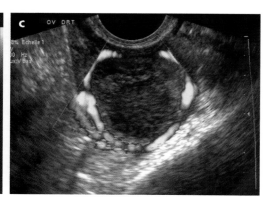

Fig. 7.37 Corpus luteum hemorrhagic cyst of first trimester of pregnancy. (a) Endovaginal view of the uterus showing an intrauterine gestational sac. (b) The right ovary contains a 32-mm corpus luteum cyst. (c) Endovaginal ultrasound with color Doppler better individualizes three different layers. A peripheral ring of intense vascularization in the theca, a middle echogenic layer without vascularization corresponding to the granulosa, and a less echogenic central portion containing blood or coagulum

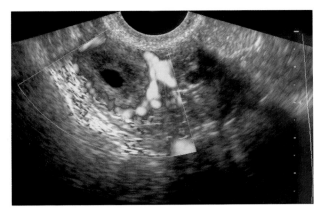

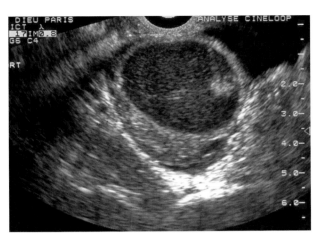

Fig. 7.38 Corpus luteum of first trimester of pregnancy. Endovaginal US with color Doppler of the right ovary shows a 28-mm right corpus luteum with three different layers. A peripheral ring of intense vascularization, a middle echogenic layer without vascularization, and an echo-free central portion. The term cyst is not applied because the lesion is <3 cm

Fig. 7.39 Corpus luteum hemorrhagic cyst of first trimester of pregnancy. Endovaginal US displays a 4.2-cm cyst less echogenic than the normal ovarian parenchyma containing a more echogenic focus corresponding probably to a clot

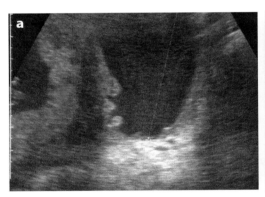
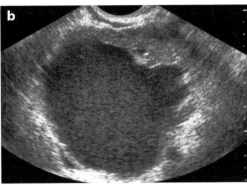
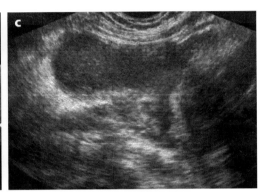

Fig. 7.40 Corpus luteum cyst of first trimester of pregnancy. (a) *Endovaginal US* displays an echogenic cystic mass of 50 mm of long axis of the left ovary with a convoluted inner border simulating endocystic vegetations and suggesting the possibility of an epithelial tumor. No color flow was detected in the protrusions. **(b)** *Endovaginal US 4 days later*: the cyst has slightly increased in size measuring 65 mm of long axis. The wall is now regular, confirming the absence of vegetations and strongly suggesting the diagnosis of a corpus luteum cyst. **(c)** Endovaginal US 17 days later: the cyst has significantly decreased in size. Although its long axis measures 55 mm, it appeared almost completely flattened definitely confirming its functional nature

7.4.2 Large Solitary Luteinized Follicle Cyst of Pregnancy (Fig. 7.40) and Puerperium

At macroscopy, the cyst resembles a typical follicle cyst except for its large size (median diameter 25 cm). On microscopic examination, it is lined by one to several layers of luteinized granulosa and theca cells that are usually indistinguishable [1]. The cells vary considerably in size and shape; focal marked nuclear pleomorphism and hyperchromasia are present. It is presumably related to hCG stimulation.

Theca lutein cysts classically occur when the hCG levels are abnormally increased. This occurs mainly in two situations: during pregnancy in the gestational trophoblastic disease and in the hyperstimulation syndrome (mainly after stimulation by FSH followed by hCG [22], more rarely in the hyperreactio luteinalis.

The theca lutein cyst is the largest of the physiologic ovarian cysts and is usually bilateral and multiple [23].

Approximately, 25–50 % of these cysts are associated with trophoblastic disease and usually disappear 2–4 months after resolution of the condition.

7.4.3 Hyperreactio Luteinalis (HL)

7.4.3.1 Definition

HL is characterized by bilateral ovarian enlargement caused by numerous follicle cysts with prominent luteinization of the theca interna cells and in some cases of the granulosa cells. These macroscopic and microscopic findings are identical to those of ovarian hyperstimulation syndrome, which is in fact an iatrogenic form of hyperreactio luteinalis.

7.4.3.2 Physiopathology

The condition is most commonly seen in association with disorders resulting in high levels of circulating hCG such as hydatidiform mole, choriocarcinoma, fetal hydrops, and multiple gestations [1].

Because HL rarely occurs in patients with otherwise normal pregnancies and normal hCG levels, the pathogenesis of the disorder is probably not related to high levels of hCG alone. Elevated levels of progesterone, prolactin, and estradiol have been found in patients with hyperreactio luteinalis and gestational trophoblastic disease.

7.4.3.3 Clinical Findings

HL may be detected during any trimester, at cesarian section, or rarely during the puerperium. The patients usually have pain, palpable adnexal masses, or both.

In approximately 15 % of cases unassociated with trophoblastic disease, there has been virilization of the patient but not the female infant, probably because the androgens produced by the cysts are aromatized to estrogens by the placenta.

HL typically regresses in the postpartum period but sometimes requires as long as 6 months. Exceptional cases regress spontaneously during pregnancy. In cases associated with trophoblastic disease, gradual regression occurs 2–12 weeks after uterine evacuation.

Because HL is self limited, operative intervention is needed only to control hemorrhage and reduce ovarian size in order to diminish androgen production in virilized patients.

7.4.3.4 Macroscopic and Radiological Findings

They are reported in Table 7.15.

7.4.3.5 Ultrasound (Figs. 7.41 and 7.42)

Bilateral enlargement, relatively symmetrical, is usually observed. Both ovaries contain multiple cysts measuring from some millimeters up to 3 cm that in fact are related histologically to follicles. These follicles are anechoic, but can be more or less echoic when

Table 7.15 Findings in hyperreactio luteinalis

Common findings
Thin-walled cysts
Bilateral enlargement
Clear or hemorrhagic fluid
Uncommon findings
Rupture or torsion

they contain a hemorrhagic fluid. The follicles occupy most of the ovaries with a peripheral distribution preserving only a little central echogenic part related at histology to the medullary portion. The surface of the ovary can be convoluted when the lesions are huge (>10 cm). Because of the apposition of both ovaries, it can be difficult on US examination to diagnose a bilateral lesion.

While the diagnosis can be suggested in an appropriate clinical setting, HL can be very difficult to diagnose in the cases of a normal pregnancy, especially when the lesion is huge [22].

7.4.3.6 MR (Fig. 7.41)

MR can be advocated when the lesions are huge (>10 cm) and when the complete study of the mass is more easy than with US. Moreover, in these cases, when the masses are bilateral, axial sections at the top of the masses or coronal sections better depict than US the separation of the masses.

7.4.3.7 Differential Diagnosis

The lesions can be very difficult to differentiate from a multilocular benign epithelial tumor such as serous or mucinous cystadenomas. Other multiloculated masses can also be discussed particularly endocrine tumors such as granulosa tumors or androgenic tumors as far as HL can be associated with virilizing findings.

7.4.4 Pregnancy Luteoma (PL)

PL is considerably uncommon.

PL is characterized by solid circumscribed nodules, composed of large luteinized cells, probably arising from stromal cells [1, 18]. They can be cystic [24] (Table 7.16).

PL most likely arises from hCG induced proliferations of luteinized ovarian stromal cells. However, the rarity of PL in association with trophoblastic diseases that are typically accompanied by high levels of hCG indicates that hCG is not the only factor of development. A preexisting endocrinopathy such as a hyperthecosis or a PCOS might predispose to the development of PL.

7.4.4.1 Clinical Findings

Most patients are asymptomatic.

Rarely a pelvic mass is discovered.

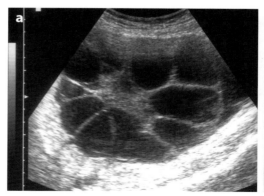
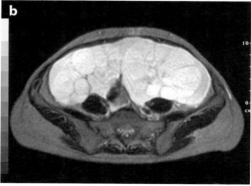

Fig. 7.41 Hyperreactio luteinalis in a pregnant woman with normal beta-hCG and a single fetus. (a) Ultrasound disclosed two enlarged ovaries with multiple large peripheral follicles. (b) T2W MR disclosed two large multiloculated masses occupying entirely the abdominopelvic cavity. Laparotomy and partial bilateral ovariectomy were performed. Pathology confirmed the diagnosis of hyperreactio luteinalis. Patients received progesterone; pregnancy follow-up and delivery were uneventful (Figures from Author's personal publication: Ghossain et al. [22])

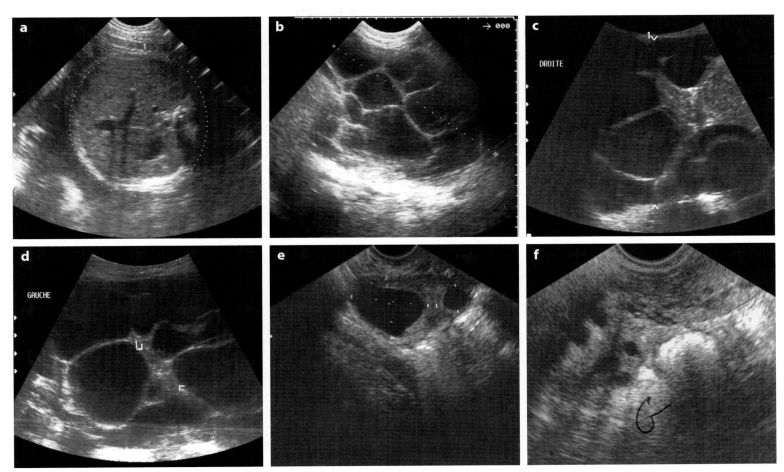

Fig. 7.42 Hyperreactio luteinalis in a normal pregnancy. *First ultrasound.* (**a**) Abdominal view of the fetus. (**b**) Multicystic ovarian mass of the right ovary composed of cysts with regular wall. (**c**) The central portion of the ovary which is echogenic seems to correspond to the medulla. (**d**) Left ovary: an identical multicystic mass with a central echogenic portion is also visualized. Three months later. (**e**) In the right ovary, the cysts have almost completely disappeared. (**f**) The left ovary is normal

Table 7.16 Macroscopic and radiologic findings of pregnancy luteoma

Bilateral (1/3 of cases)
Size (from microscopic to 20 cm, mean 6.6 cm)
Solid circumscribed nodules (may be cystic)
Multiple (1/2 of cases)
Hemorrhagic foci

In approximately 25 % of patients during the latter half of pregnancy, there is onset of virilization or exacerbation of hirsutism that was present before pregnancy. Two thirds of female infants born to virilized mothers also show virilization.

7.4.4.2 Ultrasound

In the two cases reported by Choi et al. [25], in one case, the mass was unilateral slightly hypoechoic compared to ovarian parenchyma, with small areas of hypoechogenicity and hyperechogenicity, while in the other case, the mass was bilateral with a uniformly echoic mass on one side and a mixed solid and cystic mass (related to necrosis at pathology) on the other side. In both cases, the solid portions were hypervascular on color Doppler.

7.4.4.3 MR

In a case reported by Wang et al. [24], MR in a pregnant asymptomatic woman at 27th gestational week showed bilateral multilocular cystic ovarian masses on T2WI hyperintense cystic content and hypointense thickened septa. Histological diagnosis was proved at cesarian section.

In another case reported by Kao et al. [26], US in a woman with virilization at third trimester of pregnancy showed enlarged heterogeneous ovaries. MR showed bilateral small solid nodules hypointense on T2WI, of intermediate intensity on T1WI, and of avid enhancement after gadolinium injection. Spontaneous regression of the masses was observed after delivery with normal ovaries 2 months postpartum. Virilization was present in the female newborn.

7.4.4.4 Differential Diagnosis

When multiple, metastases can be discussed [1].

When the nodule is unique, solid primary tumors composed partially or entirely of luteinized cells such as thecoma, granulosa cell tumor or steroid cell tumor can be discussed.

7.5 In Young Girls

Small ovarian follicles (≤9 mm) are common in normal premenarchal girls, sometimes exceeding 9 mm [27]. Multiple bilateral follicle cysts can be seen in juvenile hypothyroidism, prematurity, and 17 hydroxylase deficiency. In juvenile hypothyroidism, 75 % have multicystic ovaries [28].

Hypothyroidism is associated with sexual precocity related to the elevated estrogen levels, resulting from an increase secretion of pituitary gonadotrophin, and the galactorrhea due to mildly elevated levels of prolactin.

Prematurity: The cysts are associated with estradiol production. It is postulated that marked prematurity is associated with relative insensitivity of hypothalamus and interior pituitary to negative feedback by estradiol.

17-Hydroxylase deficiency: Congenital deficiency of 17-hydroxylase, an enzyme required for both cortisol and estrogen synthesis, results in low estrogen levels and secondary elevated levels of FSH and LH. Congenital adrenal hyperplasias, primary amenorrhea, and absence of sexual maturation are associated with bilateral ovarian enlargement.

Multiple cysts can be present in newborn infants due to maternal hormonal status.

7.6 Others

7.6.1 Hilus Leydig Cell Hyperplasia (HCH)

Definition: Leydig cells are mainly hilus cells typically intermingled with nonmyelinated nerves. Rarely they are located in the ovarian stroma. HCH is characterized by an increase in number and size of these cells in a nodular or less commonly diffuse arrangement. When the nodule is >1 cm, a hilus cell tumor is diagnosed.

Two types can be encountered:
- Mild HCH can occur as the result of elevated hCG (pregnancy) or LH (after menopause). Generally it is not accompanied by endocrinal disturbance except some degree of hirsutism during pregnancy.
- Severe HCH often associated with virilization and elevated serum testosterone level may occur in both pregnant and non-pregnant women.

HCH may be associated with stromal hyperplasia, stromal hyperthecosis, and stromal Leydig cell hyperplasia.

To our knowledge, no imaging documentation of this entity has been published.

References

1. Clement PB (2002) Nonneoplastic lesions of the ovary. In: Kurman RJ (ed) Blaustein's pathology of the female genital tract, 5th edn. Springer, New-York, pp 675–727
2. Outwater EK, Mitchell DG (1996) Normal ovaries and functional cysts: MR appearance. Radiology 198(2):397–402
3. Jain KA, Friedman DL, Pettinger TW, Alagappan R, Jeffrey RB Jr, Sommer FG (1993) Adnexal masses: comparison of specificity of endovaginal US and pelvic MR imaging. Radiology 186(3):697–704
4. Jain KA (1994) Prospective evaluation of adnexal masses with endovaginal gray-scale and duplex and color Doppler US: correlation with pathologic findings. Radiology 191(1):63–67
5. Okai T, Kobayashi K, Ryo E, Kagawa H, Kozuma S, Taketani Y (1994) Transvaginal sonographic appearance of hemorrhagic functional ovarian cysts and their spontaneous regression. Int J Gynaecol Obstet 44(1):47–52
6. Jain KA (2002) Sonographic spectrum of hemorrhagic ovarian cysts. J Ultrasound Med 21(8):879–886
7. Reynolds T, Hill MC, Glassman LM (1986) Sonography of hemorrhagic ovarian cysts. J Clin Ultrasound 14(6):449–453
8. Baltarowich OH, Kurtz AB, Pasto ME, Rifkin MD, Needleman L, Goldberg BB (1987) The spectrum of sonographic findings in hemorrhagic ovarian cysts. AJR Am J Roentgenol 148(5):901–905
9. Buy JN, Ghossain MA, Hugol D, Hassen K, Sciot C, Truc JB, Poitout P, Vadrot D (1996) Characterization of adnexal masses: combination of color Doppler and conventional sonography compared with spectral Doppler analysis alone and conventional sonography alone. AJR Am J Roentgenol 166(2):385–393
10. Togashi K, Nishimura K, Kimura I, Tsuda Y, Yamashita K, Shibata T, Nakano Y, Konishi I, Konishi J, Mori T (1991) Endometrial cysts: diagnosis with MR imaging. Radiology 180(1):73–78
11. Buy JN, Ghossain MA, Mark AS, Deligne L, Hugol D, Truc JB, Poitout P, Vadrot D (1992) Focal hyperdense areas in endometriomas: a characteristic finding on CT. AJR Am J Roentgenol 159(4):769–771
12. Pache TD, Wladimiroff JW, Hop WC, Fauser BC (1992) How to discriminate between normal and polycystic ovaries: transvaginal US study. Radiology 183(2):421–423
13. Yen SSC (1996) Contemporary overview. In: Adashi EY (ed) Reproductive endocrinology, surgery, and technology. Lippincott-Raven, Philadelphia, pp 1117–1126
14. Hughesdon PE (1982) Morphology and morphogenesis of the Stein-Leventhal ovary and of so-called "hyperthecosis". Obstet Gynecol Surv 37(2):59–77
15. Yeh HC, Futterweit W, Thornton JC (1987) Polycystic ovarian disease: US features in 104 patients. Radiology 163(1):111–116
16. Mitchell DG, Gefter WB, Spritzer CE, Blasco L, Nulson J, Livolsi V, Axel L, Arger PH, Kressel HY (1986) Polycystic ovaries: MR imaging. Radiology 160(2):425–429
17. Young RH, Scully RE (1984) Fibromatosis and massive edema of the ovary, possibly related entities: a report of 14 cases of fibromatosis and 11 cases of massive edema. Int J Gynecol Pathol 3(2):153–178
18. Scully RE, Young RH, Clement PB (1998) Tumor-like lesions. In: Rosai J, Sobin LH (eds) Tumors of the ovary, maldeveloped gonads, fallopian tube, and broad ligament, vol 23. Armed Forces Institute of Pathology, Washington, pp 409–450
19. Bazot M, Salem C, Cortez A, Antoine JM, Darai E (2003) Imaging of ovarian fibromatosis. AJR Am J Roentgenol 180(5):1288–1290
20. Nagamani M (1996) Polycystic ovary syndrome variants: hyperthecosis. In: Adashi EY (ed) Reproductive endocrinology, surgery, and technology. Lippincott-Raven, Philadelphia, pp 1257–1269
21. Rousset P, Gompel A, Christin-Maitre S, Pugeat M, Hugol D, Ghossain MA, Buy JN (2008) Ovarian hyperthecosis on grayscale and color Doppler ultrasound. Ultrasound Obstet Gynecol 32(5):694–699
22. Ghossain MA, Buy JN, Ruiz A, Jacob D, Sciot C, Hugol D, Vadrot D (1998) Hyperreactio luteinalis in a normal pregnancy: sonographic and MRI findings. J Magn Reson Imaging 8(6):1203–1206
23. Sutton CL, McKinney CD, Jones JE, Gay SB (1992) Ovarian masses revisited: radiologic and pathologic correlation. Radiographics 12(5):853–877
24. Wang HK, Sheu MH, Guo WY, Hong CH, Chang CY (2003) Magnetic resonance imaging of pregnancy luteoma. J Comput Assist Tomogr 27(2):155–157
25. Choi JR, Levine D, Finberg H (2000) Luteoma of pregnancy: sonographic findings in two cases. J Ultrasound Med 19(12):877–881
26. Kao HW, Wu CJ, Chung KT, Wang SR, Chen CY (2005) MR imaging of pregnancy luteoma: a case report and correlation with the clinical features. Korean J Radiol 6(1):44–46
27. Cohen HL, Eisenberg P, Mandel F, Haller JO (1992) Ovarian cysts are common in premenarchal girls: a sonographic study of 101 children 2–12 years old. AJR Am J Roentgenol 159(1):89–91
28. Riddlesberger MM Jr, Kuhn JP, Munschauer RW (1981) The association of juvenile hypothyroidism and cystic ovaries. Radiology 139(1):77–80

29. Kanso HN, Hachem K, Aoun NJ, Haddad-Zebouni S, Klein-Tomb L, Atallah D, Buy JN, Ghossain MA (2006) Variable MR findings in ovarian functional hemorrhagic cysts. J Magn Reson Imaging 24(2):356–61

30. Chereau A (1844) Mémoires pour servir à l'étude des maladies des ovaires. Paris: Fortin, Masson, Cie

31. Robert Y, Dubrulle F, Gaillandre L, Ardaens Y, Thomas-Desrousseaux P, Lemaitre L, Dewailly D (1995) Ultrasound assessment of ovarian stroma hypertrophy in hyperandrogenism and ovulation disorders: visual analysis versus computerized quantification. Fertil Steril 64:307–312

32. Goldzieher JW (1981) Polycystic ovarian disease. Fertil Steril 35(4):371–94

33. Adashi EY, Rocks JA, Rosenwaks Z (eds) (1996) Reproductive endocrinology, surgery, and Technology (Vol 1). Lippincot-Raven Pubishers, Philadelphia, NY

Ovarian Infertility

8

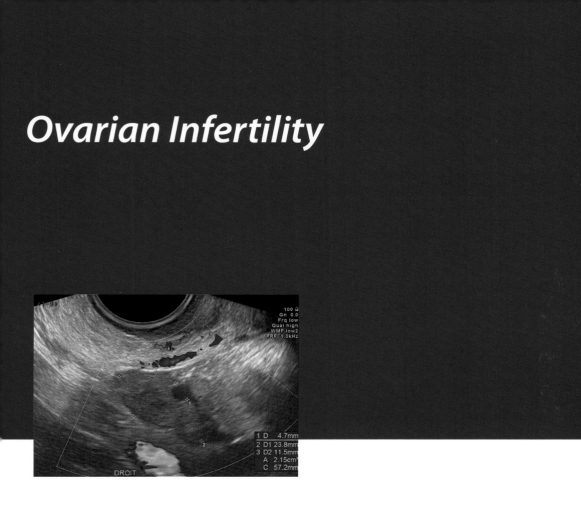

Contents

Infertility is defined as 12 months or more of unprotected intercourse without pregnancy. It is primary when there is no previous pregnancy. It is secondary when fertility problems occur in a couple that has conceived on their own and had a child in the past. A standard infertility evaluation is made with a series of test [1] which are reported in Table 8.1.

Female infertility after 35 years old increases with age. The most common causes are ovulation problem, followed by tubal problems (previous PID, previous tubal pregnancy). More uncommonly it may be related to abnormal function of the hypothalamic-hypophyseal axis, to adrenal dysfunction, to metabolic disease, and to multiple pelvic disorders which can involve the different compounds of the Muller duct and the secondary Mullerian system. Moreover, in some of these entities like in PCOD, different factors can be associated. In some cases, the cause of infertility is unexplained.

Etiological diagnosis of infertility is mainly based on clinical and biological findings. However, imaging modalities, particularly ultrasound, occupy an important place in the detection and characterization of a pathologic process of the pelvic organs. This modality is also particularly appropriate to evaluate the ovarian function. MR can provide additional informations in the evaluation of infertility.

Ovarian infertility is related to three different causes: ovulation disorders which may be related to ovarian or to hypothalamic and

Table 8.1 Diagnostic evaluation of infertility

1. Male factor (semen analysis)
2. Ovulatory and luteal function (serum progesterone)
3. Cervical factor (postcoital test (PCT))
4. Uterine factor (HSG and/or hysteroscopy, ultrasound)
5. Tubal factor (HSG and coelioscopy)
6. Endometriosis or other pelvic pathology (coelioscopy)

J.N. Buy, M. Ghossain, *Gynecological Imaging*,
DOI 10.1007/978-3-642-31012-6_8, © Springer-Verlag Berlin Heidelberg 2013

hypophyseal dysfunction or endocrine disorders, endometriosis in which the factors responsible for sterility are multiple, and periovarian adhesions. When ovarian infertility is suspected, the first step in the work-up is to evaluate the ovarian reserve.

8.1 Evaluation of Ovarian Reserve

8.1.1 Work-Up for Infertility

Evaluation of ovarian reserve is part of every work-up for infertility. It is made at day 3 of the menstrual cycle and comprises day-three blood test and an antral follicle count with endovaginal sonography (Table 8.2).

Table 8.2 Ovarian reserve screening tests

Biological findings at day 3
FSH (normal <10 mIU/ml)
Estradiol (E2) (normal 25–75 pg/ml)
AMH[a] (normal between 1 and 3 ng/ml)
US findings at day 3: antral follicle count (AFC) (between 2 and 8 mm)

[a]AMH anti-Mullerian hormone is a substance produced by the granulosa cells first in primary follicles. It is highest in preantral and antral follicles <4 mm diameter

8.1.2 Biological Findings

FSH >10 mIU/ml or normal FSH associated with an elevated estradiol level indicates a reduced ovarian reserve. A level >20 is usually correlated with a very poor response to stimulation. However, a significant number of woman with normal FSH have a reduced egg supply.

AMH blood level is thought to reflect the size of the remaining egg supply or ovarian reserve. A low level <1 ng/ml expresses a decrease of this reserve. With increasing female age, the size of their pool of remaining microscopic follicle decreases. Likewise their blood AMH levels and the number of ovarian antral follicles visible on ultrasound decrease. Women with many small follicles such as PCOD have high AMH, and women who have few remaining follicles have low levels of AMH. However, AMH levels do not reflect egg quality.

8.1.3 Basal Antral Follicle Count

The basal antral follicle count test is a transvaginal ultrasound test that measures a woman's ovarian reserve, or her remaining egg supply. The ovarian reserve reflects her fertility potential.

The basal antral follicle count, along with the woman's age and cycle day 3 blood work levels, is considered one of the best indicators

Table 8.3 Antral follicle count

<4	Extremely low count	Very poor response to stimulation
4–6	Low count	Poor response to stimulation drug
7–10	Reduced count	Higher than average rate of IVF cancelation
11–15	Intermediate count Good count	Response to stimulation usually adequate
16–30	Normal antral count	Excellent response to stimulate
>30	High count	Risk of overstimulation

for estimating ovarian reserve and the woman's chance for pregnancy with in vitro fertilization. The antral follicles are a good predictor of the number of mature (dominant) follicles in woman's ovaries that can be stimulated by medications leading up to IVF.

The results of basal antral follicle count and correlation with response to stimulation are reported in Table 8.3.

8.2 Causes of Ovarian Infertility

8.2.1 Ovulation Disorders

There are two main types of ovulation disorders: anovulation and dysovulation.

In anovulation corpus luteum is absent. In dysovulation, ovulation is irregular; the presence of corpus luteum is possible.

These ovulation disorders typically result in oligomenorrhea, or even amenorrhea, or dysfunctional uterine bleeding. These abnormalities can be ovarian in origin, secondary to abnormalities of the hypothalamus and/or hypophysis, or both.

8.2.1.1 Functional Abnormalities

PCOD

PCOD Fig. 8.1 (different factors arising from the ovary, the hypothalamo-hypophyseal axis and metabolic disease, are responsible for PCOD) (see Chap. 7)
It is a very common cause of anovulation, or oligoovulation and infertility.

While in the typical cases morphologic findings of PCOD can be very suggestive, in most of the cases, the diagnosis is based on an association of clinical, biological, and imaging findings.

LUF Syndrome [2]

Definition: A relatively mature follicle receives just enough LH to cause progesterone production, but not enough to cause egg release by the follicle.

It is a very uncommon cause.

Fig. 8.1 Bilateral PCOD. Twenty-nine-year-old woman; oligomenorrhea, hirsutism. In the plasma, androstenedione level was increased. EVS of the right (**a**) and left (**b**) ovaries depict: (1) A bilateral enlargement of ovaries which have a surface of 9 and 9.5 cm2, respectively. They contain about 30 antral follicles measuring from 2 to 8 mm. Some of them have a thickened wall related to luteinization of their wall (*arrow* in **b**). (2) No dominant follicle is visualized. (3) In the right ovary, stroma looks hyperechogenic (**a**). These findings associated to the clinical and biological findings allow to make the diagnosis of PCOD

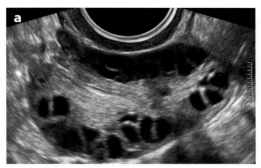
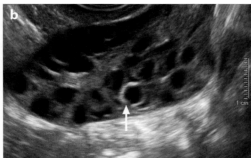

8.2.1.2 Primary Ovarian Insufficiency (POI)

This syndrome is also called premature ovarian failure (POF); however, primary ovarian insufficiency is preferred over premature ovarian failure because this last term implies a totally menopause situation.

In primary ovarian insufficiency, the ovary fails to respond to appropriate gonadotropin stimulation provided by the hypothalamus and the pituitary.

POI is often preceded by a period of variable duration of impaired ovarian reserve with shortening of menstrual cycle, followed by oligomenorrhea, vasomotor symptoms which may

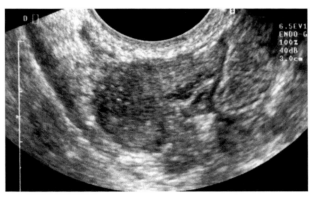

Fig. 8.2 Ovarian Insufficiency. Thirty-year-old woman with disseminated erythematous lupus, secondary infertility, antiphospholipid antibodies. Evs (**a**): the right ovary has a small size with a thin cortex without any follicle. Left ovary was normal

appear long before menstrual irregularity [3]. During this period, women retain ovarian function, and despite lower fecundability, pregnancy may occur.

Table 8.4 Primary ovarian insufficiency

Clinical and biological findings
Women younger than 40 years
Amenorrhea
Low level estrogens
High FSH level
Low AMH level
Ultrasound
Low antral follicle count

Table 8.5 Primary ovarian insufficiency etiology

1. Genetic causes
1.1. Gonadal dysgenesis
Turner's syndrome
46XX gonadal dysgenesis
46XY gonadal dysgenesis
1.2. X-fragile syndrome (caused by premutation of the FMR1 gene)
1.3. Other genetic causes
2. Autoimmune disease (associated polyendocrinopathy)
3. Infection (viral oophoritis)
4. Iatrogenic (chemotherapy, radiotherapy, surgery, embolization)
5. SORG (syndrome ovary resistant to gonadotrophs)

Definition

Primary ovarian insufficiency (POI) is a condition diagnosed on the following features (Table 8.4).

Etiology

The different ovarian etiologies are reported in Table 8.5.

An example of abnormal ovary is illustrated in autoimmune disease (Fig. 8.2).

On EVS, in case of premature menopause, the ovaries can look smaller compare to the usual size for age, with few or with no follicle (Figs. 8.3 and 8.4).

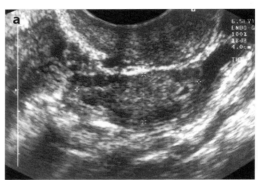

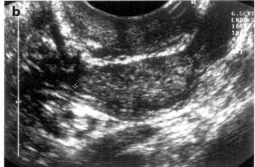

Fig. 8.3 Thirty-year-old woman with irregular menstrual cycles, infertility, AMH <1 ng/ml. Familial history of premature menopause. EVS of the right (**a**) and the left (**b**) ovaries depict ovaries of small size without any ovarian follicle

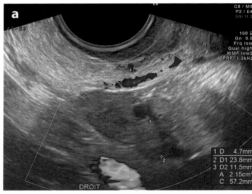

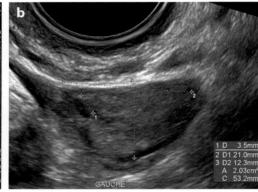

Fig. 8.4 Primary ovarian Insufficiency. Forty-year-old woman, Infertility, FSH 15 mUI/ml. AMH 0.70 ng/ml. EVS depicts bilateral small ovaries; surface of the right one (**a**) is 2.15 cm^2 and of the left one (**b**) is 2 cm^2. Only one antral follicle is visualized in both ovaries

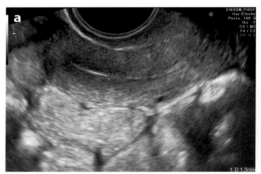

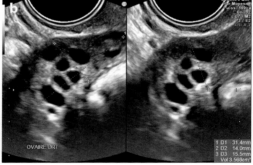

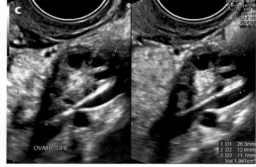

Fig. 8.5 Functional hypothalamic insufficiency. Thirty-nine-year-old woman. Secondary amenorrhea, anorexia nervosa, and weight loss. Longitudinal EVS (**a**) displays an overall small uterus with an atrophic endometrium. EVS of the right (**b**) and left (**c**) ovaries depicts normal size ovaries, with a normal follicle count

8.2.1.3 Hypothalamo-Hypophyseal Causes of Anovulation-Dysovulation

Hyperprolactinemia

Prolactin is secreted by the pituitary gland. The hypothalamic control of prolactin secretion is primarily inhibitory. The hypothalamic factor that inhibits prolactin secretion is the neurotransmitter the dopamine. The prolactin releasing factor (PRF) secreted by the hypothalamus stimulates the production of prolactin. Thyroid releasing factor (TRF) can also have this effect.

Effects of prolactin on the ovary:

1. Hyperprolactinemia suppresses LH pulsatile secretion.
2. Perfusion studies of human varies in vitro reveal a direct suppressive effect of the PRL on progesterone and estrogen secretion [4].

3. The prolactin can inhibit estrogen formation by antagonizing the stimulatory effects of FSH on aromatase activity (which allows conversion of androstenedione in estrone) and by direct inhibition of aromatase synthesis [5].
4. *Both ACTH and PRL stimulate adrenal androgen secretion.*

The common causes of hyperprolactinemia are reported in Table 8.6.

In the ovary, the prolactin binds with the membrane of the cell of the internal theca and induces a hypersecretion of androgens.

Functional Hypothalamic Amenorrhea (Fig. 8.5)

The pattern of multifollicular encountered in PCOD is not specific and must be distinguished from the multifollicular ovary (MFO)

Table 8.6 Common causes of hyperprolactinemia

1. Pituitary tumors Prolactinomas Other macroadenomas (hyperprolactinemia results in this case from deprivation of dopamine inhibition) **2. Hypothyroidism**, inducing an increased TRH resulting in increased TSH and prolactin **3. Ingestion of certain drugs** including phenothiazines, alpha-methyldopa, certain tranquilizers, and oral contraceptives

Table 8.7 Multifollicular ovaries (MFO)

1. Particular profile 2. Absence of clinical and biological findings of hyperandrogenism 3. Ovaries of normal shape and of normal or slightly enlarged size Follicles (≥6) of different sizes from 4 to 10 mm in diameter Normal stroma 4. Small uterus with atrophic endometrium (related to estrogen deficiency) 5. Disappearance of the abnormalities after correction of the functional disorders or treatment with LHRH

related to hypothalamic insufficiency. In this case, the profile is particular (anorexia nervosa, excess of physical training, drugs). The main findings of MOF [6] are reported in Table 8.7.

Organic Causes of Hypogonadotropic Hypogonadisms

Hypophyseal Adenoma

MR can be helpful to detect an adenoma and to evaluate its extension.

Genetic Hypothalamic Dysfunction

This syndrome called Kallmann's syndrome associates hypogonadic hypogonadism with anosmia. Abnormalities in various genes have been shown to disrupt the ability of the hypothalamus to produce gonadotrophin releasing hormone (GnRH) which in turn causes the pituitary to fail to release sufficient levels of follicle-stimulating hormone (FSH) and luteinizing hormone (LH). LH and FSH have a direct action on the ovaries.

8.2.1.4 Other Causes of Anovulation-Dysovulation

Hypothyroidism

Thyroid disease may cause:

Anovulation and irregular menstruations, LPD, Hyperprolactinemia.

8.2.2 Another Functional Disorder, but Not Related to Anovulation: Luteal Phase Defect (LPD)

Definition: LPD was described by Jones [7] as a defect in corpus luteum production of progesterone or in endometrial response to progesterone stimulation.

The luteal phase is <11 days.

In many of these cases, the egg is fertilized by sperm, so that the conception takes place.

However, the conceptus is unable to implant and is lost during menstruation.

8.2.3 Endometriosis

Multiple factors, ovarian, tubal, peritoneal, and subperitoneal, can be responsible for infertility.

In the ovary, the main factors of infertility are anovulation, LPD, and LUFS.

8.2.4 Periovarian Adhesions

Pelvic adhesions mainly develop after surgery, pelvic inflammatory disease, and endometriosis. These adhesions can be located between the ovary and the peritoneum particularly the ovarian fossa, or between the ovary and the neighboring ligaments or organs.

Although diagnosis of adhesions can be highly suggested in some cases on the different imaging modalities, this diagnosis can be very difficult to perform.

When extensive, these adhesions may be a cause of infertility. However, when these adhesions are associated with other lesions in the pelvis (like hydrosalpinx), it can be difficult or even impossible to ascertain that adhesions are the main cause of infertility.

References

1. Guzick DS (1996) Human infertility: an introduction. In: Adashi EY, Rock JA, Rosenwaks Z (eds) Reproductive endocrinology, surgery, and technology. Lippincott, Philadelphia, pp 1897–1913, Chap 101
2. Koninckx PR, De Moor P, Brossens A (1980) Diagnosis of the luteinized unruptured follicle syndrome by steroid hormone assays on peritoneal fluid. Br J Obstet Gynaecol 87:929–934
3. Nelson LM, Anasti JN, Flack MR (1996) Human infertility: an introduction. In: Adashi's reproductive endocrinology, surgery, and technology. Lippincott, Philadelphia, pp 1393–1410, Chap 71
4. Mc Natty KP (1979) Relationship between plasma prolactin and the endocrine microenvironment of the developing human antral follicle. Fertil Steril 32:433–438
5. Krasnow JS, Hickey GJ, Richards JS (1990) Regulation of aromatase mRNA and estradiol biosynthesis in rat ovarian granulose and luteal cells by prolactin. Mol Endocrinol 4:13–21
6. Adams J, Franks S, Polson DW et al (1985) Multifollicular ovaries: clinical and endocrine features and response to pulsatile gonadotropin releasing hormone. Lancet 21–28:1375–1379
7. Jones GS (1949) Some newer aspects of management of infertility. JAMA 141:1123

Surface Epithelial-Stromal Tumors of the Ovary

9

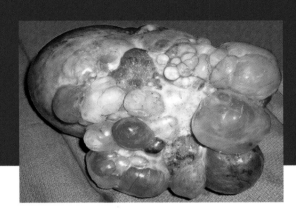

Contents

J.N. Buy, M. Ghossain, *Gynecological Imaging*,
DOI 10.1007/978-3-642-31012-6_9, © Springer-Verlag Berlin Heidelberg 2013

9.1 Introduction

Surface epithelial-stromal tumors of the ovary account for 50–55 % of all ovarian tumors and their malignant forms for approximately 90 % of all ovarian cancer [1].

9.1.1 Definitions

These tumors are so designated because most of them are considered to be derived from the surface epithelium of the ovary and the adjacent ovarian stroma or from surface epithelial inclusions lying in the ovarian cortex [1, 2].

9.1.1.1 Surface Epithelium of the Ovary

It is a simple focally pseudostratified layer.

The cells vary from flat to cuboidal to columnar, and several types may be seen in different areas of the same ovary.

The cells are separated from the stroma by a basement membrane.

9.1.1.2 Superficial Epithelium Inclusion (SEI) Glands

They arise from cortical invaginations of the surface epithelium and have lost their connection with the surface [1]. They are lined by a single layer of columnar cells which may be ciliated, mimicking tubal (endosalpingeal) epithelium. Less frequently, SEI glands are lined by other Mullerian cell types (endometrioid, mucinous) or by nonspecific columnar or flattened cells [3, 4].

9.1.1.3 Stroma

The spindle-shaped stromal cells, which have scanty cytoplasm, are typically arranged in whorls or a storiform pattern.

Stroma cells are separated by a dense reticulin network and a variable amount of collagen.

9.1.2 General Histologic Features

The surface epithelial-stromal tumors of the ovary present two components: an epithelial component and a stromal component.

On the other hand, all these tumors can be benign, borderline (atypical proliferative), or malignant (carcinomas).

9.1.2.1 The Epithelial and Stromal Components

Epithelial Component

According to the epithelial cell type, there are three major types depending on whether the epithelium is serous mimicking the fallopian tube epithelium, mucinous mimicking the endocervical epithelium or the intestinal epithelium, or endometrioid recapitulating the endometrial lining [5]. More rare types are Brenner tumors which are characterized by an epithelium of urothelial type [1] and clear cell tumors which are characterized by abundant cytoplasmic glycogen [1] and exceptionally squamous cell tumors.

Beside these six types, they are undifferentiated epithelial tumors and mixed epithelial tumors [6]. Since most of the tumors in the surface-epithelial category have a similar origin, it is not surprising that admixtures of the various subtypes often occur [1]. According to the WHO, mixed epithelial tumors are those in which different tumor types are recognizable on gross examination, and those in which one or more components other than the predominant component account for at least 10 % of the tumor on microscopic examination.

Stromal Component

Stroma is present in variable amounts in all the subtypes. When the stroma occupies an area greater than that of the cysts and their contents, the suffix fibroma is added to the diagnostic designation, for example, serous adenofibroma [1]. However, a lot of pathologists use the suffix fibroma as soon as the stromal component is macroscopically evident.

9.1.2.2 Benign, Borderline (Atypical Proliferative), or Malignant (Carcinomas)

Benign Tumors

They consist of a unstratified epithelial proliferation with morphology close to the normal epithelial type, without any invasion of the basement membrane.

Borderline or Atypical Proliferative Tumors

The authors of the WHO classification defined a borderline tumor as:
1. "One that has some, but not all of the morphologic features of malignancy."
   This include in varying combinations:
   - Stratification of epithelial cells
   - Apparent detachment of cellular clusters from their sites of origin
   - Mitotic and nuclear abnormalities intermediate between those of clearly benign and unquestionably malignant tumors of a similar cell type
2. "On the other hand, obvious invasion of the adjacent stroma is lacking."

They also indicated that the histologic diagnosis must be based exclusively on an examination of the ovarian tumor without consideration of whether spread beyond the ovary has taken place.
   However:
- Tumors without stromal invasion with clear-cut malignant nuclear features should be regarded as *intraepithelial carcinoma* irrespective of whether stromal invasion is identified [7].
- Conversely, borderline tumors may show *microinvasion*. The more common type is characterized by isolated cells with abundant eosinophilic cytoplasm that appear budding from the epithelium into the superficial stromal cores of the papillae. Less commonly, the lesion is characterized by a haphazard infiltrative pattern of small nests of cells forming micropapillae, often surrounded by a clear space and associated with an identifiable stromal response. Occasionally, the nests display a cribriform pattern.
   In either case, the invasion is limited in extent and should occupy a total area of no more than 10 mm^2 with no single focus exceeding 3 mm.

For mucinous lesions, the differential diagnosis of borderline and invasive mucinous tumors is more difficult than that of the serous type:

- Extensive sampling is especially critical since the most atypical degree of epithelial proliferation may be localized to a small portion of the tumor.
- Because these tumors (most often of intestinal type, more rarely of endocervical type) often contain small glands and cysts surrounded by stroma. It may be difficult or even impossible to determine in some cases whether the location of these structures reflects an innocuous intrusion of tumor cells into the stroma or aggressive invasion [1].

Malignant Tumors (Carcinomas)

Except for the intraepithelial carcinomas, in all the different types of carcinoma, the cellular proliferation invades the underlying stroma and induces stroma reaction [5] which have three main components:

- Stromal proliferative reaction referred as desmoplasia
- Inflammatory reaction
- Angiogenesis, that is, new formation of endothelial type vessels induced by a tumor angiogenesis factor (TAF) produced by neoplastic cells

Angiogenesis plays an important role in the diagnosis. The ovarian carcinomas have been shown to have higher microvessel density (MVD) than benign ovarian neoplasms [8–10], but some authors have found no difference in MVD in borderline tumors versus carcinomas [11]. This angiogenesis is responsible for an increase in size and number of small vessels with an increase in size of the feeding vessels. These vessels are very particular to malignant tumors [12] and therefore are one of the clues in the diagnosis of carcinomas on the different imaging modalities.

A particular form is micropapillary serous carcinoma (MPSC) [13, 14]. It is a well-differentiated serous carcinoma usually purely intraepithelial [15]. The architecture is different from a borderline tumor. The distal papillary branches are thin and delicate and emanate abruptly from thick more centrally located papillae without intervening branches of successive intermediate size, unlike the hierarchical branching pattern of borderline tumors.

- Cytologic features are different from a usual carcinoma. There is mild to moderate nuclear atypia unlike a conventional carcinoma.
- In some cases, invasion has been reported. Because micropapillary and cribriform pattern may be focally present in borderline, an area of 5 mm in diameter of a confluent micropapillary pattern is required for the designation of MPSC.
- The neoplastic cells have direct access to the peritoneal cavity and may exfoliate and implant on peritoneal surfaces accounting for the strong association with invasive implants.

General Considerations for Benign, Malignant, and Borderline Tumors

For a cellular type, there is a continuum in the macroscopic aspect between benign borderline and malignant tumors. Papillary projections are present in benign serous, borderline, and carcinomas. Most of mucinous tumors (benign, borderline, and malignant) are multiloculated cystic masses.

Some macroscopic characteristics, and their corresponding radiologic aspects, can be observed on the different imaging modalities. The benign tumors (serous cystadenoma, mucinous cystadenoma) are mainly or exclusively cystic with the exception of the uncommon Brenner tumor that is solid and looks like an ovarian fibroma. The borderline tumors are mainly cystic but contain a high proportion of papillary projections. The carcinomas may be mainly cystic, mixed, or mainly solid.

Preoperative diagnosis of benign versus borderline and malignant tumor of the ovary is one of the major problems encountered in ovarian tumors. The surgical approach (laparoscopy versus laparotomy) and the surgical treatment are completely different according to the nature and extension of the tumor [16, 17].

Cystectomy or ovariectomy is performed in most benign tumors.

Adnexectomy is performed in most borderline tumors and carcinomas stage I, particularly in young women, followed or not by chemotherapy [18] *stage 1*.

Bilateral adnexectomy with total hysterectomy and omentectomy is performed in carcinomas, eventually associated with lymphadenectomy and more extensive histologic specimens, followed or not by chemotherapy [18] *stage 1*.

9.1.3 Frequency and Classification

The frequency of surface epithelial-stromal tumors versus total ovarian tumors is reported in Fig. 9.1 [1, 19].

Classification of these tumors according to WHO is reported in Table 9.1. The most common tumors encountered in clinical practice are reported in Table 9.2.

The frequency of epithelial surface stromal tumors related to histologic type is reported in Table 9.3 [15].

The age-specific incidence of ovarian epithelial cancer rises precipitously from approximately 20–80 years [20]. The chance that a primary ovarian epithelial tumor is borderline or malignant in a patient under the age of 40 years is approximately 1 in 10; beyond that age, it rises to 1 in 3.

9.1.4 Risk Factors

Worldwide, ovarian cancer is the sixth most common cancer in women [21] and the most common cause of death from gynecologic cancer [21]. The lifetime risk for ovarian cancer in the general population is 1.3 %.

9.1.4.1 Familial and Hereditary Carcinoma of the Ovary

Approximately 7 % of women with ovarian epithelial cancer have one or more relatives with the disease (familial ovarian cancer) [1]. These women are estimated to have a risk for the development of ovarian cancer over three times that of women without a family history.

One to three percent of ovarian cancer patients have a germ-line genetic abnormality that greatly increases their risk of development of ovarian cancer (hereditary ovarian cancer) [22].

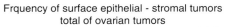

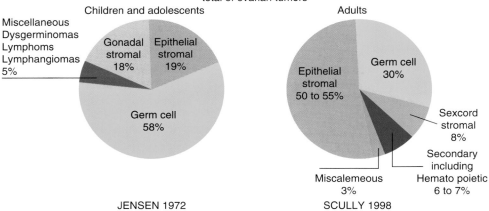

Fig. 9.1 Frequency of surface epithelial-stromal tumors total of ovarian tumors

Table 9.1 World Health Organization histological classification of surface epithelial-stromal tumors

1 Serous tumors
1.1 Benign
  1.1.1 Cystadenoma and papillary cystadenoma
  1.1.2 Surface papilloma
  1.1.3 Adenofibroma and cystadenofibroma
1.2 Of borderline malignancy (of low malignant potential)
  1.2.1 Cystic tumor and papillary cystic tumor
  1.2.2 Surface papillary tumor
  1.2.3 Adenofibroma and cystadenofibroma
1.3 Malignant
  1.3.1 Adenocarcinoma, papillary adenocarcinoma, and papillary cystadenocarcinoma
  1.3.2 Surface papillary adenocarcinoma
  1.3.3 Adenocarcinofibroma and cystadenocarcinofibroma (malignant adenofibroma and cystadenofibroma)
2 Mucinous tumors, endocervical-like, and intestinal types
2.1 Benign
  2.1.1 Cystadenoma
  2.1.2 Adenofibroma and cystadenofibroma
2.2 Of borderline malignancy (of low malignant potential)
  2.1.1 Cystic tumor
  2.1.2 Adenofibroma and cystadenofibroma
2.2 Malignant
  2.2.1 Adenocarcinoma and cystadenocarcinoma
  2.2.2 Adenocarcinofibroma and cystadenocarcinofibroma (malignant adenofibroma and cystadenofibroma)
3 Endometrioid tumors
3.1 Benign
  3.1.1 Cystadenoma
  3.1.2 Cystadenoma with squamous differentiation
  3.1.3 Adenofibroma and cystadenofibroma
  3.1.4 Adenofibroma and cystadenofibroma with squamous differentiation
3.2 Of borderline malignancy (of low malignant potential)
  3.2.1 Cystic tumor
  3.2.2 Cystic tumor with squamous differentiation
  3.2.3 Adenofibroma and cystadenofibroma
  3.2.4 Adenofibroma and cystadenofibroma with squamous differentiation
3.3 Malignant
  3.3.1 Adenocarcinoma and cystadenocarcinoma
  3.3.2 Adenocarcinoma and cystadenocarcinoma with squamous differentiation
  3.3.3 Adenocarcinofibroma and cystadenofibroma with squamous differentiation (malignant adenofibroma and cystadenofibroma with squamous differentiation)
  3.3.4 Adenocarcinofibroma and cystadenocarcinofibroma with squamous differentiation (malignant adenofibroma and cystadenofibroma with squamous differentiation)

Table 9.1 (continued)

3.4 Epithelial-stromal and stromal
  3.4.1 Adenosarcoma, homologous, and heterologous
  3.4.2 Mesodermal (Mullerian) mixed tumor (carcinosarcoma), homologous, and heterologous
  3.4.3 Stromal sarcoma
4 Clear cell tumors
4.1 Benign
  4.1.1 Cystadenoma
  4.1.2 Adenofibroma and cystadenofibroma
4.2 Of borderline malignancy (of low malignant potential)
  4.2.1 Cystic tumor
  4.2.2 Adenofibroma and cystadenofibroma
4.3 Malignant
  4.3.1 Adenocarcinoma
  4.3.2 Adenocarcinofibroma and cystadenocarcinofibroma (malignant adenofibroma and cystadenofibroma)
5 Transitional cell tumors
5.1 Brenner tumor
5.2 Brenner tumor of borderline malignancy (proliferating)
5.3 Malignant Brenner tumor
5.4 Transitional cell carcinoma (non-Brenner type)
6 Squamous cell tumors
7 Mixed epithelial tumors (specify types)
7.1 Benign
7.2 Of borderline malignancy (of low malignant potential)
7.3 Malignant
8 Undifferentiated carcinoma

Table 9.2 Simplified histological classification

Benign
  ▪ Serous cystadenoma (or cystadenofibroma)
  ▪ Mucinous cystadenoma (or cystadenofibroma)
  ▪ Brenner tumor
Borderline
  ▪ Serous borderline
  ▪ Mucinous borderline
Malignant
  ▪ Serous (including papillary carcinoma)
  ▪ Mucinous
  ▪ Endometrioid
    – Adenocarcinoma
    – Mesodermal mixed tumors
  ▪ Clear cell
  ▪ Urothelial (Brenner)
  ▪ Mixed (composite)
  ▪ Poorly or undifferentiated

Table 9.3 Approximate distribution of surface epithelial tumors (% of all ovarian surface epithelial tumors) and among them (% of benign, borderline and carcinomas in each cellular type) according to Seidman [14]

	Benign (%)	Borderline (%)	Carcinoma (%)	Total (%)
Serous	31	5	17	53
Mucinous	23	4	4	31
Endometrioid	–	0.5	6	6
Clear cell	–	0.2	2.4	3
Transitional	3	–	–	3
Undifferentiated	–	–	2	2
Mixed	0.5	0.1	2	2
Total	57	10	33	100

Hereditary predisposition to ovarian cancer:

(a) Cell cycle regulation:

The cell cycle is tightly regulated by a large number of genes and their respective proteins in a complex interrelated series of events. Neoplastic cells manifest deregulated growth, division, and senescence by a variety of mechanisms [15].

- Proto-oncogenes are normal cellular growth control genes that when mutated, amplified, or overexpressed, facilitate malignant behavior and are then designated oncogenes. Oncogenes exert their growth-promoting effects through several pathways that often include growth factors and their cell-surface receptors. Oncogenes that have been studied extensively in ovarian cancer include C-erbB-2 (HER2/neu), C-erbB-1 (EGFR), C-myc, and K-ras.

- Tumor suppressor genes normally inhibit all growth through a variety of growth regulatory pathways and when mutated lose this inhibitory effect, thus promoting cell growth. Important suppressor genes in ovarian cancer include p53, BRCA1, and BRCA2. Mutation of the p53 tumor suppressor gene located on the short arm of chromosome 17 is observed in approximately 50–60 % of ovarian cancers.

(b) There are three hereditary syndromes that predispose to ovarian cancer:

- The breast-ovarian cancer syndrome [23], is caused by mutations in the tumor suppressor gene BRCA1 and BRCA2. Both BRCA1 and BRCA2 are transmitted in an autosomal dominant fashion. The gene is in chromosome 17 at locus 21. Approximately 10 % of women with ovarian cancer and 7 % of breast cancer cases [24] are carriers of breast/ovarian cancer susceptibility gene. The lifetime risk for ovarian cancer in the general population is 1.3 %, whereas estimates for gene carriers range from 10 to 60 % [25]. The proportion of cases of ovarian cancer resulting from such a gene decreases with age.

- Lynch syndrome II [26, 27] is a subtype of hereditary nonpolyposis colon cancer, in which cancer may appear in the colon most often right-sided [28] ovary, endometrium, and occasionally other organs with variable degrees of frequency [29]. The relative risk of ovarian cancer in these families is 3.5 %.

- Site-specific ovarian cancer [30] is the least common of the three hereditary cancer syndromes, characterized by an increased risk of ovarian cancer. Most families with the syndrome are linked to mutation in the BRCA1 gene.

Clinicopathologic features of familial ovarian cancers versus sporadic ovarian cancers:

- Age: younger [24]
- Stage: similar

- Pathology: essentially papillary serous carcinomas
- Prognosis (for BRCA-associated familial cases): better

9.1.4.2 Putative Histopathologic Precursor Lesions

Endometriosis is the best documented precursor of ovarian carcinoma. Approximately 6 % of all ovarian carcinomas are associated with endometriosis [15] mainly endometrioid and clear cell carcinoma.

9.1.5 Detection, Clinical Findings, and Physical Examination

Ovarian carcinoma often is called the silent killer because usually the disease is not detected until an advanced stage [31].

(a) Over one fourth of patients with ovarian tumors are asymptomatic [32]. The ovarian mass is discovered during a routine pelvic examination, better associated with an EVS examination.

(b) The most common initial manifestations are unspecific:

- Abdominal pain or discomfort, abdominal swelling, a feeling of pressure in the pelvis
- Urinary symptoms and mainly a feeling of pressure on the bladder or a pseudocystitis may wrongly orient the diagnosis to a urinary problem
- Gastrointestinal symptoms, mainly with modification of the feces habit, with diarrhea or constipation can wrongly be misdiagnosed as a colitis and delay the diagnosis
- In occasional cases, abnormal vaginal bleeding, particularly if the tumor is malignant or associated with a luteinization of the stroma (Table 9.4)

(c) Unfortunately, carcinoma of the ovary can be discovered at a late stage with ascites or even with pleural effusion (mostly the right side).

(d) Complications are rare: torsion, rupture, hemorrhage, infection.

(e) Occasionally, paraendocrine and paraneoplastic manifestations are the first symptoms (Table 9.4).

Physical examination is of little value at the very beginning at least when the tumor is of a small size.

Table 9.4 Endocrine, paraendocrine, paraneoplastic, and other syndromes

- **Unusual endocrine and paraendocrine syndromes**
  Chorionic gonadotropin production (B, Bo, M)
  Hypercalcemia (M)
  Cushing's syndrome (M)
  Zollinger-Ellison syndrome (mucinous: B, Bo, & M)
- **Paraneoplastic syndromes**
  Subacute cerebellar degeneration (M)
  Dermatomyositis polymyositis (M)
  Rheumatoid-like polyarthritis and palmar fasciitis
  Autoimmune hemolytic anemia
  Disseminated intravascular coagulation (M)
- **Heritable and other congenital syndromes**
  Peutz-Jeghers syndrome (mucinous: B, Bo, & M)
- **Other syndromes**
  Meigs' syndrome (Brenner)
  Pseudo-Meigs (M primary or secondary)

B benign, *Bo* borderline, *M* malignant

Table 9.5 Characterization of tumors with papillary projections [36]

	Benign	Borderline	Malignant
Papillary projections			
Topography	Endocystic Exocystic (exceptional) Localized Disseminated (uncommon)	Endocystic Exocystic (70%) Localized Disseminated	Endocystic Exocystic (less common) Localized Disseminated
Size	Unique or small group <5 mm	Around 1 cm	>2 cm
Morphologic findings	– Round or mushroom – Short base of implantation – Regular surface – Homogeneous – Macrocalcification	– Sessile – Broad base of implantation – Irregular surface	– Sessile – Broad base of implantation – Irregular surface – Degenerative changes – Hemorrhage and necrosis on the surface
Associated findings			
Cystic content	Serous fluid	Nonserous fluid Detachment of cells in the fluid	
Normal ovarian parenchyma **Irregular solid tissue**	Visualized Absent	Visualized Absent	Not Visualized Present

9.2   Principles of Imaging Characterization

Preoperative characterization of ovarian tumor is of utmost importance as much as frozen sections have major limitations. If this procedure is accurate enough to exclude the presence of a benign pathology [33], a diagnosis of borderline can be made solely on frozen sections with a sensitivity of 64 % in serous and 31 % in mucinous [34].

Pathologic diagnosis is as much difficult as the volume of the mass is important [35]. Also, sensitivity of frozen section was only of 81 % in early stage ovarian cancer [34].

Preoperative characterization is rarely suggested on the clinical findings, except in cases of extension outside the ovary.

The diagnosis of benignity versus borderline and carcinoma is based on four different types of findings:
1. Uni- or bilaterality
2. Macroscopic and imaging findings
3. Vascular findings
4. Extension

In some cases, with EVS and color Doppler, these findings are highly suggestive of benign, borderline, or malignant tumor. They can be even suggestive of a specific type of epithelial tumor. In other cases, CT or MR will improve this characterization. In other cases, the diagnosis is difficult or even impossible to suggest on the different imaging modalities. Particularly in these difficult cases, association with the results of the tumor markers is very useful.

9.2.1   Uni- or Bilaterality

Benign tumors are most commonly unilateral.

Borderline tumors are bilateral in roughly one-third of serous tumors while mucinous tumors are almost always unilateral.

Serous and undifferentiated carcinomas are commonly bilateral while mucinous, endometrioid, and clear cell carcinomas are most commonly unilateral.

Table 9.6 Characterization of an ovarian epithelial tumor with a solid component

	Benign	Borderline	Malignant
Morphologic characters of the solid component	– Homogeneous – Regular contour	Absent	– Degenerative changes – Necrosis – Hemorrhage – Irregular contour

Ovarian metastases can have a pattern very similar to a primary ovarian carcinoma and are bilateral in 70–80 % of cases. Except the cases of serous and undifferentiated carcinoma, this criterion of bilaterality can be helpful to orient the diagnosis.

9.2.2   Macroscopic and Imaging Findings

At macroscopy, in benign, borderline, and malignant tumors, four main structures can be studied: papillary projections, solid components, septa, and wall.

9.2.2.1 Papillary Projection

Papillary projection (sometimes called vegetation) is defined as a tissue proliferation contiguous with the inner wall (endocystic) or rarely with the outer wall (exocystic). They can be also present on septa. The epithelial proliferation is contiguous with the epithelial cell type of the wall. The papillary projections have a vascular axis that is more or less perpendicular to the wall so that size of the vessels tapers progressively toward the surface of the papillary projections (Table 9.5).

9.2.2.2 Solid Component

Solid component is defined as a portion of tissue which is adjacent to the cystic portions or which contains a cystic portion. This solid tissue has no vascular axis; the vessels are irregularly distributed at the periphery and in the central portion. Their morphologic features are displayed in Table 9.6.

9.2.2.3 The Septa

Table 9.7 Characterization of multiloculated epithelial tumor

	Benign	Borderline and malignant
Morphologic characters of septa	Thin and regular Few	Thick and irregular Numerous and gathered

9.2.2.4 The Wall

Table 9.8 Characterization of the wall of the tumor

	Benign	Borderline and malignant
Morphologic characters of the wall	Thin <3 mm Regular	**Thick >3 mm Irregular**

9.2.2.5 Macroscopic Findings Related to Histological Types

Some macroscopic findings of carcinoma can be related to the histological type (Table 9.9).

Table 9.9 Macroscopic findings of carcinoma related to the histological type

	Cystic with vegetation	Cystic with tissular portion	Mixed or mainly solid	Multilocular
Serous	+++	+	+	+
Mucinous	+	+	+	+++
Endometrioid	++	++	++	+
Clear cell	+++	+++	+	+

Cystic: more than two-thirds of the mass is cystic
Mainly solid: more than two-thirds of the mass is tissular
+ uncommon, +++ common

Although it is difficult on the basis of macroscopic findings to relate them to a specific histologic type, some macroscopic presentations are more common and more suggestive of one or some histological types.

(a) The cystic form with vegetation is the most common form of serous carcinoma [37]. However, this macroscopic presentation can be also observed in clear cell carcinoma [38] and other types.

(b) The cystic form with tissular portion is the usual form of presentation of endometrioid carcinoma [39] but can also be seen in serous carcinoma. A unilocular cyst with one or more nodules protruding into the lumen is a typical appearance of a clear cell carcinoma [40].

(c) The predominantly multiloculated cystic form, which can be associated with a small tissular portion or vegetation [38], is the usual form of presentation of mucinous carcinomas.

(d) The mainly solid tumors cannot be related to a specific type.

(e) Focal or diffuse calcific deposits related to psammoma bodies suggest a serous cystadenocarcinoma [41, 42]. They are present in approximately 30 % of serous carcinoma [43].

(f) Recognizable small foci of endometriosis or an endometriotic cyst may be present within an endometrioid carcinoma [41].

(g) Surface papillary carcinoma: A serous tumor may be entirely exophytic, but most often, the underlying ovary is focally replaced by neoplastic tissue. It may appear as plaques or polypoid excrescences occupying part of the external surface of the ovary [41].

9.2.3 Vascular Findings

Vasculogenesis and tumor neovascularization are responsible for the production of new capillaries in the stroma of the tumor. These capillary vessels are responsible for abnormal development of arterial and venous vessels that are displayed on the different imaging modalities.

9.2.3.1 On Doppler

Based on a standard technique [44], ultrasound combined with color Doppler has been proven to be a valuable tool to characterize epithelial tumors (Table 9.10).

In papillary projection >1 cm, vessels are displayed in carcinoma mainly at the base and in some borderline tumors while they are absent in benign tumors.

In papillary projection <1 cm, vessels are not displayed even in the case of carcinoma.

Table 9.10 Vascular findings

	Benign	Borderline	Malignant
Ultrasound Color Doppler			
Papillary projections >1 cm	Absent	Present	Present
Papillary projections <1 cm	Absent	Absent	Absent
Solid tissue	Few regular vessels		Prominent irregular vessels
Spectral Doppler Resistivity index			<0.4 (high specificity, low sensitivity)
DCT & DMR Arterial vessels	Absent		Present with specific morphologic features
Venous phase	Slight uptake	Moderate uptake	High uptake
Hemorrhage and necrosis	Absent		Present
Time-intensity curve	Slow and low contrast uptake	Intermediate findings	Rapid and high contrast uptake with sometimes washout

In a solid component, vessels can be large and prominent in carcinomas while vascularization is poor and made up of tiny vessels in benign tumors.

Considering spectral Doppler analysis, a resistivity index <0.4 is highly specific of malignant tumors if corpus luteum cyst is excluded; however, sensitivity is low [44].

9.2.3.2 Dynamic CT (DCT) and Dynamic MR (DMR)

1. At the arterial phase, characters of the vessels in solid portions are fundamental for the diagnosis.

   In malignant tumors, vessels are clearly depicted. They are thin and tortuous without any origin and without a well-defined end. On the next phase, they disappear in some areas of the tumor and appeared in other territories owing to different velocities according to the different characters of the stroma of the tumors (Table 9.11) [45].

Table 9.11 Tumoral vessels in a malignant solid component: morphologic findings and hemodynamic features

At the arterial phase
– They are visualized
– They are thin and tortuous
– Without an origin and a well-defined end
– Disappear in some areas of the tumor on the next step and appear in other territories owing to different velocities according to the different characters of the tumor
At the venous phase
– A significant contrast uptake is present
At the late phase
– Some washout can be displayed

In benign tumors, vessels are usually not depicted. Exceptionally, few thin regular vessels can be displayed.

In borderline tumors, characters of the vessels are intermediate between benign and carcinoma [44]. Usually, tiny vessels can be demonstrated. However, in mucinous tumors, because of the architecture of the tumor, these vessels are not demonstrated in most tumors.

2. At the venous phase and on the following sequences, contrast uptake in the interstitial space precisely evaluated with time-intensity curve is displayed.

   In malignant tumors, a significant contrast uptake is usually displayed at an early phase, which usually slightly increases on the following phases.

   In benign tumors, contrast uptake at the early phase is very low and only slightly increases on the following sequences.

   In borderline tumors, contrast uptake (when it can be measured in solid portion or papillary projections) is usually intermediate between carcinoma and benign tumors, which allows in most of cases to distinguish a carcinoma from a borderline tumor [45].

9.2.4 Extension

Different types of extension are possible:
- Pelvic extension
- Peritoneal extension
- Lymph nodes
- Metastases

9.2.4.1 Extensions Related to Histological Types

Some pattern can be related to the histological type.
(a) Serous carcinoma gives rise early to peritoneal metastases with rarely calcified deposits (psammoma bodies) that are specific for this type of tumor.
(b) Mucinous carcinomas, even when reaching a large size, stay for a long time confined to the ovary (Stage I).
(c) Endometrioid carcinoma is the most common tumor which is associated with endometrial carcinoma (20–30 % of cases) [46]. When carcinoma of the ovary and the uterus is associated, endometrioid carcinoma represents 50–60 % of cases [47, 48].
(d) Association of slightly enlarged ovaries or ovaries of macroscopic normal aspect with carcinomatosis is mainly observed in undifferentiated ovarian carcinoma.

9.3 Serous Tumors

9.3.1 Benign Serous Cystadenoma

9.3.1.1 General Features

They are the most common epithelial tumors and represent 31 % benign, 5 % borderline, and 17 % malignant of all epithelial tumors (Table 9.3).

They are most common in the reproductive age group although not uncommon in perimenopausal women [49].

They are usually inferior to 10 cm. Bilaterality is present in 12–23 % of cases [50].

Tumoral markers CA 125 and CA 19-9 are normal.

9.3.1.2 Pathology [49, 50]

Macroscopy

Different forms may be present (Table 9.12).
(a) *The unilocular form* (the majority) [51] (Fig. 9.2) with:
   - Thin regular wall
   - Watery fluid content, occasionally more stringy mucinous material and exceptionally hemorrhagic [52]
(b) *The multilocular form with thin regular septa.*
(c) *The cystic form with papillary projections.*
   The lining of the cyst may have coarse papillary projections; such papillary projections rarely cover the entire surface of the

Table 9.12 Macroscopical forms of serous benign tumors

Cystic unilocular
Cystic multilocular
Cystic with papillary projections
Cystic with solid tissue (cystadenofibroma)
Cystic with solid tissue and papillary projections
Serous surface papillary adenofibromas

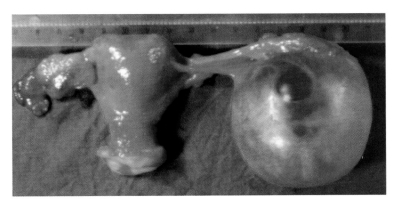

Fig. 9.2 Unilocular serous cystadenoma. Unilocular ovarian cyst with a thin regular wall

cyst (Fig. 9.3). Occasionally small papillary excrescences may be found on the surface of the cyst [49, 50].

(d) *The cystic form with solid tissue (cystadenofibroma):*
The solid tissue may have degenerative cystic changes and macrocalcifications.
It is very suggestive of benignity when:
- Its limits are regular.
- It looks homogeneous.

Degenerative changes (edema, calcification) are possible, but hemorrhage and necrosis are usually absent.

Serous adenofibromas and cystadenofibromas are typically hard predominantly solid fibromatous tumors that contain glands or cysts filled with clear fluid. The cysts linings may bear polypoids excrescences, and their presence in combination with the hard consistency of the stromal component may lead to an erroneous gross impression of carcinoma, particularly when the tumors are bilateral in postmenopausal women [49].

(e) *Papillary projections (Fig. 9.3) and solid tissue can be associated.*

(f) *Serous surface papillary adenofibromas* appear as warty excrescences, which are usually limited in extent, but may be widespread on the outer surface of one or both ovaries.

Microscopy

The Epithelium

There is a broad spectrum of epithelial proliferation that is manifested by variation in the prominence and complexity of the papillae, from a simple, single layer and blunt papillae to focal stratification and detachment of cell clusters approaching the degree of proliferation seen in borderline tumors. Identification of these features in 10 % of the histologic material is the boundary between benign and borderline tumors, but this is an equal and arbitrary and artificial division in an otherwise smooth morphologic continuum.

Cystadenomas are generally lined by a single layer of flattened to cuboidal cells with uniform basal nuclei. The epithelial cells can be pseudostratified and tubal type (Fig. 9.3) with the characteristic elongated (secretory cell) or rounded (ciliated cell) nuclei. In large cysts, the epithelium often becomes attenuated.

Although the cells produce mucin that is secreted into the cystic spaces, they do not contain the basophilic cytoplasmic vacuoles characteristic of mucinous neoplasms.

The Stroma

The stroma is dense and fibrous [49] (Fig. 9.4). Edema is sometimes present. When the stroma is highly cellular and fibrous, the tumor can be designated as an adenofibroma.

Psammoma bodies (sand in Greek) can be present in the stroma. They are round to oval calcifications with concentric laminations measuring 5–100 μm in diameter, thought to be secondary to intracellular accumulations of hydroxyapatite – $Ca_{10} (PO_4) 6(OH)_2$ – in cells that undergo dystrophic calcification related to cellular degeneration [53–56]. Large extracellular psammoma bodies result from fused calcified bodies that have been extruded from calcified cell [57].

They are present in the stroma in 15 % of cystadenomas [50], but they can be encountered in other etiologies (Table 9.13).

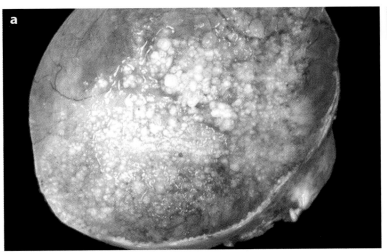
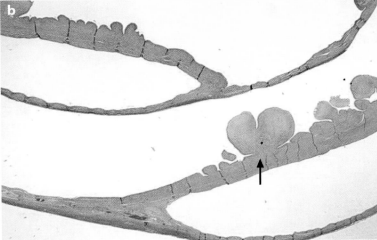

Fig. 9.3 (a) **Macroscopic specimen: multiple small papillary projections.** (b) Microscopy: papillary projections are of small size, with a regular surface, forming acute angles with the wall of the cyst; this pattern is very suggestive of their benign nature

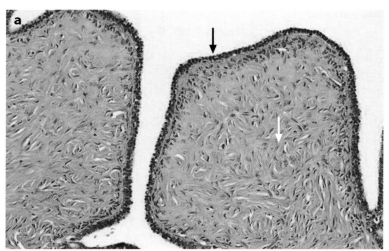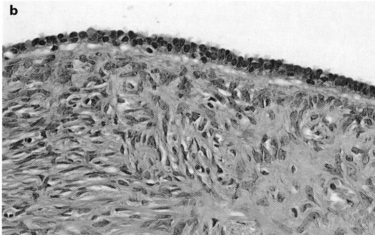

Fig. 9.4 Microscopy (**a** and **b**) (at a higher magnification): two layers of serous type cells are present (*black arrow* in **a**). Under the basal lamina, the stroma is dense and fibrous (*black arrow* in **b**). These findings are typical for benign serous cystadenoma

Table 9.13 Etiology of psammoma bodies

Serous ovarian tumors	
– Benign	15 %
– Borderline	50 %
– Carcinoma	25 %
Surface epithelial inclusion (SEI) glands or cysts	
Within lumen or adjacent stroma	
Endosalpingiosis	
Benign glands lined by tubal-type epithelium involving the peritoneum	
Carcinoma of the endometrium	
Serous or clear cell	
Chronic salpingitis	

Table 9.14 Macroscopic and common imaging findings of cystadenoma

– Bilateral (12–23 %)
– Cystic uni- or multilocular
– Watery fluid (mucinous fluid uncommon)
– Endocystic papillary projections (exocystic uncommon)
    * Localized (<50 % of the surface)
    * Size (2–23 mm; mean 9 mm)
    * Short base, acute angle with the wall, regular surface
– Thin and regular wall and septa
– Psammoma bodies in the stroma in 15 % of cases
– Solid tissue usually absent
– Normal ovarian parenchyma pushed toward the periphery

9.3.1.3 Imaging Findings

Macroscopic and Common Imaging Findings

Macroscopic and common imaging findings on US CT MR are summarized in Table 9.14.

Unilocular Purely Cystic Form

Ultrasound is the modality of choice to display a purely cystic form.

The cysts are usually round with a thin regular wall [58] or no visible wall, anechoic or slightly echogenic, with a good sound transmission [59] (Fig. 9.5). During the reproductive age year, when the cyst is <8 cm in diameter and the differential diagnosis with a functional cyst is not possible, a control with US after the next period is necessary.

Conversely, a cyst inferior to 3 cm must not be necessarily considered as a functional cyst (Fig. 9.6).

Rarely, content of the cyst is echogenic related to hemorrhage and can simulate a functional hemorrhagic cyst (Fig. 9.7).

During perimenopause and after menopause, surface epithelium inclusion (SEI) cysts may be visible on gross inspection of the ovary, although most of them are appreciable only on microscopic

examination; SEI cysts greater than 1 cm in diameter are designated cystadenomas [60].

SEI glands and cysts are usually multiple scattered singly or in small clusters throughout the superficial cortex, less commonly extend into the deeper cortical or medullar stroma. They are typically lined by a single layer of columnar cells. Psammoma bodies may be present within the glands, the cysts, or the adjacent stroma.

While the diagnosis of benignity of purely cystic mass is almost certain, the diagnosis of location of the nature of the mass ovarian (functional or tumoral) or its location (ovarian or extraovarian) is one of the most common problems encountered in gynecological practice (Table 9.15).

Multilocular Cystic Form

More rarely, serous cystadenoma is multilocular. Usually, the wall is thin and regular. The septa are usually thin (<3 mm) and regular, and not numerous. The loculi contain anechoic (Fig. 9.8) or echoic liquids. These findings are highly suggestive of a benign mass.

In this case, differential diagnosis is only discussed with other benign multilocular cystic masses, mainly with mucinous cystadenoma, more rarely with endometriosis and peritoneal pseudocyst (Table 9.23 in mucinous tumor).

Fig. 9.5 A TES: the cyst is unilocular anechoic with a thin regular wall without papillary projection. It measures 6 cm in its long axis. *Laparotomy* with left adnexectomy was performed. *Pathology*: serous cystadenoma

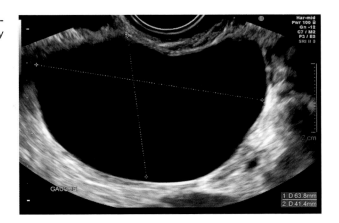

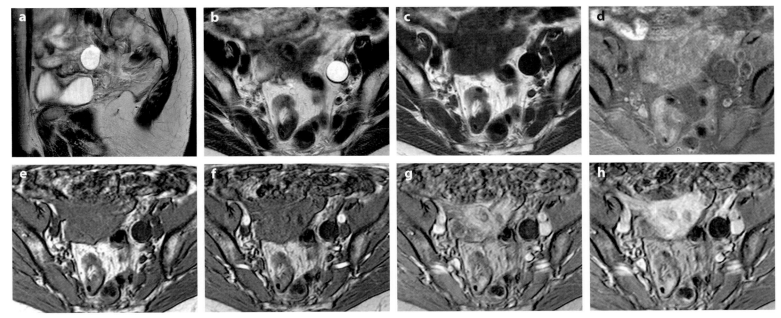

Fig. 9.6 MR with sagittal (**a**), axial T2 (**b**), axial T1 (**c**), and fat suppression (**d**) display a unilocular left ovarian cystic mass with a thin regular wall with a high signal intensity on T2, a signal intensity as urine on T1 and fat suppression typical for serous fluid. DMR without injection (**e**) at the arterial phase (**f**), at the venous phase (**g**), and on the delayed (**h**) does not demonstrate any abnormal contrast uptake in the wall of the cyst. The benign character of the mass is obvious. However, a functional ovarian cyst must be discussed. Follow-up did not demonstrate disappearance of the cyst. At pathology, an ovarian cystadenoma was diagnosed

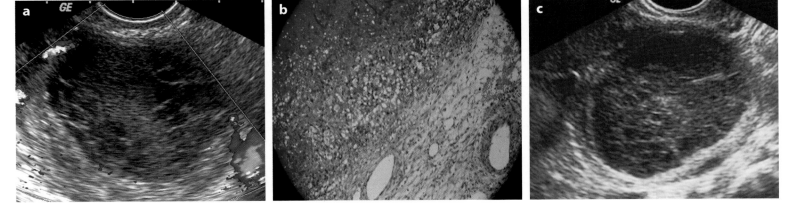

Fig. 9.7 *Serous cystadenoma* EVS (**a**) Mixed echogenic mass with a fishnet appearance without any vessel on color Doppler confirming its cystic nature; the pattern suggested the possibility of a FHC. Because of the persistence of the mass, a celioscopy was performed with resection of the cyst. At histology (**b**), the epithelium of the cyst is abrased but still recognizable. At pathology: serous cystadenoma. *Functional hemorrhagic cyst* EVS (**c**) Ovarian cystic mass with an identical fishnet appearance typical for a FHC.

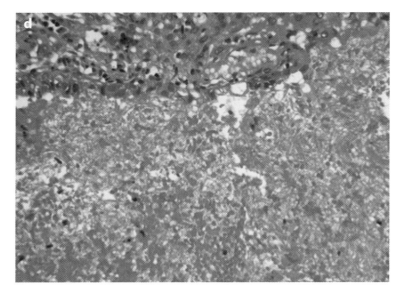

Fig. 9.7 (*continued*) At histology (**d**), the diagnosis of FHC was confirmed; the cyst is lined by granular cells

Table 9.15 Differential diagnosis of purely unilocular ovarian cystic masses

Common
Serous cystadenoma
Functional ovarian cyst
Cumulus oophorus
Regression or disappearance after the next periods or sometimes after prescription of a birth control
Hydrosalpinx
Tubular shape, tubal folds, and plicae
Paraovarian cyst
When in contact with the ovarian parenchyma, differential diagnosis may be difficult or even impossible
Uncommon
Mucinous cystadenoma
Rarely unilocular
Peritoneal inclusion cyst
Rarely unilocular, usually not round and encompasses to adjacent organs
Mature cystic teratoma
In the pediatric age where the unilocular cystic form is frequent
Granulosa cell tumor
Exceptionally unilocular (juvenile and adult)
Tarlov cyst

On conventional US, when the echogenic loculi are difficult to identify as cystic or tissular, absence of color flow on color Doppler classifies these echogenic portions as cystic or related to poorly vascularized benign connective tissue and rules out the possibility of malignant tissue. However, color flow could not be detected in papillary projection <1 cm even if malignant (Table 9.10).

MR and CT in Cystic Forms

In purely cystic forms, MR and CT are unnecessary. However, in some situations (virgin and obese patient, voluminous tumor), MR or CT in case of contraindication to MR can be performed.

In the unilocular form, signal intensity of the cystic content on the different sequences on MR and density on CT is usually close to urine (Fig. 9.9). In the multilocular form, usually the different loculi have the same signal intensities (Fig. 9.10).

Sometimes, the hemorrhagic content can be depicted on T1W images [61] (Fig. 9.11); this hemorrhagic content can have a fluid level. Simple cysts may have intermediate signal on T1W image that may reflect high protein content.

Cystic Form with Papillary Projections

The presence of papillary projections at pathology most often identifies the mass as an ovarian surface epithelial-stromal neoplasm [62]. However, papillary projections may also be encountered in very uncommon other tumors (Table 9.16).

Papillary projections were present in 66 % of cases of cystadenomas in our series [59]. Detection of papillary projections in a cystic mass always requires surgery [62].

While macroscopic detection and characterization of exocystic papillary projections is easily performed during laparoscopy or laparotomy, an attempt to characterize preoperatively endocystic locations by US is fundamental especially in young women. This will determine the technical approach and the type of surgery (cystectomy vs. more aggressive surgery).

Ultrasound of Papillary Projection

Papillary projections appear as an echogenic structures, round, finger-like shape or with a mushroom appearance, unique or multiple, well separated from each other, or gathered as a small group. They lie most often on the inner wall, more rarely on septa, uncommonly on the outer wall in case of benign tumor [49].

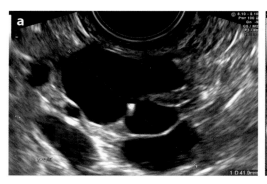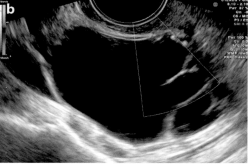

Fig. 9.8 Multilocular serous cystadenoma. Sixty-three-year-old woman without hormonal replacement. At a routine examination, an ovarian mass was discovered. EVS (**a**) and with color Doppler (**b**) display a multilocular cystic ovarian mass with thin and regular wall and septa without any papillary projection. A prospective diagnosis of benign epithelial and stroma ovarian mass more likely related to a serous cystadenoma rather a mucinous one was made

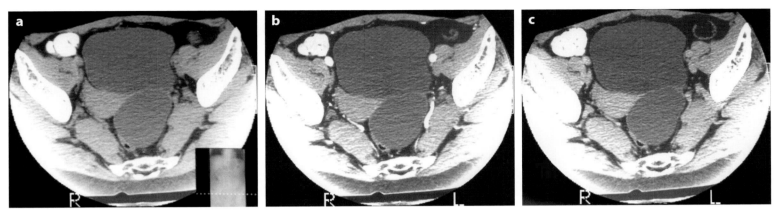

Fig. 9.9 Serous cystadenoma on CT. Forty-year-old woman. DCT without injection (**a**), at the arterial phase (**b**), at the venous phase(**c**): Left ovarian unilocular cyst with a regular wall, without any papillary projection; content of the cyst is close to urine. No abnormal vessel is shown at the arterial phase, and no abnormal contrast uptake is visualized at the venous phase. Prospective diagnosis: benign ovarian cyst; during reproductive age year, two main diagnoses must be suggested: serous cystadenoma and functional cyst. A control with US is necessary after the next period; final diagnosis: serous cystadenoma

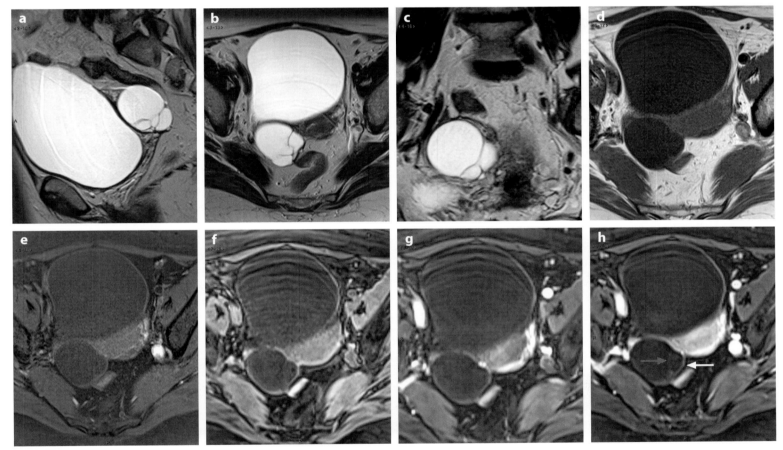

Fig. 9.10 Multilocular serous cystadenoma. MR sagittal T2 (**a**), axial T2 (**b**), and coronal T2 (**c**) display multilocular cystic mass which is roughly round in the three different planes, which allows to rule out a hydrosalpinx. On these previous sequences and on axial T1 (**d**), content of the cyst has a signal intensity close to urine on the different sequences. DMR with fat suppression without injection (**e**), at the arterial phase (**f**), at the venous phase (**g**), and on the delayed (**h**) display a low and progressive contrast enhancement in the wall (*white arrow*) and the septa (*red arrow*). Prospective diagnosis: serous cystadenoma which was confirmed at pathology

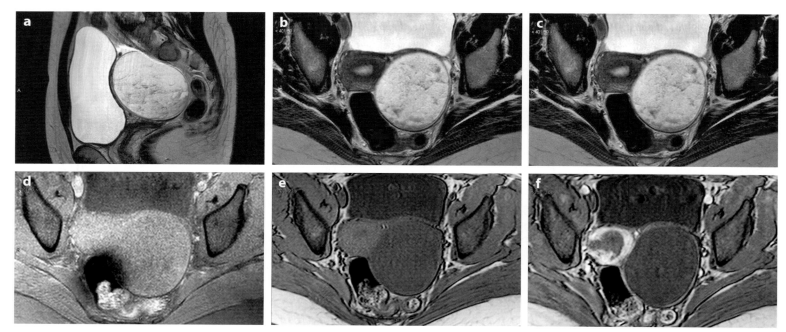

Fig. 9.11 Hemorrhagic serous cystadenoma. MR sagittal T2 (**a**), axial T2 (**b**), axial T1 (**c**), and fat suppression (**d**) display a left ovarian mass slightly heterogeneous with a signal close to adipose tissue on T1 an intermediate signal on fat suppression and a high signal on T2. DMR without injection (**e**) at the arterial phase (**f**), at the venous phase (**g**), and on the delayed (**h**) one confirms the cystic nature of the mass, with a ring sign at the arterial phase, which is only a finding of an ovarian mass. Prospective diagnosis: a functional hemorrhagic cyst was suggested; a control of the mass after the next period was proposed. In fact, the patient was operated in the following days. At pathology, a serous cystadenoma with a hemorrhagic content was diagnosed

Table 9.16 Etiology of papillary projections at pathology

| **Epithelial ovarian tumors** |
| – Benign |
| – Borderline |
| – Malignant |
| **Non-epithelial ovarian tumors** |
| – Germinal cell tumors (embryonal carcinoma, yolk sac tumor) |
| – Sex cord stroma cell tumor (retiform pattern of Sertoli-Leydig cell tumor) |
| **Extraovarian epithelial tumors** |
| – Broad ligament and paraovarian tumors |
| – Mesonephric and paramesonephric cysts |
| – Tubal carcinoma |

Detection of Papillary Projection
False Negative Case

(a) When papillary projections are of small size (Fig. 9.12), US is usually more accurate than MR and even more than CT to detect them [62]; although in some cases, they can be detected on MR as well (Fig. 9.13).

(b) However, these papillary projections can be missed on ultrasound especially when small <2 mm in diameter and when the diameter of the cyst is >10 cm [63].

(c) Exocystic papillary projections are difficult to detect on US.

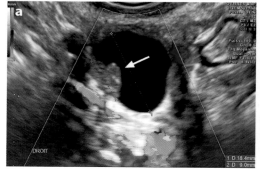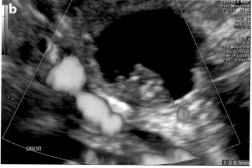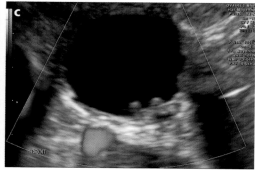

Fig. 9.12 Cystadenoma with papillary projections less than 1 cm in size. Sixty-two-year-old woman. During routine ultrasound examination, a right ovarian mass is discovered; (**a**) EVS Unilocular cystic ovarian mass containing endocystic papillary projection of 9 mm with obtuse angles with the wall suggesting the possibility of a carcinoma or borderline (*arrow*). (**b**) Small hyperechogenic foci very likely related to tiny calcifications are visualized mainly on the top of the papillary projection. Absence of flow on color Doppler (**b**). (**c**) Papillary projections of 1–2 mm in diameter are displayed adjacent to the largest one. Prospective diagnosis: on the basis of ultrasound findings, characterization is indeterminate.CA 125 is normal. Association of these findings suggests the possibility of a benign or borderline tumor. At microscopy: serous cystadenoma

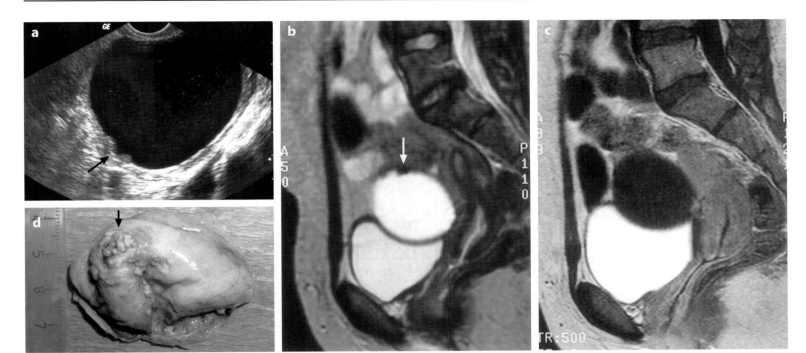

Fig. 9.13 Serous cystadenoma small papillary projection visualized on US and MR. EVS (**a**); unilocular cystic mass containing small papillary projections (2 mm in size) (*arrow*). Their size is very suggestive of benign tumor. MR sagittal T2 (**b**) displays these papillary projections as well (*arrow*), while they are not visualized on sagittal T1 (**c**). Macroscopic specimen (**d**): a focus of small papillary projections (*arrow*) which are much more numerous than on the imaging modalities is displayed

False Positive (Table 9.11)

Papillary projections can be confused with other echogenic foci:

- Tubal folds or plicae in a hydro or pyosalpinx (Fig. 9.14): The usual tubular shape of the tube with infoldings and the usual finger-like shape of the plicae (although contrast medium diffuses in it) may help to make the differential diagnosis. However, it must be outlined that in chronic salpingitis, the term papillary tufts is used [64] which outlines the pathologic boundaries between a papillary projection of a serous ovarian tumor and blunt papillae of a chronic salpingitis.
- Cumulus oophorus in a functional cyst (Fig. 9.15).
- Clots in endometriomas [65] (Fig. 9.16) [66] and functional hemorrhagic cysts (Fig. 9.17).
- Rokitansky protuberance in dermoid cysts [66] (see Figs. 10.40 and 10.41).
- Mucin accumulation in mucinous tumors (Fig. 9.18).
- Small intracystic projections in tubo-ovarian abscess [62] (Table 9.17).

When the differential diagnosis between papillary projection versus clot or echogenic loculus cannot be established, MR performed before and after contrast displays diffusion of contrast medium in the papillary projection [62] or tissular portion [61], while no contrast enhancement is visualized in a clot or echoic loculus.

Characterization of Papillary Projection

Although a definite diagnosis of benign, borderline, or malignant papillary projection can only be made at microscopy, three main factors can help to orient the diagnosis: age of the patient, tumoral markers, and morphological and vascular findings on ultrasound (Tables 9.5 and 9.10).

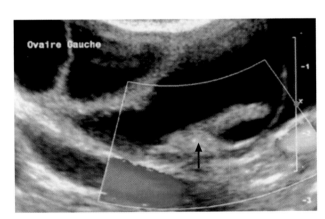

Fig. 9.14 Plica in a hydrosalpinx. In a tubular shape cystic adnexal mass related to a hydrosalpinx, localized tissular portion can simulate a papillary projection. When the digitiform shape and the oblique orientation are present like in this case, these morphologic findings are very helpful to distinguish it from a papillary projection in an ovarian cyst and to diagnose a plica (*arrow*). However, in some cases, the plicae can be smaller and round, impossible to distinguish from an endocystic papillary projection

Likelihood of malignancy increases with age. Carcinoma is very uncommon before 30 years, while borderline tumors are possible.

Ultrasound pattern favoring benign papillary projections are summarized in Tables 9.5 and 9.10 [67].

- Topography
  Benign papillary projections never cover the entire inner surface of the tumor [50]. They usually cover less than 50 % of the surface of the cyst.
- Size
  Benign papillary projections (not solid tissue) measure from 2 to 23 mm (mean 9 mm). Papillary projections measuring less than 5 mm are very suggestive of benignity [49, 58, 68] (Figs. and 9.20).

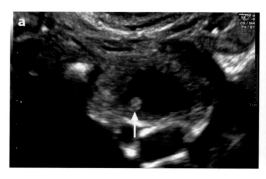
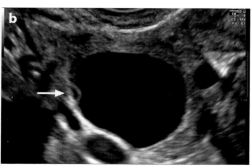

Fig. 9.15 Cumulus oophorus simulating a papillary projection. (**a**) EVS displays in a unilocular an echogenic cyst against the inner wall an echogenic focus resembling a papillary projection (*arrow*). (**b**) EVS performed in a plan perpendicular to the previous one displays a typical cumulus oophorus (*arrow*) in a functional cyst

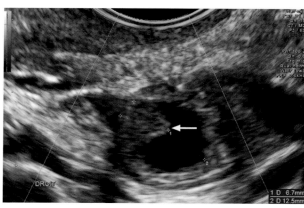

Fig. 9.16 Clot in an endometrioma simulating a papillary projection. EVS: In an ovarian low echogenic cyst, a localized echogenic portion protruding in the cystic cavity (*arrow*) is very suggestive of papillary projection. At surgery it was in fact a clot in an endometrioma

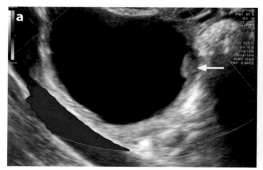
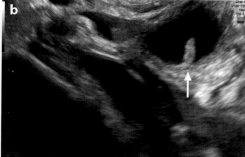

Fig. 9.17 Clot in a functional hemorrhagic cyst simulating a papillary projection. EVS with color doppler on transverse section (**a**) displays against the inner wall of the cyst an echogenic focus without any vessel which looks like a papillary projection (*arrow*). On oblique section (**b**), this echogenic focus appears with an elongated shape perpendicular to the wall (*arrow*); a plica in a hydrosalpinx or a clot in a functional ovarian cyst was discussed. Disappearance of the cyst after the next period confirmed the diagnosis of functional hemorrhagic cyst

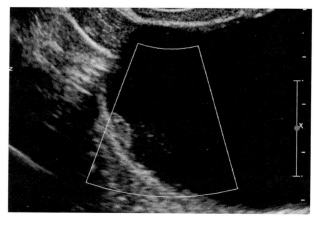

Fig. 9.18 Mucinous cystadenoma. A Unilocular cystic ovarian mass containing its inner wall, an echogenic focus (*arrow*) which looks like a papillary to projection. At macroscopy, this focus was in fact related to an accumulation of mucin

Table 9.17 False positive diagnosis of papillary projections

Common
– Clot in endometriosis and functional hemorrhagic cyst
– Tubal folds or plicae in hydrosalpinx (persistent normal or blunting)
– Echogenic foci in a cystadenoma, serous, and especially mucinous
– Cumulus oophorus in a functional cyst
Uncommon
– Rokitansky protuberance in dermoid cyst
– Mucin in a mucinous cystadenoma
– Debris in a tubo-ovarian abscess

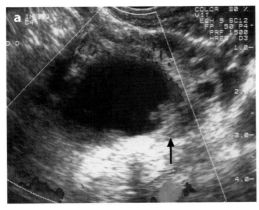
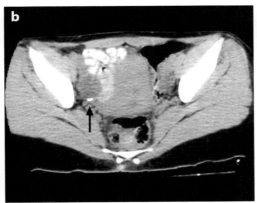
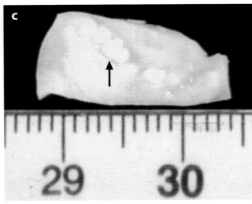

Fig. 9.19 *Serous cystadenoma with vegetations.* A 20-year-old woman. (a) *Endovaginal US with color Doppler*: sagittal view disclose a 4 cm right ovarian cyst with a group of vegetations, measuring 5 mm at the base of implantation without any color flow (*arrow*). (b) *CT scan without contrast* demonstrates a calcification at this level (*arrow*). (c) *Pathologic specimen.* Endocystic vegetations individually measuring 1–2 mm with regular surface are visualized (*arrow*). *Pathology*: serous cystadenoma (Figures (a, c) from Author's personal publication: Hassen et al. [36])

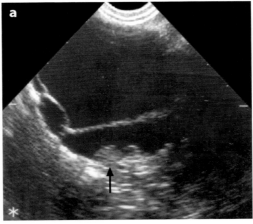
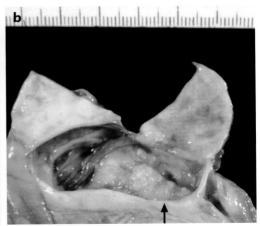

Fig. 9.20 *Serous cystadenoma with vegetations.* A 42-year-old woman with a right pelvic mass. (a) *Endovaginal US*: bilocular right cystic mass measuring 6 cm in its largest axis. Small endocystic vegetations inferior to 5 mm (*arrow*) with regular surface are visualized. (b) *Pathologic specimen*: a group of endocystic vegetations is visualized in one loculation (*arrow*). *Pathology*: serous cystadenoma (Figures from Author's personal publication: Buy et al. [45])

- Shape
  Benign papillary projection usually have a round, or mushroom appearance with a short base of implantation (Figs. 9.21 and 9.22), and a regular surface [58], without any degeneration.
- Structure
  It can appear as an association of multiple echogenic points, some of which are more echogenic than the other ones (Figs. 9.12 and 9.23).
- Macrocalcification
  Rare but always associated to benign vegetation (Hassan, Buy AJR). When macrocalcification is present (Fig. 9.24) [69], it is easily depicted on CT.
- Associated findings
  Cystic content is usually anechoic.
  Ovarian parenchyma (when the masses <10 cm) is pushed away to the periphery.
  Solid tissue is usually absent.
  Color Doppler (Table 9.10)
  When the vegetation is >1 cm, color Doppler demonstrates vessels in malignant vegetation but not in benign vegetation (Figs. 9.21, 9.22, and 9.25) [59].
  When the vegetations are <1 cm, color flow is absent in malignant vegetation as well as in benign vegetation, and differentiation between them is not possible.

MR and CT of Papillary Projection

While US is superior to MR in the ability to detect small papillary projections, in some cases small papillary projections can be demonstrated on MR as well (Fig. 9.13). On MR, papillary projections are well depicted on T2-weighted images with signal intensity usually intermediate between muscle and adipose tissue. On T1-weighted images, these structures can be difficult or impossible to visualize because their signal intensity is very close to the cystic content [70] (Fig. 9.25).

On CT without injection, papillary projections are usually not visualized or hardly depicted except if calcified (Fig. 9.19).

Findings on DMR or DCT are summarized in Table 9.10:
- At the arterial phase, absence of vessel or few tiny vessels is displayed in the papillary projections.
- At the parenchymal phase, a slight uptake is seen.
- At the delayed phase, papillary projections are better depicted; indeed, a slight increase of contrast uptake is displayed in the papillary projections as well as in the regular wall [71] and in the septa [62, 72] (Figs. 9.25 and 9.26).

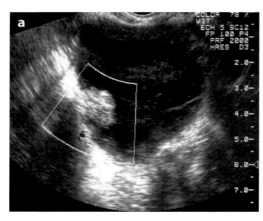
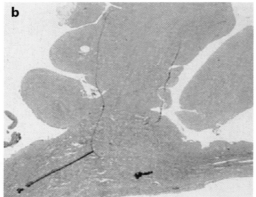
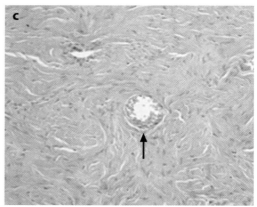

Fig. 9.21 *Serous cystadenoma with papillary projection.* A 22-year-old woman with pelvic pain. (**a**) *Endovaginal US with color Doppler*: in a left 7 cm ovarian cyst with slightly echogenic fluid, several endocystic vegetations are displayed. The largest one measuring 18 mm of longer axis has regular surface and a narrow base of implantation, forming an acute angle with the cyst wall. Color Doppler does not visualize any vessel in the vegetation. (**b**) *Pathologic specimen*: perpendicular section through the wall of the vegetation. The mushroom appearance with a narrow base of implantation and a regular surface is clearly depicted. (**c**) *Microscopic examination* (×20) demonstrates only few vessels in the connective tissue, with a small diameter, the largest ones measuring from 5 to 10 μ (*arrow*). *Pathology*: serous cystadenoma (Figures (**a**, **c**) from Author's personal publication: Buy et al. [8])

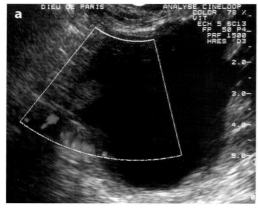
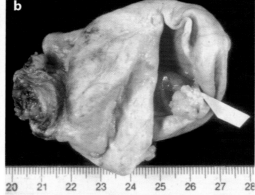

Fig. 9.22 Serous cystadenoma with endocystic papillary projection. A 56-year-old woman. (**a**) EVS displays an endocystic papillary projection with a short base of implantation and a regular surface very suggestive of benignity. Absence of color flow in this papillary projection measuring 1.2 cm is very much in favor of benignity. (**b**) Macroscopic specimen confirms the short pedicle of the papillary projection. Prospective diagnosis: serous cystadenoma which was confirmed at microscopy

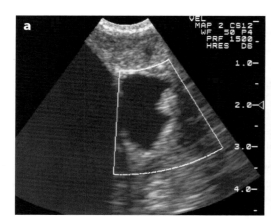
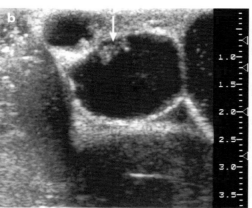
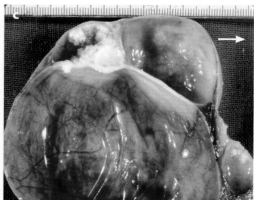

Fig. 9.23 Left serous cystadenofibroma and right serous cystadenoma. (**a**) EVS multilocular cystic mass with endocystic vegetations. Individually the vegetations measure from 1 to 3 mm but they form groups measuring up to 5 mm (*arrow*). (**b**) Ultrasound of the pathologic specimen gives more detail about the structure of the papillary projection (*arrow*). (1) It is composed of a gathering of multiple echogenic foci, some of which are more echogenic than the others. (2) The base of the papillary projection is separated from the wall by a line which is less echogenic than the wall itself. (**c**) Pathologic specimen of the right ovary (1) confirms that the papillary projection is composed of multiple tiny round structures gathered one against the other. (2) At the base of implantation the wall has the same thickness as in areas devoid of papillary projections and the papillary projections seem to be separated from the wall by a clear line

Fig. 9.24 Serous cystadenoma with calcified vegetations. A 65-year-old woman with a left ovarian mass. (**a**) *Endovaginal US, coronal view*: endocystic vegetations containing hyperechogenic foci with sharp acoustic shadowing. The content of the cyst is anechoic. (**b**) *CT scan without contrast*: calcifications are clearly displayed. *Prospective diagnosis*: serous cystadenoma. *Laparotomy* with cystectomy was performed. *Pathology*: serous cystadenoma

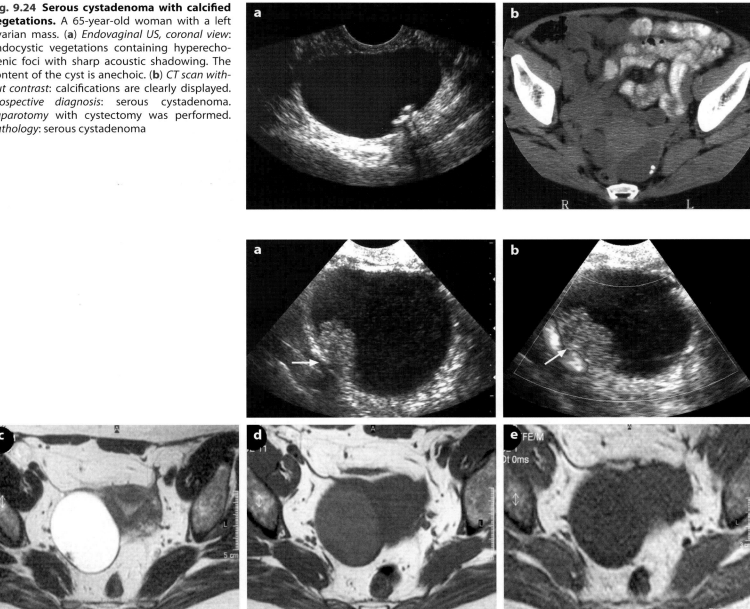

Fig. 9.25 *Serous cystadenoma with papillary projection.* A 58-year-old woman with a right ovarian mass discovered at a routine gynecologic examination. CA-125 35 IU/ml (normal: ≤35 ml). (**a**) *Endovaginal US*: right cystic ovarian mass of 6 cm contains a 2.5 cm endocystic papillary projection with a broad base of implantation (*arrow*). Malignancy is suggested. (**b**) *Color Doppler* does not visualize any vessel in the papillary projection (*arrow*) and suggests the diagnosis of benignity (*arrow*). However, because of the difficulty of characterization MR is performed. (C) *MR Axial T2*: Papillary projection with a signal intensity comprised between pelvic muscles and adipose tissue is clearly visible in the hyperintense fluid. (**d**) *Axial T1*: Signal intensity of the ovarian cyst is slightly superior to pelvic muscles. Endocystic papillary projection is not visible. DMR without injection (**e**) *at the arterial phase*

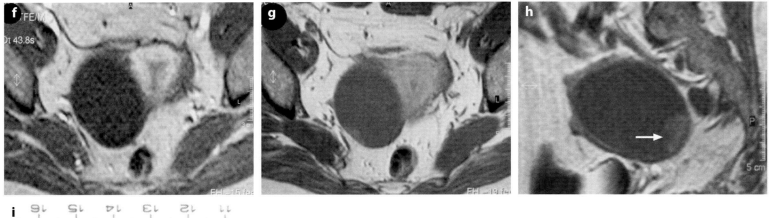

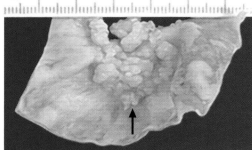

Fig. 9.25 (*continued*) (**f**) and *parenchymal phase* (**g**) does not demonstrate the papillary projection. On the delayed *sagittal* (**h**): the papillary projection is visible with a signal intensity comprised between pelvic muscles and adipose tissue (*arrow*). These vascular findings are typical for benign papillary projections; prospective diagnosis: serous cystadenoma which was confirmed at microscopy (**i**) *Specimen of the right ovarian cyst*: the vegetation seen on US corresponds in fact to a group of gathered small endocystic papillary projections (Figures (**a**, **b**, **i**) from Author's personal publication: Hassen et al. [36])

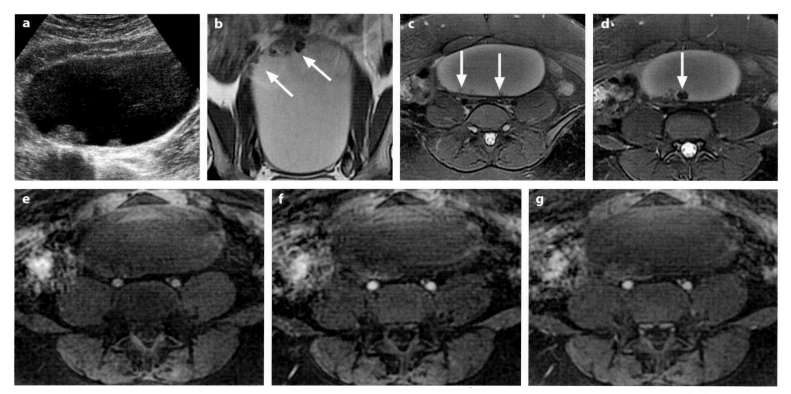

Fig. 9.26 *Serous cystadenoma with vegetations in a 21-year-old woman.* (**a**) TAS (virgin woman) discloses a large anechoic cyst with vegetations. One vegetation looks large with a transverse diameter reaching 2 cm but at MR imaging and gross anatomy it was constituted of an agglomerate of smaller vegetations. No color flow could be detected in these vegetations on trans-abdominal ultrasound. (**b**) Coronal T2W and (**c**, **d**) axial T2W-FS images disclose papillary projections of different size, gathered in the *upper right* part of the cyst. The largest one (*arrow* in **d**) reaches 11 mm and seems to have a regular surface and an acute angle at the base of implantation. DMR before injection (**e**), at 25 s (**f**), 70 s (**g**),

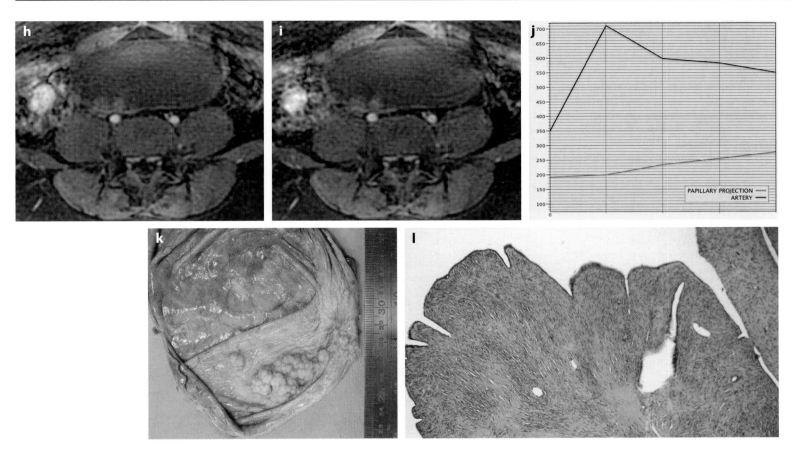

Fig. 9.26 (*continued*) 125 s (**h**) and 240 s (**i**) before injection with corresponding time-intensity curves (**j**) show a low and slow uptake in the largest vegetation, typical of benign tissue. Prospective diagnosis: serous cystadenoma. Photography of the surgical specimen (**k**) shows large vegetations in the upper part of the cyst and numerous granular vegetations non-visualized on US and MR covering the entire inner wall. Microscopy of vegetations (**l**) shows well delineated papillae with a single layer epithelium typical of benign cystadenoma and abundant fibrous stroma with rare vessels explaining the low and slow contrast uptake

Cystic Form with Solid Tissue (Cystadenofibroma)

Uncommonly, cystadenomas contain a significant component of solid tissue and in these cases are designated as cystadenofibromas.

On US, one or more echogenic portions usually homogeneous and well limited protruding in a cystic portion are present (Fig. 9.27).

On MR, fibrotic tissue appears with characteristic low signal intensity close to pelvic muscle on T2 (Fig. 9.28). In the bilateral and voluminous masses, MR is more appropriate than US to diagnose these tumors (Fig. 9.29).

On CT, density of the solid tissue is close to pelvic muscle; macrocalcifications are well displayed (Fig. 9.30).

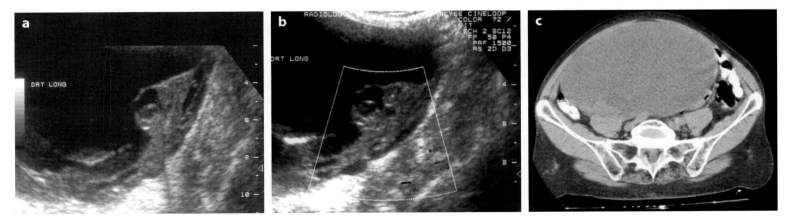

Fig. 9.27 *Serous cystadenofibroma.* A 80-year-old woman with a history of hysterectomy and right adnexectomy. (**a**) *Endovaginal US*: left ovarian cyst with a 3 cm tissular portion against the inner wall containing cystic degenerative changes. (**b**) *Color Doppler* does not demonstrate any vessel in the tissular portion. (**c**) *CT scan without contrast*: the tissular portion lying in the posterior right part of the cyst looks regular.

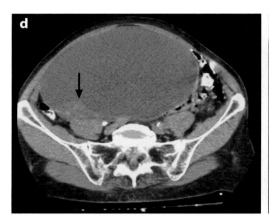

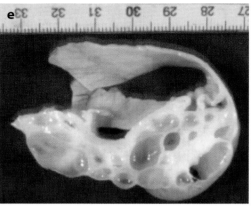

Fig. 9.27 (continued) (**d**) CT after contrast: slight contrast uptake in the tissular portion is visualized (arrow). (**e**) Pathologic specimen: tissular portion with cystic portions

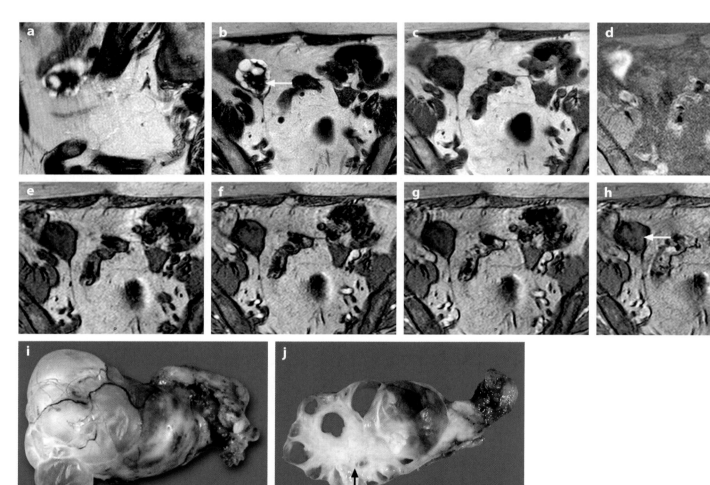

Fig. 9.28 Right ovarian cystadenofibroma. MR sagittal T2 (**a**) axial T2 (**b**) axial T1 (**c**) and fat suppression (**d**) display a mixed ovarian mass. On T2, solid tissue has a low intensity of a fibrous tissue (arrow). Signal intensity of the cysts on T2, T1, and fat suppression corresponds to clear fluid. DMR without injection (**e**), at the arterial phase (**f**), at the venous phase (**g**), and on the delayed phase (**h**) does not display any vessel in the tissular portion at the arterial phase, a slight contrast uptake at the venous phase which slightly increases on the delayed (arrow). These findings are typical for benign fibrous tissue. Prospective diagnosis: cystadenofibroma. Macroscopy (**i**, **j**) fibrous tissue (arrow) with cysts containing serous fluid. Microscopy: cystadenofibroma

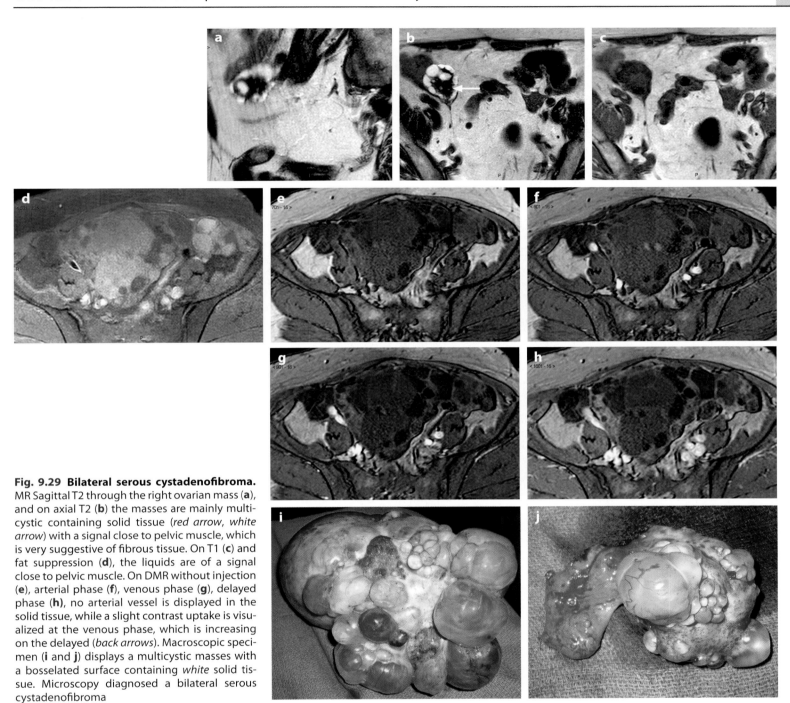

Fig. 9.29 Bilateral serous cystadenofibroma. MR Sagittal T2 through the right ovarian mass (**a**), and on axial T2 (**b**) the masses are mainly multi-cystic containing solid tissue (*red arrow*, *white arrow*) with a signal close to pelvic muscle, which is very suggestive of fibrous tissue. On T1 (**c**) and fat suppression (**d**), the liquids are of a signal close to pelvic muscle. On DMR without injection (**e**), arterial phase (**f**), venous phase (**g**), delayed phase (**h**), no arterial vessel is displayed in the solid tissue, while a slight contrast uptake is visualized at the venous phase, which is increasing on the delayed (*back arrows*). Macroscopic specimen (**i** and **j**) displays a multicystic masses with a bosselated surface containing *white* solid tissue. Microscopy diagnosed a bilateral serous cystadenofibroma

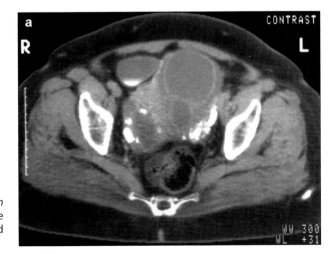

Fig. 9.30 *Bilateral serous cystadenofibroma.* A 66-year-old woman. (**a**) *CT scan with contrast*: pelvic mass containing cystic portions and tissular portions with multiple macrocalcifications very suggestive of benignity. *Laparotomy* with hysterectomy and bilateral adnexectomy was performed. *Pathology*: bilateral cystadenofibroma

More than the morphologic characters, the vascular characters are essential to make the diagnosis (Table 9.10). Indeed, the more the solid tissue is prominent, the more the characters of the vessels (Doppler, DMR, DCT) and the contrast uptake (low contrast uptake on DCT and DMR) are helpful to distinguish benign tumors from borderline and carcinomas (Figs. 9.27 and 9.31). Diffusion sequences on MR display a low signal very suggestive of a benign tumor.

They may contain degenerative cystic changes or macrocalcifications, but never hemorrhage and necroses [49] (Table 9.18).

Table 9.18 Differential diagnosis of cystadenofibroma

Common
Subserous leiomyoma
In case of degenerative changes when the normal ipsilateral ovary is not displayed
– Fibrous tissue: US areas of attenuation MR, low signal on T2
– Peripheral ring of regular vessels on Doppler, DMR, and DCT
– Early and equal to myometrium contrast uptake on DMR and DCT
Mainly solid benign ovarian tumors containing fibrous tissue (which may display degenerative changes)
Fibrothecoma and Brenner tumor
– Fibrous tissue: US areas of attenuation MR, low signal on T2
– Absence of vessels on Doppler, DMR, DCT (arterial phase)
– Late and slight contrast uptake on DMR, DCT
– In Brenner tumor, psammoma-like calcifications are numerous and association with a mucinous cystadenoma
Uncommon
Uncommon form of borderline with tissular portion
Sclerosing stromal tumor

Psammoma Bodies

They can be seen in the different previous forms.

The radiologic appearance of psammoma bodies depends on the size of the neoplastic mass and the concentration of calcifications [73]. Usually, they are inconspicuous [49].

On CT, they are less dense than most of calcifying masses and usually appear as a hazy, cloud-like aggregation only slightly denser than soft tissue. In some cases, they form aggregates of calcification, resulting in dense macrocalcifications (Fig. 9.30). They are more difficult to detect on US and are not visible on MR.

Among ovarian tumors, true psammomatous calcifications are a finding of the serous type. However, some rare ovarian tumors such as Brenner tumor, thecoma, virilizing lipid cell tumors, and gonadoblastoma may contain dystrophic calcifications that mimic true psammomatous calcifications (Table 9.13).

Association of Different Findings

Association of papillary projections, solid tissue, and calcifications in the same tumor is possible.

Association with Another Tumor (Collision Tumors)

Definition

A collision tumor of the ovary is an uncommon ovarian neoplasm where there is co-existence of two adjacent but histologically distinct tumors with no histologic admixture at the interface.

This association is very uncommon in the serous type. Association of a serous tumor with a Brenner tumor or a dermoid cyst has been reported.

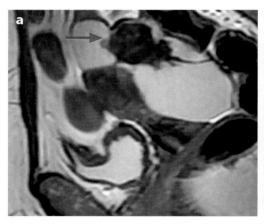 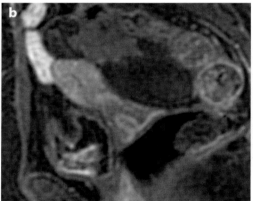 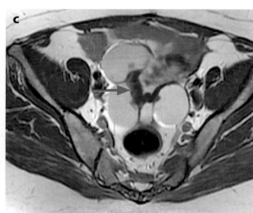

Fig. 9.31 *Serous cystadenofibroma in a 45-year-old woman.* Sagittal T2 (**a**) and axial T2 (**c**) show a large multilcular mainly cystic ovarian mass containing a solid portion (*red arrows* in **a** and in **c**) with lobulated borders. On the delayed sequence (**b**) performed after DMR, this solid tissue enhances moderately.

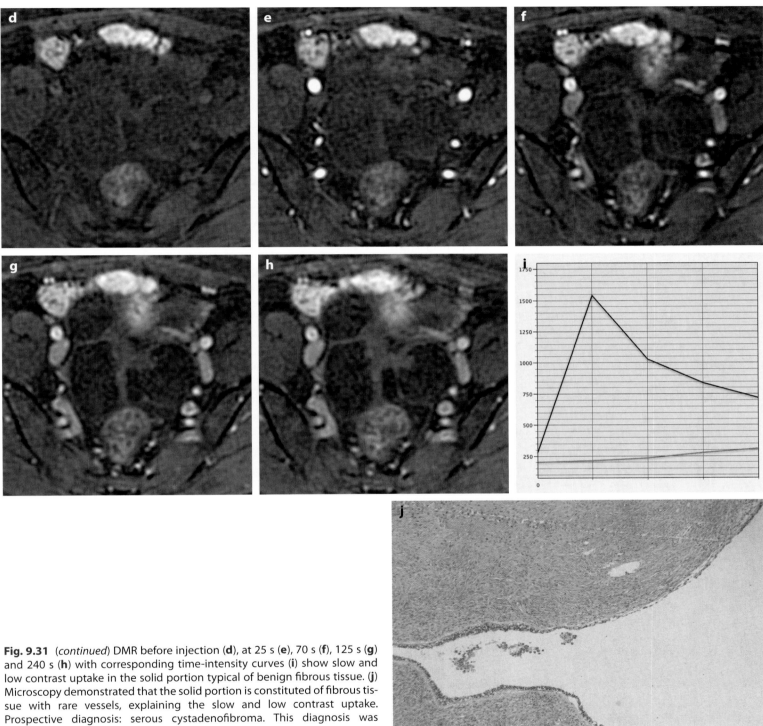

Fig. 9.31 (*continued*) DMR before injection (**d**), at 25 s (**e**), 70 s (**f**), 125 s (**g**) and 240 s (**h**) with corresponding time-intensity curves (**i**) show slow and low contrast uptake in the solid portion typical of benign fibrous tissue. (**j**) Microscopy demonstrated that the solid portion is constituted of fibrous tissue with rare vessels, explaining the slow and low contrast uptake. Prospective diagnosis: serous cystadenofibroma. This diagnosis was confirmed at microscopy

9.3.2 Borderline Serous Tumors or Atypical Proliferative Serous Tumors (APST)

9.3.2.1 General Features

They account for 5 % of all epithelial tumors (Table 9.3). They are bilateral in 37 % [50]. Tumoral marker CA 125 is elevated in 75 % of patients [74].

9.3.2.2 Pathology

Macroscopy (Fig. 9.32)

They are:

- Uni- or multilocular.
- Their content is watery or may contain a thick mucinous fluid which should not lead to an erroneous gross diagnosis of a mucinous cystic tumor [49, 58].
- Papillae (papillary protuberance) are nearly always present on the internal surfaces and are present on the external surfaces in as many as 70 % of cases (Seidman). Exophytic papillae are more often found in patients who also have peritoneal implants [75].

  Occasionally, the entire tumor consists of an exophytic papillary surface lesion unassociated with internal cystic papillary projections [76]. Papillae are greater, more exuberant than in the benign form [77]. Their mean size is intermediate between benign and malignant papillary projections. Their morphologic characters can look like either benign or malignant papillae. They can form polypoid structures resembling grapes that range from 1 to 10 mm in greatest dimension and may not be distinguishable from markedly papillary cystadenomas [76] (Fig. 9.33). Frequently, they form broad-based structures covering portions of the cyst lining on the serosa of the ovary [58] and can be indistinguishable from papillary of serous cystadenocarcinomas [76]. Necrosis is absent [58].

- A solid fibromatous component can be present [49].
- The wall and the septa can be thickened.

Microscopy [50] (Figs. 9.34 and 9.35)

APST display:

(a) Hierarchical branching with successively smaller papillae emanating from larger more centrally located papillae
(b) Extensive epithelial stratification and tufting
(c) Detachment of cell clusters
(d) Cells with features of epithelial and mesothelial differentiation:
  - Ciliated cells resembling those of the fallopian tube are present in about one-third of cases.
  - Hobnail-type cells may be present.
  - Attenuated epithelium resembling mesothelium.
  - Cells with abundant eosinophilic cytoplasm and rounded nuclei resembling hyperplasic mesothelial cells.
  - Nuclei basely located.
  - Chromatin is usually fine, but nucleoli sometimes prominent mitoses rarely exceed 4 per 10 MF.

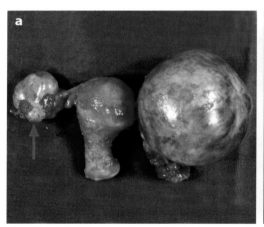
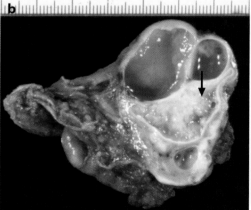
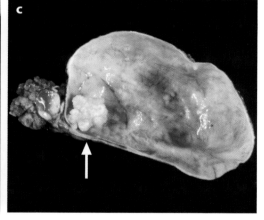

Fig. 9.32 Bilateral borderline serous tumor with vegetations size of vegetation suggestive of malignancy. Macroscopic specimen of the right and left ovaries (**a**) displays a bilateral ovarian mass with exocystic papillary projections (*arrow*). Macroscopic specimen of the *right* (**b**) and *left* (**c**) opened ovaries: small vegetations in the right ovary are displayed (*arrow* in **b**). A larger vegetation in the left ovary is depicted (*arrow* in **c**)

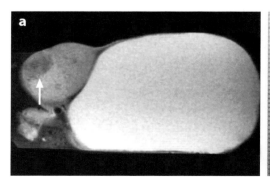
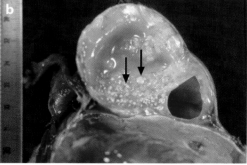

Fig. 9.33 Borderline serous tumor with a very unusual presentation of vegetations. Bridge pattern. (**a**) In vitro MR study: vegetations are clearly seen (*T*).The endocystic vegetations are depicted against the inner wall of the cyst (*arrow*) and as a very unusual pattern as a bridge between two portions of the inner wall. (**b**) Pathologic specimen: multiple small endocystic papillary projections (*arrows*) (Figure (**a**) from Author's personal publication: Ghossain et al. [70])

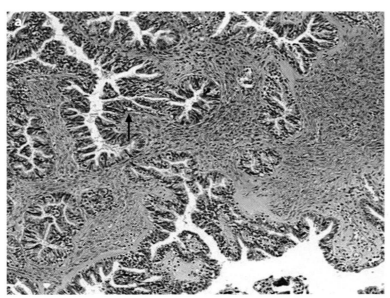

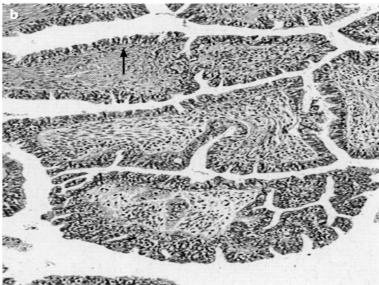

Fig. 9.34 Serous borderline tumor at microscopy. Papillar pattern with hierarchical branching (*arrow* in **a**); stratification of lining epithelial cells without stromal invasion (*arrow* in **b**)

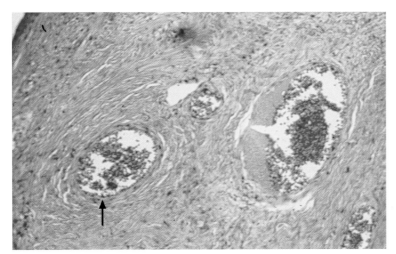

Fig. 9.35 In the papillary projection, vessels (*arrow*) are more numerous per unit of field and are larger than in a benign vegetation, but are usually smaller and less numerous than in a malignant vegetation

Table 9.19 Macroscopic and common imaging findings of serous borderline tumors

– Bilateral (37 %)
– Cystic uni- or multilocular
– Watery or mucinous fluid content
– Papillary projections:
* Endocystic and/or exocystic (common)
* Can be disseminated
* Size (2–30 mm; mean 6)
* Broad base with irregular surface or short base with regular surface
– Thick or thin wall and septa
– Psammoma bodies can be present
– Solid tissue usually absent
– Normal parenchyma pushed toward the periphery
– Associated lesions
* Peritoneal endosalpingiosis (40 % of patients)
* Peritoneal implants (40 % of patients)
* Lymph nodes

Microinvasion

The more common type is characterized by isolated cells with abundant eosinophilic cytoplasm that appear to budding from the epithelium into the superficial stromal cores of the papillae.

Less commonly, the lesion is characterized by a haphazard infiltrative pattern of small nests of cells forming micropapillae, often surrounded by a clear space and associated with an identifiable stromal response. Occasionally, the nests display a cribriform pattern. In either case, the invasion is limited in extent and should occupy a total area of no more than 10 mm² with no single focus exceeding 3 mm.

9.3.2.3 Imaging Findings

Macroscopic and common imaging findings on US, CT, and MR are summarized in Table 9.19.

1. The tumor is mainly cystic unilocular or multilocular in 30 % of cases [74].
2. The cystic content on US is most often diffusely slightly echogenic [78]. On MR, signal intensity of the liquid is close to pelvic muscle on T1 and close to urine on T2. On CT, density of the liquid is higher than that of urine. On MR and US, desquamation of cells can be visualized in the cystic content.
3. Ovarian parenchyma (when the mass is <10 cm) is pushed toward the periphery.
4. Papillary projections are always present.
   Characterization on US [67], MR, and CT is based on (Table 9.5):
   • Topography: They can cover the entire inner surface of the tumor [50] and usually cover more than 50 % of the surface of the cyst. They are endocystic and commonly exocystic.
   • Size: Papillary projections (without solid tissue) usually measure from 2 to 30 mm (mean 1.2 mm).

- Shape: They can have a broad base of implantation and an irregular surface as in carcinoma or make an acute angle with the wall like a benign papillary projection.

On US (Figs. 9.36 and 9.37), they look more echogenic than the low echogenic cystic content. On color Doppler, according to Pascual [78] and Emoto [79], borderline serous tumors have more vascularization than their benign counterpart. In papillary projections with a size >1 cm, color Doppler can detect vessels mainly at the base [59], while color flow is absent in papillary projections <1 cm. Spectral analysis is not very helpful in characterization [59, 78].

On MR (Figs. 9.36, 9.37, and 9.38), they appear with a signal close to pelvic muscle on T1 and with an intermediate signal between pelvic muscle and adipose tissue on T2 [70].

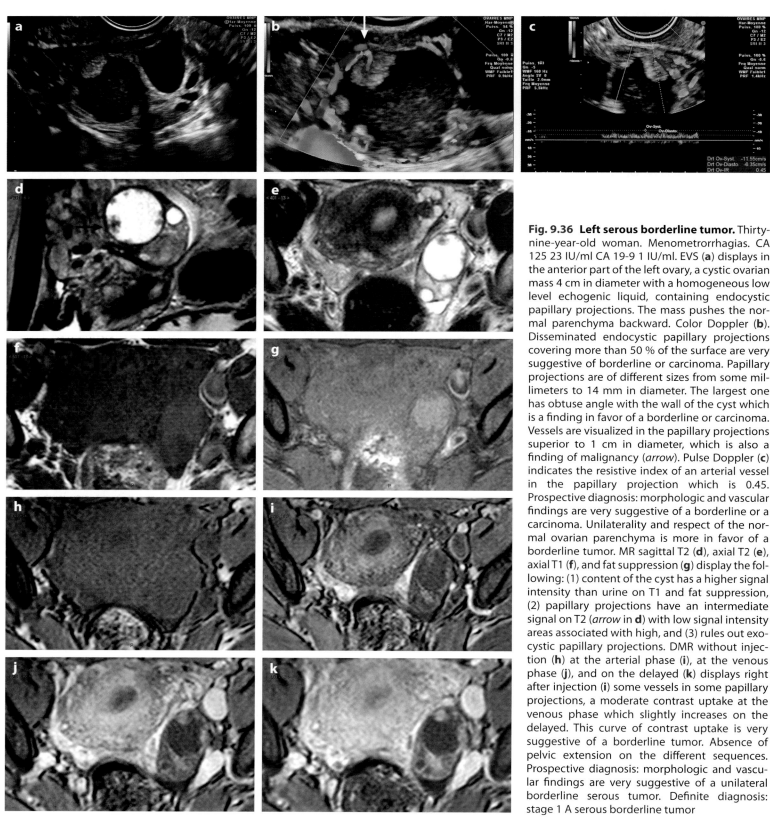

Fig. 9.36 Left serous borderline tumor. Thirty-nine-year-old woman. Menometrorrhagias. CA 125 23 IU/ml CA 19-9 1 IU/ml. EVS (**a**) displays in the anterior part of the left ovary, a cystic ovarian mass 4 cm in diameter with a homogeneous low level echogenic liquid, containing endocystic papillary projections. The mass pushes the normal parenchyma backward. Color Doppler (**b**). Disseminated endocystic papillary projections covering more than 50 % of the surface are very suggestive of borderline or carcinoma. Papillary projections are of different sizes from some millimeters to 14 mm in diameter. The largest one has obtuse angle with the wall of the cyst which is a finding in favor of a borderline or carcinoma. Vessels are visualized in the papillary projections superior to 1 cm in diameter, which is also a finding of malignancy (*arrow*). Pulse Doppler (**c**) indicates the resistive index of an arterial vessel in the papillary projection which is 0.45. Prospective diagnosis: morphologic and vascular findings are very suggestive of a borderline or a carcinoma. Unilaterality and respect of the normal ovarian parenchyma is more in favor of a borderline tumor. MR sagittal T2 (**d**), axial T2 (**e**), axial T1 (**f**), and fat suppression (**g**) display the following: (1) content of the cyst has a higher signal intensity than urine on T1 and fat suppression, (2) papillary projections have an intermediate signal on T2 (*arrow* in **d**) with low signal intensity areas associated with high, and (3) rules out exocystic papillary projections. DMR without injection (**h**) at the arterial phase (**i**), at the venous phase (**j**), and on the delayed (**k**) displays right after injection (**i**) some vessels in some papillary projections, a moderate contrast uptake at the venous phase which slightly increases on the delayed. This curve of contrast uptake is very suggestive of a borderline tumor. Absence of pelvic extension on the different sequences. Prospective diagnosis: morphologic and vascular findings are very suggestive of a unilateral borderline serous tumor. Definite diagnosis: stage 1 A serous borderline tumor

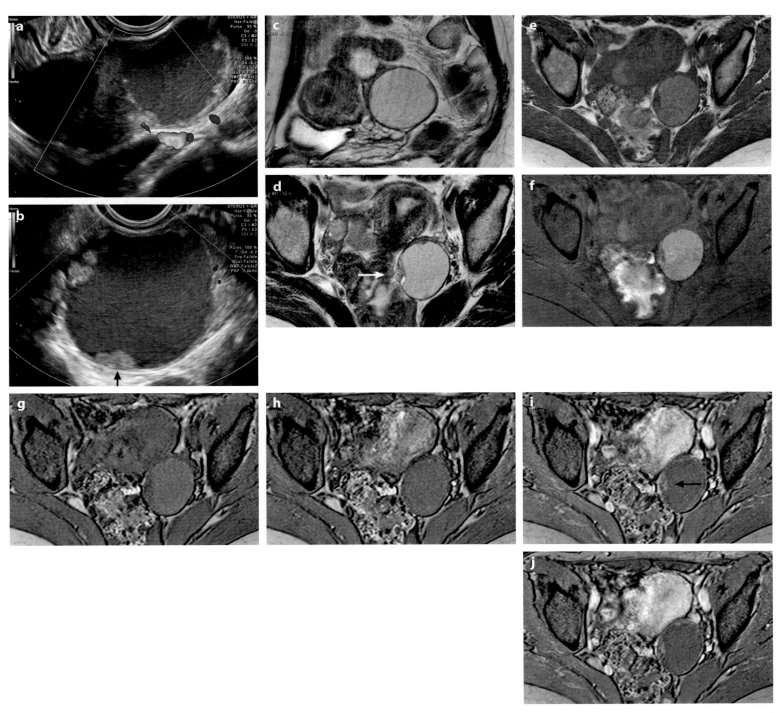

Fig. 9.37 ATP serous tumor. A 56-year-old woman. CA 125: 58 IU/ml. US (**a**) 5 cm unilocular cystic left ovarian mass containing a liquid with a ground glass pattern with disseminated endocystic papillary projection. Normal parenchyma is pushed toward the periphery. (**b**) The largest papillary projection measuring 11 mm in diameter has a broad base forming an obtuse angle with the wall of the cyst without any flow on color Doppler (*arrow*). The topography disseminated the papillary projections, the broad base of the largest one although no color flow is present, the aspect of the liquid with a ground glass pattern, and respect of the normal ovarian parenchyma are very suggestive of a borderline tumor. MR sagittal T2 (**c**) displays a cystic ovarian mass respecting the normal ovarian parenchyma containing endocystic papillary projections; on axial T2 (**d**) on the medial border, the largest papillary projection has an endocystic component with a broad base of implantation and overall an exocystic component (which was not depicted on US) very suggestive of borderline tumor (*arrow*). MR axial T1 (**e**) and fat suppression (**f**): content of the cyst with an intermediate signal is not watery like in a usual cystadenoma. DMR without injection (**g**) at the arterial phase (**h**), the venous phase (**i**), and on the delayed (**j**). No vessel is displayed in the papillary projection at the arterial phase. A slight contrast uptake is visualized at the venous phase (*arrow*) which slightly increases on the delayed. Prospective diagnosis: borderline serous tumor. At microscopy: borderline serous tumor

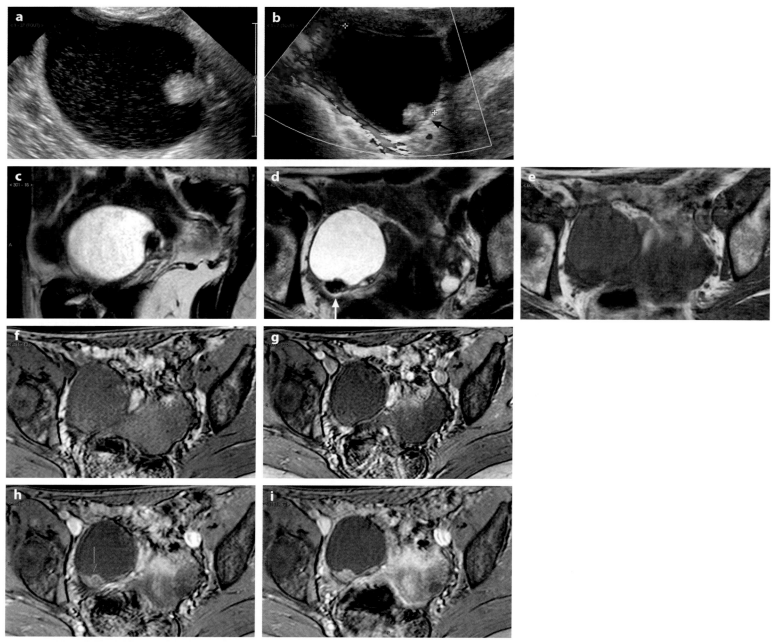

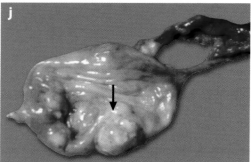

Fig. 9.38 Serous borderline tumor. Fifty-four-year-old woman. During a check up for microscopic hematuria, an ovarian mass is discovered during an ultrasound examination. CA 125: 11 IU/ml, *CA 19-9 : 23 UI/ml. EVS (**a**) displays a 5 cm right cystic ovarian mass; content of the cyt has a ground glass pattern. On (**b**) performed with color Doppler, the largest vegetation of 12 mm makes an obtuse angle with the wall and does not contain any vessel (*arrow*). MR sagittal T2 (**c**) and axial T2 (**d**) depict a cystic ovarian mass presenting posteriorly an endo- and exocystic papillary projection (*arrow* in **d**). Normal ovarian parenchyma is visualized around the papillary projection on (**e**). On axial T1 (**e**), content of the cyst has a signal close to pelvic muscles different from clear fluid. DMR without injection (**f**) at the arterial phase (**g**) displays small vessels in the vegetation. At the venous phase (**h**), a slight contrast uptake is depicted in the papillary projection (*red arrow*), which steadily increases on the delayed sequence (**i**). Macroscopic specimen (**j**) demonstrates the endo- and exocystic papillary projection (*white arrow*). Microscopy: serous borderline tumor

On CT without injection, they may be not visible (Fig. 9.39) because their density is close to the cystic content.

On DMR and DCT, at the arterial phase, tumoral vessels can be visualized (Fig. 9.40). Contrast uptake is displayed at the venous phase (Fig. 9.41) which slightly increases on the delayed phase (Figs. 9.39 and 9.42). This contrast diffusion can be

significant while vessel cannot be detected on color flow (Fig. 9.37).

5. Wall and septa can be thick and irregular or thin and regular.
6. Solid tissue is usually absent. Uncommonly, the tumor contains a significant component of fibrous tissue like in a benign serous cystadenofibroma (Fig. 9.43).

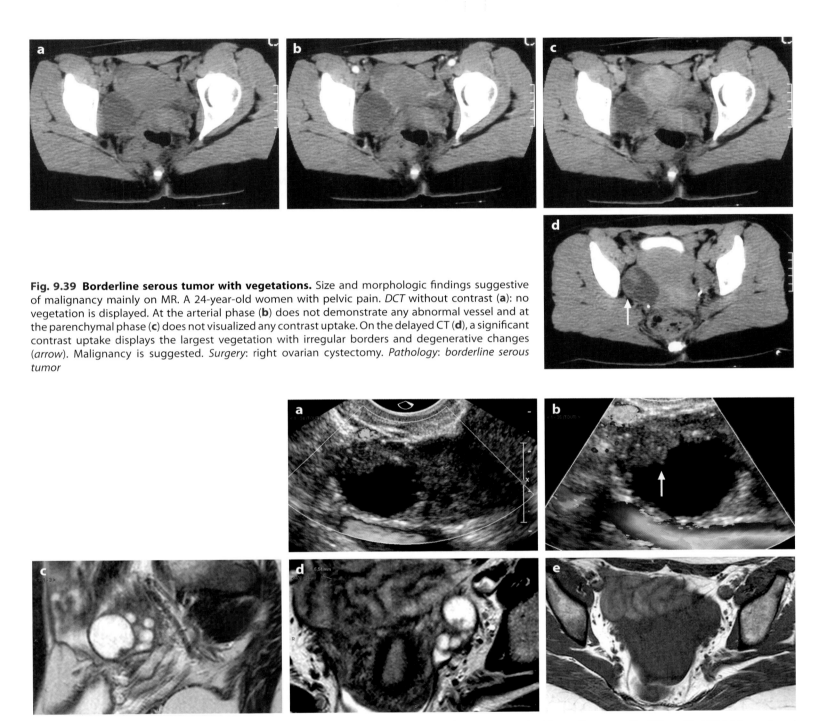

Fig. 9.39 Borderline serous tumor with vegetations. Size and morphologic findings suggestive of malignancy mainly on MR. A 24-year-old women with pelvic pain. *DCT* without contrast (**a**): no vegetation is displayed. At the arterial phase (**b**) does not demonstrate any abnormal vessel and at the parenchymal phase (**c**) does not visualized any contrast uptake. On the delayed CT (**d**), a significant contrast uptake displays the largest vegetation with irregular borders and degenerative changes (*arrow*). Malignancy is suggested. *Surgery*: right ovarian cystectomy. *Pathology*: borderline serous tumor

Fig. 9.40 Serous borderline tumor of the left ovary. Color Doppler sagittal (**a**) and transverse (**b**) display in the left ovary a 2 cm cyst pushing the normal ovarian parenchyma toward the periphery. The cyst contains endocystic papillary projections, the largest one measuring 6 mm without color flow, associated with smaller ones. On MR sagittal T2 (**c**) (*arrow*) and axial T2 (**d**), the largest papillary projection has obtuse angles with the inner wall of the cyst. On T1 (**e**), content of the cyst has a signal intensity close to pelvic muscle which does not correspond to clear fluid.

9.3.2.4 Particular Form: Serous Surface Papillary Borderline Tumor (SSPBT)

Definition: (1) surface lesions, (2) usually entirely solid, (3) papillary architecture with an internal branching, (4) with or without peritoneal extension

The Masses: On US (Fig. 9.44), papillary projections on the surface of the ovary are better displayed because of the peritoneal fluid associated with the ovarian lesions.

On MR (Fig. 9.45), six cases were reported by *Tanaka* (age range 26–58 years; mean 43 years) [83]. The masses have a sea anemone-like shape, with irregular nodular or papillary margins.

On T2, sharp demarcation from the low intensity of the superficial cortex of the normal ovary is displayed.

All masses were almost entirely solid and showed a very particular hyperintense papillary architecture with hypointense internal branching [83].

On T1, the tumors showed intermediate signal intensity [84].

After contrast enhancement, the tumors were enhanced as much as the ovaries [84].

CT showed ill-defined solid ovarian masses and failed to show normal ovaries inside the masses [84].

Extension [83]: Five patients had peritoneal implants, and two had lymph node enlargement, and all tumors were accompanied by ascites. In all cases, contralateral ovaries had cystic masses with mural nodules or mixed solid and cystic masses, of which the solid part was similar to the contralateral mass.

Prognosis: It is far better than that of serous surface papillary adenocarcinoma (SSPC).

Differential diagnosis: Exceptionally peritoneal inclusion cyst may have papillary projections and may simulate a borderline surface papillary tumor (Fig. 9.46).

9.3.2.5 Rupture

Exceptionally, a borderline serous tumor can rupture at time of presentation and be accompanied with ascites [85].

9.3.2.6 Recurrence

When cystectomy for borderline serous tumors has been performed, recurrence of the same tumor can occur in the same ovary (Fig. 9.47).

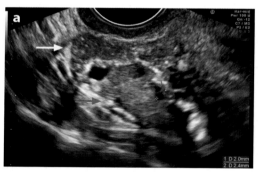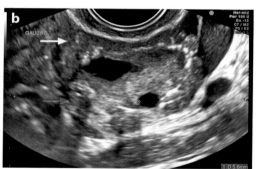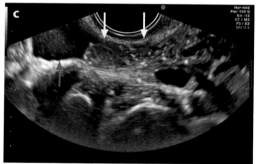

Fig. 9.44 Borderline surface papillary tumor. Thirty-nine-year-old woman. US examination performed for menorrhagia. Transverse EVS at the level of the right ovary (**a**) and of the left ovary (**b**) display multiple hyperechogenic foci on the outer cortex of both ovaries (*black arrows*) surrounded by echogenic tissue (*white arrows*). Transverse EVS through the Douglas (**c**) depicts echogenic tissue (*white arrows*) associated with echogenic fluid (*black arrow*). Prospective diagnosis: endometriosis was suggested. Final diagnosis: borderline surface papillary tumor. At microscopy, calcifications were displayed in the papillary projections

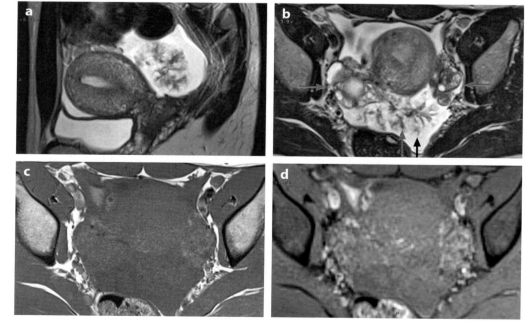

Fig. 9.45 Surface serous borderline tumor. MR sagittal T2 (**a**) and axial T2 (**b**) display in contact with the periphery of the outer cortex without invading the parenchyma of the underlying ovaries (*green arrows*) a bilateral pelvic mass. On the *right*, the mass is almost entirely solid and shows a very particular hyperintense papillary architecture (*black arrow*) with hypointense internal branching (*red arrow*). On the *left*, the mass is much smaller with a less characteristic appearance. Ascites is present in the posterior pelvis. Axial T1 (**c**) with fat suppression (**d**). The masses cannot be individualized from ovaries, and pelvic ascites look hypointense like pelvic muscles.

Fig. 9.45 (*continued*) DMR without injection (**e**) at the arterial phase (**f**) displays multiple arterial vessels in the tumors with a contrast uptake slightly superior to that of ovarian parenchyma at the venous phase (**g**) and on the delayed (**h**)

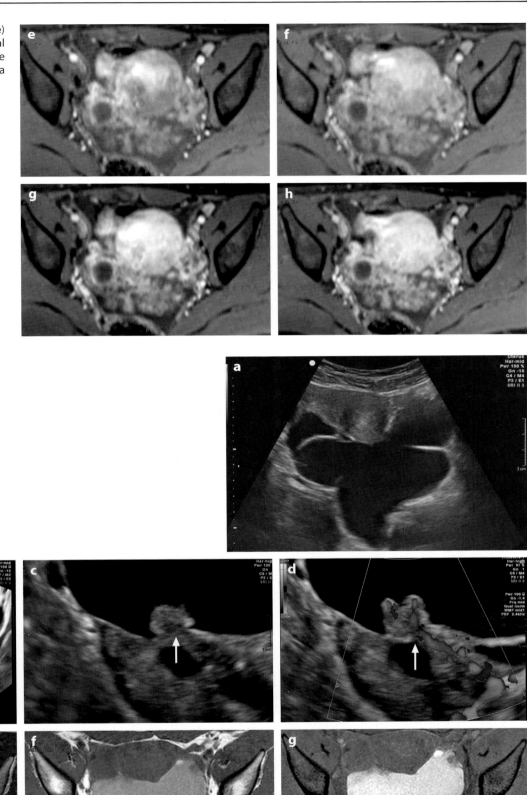

Fig. 9.46 Peritoneal inclusion cyst with papillary projections. Simulating a papillary surface serous tumor. Forty-four-year-old woman. Previous polymyomectomy 4 years ago. For some months, abdominal swelling. Pelvic mass at clinical examination. Transverse TAS (**a**) displays a collection in the Douglas, which follows the lateral walls of the pelvis. Transverse EVS (**b**) shows an echogenic collection, with papillary projection (*arrow*) at the surface of the left ovary. Transverse EVS (**c**) of the right ovary also displays a papillary projection (*arrow*) forming an obtuse angle with the surface of the ovary; on color Doppler (**d**), a large vessel penetrates at its base (*arrow*). MR axial T2 (**e**) depicts a large posterior collection, with papillary projections at the surface of both ovaries (*arrows*) and against the posterior face of the uterus. On T1 (**f**) and on fat suppression (**g**), the liquid has a high signal suggesting either hemorrhage of a high protein content.

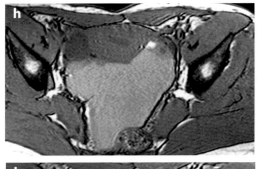

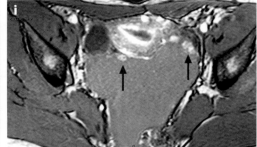

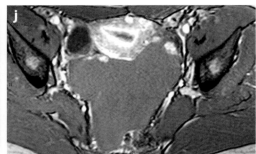

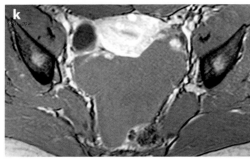

Fig. 9.46 (*continued*) On DMR without injection (**h**) and at the arterial phase (**i**) depict vessels in the papillary projections (*arrows*), with a high contrast uptake at the venous phase (**j**) and on the delayed (**k**), associated with a high contrast uptake on the right parietal peritoneum. Prospective diagnosis: surface borderline tumor. Surgery: an inclusion peritoneal cyst and encasing and hiding both adnexa is subperitoneal. Resection of the collection and bilateral adnexectomy. Microscopy: benign peritoneal inclusion cyst

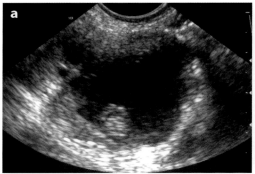

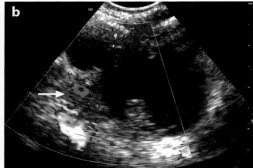

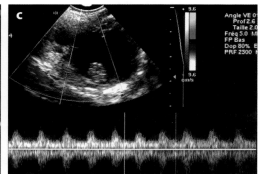

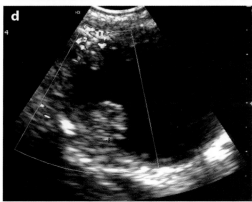

Fig. 9.47 *Recurrence* **of a right borderline serous tumor simulating a carcinoma.** A 21-year-old women. Right ovarian cystectomy 3 years ago for borderline papillary serous tumor. During a routine examination, a right ovarian mass is discovered. CA 125 is normal. TVS (**a**): a right ovarian cystic mass contains multiple vegetations. The largest one measures 2.5 cm and has a broad base of implantation; its surface is regular. Morphologic findings strongly suggest malignancy. Color Doppler (**b**) visualizes unusual large vessels (*arrow*) for a borderline tumor making the diagnosis of carcinoma very likely. At spectral analysis (**c**); RI 0, 56 IP-0, 83 peak systolic velocity 8 cm/s. Color Doppler of another 1 cm vegetation (**d**) with degenerative changes does not visualize any vessel. Surgery: right adnexectomy and multiple peritoneal biopsies. Pathology: papillary serous borderline tumor

9.3.3 Malignant Serous Tumors

9.3.3.1 Serous Carcinomas

General Features

They account for 17 % of all ovarian tumors (Table 9.3).

Seventy to eighty percent are present in FIGO stage II or higher. Two-thirds are bilateral (for stage 1A, 40 % are bilateral).

Tumoral markers (CA 125 >35 IU/ml) are usually frankly elevated in about 90 % of patients [50].

Pathology

Macroscopy [50] (Fig. 9.48)

Four patterns could be described:

(a) Mainly cystic containing serous, turbid, or bloody fluid, uni- or multilocular with soft friable papillae filling the cyst cavities. The papillae can be small or large with prominent vessels in their stromal core [49]. The external surface may be smooth or lobulated and sometimes displays surface papillae.

(b) Mixed.

(c) Entirely solid with less obvious papillae and may be soft or firm depending on the character of stroma tumor. Hemorrhage and necrosis are often present.

(d) The tumor can be entirely exophytic (*serous surface carcinoma*), but most often, the underlying ovary is at least focally replaced by neoplastic tissue as well [49]. Serous surface carcinomas appear as velvety patches or hard plaques on the ovarian surface. At microscopy, they usually invade the underlying stroma [49].

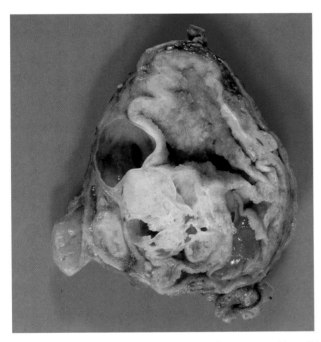

Fig. 9.48 Serous cystadenocarcinoma. Mixed pattern with solid mass associated with degenerative changes

Microscopy [50] (Fig. 9.49)

Typical serous carcinomas display complex papillary and solid patterns.

A frequent and quite characteristic pattern is a lacelike or labyrinthine pattern. This pattern may be focal, but often predominates, and is characterized by extensive bridging and coalescence of papillae resulting in slit-like spaces between the papillae. Necrosis is often pronounced.

Marked nuclear atypia and numerous mitoses are usually present.

A glandular pattern is not necessarily diagnostic of endometrioid differentiation, and the distinction between a high-grade serous carcinoma and an endometrioid carcinoma may be very difficult.

Psammoma bodies are present in 25 % of cases.

Imaging Findings

Macroscopic and Common Imaging Findings

Macroscopic and common imaging findings on US, CT, and MR are reported in Table 9.20.

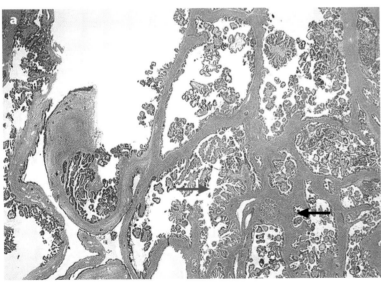 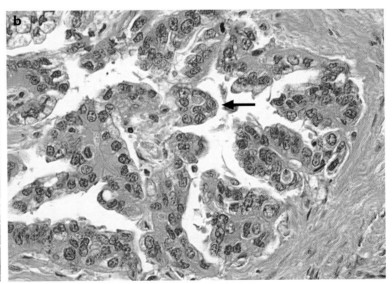

Fig. 9.49 Serous cystadenocarcinoma. (**a**) Irregular glands with different sizes and shapes (*black arrow*) with papillary patterns (*green arrow*). (**b**) glands and papillae are lined by atypical cells (*arrow*)

Table 9.20 Macroscopic and common imaging findings of serous carcinomas on US, CT and MR

- Bilateral (two-thirds of cases)
- Size <10 cm
- Cystic component: uni- or multilocular – watery or mucinous fluid
- Papillary projections
  * Endocystic and or exocystic (common)
  * Disseminated
  * Size (5–45 mm: mean 32 mm)
  * Broad base, irregular surface
- Solid tissue with irregular limits
  * Degenerative changes (necrosis)
  * Tumoral vessels
- Wall and septa: thick and irregular
- Psammoma bodies in 25 % of cases
- Normal parenchyma not visualized
- Extension
  * Peritoneal
  * Lymph nodes

The Cystic Pattern with Papillary Projections [67] (Table 9.5)

This pattern of presentation is usually discovered at a stage with extension beyond the ovary; exceptionally, the tumor is diagnosed at a stage 1A (Fig. 9.50).

Cystic Content

The cystic content on US is slightly echogenic, on CT with a density a little more than urine, on MR with a signal equal to pelvic muscle, and equal to urine on T1 and T2.

Papillary Projection

They are endocystic and can be exocystic (Fig. 9.51).

- Topography:
  They can cover the entire inner surface of the tumor [50] and usually cover more than 50 % of the surface of the cyst (Fig. 9.52).
- Size:
  Papillary projections (without solid tissue) usually measure from to 2–45 mm (mean 1.2 cm).
- Shape:
  They typically and commonly have a broad base of implantation and an irregular surface (Fig. 9.53). Rarely, an acute angle with the wall like a benign papillary projection is present.
- Pattern:
  On US, they look more echogenic than the low echogenic cystic content. On MR, they appear with a signal close to pelvic muscle on T1 and with an intermediate signal between pelvic muscle and adipose tissue on T2.
  On CT without injection, they are barely visible because their density is close to the cystic content.
- Vascular findings
  Detection of color flow confirms the tissular nature of the echogenic portion and definitely rules out a clot or accumulation of mucin. Vessels are larger at the base and taper progressively toward the tip of the vegetation, with a direction more or less perpendicular to the wall. They are never displayed lining the tip of the vegetation unlike the inner lining of solid tissue.

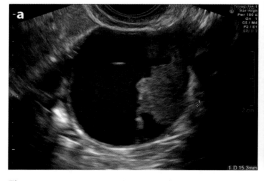 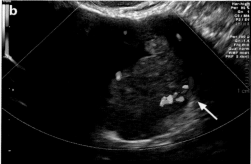 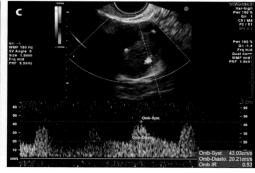

Fig. 9.50 Serous carcinoma of the left ovary stage 1A. Fifty-nine-year-old woman without hormonal treatment. During routine examination. EVS (**a**) displays a 5 cm left ovarian mass containing a 3 cm echogenic endocystic papillary projection with a more echogenic band at the top (very likely related to necrosis) and a cystic portion with a low level echogenicity. Color Doppler (**b**) depicts typical tumoral vessels at the base of the solid tissue, very suggestive of carcinoma (*arrow*). Pulsed Doppler (**c**) shows a very high peak systolic velocity of 43 cm/s very suggestive of carcinoma while the resistive index of 0.53 wrongly would classify the tumor as benign. Prospective diagnosis: carcinoma of the ovary. CA 125 performed after US: 50 IU/ml. Surgery: Hysterectomy with bilateral adnexectomy, omentectomy, multiple peritoneal biopsies, and lymphadenectomy. Absence of extraovarian extension. Pathology: serous carcinoma containing some areas of necrosis of grade 2. Association with some endometrioid components. Stage 1 A

Fig. 9.51 Less differentiated serous carcinoma stage I C. A 52-year-old woman with abdominal pain. CA 125 CA19-9 normal. EVS of the right ovarian mass (**a**, **b**) displays a mixed ovarian mass within the anterior part of the cystic portion an endocystic and exocystic papillary projection (*black arrow*) with few color flow without registration on pulsed doppler. Because of the paucity of vascularization a borderline tumor is first suggested. EVS (**c**, **d**) of the left ovarian mass depicts an echogenic mass with multiple areas with sound attenuation (*arrow*) containing rare tiny vessels. A fibrothecoma could be discussed. CT scan (**e**, **f**) without injection and at the arterial phase with MIP reformation displays in the left ovarian mass arterial tumoral vessels typical for a malignant tumor (*black arrow* in **f**). CT falsely rules out an extraovarian extension. MR sagittal T2 of the right ovarian mass (**g**) shows the endocystic and exocystic papillary projection (*arrow*). Axial T2 (**h**) of the left ovary shows a tissular mass with an intermediate signal.

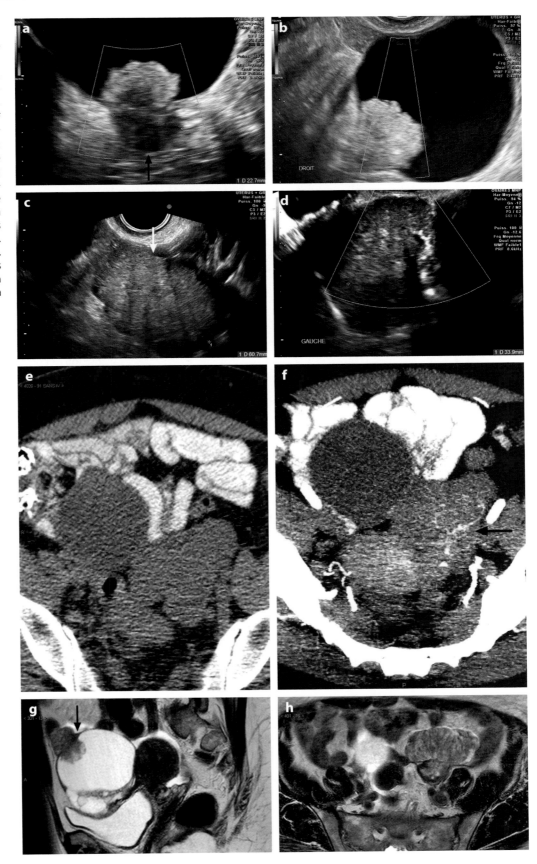

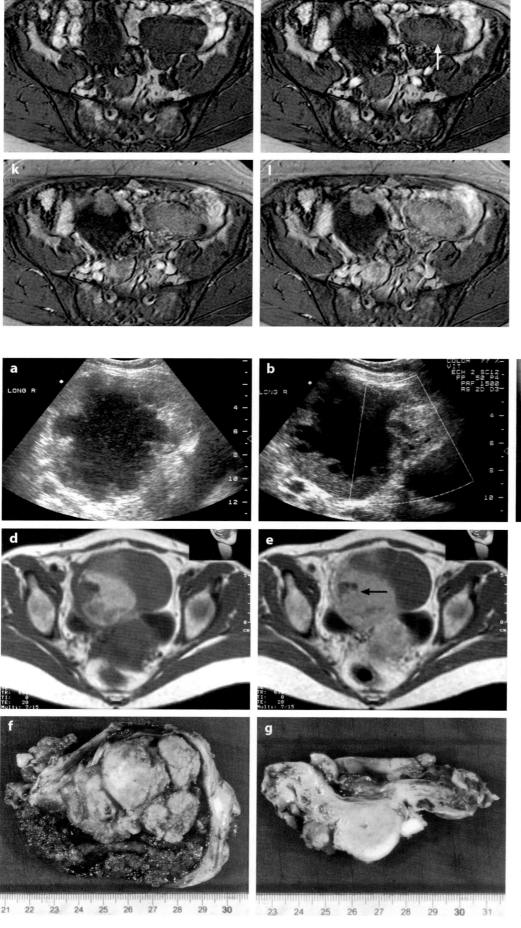

Fig. 9.51 (*continued*) DMR without injection (**i**) at the arterial phase (**j**) displays arterial tumoral vessels (*arrow*) (not as well as DCT) and shows at the venous phase (**k**) a significant contrast uptake, which slightly increases on the delayed sequence (**l**). CT and MR prospective diagnosis: bilateral ovarian carcinoma without any extraovarian extension. Surgery: usual protocol for ovarian carcinoma. Multiple small nodules <2 mm on the serosa of the rectum were missed with the three techniques. Pathology: bilateral less differentiated serous carcinoma

Fig. 9.52 Mixed half cystic half solid tumor. A 54-year-old women with pelvic pain. TVS (**a**) displays a 10 cm mixed ovarian mass with a tissular component and disseminated large endocystic papillary projections with irregular borders typical for a malignant tumor. On color Doppler (**b**), large vessels are visualized in the tissular portion. MR sagittal T2 (**c**): displays the tissular portion of intermediate signal (*white arrow*) and in the cystic portion the disseminated papillary projections (*black arrow*). Axial T1 without contrast (**d**) and with contrast (**e**). Contrast uptake is visualized in the solid portion without any contrast uptake a focus in the anterior part related to necrosis (*arrow*). Pathologic specimens (**f** and **g**) display a large portion of solid tissue associated with multiple large papillary projections with necrosis on the surface typical for a carcinoma. Pathology: papillary right ovarian carcinoma; stage I

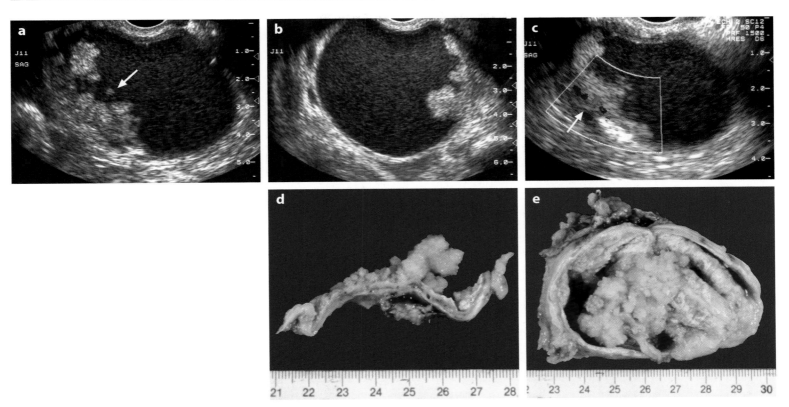

Fig. 9.53 Cystic form with papillary projections typical for malignancy. A 40-year-old women with right pelvic mass discovered on an ultrasound examination. CA 125: 163 IU/ml. TVS of right ovary on a longitudinal (**a**) and coronal (**b**) sections demonstrates a 7 cm cystic mass containing endocystic vegetations, the largest one >2 cm, with a broad base of implantation and an irregular surface typical of malignancy. The cystic content is low echogenic like in an endometrioma, with some desquamated cells in the fluid (*arrow*). Color Doppler (**c**) visualizes large vessels at the base of the vegeta- tion (*arrow*) confirming the diagnosis of malignancy. At macroscopy of the right ovary (**d**), multiple vegetations, some of which are confluent, are visualized. Section through a large vegetation (**e**) displays its broad base of implantation with an irregular surface (*arrow*), associated with contiguous multiple small vegetations. *Pathology*: (1) serous carcinoma of the right ovary; Stage IIIc. (2) Extension to the serosa of the left ovary and to the right obturator lymph node and of the greater omentum were missed on US (Figures (**a, c, d**) from Author's personal publication: Hassen et al. [36])

Visualization of vessels in a papillary projection >1 cm highly suggests the diagnosis of malignancy while color flow in vegetation >1 cm is usually not observed in benign tumor [59].

Spectral analysis has been proposed by some authors to characterize these tumors. A resistive index <0.40, a pulsatility index <1, and a peak systolic velocity >15 cm/s are considered by some authors as very suggestive of malignancy (Delmas). In fact, their specificity particularly the specificity of RI is high, but their sensitivity is low [59]. This is the reason why these parameters are rarely taken in account.

On DMR and DCT, at the arterial phase, tumoral vessels can be visualized (Fig. 9.54). Contrast uptake is displayed at the venous phase and on the delayed phase (see later solid tissue). On MR, in their superficial part, which can be the site of hemorrhage or necrosis, absence of contrast enhancement can be visualized.

Wall and Septa

The wall and the septa look thick and irregular. On US, they appear echogenic containing vessels on color Doppler. On MR, they appear with low signal intensity on T2 and enhance after contrast injection. On CT, they enhance after injection.

The differential diagnosis of true papillary projections has been already reported in Table 9.17 and the differential diagnosis of a cystic tumor containing true papillary projections in Table 9.16.

The Mixed Pattern and the Predominantly Solid Pattern

Solid tissue can have regular or irregular limits. Commonly, it has degenerative changes particularly hemorrhage and necrosis. Uncommonly, primary malignant tumors are entirely solid.

On US, solid tissue appears clearly more echogenic than the cystic content. It can be associated with a significant cystic component or represent the major part of the tumor. Morphologic findings suggestive of malignancy are:

- Irregular limits.
- Anechoic or less echogenic areas related to degenerative changes; however, this last finding is not specific and can also be seen in benign tumors.
- Usually in primary malignant tumor, in the absence of calcification, attenuation of the US beam is not depicted unlike what is commonly observed in benign tumors with a predominant fibrous component (fibrothecoma, Brenner tumor) and in dermoid cyst.

However, attenuation can be visualized in some metastases (Krukenberg) and exceptionally in primary carcinomas (Figs. 9.51 and 9.55 see mucinous carcinomas).

It must be outlined that the best findings of malignancy are morphologic findings associated with vascular findings.

On color Doppler, multiple irregular vessels are visualized in the central part and at the periphery of the echogenic portions with an irregular distribution [59, 86, 87] (Fig. 9.56).

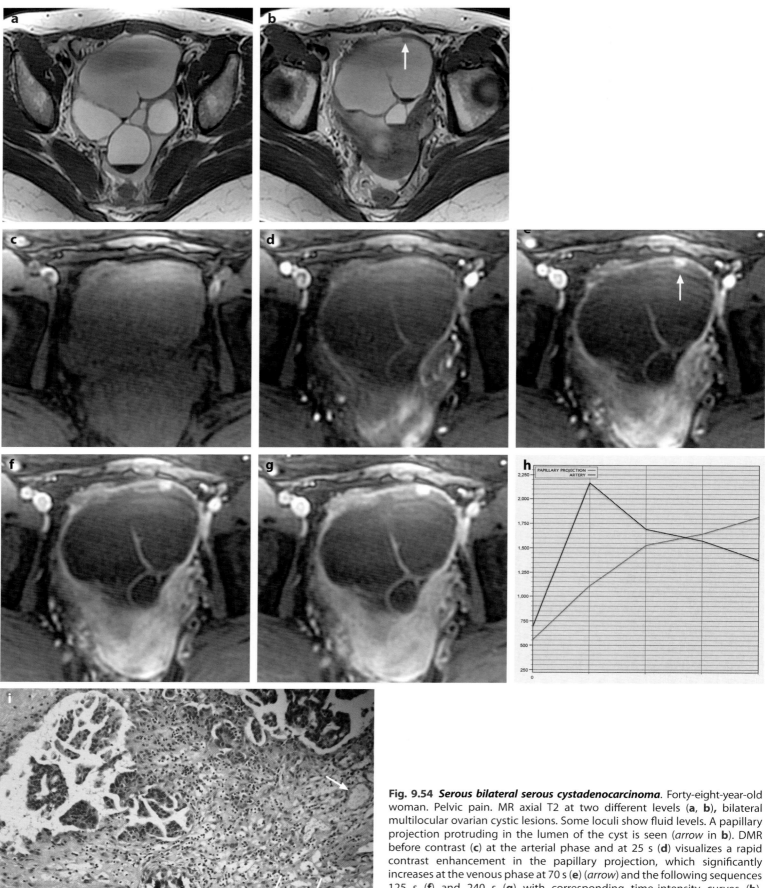

Fig. 9.54 *Serous bilateral serous cystadenocarcinoma*. Forty-eight-year-old woman. Pelvic pain. MR axial T2 at two different levels (**a**, **b**), bilateral multilocular ovarian cystic lesions. Some loculi show fluid levels. A papillary projection protruding in the lumen of the cyst is seen (*arrow* in **b**). DMR before contrast (**c**) at the arterial phase and at 25 s (**d**) visualizes a rapid contrast enhancement in the papillary projection, which significantly increases at the venous phase at 70 s (**e**) (*arrow*) and the following sequences 125 s (**f**) and 240 s (**g**) with corresponding time-intensity curves (**h**). Prospective diagnosis: borderline tumor or carcinoma. Surgery: the usual protocol for ovarian carcinoma. (**i**) At microscopy, a bilateral serous carcinoma is diagnosed. In the papillary projection, tumor cells and marked vascularization are present (*arrows*) explaining the rapid and high contrast uptake

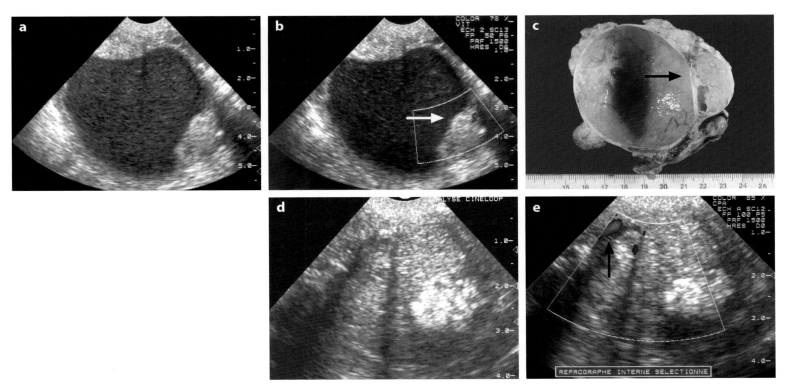

Fig. 9.55 Very atypical bilateral mucinous carcinoma with necrotic tissular portion. A 51-year-old women with pelvic pain. CA 125: 38 IU/ml. CA 19-9 was not performed. (1) Right ovary. TVS (**a**) with color Doppler (**b**) of the right ovary; 8 cm ovarian mass presenting a low echogenic homogeneous cystic component with a more echogenic focus measuring 2.8 cm in its inner part. Only a small vessel is visualized at the periphery of this echogenic focus (*arrow*), suggesting a possibility of solid tissue. (**c**) Pathologic specimen of the right ovary: a tissular portion occupied almost entirely by necrosis (which corresponded to the echogenic focus) (*arrow*). Exocystic vegetations were not visualized on US. Tiny multiple endocystic vegetations are visualized. (2) Left ovary. TVS (**d**) with color Doppler (**e**) left ovarian: 5 cm echogenic mass with acoustic shadowings containing a highly echogenic focus with few vessel on color Doppler (*arrow*). In fact at pathology, the mass was halfly cystic halfly solid with important necrotic changes. Prospective diagnosis: An epithelial-stromal tumor is the first possibility without being able to make any conclusion about its benign or malignant nature. Microscopy: bilateral mucinous carcinoma; stage Ib

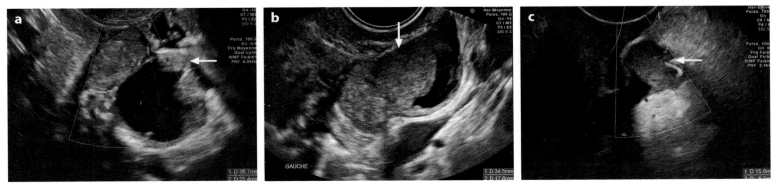

Fig. 9.56 Bilateral serous ovarian carcinoma. Fifty-one-year-old woman. In the follow-up of a canalar breast carcinoma treated 15 years before, a US is performed. Multiple stimulations of ovulation have been performed. EVS (**a**) displays a 4 cm right mixed ovarian mass with solid tissue containing tumoral vessels and endocystic papillary projections with a small vessel (*arrow*); the presence of papillary projections excludes the possibility of metastases and signifies the tumor is a primary epithelial and stromal malignant tumor. EVS (**b**) displays a 3.5 cm left mixed ovarian mass composed mainly of solid tissue (*arrow*). EVS (**c**) depicts solid tissue with an abnormal vessel in the Douglas pouch typical for a peritoneal metastases (*arrow*). CA 125 performed after US: 302 IU/ml. Prospective diagnosis: bilateral primary ovarian carcinoma with peritoneal metastases in the Douglas pouch. Surgery: total hysterectomy, bilateral adnexectomy, omentectomy, and lomboaortic curettage. Pathology: bilateral serous carcinoma grade 3. Peritoneal metastases in the Douglas pouch confirmed, with false negative on the omentum. False negative of metastases on the lomboaortic curettage only diagnosed at microscopy

On CT, without injection solid tissue is depicted with a density between 20 and 30 HU; on MR, the solid tissue usually appears on T2 with an intermediate signal (between pelvic muscle and adipose tissue) very characteristic of its malignant nature while on T1, its signal is close to pelvic muscle like benign fibrous tissue; degenerative changes can be seen. Calcifications are better displayed on CT. Multiple calcifications related to psammoma bodies can be seen through the mass (Figs. 9.57, 9.60, and 9.61).

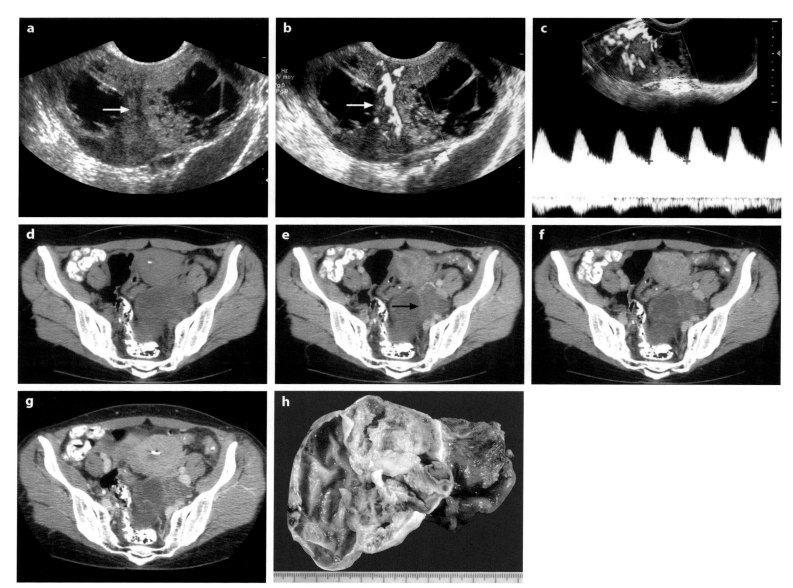

Fig. 9.59 A 44-year-old women with pelvic mass. Transversal EVS (**a**) and color Doppler (**b**): partly cystic and partly solid 9 cm tumor. The echogenic portion has an irregular border. The central portion contains a low echogenic line (*arrow*) related to large vessels on color Doppler (**b**) (*arrow*) typical for a malignant tumor. Spectral analysis (**c**) shows an RI 0.49; PI 0.72; PVS 37 cm/s. DCT without contrast (**d**) at the arterial phase (**e**) and the parenchymal phase (**f**), and on the delayed (**g**); although it demonstrates tumoral vessels (**e**) (*arrow*) and an early contrast uptake (**f**) (in the anterior part of the masses), very suggestive of malignant tumor, US and Doppler are in this case more demonstrative. Only a slight contrast uptake at the venous phase and on the delayed is visualized. Overall, CT did not demonstrate any extension. Preoperative diagnosis: stage 1a carcinoma. Surgery: although the tumor seemed to be localized to one ovary, a usual protocol of surgery was performed. Pathologic specimen (**h**): mixed ovarian mass. Tissular portion has irregular borders and degenerative changes. Microscopy: serous carcinoma stage Ia

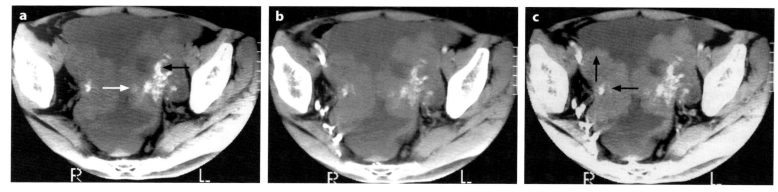

Fig. 9.60 Calcified bilateral serous ovarian carcinoma related to calcospherities. DCT before contrast (**a**) displays a bilateral ovarian tissular mass containing multiple tiny (*white arrow*) and dense conglomerates (*black arrow*) typical for calcospherites. At the arterial phase 20 s (**b**) and mainly 30 s after injection (**c**) fine irregular arterial vessels (*arrows*) typical for malignant tumors are visualized

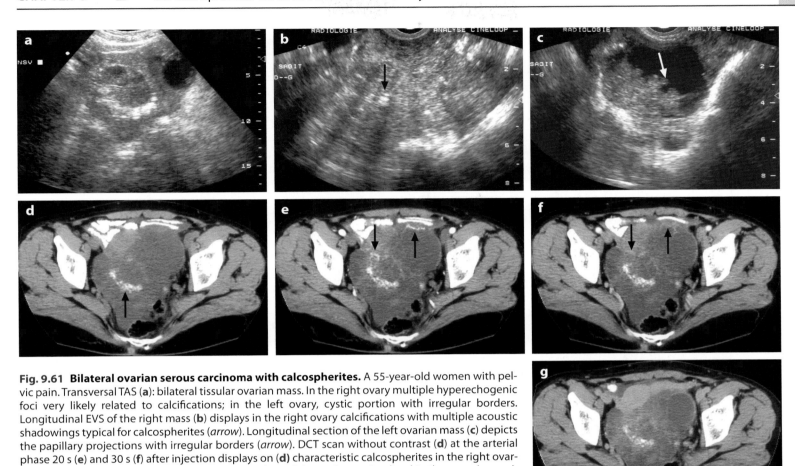

Fig. 9.61 Bilateral ovarian serous carcinoma with calcospherites. A 55-year-old women with pelvic pain. Transversal TAS (**a**): bilateral tissular ovarian mass. In the right ovary multiple hyperechogenic foci very likely related to calcifications; in the left ovary, cystic portion with irregular borders. Longitudinal EVS of the right mass (**b**) displays in the right ovary calcifications with multiple acoustic shadowings typical for calcospherites (*arrow*). Longitudinal section of the left ovarian mass (**c**) depicts the papillary projections with irregular borders (*arrow*). DCT scan without contrast (**d**) at the arterial phase 20 s (**e**) and 30 s (**f**) after injection displays on (**d**) characteristic calcospherites in the right ovarian mass (*arrow*). At the arterial phase (**e**) tumoral arterial vessels are visualized in the mass (*arrows*); high velocity in these arterial vessels illustrated by the wash-out on the next sequence (**f**) is characteristic for a malignant tumor. On the delayed (**g**) contrast uptake is displayed in the solid tissue; a peritoneal implant (*arrow*) with ascites is associated

Table 9.21 Differential diagnosis of mainly tissular or mixed patterns

Common
1. Subserous leiomyoma with degenerative changes when the normal ipsilateral ovary is not displayed
Fibrous tissue: US areas of attenuation, MR low signal on T2
Peripheral ring of regular vessels on Doppler, DMR, DCT
Early and equal to myometrium contrast uptake on DMR, DCT
2. Cystadenofibroma and benign ovarian tumors containing fibrous tissue with degenerative changes: fibrothecoma and Brenner tumor
Fibrous tissue: US areas of attenuation MR low signal on T2
Absence of vessels on Doppler, DMR, DCT (arterial phase)
Late and slight contrast uptake on DMR, DCT
Brenner: psammoma-like calcifications, association with a mucinous cystadenoma
3. Secondary tumors
Metastases: previous etiology, history, routes of dissemination, bilateral multinodular, particular aspects (Krukenberg)
4. Lymphoma
Bilateral, homogeneous, few vessels
Uncommon
1. Solid forms of ovarian abscess (actinomycosis)
2. Malignant germ cell
3. Sex cord stroma cell tumor (fibrosarcoma, Sertoli-Leydig tumor)
4. Tubal carcinoma
5. Broad ligament malignant tumor
6. Borderline with solid tissue
7. Sclerosing stromal tumor

Extension

See Sect. 9.10.

9.3.3.2 Particular and Uncommon Patterns

Micropapillary Serous Carcinoma (MPSC)

Pathology [89, 90]

It is a well-differentiated serous carcinoma usually purely *intra-epithelial* [50], *but the architecture is different from a borderline*: The distal papillary branches are thin and delicate and emanate abruptly from thick more centrally located papillae without intervening branches of successive intermediate size, unlike the hierarchical branching pattern of borderline tumors.

Cytologic features are different from a usual carcinoma: mild to moderate nuclear atypia unlike a conventional carcinoma.

In some cases, invasion has been reported. Because micropapillary and cribriform pattern may be focally present in borderline, an area of 5 mm in diameter of a confluent micropapillary pattern is required for the designation of MPSC.

The neoplastic cells have direct access to the peritoneal cavity and may exfoliate and implant on peritoneal surfaces accounting for the *strong association with invasive implants*.

General Features [50]
Bilateral in 64 % of cases
Stage 1 in 45 % of cases

Gross Findings
- Tumor growing exophytic from the surfaces of the ovaries, with slight to moderate invasion of the underlying parenchyma in 54 % of cases. This is the reason why these tumors have also been designated *serous surface carcinomas* (SSC or SSPC) [49, 91].
- Mean tumor size is 8.5 cm long.

- Papillary and cystic appearance resembling APSTs and little if any necrosis.
- Peritoneal implants commonly invasive.

Imaging Findings
1. In some cases, the tumor over the surface of the ovary is clearly seen (Figs. 9.57 and 9.62).
2. In other cases, the predominant pattern is a malignant process of the peritoneum, while the ovaries look normal on the imaging modalities (Fig. 9.63).

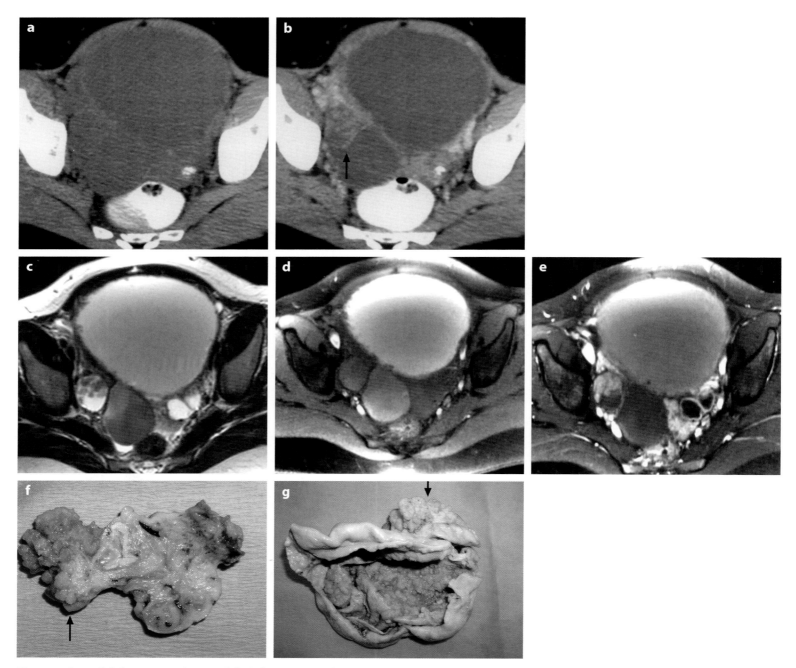

Fig. 9.62 *Superficial serous carcinoma of the left ovary.* (**a** and **b**): CT scan without (**a**) and after (**b**) contrast. Bilateral ovarian mass. On the left, an irregular tissular portion is visualized on the inner part of the mass. On the right, typical ovarian carcinoma. (**c**, **d**, and **e**) MR with T2 (**c**), fat suppression before (**d**), and after contrast (**e**) (*arrow*). On the left ovary, a superficial irregular excrescence is visualized on the medial part of the left ovary (*arrow*) which contains follicular cysts. Typical right ovarian carcinoma. (**f**) Pathologic specimen of the left ovary. A large tissular excrescence is seen arising from the surface of the left ovary. Magnified view after removing part of the mass shows an almost normal ovary with a corpus luteum cyst. (**g**) Pathologic specimen of the right ovary showing numerous endocystic and exocystic vegetations (*arrow*)

Psammocarcinoma

Definition

A rare variant of serous carcinoma that appears to arise as often in the peritoneum as in the ovaries [53].

Microscopy [53]

It is a carcinoma with destructive invasion of ovarian stroma. Epithelial cells are arranged in small nests and papillae.

Unlike a usual serous carcinoma, there are no areas of solid epithelial proliferation.

At least 75 % of papillae or nests are associated with *psammoma body formation.*

There is no more than moderate nuclear atypia, no mitotic figures.

Follow-Up

Although psammocarcinomas are usually discovered at a stage III, psammocarcinoma has a much slower evolution than the usual serous carcinoma and a relatively favorable prognosis [53].

Macroscopy

Ovarian carcinoma may be solid, cystic, or mixed (mean size is 11 cm).

Peritoneal carcinoma appears as a mass of 4–19 cm or multiple nodules from several millimeters to 2.5 cm.

Imaging Findings

MR Findings (Fig. 9.64)

Psammomas appear as low signal intensity areas in the ovarian tumors on T1 and T2; however, these findings are not specific for calcifications and could be misdiagnosed as fibrous tissue.

Peritoneal implants are visualized as thickening of the peritoneum with high signal intensity on diffusion and with a significant contrast uptake on DMR.

CT Findings

CT much better than US and MR allows to highly suggest the diagnosis of psammocarcinoma.

Tiny calcifications in both ovaries and over the peritoneum associated with findings of malignancy in the ovaries and the peritoneum are very suggestive of psammocarcinoma (Figs. 9.65 and 9.66).

Evolution

Late in the evolution, metastases can be displayed (Fig. 9.67) (see Sect. 9.12).

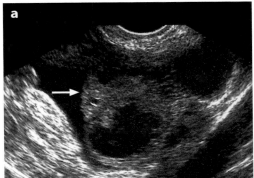
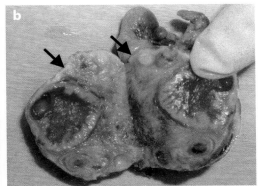

Fig. 9.63 Micropapillary serous carcinoma. A 35-year-old woman with pelvic pain. CA 125 335 IU/ml. EVS of the right ovary (**a**); size of the ovary is normal, it contains a corpus luteum cyst. Surface of the ovary is thickened and irregular (*arrow*). Pelvic ascites is present. Macroscopic specimen (**b**) displays at the surface of the ovary small papillary projections (*arrow*). Ovary contains a corpus luteum cyst and small corpora albicantia. Pathology: micropapillary serous carcinoma with peritoneal extension

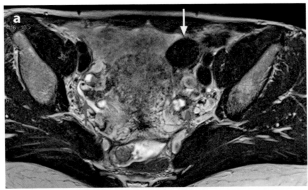

Fig. 9.64 *Ovarian and peritoneal psammocarcinoma*. A 42-year-old woman with abdominal pain for 1 year associated with meteorism. Right pelvic pain for a week. US: Calcified mass on the anterior part of the fundus suggested the possibility of a subserous leiomyoma. Ovarian calcifications. CA125 CA19-9 ACE normal. (1) *Ovary.* On MR axial T2 (**a**) low signal intensity foci in both ovaries (*red arrows*) which were proven to be calcifications on CT; low intensity left anterior pelvic mass (*white arrow*). (2) Peritoneal extension to the greater omentum. MR coronal T2 (**b**) and axial T2 (**c**): mass of the greater omentum of intermediate signal (*white arrow*) containing low intensity areas suspected to be related to calcifications (*red arrow*) surrounded by peritoneal ascites (*blue arrow*).

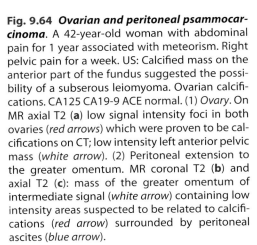
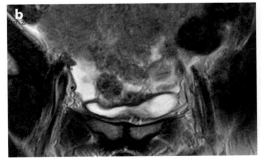
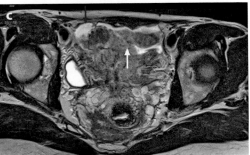

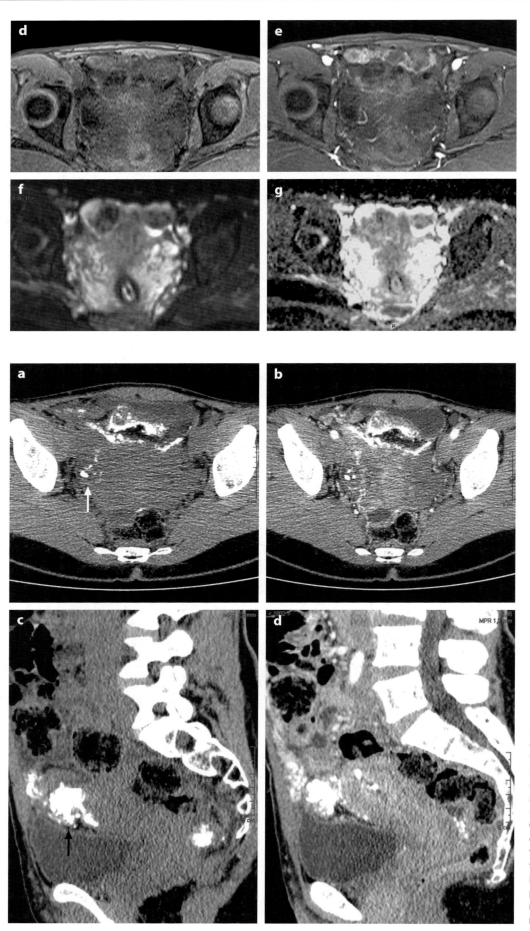

Fig. 9.64 (*continued*) On axial T1 without injection (**d**) and at the arterial phase (**e**) peripheral and central tumoral vessels are visualized. On diffusion (B0) (**f**) (B1000) (**g**) from outside to inside peritoneal fluid, high signal implants and calcified portion are visualized. Prospective diagnosis: implants with a tissular component surrounded with ascites, with bilateral ovarian low intensity foci of undetermined origin. CT is performed to precise the diagnosis (see Fig. 9.65)

Fig. 9.65 *Ovarian and peritoneal psammocarcinoma.* (Same patient as in Fig. 9.4 (1) *Ovary*. CT without contrast (**a**) and at the arterial phase (**b**) both ovaries mainly the right one containing calcifications related to psammoma calcifications at pathology (*arrow*). (2) *Peritoneal extension.* (1) *Serosa of the uterus and in the pouch of Douglas.* CT with sagittal reformation without contrast (**c**) displays a calcified round mass on the serosa of the uterus (*black arrow*) (more suggestive of peritoneal implant than a subserous leiomyoma) and in the Douglas's pouch (*red arrow*) with a thin peripheral enhancement at the arterial phase (**d**) related to peritoneal implants containing psammomas at pathology.

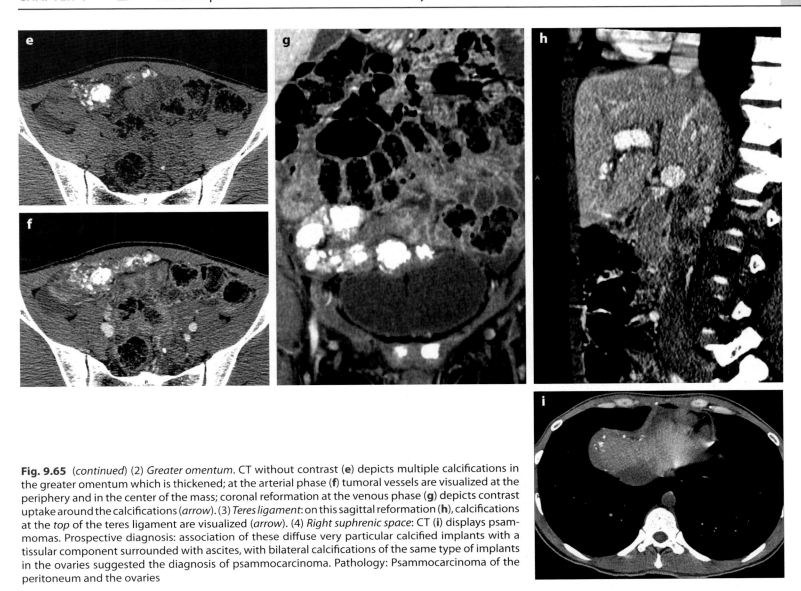

Fig. 9.65 (*continued*) (2) *Greater omentum*. CT without contrast (**e**) depicts multiple calcifications in the greater omentum which is thickened; at the arterial phase (**f**) tumoral vessels are visualized at the periphery and in the center of the mass; coronal reformation at the venous phase (**g**) depicts contrast uptake around the calcifications (*arrow*). (3) *Teres ligament*: on this sagittal reformation (**h**), calcifications at the *top* of the teres ligament are visualized (*arrow*). (4) *Right suphrenic space*: CT (**i**) displays psammomas. Prospective diagnosis: association of these diffuse very particular calcified implants with a tissular component surrounded with ascites, with bilateral calcifications of the same type of implants in the ovaries suggested the diagnosis of psammocarcinoma. Pathology: Psammocarcinoma of the peritoneum and the ovaries

Fig. 9.66 Peritoneal psammocarcinoma. A 57-year-old woman. Abdominal pain for 6 months; abdominal mass at the level of the umbilicus; CA 125 at 485 IU/ml. CT without injection (**a**, **b**) displays a round abdominal mass against the parietal abdominal peritoneum containing at its periphery dense calcifications.

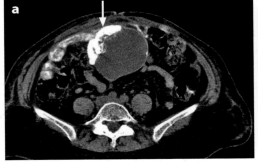

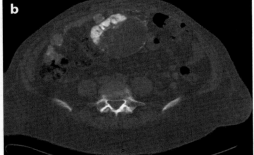

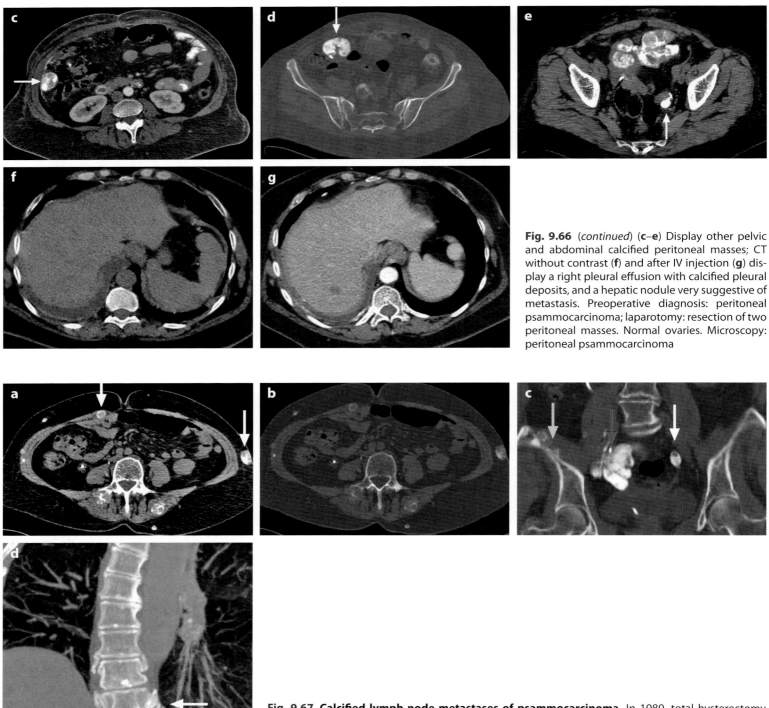

Fig. 9.66 (*continued*) (**c–e**) Display other pelvic and abdominal calcified peritoneal masses; CT without contrast (**f**) and after IV injection (**g**) display a right pleural effusion with calcified pleural deposits, and a hepatic nodule very suggestive of metastasis. Preoperative diagnosis: peritoneal psammocarcinoma; laparotomy: resection of two peritoneal masses. Normal ovaries. Microscopy: peritoneal psammocarcinoma

Fig. 9.67 Calcified lymph node metastases of psammocarcinoma. In 1989, total hysterectomy with bilateral adnexectomy for serous borderline tumor. In 1999, right subclavian calcified lymphadenopathy; at pathology, metastases from an adenocarcinoma. In 2003, recurrence of a right subclavian lymphadenopathy. CT without injection (**a** and **b**) displays metastases in the abdominal wall and in the subcutaneous tissue (*arrows*). On (**c**), metastatic calcified left iliac lymph node (*white arrow*) and a right pelvic calcified mass (*red arrow*) are visualized. Metastases to the right ilium (*yellow arrow*). On (**d**), metastases to the left eleventh rib is displayed (*arrow*)

9.4　Mucinous Tumors

Mucinous tumors account for 31 % of all epithelial ovarian tumors and are second in frequency after serous epithelia tumors; 23 % are benign, 4 % borderline, 4 % carcinomas (Table 9.3). They are characterized by glands and cysts lined by epithelial cells, some of which contain abundant intracytoplasmic mucin.

These tumors can be associated with:

(a) Another ovarian tumor:
- Dermoid cysts in 3–5 % of cases
- Brenner tumor

(b) A mucinous tumor of another organ especially mucinous tumor of the appendix that is almost always accompanied by pseudomyxoma peritonei.

(c) A mucinous adenocarcinoma of the uterine cervix, particularly those of adenoma malignum. This association may occur in patients with Peutz-Jeghers syndrome.

(d) Among the ovarian tumors with functioning stroma, mucinous ovarian tumors are among the most common neoplasms. The most common clinical syndromes are those caused by the secretion of steroid hormones that are probably produced predominantly by the stroma within or surrounding the tumor.

9.4.1　Benign Mucinous Tumors

9.4.1.1　General Features

They account for 23 % of all epithelial ovarian tumors (Table 9.3).

Most of them occur during the third to fifth decade [92]. They are bilateral in 2–5 % of the cases [93, 94].

9.4.1.2　Pathology

Macroscopy (see Table 9.22) (Fig. 9.68)

Microscopy [93] (Fig. 9.69)
They are lined by a single layer of uniform tall columnar cells with clear or basophilic cytoplasm and small basal hyperchromatic nucleoli.

Goblet cells are almost always present and indicate gastrointestinal differentiation. Rarely, endocervical mucinous epithelium predominates, usually associated with a papillary architecture.

More complex cystadenomas have multiple locules that may be similar or of widely varying size, some of which display a peripheral arrangement of small acini or daughter cysts that may create a pseudoinvasive pattern.

The complexity of glandular and papillary arrangement may be quite florid, and the presence or absence of invasion is difficult to assess.

Table 9.22 Macroscopic and radiologic findings of benign mucinous tumors

Common
– Cystic usually superior to 10 cm
– Convoluted surface
– Multiloculated (usually less numerous loculi than in borderline or carcinoma)
– Regular thick wall (2–3 mm), collagenous, acellular, sometimes with dystrophic calcification
– Regular septa
– Containing liquids of different nature: thick stringy, watery, hemorrhagic
Uncommon
– Small
– Unilocular

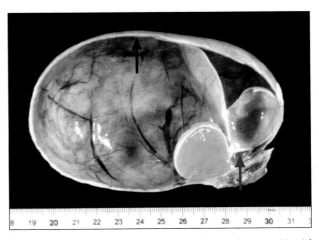

Fig. 9.68 Macroscopic specimen. Multilocular cystic mass. Liquids of different natures, with *yellow thick* material in one loculation, while clear fluid and hemorrhagic fluid were eliminated at the opening of the tumor. Three thick and regular wall (*black arrow*) and septa (*blue arrow*)

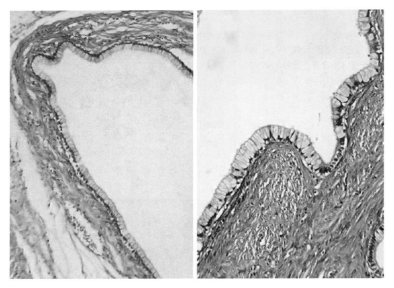

Fig. 9.69 Mucinous epithelium: (1) on the left of endocervical type and (2) on the right with goblet cells of intestinal type

9.4.1.3 Imaging Findings

The Macroscopic and Radiologic Findings

The macroscopic and radiologic findings of benign mucinous tumors are summarized in Table 9.22. These tumors are often >10 cm and in some cases may fill the abdominopelvic peritoneal cavity; in this last case, CT is much more appropriate than US and MR for a complete study of the tumor [93–95].

The Multilocular Form

Wall and Septa

On US, they are echogenic and regular with vessels on color Doppler. On MR, they appear with a low signal on T2. On the DMR (Fig. 9.70) and on the DCT at the arterial phase, regular vessels can be displayed. At the venous phase, contrast uptake is depicted which progressively increases on the delayed phases.

Rarely, calcifications may be present in the wall or in the septa. CT is the best method to display them (Fig. 9.71).

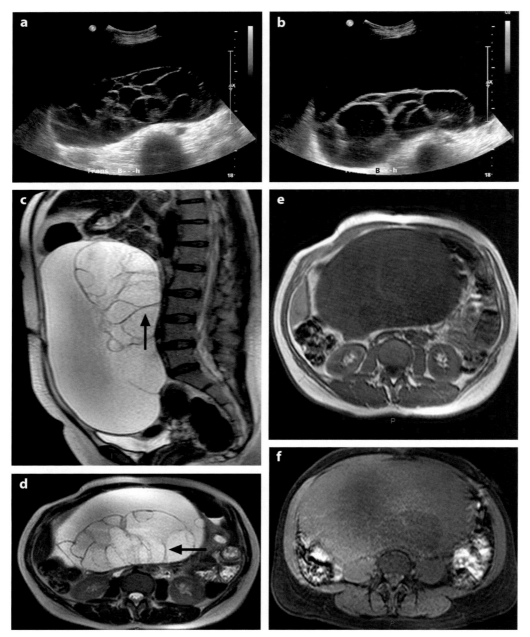

Fig. 9.70 Mucinous cystadenoma. Fifty-year-old woman with increase volume of the abdomen falsely considered clinically as ascites. CA 125 and CA 19-9 are normal. EVS transverse (**a**) and longitudinal (**b**) sections display a left multiloculated cystic mass, containing liquids of different echogenicities, very suggestive of mucinous tumor. Because of the large volume of the tumor, MR is indicated. MR sagittal T2 (**c**), axial T2 (**d**), axial T1 (**e**), and fat suppression (**f**) display loculi of different signal intensities separated by regular septa (*arrows*).

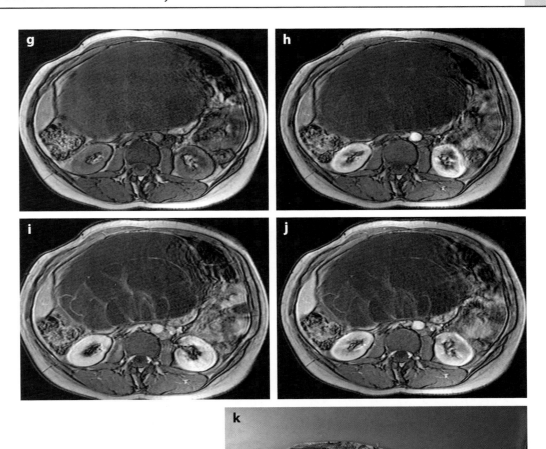

Fig. 9.70 (*continued*) DMR without injection (**g**) at the arterial phase (**h**), at the venous phase (**i**), and on the delayed (**j**) rules out findings of malignancy. Prospective diagnosis: mucinous cystadenoma. Although association with normal tumoral markers in a tumor of that volume reinforced the diagnosis of benignity, a laparotomy with a usual protocol of ovarian carcinoma was performed. Pathologic specimen (**k**) does not visualize any finding of malignancy. Microscopy: mucinous cystadenoma of endocervical type. Laparotomy: total hysterectomy, bilateral adnexectomy, and omentectomy. Microscopy: mucinous cystadenoma (type not precised)

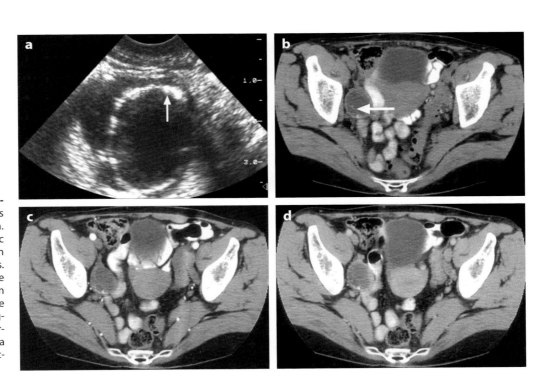

Fig. 9.71 *Mucinous cystadenoma with calcifications.* A 59-year-old woman with pelvic mass discovered on a routine clinical examination. Normal CA 125. (**a**) *EVS*: multiloculated right cystic ovarian mass with multiple hyperechogenic foci in the wall and septa very likely related to calcifications. (**b**) CT scan without contrast confirms the presence of calcifications (*arrow*). (**c** and **d**) Dynamic CT scan at the arterial phase (**c**) and the parenchymal phase (**d**) demonstrates the absence of findings of malignancy. Celioscopy with right ovariectomy was performed. Pathology: mucinous cystadenofibroma with more or less thick calcifications in the connective tissue

When the septa are numerous and gathered in a part of the tumor, after contrast, they can simulate a solid tissue, and differentiation from a borderline or malignant tumor is difficult (Fig. 9.72).

Loculi

On US (Figs. 9.70 and 9.73), they have different echogenicities from anechoic to echogenic.

Hyperechogenic foci floating in the liquid are very particular to mucinous cystadenoma (Figs. 9.74, 9.75, and 9.76).

Sometimes, they display a ground glass pattern quite similar to endometriosis (Figs. 9.77 and 9.78).

On MR (Figs. 9.78 and 9.79), on T1, usually at least one loculation has an intermediate signal related to a hemorrhagic or mucinous content; on fat suppression, signal intensity can be very high like endometriosis. On T2, they have different signal intensities with an intermediate signal, between pelvic muscle and adipose tissue, (blood) to a signal superior to urine (mucinous content).

On CT, they appear with different signal intensities [96, 97].

Very uncommonly, a fluid level due to a hemorrhagic content can be depicted (Fig. 9.80).

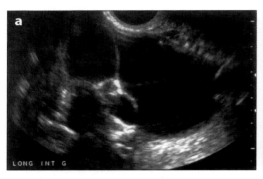
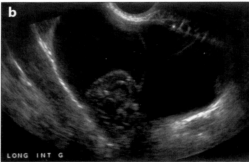
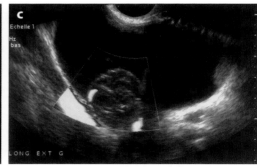

Fig. 9.72 Mucinous cystadenoma. EVS (**a**) displays a multilocular cystic mass containing liquids of different signal intensities. (**b**) In one part of the tumor, a round echogenic portion suggests two possibilities, solid tissue or more likely gathered septa. Color Doppler (**c**) displays some regular vessels at the periphery and a small one in the center. Prospective diagnosis: a mucinous tumor is diagnosed; benign tumor is first suggested; because of the gathered septa, a borderline tumor cannot be excluded. Laparotomy: left ovarian cystectomy. Microscopy: mucinous cystadenoma

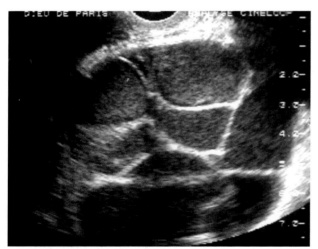

Fig. 9.73 Multilocular mucinous cystadenoma. Forty-year-old woman. Increase size of the abdomen. CA 125 and CA 19-9 normal. US displays a multilocular cystic mass with regular wall and septa containing liquids of different echogenicities, without papillary projection or solid tissue. Prospective diagnosis: mucinous cystadenoma. Laparotomy: right adnexectomy. Microscopy: mucinous cystadenoma

Fig. 9.74 Endocervical mucinous cystadenoma. Forty-five-year-old woman. Left pelvic pain. EVS transverse (**a**) and sagittal (**b**) display a unilocular ovarian cystic mass containing a low level echogenic fluid with very particular hyperechogenic foci floating in the cyst (*arrow*) characteristic for a mucinous cystadenoma. In the dependent portion of the cyst, lying in the wall, a hyperechogenic band (*arrow*) was related to calcifications at pathology. Prospective diagnosis: mucinous cystadenoma. Celioscopy: right ovarian cystectomy. Microscopy: endocervical type of mucinous cystadenoma

Fig. 9.75 Unilocular mucinous cystadenoma. Forty-nine-year-old woman. Abdominal pain. EVS (**a**) displays an 8 cm unilocular ovarian cyst, pushing the normal ovarian parenchyma toward the periphery. Content of the cyst is slightly echogenic; very particular multiple echogenic foci in the wall of the cyst are very suggestive of mucinous tumor (*arrow*). On (**b**), echogenic material is present in the dependent part of the cyst (very likely related to mucin) (*arrow*). Prospective diagnosis: benign ovarian cyst. Celioscopy: cystectomy. Microscopy: mucinous cystadenoma (cellular type not precised)

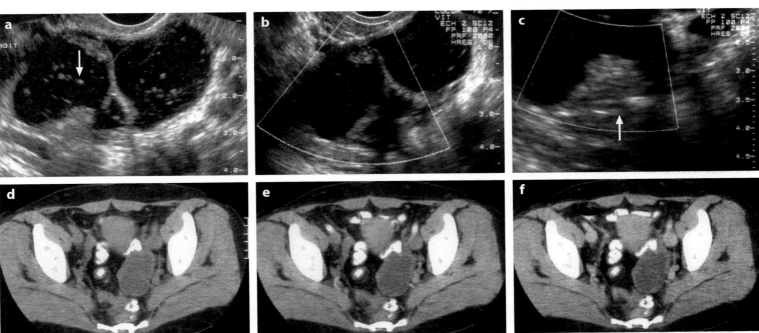

Fig. 9.76 *Multilocular mucinous cystadenoma.* A 53-year-old-woman with pelvic mass at physical examination. (**a**) *EVS*: multiloculated cystic mass containing echogenic portions against the inner wall and septum with floating echogenic material very suggestive of mucinous tumor (*arrow*). (**b** and **c**) *EVS with color Doppler*: no color flow in the echogenic portions (*arrow*) allowing to rule out a malignant tissular portion. (**d**, **e**, and **f**) *DCT scan without contrast* (**d**), *at the arterial phase* (**e**), *and at the parenchymal phase* (**f**): no abnormal vascularization or contrast uptake is seen in the echogenic portions confirming the absence of malignancy and the absence of tissular portion. Prospective diagnosis: a mucinous cystadenoma is suggested first; a borderline cannot be excluded. *Laparotomy*: total hysterectomy with bilateral adnexectomy. *Pathology*: multilocular mucinous cystadenoma without vegetation or solid portion

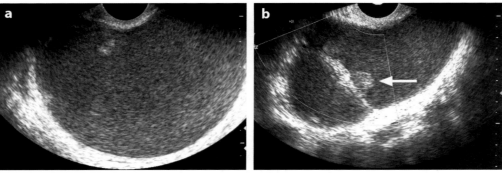

Fig. 9.77 Multilocular mucinous cystadenoma resembling an endometrioma. A 48-year-old woman. *EVS* (**a**): right ovarian bilocular cyst containing uniform low level echoes with ground glass pattern very suggestive of endometrioma. Color Doppler (**b**) displays a bilocular pattern with an echogenic foci without color flow (*arrow*), misinterpreted as a clot. Prospective diagnosis: endometrioma. MR was performed to evaluate extension. *Surgery*: bilateral adnexectomy. *Pathology*: right mucinous cystadenoma

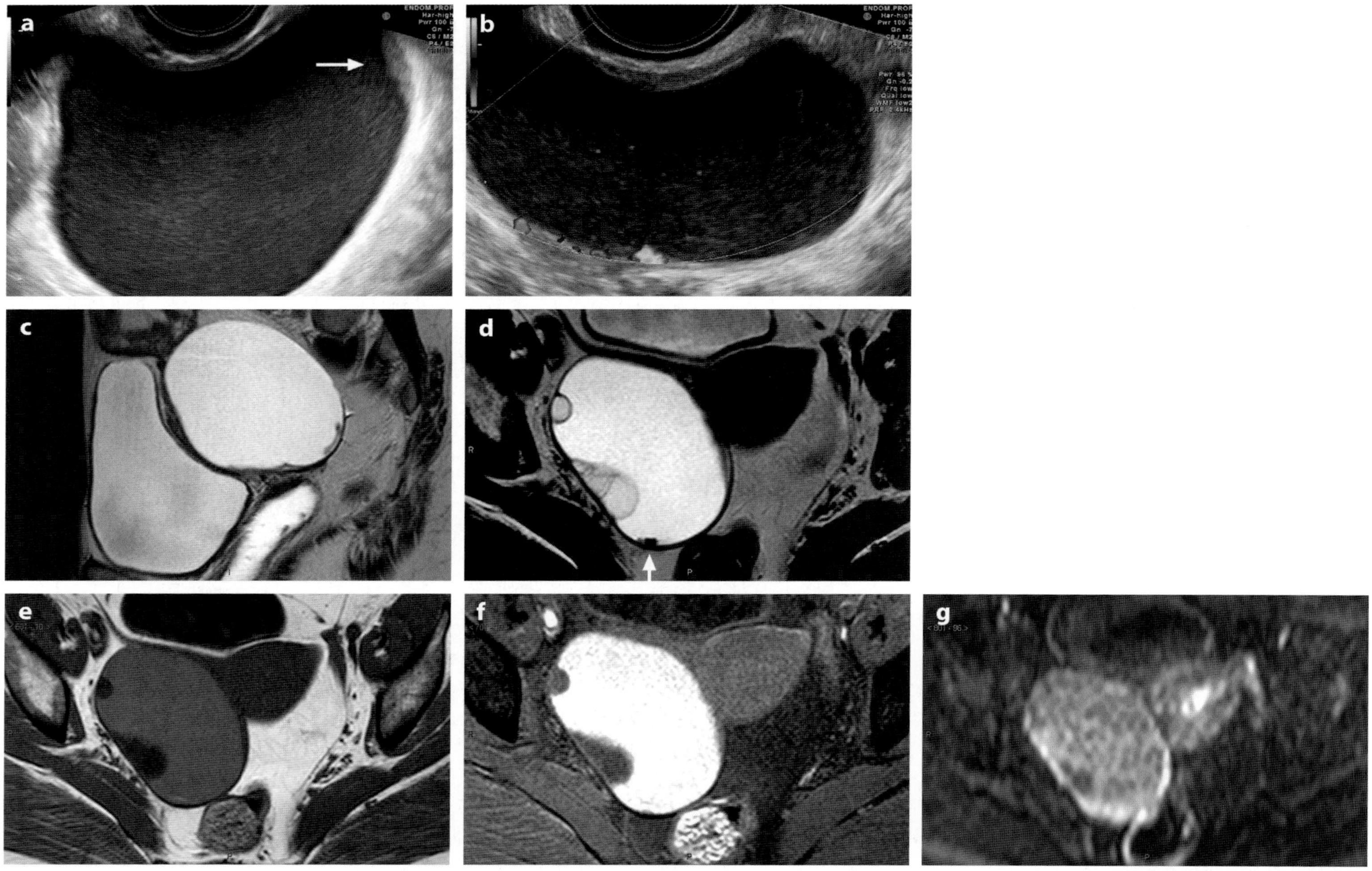

Fig. 9.78 Multilocular mucinous cystadenoma of endocervical type. Forty-two-year-old woman, with a known left ovarian cyst followed for 1 year. Right pelvic pain. CA 125 and CA 19-9 normal. US (**a**) displays a right ovarian cystic mass with a ground glass pattern; an echogenic deposit is visualized in the dependent portion of the cyst (*arrow*). On color Doppler (**b**), no vessel is demonstrated in this mass with few vessels in the wall, which rules out an abscess. Some echogenic foci are visualized in the middle part of the cystic content which could be related to clots or aggregation of mucinous deposits. Prospective diagnosis: two diagnoses can be discussed, endometriosis, mucinous cystadenoma. MR sagittal T2 (**c**) and axial T2 (**d**) display a 10 cm left multilocular ovarian mass containing liquids of different nature, with a thin wall and thin and regular septa without any papillary projection. Some septa gathered in the upper pole of the tumor are very suggestive of mucinous tumor. Deposits in the dependent part of the cyst (**d**) could be related to clots or mucin (*arrow*). On axial T1 (**e**) and with fat suppression (**f**), liquids appear with different signals; on T1, the most important loculation has an intermediate signal which is different from the typical high signal intensity of endometriosis. Diffusion b1000 (**g**) fluid is of low intensity.

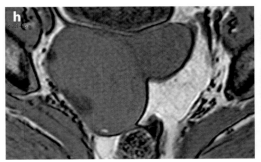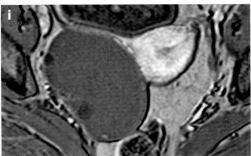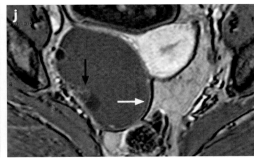

Fig. 9.78 (*continued*) DMR without injection (**h**) at the arterial phase (**i**); regular vessels are visualized in the septa, with a progressive increase of the contrast enhancement in the septa and in the wall at the venous phase (**j**) (*black* and *white arrows*, respectively). Prospective diagnosis: mucinous cystadenoma. Diffusion sequence (b1000) and DMR display a blurring of the posterior border of the ovarian mass in contact with the sigmoid very suggestive of adhesion. Coelioscopy: pelvic peritoneal adhesions in the ovarian fossa and in the Douglas right adnexectomy. Microscopy: endocervical mucinous cystadenoma

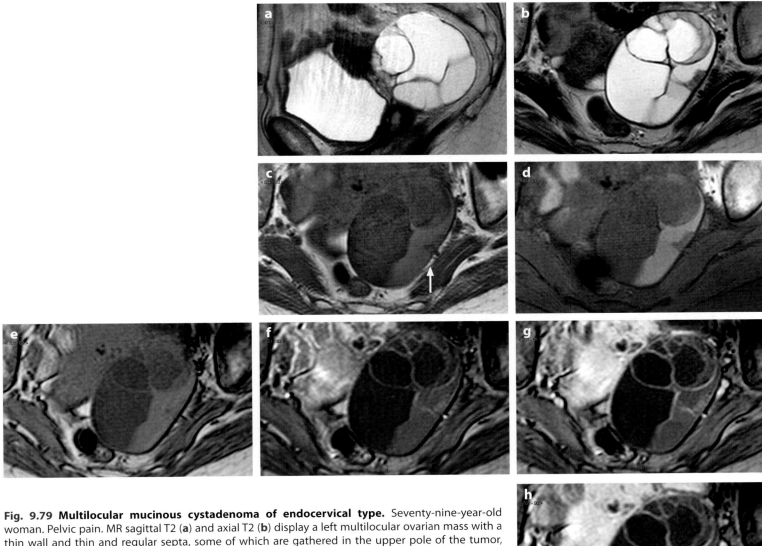

Fig. 9.79 Multilocular mucinous cystadenoma of endocervical type. Seventy-nine-year-old woman. Pelvic pain. MR sagittal T2 (**a**) and axial T2 (**b**) display a left multilocular ovarian mass with a thin wall and thin and regular septa, some of which are gathered in the upper pole of the tumor, without any papillary projection. Liquids are of different nature. On axial T1 (**c**) and with fat suppression (**d**), liquids appear with different signals; a lateral loculation has an intermediate signal (*arrow*). DMR without injection (**e**) at the arterial phase (**f**), regular vessels are visualized in the septa, with a progressive increase of the contrast enhancement in the septa at the venous phase (**g**) and on the delayed (**h**). Prospective diagnosis: mucinous cystadenoma. Surgery: left adnexectomy with peritoneal washings. Microscopy: mucinous cystadenoma of endocervical type. Immunohistochemistry: CK7++, CK20+ are in accordance with an ovarian origin

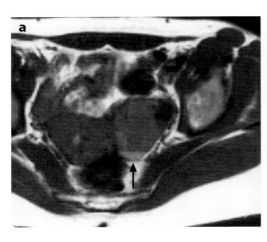

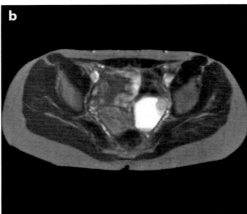

Fig. 9.80 Mucinous cystadenoma with a hemorrhagic level. A 24-year-old woman with pelvic pain. (**a**) Transverse axial T1 MR: left ovarian multilocular cystic mass with a fluid level in the largest loculation. The fluid in the dependent portion has a high signal intensity (*arrow*) comprised between pelvic muscles and adipose tissue. (**d**) Axial MR SE T2-weighted image: the liquid in the dependent portion has a signal intensity lower that the one in the dependent portion. *Laparotomy* with left cystectomy was performed. *Pathology*: left multilocular mucinous cystadenoma. The liquid of the cyst contained necrotic material rich in red blood cells and polynuclear white cells

More Rarely, the Mass Is Unilocular

On US, the liquid is echogenic which is usually different from the non-echogenic cystic content of a serous cystadenoma.

Uncommonly, the content on US is so viscous that it can mimic solid tissue (Fig. 9.81). Color Doppler in demonstrating the absence of color flow in the echogenic portion can highly suggest the cystic nature of this component DCT (Fig. 9.81), or DMR can definitely prove the cystic nature of the tumor.

On MR, on T1, signal intensity of the liquid is superior to urine (Fig. 9.82).

Rarely, the borders of the mass are so convoluted that it may let discuss a possibility of a hydrosalpinx (Fig. 9.83).

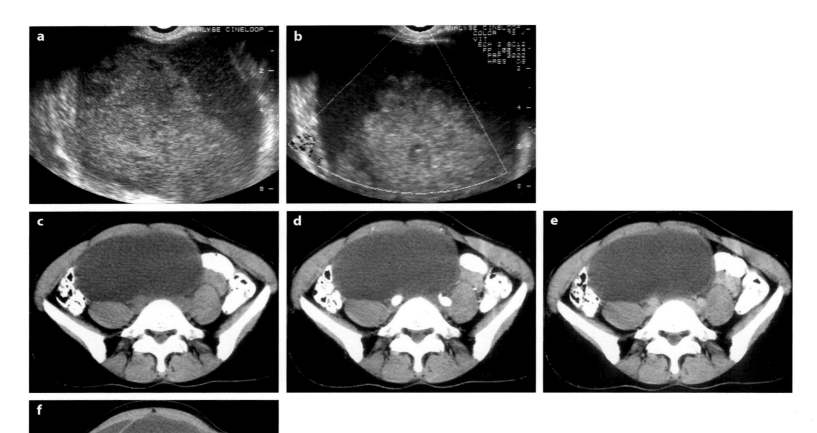

Fig. 9.81 *Multilocular mucinous cystadenoma.* A 35-year-old woman with abdominopelvic mass. CA 125: 48 IU/ml (normal <35 IU/ml). (**a**) *Endovaginal US*: huge echogenic portion with an irregular surface lying against the inner wall of the cyst suggesting a malignant tumor. (**b**) *Endovaginal US with color Doppler*: no vessel is displayed in the entire echogenic portion, allowing to rule out the diagnosis of a malignancy. (**c–f**) *DCT scan without contrast* (**c**), at the *arterial phase* (**d**), at the *parenchymal phase* (**e**), and *delayed scan* (**f**) demonstrate absence of vegetation or tissular portion in the ovarian tumor. Prospective diagnosis: benign epithelial tumor. *Laparotomy* with right ovarian cystectomy and left ovarian biopsy was performed. *Pathology*: Mucinous cystadenoma (Figures (**a**, **b**) from Author's personal publication: Buy et al. [8])

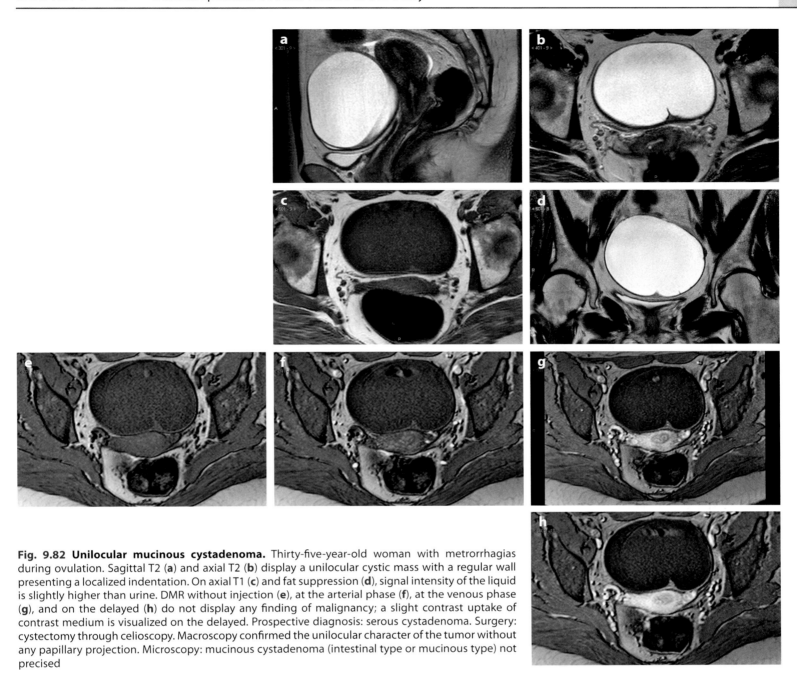

Fig. 9.82 Unilocular mucinous cystadenoma. Thirty-five-year-old woman with metrorrhagias during ovulation. Sagittal T2 (**a**) and axial T2 (**b**) display a unilocular cystic mass with a regular wall presenting a localized indentation. On axial T1 (**c**) and fat suppression (**d**), signal intensity of the liquid is slightly higher than urine. DMR without injection (**e**), at the arterial phase (**f**), at the venous phase (**g**), and on the delayed (**h**) do not display any finding of malignancy; a slight contrast uptake of contrast medium is visualized on the delayed. Prospective diagnosis: serous cystadenoma. Surgery: cystectomy through celioscopy. Macroscopy confirmed the unilocular character of the tumor without any papillary projection. Microscopy: mucinous cystadenoma (intestinal type or mucinous type) not precised

Fig. 9.83 Unilocular mucinous cystadenoma.
Fifty-three-year-old woman. Sagittal (**a**) and axial (**b**) T2 display a unilocular cystic mass, with convoluted inferior border which lets discuss a possibility of hydrosalpinx. Visualization of the normal right ovary, while a normal left ovary independent of the mass is not visualized, and the fact as the tumor is completely surrounded by a low intensity rim is in favor of an ovarian origin.

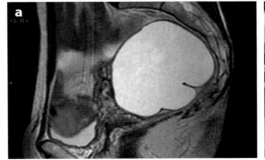
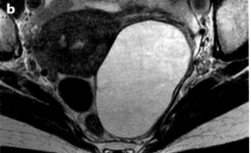

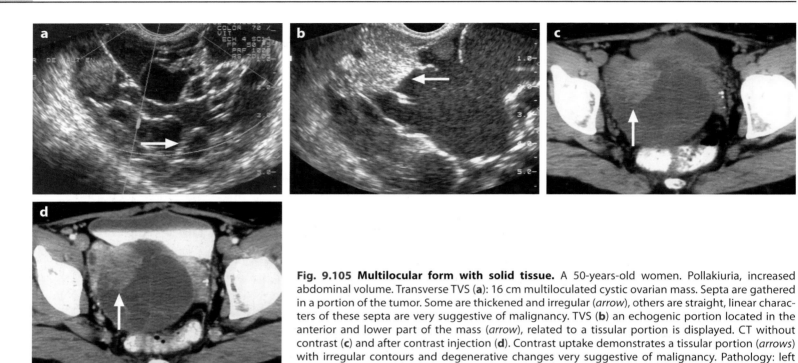

Fig. 9.105 Multilocular form with solid tissue. A 50-years-old women. Pollakiuria, increased abdominal volume. Transverse TVS (**a**): 16 cm multiloculated cystic ovarian mass. Septa are gathered in a portion of the tumor. Some are thickened and irregular (*arrow*), others are straight, linear characters of these septa are very suggestive of malignancy. TVS (**b**) an echogenic portion located in the anterior and lower part of the mass (*arrow*), related to a tissular portion is displayed. CT without contrast (**c**) and after contrast injection (**d**). Contrast uptake demonstrates a tissular portion (*arrows*) with irregular contours and degenerative changes very suggestive of malignancy. Pathology: left mucinous carcinoma; stage I

Fig. 9.106 Multiloculated cystic form. A 48-year-old women with abdominopelvic mass. (**a** and **b**) EVS: 17 cm left ovarian multiloculated cystic mass containing liquids of different echogenicities. The septa are gathered in a portion of the tumor; some look thick and irregular (*arrow*). DCT without contrast (**c**) at the arterial phase (**d**) and at the venous phase (**e**) does not demonstrate any abnormal vessel and early contrast uptake. Some septa are thick and irregular (*arrow*) No tissular portion is visualized. Prospective diagnosis: a mucinous tumor is suggested; because of the character of the septa, a borderline tumor is most likely. Pathology: left mucinous cystadenocarcinoma; stage I

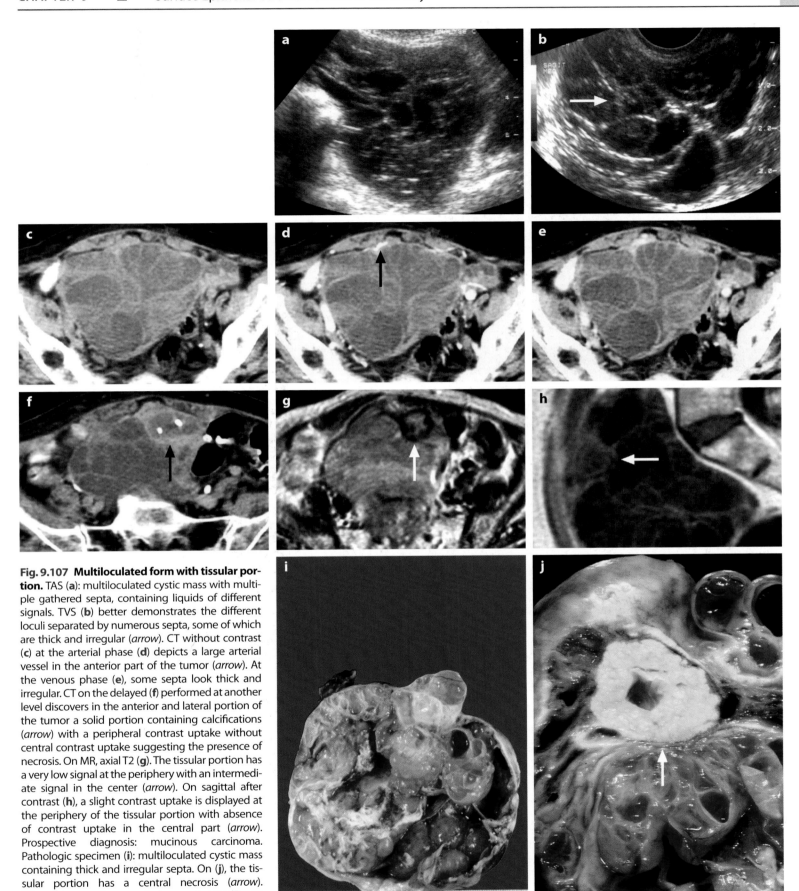

Fig. 9.107 Multiloculated form with tissular portion. TAS (**a**): multiloculated cystic mass with multiple gathered septa, containing liquids of different signals. TVS (**b**) better demonstrates the different loculi separated by numerous septa, some of which are thick and irregular (*arrow*). CT without contrast (**c**) at the arterial phase (**d**) depicts a large arterial vessel in the anterior part of the tumor (*arrow*). At the venous phase (**e**), some septa look thick and irregular. CT on the delayed (**f**) performed at another level discovers in the anterior and lateral portion of the tumor a solid portion containing calcifications (*arrow*) with a peripheral contrast uptake without central contrast uptake suggesting the presence of necrosis. On MR, axial T2 (**g**). The tissular portion has a very low signal at the periphery with an intermediate signal in the center (*arrow*). On sagittal after contrast (**h**), a slight contrast uptake is displayed at the periphery of the tissular portion with absence of contrast uptake in the central part (*arrow*). Prospective diagnosis: mucinous carcinoma. Pathologic specimen (**i**): multiloculated cystic mass containing thick and irregular septa. On (**j**), the tissular portion has a central necrosis (*arrow*). Microscopy: mucinous cystadenocarcinoma (Figure (**b**) from Author's personal publication: Buy et al. [8])

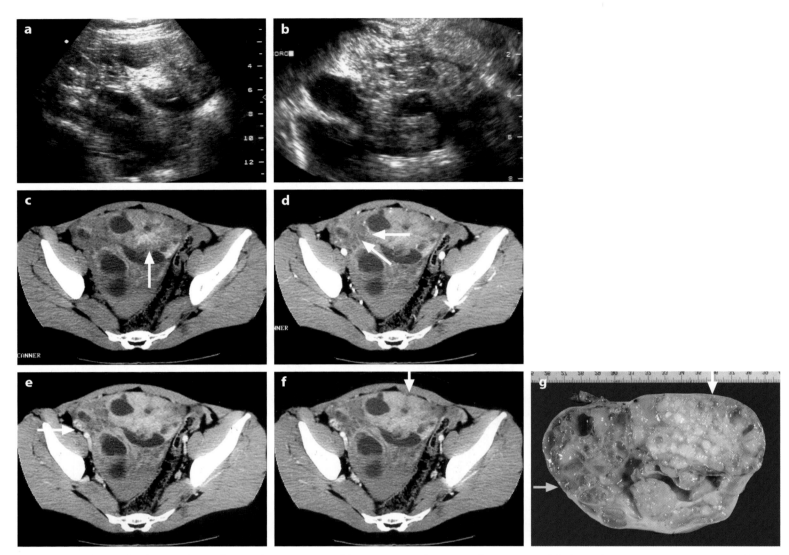

Fig. 9.108 Multilocular form with tissular portion. A 31-year-old women with amenorrhea and abdominopelvic mass. CA 125: 54 IU/ml. TAS (**a**) displays a mixed ovarian mass containing a hyperechogenic focus in its anterior portion without acoustic shadowing. EVS (**b**) depicts multiple hyperechogenic foci and cystic portions in the mass. DCT without contrast (**c**) displays a mixed right ovarian mass, containing several loculi and in its solid tissue multiple calcifications. At the arterial phase (20 s after injection) (**d**), tumoral arterial vessels (*arrows*) typical for a malignant tumor are visualized. At 30 s after injection (**e**), the right ovarian artery appears enlarged; contrast in some arterial vessels decreases, while contrast appears in some other vessels. At the venous phase (**f**), a significant contrast uptake in a tissular portion is demonstrated (*arrow*). Prospective diagnosis: carcinoma of the ovary. Pathologic specimen (**g**): (1) Solid tissue in the anterior and left portion of the mass (*white arrow*). (2) Cystic portion with numerous and gathered septa is displayed (*yellow arrow*). Microscopy: *Mucinous cystadenocarcinoma*

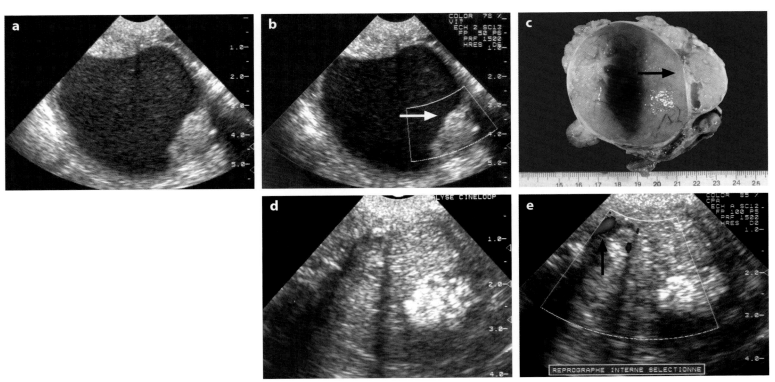

Fig. 9.109 Very atypical bilateral mucinous carcinoma with necrotic tissular portion. A 51-year-old women with pelvic pain. CA 125: 38 IU/ml. CA 19-9 was not performed. (1) Right ovary. (**a** and **b**) TVS (**a**) with color Doppler (**b**) of the right ovary; 8 cm ovarian mass presenting a low echogenic homogeneous cystic component with a more echogenic focus measuring 2.8 cm in its inner part. Only a small vessel is visualized at the periphery of this echogenic focus (*arrow*), suggesting a possibility of solid tissue. (**c**) Pathologic specimen of the right ovary: a tissular portion occupied almost entirely by necrosis (which corresponded to the echogenic focus) (*arrow*). Exocystic vegetations were not visualized on US. Tiny multiple endocystic vegetations are visualized. (2) Left ovary. (**d** and **e**) TVS (**d**) with color Doppler (**e**) left ovarian: 5 cm echogenic mass with acoustic shadowings containing a highly echogenic focus with few vessel on color Doppler (*arrow*). In fact at pathology, the mass was halfly cystic halfly solid with important necrotic changes. Prospective diagnosis: an epithelial-stromal tumor is the first possibility without being able to make any conclusion about its benign or malignant nature. Microscopy: bilateral mucinous carcinoma; stage Ib

The Mainly Solid Pattern

In uncommon cases, the tumor is mainly solid. While in these forms, CT (Fig. 9.110) or MR displays typical vascular findings of malignancy, vascularization is not as well demonstrated on US.

Differential Diagnosis

Whatever the imaging modality used, the differential diagnosis (Table 9.7) of mucinous carcinoma with borderline and even in some cases of benign mucinous tumor can be very difficult [118]. This is particularly true in ultrasound because of the frequent important volume of the mass which is impossible to analyze completely with endovaginal ultrasound and which is difficult to correctly analyze with suprapubic examination. The other differential diagnoses are reported in Table 9.26.

The most difficult problem in the differential of mucinous carcinoma of the ovary is their distinction from metastasis (intestinal, appendiceal, uterine cervix).

Metastatic mucinous carcinomas are much more common than primary mucinous carcinoma. They can have very similar morphologic features. However, location seems to be a very interesting finding to differentiate them. In a series, among bilateral tumors,

6 % were primary and 94 % metastatic (Seidman). Other findings suggesting metastatic lesions are:

- Previous history of one of these tumors
- Dissemination along different pathways as that of primary ovarian tumors

Table 9.26 Differential diagnosis of mucinous carcinoma

Common
Metastatic mucinous carcinoma
Differential diagnosis is based on bilaterality (6 % for primary; 94 % for secondary), history of previous mucinous carcinoma, and different routes of dissemination
Etiologies are:
From GI tract
Colon
Intestinal (60 % of cases)
Appendix
Biliary tract
Pancreas
From endocervix or uterus
APMT
Their gross appearance can be very similar
Uncommon
Very rare malignant tumors with a mucinous component:
Hypercalcemic type of small cell carcinoma
The rare form of mucinous carcinoid tumor

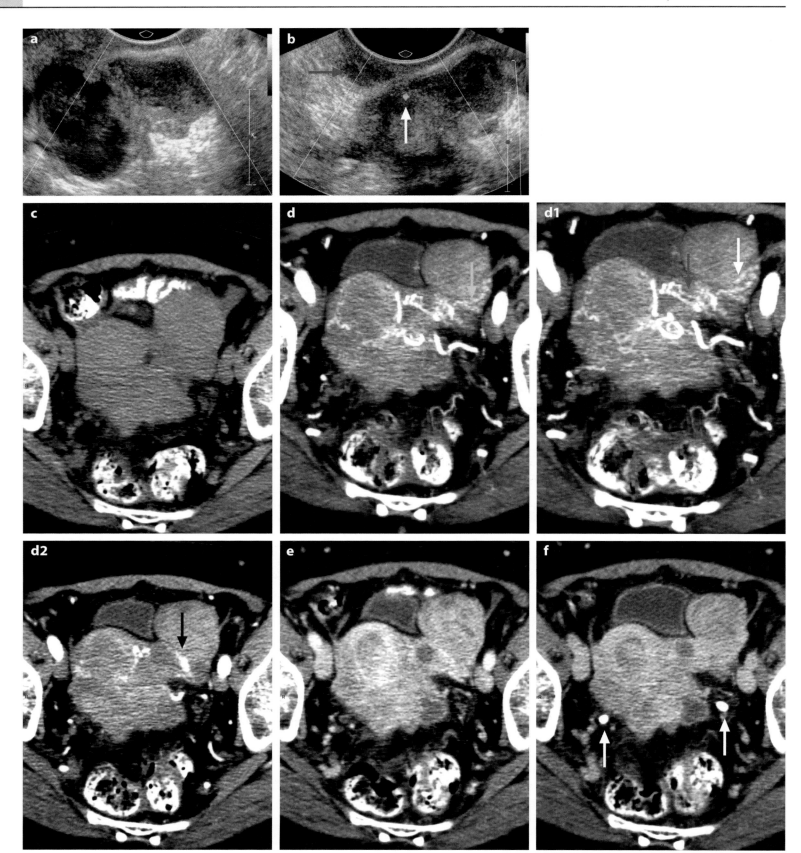

Fig. 9.110 Unusual mainly solid bilateral mucinous carcinoma stage IIIc. Sixty-eight-year-old woman; metrorrhagias. CA 125: 436 IU/ml. CA 19-9: 497 IU/ml. EVS (**a**) displays a mainly solid ovarian mass 6 cm in diameter, in contact with the left lateral border of the uterus. On color Doppler (**b**), only a tiny vessel is displayed in the solid tissue (*white arrow*). Left ovary is not clearly visualized. Ascites is present above the mass (*red arrow*). DCT of the left ovary without contrast (**c**) at the arterial phase at three different levels (**d**, **d1**, **d2**) depicts in **d** in the ovary tumoral vessels (*arrow*), in **d1**, tumoral vessels in the ovary (*white arrow*) and irregular vessels in the mesosalpinx (*red arrow*) and in **d2**, a significant enlarged artery in the mesovarium (*arrow*) typical for a malignant ovarian tumor. At the venous phase (**e**) and on the delayed 4 mm after injection (**f**), a significant contrast uptake is visualized in the tissular portions while absence or few contrast uptake is visualized in the portions with degenerative changes. In (**f**), relationships with the ureters are depicted (*arrows*).

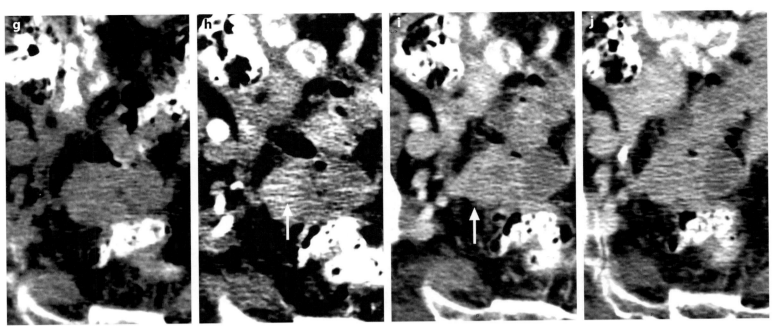

Fig. 9.110 (*continued*) DCT of the right ovary without contrast (**g**) at the arterial phase (**h**) displays tiny tumoral arterial vessels (*arrow*) very suggestive of the same type of tumor. At the venous phase (**i**), a higher contrast uptake than usually is displayed in the central part of the ovary (*arrow*) while a diffuse contrast uptake is visualized on the delayed (**j**). Extension outside the ovary was identified (see chapter extension Fig. 9.165). Prospective diagnosis: bilateral ovarian carcinoma. Laparotomy: bilateral ovariectomy. Important extension outside the ovary making hysterectomy impossible. Pathology: bilateral mucinous cystadenocarcinoma

9.4.3.4 Collision Tumors

Mucinous tumors can be associated with another type of ovarian tumor, particularly a mature cystic teratoma or a Brenner tumor.

9.5 Endometrioid Tumor

9.5.1 Endometrioid Adenocarcinomas

9.5.1.1 General Features

They account for 6 % of all epithelial tumors (Table 9.3).
They are diagnosed at stage 1 in 43 % of cases [119]. About 13 % of early stages (stages I and II) are bilateral.
Particular clinical findings are:
- Abnormal vaginal bleeding is also frequent; this is in part related to the association with endometrial hyperplasia and carcinoma.
- Another clinical association is breast cancer in 7 % of cases [120].

9.5.1.2 Pathology [121]

Macroscopy

They have a smooth surface. Three different patterns may be observed:
- Most often, they are solid and cystic, with the cysts containing friable soft masses and bloody fluid. Cysts occasionally contain mucus or greenish fluid.
- Less commonly, the tumor is solid with extensive hemorrhage and necrosis.
- Tumors arising in endometriosis may display gross findings of an endometriotic cyst containing chocolate-colored fluid, with a solid nodule in the wall reflecting the focus of malignant transformation.

Microscopy

(a) Well-differentiated endometrioid adenocarcinomas account for the majority of cases and are characterized by invasive round or oval tubular glands (Fig. 9.69) lined by stratified non-mucin containing tall columnar epithelium with sharp luminal margins; a confluent or cribriform proliferation may be present.
A villoglandular pattern also occurs.
Mitotic figures are commonly seen.
Squamous differentiation is present in up to 50 % of cases.
Areas of atypical proliferative (borderline) tumors are commonly associated.
Luteinized stromal cells are present in 12 % of cases.
(b) Moderately or poorly differentiated endometrioid carcinomas display solid growth and complex glandular and microglandular patterns. Nuclear pleomorphism and mitotic activity are marked, and necrosis and hemorrhage are often prominent.
(c) One-third of ovarian carcinomas classified as endometrioid based on the predominant epithelial component are mixed with a clear cell component in 20 % and a serous component in 10 %.

9.5.1.3 Imaging Findings

1. *The mainly solid and cystic form* (Fig. 9.111)
   Two main patterns may be encountered.
   The mainly solid (Fig. 9.112)
   The cystic form with solid tissue or papillary projections (Fig. 9.113)

2. *Less commonly, tumor is solid with extensive hemorrhage and necrosis* (Fig. 9.114).

On US, MR, and CT, findings of malignancy are the same as those described previously described concerning morphological and vascular findings (Tables 9.6, 9.10, and 9.11).

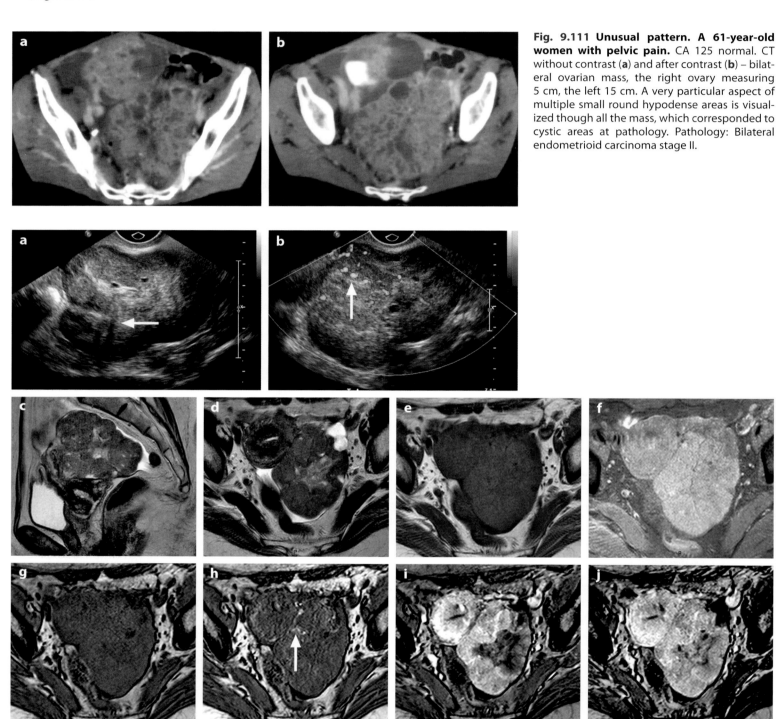

Fig. 9.111 Unusual pattern. A 61-year-old women with pelvic pain. CA 125 normal. CT without contrast (**a**) and after contrast (**b**) – bilateral ovarian mass, the right ovary measuring 5 cm, the left 15 cm. A very particular aspect of multiple small round hypodense areas is visualized though all the mass, which corresponded to cystic areas at pathology. Pathology: Bilateral endometrioid carcinoma stage II.

Fig. 9.112 Endometrioid carcinoma of the left ovary. EVS (**a**) displays a 7 cm left solid ovarian mass with lobulated contours, containing some acoustic shadowings (*arrow*).On color doppler (**b**) some vessels are visualized in the mass (*arrow*), without peripheral vascularization as in a leiomyoma. MR sagittal T2 (**c**) and axial T2 (**d**) depict a left solid ovarian mass with an intermediate signal and central degenerative changes. On axial T1 (**e**) and fat suppression (**f**), no hemorrhage is displayed in the central part of the mass. DMR without injection (**g**) and at the arterial phase (**h**) depicts multiple arterial tumoral vessels in the mass (*arrow*); at the venous phase (**i**) there is a high contrast uptake at the periphery of the mass with a central diffusion of contrast uptake in the central portion on the delayed (**j**). Prospective diagnosis: Malignant tumor of the left ovary. Absence of extraovarian extension. At operation a usual protocol for ovarian carcinoma was performed. Pathology: endometrioid carcinoma Stage 1A

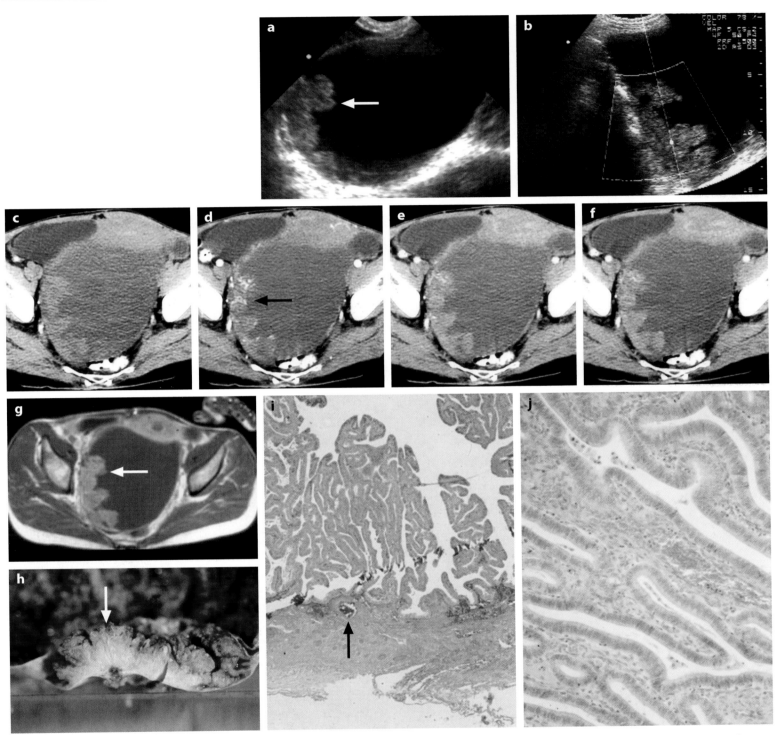

Fig. 9.113 Endometrioid carcinoma stage 1 cystic form with vegetations. A 74-year-old women with metrorrhagia and increased abdominal girdle. EVS (**a**): A 15 cm right ovarian cystic mass with endocystic vegetations is displayed. The papillary projections have a broad base of implantation and an echogenic band at their surface related to degenerative changes (hemorrhagia and necrosis at pathology) (*arrow*). Color Doppler (**b**) displays vessels in the papillary projections; (**d**) CT scan without contrast (**c**) at the arterial phase (**d**) displays a wide papillary projection with an irregular surface with characteristic tumoral vessels thin and irregular (*arrow*) appearing at the same time as in the iliac arteries. A wash-out in the vessels is visualized 30 s after injection (**e**) with an increase in contrast uptake 40 s after injection (**f**); MR T1 after contrast (**g**) visualizes contrast uptake in the papillary projections with areas of necrosis (*arrow*). Pathologic specimen (**h**) demonstrated disseminated vegetations all over the inner wall associated with the wide vegetation at the surface of this last one; hemorrhagia and necrosis are seen at the surface (*arrow*) while large vessels are visualized at the base. Microscopy (low magnification) (**i**) visualized large vessels at the base of vegetations (*arrow*). Microscopy (high magnification) (**j**) displays a tubal architecture typical for endometrioid carcinoma

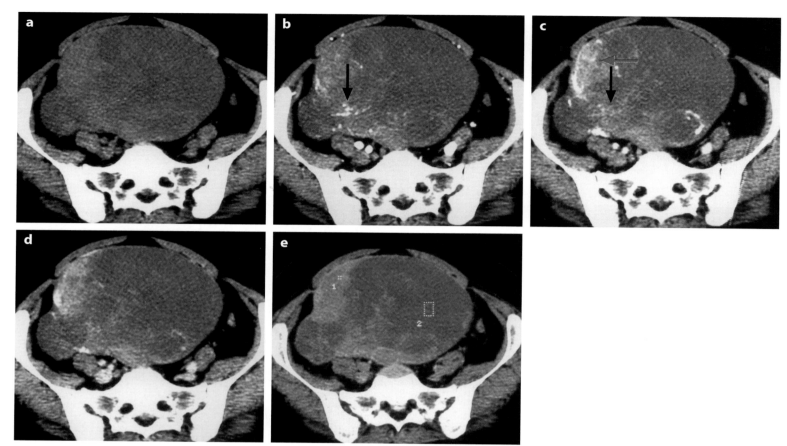

Fig. 9.114 Endometrioid carcinoma of the right ovary mainly solid tumor with degenerative changes, stage II. A 51-year-old women with vaginal hysterectomy 1 year before for uterine fibroids. Abdominopelvic mass with dysuria and constipation. CA 125: 400 IU/ml. DCT without contrast (**a**), at the arterial phase 20 s (**b**) and 30 s (**c**), at the venous phase (50 s), and the delayed CT scan (**e**) (4 mm): tumoral vessels appear in some parts of the tumor 20 s after injection (**b**) (*arrow*). Ten seconds after (**c**), a wash out in these vessels (*black arrow*) is visualized while other vessels in other parts of the tumor are opacified (*red arrow*) due to their different velocities, which is a typical hemodynamic finding of a malignant tumor. On (**d**). On the delayed CT scan (**e**), contrast accumulation in the tissular portions is displayed while absence of contrast is noted in parts of the tumor with ill-defined borders. Prospective diagnosis: carcinoma of the ovary. Macroscopy: The tumor looked completely solid with hemorrhagic changes and sheets of edema, without any cystic component. Microscopy: endometrioid carcinoma; stage II with 5 cm tumoral nodule in the superior part the anterior rectum

9.5.1.4 Association

Uterine Endometrial Carcinoma

Association with uterine endometrial carcinoma is present in 14 % of cases (Figs. 9.115 and 9.116). Endometrial hyperplasia is also frequent (see Chap. 22, Sect. 22.4.1).

As both tumors are often well differentiated endometrioid adenocarcinomas, they resemble each other, and excluding the possibility that the ovarian tumor is metastatic can be a problem. Diagnosis of a primary endometrial with ovarian metastases is based on three findings:

(a) Carcinoma of the endometrium of high grade and $\geq$ to stage 1B and tumor within the fallopian tube
(b) Ovarian bilaterality (primary ovarian is bilateral in 13 % of stages I and II)
(c) Ovarian surface involvement [119, 120]

Endometriosis

At pathology, 15–20 % of endometrioid carcinomas are associated with endometriosis.

- Endometrial carcinoma (mainly clear cell and endometrioid) (see Chap. 22, Sect. 22.4.1) can be associated with an endometriotic cyst in the same or contralateral ovary or endometriosis elsewhere [121]. In these cases, on MR, diagnosis of this association is easy.
- Epithelial carcinoma can arise in an endometriotic cyst and displays a thickening of the cyst wall or a nodule or a papillary projection protruding into the cyst. On MR, such cases have been reported by Tanaka [122].

While at pathology, these nodules or papillary projections contained malignant epithelial tissue associated with endometriotic tissue; on MR, content of the cyst was not typical for endometriosis in the documented cases [122].

Moreover, this author reports in the same series benign nodules at pathology as fibrosis or polyps inside an endometrial cyst. Of these cases, one documented on MR has typical findings of endometrial cyst.

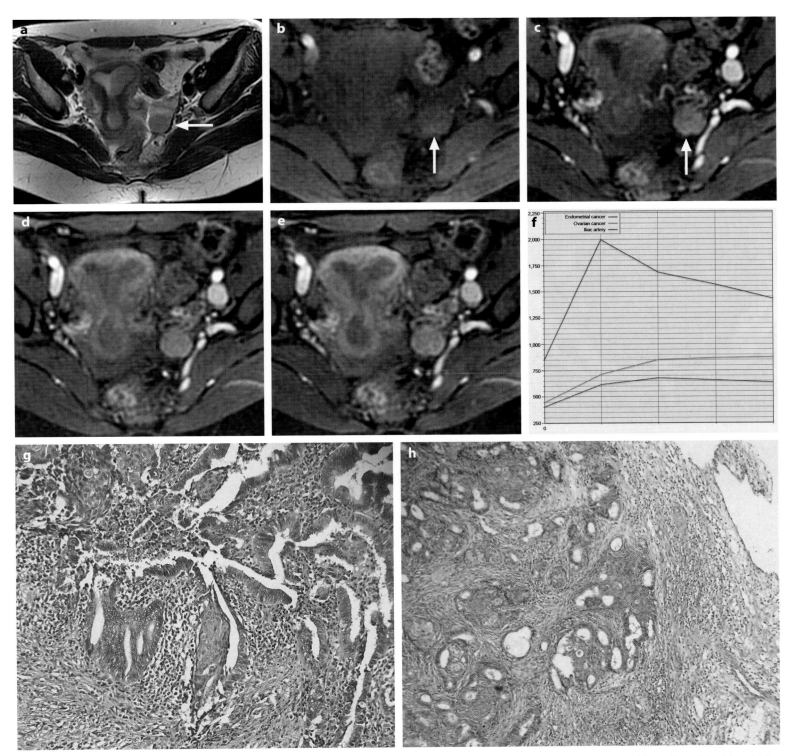

Fig. 9.115 Endometrioid ovarian carcinoma and synchronous endometrial carcinoma. (a) Axial T2 shows (a) a rounded mass of 2 cm of intermediate signal in the left ovary (*arrow*) and (b) an endometrial lesion of intermediate signal (of the same signal intensity) in the left part of the endometrial cavity extending into the endocervical. (b-f) DMR at early arterial phase (b) displays arterial vessels in the ovarian mass (*arrow*), contrast uptake at the venous phase (c) (*arrow*), (d) and late phase (e) with a similar enhancement in the endometrial and ovarian lesions. The corresponding curves are displayed in (f). (g and h) Histology of the surgical specimens show similar endometrioid carcinoma of the endometrium (g) and endometrioid carcinoma of the ovary (h)

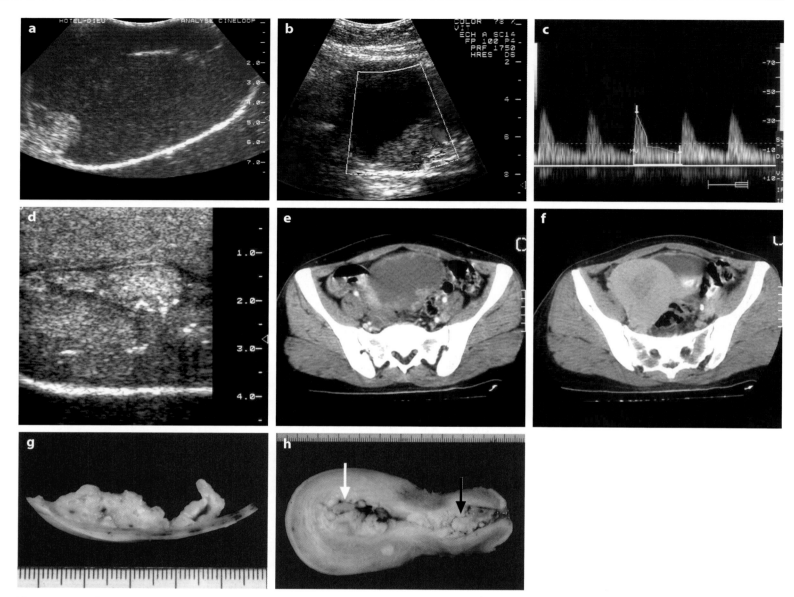

Fig. 9.116 Endometrioid carcinoma with left ovarian location and double uterine location in the corpus and in the cervix. A 48-year-old women with metrorrhagia. TAS (**a**) with color Doppler (**b**): In a cystic tumor, a broad base papillary projection with vascularization is very suggestive of malignancy. On pulse Doppler (**c**), the resistive index is high. In vitro US study of the uterus (**d**): A hyperechogenic mass occupies the central portion of the uterine body. DCT scan at the arterial phase (**e**) displays arterial vessels typical for carcinoma. Delayed CT scan through the corpus of the uterus (**f**): Ill-defined hypodense lesions are seen in the endometrium extending into the myometrium. Pathologic specimen of the ovary (**g**): A vegetation with a broad base of implantation is visualized. Pathologic specimen of the uterus (**h**): Uterine tumor of the endometrium extending into the myometrium at the level of the fundus (*white arrow*). Other location in the uterine cervix (*black arrow*). Pathology: endometrioid carcinoma of the left ovary, the uterine fundus, and the cervix

9.5.2 Endometrioid Adenofibromas

9.5.2.1 General Features

It is an exceptional tumor.

9.5.2.2 Pathology [121]

Macroscopy

The external surface is smooth.
The tumor is fibrous, often mixed with cystic areas creating a honeycomb appearance similar to a serous cystadenofibroma. The cysts contain clear or yellowish fluid.

Microscopy

(a) Common pattern:
   Architecture
   The epithelial elements are arranged in branching tubular nests and cysts and usually resemble those of a proliferative endometrium.
   Cell proliferation
   The epithelium is columnar with oval nuclei and basophilic cytoplasm.
(b) Sometimes:
   The nuclei resemble those of an atrophic endometrium.
   Secretory changes and focal squamous differentiation may be present.

9.5.2.3 Imaging Findings

A case of cystadenofibroma arising in an endometriotic cyst is reported (Fig. 9.117). The content of the cyst was not quite typical of endometriosis on MR (hyperintense on T1, T1FS, and T2) but with vascularized papillary projections.

9.5.2.4 Association

Occasionally, they are associated with endometriosis.

9.5.3 Atypical Proliferative Endometrioid Tumors

9.5.3.1 General Features

They account for only 0.5 % of epithelial tumors (Table 9.3).

9.5.3.2 Pathology [121]

Macroscopy

The characteristic gross appearance is mixed. The cyst fluid is usually hemorrhagic and necrosis is common.

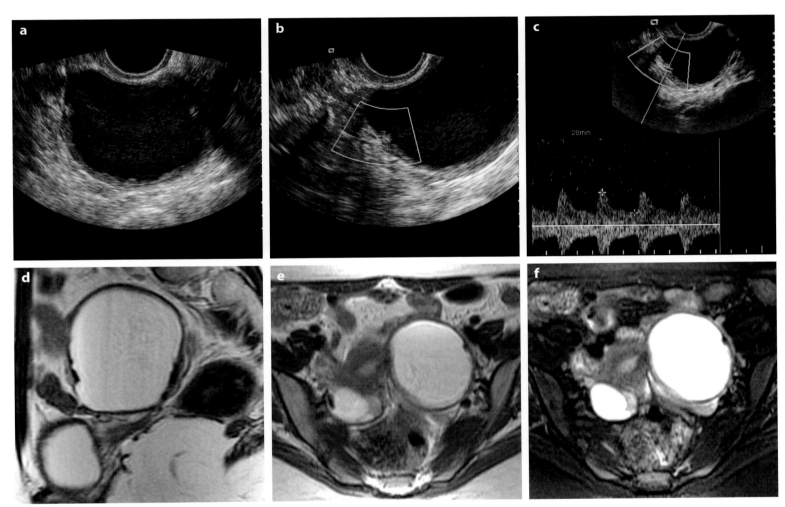

Fig. 9.117 Endometrioid cystadenoma arising in an endometrioid cyst in a 29-year-old woman. (a) Ultrasound disclosed a 7 cm left ovarian cyst with homogeneous hypoechoic ground glass pattern and several small papillary projections. (b) Color Doppler showed flow at the base of the biggest papillary projection that measured 6.4 mm but not flow inside the papillary projection. (c) Spectral Doppler demonstrates a resistivity index of 0.63. The ultrasound pattern suggests an endometrioma, but the wall protrusions were more suggestive of papillary projections than peripheral clots. (d–i) Sagittal (d) and axial (e) T2W images show small papillary projections (or clots). Axial T2WFS (f),

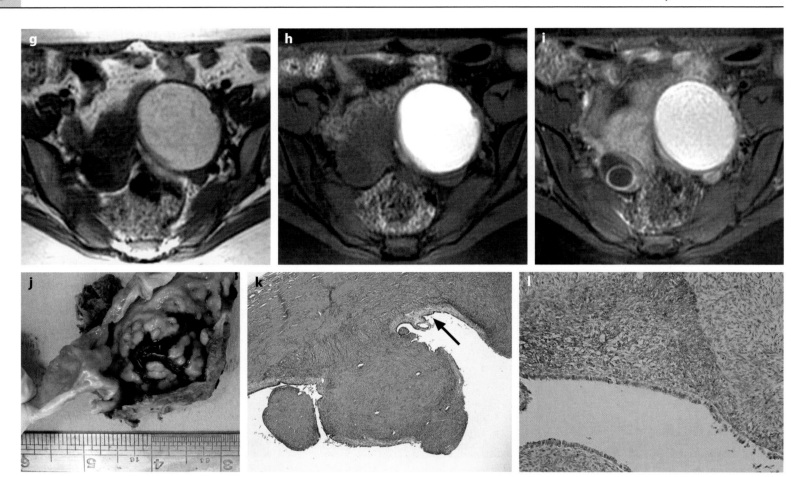

Fig. 9.117 (*continued*) T1W (**g**), and T1WFS (**h**) images show a left intracystic papillary projection on all sequences. However, on T1WFS image after gadolinium injection (**i**), the papillary projection is almost not visible because it enhanced and its signal intensity became close to that of the hemorrhagic cystic content; this ruled out a clot. A corpus luteum and a simple follicle are displayed in the right ovary. The signal of the cystic content is hyperintense on T2, T1, and T1FS images compatible with endometrioma but not fully typical because no low or intermediate signal intensity on T2. (**j**) Macroscopy of the surgical specimen shows small infracentimetric papillary projections along a surface of 4 cm. Chocolate blood is still stuck to the wall. (**k** and **l**) The cyst wall shows papillary processes with dense fibrous stroma underlying a regular columnar epithelium. In some areas, endometrial stroma is observed beneath the epithelium (*arrow* in **k**) that stains positively (*brown*) with anti-CD10 antibody (**l**), consistent with typical endometriosis and raising the hypothesis of an adenofibroma arising in an otherwise endometriotic cyst

Microscopy

Architecture
The glandular/papillary proliferation displays varying degrees of glandular complexity and crowding:

- Epithelial stratification.
- Tufting and bridging may be present.
- Mild to moderate cytologic atypia.

Stroma

Periglandular cuffing surrounds the glandular elements characterized by stromal cellularity around the glandular elements. However, these areas lack the mitoses and atypia of adenosarcoma.

Cytology
Severe cytologic atypia is present. A confluent epithelial proliferation that exceeds 5 mm warrants the diagnosis of carcinoma

9.5.3.3 Imaging Findings

A case is reported hereby that cannot be differentiated from an endometrioid carcinoma (Fig. 9.118).

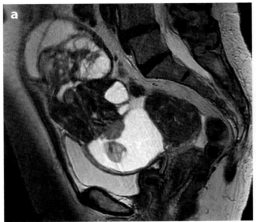
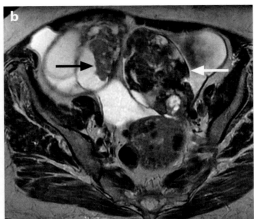
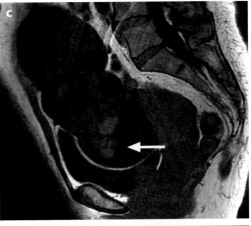
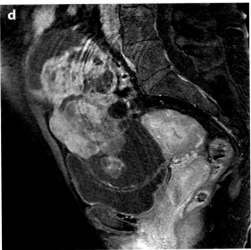

Fig. 9.118 Atypical proliferative endometrioid tumor of the left ovary. MR sagittal T2 (**a**) and axial T2 (**b**) display a mixed solid and cystic mass. While most of the solid tissue situated in the left part of the mass is of low signal suggesting a predominance of fibrous tissue (*white arrow*), in the right part of the mass, solid tissue of intermediate signal suggests a possibility of carcinoma (*black arrow*). Axial T1 (**c**) displays some hemorrhage (*arrow*) which is more common in malignant than in benign ovarian tumors. Sagittal T2 (**d**) displays a significant contrast uptake in the solid portions, with numerous areas of degenerative changes. Prospective diagnosis: carcinoma. Pathology: presence of two foci of 0.5 cm of poorly differentiated endometrioid carcinomas in an atypical proliferative endometrioid tumor

9.6 Clear Cell Tumors

The Mullerian nature of clear cell tumors of the ovary is supported by:
- The close association with endometriosis
- Their frequent association with endometrioid carcinoma
- The occurrence of identical tumors in the endometrium
- Their origin in vaginal adenosis in DES exposed women

9.6.1 Clear Cell Carcinomas

9.6.1.1 General Features [123]

Clear cell carcinoma is a very uncommon tumor accounting for 2.4 % of all epithelial tumors (Table 9.3).

It is the most common epithelial ovarian neoplasm to be associated with paraneoplastic hypercalcemia.

Half of patients present with stage I, 15 % with stage II.

Four percent of stage I are bilateral.

9.6.1.2 Pathology [123]

Microscopy

The most common patterns are:
(a) The solid pattern characterized by sheets of polyhedral cells with abundant clear cytoplasm.

(b) The tubulopapillary pattern (Fig. 9.119); the cells are often columnar with a hobnail appearance. The fibrovascular cores are often hyalinized. The hyalinized and homogeneous stromal fibrosis is a very characteristic feature of this tumor.

The most common cell types are:
- Clear cell typically rounded or polyhedral
- Hobnail cells (Fig. 9.120) containing bulbous dark nuclei that protrude into lumens beyond the apparent cytoplasmic limit of the cells

9.6.1.3 Imaging Findings

Common Macroscopic and Radiologic Findings

(a) They are most often predominantly cystic unilocular (Figs. 9.121, 9.122, and 9.123) or sometimes multilocular containing one more polypoid nodules protruding into the lumen. The cyst lumen may contain serous or mucinous fluid. In case in which the tumor has a region arising in an endometriotic cyst, the cystic content may be chocolate color. The external surface is often shaggy due to adhesions, which in some cases are related to associated endometriosis.

(b) Less commonly, the mass is solid (Figs. 9.124 and 9.125) and fibrous with a honeycomb cut surface.

On US, MR, and CT, morphologic and vascular findings of the nodules are the same as for other carcinomas described previously (Tables 9.6, 9.10, and 9.11).

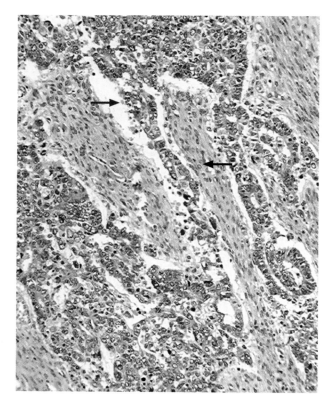

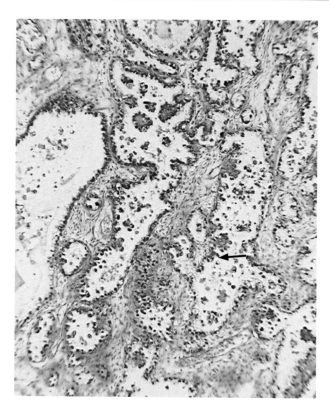

Fig. 9.119 Clear cell carcinoma. Overview of the proliferation of epithelial cells (*blue arrow*) within stroma (*black arrow*)

Fig. 9.120 Clear cell carcinoma. Proliferation of epithelial cells with hobnail cells (*arrow*) characteristic for clear cell carcinoma

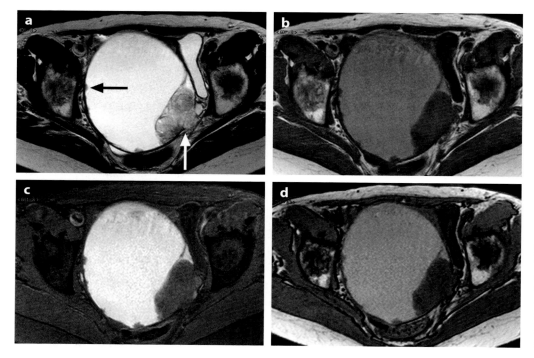

Fig. 9.121 Clear cell carcinoma stage 1a. Sixty-year-old woman. Left pelvic pain, common urge to urinate. CA 125: 9 IU/ml. MR axial T2 (**a**) displays a left 12 cm unilocular cystic ovarian mass containing solid tissue which seems to go beyond the capsule (*white arrow*) and multiple endocystic papillary projections (*black arrow*). Content of the cyst is of intermediate signal on T1 (**b**) and high on fat suppression (**c**). DMR without injection (**d**)

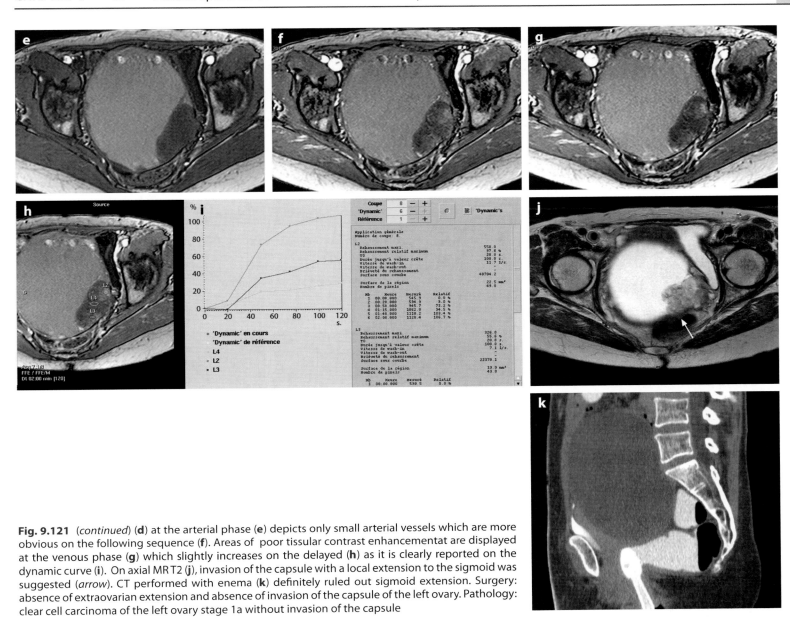

Fig. 9.121 (*continued*) (**d**) at the arterial phase (**e**) depicts only small arterial vessels which are more obvious on the following sequence (**f**). Areas of poor tissular contrast enhancementat are displayed at the venous phase (**g**) which slightly increases on the delayed (**h**) as it is clearly reported on the dynamic curve (**i**). On axial MR T2 (**j**), invasion of the capsule with a local extension to the sigmoid was suggested (*arrow*). CT performed with enema (**k**) definitely ruled out sigmoid extension. Surgery: absence of extraovarian extension and absence of invasion of the capsule of the left ovary. Pathology: clear cell carcinoma of the left ovary stage 1a without invasion of the capsule

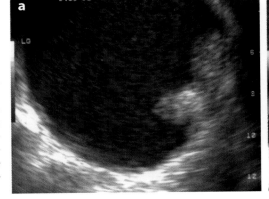
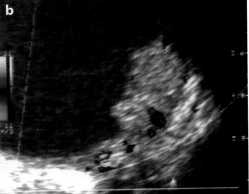

Fig. 9.122 Clear cell carcinoma stage 1a. A 55-year-old women with pelvic mass. EVS (**a**) displays a 15 cm unilocular left cystic ovarian mass containing a large papillary projection with obtuse angles with the inner wall, with large vessels at the base on color Doppler (**b**) very suggestive of carcinoma. The ground glass pattern of the cystic content is particularly seen in case of borderline or carcinoma.

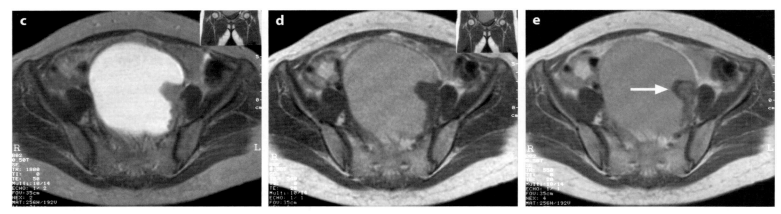

Fig. 9.122 (*continued*) Axial MR (**c**) the vegetation appears clearly with a in a cystic content. Axial MR T1 (**d**) the content of the cyst has a signal comprised between pelvic muscle and adipose tissue. The endocystic vegetations appear with a signal close to pelvic muscle. Axial MR T1 after contrast injection (**e**) contrast uptake is visualized in most of the vegetation while no uptake is depicted at the surface owing to necrosis at pathology (*arrow*). This aspect is characteristic for a malignant tumor. Surgery: absence of extraovarian extension. Pathology: clear cell carcinoma

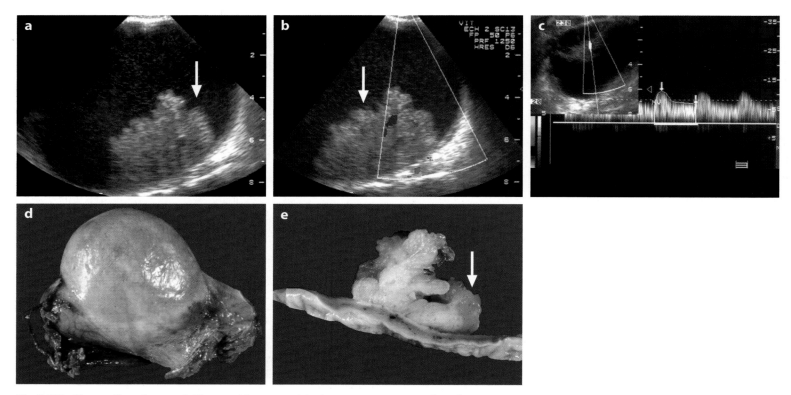

Fig. 9.123 Clear cell carcinoma. A 40-year-old women with a latero-uterine mass discovered at a routine examination. CA 125 normal. EVS (**a**): 11 cm right ovarian mass. The largest vegetation measures 5 cm and is echogenic. Its irregular and more echogenic surface (*arrow*) related to necrosis is depicted on the specimen (**e**) (*arrow*). Color Doppler (**b**) visualizes few vessels in the vegetation. At pulsed Doppler (**c**), the resistive index is 0.40. At surgery, the right mainly cystic ovarian tumor was removed (**d**). Extension outside the ovary was absent .Pathologic specimen (**e**) of a longitudinal section of the vegetation visualizes necrosis at its surface. At microscopy: papillary clear cell carcinoma stage Ia

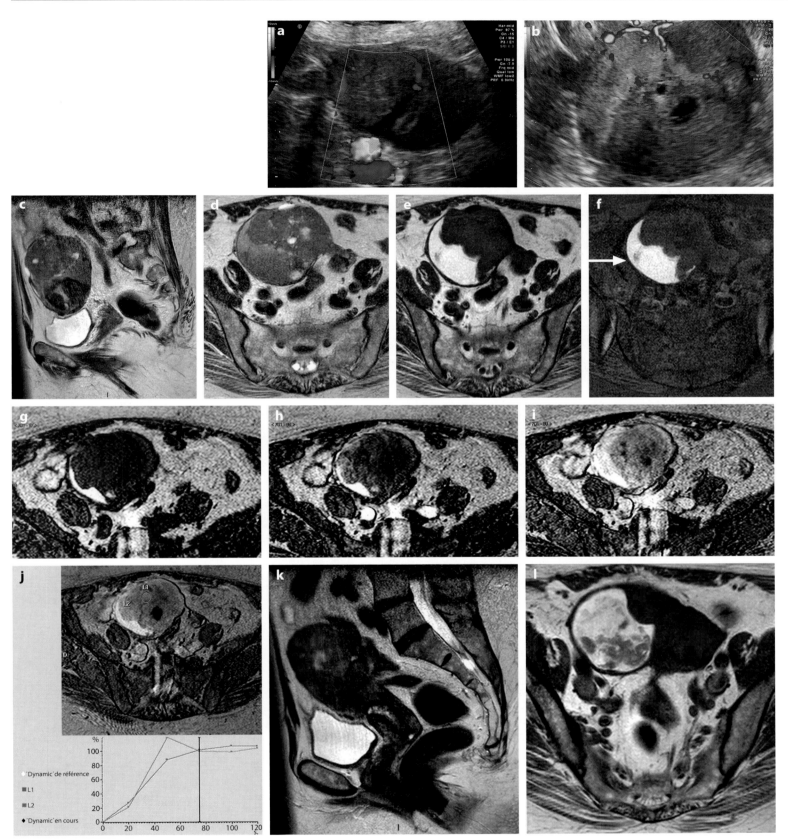

Fig. 9.124 Clear cell carcinoma associated with subperitoneal endometriosis. EVS with color Doppler (**a**) and (**b**) depicts a right solid ovarian mass with a peripheral and central vascularization. MR sagittal (**c**) and axial T2 (**d**) depict a solid ovarian mass with an overall intermediate signal containing some cystic areas in its upper two-thirds and a low signal in its lower third. On T1 (**e**) and fat suppression (**f**), hemorrhage is visualized in the lateral part of the mass (*arrow*). DMR without injection (**g**) and at the arterial phase (**h**) depicts arterial tumoral vessels in the right part of the mass, with contrast uptake at the venous phase (**i**) at the maximum at 50 s in the lateral portion as it is reported in the curve (**j**). On sagittal (**k**) and axial T2 (**l**), attraction of the rectosigmoid junction to the torus of the uterus (*arrow*) was suspected to be related to endometriosis. Prospective diagnosis: carcinoma of the right ovary. Absence of extraovarian extension. At operation, right ovarian tumor; absence of extension. Endometriosis at the rectosigmoid junction. Pathology: clear cell carcinoma stage 1a

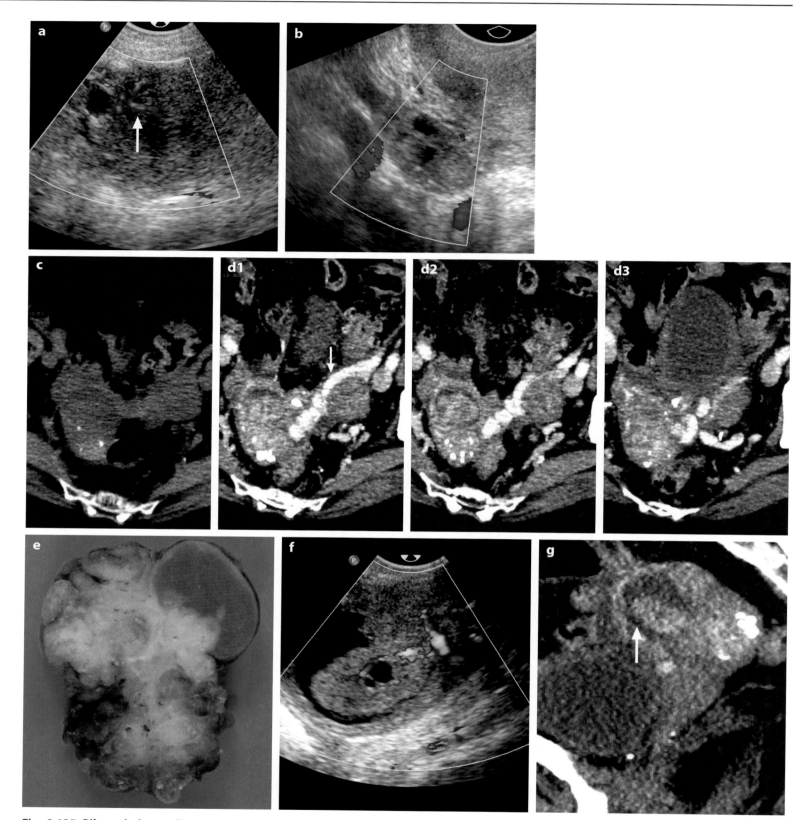

Fig. 9.125 Bilateral clear cell ovarian carcinoma stage IIIc. Seventy-six-year-old woman. Absence of hormonal treatment. Left pelvic pain, alternation of constipation and diarrhea. (1) Ovaries. EVS and color Doppler of the left ovary (**a**) display a mainly solid ovarian mass with some degenerative changes, with large vessels at its anterior and lateral portion (*arrow*), very suggestive of carcinoma. EVS and color Doppler of the right ovary (**b**) depict a slightly enlarged ovary containing two small cysts, without any vessel; characterization is not possible. DCT without injection (**c**) at the arterial phase at three different levels (**d1, d2, d3**) displays arterial tumoral vessels in both ovaries with a very early venous drainage in the ovarian vein (*arrow* on

d1) on the left side, reflecting the malignant character of the ovarian tumors. Macroscopic specimen (**e**): whitish tumor, with a cystic portion and exophytic papillary projections. Microscopy: bilateral clear cell carcinoma. (2) Uterus. Longitudinal EVS of the uterus with color Doppler (**f**) displays a polyp of the endometrium with an anterior irregular border containing a vascular pedicle. On CT at the arterial phase with sagittal reformation (**g**), the polyp contains irregular arterial vessels. On its surface are visualized some tiny nodules (*arrow*). Two possibilities were discussed: a benign endometrial polyp, or a secondary endometrial location.

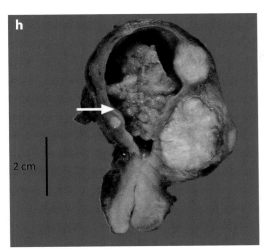

Fig. 9.125 (*continued*) Macroscopic specimen (**h**) displays several small nodules at the surface of the endometrial polyp (*arrow*). At pathology: secondary location on a glandular cystic polyp. At surgery, this patient had also metastatic peritoneal implants

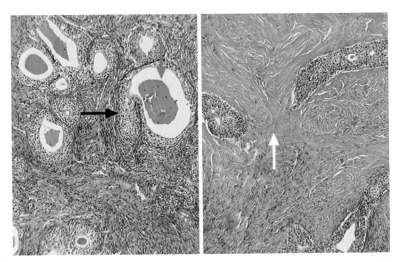

Fig. 9.126 (1) Proliferation of transitional cell types (*black arrow*), (2) hyalinized areas (*green arrow*), and (3) fibrosis (*white arrow*)

Differential Diagnosis

The main differential diagnoses are listed in Table 9.27.

Table 9.27 Differential diagnosis of clear cell carcinoma

Germ cell tumors
– Dysgerminomas
– Yolk sac tumor
– Struma ovarii
Endometrioid carcinoma (with secretory changes)
Metastases (rare)
Other ovarian clear cell tumors
– Atypical proliferative clear cell tumors (rare)
– Clear cell adenofibroma (Exceptional)

9.6.1.4 Association

Thirty to thirty-five percent of ovarian clear cell carcinomas are associated with endometriosis either in the involved ovary or elsewhere in the pelvis (Fig. 9.124) or the abdomen (1) This type of association is similar to that encountered in case of ovarian endometrioid carcinoma associated with endometriosis (see Sect. 9.5.1.4).

9.6.2 Atypical Proliferative Clear Cell Tumors

They are rare, accounting for 0.2 % of epithelial tumors.
Their macroscopic appearance is similar to that of the clear cell adenofibroma.

9.6.3 Clear Cell Adenofibroma

They are exceptional. Cut surface has a fine honeycomb appearance with minute cysts embedded in firm rubbery stroma.

9.7 Transitional Cell Tumor: Brenner Tumor

They are almost always benign. Borderline and malignant forms represent 2–5 % of these tumors [124–126].

9.7.1 Benign Transitional Cell Tumor

9.7.1.1 General Features

Most benign forms have been encountered in the fourth through eight decades with a peak frequency in the late forties. They account for 3 % of all epithelial tumors (Table 9.3).
They are very particular benign epithelial tumors. Indeed, they are mainly solid resembling macroscopically ovarian fibroma.

9.7.1.2 Pathology

Microscopy (Fig. 9.126)

Brenner tumors are characterized by:
(a) Sharply demarcated epithelial nests, most or all of which are transitional type resembling the epithelial lining cells of the urinary bladder. The nests often become cystic.
(b) Occasionally, metaplastic endocervical epithelium lines the cystic nests. The metaplastic mucinous component may occasionally form the dominant part of the tumor and may account for the association of Brenner tumor with mucinous cystadenoma.
(c) The major component of the tumor is stroma that varies from one resembling ovarian cortical stroma to densely fibrous.

Hyalinized areas are common, and dystrophic calcification is present in 50 % of cases.

Common Macroscopic and Radiologic Findings

One-half to two-thirds are less than 2 cm [127].

They are bilateral in 7 % of the cases [128].

Most of the tumors are solid and fibrous, firm with a gray-white whorled cut surface.

Degenerative Changes

- Calcifications are present in 50 % of the cases [129]. Rarely, the tumor is massively calcified [127]. Degenerative cystic changes can be observed. Often, they form scattered microcysts; large cysts are occasionally present and may predominate [127].

9.7.1.3 Imaging Findings

Homogeneous Pattern

Ultrasound: The mass looks echogenic equal or less than myometrium [130, 131] with acoustic shadowing related to fibrous tissue. This pattern is typical for a benign mass and is only present in Brenner tumor, ovarian fibroma, and subserous leiomyoma (Fig. 9.127).On Doppler, like in ovarian fibroma, vessels are very rare and scattered. Unlike pedunculated subserous leiomyoma, no peripheral ring of vascularization is observed.

Uncommonly, the tumor is connected to the ovary by a small pedicle (Fig. 9.128).

On MR: On T1-weighted images, signal intensity is close to pelvic muscle.

On T2-weighted images, signal intensity is close to pelvic muscle [132]; this signal intensity is significantly lower than other nonfibrous ovarian tumors. The low signal intensity seen on T1- and T2-weighted images is due to abundant fibrotic tissue [132, 133].

On CT, when the mass is small, <3 cm in diameter, it may be not visualized on CT. When it is >3 cm on the noncontrast CT, the mass is well delineated. Density of the mass is less or equal to myometrium.

On DMR (Fig. 9.129) *and DCT* (Figs. 9.130 and 9.131), findings are identical to those observed in ovarian fibroma [134]:

- At the arterial phase, no vessel is seen inside the mass.
- At the parenchymal phase, no early contrast uptake or a slight contrast uptake is seen.
- On the delayed scan, a mild or moderate contrast enhancement [135] less than myometrium is noted. This slow diffusion is related to the particular type of rare scattered vessels as in ovarian fibroma.

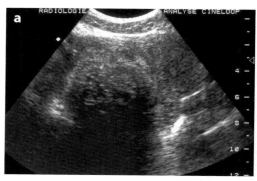
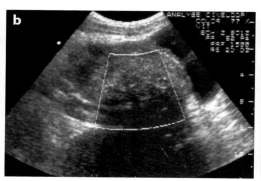
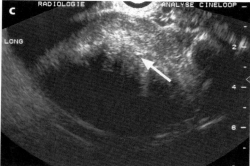

Fig. 9.127 Brenner tumor. A 47-year-old woman. (a) *TAS*: echogenic mass with strong attenuation and a broad ill-defined acoustic shadowing. *TAS with Doppler*: no vessel is seen in the mass. (**b**) On EVS, multiple areas of acoustic shadowing are displayed. (**c**) Tiny echogenic foci are present in the tumor (*arrow*). Prospective diagnosis: ovarian fibroma or Brenner tumor. *Surgery*: left adnexectomy. *Pathology*: Brenner tumor

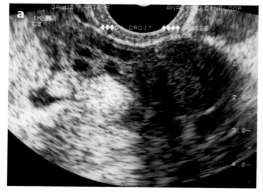
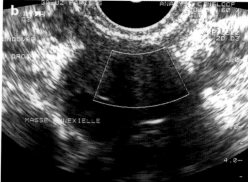

Fig. 9.128 Pedunculated Brenner tumor. A 30-year-old woman with right large ovary on a routine physical examination. (**a**) *Endovaginal US*: 2–3 cm echogenic mass with acoustic shadowing arising from the right ovary almost pedunculated resembling an ovarian fibroma. (**b**) *Endovaginal US with color Doppler*: vessels are seen in the echogenic portions proving the tissular nature. The scarcity of the vessels is typical of ovarian fibroma and Brenner tumor. *Celioscopy*: right ovarian tumorectomy was performed. *Pathology*: Brenner tumor

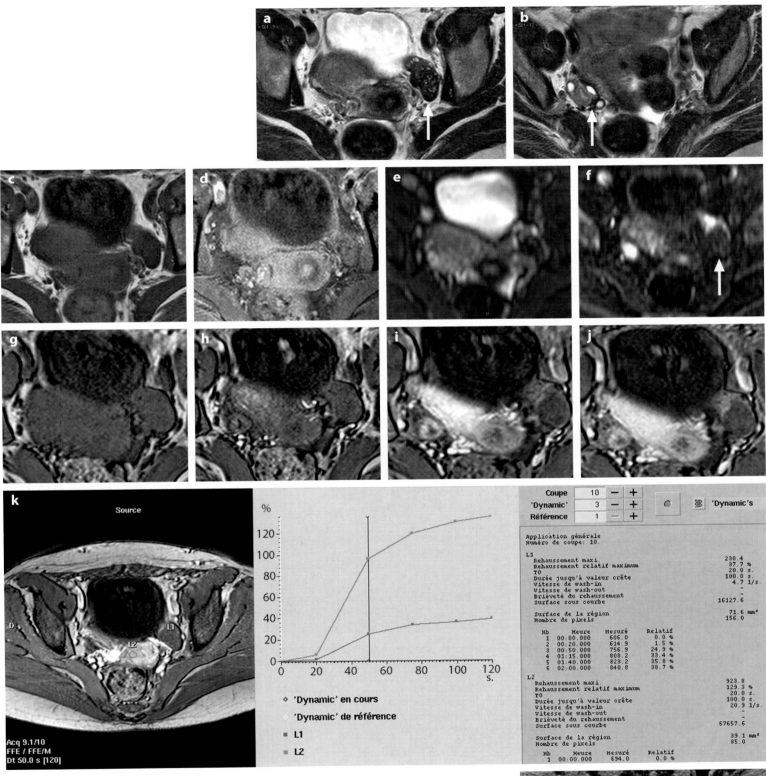

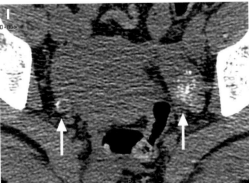

Fig. 9.129 Bilateral Brenner tumor. Thirty-six-year-old woman. During a routine US, a left ovarian mass is discovered. MR axial T2 (**a** and **b**) displays on (**a**) a mass of the left ovary containing low intense fibrous tissue (*arrow*) associated with multiple cystic cavities. On (**b**), a low intense area in the right ovary missed on a prospective study is seen (*arrow*); on T1 (**c**) and fat suppression (**d**), the left ovarian mass appears with a signal close to pelvic muscles. On diffusion using bo (**e**) and b1000 (**f**), the mass has a low intensity (*arrow*). On DMR without injection (**g**) at the arterial phase (**h**), at the venous phase (**i**), and on the delayed (**j**), a slight contrast uptake is visualized at the venous phase which slightly increases on the delayed. ROC curve (part of the figure **k**) illustrates a very low and slightly progressive contrast enhancement in the tumor (*red curve*) compare to a relativey rapid and high contrast enhancement in the myometrium (*green curve*). CT without injection (**l**) displays (**1**) in the left ovarian mass, multiple tiny calcifications (*arrow*), very suggestive of a Brenner tumor and (**2**) in the right ovary, a curvilinear calcification (*arrow*) in the area of low intensity on MR. Prospective diagnosis: bilateral benign Brenner tumor. Surgery: a left ovariectomy was performed; the right ovary was not verified. Pathology: benign left Brenner tumor

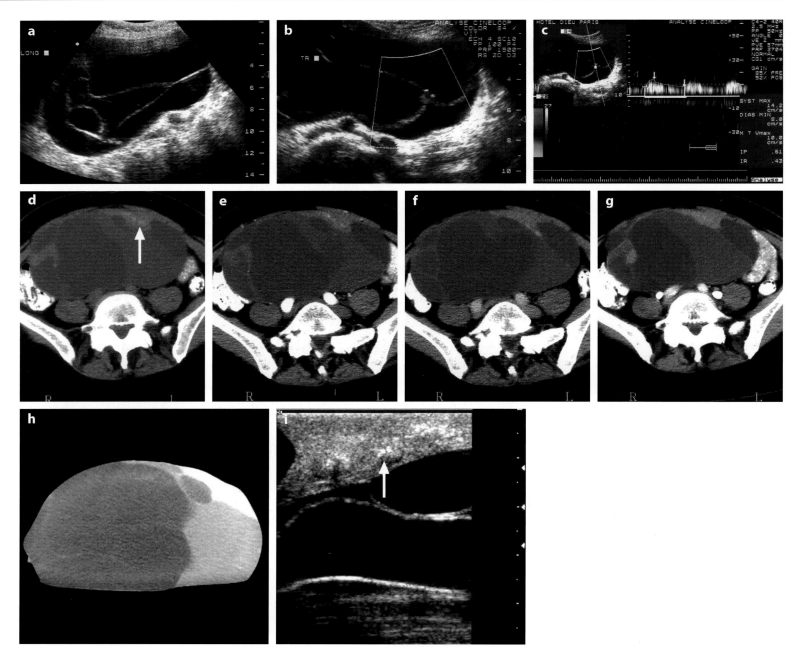

Fig. 9.130 Mucinous cystadenoma containing a Brenner tumor.
A 67-year-old woman with a pelvic mass. TAS (**a**) multiloculated cystic mass with fine septa. A mucinous cystadenoma is first suggested. No solid portion was detected by US. TAS with color Doppler (**b**) vessels are seen in the septa, with on pulsed Doppler (**c**) a RI of 0.43. DCT at the level of a solid portion without contrast (**d**) at the arterial phase (**e**), at the parenchymal phase (**f**), and delayed scan (**g**) displays in the multilocular cystic solid tissue. This portion has regular contour, with no abnormal vessels, no early contrast uptake, and slight contrast uptake on the delayed CT, suggesting fibrous tissue. Tiny and low dense calcifications, very particular to the Brenner tumor, are visualized in the tissular portion in (**d**) (*arrow*). CT of the pathological specimen (**h**) demonstrates the solid portion containing diffuse calcifications. Ultrasound of the pathological specimen (**i**) depicts tiny calcifications (*arrow*) particular to the Brenner tumor

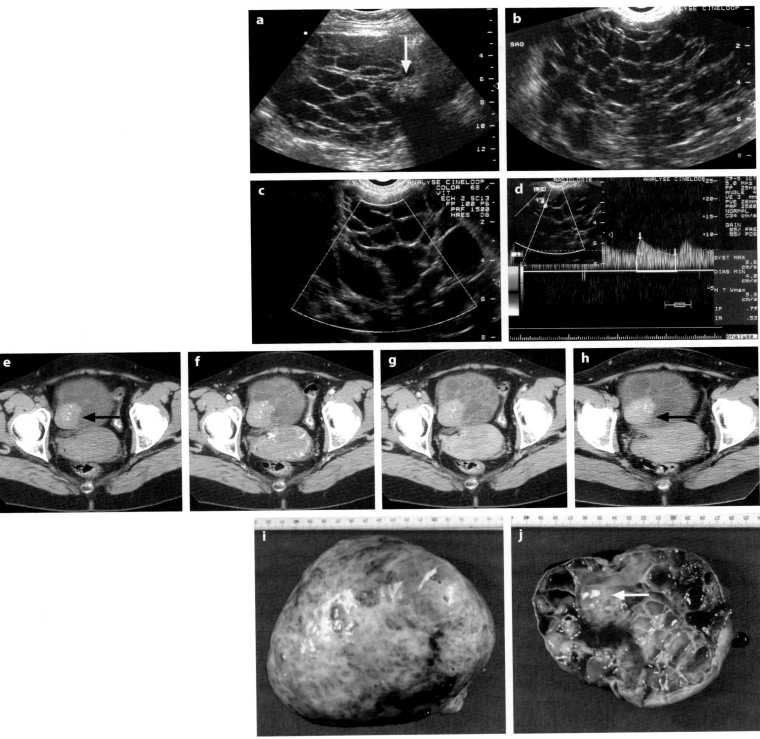

Fig. 9.131 Mucinous borderline cystadenoma containing a Brenner tumor. Pelvic mass in a 57-year-old woman. TAS longitudinal section (**a**): Multiloculated 17 cm cystic mass with numerous septa containing an echogenic 3.5 cm nodule with tiny hyperechogenic foci and a broad sharp acoustic shadowing (*arrow*). On EVS (**b**), the septa are numerous and gathered and some are thick and irregular; these findings suggest the possibility of a borderline tumor or a carcinoma. Color Doppler (**c**) visualizes vessels in the septa. Spectral analysis of one of the arteries (**d**) shows an RI of 0.53, a PI of 0.79, and a PSV of 8.6 cm/s. DCT without contrast (**e**) well depicts the solid regular nodule containing calcifications at the lower part of the multiloculated cystic mass (*arrow*). At the arterial phase (**f**) in the solid mass, no tumoral vessel is visualized. At the parenchymal phase (**g**), absence of contrast uptake while on the delayed a small contrast uptake is visualized (**h**) (*arrow*). The characters of the calcifications associated with benign solid tissue first suggest the diagnosis of a Brenner tumor, while the characters of the septa are very suggestive of a borderline tumor or a carcinoma. *Laparotomy*: total hysterectomy and bilateral adnexectomy. Macroscopic specimen (**i**) and a transverse section of the tumor (**j**) show the solid nodule with calcifications (*arrow*) which corresponds on microscopy at a benign Brenner tumor and the multiloculated cystic mass which corresponds at microscopy to a borderline mucinous tumor

Table 9.28 Differential diagnosis of homogeneous tissular mass

Unilateral:
Common:
Brenner tumor
Ovarian fibroma thecoma
Pedunculated subserous uterine leiomyoma
Uncommon:
Sertoli-Leydig cell tumor, granulosa cell tumor
Bilateral:
Lymphoma
Metastases : Krukenberg tumors, carcinoid, breast carcinoma
Exceptionally:
Primary carcinoma
Recurrence of carcinoma

Differential Diagnosis of the Homogeneous Pattern

They are listed in Table 9.28.

Unilateral:

(a) Uterine subserous leiomyoma of the uterus that usually presents a rich peripheral and central vascularization at the arterial phase and early significant contrast uptake

(b) Ovarian fibroma that in most of the cases cannot be distinguished from a Brenner tumor [136–138]

(c) Low intensity endometriomas on T1- and T2-weighted images

Bilateral:

Metastasis or lymphoma can be discussed [139]. Krukenberg tumor is usually associated with other findings of primary malignancy. Primary lymphoma and Krukenberg tumors usually have no calcification [135].

Pattern with Degenerative Changes

With Calcifications

Ultrasound

When multiple echogenic foci are depicted, these foci are sometimes difficult to relate to calcifications. In these cases, the mass can also mimic an ovarian fibroma or pedunculated subserous leiomyoma [140] (Figs. 9.130 and 9.131).

CT

CT is the best modality to detect calcifications [141]. These calcifications are very peculiar and resemble psammomatous calcifications [142] (Fig. 9.130). Rarely, a round peripheral focus of calcification can be present [140].

This form can also be difficult to distinguish from a pedunculated subserous leiomyoma [143]. However, dystrophic-type calcification in leiomyoma usually has a mottled appearance with curvilinear rim or whorled or streaked appearances [144] quite different from those of a Brenner tumor.

MR

Calcifications are not visualized. Exceptionally, the hyposignal due to calcifications makes the tumor look like a bowel.

With Degenerative Cystic Changes

Degenerative cystic can be observed [145]. In these cases, the mass can be difficult to distinguish, not only from ovarian fibroma and subserous leiomyoma, but also from a malignant ovarian tumor and particularly from the very uncommon malignant Brenner tumor which contains cystic areas with necrosis [146].

Diffusion of gadolinium in the solid portion does not allow making the differential with a malignant tumor [135, 147]. DMR or better DCT is helpful to exclude malignancy mainly on the basis of absence of the classical vascular findings of malignancy (Tables 9.10 and 9.11).

9.7.1.4 Association

Association [127] with other types of tumor in the ipsilateral ovary occurs in 30 % of cases:

- Ten to twenty-five percent appear as small, firm nodules in the wall of a mucinous cystadenoma (Fig. 9.130).
- Fewer are found in the wall of a serous cystadenoma or dermoid cyst.
- Rare examples are associated with mucinous cystadenocarcinomas or borderline mucinous tumor [148] (Fig. 9.131).
- Association with a simple cyst has been reported [132, 133, 149, 150].

When associated with a mucinous tumor, differential diagnosis with a pure mucinous tumor containing a solid portion (borderline or rarely malignant) can be quite difficult. Vascular findings can be helpful to make the differential diagnosis (Tables 9.10 and 9.11).

9.7.1.5 Overall Differential Diagnosis

1. When the mass is mainly tissular with a suspicion of predominantly fibrous component, it is always benign. Three main differential diagnoses must be considered: an ovarian fibroma, a Brenner tumor, and a subserous leiomyoma (Table 9.28).

   The findings used to make the differential between a Brenner tumor or an ovarian fibroma and subserous leiomyoma are:
   - Visualization of a normal ipsilateral ovary in leiomyoma
   - A rich peripheral and central vascularization at the arterial phase in leiomyomas associated with early significant contrast uptake

2. When degenerative changes are present, the main differential is a malignant tumor. Among these malignant tumors, the very uncommon malignant Brenner tumor must be discussed. Differentiation is made on classical findings of malignancy.

3. When associated with a mucinous tumor, the differential diagnosis with purely mucinous tumor containing a tissular portion is not possible, except in the cases where these tissular portions contain calcifications very suggestive of Brenner tumor. In case the mucinous tumor is borderline or malignant, vascular findings are helpful.

9.7.2 Atypical Proliferative Transitional Cell Tumors

9.7.2.1 General Features

Borderline Brenner tumors are very uncommon. Mean age is 59 years.

9.7.2.2 Pathology

Macroscopy

- Always unilateral.
- Larger than their benign counterpart.
- Usually cystic.
- Friable papillary or polypoid masses project into the cysts lumens.
- Usually, a benign Brenner component with a more solid and fibrous cut surface is present.

Microscopy

The intracystic papillary component is composed of transitional-type epithelium resembling low-grade noninvasive papillary transitional cell neoplasms of the urinary tract.

9.7.2.3 Imaging Finding

Rare cases have been reported (Fig. 9.132).

9.7.3 Transitional Cell Carcinomas

9.7.3.1 General Features

Malignant Brenner tumors have malignant cells resembling invasive transitional carcinoma of the urinary bladder [146].

They are very uncommon tumors.

9.7.3.2 Pathology

Gross Appearance

They are typically solid and cystic.

Cysts may contain polypoid mural nodules. Cyst fluid is watery or mucinous.

Hemorrhage and necrosis may be prominent.

Foci of gritty calcifications may be present.

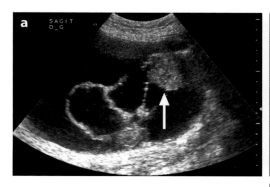
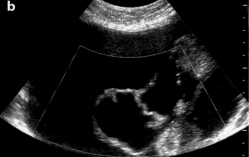
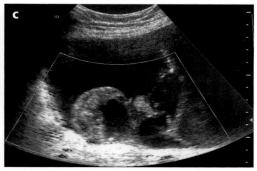
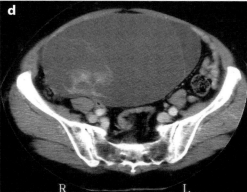
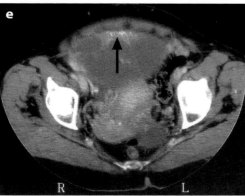
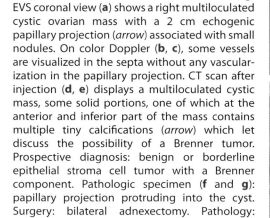
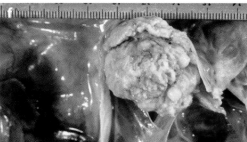
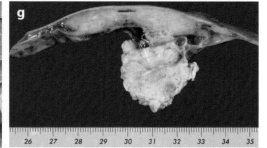

Fig. 9.132 Borderline Brenner tumor. A 72-year-old woman with abdominal swelling. EVS coronal view (a) shows a right multiloculated cystic ovarian mass with a 2 cm echogenic papillary projection (arrow) associated with small nodules. On color Doppler (b, c), some vessels are visualized in the septa without any vascularization in the papillary projection. CT scan after injection (d, e) displays a multiloculated cystic mass, some solid portions, one of which at the anterior and inferior part of the mass contains multiple tiny calcifications (arrow) which let discuss the possibility of a Brenner tumor. Prospective diagnosis: benign or borderline epithelial stroma cell tumor with a Brenner component. Pathologic specimen (f and g): papillary projection protruding into the cyst. Surgery: bilateral adnexectomy. Pathology: borderline Brenner tumor

Microscopy

The histologic patterns are often mixed with other types of carcinoma, most often serous; 10 % of carcinomas are pure.

More than 50 % of the tumor should display the patterns of TTC for a diagnosis of TTC. A diagnosis of malignant Brenner tumor is warranted when a benign or atypical Brenner component is identified.

The characteristic feature is thick blunt and often papillary folds with fibrous cores lined by transitional-type epithelium resembling urothelium.

Stroma invasion is characterized by haphazard infiltrative growth of epithelium at the base of the papillae into the cyst wall or extensive areas of solid proliferation.

9.7.3.3 Imaging Findings (Fig. 9.133)

Sugimura et al. [147] reported MR findings of a malignant Brenner tumor composed of complicated cysts and tissular component. On T1W images, the cystic component appeared with a low signal and shape margins. On T2W images, the signal intensity of the cystic component was similar to that of fat; the solid component had intermediate signal intensity. After injection, a marked patchy enhancement of the tissular portion was observed.

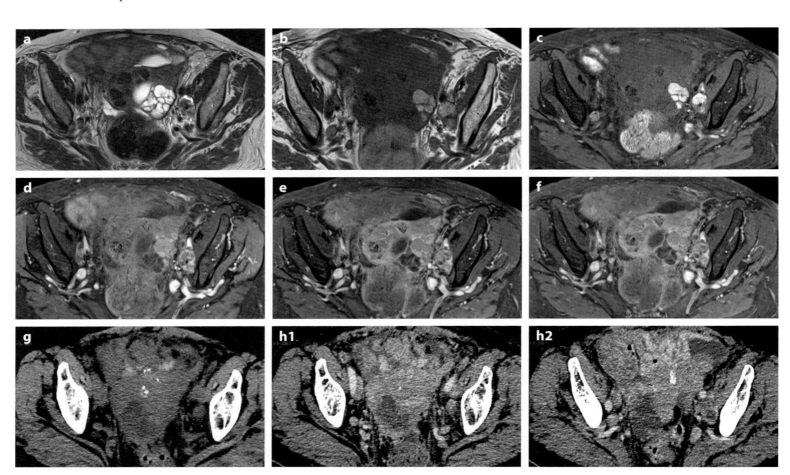

Fig. 9.133 Malignant Brenner tumor. MR findings. (1) Tumor of the left ovary: MR axial T2 (**a**) depicts a left ovarian mass containing cystic portions and solid tissue with low intensity areas. On axial T1 (**b**) and fat suppression (**c**), hemorrhage is visualized in the cystic portions. On DMR at the arterial phase (**d**) and at the venous phase (**e** and **f**) depicts some thin arterial vessels in the solid tissue, associated with contrast uptake. (2) Extension. Peritoneal infiltration of the omentum and left iliac lymph node metastasis are depicted. CT findings. DCT without injection (**g**) depicts tiny calcifications in the anterior part of the mass, suggestive of a Brenner tumor associated with larger and denser calcifications in the central part of the mass. At the arterial phase (**h1** and **h2**), tumoral vessels are visualized in the mass, the omentum, and iliac lymph node

9.8   Other Epithelial and Mixed Tumors

9.8.1   Mixed Epithelial Tumors (Figs. 9.134 and 9.135)

Definition: These are the presence of two epithelial cell types in an ovarian neoplasm comprising at least 10 % of the tumor.

However, it is more convenient to classify tumors based solely on the predominant component.

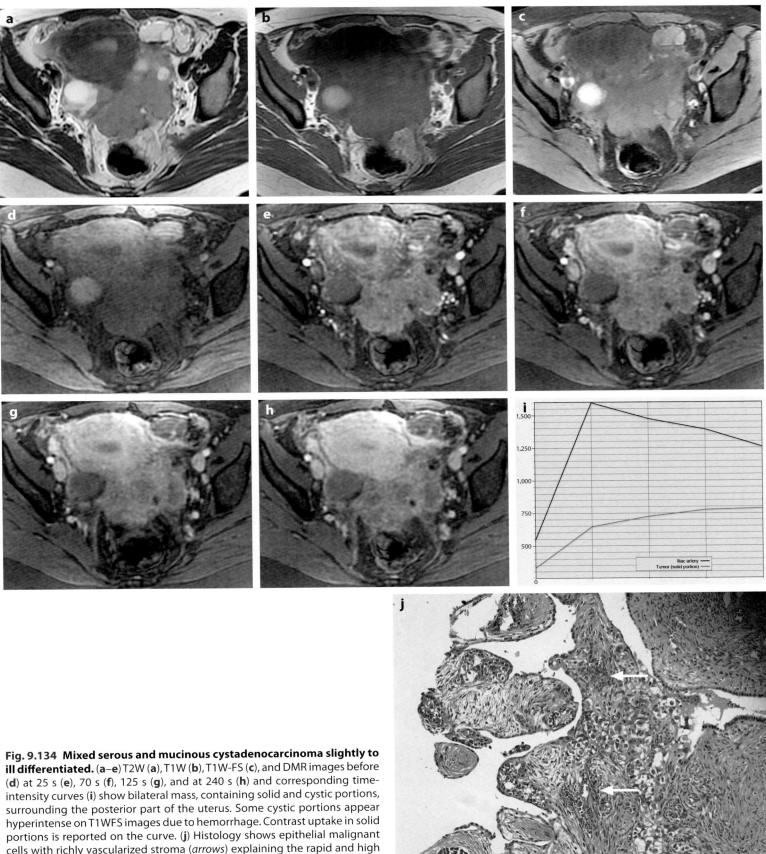

Fig. 9.134 Mixed serous and mucinous cystadenocarcinoma slightly to ill differentiated. (a–e) T2W (a), T1W (b), T1W-FS (c), and DMR images before (d) at 25 s (e), 70 s (f), 125 s (g), and at 240 s (h) and corresponding time-intensity curves (i) show bilateral mass, containing solid and cystic portions, surrounding the posterior part of the uterus. Some cystic portions appear hyperintense on T1WFS images due to hemorrhage. Contrast uptake in solid portions is reported on the curve. (j) Histology shows epithelial malignant cells with richly vascularized stroma (*arrows*) explaining the rapid and high contrast uptake

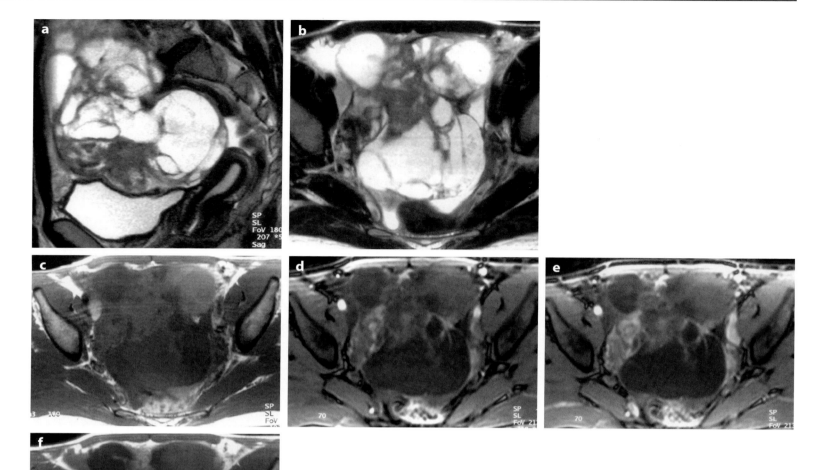

Fig. 9.135 Composite tumor. A 45-year-old woman – CA 125 185 IV/ml. Sagittal (**a**) and axial T2 (**b**) display a multilocular cystic mass with a low intensity portion in the right and lower part of the mass. DMR without contrast (**c**) at the arterial phase (**d**) demonstrates arterial tumoral vessels with early contrast uptake (**e**) in the solid portion, situated in the right and lower part of the mass, typical for a malignant tumor. The tissular portion with irregular borders, containing degenerative changes, is clearly depicted on the delayed MR (**f**). Pathology: composite tumor (endometrioid and clear cell carcinoma) stage Ia

9.8.2 Undifferentiated Tumors (Figs. 9.136 and 9.137)

Definition: They do not present identifiable features of any of the cell types.

There are three types:

- Undifferentiated carcinoma (Fig. 9.138)
- The hypercalcemic type of small cell carcinoma (Fig. 9.139)
- The pulmonary type of small cell carcinoma

In all cases, it is important to exclude metastatic tumor particularly from the lungs.

9.8.3 Tumors with Sarcomatous Component

9.8.3.1 Malignant Mixed Mullerian Tumor (MMMT)

MMMTS are unusual neoplasms occurring mostly in uterus. In the ovary, they are very rare and represent less than 1 % of all ovarian malignancies; in the salpinx, they are even rarer than those of the ovary [151].

Malignant mixed Mullerian tumor is composed of derivatives of Mullerian mesoderm, a primitive structure that gives rise to the stroma and epithelium of the endometrium [152].

These tumors are composed of carcinomas (of various Mullerian types) and sarcoma-like tissue that may be homologous (characterized by tissue type native of the ovary) or heterologous (containing foreign tissue such as cartilage, skeletal muscle, osteoid, and adipose tissue) [153].

Although these neoplasms often contain non-endometrioid epithelial and stromal elements, they are classified as endometrioid because of their close similarity to their more common counterparts in the endometrium [153].

They usually involve postmenopausal women [154] with low parity [154, 155].

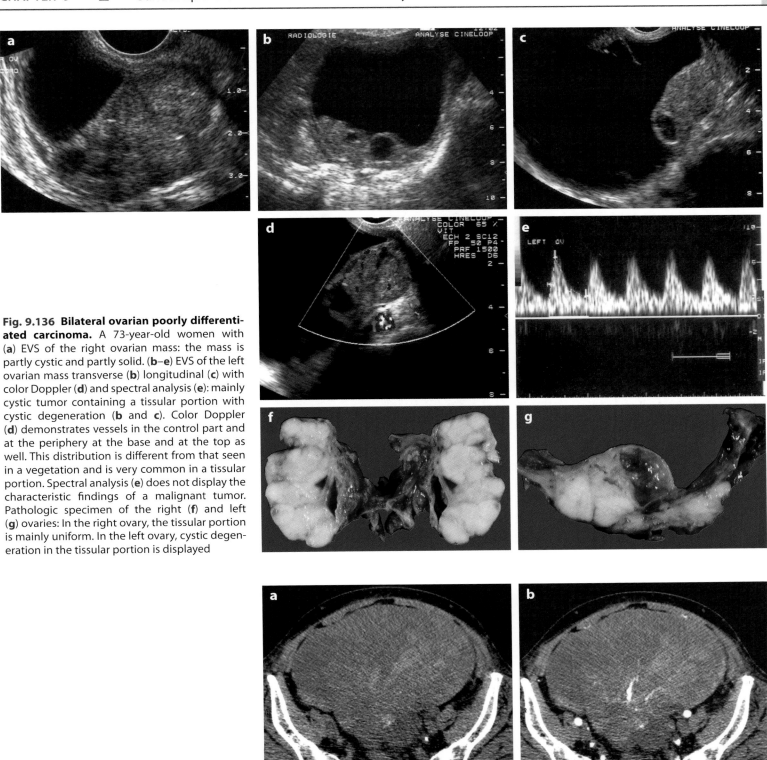

Fig. 9.136 Bilateral ovarian poorly differentiated carcinoma. A 73-year-old women with (**a**) EVS of the right ovarian mass: the mass is partly cystic and partly solid. (**b–e**) EVS of the left ovarian mass transverse (**b**) longitudinal (**c**) with color Doppler (**d**) and spectral analysis (**e**): mainly cystic tumor containing a tissular portion with cystic degeneration (**b** and **c**). Color Doppler (**d**) demonstrates vessels in the control part and at the periphery at the base and at the top as well. This distribution is different from that seen in a vegetation and is very common in a tissular portion. Spectral analysis (**e**) does not display the characteristic findings of a malignant tumor. Pathologic specimen of the right (**f**) and left (**g**) ovaries: In the right ovary, the tissular portion is mainly uniform. In the left ovary, cystic degeneration in the tissular portion is displayed

Fig. 9.137 Poorly differentiated left ovarian carcinoma. CT without injection (**a**) at the arterial phase (**b**) displays typical arterial tumoral vessels.

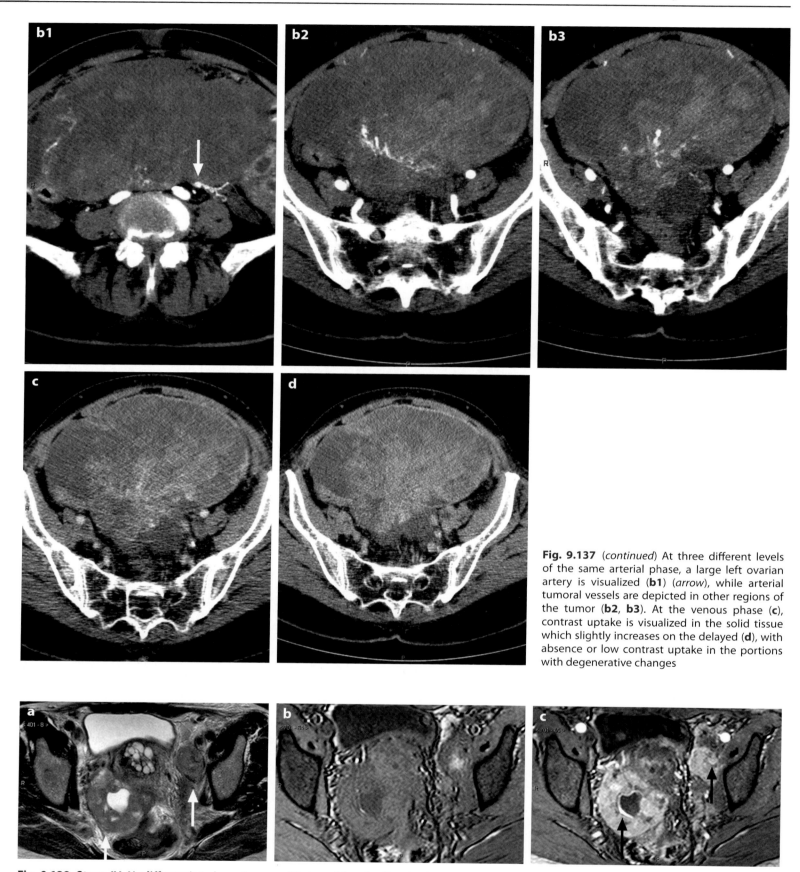

Fig. 9.137 (*continued*) At three different levels of the same arterial phase, a large left ovarian artery is visualized (**b1**) (*arrow*), while arterial tumoral vessels are depicted in other regions of the tumor (**b2**, **b3**). At the venous phase (**c**), contrast uptake is visualized in the solid tissue which slightly increases on the delayed (**d**), with absence or low contrast uptake in the portions with degenerative changes

Fig. 9.138 Stage IV. Undifferentiated carcinoma with transitional cell carcinoma component. Forty-three-year-old woman. Lumbar pain. CA 125 1,200 IU/ml. Sus-clavicular lymph node first biopsy demonstrated a malignant urothelial carcinoma. After surgery, ovariectomy, and lymph node curettage, undifferentiated carcinoma. *MR.* (1) Ovarian masses. MR axial T2 (a) displays a bilateral ovarian mass with the same morphologic features: there are tissular with cystic components (*arrows*). DMR of the right ovarian mass without injection (**b**) at the arterial phase (**c**) displays tumoral vessels in the masses (*arrows*).

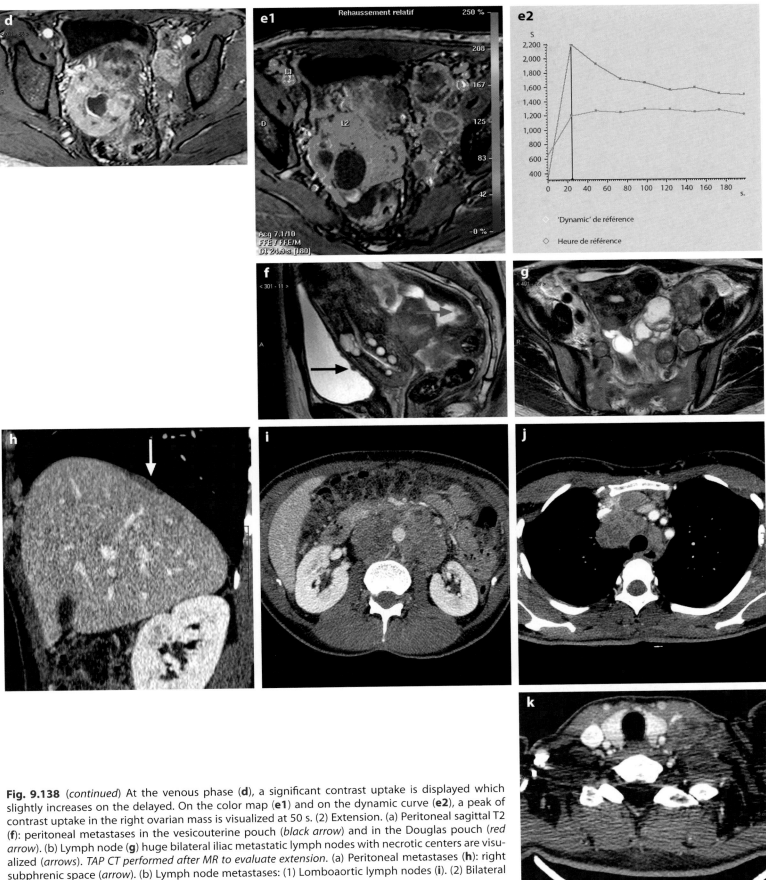

Fig. 9.138 (*continued*) At the venous phase (**d**), a significant contrast uptake is displayed which slightly increases on the delayed. On the color map (**e1**) and on the dynamic curve (**e2**), a peak of contrast uptake in the right ovarian mass is visualized at 50 s. (2) Extension. (a) Peritoneal sagittal T2 (**f**): peritoneal metastases in the vesicouterine pouch (*black arrow*) and in the Douglas pouch (*red arrow*). (b) Lymph node (**g**) huge bilateral iliac metastatic lymph nodes with necrotic centers are visualized (*arrows*). *TAP CT performed after MR to evaluate extension.* (a) Peritoneal metastases (**h**): right subphrenic space (*arrow*). (b) Lymph node metastases: (1) Lomboaortic lymph nodes (**i**). (2) Bilateral mediastinal lymph nodes (**j**). (3) Left cervical metastatic lymph node (**k**)

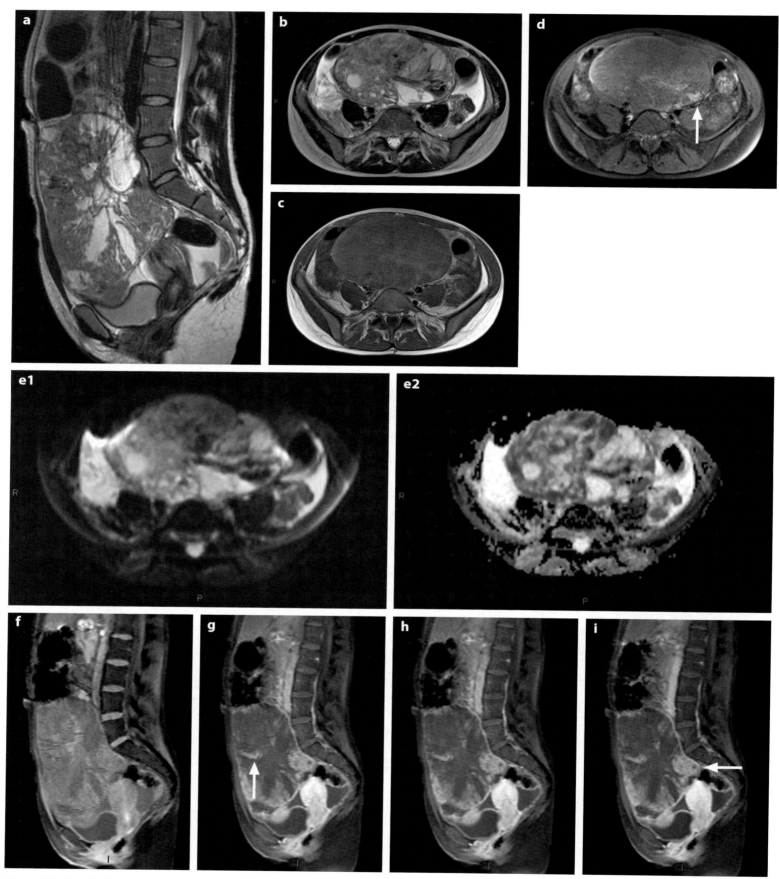

Fig. 9.139 Small cell carcinoma with hypercalcemia. MR sagittal (**a**) and axial T2 (**b**) display a huge well-delineated mixed ovarian mass, with tissular portions of intermediate signal, with cystic portions. On axial T1 (**c**) and fat suppression (**d**) areas of hemorrhage are displayed (*arrow*). On diffusion (**e1**) and ADC map (**e2**), areas of hyperintense signal are visualized; on DMR without injection (**f**) and at the arterial phase (**g**), large tumoral arterial vessels are depicted (*arrow*). At the venous phase (**h**) and on the delayed (**i**), intense contrast uptake is visualized in the tissular portions located mainly at the periphery (*arrow*). Prospective diagnosis: malignant ovarian tumor without extraovarian extension. Surgery: total hysterectomy, bilateral adnexectomy, and omentectomy. Pathology: small cell carcinoma with hypercalcemia of the right ovary stage 1a

Gross and Microscopy

The gross and microscopic features of ovarian MMMTS resemble its more common uterine counterpart [156].

The tumor is typically large [153], may be predominantly cystic or solid, and commonly containing areas of necrosis and hemorrhage. Rarely, it arises in an endometrioid cyst.

Imaging Modalities (Figs. 9.140 and 9.141)

They are aggressive, bilateral, large, usually more than 10 cm [154, 157] mixed (solid and cystic), sometimes with a central low-attenuation [158] or multiseptated, thick-walled cystic tumors.

Smith et al. [158] reported the CT findings of uterine MMMTS as a large heterogeneous mass up to 30 cm in maximum diameter with central low attenuation.

Differential Diagnosis

The most common forms which are homologous are indistinguishable macroscopically from purely carcinoma.

The heterologous form is mainly represented by chondrosarcoma and fibrosarcoma. These forms can be confused most often with immature teratomas (Table 9.29) (see Chap. 10).

Table 9.29 Differential diagnosis between malignant mesodermal mixed tumors (MMMT) and immature teratoma

	MMMT	Immature teratoma
Age	Menopausal	Young
Germ layer	Monodermal	All three layers
Neuroectodermal tissue	Rare (minor component when present)	Predominant

Spread

They are usually found at an advanced stage in postmenopausal women [154, 155, 157, 159]. Over 90 % of these tumors have spread beyond the ovary at the time of diagnosis, with 60 % stage III and 10 % stage IV [160, 161].

Ascites is frequent with peritoneal seeding and direct invasion [162].

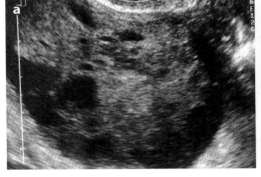 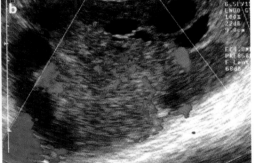

Fig. 9.140 MMMT with heterologous sarcomatous component. EVS without (**a**) and with color Doppler (**b**) displays a right ovarian mass with a significant solid portion associated with degenerative changes. Large arterial vessels are displayed in the solid tissue. Prospective diagnosis: ovarian malignant tumor. Microscopy: MMMT. The epithelial component comprises at the level of the intracystic component glands with cylindrical or cuboidal cells, hobnail cells, and foci of undifferentiated cells. The stromal component comprises areas of heterologous sarcoma, particularly with chondroid differentiation, with a fibrosarcomatous component

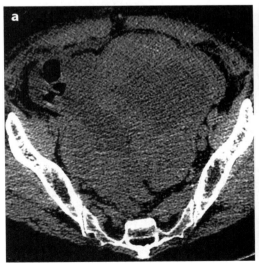 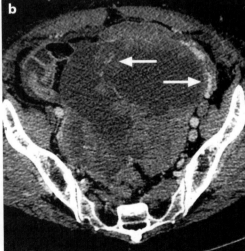 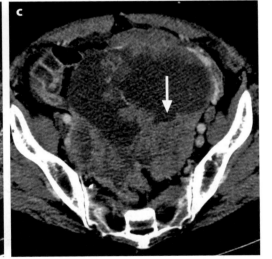

Fig. 9.141 MMMT. DCT without injection (**a**) at the arterial phase (**b**) depicts a mixed large ovarian mass containing large tumoral arterial vessels at the periphery of the mass with smaller tortuous vessels in the central part of the mass (*arrows*), typical for a malignant tumor. At the venous phase (**c**), a significant contrast uptake is depicted in the solid parts of the mass (*arrow*).

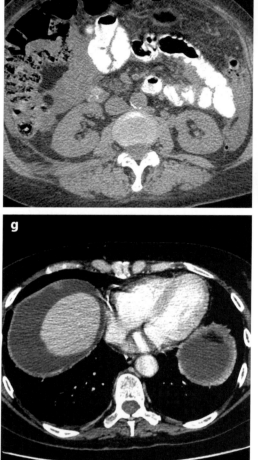

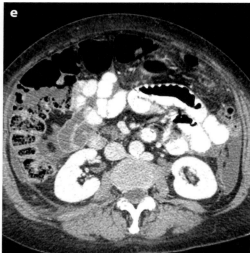

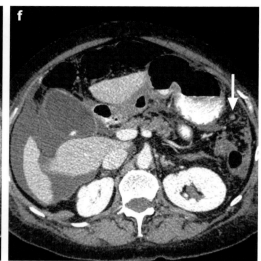

Fig. 9.141 (*continued*) CT without (**d**) and after injection (**e**) at the level of the omentum and of the gastrocolic ligament (**f**) (*arrow*) display nodules and some infiltration with an increase of vascularization related to peritoneal metastases. Ascites in both subphrenic spaces with a nodular peritoneal implant is visualized in (**g**). Prospective diagnosis: ovarian carcinoma stage IIIc. At microscopy: MMMT

Mixed Epithelial and Stromal Adenosarcoma

This tumor is very uncommon. It contains a benign epithelial component and a malignant sarcomatous component.

Endometrioid Stromal Sarcoma

Although this tumor is purely of mesenchymal origin, it is mentioned here with other ovarian sarcoma. This tumor is also very uncommon. There is no epithelial component with a sarcomatous stromal component mimicking endometrial stroma.

9.9   Particular Presentations

9.9.1   Carcinomas of Small Size (<4-cm) and Peritoneal Carcinomatosis (Fig. 9.142)

Carcinoma of the ovary can be detected lately at a stage of diffuse abdominopelvic carcinomatosis while the ovaries are of small size or even are not recognizable because they are included in peritoneal metastases.

The following abnormalities can be observed:

- Increased size related to the age. The volume of the ovary decreases significantly in perimenopause and mainly after menopause. The mean ovarian volume in premenopausal woman is 4.9 ± 0.03 cm³ and in postmenopausal woman 2.2 ± 0.01 cm³ [163]. An increase in size of the ovarian volume reported to the age is a nonspecific finding but much draw the attention to the possibility of a small ovarian carcinoma.
- Modification of the usual oval shape.
- Irregularity of the surface.
- Inhomogeneous pattern related to degenerative changes. These degenerative changes must not be confused with inclusion cysts which are particularly common in postmenopausal women.

These different abnormalities are not specific but at least should draw the attention to the possibility of ovarian cancer particularly in women in perimenopause or after menopause especially when presenting one or more risk factors of ovarian cancer.

This form is mainly observed in undifferentiated carcinomas [164]. Ultrasound study of this form is limited. The identical echogenicity of ovarian tumors and peritoneal metastasis makes identification of the ovaries difficult. CT scan visualizes the tissular lesions and evaluates the extension. In this form, CT scan appears more accurate than MR. The main differential diagnosis includes primary serous carcinoma of the peritoneum (PSCP) and well-differentiated papillary mesothelioma and peritoneal tuberculosis.

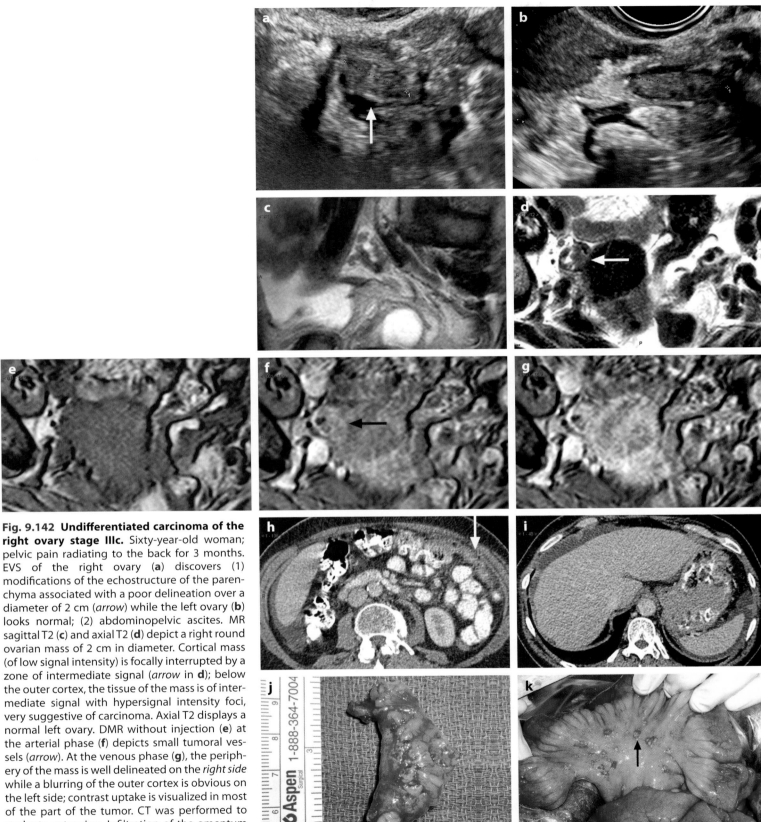

Fig. 9.142 Undifferentiated carcinoma of the right ovary stage IIIc. Sixty-year-old woman; pelvic pain radiating to the back for 3 months. EVS of the right ovary (**a**) discovers (1) modifications of the echostructure of the parenchyma associated with a poor delineation over a diameter of 2 cm (*arrow*) while the left ovary (**b**) looks normal; (2) abdominopelvic ascites. MR sagittal T2 (**c**) and axial T2 (**d**) depict a right round ovarian mass of 2 cm in diameter. Cortical mass (of low signal intensity) is focally interrupted by a zone of intermediate signal (*arrow* in **d**); below the outer cortex, the tissue of the mass is of intermediate signal with hypersignal intensity foci, very suggestive of carcinoma. Axial T2 displays a normal left ovary. DMR without injection (**e**) at the arterial phase (**f**) depicts small tumoral vessels (*arrow*). At the venous phase (**g**), the periphery of the mass is well delineated on the *right side* while a blurring of the outer cortex is obvious on the left side; contrast uptake is visualized in most of the part of the tumor. CT was performed to evaluate extension. Infiltration of the omentum with an omental cake pattern extending to the transverse colon is diagnosed (**h**) (*arrow*). Peritoneal implants with ascites are visualized in the right subhepatic space and both subphrenic spaces (**i**). Macroscopic specimen of the right ovary (**j**) displays infiltration by a tumor. Small metastatic nodules are visualized on the omentum (**k**) (*arrow*)

9.9.2 Utero-Tubo-Ovarian Carcinoma
(Figs. 9.143 and 9.144)

The carcinoma includes the ovaries, the tube, and the uterus realizing a block. The tumoral process extends sometimes to the other pelvic organs and to the pelvic sidewall realizing what surgeons call a frozen pelvis.

9.9.2.1 Ultrasound

Owing to the mainly echogenic character of these forms, of their volume, and of their undefined limits, it is very difficult to make a correct study of these lesions and even in some cases to diagnose ovarian carcinoma.

9.9.2.2 CT and MR

MR (mainly T2 and DMR sequence) better than CT allows in most of the cases to distinguish the uterus and the adnexal masses, and to evaluate loco-regional extension. In these cases, CT is very helpful to evaluate the abdominopelvic extension and eventually the thoracic extension.

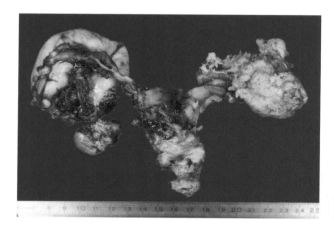

Fig. 9.143 Utero- tubo-ovarian serous carcinoma. Pathologic specimen: bilateral ovarian masses with extension to the wall of the body and the uterine cervix

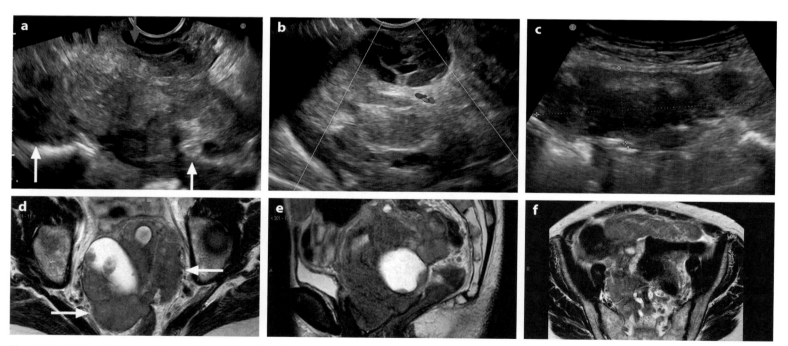

Fig. 9.144 Bilateral tubo-ovarian carcinoma invading the uterus. Transverse EVS (**a**) depicts a bilateral pelvic mass (*white arrows*) impossible to separate from the uterus (*red arrow*), realizing a pelvic block with ascites. Sagittal view with color Doppler (**b**) displays degenerative changes in the mass, with some vessels. Transverse view of the abdomen (**c**) depicts an omental cake. MR axial T2 (**d**) and sagittal T2 (**e**) confirm the presence of a bilateral malignant tubo-ovarian mass (*white arrows*) with degenerative changes and precised invasion of the uterus (*red arrow*). Massive invasion of the omentum (**f**) is depicted

9.9.3 Synchronous Tumors [165]

1. Ovarian and endometrial tumors (see Chap. 22, Sect. 22.4.1). The histology of the ovarian tumor and the carcinoma of the endometrium can also be different (Fig. 9.145).
2. Appendiceal and mucinous ovarian tumors.

3. Mucinous tumor which can be benign, borderline, or malignant [166] can be associated with a mature cystic teratoma in 5 % of cases [167] or a Brenner tumor. Patients with mucinous ovarian cystadenocarcinoma sometimes develop an independent mucinous cystadenocarcinoma of the cervix. Such tumors also have been reported in patients with Peutz-Jeghers syndrome [165].
4. Ovarian and rectal or sigmoid carcinoma (Fig. 9.146).

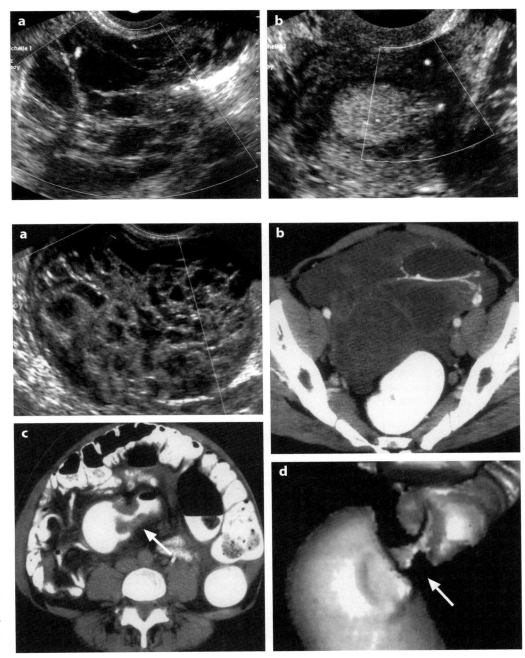

Fig. 9.145 Synchronous tumor. Endovaginal US with color Doppler (**a**): multiloculated left 6 cm ovarian mass with multiple septa gathered in some parts of the mass with regular vessels in some septa. EVS of the uterus (**b**): a 3.5 cm polyp with regular contours and a vascular pedicle are depicted, which was considered to be benign on the ultrasound findings. Surgery: total hysterectomy with bilateral adnexectomy. Pathology: left ovarian borderline mucinous tumor associated with clear cell adenocarcinoma of the endometrium

Fig. 9.146 Synchronous ovarian mucinous carcinoma of the ovary with sigmoid adenocarcinoma. TVS (**a**): multiloculated cystic mass with thick and irregular septa. With large vessels in the septa. Malignancy is suggested. DCT at the arterial phase (**b**) only depicts regular vessels in the septa. Association with a sigmoid tumor (**c** and **d**) is displayed (*arrow*)

9.9.4 Tumors with Functioning Stroma

See Chap. 13

9.9.5 Tumors Discovered on the Occasion of Complications

See Chap. 32

9.10 Extension

9.10.1 Introduction

Definite staging of ovarian cancer is surgical [168] and usually includes abdominal hysterectomy with bilateral salpingo-oophorectomy and excision of the infracolic omentum. Biopsies of pelvic and abdominal lymph nodes, surgical evaluation of multiple pelvic and abdominal peritoneal sites including the diaphragm, and cytologic tests of peritoneal fluid are required. This thorough protocol is recommended by gynecologic oncologists, as tumor stage and tumor size left after surgery are directly related to the survival of patients with ovarian cancer [168–172]. In practice, however, surgical protocol is not done in the majority of patients. As a result, up to 40 % of patients are understaged at initial laparotomy [168, 172]. Other prognostic factors include age, histology, grade, stage of disease, intraperitoneal blood loss, and prescription or not of the postoperative chemotherapy in stage I [173].

The preoperative evaluation of extension is essential for the surgical approach and the type of surgical treatment or for the indication of a presurgical treatment.

It must try to answer to three main questions:

1. Is the tumor limited to the ovary? Whatever the tumor is benign, borderline or malignant, the surgical excision is usually limited to the tumor, the ovary, or at the most the adnexa.
2. In case of malignant tumor, is there any particular extension particularly to the GI tract which lets presume of the necessity of a complementary excision with eventually a colostomy?
3. Is there any suspicion of nonresectability of the tumor with the indication of a preoperative chemotherapy? [174]

Moreover, extension of the tumor outside the ovary constitutes a positive finding of malignancy which has already been mentioned [175, 176].

Besides this information, visualization of the topography of the pelvic urethras with injection of contrast medium is essential in the preoperative staging, is more safety for the surgeon, and shortens the operation timing.

9.10.2 Different Pathways

Dissemination of ovarian carcinomas spreads through four different pathways:
- By direct locoregional extension in the pelvis
- Peritoneal extension
- Through the lymphatic system
- Hematogenous metastases (exceptional at time of presentation)

9.10.3 FIGO Staging

Extension outside the ovary is classified according to the FIGO classification (Table 9.30).

Table 9.30 FIGO Classification [177]

Stage I Growth limited to the ovaries
Ia – Growth limited to one ovary
No tumor on the external surface, capsule intact
No ascites present containing malignant cells
Ib – Growth limited to both ovaries
No tumor on the external surface, capsule intact
No ascites present containing malignant cells
Ic – Tumor either stage Ia or Ib
But with tumor on surface of one or both ovaries or with capsule ruptured
Or with ascites present containing malignant cells or with positive peritoneal washings
Stage II Growth involving one or both ovaries with pelvic extension
IIa – Extension and/or metastases to the uterus and/or the tube
IIb – Extension to other pelvic tissues
IIc – Tumor either stage IIa or IIb, but with tumor on surface of one or both ovaries or with capsule ruptured or with ascites present containing malignant cells or with positive peritoneal washings
Stage III
– Tumors involving one or both ovaries with histologically confirmed peritoneal implants outside the pelvis and/or positive retroperitoneal or inguinal lymph nodes
– Superficial liver metastases equals stage III
– Tumor is limited to the true pelvis but with histologically proven malignant extension to small bowel or omentum
IIIa – Tumor grossly limited to the true pelvis, with negative nodes, but with histologically confirmed microscopic seeding of abdominal peritoneal surfaces or histologic-proven extension to small bowel or mesentery
IIIb – Tumors of one or both ovaries with macroscopic histologically confirmed abdominoperitoneal implants not exceeding 2 cm in diameter Nodes are negative
IIIc – Peritoneal metastasis beyond the pelvis >2 cm in diameter And/or positive retroperitoneal or inguinal nodes
Stage IV Growth involving one or both ovaries with metastases to the liver or outside the peritoneal cavity
If pleural effusion is present, there must be positive cytology to allot a case of stage IV
Parenchymal (not peritoneal) liver metastasis equals stage IV

9.10.4 Imaging Modalities

Different imaging modalities, US [178–180], CT [175, 181, 182], and MR [183] can be used to evaluate preoperatively the extension of the tumor.

Recently, the Radiologic Diagnostic Oncology Group reported a prospective evaluation of preoperative staging of ovarian cancer with the three modalities [184].

US is of lower value than CT and MR for preoperative staging (except in some locations) due to lower sensitivity for identifying pelvic and retroperitoneal lymph node metastases and peritoneal implants [185] and colon and pelvic side wall invasion [184]. Both CT and MRI have their own advantages [186]. For some authors, overall staging accuracy is similar while others consider CT superior to MR to evaluate this extension [187, 188]. At present, due to cost and examination and interpretation time, contrast-enhanced CT is the primary imaging modality for ovarian cancer staging. MR should be reserved for cases in which CT findings are equivocal, in pregnant patients, or when iodinated contrast material is contraindicated [186].

9.10.5 Pelvic Extension

Pelvic extension is essential to be evaluated before surgery in order to predict the importance of the excision (ureterostomy, partial cystectomy, colostomy). The diagnosis of contiguous invasion is suggested when a lesion with identical morphologic characters to the primary tumor extends into the adjacent organs and disturbs its normal anatomy.

9.10.5.1 Uterus

In clinical practice, when the preoperative diagnosis of ovarian carcinoma is made, evaluation of extension to the uterus has no real importance for the surgeon as far as uterus is systematically removed.

However, in some cases, ovarian carcinoma can be revealed by a uterine carcinoma (endometrial or endocervical). It must outline the difficulty in this type of situation and especially when it is an endometrioid carcinoma at histology to know which the primary is. In this situation, the patient is usually treated as an ovarian carcinoma.

Evaluation of extension to the uterus can be helpful for the diagnosis in case the ovarian mass cannot be characterized as benign or malignant.

Extension to the uterus can be due to different mechanisms: (1) by contiguity and (2) by metastases to the endometrium and/or the endocervix.

Whatever the radiological modality used, extension by contiguity is diagnosed according to the findings described above. Metastatic extension to the endometrium eventually associated to extension to myometrium appears:

- In ultrasound as a echogenic lesion (Fig. 9.116) which can resemble a primary carcinoma or a benign polyp (Fig. 9.116).
- In MR (Fig. 9.147) as a tissular lesion with a signal close to pelvic muscle on T1, with a higher signal than muscle on the T2 and with contrast uptake. A lesion of the endometrium extending into the myometrium is particularly well displayed when the junctional zone, in contact with the lesion, is disrupted.
- In CT as a lesion which appears at the best on delay scans and which is less dense than uterine parenchyma and usually with irregular borders (Figs. 9.116 and 9.148).

When the extension is strictly limited to the endometrium, differentiation with a benign polyp on the different imaging modalities may be impossible (Fig. 9.145).

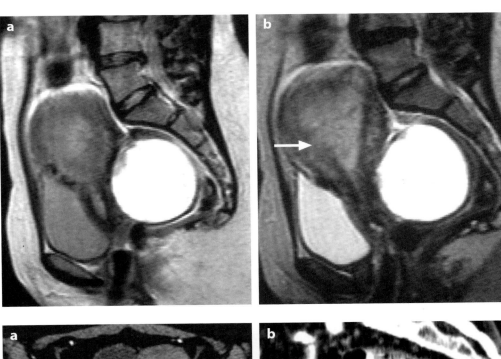

Fig. 9.147 Extension to the endometrium from an endometrioid carcinoma of the ovary. MR SAGITTAL T2 (**a** and **b**) displays (**a**) an ovarian carcinoma and (**b**) an endometrial tissular lesion, with extension to the myometrium (*arrow*)

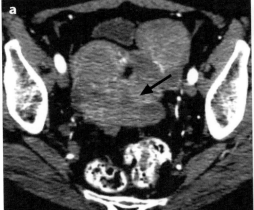

Fig. 9.148 Bilateral mucinous carcinoma extension to the cervix. CT (**a**): ovarian tumor with extension to the left border of the cervix (*arrow*). Sagittal reformation (**b**): extension to the posterior part of the cervix (*white arrow*) and through continuity to the sigmoid (*red arrow*)

9.10.5.2 Tubes (Fig. 9.149)

Tubal involvement is frequent but almost never diagnosed preoperatively.

9.10.5.3 Vagina

Extension to the vagina is rare except in case of recurrence after surgery (Fig. 9.150) (see Sect. 9.12). It has been reported preoperatively in cases of endometrioid carcinoma [189].

9.10.5.4 Bladder

It is always an extension by contiguity associated with an involvement of vesical peritoneum. On the radiological point of view, it is sometimes very difficult to distinguish peritoneal involvement from wall involvement. Ultrasound, CT using multiplanar reformation, and MR have roughly similar results.

9.10.5.5 Ureters

Only opacification (CT or MRI with contrast) can determine correctly an obstruction, its level, and eventually an invasion.

A preoperative clear visualization of the topography of the ureters and of their relationships with the pelvic organs can only be made on the delayed post IV contrast CT.

9.10.5.6 Gastrointestinal Tract

(a) The *rectosigmoid* (Fig. 9.151) is most often involved. As for the bladder, the rectosigmoid is always invaded from a peritoneal lesion. CT scan appears as the best method to diagnose this extension that is fundamental to evaluate preoperatively in order to inform the patient from the possibility of a colostomy.
   CT with opacification of the large bowel is very accurate to visualize a thickened wall, nodules extending more or less in the lumen, irregularity of the mucosa (Fig. 9.151). According to the results of this examination, endoscopy can be done.

(b) Invasion of *transverse colon*, uncommon, is usually an extension from a lesion of greater omentum. These lesions may extend to the anterior abdominal wall. Cecum may also be involved.

(c) *Small bowel* involvement is uncommon. Most often, there are only peritoneal lesions of carcinomatosis on the serous surface.

9.10.5.7 Parametrium and Pelvic Wall

Pelvic wall is uncommonly involved.

Location at the level of the umbilicus can happen exceptionally when the tumor is discovered.

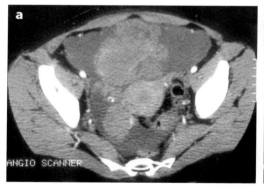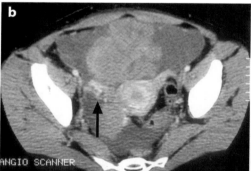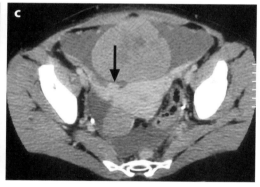

Fig. 9.149 Bilateral mixed ovarian mass with extension to the right tube. A 41-year-old women with increased abdominal volume. DCT at the arterial phase 20 s after injection (**a**) displays a bilateral ovarian carcinoma with ascites. Thirty seconds after injection (**b**), a hypervascularization of the right tube (*arrow*) is displayed. Sixty seconds after injection (**c**), two small nodules are visualized on the tube (*arrow*)

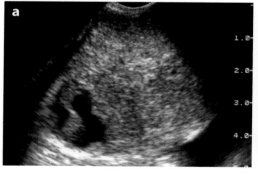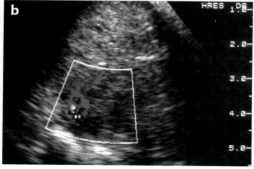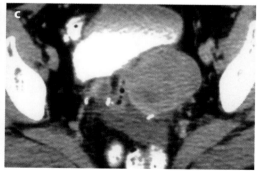

Fig. 9.150 Vaginal recurrence from an ovarian endometrioid carcinoma stage II operated 2 years before. During a routine examination, a pelvic mass is palpated in the upper vagina. Longitudinal EVS (**a**) demonstrates in the upper part of the vagina a tissular echogenic mass with a high degree of tumoral vessels on color Doppler (**b**) in the upper portion of the mass, typical for a recurrence. CT was performed to confirm the diagnosis and to evaluate abdominopelvic extension. CT scan after IV contrast (**c**): a 5 cm round tissular mass with degenerative changes is visualized in the *left middle* and left lateral portion of the fornix; it is surrounded by surgical clips. This pattern is typical for a recurrence on the vagina and is particularly seen in case of endometrioid carcinoma. A marked compression on the posterior wall of the bladder is depicted

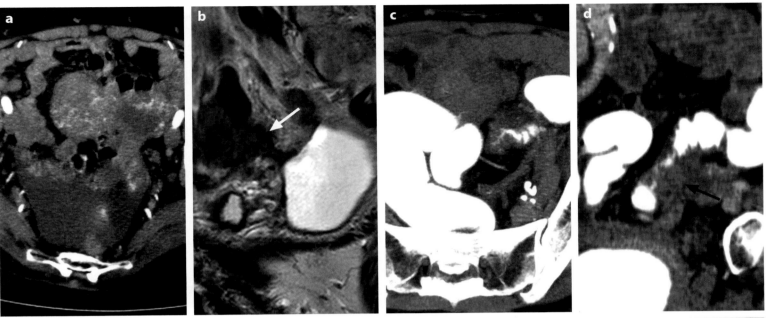

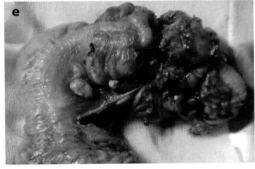

Fig. 9.151 Extension of an ovarian carcinoma to the sigmoid. DCT at the arterial phase (**a**) depicts a typical ovarian carcinoma. MR sagittal (**b**) displays a left ovarian mass, in contact with the sigmoid (*arrow*), but extension to the wall cannot be assessed. CT with enema in axial view (**c**) and in slightly oblique coronal view (**d**) demonstrates on the sigmoid over a 3 cm length a thickening of the wall associated with irregularity of the mucosa (*arrow*) related to extension to the sigmoid. On pathologic specimen confirms (**e**) nodule on the serosa, infiltration of the muscular wall, and extension to the mucosa

Frozen Pelvis

Diffuse extension to the different viscera, peritoneum, and pelvic wall results in what surgeon call a frozen pelvis. Although it is difficult preoperatively to predict the impossibility for the surgeon to proceed to complete tumoral resection, the pattern on CT is sometimes very suggestive of the frozen pelvis.

9.10.6 Peritoneal Extension

9.10.6.1 Pathophysiology

Dissemination of Cells

Ovarian cancers commonly shed cells directly in the peritoneum [190].

In the abdomen and pelvis, cells migrate in a cephalic direction. Three different mechanisms are considered responsible of this migration:

- The intraabdominal pressure in the upper abdomen is lower than in the hypogastrium [191, 192].
- Furthermore, pressure in the upper abdomen decreases further during inspiration [192].
- The rolling motion of the intestine [190].

The routes of migration (Fig. 9.152) are considered the same as those of peritoneal fluid [193–195].The cells ascend to the para-

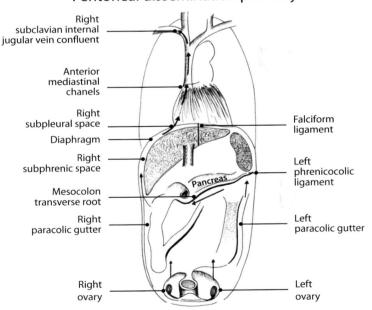

Fig. 9.152 Peritoneal dissemination pathways

colic gutters. Passage up to the shallower left gutter is slow and weak; uphold extension is limited by the left phrenicocolic ligament that continues the transverse mesocolon partially separating the paracolic gutter from the left subphrenic space. Thus, the major flow from the pelvis is up to the right paracolic gutter. This then progresses to the right subhepatic and subphrenic spaces. Direct passage across the midline to the left subphrenic space is prevented by the falciform ligament.

From the lymphatic capillaries that line the diaphragmatic peritoneum, the cells migrate into the right diaphragm [196]. Feldman [190] has demonstrated that these capillaries form a diffuse communicating network via intradiaphragmatic capillaries with a similar plexus on the diaphragm's pleural surface [190, 197]. Then, retrosternal lymphatic channels carry the bulk of peritoneal lymph to anterior mediastinal nodes. From the anterior mediastinal nodes, the main stream of peritoneal lymph proceeds to the right thoracic trunk [198, 199] and finally join admittance into the blood circulation via the right subclavian vein.

Exceptionally, the falciform ligament is crossed by the peritoneal implants. In this case, peritoneal implants of the left subphrenic space can migrate into the left hemidiaphragm, and through it, into the left pleura, causing a left pleural effusion (Fig. 9.153).

Peritoneal Fluid

The peritoneal cavity usually contains a small volume of fluid. This fluid is much like plasma and arises from the filtration of transudation of blood through capillary walls. Virtually, all the proteins present in the plasma including albumin, immunoglobulins, and clotting factors are also present in peritoneal fluid, although at somewhat different concentrations [199]. This proteinaceous pool is far from stagnant. Showenberger demonstrated in man that up to 75 % of the total body albumin passes into and out of the peritoneal

cavity at surprisingly rapid rates. If India ink is injected intraperitoneally, it is washed through the system so rapidly that diaphragmatic lymphatics and retrosternal nodes are stained black within a matter of minutes. Two different mechanisms seem to be responsible for accumulation of ascitic fluid:

- Increased production of a protein-rich fluid from the tumor-bearing surfaces of the peritoneum [194].
- Partial or complete obstruction of lymphatic vessels through which peritoneal fluid is drained. Some patients with multiple peritoneal metastases do not have ascites. Indeed, as long as the increased production of fluid is less than the drainage's system capacity to handle it, ascites would not be expected to develop. It has been demonstrated that the diaphragmatic lymphatics are the major pathways for peritoneal fluid drainage, with the omental, peritoneal lymphatics and thoracic ducts playing only a minor role [195, 200–202].

9.10.6.2 Imaging Modalities

Ultrasound Findings in Peritoneal Lesions

Many authors have assessed the usefulness of US in the detection of peritoneal deposits [178, 203].

The masses are nodular, mantle, or sheetlike or irregular.

Locations in the Douglas (Fig. 9.154), in the greater omentum especially when it has the appearance of an omental cake (Fig. 9.154), and in the right subhepatic and subphrenic space (Fig. 9.155) are well detected.

When ascites is present, peritoneal implants as small as 2–3 mm can be delineated [178].

However, implants in some locations are very difficult to detect.

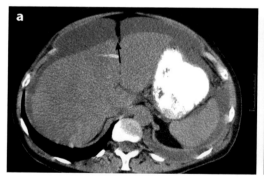
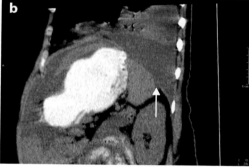

Fig. 9.153 **Carcinoma of the right ovary with very unusual case of ascites in the left subphrenic space with involvement of the left pleura.** Transverse view (**a**): ascites of both subphrenic spaces on each side of the falciform ligament (*arrow*). Sagittal reformation through the left hemidiaphragm (**b**): left subphrenic space, involvement of the left hemidiaphragm (*arrow*), left pleural effusion

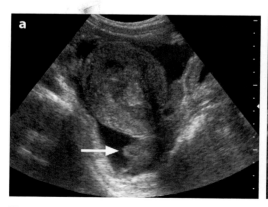
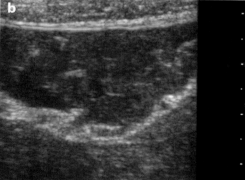
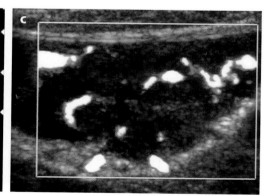

Fig. 9.154 **Peritoneal implants.** (**a**) Sagittal TAS of the uterus displays metastatic nodules in the pouch of Douglas (*arrow*). (**b** and **c**): TAS using a superficial probe without (**b**) and with Doppler (**c**) demonstrates an omental cake with a typical hypervascularization

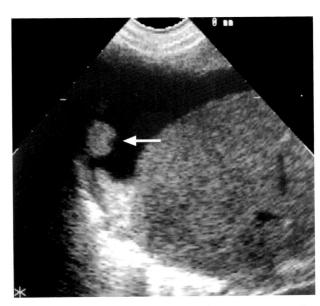

Fig. 9.155 Peritoneal nodule in the right subphrenic space associated with ascites (*arrow*)

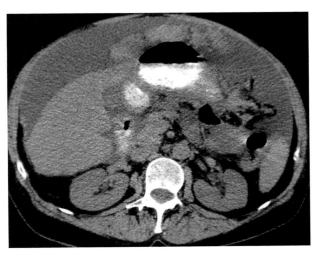

Fig. 9.156 (1) Peritoneal fluid in the lesser sac (*arrow*). (2) Involvement of the gastrocolic ligament (*arrow*)

CT Findings in Peritoneal Lesions

CT is a very appropriate method to evaluate peritoneal metastases.

Ascites is usually associated with peritoneal implants. However, ascites can be present without detectable peritoneal implants, and conversely, peritoneal implants can be present without ascites [190].

Ascites

Three different findings are very suggestive of malignant ascites:

- *Abdominopelvic ascites*: Ascites is usually most often located in the great peritoneal cavity. However, in some cases, ascites is also located to the lesser sac; among malignant causes of ascites, this topography is very suggestive of a primary ovarian carcinoma (Fig. 9.156). While pelvic ascites can be present in normal condi-

tions, in functional disorders, and even in benign tumors such as ovarian fibroma [204], abdominopelvic ascites is very suggestive of malignancy. Walkey has even outlined that significant ascites in the abdomen with no fluid in the cul de sac of Douglas is suggestive of peritoneal carcinomatosis. However, abdominopelvic ascites can also be observed in acute conditions such as torsion, rupture of functional hemorrhagic cyst, or ectopic pregnancy and in the exceptional Demons-Meigs syndrome.

- *Localized ascites*: Localized often round or oval fluid collection or limitation of fluid to one compartment was found in 25/54 (46 %) malignant ascites while no loculation was observed in benign ascites (*n* = 50) [205]. However, loculations secondary to surgical adhesions or peritonitis has already been mentioned [206].

- *Retraction of the peritoneum*: Retraction with inward displacement of parietal peritoneum in front of ascites has been found in peritoneal metastases [207] (Fig. 9.157), while it has never been observed in benign ascites.

Fig. 9.157 Peritoneal extension associated with retraction of the peritoneum by endometrioid carcinoma of the right ovary stage IIIc. A 72-year-old women with a previous history of breast carcinoma. CA 125: 685 IU/ml. DCT without contrast (**a**) at the arterial phase (**b**) utero-ovarian mass with morphologic and vascular findings of malignancy. Retraction of the parietal peritoneum (*arrow*) on the right in contact with periuterine tumoral tissue, associated with ascites is very suggestive of malignancy

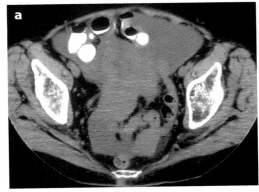
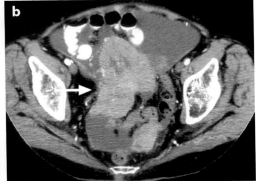

Brenner Tumors

124. Woodruff JD et al (1981) Proliferative and malignant Brenner tumors. Review of 47 cases. Am J Obstet Gynecol 141(2):118–125
125. Hallgrimsson J, Scully RE (1972) Borderline and malignant Brenner tumours of the ovary. A report of 15 cases. Acta Pathol Microbiol Scand A 233: 56–66
126. Miles PA, Norris HJ (1972) Proliferative and malignant brenner tumors of the ovary. Cancer 30(1):174–186
127. Scully RE, Young RH, Clement PB (1998) Tumors of the ovary, maldeveloped gonads, fallopian tubes and broad ligament. In: Rosai J, Sobin LH (eds) Atlas of tumor pathology, vol 3. Armed Force Institute of Pathology, Washington, DC, pp 51–168
128. Krigman H, Bentley R, Robboy SJ (1994) Pathology of epithelial ovarian tumors. Clin Obstet Gynecol 37(2):475–491
129. Seidman JD, Russel P, Kurman RJ (2002) Surface epithelial tumors of the ovary. In: Kurman RJ (ed) Blaustein's pathology of the female genital tract. Springer, New-York, pp 791–904
130. Athey PA, Malone RS (1987) Sonography of ovarian fibromas/thecomas. J Ultrasound Med 6:431–436
131. Williams AG, Mettler FA, Wicks JD (1983) Cystic and solid ovarian neoplasms. Semin Ultrasound 4:166
132. Outwater EK et al (1998) Ovarian Brenner tumors: MR imaging characteristics. Magn Reson Imaging 16(10):1147–1153
133. Ohara N, Teramoto K (2001) Magnetic resonance imaging of a benign Brenner tumor with an ipsilateral simple cyst. Arch Gynecol Obstet 265(2):96–99
134. Bazot M et al (1993) Fibrothecomas of the ovary: CT and US findings. J Comput Assist Tomogr 17:754–759
135. Moon WJ et al (2000) Brenner tumor of the ovary: CT and MR findings. J Comput Assist Tomogr 24(1):72–76
136. Outwater EK et al (1997) Ovarian fibromas and cystadenofibromas: MRI features of the fibrous component. J Magn Reson Imaging 7(3):465–471
137. Troiano RN et al (1997) Fibroma and fibrothecoma of the ovary: MR imaging findings. Radiology 204(3):795–798
138. Yamashita Y et al (1995) Adnexal masses: accuracy of characterization with transvaginal US and precontrast and postcontrast MR imaging. Radiology 194:557–565
139. Sutton CL et al (1992) Ovarian masses revisited: radiologic and pathologic correlation. Radiographics 12(5):853–877
140. Athey PA, Siegel MF (1987) Sonographic features of Brenner tumor of the ovary. J Ultrasound Med 6:367–372
141. Mitchell DG et al (1986) Polycystic ovaries: MR imaging. Radiology 160(2):425–429
142. Schultz SM, Curry TS, Voet R (1986) Psammomatous-like calcification in a Brenner tumour of the ovary. Br J Radiol 59(700):412–414
143. Buy JN et al (1991) Epithelial tumors of the ovary: CT findings and correlation with US. Radiology 178:811–818
144. Casillas J, Joseph RC, Guerra JJ Jr (1990) CT appearance of uterine leiomyomas. Radiographics 10(6):999–1007
145. Williams CO (1978) Radiologic seminar CLXXXIV: Brenner tumor of the ovary – ultrasound findings. J Miss State Med Assoc 19(9):168–169
146. Roth LM, Czernobilsky B (1985) Ovarian Brenner tumors. II. Malignant. Cancer 56(3):592–601
147. Sugimura K, Okizuka H, Imaoka I (1991) Malignant Brenner tumor: MR findings. AJR Am J Roentgenol 157(6):1355–1356
148. Osadchaia VV (1980) Borderline mixed epithelial tumor of the ovary. Arkh Patol 42(10):56–58
149. Balasa RW et al (1977) The Brenner tumor: a clinicopathologic review. Obstet Gynecol 50(1):120–128
150. Silverberg SG (1971) Brenner tumor of the ovary. A clinicopathologic study of 60 tumors in 54 women. Cancer 28(3):588–596

Other Epithelial Tumors

151. Lim SC et al (1998) Malignant mixed Mullerian tumor (homologous type) of the adnexa with neuroendocrine differentiation: a case report. J Korean Med Sci 13(2):207–210
152. Seidman JD, Russel P, Kurman RJ (2002) Surface epithelial tumors of the ovary. In: Kurman RJ (ed) Blaustein's pathology of the female genital tract. Springer, New-York, pp 791–904

153. Scully RE, Young RH, Clement PB (1998) Tumors of the ovary, maldeveloped gonads, fallopian tubes and broad ligament. In: Rosai J, Sobin LH (eds) Atlas of tumor pathology, vol 3. Armed Force Institute of Pathology, Washington, DC, pp 51–168
154. Fowler JM et al (1996) Mixed mesodermal sarcoma of the ovary in a young patient. Eur J Obstet Gynecol Reprod Biol 65(2):249–253
155. Boucher D, Tetu B (1994) Morphologic prognostic factors of malignant mixed mullerian tumors of the ovary: a clinicopathologic study of 15 cases. Int J Gynecol Pathol 13(1):22–28
156. Rosai J (1996) Female reproductive system. In: Ackerman's surgical pathology. Mosby, St Louis, pp 1319–1564
157. Dass KK et al (1993) Malignant mixed mullerian tumors of the ovary. An analysis of two long-term survivors. Am J Clin Oncol 16(4):346–349
158. Smith T, Moy L, Runowicz C (1997) Mullerian mixed tumors: CT characteristics with clinical and pathologic observations. AJR Am J Roentgenol 169(2):531–535
159. Haaften-Day C, Russell P, Brammah-Carr S (1990) Two homologous mixed mullerian tumor lines of the ovary and their characteristics. Cancer 65(8):1753–1761
160. Hanjani P et al (1983) Malignant mixed mesodermal tumors and carcinosarcoma of the ovary: report of eight cases and review of literature. Obstet Gynecol Surv 38(9):537–545
161. Morrow M, Enker WE (1984) Late ovarian metastases in carcinoma of the colon and rectum. Arch Surg 119(12):1385–1388
162. Cho SB et al (2001) Malignant mixed mullerian tumor of the ovary: imaging findings. Eur Radiol 11(7):1147–1150

Particular Forms

163. Pavlik EJ et al (2000) Ovarian volume related to age. Gynecol Oncol 77(3):410–412
164. Jones HW Jr, Jones GS (1979) Epithelial tumors of the ovary. In: Jones HW Jr, Jones GS (eds) Novak's textbook of gynecology. Saunders, Philadelphia, pp 507–558
165. Krigman H, Bentley R, Robboy SJ (1994) Pathology of epithelial ovarian tumors. Clin Obstet Gynecol 37(2):475–491
166. Buy JN et al (1989) Cystic teratoma of the ovary: CT detection. Radiology 171:697–701
167. Scully RE, Young RH, Clement PB (1998) Tumors of the ovary, maldeveloped gonads, fallopian tubes and broad ligament. Armed Force Institute of Pathology, Washington, DC, pp 239–306

Extension

168. Young RC, Perez CA, Hoskins WJ (1993) Cancer of the ovary. In: De Vita VT, Hellman S, Rosenberg SA (eds) Cancer. Principles and practices of oncology. J. B. Lippincott Company, Philadelphia, pp 1226–1263
169. Mayer AR et al (1992) Ovarian cancer staging: does it require a gynecologic oncologist? Gynecol Oncol 47(2):223–227
170. Nguyen HN et al (1993) National survey of ovarian carcinoma. Part V. The impact of physician's specialty on patients' survival. Cancer 72(12):3663–3670
171. Omura GA et al (1991) Long-term follow-up and prognostic factor analysis in advanced ovarian carcinoma: the Gynecologic Oncology Group experience. J Clin Oncol 9(7):1138–1150
172. Averette HE et al (1993) National survey of ovarian carcinoma. I. A patient care evaluation study of the American College of Surgeons. Cancer 71(4 Suppl):1629–1638
173. Puls LE et al (1997) Stage I ovarian carcinoma: specialty-related differences in survival and management. South Med J 90(11):1097–1100
174. Dauplat J (2001) Management of ovarian cancer. Cancer Radiother 5(Suppl 1):149s–161s
175. Buy JN et al (1988) Peritoneal implants from ovarian tumors: CT findings. Radiology 169(3):691–694
176. Buy JN et al (1991) Epithelial tumors of the ovary: CT findings and correlation with US. Radiology 178:811–818
177. Pecorelli S (2009) Revised FIGO staging for carcinoma of the vulva, cervix, and endometrium. Int J Gynaecol Obstet 105(2):103–104

178. Yeh HC (1979) Ultrasonography of peritoneal tumors. Radiology 133: 419–424
179. Solomon A et al (1983) Computerized tomography in ovarian cancer. Gynecol Oncol 15(1):48–55
180. Amendola MA et al (1981) Computed tomography in the evaluation of carcinoma of the ovary. J Comput Assist Tomogr 5(2):179–186
181. Mamtora H, Isherwood I (1982) Computed tomography in ovarian carcinoma: patterns of disease and limitations. Clin Radiol 33(2):165–171
182. Johnson RJ et al (1983) Abdomino-pelvic computed tomography in the management of ovarian carcinoma. Radiology 146:447–452
183. Stevens SK, Hricak H, Stern JL (1991) Ovarian lesions: detection and characterization with gadolinium-enhanced MR imaging at 1.5T. Radiology 181(2):481–488
184. Kurtz AB et al (1999) Diagnosis and staging of ovarian cancer: comparative values of Doppler and conventional US, CT, and MR imaging correlated with surgery and histopathologic analysis – report of the Radiology Diagnostic Oncology Group. Radiology 212(1):19–27
185. Lund B et al (1990) Correlation of abdominal ultrasound and computed tomography scans with second- or third-look laparotomy in patients with ovarian carcinoma. Gynecol Oncol 37(2):279–283
186. Forstner R et al (1995) Ovarian cancer: staging with CT and MR imaging. Radiology 197(3):619–626
187. Hamm B (1994) Computerized tomography and MR tomography in diagnosis of ovarian tumors. Radiologe 34(7):362–369
188. Buist MR et al (1994) Comparative evaluation of diagnostic methods in ovarian carcinoma with emphasis on CT and MRI. Gynecol Oncol 52(2): 191–198
189. Buy JN et al (1988) Tomodensitom‚trie des cancers endom‚trio‹des de l'ovaire. J Radiol 69:171–174
190. Feldman GB, Knapp RC (1974) Lymphatic drainage of the peritoneal cavity and its significance in ovarian cancer. Am J Obstet Gynecol 119(7): 991–994
191. Salkin D (1934) Intraabdominal pressure and its regulation. Am Rev Tuberc 30:436–457
192. Overholt RH (1931) Intraperitoneal pressure. Arch Surg 22:691–703
193. Meyers MA (1973) Peritoneography: normal and pathologic anatomy. Am J Roentgenol 117:353–365
194. Coates G, Bush RS, Aspin N (1973) A study of ascites using lymphoscintigraphy with 99m Tc-sulfur colloid. Radiology 107(3):577–583
195. Courtice FC, Steinbeck AW (1950) The lymphatic drainage of plasma from the peritoneal cavity of the cat. Aust J Exp Biol Med Sci 28:161–169
196. Bagley CM Jr et al (1973) Ovarian carcinoma metastatic to the diaphragm – frequently undiagnosed at laparotomy. A preliminary report. Am J Obstet Gynecol 116(3):397–400
197. Holm-Nielsen P (1953) Pathogenesis of ascites in peritoneal carcinomatosis. Acta Pathol Microbiol Scand 33:10–21
198. Rusznyak I, Foldi M, Szabo G (1967) Lymphatic and lymph circulation. Physiology and Pathology. Oxford Pergamon Press, Inc, Oxford
199. Yoffey JM, Courtice FC (1970) Lymphatics. Lymph and lymphomyeloid tissue. Edward Arnold, London
200. Allen L, Raybuck HE (1960) The effects of obliteration of the diaphragmatic lymphatic plexus on serous fluid. Anat Rec 137:25–32
201. Courtice FC, Harding J, Steinbeck AW (1953) The removal of free red blood cells from the peritoneal cavity of animals. Aust J Exp Biol Med Sci 31: 215–225
202. Raybuck HE, Allen L, Harms WS (1960) Absorption of serum from the peritoneal cavity. Am J Physiol 199:1021–1024
203. Wicks JD et al (1984) Correlation of ultrasound and pathologic findings in patients with epithelial carcinoma of the ovary. J Clin Ultrasound 12(7):397–402
204. Bazot M et al (1993) Fibrothecomas of the ovary: CT and US findings. J Comput Assist Tomogr 17:754–759
205. Walkey MM et al (1988) CT manifestations of peritoneal carcinomatosis. AJR Am J Roentgenol 150(5):1035–1041
206. Jeffrey RB (1980) CT demonstration of peritoneal implants. Am J Roentgenol 135:323–326
207. Buy JN et al (2000) Malignant tumors of the ovaries: role of imaging. J Radiol 81(12 Suppl):1833–1843
208. Guttner B et al (1991) Diagnosis and problems in follow-up of tumors with psammoma bodies. Bildgebung 58(2):83–86
209. Schwartz PE (1981) Surgical management of ovarian cancer. Arch Surg 116(1):99–106
210. Cooper C et al (1986) Computed tomography of omental pathology. J Comput Assist Tomogr 10:62–66
211. Epstein BM, Mann JH (1982) CT of abdominal tuberculosis. AJR Am J Roentgenol 139(5):861–866
212. Levitt RG, Sagel SS, Stanley RJ (1978) Detection of neoplastic involvement of the mesentery and omentum by computed tomography. AJR Am J Roentgenol 131(5):835–838
213. Dunnick NR et al (1979) Intraperitoneal contrast infusion for assessment of intraperitoneal fluid dynamics. AJR Am J Roentgenol 133(2):221–223
214. Gryspeerdt S et al (1998) Intraperitoneal contrast material combined with CT for detection of peritoneal metastases of ovarian cancer. Eur J Gynaecol Oncol 19(5):434–437
215. Low RN, Sigeti JS (1994) MR imaging of peritoneal disease: comparison of contrast-enhanced fast multiplanar spoiled gradient-recalled and spin-echo imaging. AJR Am J Roentgenol 163(5):1131–1140
216. Outwater EK et al (1996) Benign and malignant gynecologic disease: clinical importance of fluid and peritoneal enhancement in the pelvis at MR imaging. Radiology 200(2):483–488
217. Arai K et al (1993) Enhancement of ascites on MRI following intravenous administration of Gd-DTPA. J Comput Assist Tomogr 17(4):617–622
218. Bilgin T et al (2001) Peritoneal tuberculosis with pelvic abdominal mass, ascites and elevated CA 125 mimicking advanced ovarian carcinoma: a series of 10 cases. Int J Gynecol Cancer 11(4):290–294
219. Yoshimura T, Okamura H (1987) Peritoneal tuberculosis with elevated serum CA 125 levels: a case report. Gynecol Oncol 28(3):342–344
220. Sheth SS (1996) Elevated CA 125 in advanced abdominal or pelvic tuberculosis. Int J Gynaecol Obstet 52(2):167–171
221. Rao GJ et al (1996) Abdominal tuberculosis or ovarian carcinoma: management dilemma associated with an elevated CA-125 level. Medscape Womens Health 1(4):2
222. Gurgan T et al (1993) Pelvic-peritoneal tuberculosis with elevated serum and peritoneal fluid Ca-125 levels. A report of two cases. Gynecol Obstet Invest 35(1):60–61
223. Groutz A, Carmon E, Gat A (1998) Peritoneal tuberculosis versus advanced ovarian cancer: a diagnostic dilemma. Obstet Gynecol 91(5 Pt 2):868
224. Yapar EG et al (1995) Sonographic features of tuberculous peritonitis with female genital tract tuberculosis. Ultrasound Obstet Gynecol 6(2):121–125
225. Goldblum J, Hart WR (1995) Localized and diffuse mesotheliomas of the genital tract and peritoneum in women. A clinicopathologic study of nineteen true mesothelial neoplasms, other than adenomatoid tumors, multicystic mesotheliomas, and localized fibrous tumors. Am J Surg Pathol 19(10): 1124–1137
226. Chen SS, Lee L (1983) Incidence of para-aortic and pelvic lymph node metastases in epithelial carcinoma of the ovary. Gynecol Oncol 16(1):95–100
227. Rose PG et al (1989) Metastatic patterns in histologic variants of ovarian cancer. An autopsy study. Cancer 64(7):1508–1513
228. Dvoretsky PM et al (1988) Distribution of disease at autopsy in 100 women with ovarian cancer. Hum Pathol 19(1):57–63

Tumoral Markers

229. Herrmann UJ Jr, Locher GW, Goldhirsch A (1987) Sonographic patterns of ovarian tumors: prediction of malignancy. Obstet Gynecol 69(5):777–781
230. Schneider VL et al (1993) Comparison of Doppler with two-dimensional sonography and CA 125 for prediction of malignancy of pelvic masses. Obstet Gynecol 81(6):983–988
231. Bast RC Jr et al (1981) Reactivity of a monoclonal antibody with human ovarian carcinoma. J Clin Invest 68(5):1331–1337
232. Taylor KJ, Schwartz PE (1994) Screening for early ovarian cancer. Radiology 192(1):1–10
233. Jacobs I, Bast RC Jr (1989) The CA 125 tumour-associated antigen: a review of the literature. Hum Reprod 4(1):1–12
234. Sagan DL, Chebotareva ED, Evtushenko GV (1989) CA 125 in the diagnosis and evaluation of the efficacy of the treatment of cancer of the ovaries. Med Radiol (Mosk) 34(6):39–42
235. Crombach G, Zippel HH, Wurz H (1985) Experiences with CA 125, a tumor marker for malignant epithelial ovarian tumors. Geburtshilfe Frauenheilkd 45(4):205–212
236. Zurawski VR Jr et al (1988) An initial analysis of preoperative serum CA 125 levels in patients with early stage ovarian carcinoma. Gynecol Oncol 30(1): 7–14
237. Gotlieb WH et al (2000) CA 125 measurement and ultrasonography in borderline tumors of the ovary. Am J Obstet Gynecol 183(3):541–546

238. Ferguson AM, Fox H (1984) A study of the Ca antigen in epithelial tumours of the ovary. J Clin Pathol 37(1):6–9
239. Shi ZL (1989) Mucin histochemical and immunohistochemical studies of mucinous ovarian tumors. Zhonghua Bing Li Xue Za Zhi 18(3):201–203

Follow-Up and Recurrences

240. Lorigan PC, Crosby T, Coleman RE (1996) Current drug treatment guidelines for epithelial ovarian cancer. Drugs 51(4):571–584
241. Schilthuis MS et al (1987) Serum CA 125 levels in epithelial ovarian cancer: relation with findings at second-look operations and their role in the detection of tumour recurrence. Br J Obstet Gynaecol 94(3):202–207
242. Forstner R et al (1995) Ovarian cancer recurrence: value of MR imaging. Radiology 196(3):715–720
243. Patsner B et al (1990) Does serum CA-125 level prior to second-look laparotomy for invasive ovarian adenocarcinoma predict size of residual disease? Gynecol Oncol 37(3):319–322
244. Buist MR et al (1994) Comparative evaluation of diagnostic methods in ovarian carcinoma with emphasis on CT and MRI. Gynecol Oncol 52(2):191–198
245. Kenemans P et al (1993) CA 125 in gynecological pathology – a review. Eur J Obstet Gynecol Reprod Biol 49(1–2):115–124
246. Sugiyama T et al (1996) Comparison of CA 125 assays with abdominopelvic computed tomography and transvaginal ultrasound in monitoring of ovarian cancer. Int J Gynaecol Obstet 54(3):251–256
247. Crombach G, Zippel HH, Wurz H (1985) Experiences with CA 125, a tumor marker for malignant epithelial ovarian tumors. Geburtshilfe Frauenheilkd 45(4):205–212
248. Therasse P et al (2000) New guidelines to evaluate the response to treatment in solid tumors. European Organization for Research and Treatment of Cancer, National Cancer Institute of the United States, National Cancer Institute of Canada. J Natl Cancer Inst 92(3):205–216
249. Rutgers JL, Scully RE (1988) Ovarian mullerian mucinous papillary cystadenomas of borderline malignancy. A clinicopathologic analysis. Cancer 61(2):340–348
250. Young RC, Perez CA, Hoskins WJ (1993) Cancer of the ovary. In: De Vita VT, Hellman S, Rosenberg SA (eds) Cancer. Principles and practices of oncology. J. B. Lippincott company, Philadelphia, pp 1226–1263
251. Sella T et al (2001) Value of chest CT scans in routine ovarian carcinoma follow-up. AJR Am J Roentgenol 177(4):857–859
252. Ohta H et al (2001) Meningeal carcinomatosis from an ovarian primary with complete response to adjuvant chemotherapy after cranial irradiation. Int J Clin Oncol 6(3):157–162
253. Garcia EA et al (1998) Evaluation on non invasive diagnostic tests for the second look in epithelial ovarian cancer. Rev Clin Esp 198(8):502–505
254. Lund B et al (1990) Correlation of abdominal ultrasound and computed tomography scans with second- or third-look laparotomy in patients with ovarian carcinoma. Gynecol Oncol 37(2):279–283
255. Kainz C et al (1994) The diagnostic value of magnetic resonance imaging for the detection of tumor recurrence in patients with carcinoma of the ovaries. J Am Coll Surg 178(3):239–244
256. Forstner R et al (1995) Ovarian cancer: staging with CT and MR imaging. Radiology 197(3):619–626
257. Prayer L et al (1993) CT and MR accuracy in the detection of tumor recurrence in patients treated for ovarian cancer. J Comput Assist Tomogr 17(4):626–632
258. Ngan HY et al (1990) Role of CA125 and abdominal pelvic computerized axial tomogram in the monitoring of chemotherapy treatment of ovarian cancer. Cancer Invest 8(5):467–470
259. Triller J, Kraft R, Marincek B (1982) Computer tomographic-directed fine needle aspiration biopsy of pelvic masses. ROFO Fortschr Geb Rontgenstr Nuklearmed 137(4):422–427
260. Silverman PM et al (1988) CT prior to second-look operation in ovarian cancer. AJR Am J Roentgenol 150(4):829–832
261. Ferrozzi F et al (1998) Thin-section CT follow-up of metastatic ovarian carcinoma correlation with levels of CA-125 marker and clinical history. Clin Imaging 22(5):364–370
262. Gritzmann N et al (1986) Abdominal computerized tomography in the aftercare of ovarian cancers. Digitale Bilddiagn 6(4):171–175
263. Wakabayashi Y et al (1989) The accuracy of CT and tumor markers in the detection of a recurrent ovarian carcinoma. Gan No Rinsho 35(10):1127–1131

Germ Cell Tumors

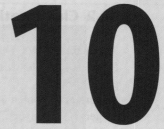

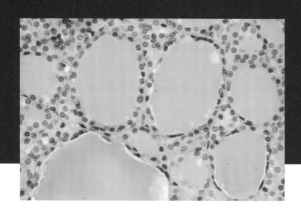

Contents

10.1 Introduction

In adults, 30% of ovarian tumors are of germ cell origin [1]; the great majority of germ cell tumors (95%) are benign and consist of mature cystic teratomas (MCT), usually designated dermoid cysts [2]. In children and adolescents, more than 60% of ovarian neoplasms are of germ cell origin, and one-third of them are malignant [2–6].

In the majority of cases, diagnosis of MCT is relatively easy and the therapeutic approach roughly univoque. However, characterization of other types of germ cell tumors and especially primary malignant tumors can be much more difficult leading in some cases to a more complex management.

While most types of germ cell tumor occur in pure form, each of them may also be mixed with one or more other types. The prognosis of a mixed germ cell tumor generally reflects that of its most malignant element, but a small focus of high malignancy does not influence the prognosis as adversely as a large component [7].

J.N. Buy, M. Ghossain, *Gynecological Imaging*,
DOI 10.1007/978-3-642-31012-6_10, © Springer-Verlag Berlin Heidelberg 2013

10.3.1.2 Macroscopy and Microscopy

The three main components of a MCT (Fig. 10.3) will be detailed separately:

1. *The wall* is regular and measures in average from 2 to 3 mm in diameter. It is composed of connective tissue lined mainly by skin [2]. This skin is lined mainly by keratinized squamous epithelium.

2. *The Rokitansky protuberance is specific of a dermoid cyst.* Almost always [7], arising from its wall and projecting into its cavity, there is a protuberance composed of a mass of tissue, which contains derivatives from 2 to 3 germ cell layers:
   (a) Number: usually single but may be multiple [2].
   (b) Size: most often comprised between 0.5 and 5 cm [11], exceptionally more than 5 cm in benign Rokitansky protuberance, like in 1/40 benign protuberances detected by CT in our series [11]. However, its size may be larger particularly in case of malignant transformation.
   (c) Content:

   – *Macroscopically*: (Fig. 10.3)
      (i) The wall of the protuberance projecting into the lumen is formed by skin and is in continuity with the inner wall of the cyst.
      (ii) Tufts of hair are radiating from the protuberance into the lumen of the cyst.
      (iii) Most often, the inner part is tissular. It contains macroscopically recognizable structures: adipose tissue (2/3 of cases) often underlining the skin, soft tissue related to other types of connective tissue, and dense elements like cartilage with or without areas of calcification (38.6%), bone (18.6%), or more rarely teeth (8%) [8]. In some cases, the protuberance is partly cystic [2]. Exceptionally, an abortive attempt to form a fetus, characterized by one or more of these complex structures is referred to as a homunculus [7].

   – *Microscopically* it usually contains derivatives from (1) the ectodermic layer (99.3%) [8]: skin and cerebromeningeal structures which can secrete cerebrospinal fluid in the cavity; (2) the mesodermic layer (73.3%) [8]: bone, cartilage, muscle, fibrous, and adipose tissue; and (3) the endodermic layer (31.9%) [8], with its derivatives from the respiratory and GI endodermal epithelium, thyroid, and salivary gland tissue. Mucinous glands can be adjacent to the protuberance and form a little mucinous cyst.

   (d) Shape and situation: Most often it lies against the inner wall of the cyst; although it has roughly the shape of a vegetation, it has different macroscopic and microscopic features which are very helpful radiologically to distinguish it from a vegetation (Table 10.3). It can also be fingerlike or look like a nodule. More rarely, it lies in a septum. Exceptionally it forms a bridge between two parts of the wall (Fig. 10.4).
   (e) Inner border: most often regular and more rarely slightly irregular
   (f) Malignant transformation: Malignant transformation occurs in 1–2% of MCT, most often in the dermoid plug but also can arise in the wall (see Sect. 10.3.3.4).

3. *The Content of the Cyst*
   According to the nature of the content, there are three different forms (Fig. 10.5):
   – Fat mixed with hair is the most common presentation. The skin which forms part of the wall secretes sebum and watery fluid more or less intermingled with hair. At body temperature, the contents are liquid but become solid at temperature below 25°C [13].
   – Purely fatty (Fig. 10.6).
   – A purely cystic content can be related to a watery fluid coming from the sweat glands. Choroid plexus formation can be prominent enough to form a cystic structure filled with cerebrospinal fluid [12]. The liquid can be gelatinous, especially when the wall contains some amount of thyroid glands.

Table 10.3 Differentiation between a Rokitansky protuberance and a vegetation

	Rokitansky protuberance	Vegetation Benign	Vegetation Borderline or malignant
Size	0.5–5 cm	Usually <1 cm	< or >1 cm
Border	Rather regular	Regular	Irregular
Content	Adipose tissue and/or other tissues	Tissular proliferation	Tissular proliferation
	Tooth, bone, cartilage, or calcifications	Macrocalcifications	
Vessels	Few	Few Thin	More numerous Larger (neovascularization)

According to Refs. [11, 30]

Fig. 10.4 Examples of two dermoid plugs. A classical dermoid plug (Rokitansky protuberance) lying against the inner border of the cyst is displayed in (**a**). An exceptional bridge shaped plug is displayed in (**b**)

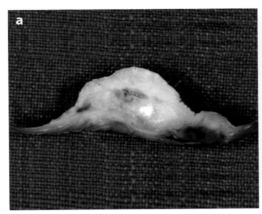
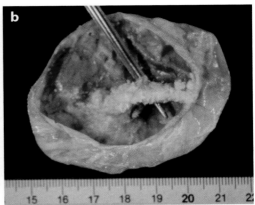

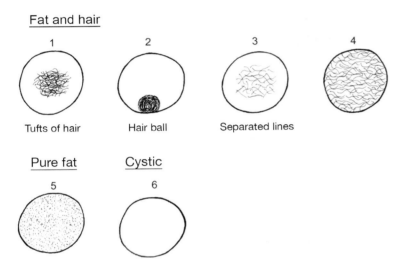

Fig. 10.5 Schematic representation of the content of the cyst

Fat and hair

1 — Tufts of hair

2 — Hair ball

3 — Separated lines

4

Pure fat

5

Cystic

6

Fig. 10.6 Dermoid cyst containing sebaceous material

10.3.2 Isolated Noncomplicated Benign Mature Cystic Teratoma

Nowadays, most MCT are discovered on ultrasound. Occasionally the lesion is discovered during a plain abdominal radiograph or during an intravenous pyelography (Fig. 10.7). The most common finding is a calcification (a) that in the typical cases has a tooth shape; exceptionally the wall of the cyst is visibly delineated by intracystic and peritoneal fat (b).

10.3.2.1 US

Pitfalls in the Diagnosis

1. Because of its property to strongly attenuate the US beam, a dermoid cyst may be confused with bowel and with a subserous leiomyoma. One must also remember that the exceptional lipoleiomyoma of the uterus may have a hyperechoic pattern that mimics a dermoid cyst.

2. Some MCT cannot be detected on US [14] because of a high position that can be related to an elongated ovarian pedicle, or because they can be hidden by bowels, or associated pelvic pathologies such as multiple myomas or dense adhesions (Fig. 10.8) [15, 16].

Conventional US and Doppler Findings

US and Doppler findings are summarized in Table 10.4.

Cystic Content

The mass is usually round in shape, exceptionally oblong [17].

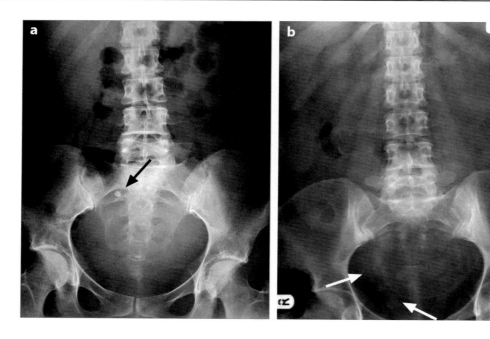

Fig. 10.7 MCT discovered on abdominal films. The most common finding is a calcification (*arrow* in **a**). Rarely the cyst wall is visible because it is silhouetted by external peritoneal fat and intracystic fat (*arrows* in **b**)

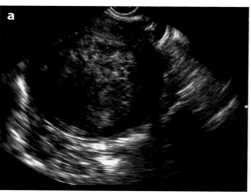 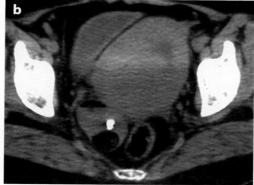

Fig. 10.8 Small MCT not detected in ultrasound because of a huge myoma. US displays a large uterine leiomyoma. CT discloses a small right dermoid cyst containing fat and calcification

Table 10.4 US and Doppler findings of mature cystic teratoma

Conventional US
A. *Content of the cyst*
Common
   1. Hyperechogenic ill-defined structure (dermoid mess) with a broad and
      ill-defined acoustic shadowing
   2. Hyperechogenic well-defined round structure (hair ball) with or
      without acoustic shadowing
   3. Hyperechogenic lines in a dark field
   4. Entirely hyperechogenic mass
   5. Fat-fluid level
Uncommon
   1. Cystic mass
   2. Echogenic mass with a nonspecific echogenicity
   3. Multiloculated
   4. Unusual floating balls
B. *Rokitansky Protuberance* (*rarely identified*)
   1. Against the inner wall
   2. Predominantly hyperechogenic
   3. May contain bright echogenic focus with sharp acoustic shadowing
C. *Wall of the Cyst* (*rarely delineated*)
   1. Regular and thin
Color Doppler
   1. Absence of flow in the cyst
   2. Absence of flow in the protuberance

Characteristic Cystic Patterns

The aspect of the cystic content depends on the nature of the liquid and the amount of hair. The most characteristic and peculiar finding of MCT is the presence in the cyst of a hyperechogenic (echogenicity superior to myometrium) element which can have different patterns.

Six main patterns can be described. Each of them can be the only pattern of representation, but more often, some of them are associated, giving the mass a very typical aspect for a dermoid cyst [18]:

1. A *hyperechogenic ill-defined structure* formed by multiple hyperechogenic and heterogenic pinpoint spots with or without a broad ill-defined acoustic shadowing [19] called by Malde et al.

[20] the dermoid mesh. It is related at pathology to fat and hair gathered as tufts (Fig. 10.5, type 1; Fig. 10.9). The shadowing is more marked with a higher-frequency transducer.

2. A *hyperechogenic well-defined round structure* without or with acoustic shadowing named on US as a hair ball. It is usually related at pathology to conglomeration of fat and hair as a ball shape (Fig. 10.5, type 2; Fig. 10.10), more rarely to conglomeration of pure fat (Fig. 10.11).

In the same tumor, with a low-frequency transducer, the hair ball can be displayed without acoustic shadowing, while a higher-frequency transducer can demonstrate an acoustic shadowing.

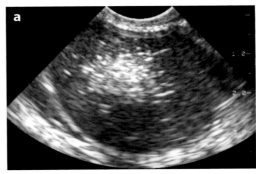
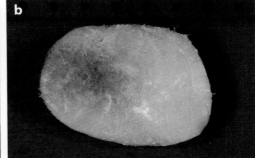

Fig. 10.9 Dermoid cyst in a 41-year-old woman with central ill-defined hyperechogenic structure. (a) Ultrasound displays an echogenic mass containing a hyperechogenic structure made of dots or lines with some sound attenuation. (b) Pathologic specimen shows that the cystic content is composed of yellow fat with a center that contains brown fat and hair

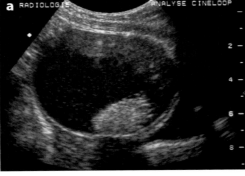
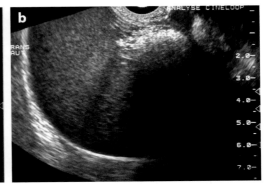

Fig. 10.10 A 50-year-old woman with a dermoid cyst that contains a hair ball and a cystic content looking like an endometrioma. (a) TAS shows a mass with a low echogenic cystic content and a hyperechoic structure with a broad acoustic shadowing in the dependent portion of the cyst. (b) On TVS with a higher-frequency transducer, the acoustic shadowing is more important

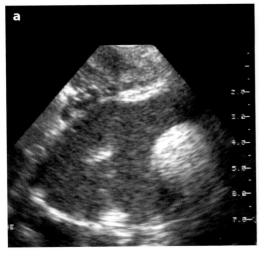
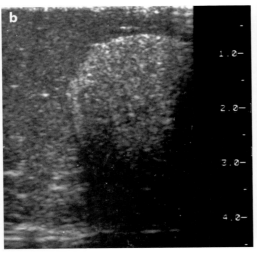
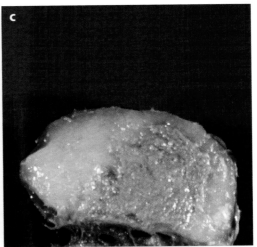

Fig. 10.11 Fat ball with US attenuation in a 44-year-old woman with a left ovarian dermoid cyst. (a) TAS shows an echogenic cystic mass that contains a round hyperechogenic mass wrongly considered as a hair ball, corresponding in fact to accumulation of fat. (b) In vitro US study shows a marked shadowing of this hyperechoic structure. (c) Pathologic specimen. Section through the cystic content shows yellow fat and brown fat without hair looking like a hair ball

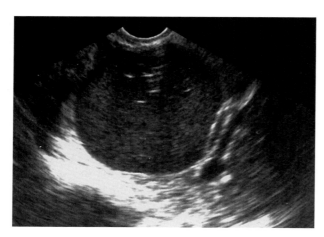

Fig. 10.12 TVU of a left 5.6×4.5-cm MCT containing hyperechogenic sparkling lines in a hypoechoic field

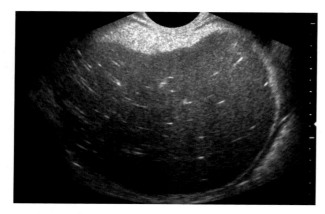

Fig. 10.13 Dermoid cyst with a low echogenic pattern containing echogenic lines and a hyperechogenic focus against the wall (corresponding to the protuberance)

3. *Hyperechogenic sparkling lines and dots* in a hypoechoic field (Figs. 10.12, 10.13, and 10.14). They are related to hair in water [19] or fat (Fig. 10.5, type 3). The presence of these hyperechogenic lines in a ground-glass pattern helps in differentiating MCT from endometrioma.

4. A *predominantly or entirely hyperechogenic mass* as in 5/23 cases of Sheth et al. series [21] (Fig. 10.15). On CT, this form corresponds to a mass containing a small amount of fat intermingled with a larger component of hair [21]. This pattern is particularly common in small dermoid cysts (<3 cm) [22] (Fig. 10.7, type 4). Sometimes this form can be confused with a hemorrhagic cyst (Fig. 10.16). CT or MR allows to make the differential diagnosis.

5. A *fluid level*
Usually the upper part is hypoechogenic, the lower part more echogenic (Fig. 10.17). Signification of this level has no clear explanation. It may be due to sedimentation, in fat that is fluid at body temperature, of cellular debris resulting from desquamation of the lining epithelium of the inner wall or simply a level between two different types of liquid like in an oil bottle.

When isolated, this finding is not specific and can represent a hemorrhagic cyst. When an echogenic mass is floating at the interface, the aspect is characteristic (Fig. 10.17). Uncommonly, the upper part of the level looks more echogenic than the lower part (Fig. 10.18); this pattern described by Sandler et al. [17] and Owre et al. [23] is considered pathognomonic for a dermoid cyst [23].

6. *Unusual floating balls*
A very uncommon presentation and at the same time very suggestive of the diagnosis of dermoid cyst is the presence in the cyst of multiple mobile spherical hyperechoic structures [24].

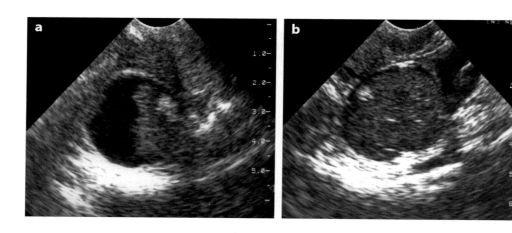

Fig. 10.14 Dermoid cyst with low echogenic cystic content and echogenic lines. (**a**) Sagittal TVS: The superior part of the cyst (*left side* of the figure) is nonechogenic, while the lower part (*right side* of the figure) is mainly low echogenic. (**b**) Transverse TVS through the lower part of the cyst demonstrates that it is diffusely low echogenic containing some hyperechoic lines

Fig. 10.15 Small dermoid cyst displayed as a hyperechogenic mass with acoustic shadowing. (a, b) Endovaginal US and **b** color Doppler: A 13-mm hyperechogenic mass with acoustic shadowing is very suggestive of a dermoid. Absence of vessel on color Doppler rules out a corpus luteum, but a corpus albicans could not be excluded. **(c, d)** CT scan is very useful in these cases and confirms the diagnosis (small cysts containing fat with a density of −90 HU)

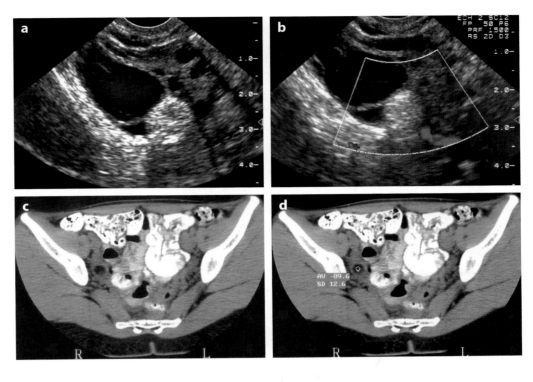

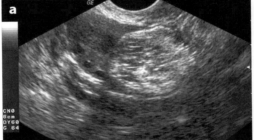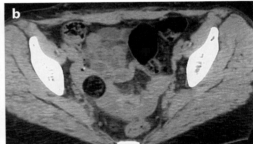

Fig. 10.16 TVU displays a 3-cm hyperechogenic mass. CT confirms the presence of a small cyst containing fat and hair

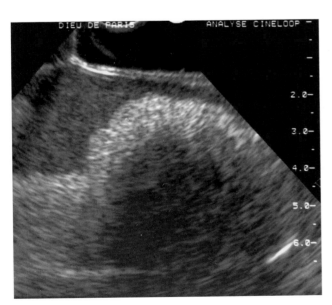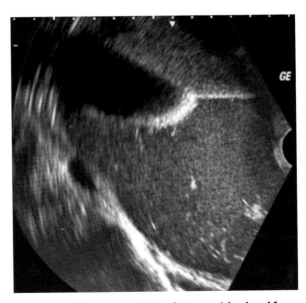

Fig. 10.17 Dermoid cyst with fat-fat level. In vitro US study: (1) Hair ball: hyperechogenic focus with broad and ill-defined acoustic shadowing. (2) Fat-fat level

Fig. 10.18 Sagittal TVU shows a MCT of 15 cm with a level formed by an upper echogenic fluid and a lower hypoechoic fluid. Hairs are seen in the hypoechoic fluid as hyperechogenic sparkle lines or foci. A hair ball is seen at the interface

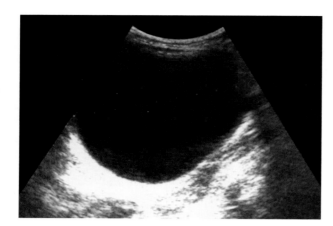

Fig. 10.19 Anechoic 8-cm MCT of left ovary in a 3-year- and 4-month-old girl. The content of the cyst was anechoic on ultrasound and clear during surgery. At pathology, the wall was slightly irregular (1–3 mm) with some hairs

Nonsuggestive Cystic Patterns

(a) *Mainly or Exclusively Anechoic*:

– Purely anechoic (Fig. 10.19). Watery fluid (Fig. 10.5, type 6) can be demonstrated as an anechoic structure like in 2/23 cases of Sheth et al. series [21] and in 7/39 in Cohen's series with enhanced sound transmission [17]. This anechoic fluid can be related to sweat glands contained in the wall or to cerebromeningeal structures in the protuberance. Differential diagnosis with a functional cyst or an epithelial tumor can be difficult.

– Mainly anechoic containing some echogenic lines (Fig. 10.20). Usually, the high echogenicity of these hair fibers in an anechoic pattern differentiates them from lower echogenic lines seen in the fishnet pattern of functional hemorrhagic cysts, but in some cases, the differential diagnosis may be difficult (Fig. 10.21).

– Mainly anechoic with an echogenic portion. This echogenic portion is difficult to characterize as a Rokitansky protuberance or a vegetation or a tissular portion (Figs. 10.22 and 10.23).

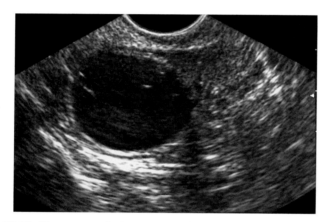

Fig. 10.20 Almost anechoic 3.1-cm right ovarian dermoid cyst in a 52-year-old woman. The content of the cyst is anechoic except for some sparkle lines representing hairs in fat

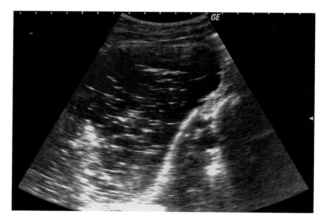

Fig. 10.21 Twenty-centimeter MCT with hyperechogenic lines in an anechoic field. TAS in an anechoic cystic portion displays multiple hyperechogenic lines that resemble the fishnet appearance of functional hemorrhagic cyst. However, the lines are not usually so echogenic in a functional hemorrhagic cyst

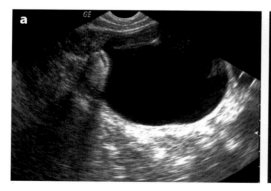
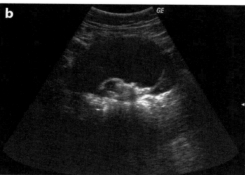
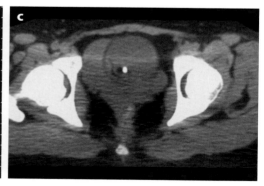

Fig. 10.22 Right 9.5-cm MCT in a 19-year-old woman. (**a**) and (**b**) Ultrasound shows a right mass composed of a large anechoic loculation (in **a**) and a smaller hyperechoic component (in **b**). (**c**) CT scan without injection discloses a right dermoid cyst with fat, hair, and calcification

Fig. 10.23 MCT with a watery cystic content.
(**a**) Sagittal TVS shows a left ovarian mass with a
purely watery cystic content and an echogenic
portion in the inferior part of the cyst. Diagnosis
of MCT is not suggested. (**b**) CT scan without
contrast. The cystic content has a mean density
of 14 HU. Identification of the protuberance with
calcifications and adipose tissue allows making a
specific diagnosis of MCT

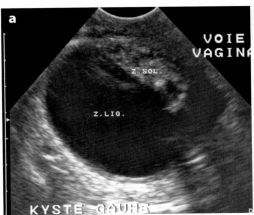

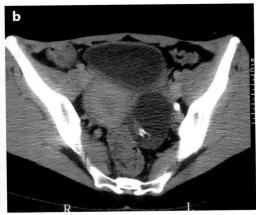

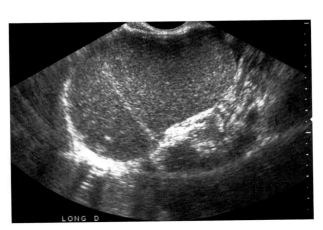

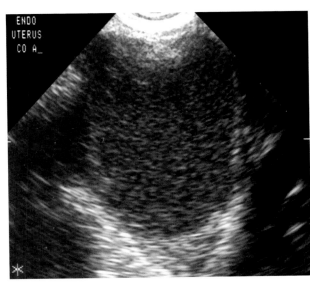

Fig. 10.24 Dermoid cyst with the cystic content resembling endometrioma   **Fig. 10.25 EVS: left ovarian MCT resembling an endometrioma.**
At pathology, content of the cyst was watery fluid

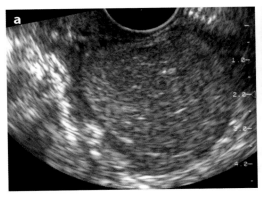

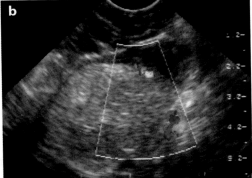

Fig. 10.26 Atypical form of MCT on US. EVS (**a**):
homogeneous echogenic form containing some
echogenic lines. Color Doppler (**b**) proves the
mass is cystic. Differential diagnosis with a functional hemorrhagic cyst or an endometrioma is
not possible

(**b**) *Hypoechoic Endometrioma-like Pattern.* A hypoechogenic portion (less than myometrium) [21] with [19] or without acoustic
shadowing. When there is no acoustic shadowing, this pattern
can be confused with an endometrioma (Figs. 10.24 and 10.25).
This low echogenicity on TVS can be depicted as anechoic on
TAS. Sheth et al. [21] has demonstrated that this pattern on US
corresponded more often on CT to low attenuation of pure fat
(Fig. 10.5, type 5).

(**c**) *Homogeneous echogenic* (equal to myometrium) containing
some hyperechogenic lines (Fig. 10.26). The main differential
diagnosis is functional hemorrhagic cyst.

(**d**) *Heterogeneous echogenic* mass (Fig. 10.27). The main differential is functional hemorrhagic cyst.

(**e**) *Exceptionally multiple hyperechogenic points* on a diffusely
echogenic background in cases of necrosis (Fig. 10.28).

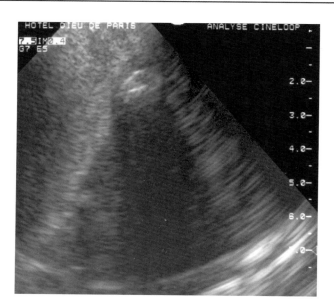

Fig. 10.38 Dermoid cyst. In vitro US study. Rokitansky protuberance: A more echogenic focus with sharp and narrow acoustic shadowing is displayed. Its echogenicity, very close to the echogenicity of the cystic content, makes its recognition difficult

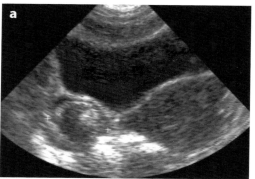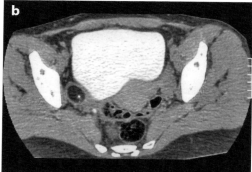

Fig. 10.39 Dermoid cyst. Unusual form of Rokitansky protuberance on US. (a) TAS: hyperechogenic focus without acoustic shadowing. Echogenicity of the cystic content is not suggestive for a MCT. (**b**) CT after contrast: a small tissular portion lying against the inner wall contains a tiny calcification related to the protuberance. Fatty content. On color Doppler, no vascularization is usually displayed in the dermoid plug

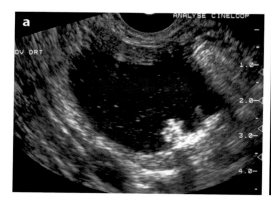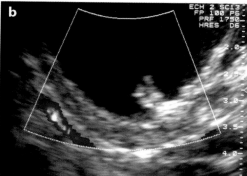

Fig. 10.40 Dermoid cyst with a Rokitansky protuberance looking like a vegetation on US. (**a**) Longitudinal TVS: A hyperechogenic focus with a narrow acoustic shadowing is considered as a vegetation in this anechoic cystic portion. (**b**) Color Doppler: No vessel is displayed in the echogenic portion. A diagnosis of epithelial tumor was suggested

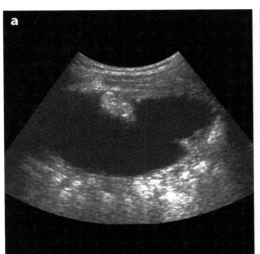
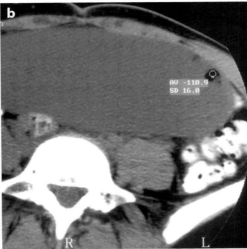
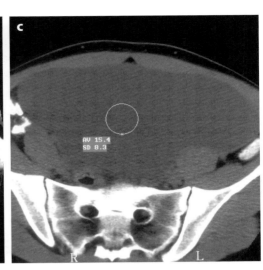

Fig. 10.41 Dermoid cyst with a Rokitansky protuberance looking like a vegetation on US. (a) TAS: unilocular anechoic cyst containing an echogenic round formation lying against the inner wall looking like an endocystic vegetation. Localized thickening of the wall. (b) CT scan displays at this level a typical protuberance containing a tooth and adipose tissue. (c) Content of the cyst is watery fluid with an overall density of 15 HU on CT

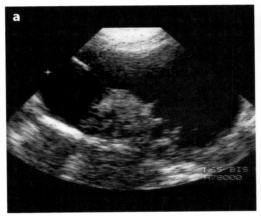
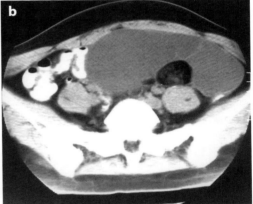

Fig. 10.42 Collision tumor. Mucinous cystadenoma and MCT. (a) Left ovarian cyst containing an echogenic portion protruding in the cyst with some attenuation. (b) CT scan confirms the diagnosis of left MCT in a multilocular cyst. Septa are thin and regular suggesting a benign mucinous cystadenoma

Wall of the Cyst

The wall was identified in 13/25 (52%) cyst in Nicolet et al. series [27].

When identified, usually one part is depicted. It is most often hypoechoic (48%); hypoechogenicity seems to be related to a wall mainly formed of fibrous tissue. It is more rarely hyperechoic; hyperechogenicity seems to be related to a thick layer of adipose tissue [27].

Association of These Different Findings

These different patterns can be associated in the same tumor and in these cases are vey suggestive of the diagnosis (Figs. 10.43 and 10.44).

Evaluation of Normal Ovarian Parenchyma

Dermoids completely surrounded by normal ovarian parenchyma have been reported [28].Usually until a certain size roughly less than 6 cm, dermoid pushes gently the normal parenchyma toward the periphery.

Color Doppler

1. On color Doppler, the absence of vessel in the tumor allows to prove its cystic nature and to rule out solid benign and malignant masses [29, 30]. However, in some cases of benign tissular ovarian masses as ovarian fibroma and Brenner tumor, vascularization is not displayed on color Doppler (Table 10.6).

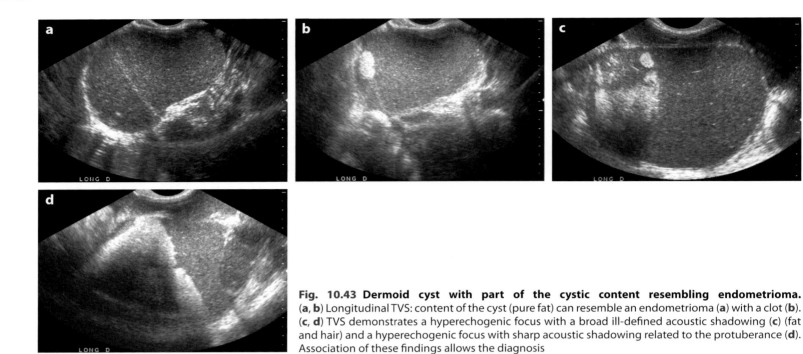

Fig. 10.43 Dermoid cyst with part of the cystic content resembling endometrioma. (**a, b**) Longitudinal TVS: content of the cyst (pure fat) can resemble an endometrioma (**a**) with a clot (**b**). (**c, d**) TVS demonstrates a hyperechogenic focus with a broad ill-defined acoustic shadowing (**c**) (fat and hair) and a hyperechogenic focus with sharp acoustic shadowing related to the protuberance (**d**). Association of these findings allows the diagnosis

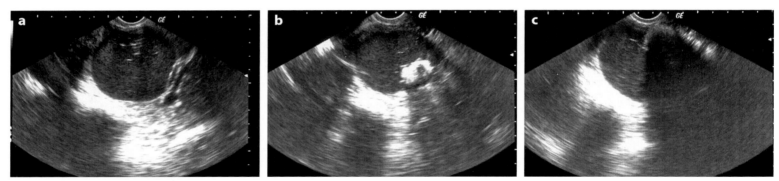

Fig. 10.44 MCT of the left ovary measuring 5.6×4.5 cm with several patterns on ultrasound: (**a**) a hypoechoic background with sparkle echogenic lines; (**b**) a hyperechoic structure with acoustic shadowing; (**c**) a broad acoustic shadowing. An association of these findings allows making with confidence the diagnosis of MCT

Table 10.6 Differential diagnosis of MCT with other echogenic masses using conventional US and color Doppler

Absence of vascularization on color Doppler:
Echogenic cystic masses
Functional hemorrhagic cyst
Endometrioma
Mucinous tumor [19]
Tubo-ovarian abscess [18]
Slight or absence of vascularization on color Doppler:
Echogenic tissular masses (slightly vascularized)
Ovarian fibroma
Brenner tumor:
High attenuation without calcification
Vascularization: slight and central
Significant vascularization on color Doppler:
Subserous leiomyoma
High attenuation without calcification
Hypervascularization: peripheral ± central
Ovarian carcinoma
Ruled out by color Doppler

2. In the dermoid plug, no vascularization is usually displayed (Fig. 10.40).
3. In the wall, vessels can be depicted in 24% of cases [31] but should not be confused with a vascularization in the protuberance (Fig. 10.45).

Other Forms

Dermoids of Small Size (<3 cm)

1. Small ovarian dermoids (<3 cm), nonpalpable, are not unusual [22, 32]. While these tumors can be missed during laparotomy [33], they can be detected on a routine ultrasound examination.
2. Although, they have structural patterns very similar to those observed for large tumors, a predominantly hyperechoic appearance with or without acoustic shadowing is commonly observed [22].

In these cases, differential diagnosis with a corpus luteum cyst [15], an endometrioma, or a simple calcification can be very difficult. CT in this case is very helpful in making a definitive diagnosis (Figs. 10.46, 10.47, 10.48, 10.49, and 10.50).

Fig. 10.45 (**a**, **b**): Dermoid cyst. Vascularization of the wall. (**a**) TVS: a small hyperechogenic focus with sharp acoustic shadowing is rarely visible because of its echogenicity close to the echogenicity of the cystic content. (**b**) TVS with color Doppler. Vessels are demonstrated in the wall of the cyst, in front of the base of the Rokitansky protuberance; on pulsed Doppler, RI is 0.61, PI 1, and peak systolic velocity 12 cm/s

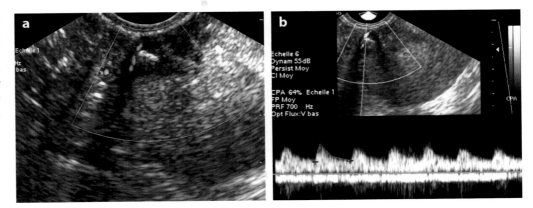

Fig. 10.46 Small dermoid cyst. (**a**) TAS: 7-mm hyperechogenic round left ovarian lesion without acoustic shadowing. Differential diagnosis with a corpus luteum cyst can be discussed. (**b**) CT scan without contrast: the fatty content with a density of −69 HU allows to make a definite diagnosis of MCT

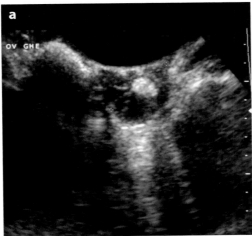
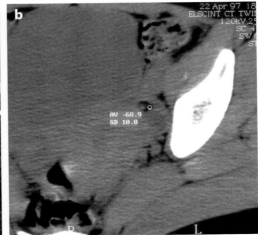

Fig. 10.47 Dermoid cyst. Unusual form of Rokitansky protuberance on US. (**a**) TAS: hyperechogenic focus without acoustic shadowing. Echogenicity of the cystic content is not suggestive for a MCT. (**b**) CT after contrast: a small tissular portion lying against the inner wall contains a tiny calcification related to the protuberance. Fatty content

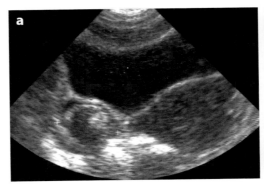
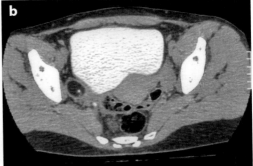

Fig. 10.48 Dermoid cyst of small size. (**a**) EVS: left ovarian mass measuring 2.5 cm with a hyperechogenic focus with broad acoustic shadowing. (**b**) CT scan without contrast: a round calcification and the fatty content (−117 UH) definitely confirm the diagnosis

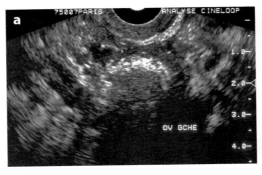
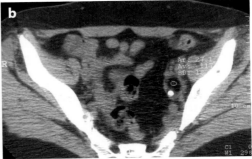

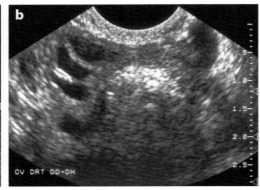

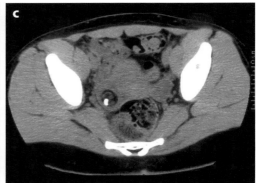

Fig. 10.49 (**a**) TAS: 2-cm hyperechogenic left ovarian mass, slightly heterogeneous with broad acoustic shadowing. (**b**) TVS: delineation with normal ovarian parenchyma is well depicted. (**c**) CT scan without contrast: a little tooth in the protuberance and fat intermingled with hair in the cyst definitely confirm the diagnosis of MCT

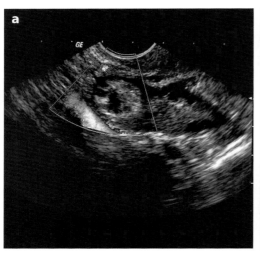

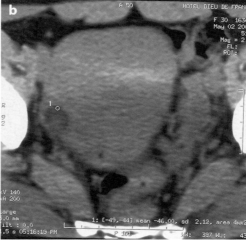

Fig. 10.50 Small MCT of 17 mm of the right ovary discovered after spontaneous abortion. EVS with color Doppler (**a**): The right ovary contains a well delneated mass, containing hyperechoic and anechoic portions; absence of color flow in the mass allows to precise its cystic nature. Although the diagnosis of dermoid cyst could be suggested in the differential diagnosis, a definite diagnosis could not not be established. On CT without contrast (**b**), presence of fat in the cyst allowed to definitely make the diagnosis of dermoid cyst hyperechoic

3. Capsi et al. [34] demonstrated that dermoids <6 cm in diameter had a very slow growth pattern. Over a roughly 3 years' period, the masses showed a growth rate of 1.8 mm/year in premenopausal women and a regression rate of 1.6 mm/year in postmenopausal women.

4. As for an impact of cystectomy performed by laparoscopy on fertility is unknown, women in this group with a desire of pregnancy might benefit from postponing operation [34, 35].

Pediatric Age

MCT accounts for about two-thirds of ovarian tumors in children [5].

In prepubertal girls, US findings are not as typical as after puberty [36]. Although MCT can show one of the findings considered as typical of ovarian teratoma, mural nodules and acoustic shadowing are seen in only 38 and 13% of lesions before puberty [36]. Approximately 10–15% are purely anechoic masses [37] (Fig. 10.51); at pathologic examination, these lesions unusually contain mural nodules less than 4 mm in diameter that are too small to be detected with TAS [37].

Pregnancy

In the past the most frequent means of diagnosis [9] were incidental at the time of delivery (Fig. 10.52). Cysts are not expected to increase significantly in size during pregnancy [35], and the incidence of torsion, hemorrhage, or rupture is not increased [8, 35].

Familial Ovarian Dermoids

Occurrence of ovarian dermoids in multiple women in the same family with a higher incidence of bilateral lesions has been reported [38]. The use of TVS in relatives of women with symptomatic dermoids may be warranted.

10.3.2.2 CT

As far as most of these tumors contain fat and hyperdense structures, CT has been proven to be the best imaging modality to detect and to characterize MCT as in 42 of 43 cases (98%) of our series [11]. Its pattern on CT is so characteristic that it is one of the diagnoses of characterization of ovarian tumors which can be made almost with certainty (Table 10.7). Their shape can be round or ovoid.

Fig. 10.51 MCT of left ovary in a 3-year- and 4-month-old girl measuring 8×7×5 cm. TAS transverse section (**a**): unilocular cyst with a regular thin wall entirely anechoic; on sagittal section (**b**) some declive echoes are displayed. While the diagnosis of a benign cyst could be established, at this age diagnosis of a dermoid cyst can only be suggested in the differential diagnosis. At macrocopy, the liquid was clear the wall was slightly irregular (1–3 mm) with some hairs

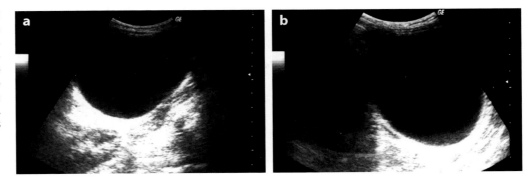

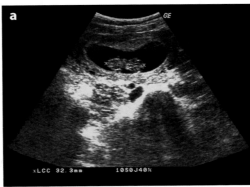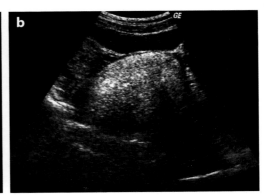

Fig. 10.52 MCT in a pregnant woman. A 26-year-old pregnant woman at 10 weeks and 2 days of amenorrhea. (**a**) Intrauterine pregnancy. (**b**) Ten-cm hyperechogenic left adnexal mass with sound attenuation suggesting a MCT. Because of the large size of the cyst, a laparoscopy with cystectomy was performed. Follow-up was uneventful with delivery of a normal girl

Table 10.7 CT findings of mature cystic teratomas

Noncontrast
A. *Content of the cyst*
Common:
    d <−20 HU (≅90%): almost specific, related to fat intermingled or not
       with hair
Uncommon:
    d >−20 HU: related to fat and large amount of hair or watery content
    Fat level
B. *Rokitansky protuberance*
Common:
    Unique
    Against the inner wall
    <5 cm
    Aspect of nodule or vegetation containing:
       Adipose tissue
       Calcification, bone, cartilage, tooth
    Regular border
Uncommon:
    Multiple
    In a septum, forming a bridge
    Irregular border
C. *Wall*
    Regular and thin
After contrast
Not very helpful
Slight contrast uptake on delayed CT in the wall, the septa and the
    protuberance

Cystic Content

Characteristic Form: Density <−20 HU

When the density is <−20 HU in at least one area of the cyst as in 93% [11] to 84% [39] of cases, the diagnosis of MCT is almost certain. Usually the mean density of the cyst is frankly negative from −40 to −148 HU (mean −109 HU) [11]. It corresponds at pathology to a fatty content more or less intermingled with hair, rarely to pure fat.

When fat is intermingled with hair, hair appears on CT as separated lines of soft tissue density in the fatty content (Fig. 10.3, type 3; Fig. 10.53), or as gathered lines forming tufts of hair (Fig. 10.3 type 1; Fig. 10.54), or as a round mass called a hair ball (Fig. 10.3, type 2; Fig. 10.55). Fat can also appear sometimes as multiple small rounded areas of low density (Fig. 10.56) [40], which can move by positional change [41].

Differential diagnosis: In very uncommon tumors such as solid mature teratoma [7], immature teratoma [7], and lipoleiomyoma [42, 43], fat can be present in some parts of the tumor.

When the content is purely fatty, it appears on CT with a density slightly inferior or equal to subcutaneous fat (−120 HU), which is almost specific for a MCT (Fig. 10.57). Only the very exceptional lipoma of the ovary [7] containing larger nodules of adipose tissue could be a differential although no such case has still been reported with an imaging modality.

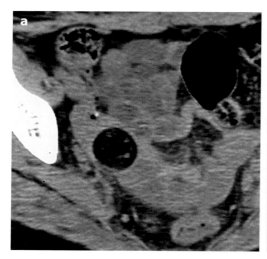

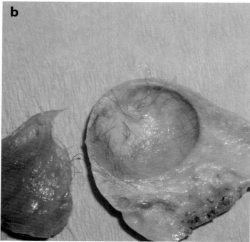

Fig. 10.53 Dermoid cyst containing scattered hairs. (a) CT scan displays a 3-cm cyst with a fatty content intermingled with dense lines corresponding to hairs. (b) View of the surgical specimen demonstrates hairs arising from the cyst wall and hairs intermingled with the fatty content that has been removed and that is solid at room temperature

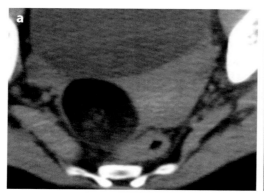

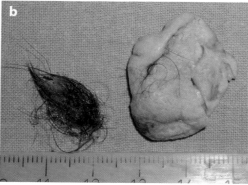

Fig. 10.54 Dermoid cyst with tuft of hairs. (a) CT scan displayed a cyst with fatty content and an irregular dense structure corresponding to hairs. (b) View of the surgical specimen shows hairs arising from the cyst wall and a tuft of hairs that has been removed from the cystic content

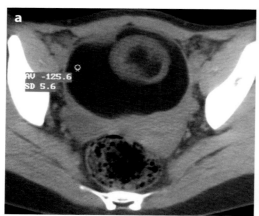

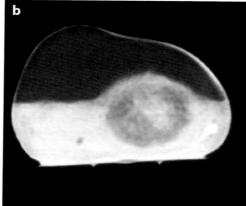

Fig. 10.55 Dermoid cysts with hair balls. Three hair-ball patterns are displayed at CT in three different dermoid cysts. (a) The cystic content is hypodense (−125 HU) and the hair ball contains a hypodense center. (b) In vitro CT study demonstrates a fluid level with an upper low-density fatty portion and a dependent high-density portion. A hair ball is floating at the interface with hair fibers intermingled with fat well depicted inside its center

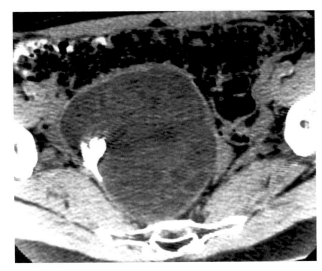

Fig. 10.56 Cystic content containing small round fatty areas

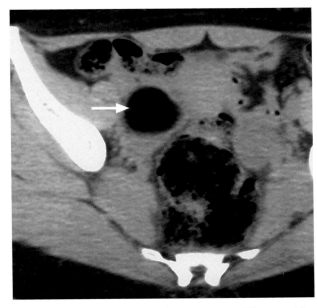

Fig. 10.57 Dermoid cyst with pure fatty content. CT scan without contrast displays a 3-cm right ovarian cyst (*arrow*) with homogeneous low-density content without hair

Exceptionally, pure fatty content may be associated with a pseudo hair-ball pattern related in fact to different types of fat (Fig. 10.58).

When a fluid level [44, 45] is present, the anterior nondependent portion has a far density, while the posterior dependent portion has a density >0 UH. Sometimes a hair ball can float at the interface (Fig. 10.59), and exceptionally two levels may be seen in the same cyst (Fig. 10.60). The high density of the dependent part has no definite explanation as it has already been mentioned on US. This finding of fat-fluid level was present in only five of 40 patients (12.5%) of Buy et al. series [11].

Nonsuggestive Pattern (Density > −20 HU)

Rarely, the density of the cystic content is ≥−20 HU, and the diagnosis of MCT on CT is not possible based on the cystic content alone because fat is not present or could not be characterized in it. These cases can be grouped in three categories:

(a) *A very large amount of hair is mixed with fat resulting in a cystic density ≥−20 HU.* In a low percentage of cases mentioned by Friedman et al. [46] and in 3/24 MCT containing fat at pathology in Guinet et al. series [39], fat mixed with hair could not be recognized on CT because the mean density was comprised between −13 and 8 HU (Fig. 10.61).

(b) *A cystic content, without fat and with a density close to water,* made of a watery fluid (Fig. 10.62), resulting from sweat glands, cerebrospinal fluid excreted from meningeal structures contained in the protuberance [12], or gelatinous fluid. In 1/25 (4%) in Guinet et al. series [39] and in 3/41 (7%) in Buy et al. series [11], attenuation around 0 HU and from 17 to 35 HU respectively corresponded to watery and gelatinous fluid.

(c) Exceptionally, the density is very high until 70 HU. We observed this pattern in some cases of gelatinous fluid (Fig. 10.63) or in dermoid cysts complicated with necrosis (Fig. 10.64). Necrosis can be isolated or secondary to torsion like in a case reported by Cederlund et al. [44].

Fig. 10.58 Fatty ball simulating a hair ball in a dermoid cyst. (**a**) CT scan without contrast shows a left ovarian cyst with a low-density fatty content and a round structure looking like a hair ball. (**b**) In vitro CT study shows a calcification within a Rokitansky protuberance and the round dense structure. At macroscopic examination, the cystic content shows yellow fat and brown fat without hair (see view of the surgical specimen in Fig. 10.11)

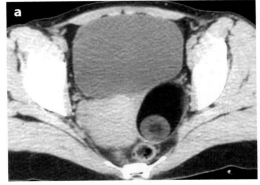
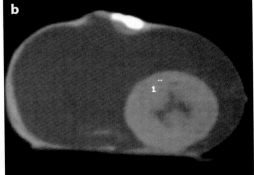

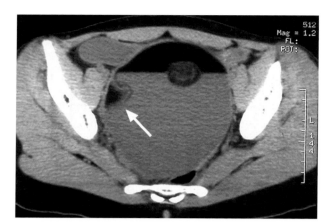

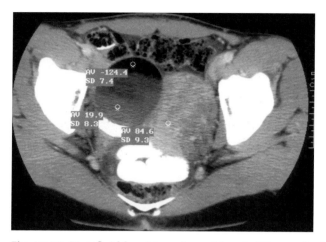

Fig. 10.59 Dermoid cyst with a hair ball floating at the interface of a fluid level. CT scan displayed a 15-cm dermoid with a fluid level and a hair ball floating at the interface. Fat is well depicted in the anterior nondependent portion of the cyst, around the hair ball, and in the adipose tissue situated in the Rokitansky protuberance (*arrow*)

Fig. 10.60 Two-fluid level in a dermoid cyst. CT scan displayed a right ovarian cyst with two levels. The anterior part has a mean density of −124 UH. The posterior part has a mean density of 19 UH. The middle part has an intermediate density. At macroscopy, the cyst contained fat intermingled with hair. No Rokitansky protuberance was present

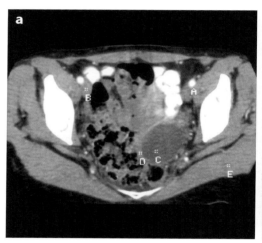

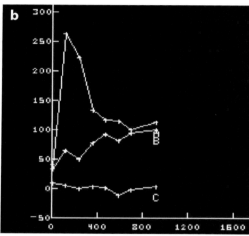

Fig. 10.61 Atypical form of MCT with no low-density content on CT. CT scan with time-density curve demonstrates that the left ovarian mass is cystic with a density close to 10 HU. Preoperative diagnosis of MCT was not suggested. At pathology, a MCT was found containing fat mixed with hair

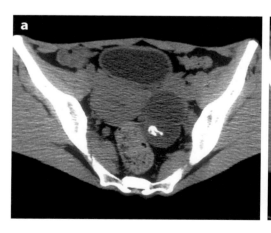

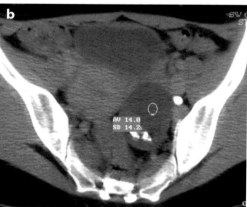

Fig. 10.62 MCT with a watery cystic content. CT scan without contrast. The cystic content has a mean density of 14 HU. Identification of the protuberance with calcifications and adipose tissue allows making a specific diagnosis of MCT

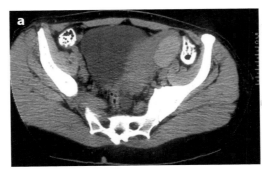
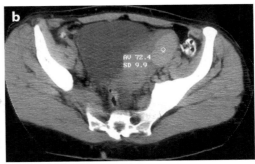

Fig. 10.63 MCT or struma ovarii with very high-density cystic content. CT scan without contrast shows homogeneous unilocular cyst with a regular wall and a density of 72 HU. Diagnosis of MCT was not suggested prospectively. At macroscopy, the cyst contained a gelatinous fluid. At microscopy, the wall contained dense connective tissue intermingled with a loosely connective tissue with thyroid vesicles. In some slides, glial tissue was demonstrated. A final diagnosis of pluritissular MCT was established

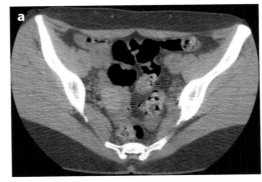
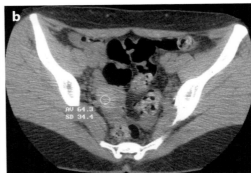

Fig. 10.64 MCT complicated with necrosis in a 29 years old woman. CT scan without contrast demonstrates a right ovarian mass with homogeneous mean density of 64 HU. On macroscopy, consistency of the cystic content was brown and pasty. On microscopy the cyst was filled with keratinized material mixed with eosinophilic proteic substance containing a polypoid mass entirely occupied by necrosis, containing some cells filled with hemosiderin

Rokitansky Protuberance

Detection

While the Rokitansky protuberance is most often overlooked on US, CT is the best modality to detect it (Fig. 10.65). Indeed, on CT, there is an excellent contrast between the content of the cyst and the Rokitansky protuberance that frequently contains tooth, calcification, or adipose tissue. In Buy et al. [11] series of 43 dermoid cyst, one or two protuberances in the same dermoid (total 43) were present at pathology in 36/43 (84%) cysts. CT detected 40/41

(98%) of benign dermoid plugs present at pathology and 2/2 dermoid plugs with malignant transformation.

Characterization

Even when a mural nodule is detected on US, the Rokitansky protuberance can be confused with a vegetation, a clot, or a hair ball, while on CT its aspect is very characteristic (Fig. 10.66). It is even better demonstrated on CT than on MR (Fig. 10.67)

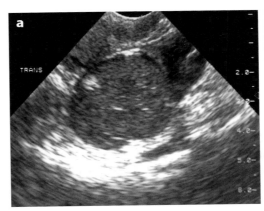
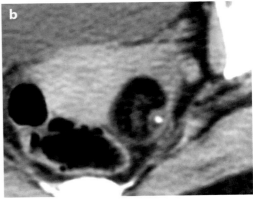

Fig. 10.65 Dermoid cyst with Rokitansky protuberance overlooked on US and detected on CT. (a) Transverse TVU of a dermoid cyst shows an echoic content with sparkle lines and a hyperechoic focus with shadowing, situated on the internal wall of the cyst, representing probably tufts of hairs. (b) On CT, a Rokitansky protuberance containing adipose tissue and a calcification is well demonstrated on the lateral wall of the cyst

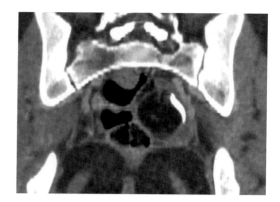

Fig. 10.72 Dermoid cyst with a Rokitansky protuberance appearing as an elongated calcification. (a) On IVP, the elongated calcification is outside the ureter. (b–d) CT scan after contrast (b) and with coronal reformation (c, d).The calcification in the protuberance looks like a canine tooth

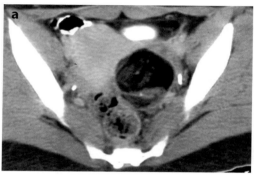
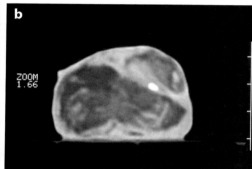

Fig. 10.73 Dermoid cyst with a Rokitansky protuberance in a septum. (a) In vivo CT scan: Rokitansky protuberance appears as a band of tissue containing a calcification. Soft tissue in contact is difficult to characterize. (b) In vitro study of the pathologic specimen

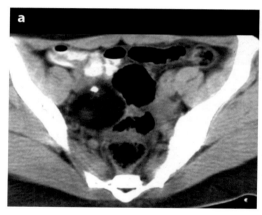
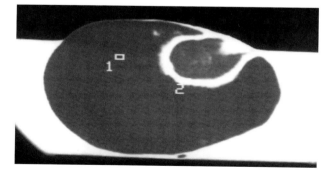

Fig. 10.74 Dermoid cyst containing a Rokitansky protuberance with a bridge shape. (a) CT scans without contrast. The Rokitansky protuberance is clearly depicted against the wall and extends as a bridge to another part of the cyst wall. A calcification is also displayed. (b) Pathologic specimen demonstrates nicely the protuberance

Structure

The wall of the protuberance clearly appears as a regular soft tissue density against the fatty content and forms with the inner wall of the cyst variable perpendicular acute or obtuse angles, which is not in agreement with previous descriptions [11, 25] (Figs. 10.75 and 10.76). Tufts of hair radiating from the wall of the protuberance into the cystic content can be demonstrated (Fig. 10.76).

The content is most often tissular. Beneath the wall, adipose tissue is usually visualized either as a rim or occupying a more important component (Figs. 10.75, 10.76, and 10.77). Nonadipose connective tissue appears as a soft tissue density. Hyperdense structures related to bone, tooth, cartilage, or calcification are commonly present allowing in most of the cases a specific diagnosis. These hyperdense structures can occupy the entire protuberance (Fig. 10.78). Not uncommonly a small mucinous cyst is visualized adjacent to the protuberance sometimes in the cyst wall. Protuberances with an almost entirely cystic content are rare (Figs. 10.79 and 10.80).

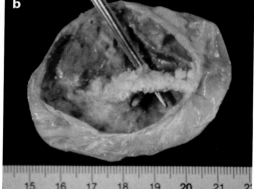

Fig. 10.75 In vitro CT study of the Rokitansky protuberance of a dermoid cyst. The surgical specimen is immerged in water. The wall is clearly visible and forms on one side an acute angle with the wall of the cyst and a perpendicular angle on the other side. A large amount of adipose tissue is present in the Rokitansky protuberance with a density very close to the fatty cystic content

Fig. 10.76 In vivo (**a**) and in vitro (**b**) CT studies of a dermoid cyst with a Rokitansky protuberance. CT scan demonstrates at the best the Rokitansky's protuberance. It appears as a 3- cm tissular portion with a regular border forming with the inner wall of the cyst variable angles. The architecture is very clearly depicted: wall, adipose tissue, tooth, and tuft of hairs

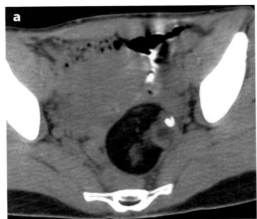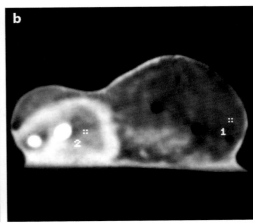

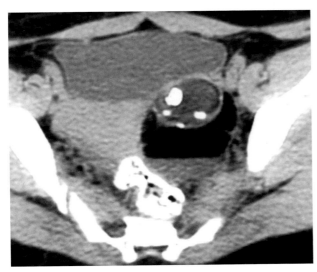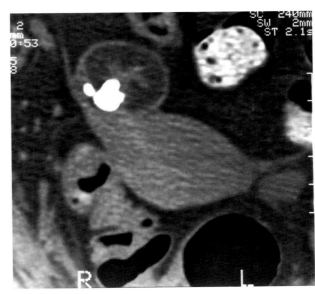

Fig. 10.77 CT of dermoid cyst with Rokitansky protuberance and fat level. The Rokitansky protuberance has a well-defined wall and contains calcifications and a thin rim of adipose tissue. Fat displayed as fat level is well visualized in the adjacent cystic content

Fig. 10.78 Dermoid cyst anterior to the broad ligament with a Rokitansky protuberance almost entirely calcified. On CT, the Rokitansky protuberance appears almost entirely occupied by teeth. A tuft of hairs is nicely depicted, arising from its wall that is imperceptible

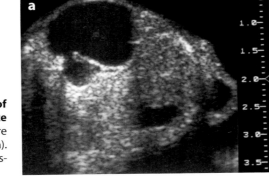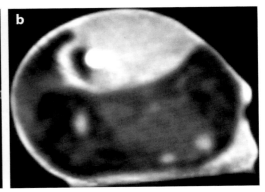

Fig. 10.79 In vitro US (a) and CT (b) studies of a MCT containing a Rokitansky protuberance with a mainly cystic content. The cystic nature of the protuberance is better displayed on US (**a**). Adipose tissue and calcification are better displayed on CT (**b**)

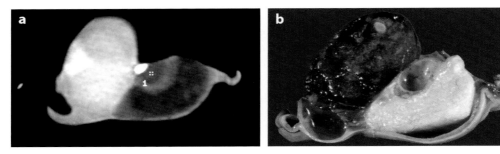

Fig. 10.80 Dermoid cyst with Rokitansky protuberance having a cystic content. (a) In vitro CT study: A typical dermoid cyst is displayed with fat and calcifications. The protuberance appears clearly with a focal hyperdense structure (related to cartilage at pathology), skin, and a cystic content close to 0 HU. **(b)** Pathologic specimen. Protuberance with a cystic content, cartilage, and its wall formed by skin is seen adjacent to a fatty cystic content with a loculation having a mucinous content

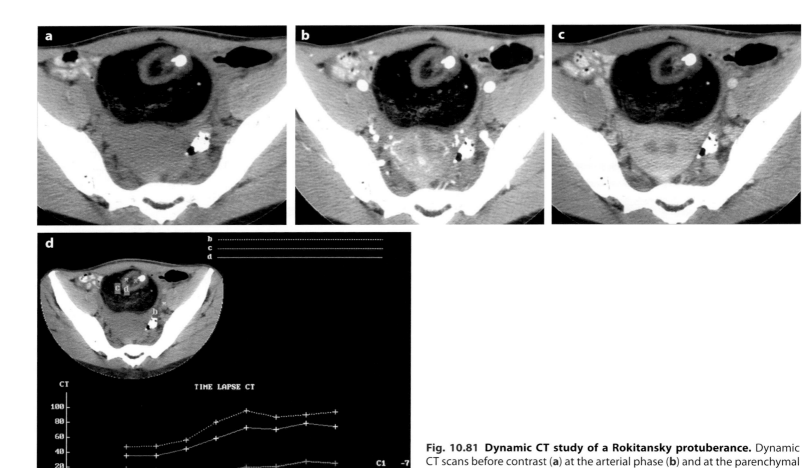

Fig. 10.81 Dynamic CT study of a Rokitansky protuberance. Dynamic CT scans before contrast (**a**) at the arterial phase (**b**) and at the parenchymal phase (**c**) with time-density curve (**d**). A typical dermoid cyst with fatty content and a Rokitansky protuberance is displayed

Inner Border

Inner border: regular or irregular

Vascularization

In most of the cases, this tissular portion is slightly vascularized. During the DCT, at the arterial phase, no vessel is visualized in the protuberance (Fig. 10.81), or small vessels are displayed. At the venous phase a moderate contrast uptake is visualized in the wall and in the protuberance. Diffusion of contrast medium is mainly seen on the delayed CT. In uncommon cases, when the protuberance contains a large portion of thyroid tissue, a high contrast uptake can be visualized at the arterial phase. In the exceptional cases of malignant transformation, at the arterial phase, tumoral vessels can be displayed in the protuberance; a significant contrast uptake can be seen at the venous phase (Table 10.8).

The Wall of the Cyst

CT much better than US depicts the entire wall. On noncontrast CT, it is clearly visualized; it is regular and thin measuring 2–3 mm. Rarely, calcifications are visualized in a part or all around the wall (Fig. 10.82).

On dynamic CT (Fig. 10.81), regular vessels are visualized at the arterial phase and slight contrast uptake is displayed at the parenchymal phase. This diffusion is also observed on delayed CT.

Analysis of the regularity of the entire wall and of the protuberance is fundamental. Indeed, carcinomas and carcinoids arise in the wall or in the protuberance. They can be detected on CT as a local-ized thickening of the wall (case 1 of Felberg et al.) [45] with eventually extracapsular extension (case 4 of Friedman) [46], which cannot be appreciated on US. Diffuse thickening of the wall with hemorrhage is very suggestive of torsion [47].

Association of These Findings

Association of one to five (mean three) of these CT findings (i.e., fat, hair, calcification in the wall or septa, fat-fluid level, Rokitansky nodule) allowed a definite preoperative diagnosis of benign ovarian cystic teratoma in 37 of 38 (97%) patients and 40 of 41 (98%) tumors [11].

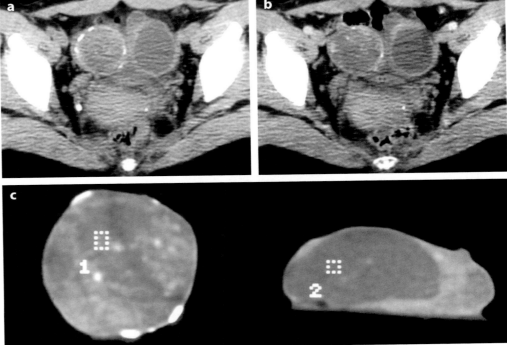

Fig. 10.82 Bilateral atypical MCT on CT with calcifications. (**a**, **b**) CT scan without (**a**) and after (**b**) contrast. Bilateral ovarian mass with calcifications in the wall of the right one. Density of the cystic content in the right one is close to pelvic muscle, while density in the left one is close to urine. A slight contrast uptake is visualized in the wall of both masses. (**c**) In vitro CT study: right ovary: Calcifications are depicted not only in the wall but also in the cystic content; mean density of the cysts is 20 HU. Left ovary: A density close to 0 HU is displayed. Preoperative diagnosis was not suggested. At pathology, content of the right MCT was mastic, and content of the left one was watery fluid

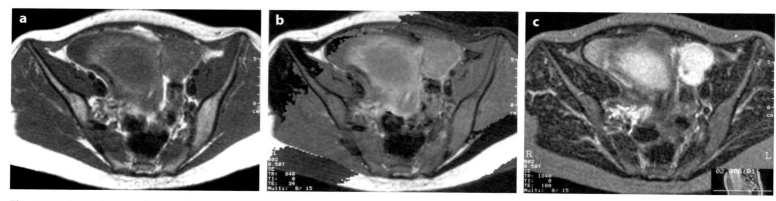

Fig. 10.90 MCT with a watery cystic content. Axial MR T1-weighted image (**a**) with fat suppression (**b**) and T2-weighted image (**c**). The cystic content has a signal identical to water on the different sequences. Diagnosis of MCT could not be established on MR

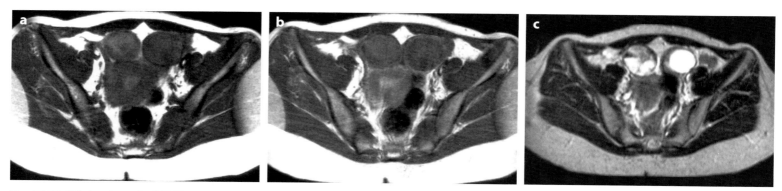

Fig. 10.91 Bilateral atypical MCT on MR. (**a**) On T1 weighted images, signal intensity of the cystic content is heterogeneous with intermediate and low signal intensity on the right and homogeneous with low signal intensity on the left. (**b**) After injection, a slight contrast uptake is visualized in the wall of the cysts. (**c**) On T2-weighted images, signal intensity is heterogeneous with low and high intensity signals in both masses. Preoperative diagnosis was not suggested. At pathology, content of the right MCT was mastic, and content of the left one was watery fluid

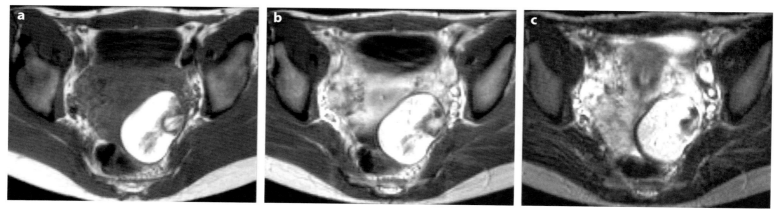

Fig. 10.92 Dermoid cyst with Rokitansky's protuberance on MR. T1-weighted images (**a**), after gadolinium (**b**), and T2-weighted image (**c**). The wall of the protuberance has a signal close to pelvic muscle on T1 and T2. No significant contrast uptake is visualized after gadolinium injection. Adipose tissue has a signal close to subcutaneous adipose tissue on T1 and T2. Tufts of hair emerging from the protuberance are clearly depicted within the cystic content. The low signal focus in the protuberance on T1 and T2 weighted images corresponds to a tooth that was better visualized on CT

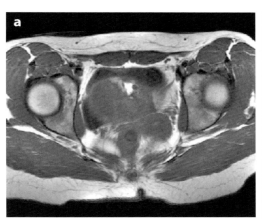
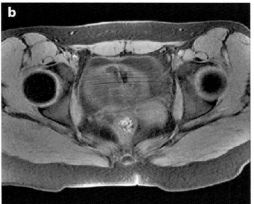
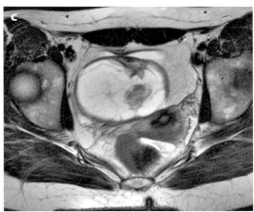
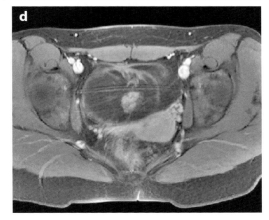

Fig. 10.93 MCT in a 16 years old girl. T1-weighted image (**a**) displays a MCT with a watery low intensity cystic content and a Rokitansky protuberance containing a high signal intensity area with a low signal intensity after fat-suppression (**b**) corresponding to adipose tissue. After injection (**d**), a second protuberance that is barely seen before injection, markedly enhance containing glial tissue on pathology. On T2-weighted image (**c**), the cystic content appears hyperintense while the two protuberance appear hypointense

Other Finding: Reversed Chemical Shift Artifact (Fig. 10.94)

Reversed chemical shift artifact (when compared to bladder) at the boundaries of the cyst (and/or within it) has been reported [48] especially on T2 W image because of narrow band-width chosen to increase signal over noise ratio [56].

Diffusion

Recently, diffusion-weighted imaging (DWI) and the calculated apparent diffusion coefficient (ADC) have been used in an attempt to differentiate benign and malignant ovarian masses. Nakayama [49] has reported the usefulness of diffusion sequences in the diagnosis of mature cystic teratoma. On quantitative and qualitative analyses, MCT tended to have higher signal intensity and areas of lower ADC values than endometrial cysts and other benign and malignant neoplasms. Indeed almost all dermoid cysts contain keratinoid substance which is a scleroprotein that originates from the cytoskeletal structure of the epidermis. The restricted Brownian movement of water molecules within the keratoid substance results in a high signal on DWI and a low ADC values.

10.3.2.4 Association of Different Imaging Modalities

Association of different imaging modalities (US, CT and MR) allow to make the diagnosis in difficult cases (Fig. 10.95).

10.3.3 Other Forms

10.3.3.1 Bilaterality and Multiplicity

Bilaterality (Figs. 10.96 and 10.97). is present in about 15% cases [7]. This is the reason why some surgeons used to perform systematically a controlateral ovariotomy. A considerable improvement in the detection of small dermoids by US, CT and MR allows nowadays to precise with accuracy the presence or absence of a controlateral MCT.

Dermoids can be multiple in the same ovary (Figs. 10.98 and 10.99). Until four MCT have been identified at pathology in the same ovary.

On ultrasound diagnosis of multiplicity and delineation of the different dermoids can be quite difficult. CT and MR are suitable in these cases for a preoperative evaluation especially in young women where coelioscopy is planned.

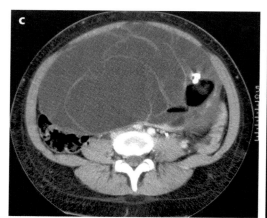
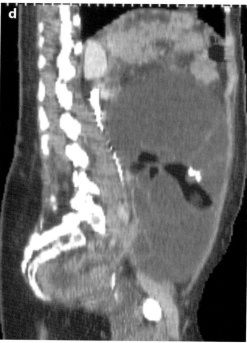

Fig. 10.104 (*continued*) (**c**, **d**) CT scan with sagittal reformation confirms the presence of a MCT in a multiloculated cystic mass suggestive of mucinous cystadenoma

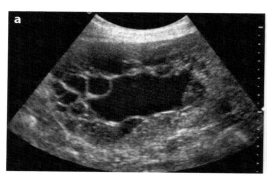
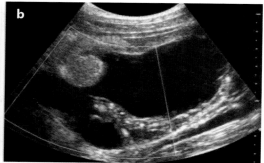

Fig. 10.105 Collision tumor. Mucinous cystadenoma with MCT and Leydig cells hyperplasia. A 28-year-old woman in the second trimester of pregnancy (21 weeks of amenorrhea). TAS (**a**) with Color Doppler (**b**) displays a 10 cm right ovarian multilocular cyst with regular walls. A 2 cm echogenic nodule is visualized in the right and anterior portion of the cyst (**a**) with no color flow (**b**). Vessels are only displayed in the septa. The preoperative diagnosis was not performed. At pathology, there was a multilocular mucinous cystadenoma associated with a 2 cm MCT and Leydig cells hyperplasia

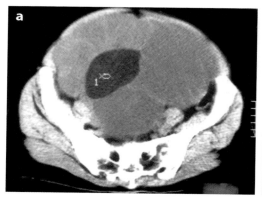
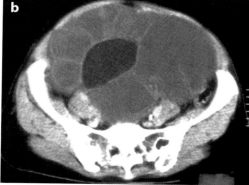

Fig. 10.106 Collision tumor. MCT in a borderline mucinous tumor. CT scan without contrast (**a**) and after contrast (**b**). An MCT is seen in a multilocular cyst suggesting an association with a mucinous tumor. After contrast (**b**) the septa are numerous and overall irregular ill defined. A borderline or malignant tumor was suspected. At surgery and pathology, there was an MCT associated with a borderline mucinous tumor without any extension (Figures from Author's personal publication: Buy et al. [11])

CT

Findings of MCT

Identification of a fatty content or a Rokitansky protberance is clearly demonstrated in our cases and in MASLIN's case report [79]. However these findings are not clearly described in a larger series performed with CT or MR or both [76].

Findings suggesting malignancy

In a retrospective study performed with CT or MR or both, a soft tissue component was identified in 9/11 cases [80].

CT seems to be the best modality to detect a malignant transformation either in the Rokitansky protuberance or in the wall.

1. The Rokitansky protuberance. Findings of malignant transformation in the Rokitansky protuberance have been reported as a cauliflower shape (Fig. 10.113), irregular borders, a size > 5 cm, obtuse angles with the inner wall of the cyst, soft tissue density like in malignant tumor (which may contain a tooth) (Fig. 10.114), a dermoid plug extending in and outside the cyst (Feldberg, case 1) [45] and a significant contrast uptake [80] with tumoral vessels on the dynamic CT [11]. However margins can be smooth as in 5/9 of PARK's series [80] and an acute angle can be observed as in 1/9 cases [80]. Although contrast enhancement raises the possibility of malignant transformation, this finding does not always necessarily indicate malignancy [81].

2. A mass arising in the wall with extracapsular extension.

3. *Remote extension: In many cases, the tumor has already thread to adjacent organs or* throughout the abdomen [7] (Figs. 10.114 and 10.115).

MR

Kido et al. [82] reported the MR appearance of six dermoid cysts with malignant transformation. Size of the tumors ranged from 10 to 32 cm.

Because of the presence of fat ($n=6$) with a fluid level ($n=5$) a diagnosis of MCT was performed in all cases.

Diagnosis of malignant transformation was not performed in a case of in situ carcinoma and was suggested in 5/6 cases. Solid tissue from 3.5 to 15 cm was displayed in five cases with an intermediate to low signal intensity on T1 weighted images, and with an intermediate to high signal intensity on T2 W images. In two of these performed with contrast enhancement, a contrast uptake was displayed. The growth pattern of this tissue was nodular in one (with contrast uptake) and diffuse and transmural in four. In three of these four tumors with transmural extension, the solid tissue grew outside the tumor and extensively invaded the adjacent structures, including uterus, vagina and the pouch of Douglas.

10.3.3.5 Parasitic Ovarian Dermoid Tumor of the Omentum

The etiology of omental teratomas is poorly understood. Three main theories have been proposed [83]:

1. Primary teratoma of the omentum originating from germ cells arrested at the level of the dorsal mesentery.
2. Teratoma developing in supernumerary ovary of the omentum.
3. Autoamputation of ovarian dermoid secondary to torsion and reimplantation of ovarian teratoma on the omentum.

Abdominal pain and a mobile round abdominal mass are the usual clinical findings of presentation.

CT suggests the diagnosis of MCT, but may [84] or may not [83] recognize the omental location of the tumor.

Exceptionally, primary omental immature teratoma has been reported [85, 86].

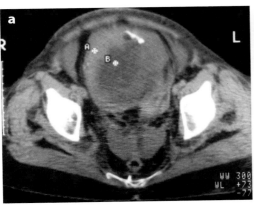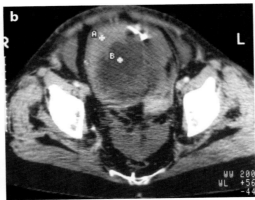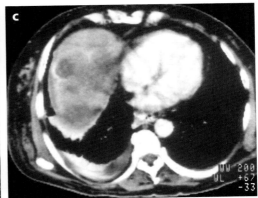

Fig. 10.114 Malignant transformation in a MCT. A 65-year-old woman with abdominal pain and weight loss (CA 125: 580 IU/ml). (**a, b**) **CT** scan before (**a**) and after contrast (**b**) displays a large irregular tissular portion with contrast uptake containing a tooth and suggesting a malignant transformation in a MCT. Small pelvic ascites is also present. (**c**) Hepatic metastases and right pleural secondary effusion are displayed on abdominal CT (Figure (**b**) from Author's personal publication: Buy et al. [11])

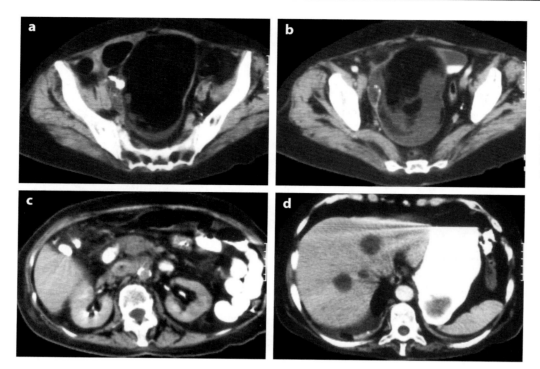

Fig. 10.115 Malignant transformation in a MCT 69 years old woman with abdominal pain. (a, b) CT scan before (a) and after contrast (b) displays a 20 cm right ovarian mass containing fat and calcifications corresponding to a MCT. The protuberance is large and irregular (with a slight contrast uptake), protruding into the cyst. (c, d) Lombo-aortic lymph modes and hepatic metastases are displayed on higher slices. At pathology an epidermoid carcinoma in the protuberance with necrosis in the cyst and secondary infection I was diagnosed

10.4 Other Teratomas

Teratomas other than MCT are the following:
– Immature cystic teratoma
– Mature solid teratoma.
– Monodermal and highly specialized teratomas
  Struma ovarii
  Carcinoids
  Other monodermal and highly specialized teratomas

10.4.1 Immature Teratoma

10.4.1.1 Definition

The immature teratoma is a malignant form of teratoma. It is composed of tissues derived from the three germ cell layers (ectoderm, mesoderm, and endoderm) and, in contrast to the very much more common mature teratoma it contains immature tissues that resembles those of the embryo [2, 7]. The amount of immature tissue varies from rare foci to a predominant component (7 Scully page 268)

Mature tissues are frequently present and sometimes may predominate. In these cases, differentiation from mature teratoma may be difficult and their separation rests exclusively on their microscopic appearance [2, 7].

10.4.1.2 Frequency and Age Distribution

They represent less than 1% of all ovarian cancers. The peak incidence is in the second decade. No case has been reported after menopause [7].

10.4.1.3 Gross Examination

Immature teratomas usually appear as predominantly unilateral solid, lobulated masses that contain numerous small cysts.

Soft tissue which is usually composed predominantly of immature neural tissue is often conspicuous and may be the site of necrosis and hemorrhage.

Occasionally, it may be prominently cystic, unilocular, multilocular, with solid areas present in the cyst wall [2, 4, 8, 87, 88] (Fig. 10.116).

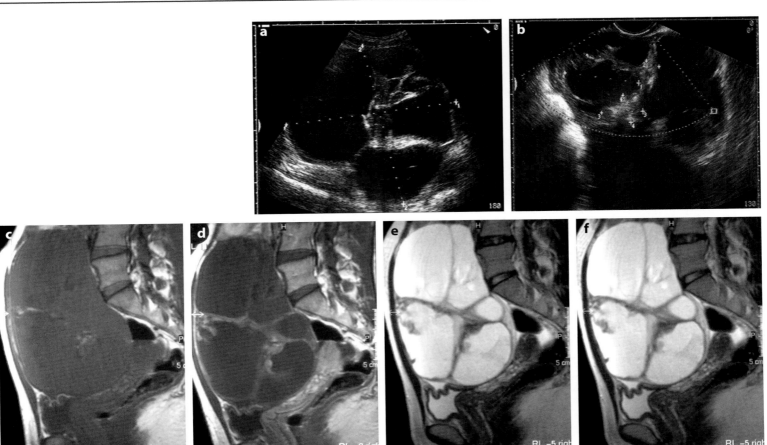

Fig. 10.116 Immature teratoma with cystic form. A 29-year-old woman with urinary compression symptoms and a large pelvic abdominal mass. CA 125: 76 IU/ml. CA 19–9: normal. (**a, b**) TAS (**a**) with Color Doppler (**b**) displays a multicystic ovarian mass with thickened septa vascularized on Color Doppler. (**c–e**) Sagital MR T1-weighted before (**c**), after (**d**) gadolinium injection and T2-weighted (**e, f**) images. On T1-weighted images, hyperintense signal in the septa was not characterized as fatty tissue because no fat suppression was performed. Adipose tissue was visualized in these septa at pathology. After injection high contrast uptake is seen in the septa (**d**) which look thickened and irregular and with a low intensity on T2 (**e, f**)

Two findings may be very suggestive of teratoma:
- The solid tissue may include cartilage bone.
- The cysts may contain sebaceous material and hair. Clear fluid mucus or colloid can also be present.

Capsular rupture som etimes with herniation of tumor through the defect is seen in almost half the cases [86, 87].

10.4.1.4 Microscopic Examination and Grading

Most or all of the immature tissue is composed of immature neuroectodermal tissue.

Immature or embryonal epithelium of various types, as well as immature mesenchymal elements such as cartilage and skeletal muscle are also frequent.

According to the importance of immature neuroepithelium grading is as follows [90]

Grade 1: Rare foci of immature neuroepithelium occupying less than one low power microscopic field (X40, LPFs) in any slide

Grade 2: one to three LFPs in any slide

Grade 3 more than three LFPs in any slide

10.4.1.5 Differential Diagnosis

Differential Diagnosis: Malignant mixed Müllerian tumor (MMMT) is composed of derivatives of Müllerian mesoderm, a primitive structure that gives rise both to the stroma and epithelium of the endometrium. The monodermal origin of malignant mixed Müllerian mesodermal tumor distinguishes it from teratoma. The lumen is composed of sarcomatous and carcinomatous tissue. Derivatives of the three germ layers are absent. Neuroectodermal derivatives, prominent in solid immature teratoma are never seen. The tumor occurs most frequently in posmenopausal woman [2].

10.4.1.6 Clinical Findings

Clinical Findings: The clinical presentation is typically that of abdominal or pelvic pain [7, 91].

10.4.1.7 Biological Markers

Biological Markers: AFP is elevated [77]. Other markers can be elevated: HCG, CA-125 et CA-19-9 [77].

10.4.1.8 Imaging Modalities (Table 10.11)

Table 10.11 Findings of immature teratoma on US CT and MR

1. Findings of teratoma
 – **Most commonly solid or predominantly solid containing small cysts**
  – Irregular solid tissue containing punctuate foci of adipose tissue and calcifications better displayed on CT
  – Degenerative changes (necrosis, hemorrhage)
  – Malignant vascularization: on color Doppler Dynamic MR dynamic CT
  – Significant contrast uptake at the venous phase (DMR, DCT)
  – Small cysts contain mucinous, serous, bloody fluid or hair [7]
 – **Uncommonly predominantly cystic uni or multilocular**
  – On MR, signal intensities identical to aqueous fluid
  – Different from fatty fluid in MCT [93]+++
2. Capsular rupture (almost 50%)
3. Extension outside the ovary
 – Ascites peritoneal implants
 – Lymph nodes Liver
4. Association:
 – In the same ovary: Dermoid cyst (25%); other germ cell tumors
 – In the contralateral ovary: Dermoid cyst (10%)
 – Bilateral 1%

Table 10.12 US CT and MR findings in struma ovarii

A. Predominantly solid with cystic areas, Rarely unilocular or multilocular cystic masses
B. Characteristics of the solid part
 1. *Morphologic findings*
  – Solid tissue with regular limits
  – US
  – CT dense Calcifications
  – MR High signal intensity on T2 very suggestive
 2. *Vascular findings*
  – Endocrine type of vascularisation: on color Doppler
  – Regular vessels with high contrast uptake at the arterial phase on the dynamic CT or MR
  – High contrast uptake at the venous phase
C. Characteristics of the cystic part
 In the tumor or at the periphery giving a particular lobulated outer wall
 Different cystic cavities with different signal intensities on T1 and T2
 Cavities with low signal(equal to muscle) or with signal void on T2 very suggestive
D. Associated tumors
 Common dermoid cysts (50%)
 Uncommon: Solid carcinoid (strumal carcinoid)
 Brenner, Mucinous cystadenoma

Ultrasound

In the predominantly solid form, the mass is of mixed echogenicity. Tumoral vessels can be displayed in the tissular portion with a low resistivity index.

In the predominantly cystic form the mass is multilocular, the different loculi being separated by thickened irregular septa which are vascularized on Color Doppler (Fig. 10.116). Differentiation with other multiloculated masses especially mucinous tumor/seems to be impossible.

CT

In the predominantly solid form, the mass contains solid portions of soft tissue density with less dense areas and denser areas related to hemorrhage.

Calcifications scattered throughout the tumor and foci of adipose tissue are better displayed than on MR [92] and highly suggest the diagnosis of teratoma.

On the dynamic CT scans typical tumoral vessels at the arterial phase and contrast uptake at the parenchymal phase strongly suggest the diagnosis of malignant ovarian tumor (Fig. 10.117).

To our knowledge no case on CT of the predominantly cystic form has been reported.

MR

The solid component:

On T1 signal intensity is low (= uterus)

On T2 signal intensity is equal or slightly higher than myometrium

On contrast-enhanced images heterogeneously high intensity identical or higher than myometrium

Fatty contents are usually scattered throughout the solid component as small punctuate foci of less than 1 cm in diameter [93]. More rarely fatty fluid can be observed as in two out of ten cases of Yamaoka's series [93].

Predominant fluid content exhibited signal intensities similar to simple fluid in 9/10 cases besides the usual findings of a mixed mass, the advantage of MR is to better display the areas of hemorrhage on T1-weighted images. However calcifications can be overlooked.

In the predominantly cystic form (Fig. 10.116), differential diagnosis with other multiloculated cystic masses especially mucinous borderline or carcinoma is very difficult. However, adipose tissue contained in the septa or in the wall might be displayed.

10.4.1.9 Immature Teratoma Can Be Associated with Dermoid Cysts

In a series of 350 cases of immature teratomas and 10 cases of dermoid cysts [57], 26% of the former contained at least one grossly visible dermoid cyst, 10% of them were associated with a contralateral dermoid cyst.

In the same series 2.6% of immature teratoma were preceded 3 years before (in average) by a cystectomy of a dermoid cyst on gross examination in the same ovary (two of those had slightly immature foci). In the same series, to evaluate the importance of the presence of these immature foci, ten *macroscopic dermoid cysts* (seven cystectomies), *with foci of immature tissue at microscopy* were studied. Follow up in 9/10 cases revealed no recurrence 11 months to 7 years post operatively. This is the reason why

1. Yannai Inbar considers that the finding of one or more microscopic foci of immature teratoma in the wall of a dermoid cyst seems to be associated with little if any increased risk of the subsequent appearance of an immature teratoma
2. According to Scully, while the presence of any immature tissue (even rare foci) warrants a diagnosis of immature teratoma, the rare otherwise typical dermoid cyst containing immature foci is considered as dermoid cyst (Scully [7, p 267]).

Immature teratoma can be associated with other forms of malignant germ cell tumor in the same ovary.

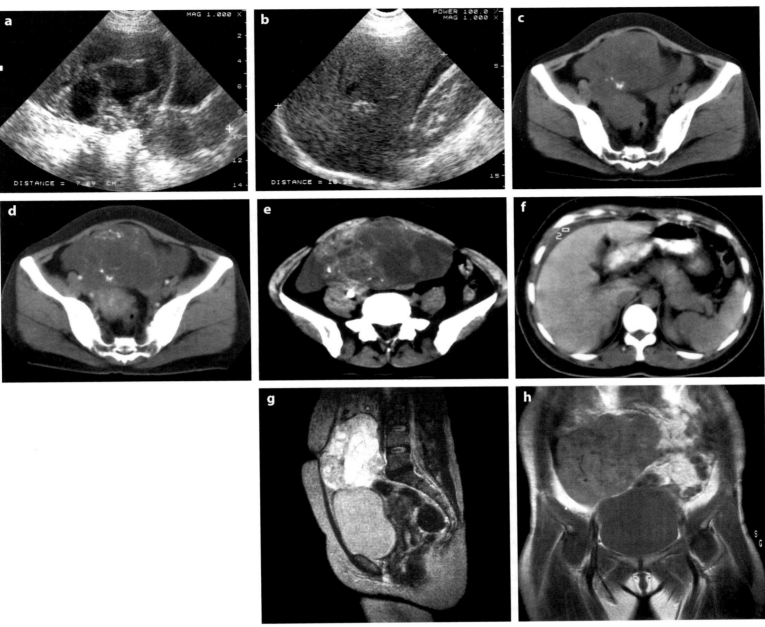

Fig. 10.117 Immature teratoma characterized on CT. Usual form with major solid component. A 39-year-old woman with pelvic abdominal mass. CA 125, CA 19–9 and Alpha-foetoprotein were normal. (**a**) TAS shows a pelvic mass with mixed echogenicity. (**b**) US of the subhepatic space shows peritoneal echogenic fluid. (**c**) CT scan without contrast showed a mixed mass containing tiny calcifications and fat suggesting a teratoma. (**d**) Dynamic CT at the arterial phase shows tumoral vessels very suggestive of malignancy. (**e**) Dynamic CT at the parenchymal phase. The mass looks solid with cystic portions separated by irregular septa. (**f**) CT of the abdomen demonstrated an abdominal ascites without peritonal implant. (**g**) Sagital MR T2-weighted image well displays the different solid and cystic components of the mass. (**h**) Coronal MR T1-weighted image. Abnormal vessels are suggestive of a malignant tumor, but diagnosis of immature teratoma could not be established. Slightly hyperintense foci which were proven to represent extensive hemorrhage at pathology are depicted

Extension

Rarely, immature teratoma are associated with peritoneal implants composed exclusively or mainly of mature glial tissue (peritoneal gliomatosis) [89, 94]. These implants can be extensively calcified [95].

Similar glial tissue is sometimes encountered in pelvic and paraaortic lymphnodes.

Metastatic liver lesions may contain fat and calcification [96]. After chemotherapy, retroconversion of immature to mature tissue in metastasis have been described [96, 97]. The lesions can increase in size and has been described as the growing teratoma syndrome [98]. The margins of the lesions become better circumscribed. Calcification with fatty areas and cystic changes can appear.

Prognosis

The two most common important factors of prognosis are the stage [99] and the histologic grade [100].

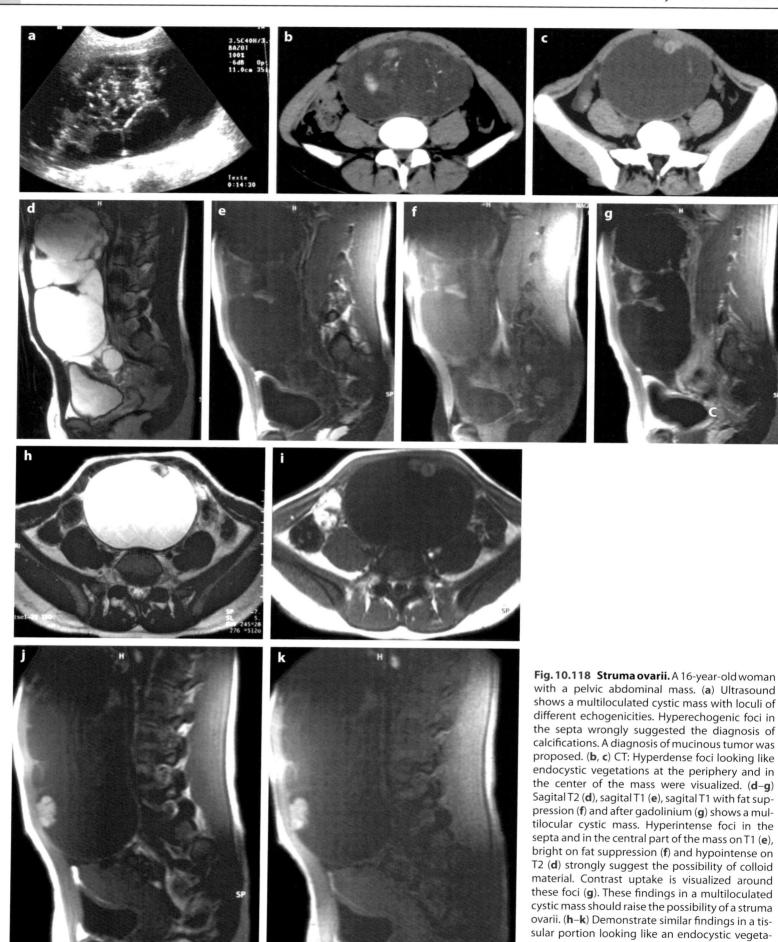

Fig. 10.118 Struma ovarii. A 16-year-old woman with a pelvic abdominal mass. (**a**) Ultrasound shows a multiloculated cystic mass with loculi of different echogenicities. Hyperechogenic foci in the septa wrongly suggested the diagnosis of calcifications. A diagnosis of mucinous tumor was proposed. (**b**, **c**) CT: Hyperdense foci looking like endocystic vegetations at the periphery and in the center of the mass were visualized. (**d–g**) Sagital T2 (**d**), sagital T1 (**e**), sagital T1 with fat suppression (**f**) and after gadolinium (**g**) shows a multilocular cystic mass. Hyperintense foci in the septa and in the central part of the mass on T1 (**e**), bright on fat suppression (**f**) and hypointense on T2 (**d**) strongly suggest the possibility of colloid material. Contrast uptake is visualized around these foci (**g**). These findings in a multiloculated cystic mass should raise the possibility of a struma ovarii. (**h–k**) Demonstrate similar findings in a tissular portion looking like an endocystic vegetation. At pathology, the diagnosis of a pure struma ovarii was confirmed

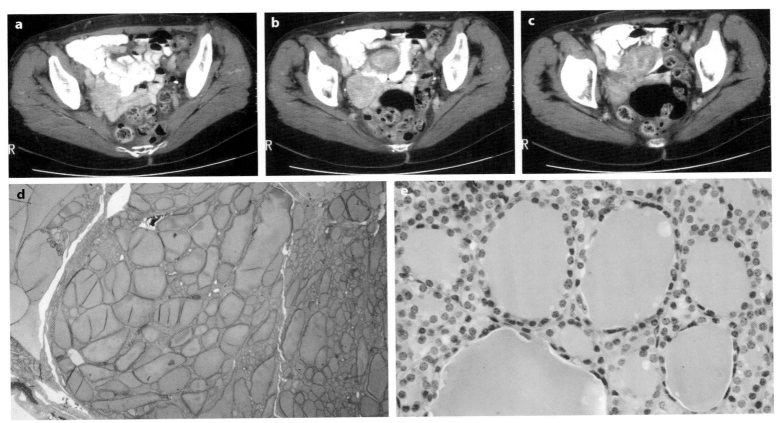

Fig. 10.119 Struma ovarii. A 58-year-old woman with lumbar pain. CT scan demonstrates retroperitoneal lymph modes (which were proved to be a scleronodular Hodgkin's disease) and a right pelvic mass wrongly considered as a subserous leiomyoma. (**a, b**) CT scan with IV contrast. A 4 cm right pelvic mass simulating a subserous leiomyoma is depicted. However left and a normal right ovary are not visualized. (**c**) Section immediately below: visualization of the right uterine vessels medial to the mass could have suggested that the mass was ovarian in origin. At the anterior part of the mass, a triangular shaped structure should have suggested a lombo-ovarian ligament coming toward the mass, which would have proved its ovarian nature. (**d, e**) Microscopic examination demonstrates multiple colloid vesicles typical for struma ovarii

Scintigraphy

Using I-123 NaI, contrast uptake in the pelvic mass can specifically diagnose a struma ovarii even in case of non functional struma [118] (Fig. 10.120, 10.121, 10.122, and 10.123).

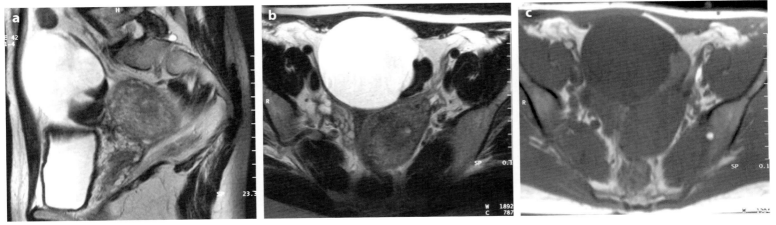

Fig. 10.120 Struma ovarii. A 39-year-old woman. (**a–d**) Axial T2 (**a**), sagital T2 (**b**), axial T1 (**c**) and sagital T1 fat suppression (**d**) MR images. Multiloculated left cystic mass measuring 7 cm and containing: Loculi separated by regular and thin septa with a signal close to urine on the different sequences. In the left part of the mass, a loculation with an intermediate signal on T1 (**c**) which stays bright on fat suppression (**d**) and with a very low signals on T2-weighted images (**a, b**). This signal characteristics can be seen in endometriosis and struma ovarii. A struma ovary was diagnosed at pathology

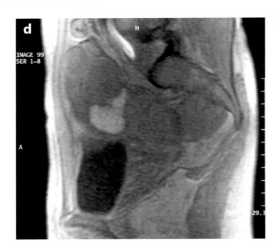

Fig. 10.120 (*continued*)

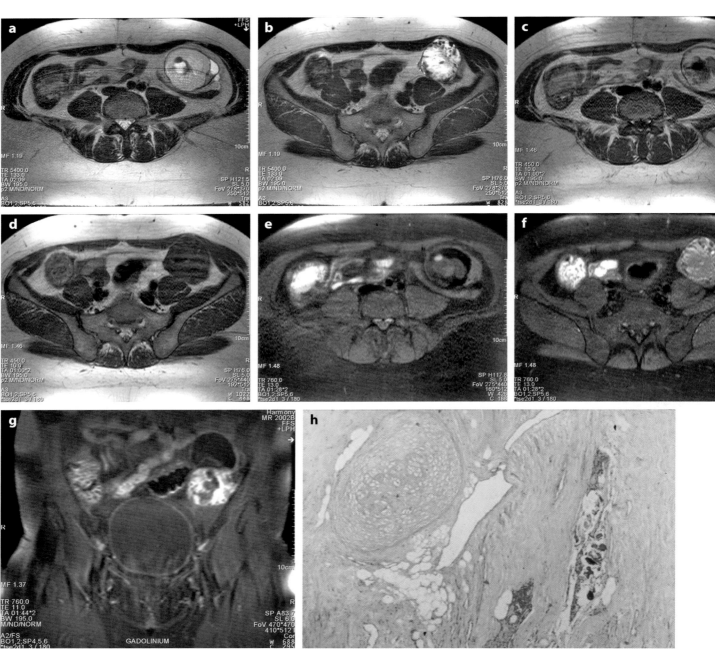

Fig. 10.121 Struma ovarii associated with a dermoid cyst: a and **b** (Axial T2), **c** and **d** (Axial T1), **e** and **f** (axial T1 fat suppression after injection) **g** (coronal fat suppression after injection) **h** and **i** (microscopy). A **c** and **e** display a typical dermoid cyst which is associated with a mass of high signal intensity on T1 (**b**) low intensity on T2 (**d**) and with a high contrast uptake on T1 fat suppression with injection (**f**). Coronal T1 after injection displays the two components of the mass in the left ovary. Microscopic examination displays a dermoid cyst (**h**) and colloid vesicles contained in the struma ovarii (**i**)

Fig. 10.121 (continued)

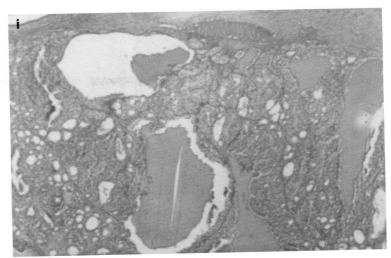

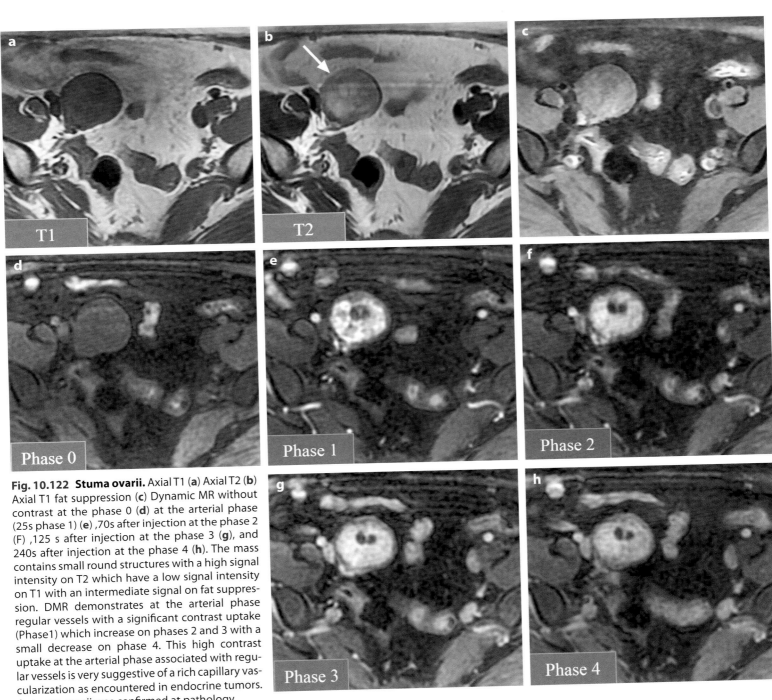

Fig. 10.122 Stuma ovarii. Axial T1 (**a**) Axial T2 (**b**) Axial T1 fat suppression (**c**) Dynamic MR without contrast at the phase 0 (**d**) at the arterial phase (25s phase 1) (**e**) ,70s after injection at the phase 2 (**F**) ,125 s after injection at the phase 3 (**g**), and 240s after injection at the phase 4 (**h**). The mass contains small round structures with a high signal intensity on T2 which have a low signal intensity on T1 with an intermediate signal on fat suppression. DMR demonstrates at the arterial phase regular vessels with a significant contrast uptake (Phase1) which increase on phases 2 and 3 with a small decrease on phase 4. This high contrast uptake at the arterial phase associated with regular vessels is very suggestive of a rich capillary vascularization as encountered in endocrine tumors. A struma ovarii was confirmed at pathology

Pathology

Microscopy

These tumors closely resemble neoplasms of the central nervous system [7, 119–121]. They have been classified [7] as:

Special stains for neural tissue, immunocytochemical staining for glial fibrillary acid protein (GFAP) and neurofilaments are helpful for the diagnosis.

(c) Anaplastic

140. Kurman RJ, Norris HJ (1976) Endodermal sinus tumor of the ovary: a clinical and pathologic analysis of 71 cases. Cancer 38:2404–2419
141. Langley FA, Govan AD, Anderson MC, Gowing NF, Woodcock AS, Harilal KR (1981) Yolk sac and allied tumours of the ovary. Histopathology 5:389–401
142. Kawai M, Furuhashi Y, Kano T et al (1990) Alpha-fetoprotein in malignant germ cell tumors of the ovary. Gynecol Oncol 39:160–166
143. Clement PB, Young RH, Scully RE (1987) Endometrioid-like variant of ovarian yolk sac tumor. A clinicopathological analysis of eight cases. Am J Surg Pathol 11:767–778
144. Levitin A, Haller KD, Cohen HL, Zinn DL, O'Connor MT (1996) Endodermal sinus tumor of the ovary: imaging evaluation. AJR Am J Roentgenol 167:791–793
145. Yamaoka T, Togashi K, Koyama T et al (2000) Yolk sac tumor of the ovary: radiologic-pathologic correlation in four cases. J Comput Assist Tomogr 24:605–609
146. Kurman RJ, Norris HJ (1976) Endodermal sinus tumor of the ovary: a clinical and pathologic analysis of 71 cases. Cancer 38:2404–2419, JID – 0374236
147. Huntington RWJ, Bullock WK (1970) Yolk sac tumors of the ovary. Cancer 25:1357–1367
148. Jimerson GK, Woodruff JD (1977) Ovarian extraembryonal teratoma. I. Endodermal sinus tumor. Am J Obstet Gynecol 127:73–79
149. Talerman A, Haije WG, Baggerman L (1978) Serum alphafetoprotein (AFP) in diagnosis and management of endodermal sinus (yolk sac) tumor and mixed germ cell tumor of the ovary. Cancer 41:272–278
150. Romero JA, Kim EE, Tresukosol D, Kudelka AP, Edwards CL, Kavanagh JJ (1995) Recurrent ovarian endodermal sinus tumor: demonstration by computed tomography, magnetic resonance imaging, and positron emission tomography. Eur J Nucl Med 22:1214–1217

Choriocarcinoma

151. Bazot M, Cortez A, Sananes S, Buy JN (2004) Imaging of pure primary ovarian carcinoma. AJR Am J Roentgenol 182:1603–1604

Embryonal Carcinoma

152. Neubecker RD, Breen JL (1962) Embryonal carcinoma of the ovary. Cancer 15:546
153. Kurman RJ, Norris HJ (1976) Embryonal carcinoma of the ovary: a clinico-pathologic entity distinct from endodermal sinus tumor resembling embryonal carcinoma of the adult testis. Cancer 38:2420–2433

Mixed Germ Cell

154. Gershenson DM, Del Junco G, Copeland LJ, Rutledge FN (1984) Mixed germ cell tumors of the ovary. Obstet Gynecol 64:200–206
155. Kurman RJ, Norris HJ (1976) Malignant mixed germ cell tumors of the ovary. A clinical and pathologic analysis of 30 cases. Obstet Gynecol 48:579–589

Sex Cord-Stromal Tumors

11

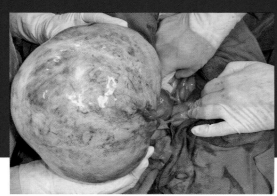

Contents

11.1 Introduction

It comprises neoplasms that contain cells of the follicular wall (granulosa cells, theca cells, and their luteinized derivates), as well as fibroblasts of stromal origin, singly or in various combinations and in varying degrees of differentiation [1, 2]. More rarely, these tumors arise from Leydig cells mainly located in the hilus of the ovary. Uncommonly, tumors can contain Sertoli cells, (which are not present in the normal ovary) isolated or less exceptionally associated with other cells types mentioned above.

Most sex cord-stromal tumors are composed of ovarian cell types (granulosa-stromal cell tumor). Very uncommonly, Sertoli-stromal cell tumors contain only cells of testicular type. Exceptionally cells of both gonads coexist (gynandroblastomas).

11.2 Embryology

11.2.1 The Indifferent Gonad

A mesodermal origin: on the medial aspect of the urogenital ridge, proliferation of cells of the coelomic epithelium and the underlying mesenchyme gives rise to the gonadal ridge. Soon fingerlike epithelial cords called primary sex cords grow into the underlying mesenchyme.

An endodermal origin: primordial germ cells originate in the wall of the yolk sac near the origin of the allantois. They migrate along the dorsal mesentery of the hindgut to the gonadal ridges into the underlying mesenchyme and become incorporated in the primary sex cords.

11.2.2 Development of Testes

In the presence of a gene called the SRY (the sex-determining region Y), the indifferent gonad differentiates in an anatomically distinct testis by day 44.

The prominent sex cords loose their connections with the coelomic epithelium because of the development of the tunica albuginea. They develop into seminiferous tubules which extend into the medulla, and their ends anastomose to form the rete testis. The walls of seminiferous tubules are composed of cells of Sertoli derived from the coelomic epithelium and spermatogonia derived from the primordial germ cells. They are separated by the mesenchyme which gives rise to the interstitial cells of Leydig.

11.2.3 Development of Ovaries

The primary sex cords do not become prominent, but they extend into the medulla and form a rudimentary rete ovarii in the hilus of the ovary.

Secondary sex cords extend from the coelomic epithelium into the underlying mesenchyme. Primitive germ cells are incorporated into them. At about 16 weeks, the cortical cords begin to break up into isolated cell clusters called primordial follicles, which consist of an oogonium derived from a primordial germ cell, surrounded by a single layer of pregranulosa cells derived from the cortical cords. The mesenchyme surrounding the follicles forms the ovarian stroma.

11.3 Definitions

11.3.1 Sex Cords

- In the developing testis by the fifth week of the embryonic life, the sex cords are formed by slender columns of primitive Sertoli cells.
- In the developing ovary by the twelfth week of the embryonic life, there are not real sex cords but instead packets of small pregranulosa cells enveloping germ cells.
- For that reason, the term "sex cord-stromal tumors" has been considered inappropriate. However, this term which has been adopted by the WHO has the advantage of acknowledging the presence in these neoplasms of derivates of either or both the sex cords.

11.3.2 Cells That Are Present in the Normal Ovary

11.3.2.1 Stroma

It is composed of stromal cells separated by a dense reticulin network and a variable amount of collagen.

11.3.2.2 Stromal Cells

Spindle-shaped stromal cells which resemble fibroblasts:
- Luteinized stromal cells
- Enzymatically stromal cells
- Decidual cells
- Endometrial stromal cells
- Smooth muscle cells
- Fat cells
- Stromal Leydig cells

11.3.2.3 Granulosa Cells

Theca Cells

Theca cells differentiate continuously from the stromal cells at the periphery of developing follicles from fetal life to the termination of the menopause.
- Theca interna: well-defined layer of the antral follicle outside the granulose. It contains abundant reticulin.
- Theca externa: ill-defined layer surrounding the theca interna and merging imperceptibly with the adjacent ovarian stroma
- Hilus cells: ovarian hilus cells are morphologically identical to testicular Leydig cells except for having a female chromatin pattern.

11.3.3 Cells Which Are Present in the Normal Testis and Which Can Be Present in Ovarian Tumors

- Sertoli cells: supporting epithelial cells of the seminiferous tubules
- Leydig cells: in the interstitial spaces between the tubules. In the ovary, ovarian hilus cells (hilar Leydig cells) are morphologically identical to testicular Leydig cells.

11.4 Frequency (Fig. 11.1)

This category accounts for approximately 8 % of all primary ovarian tumors [3].

Tumors in the thecoma-fibroma group represent roughly 87 % of these tumors, granulosa cell tumors 12 %, steroid cell tumors 1 %, Sertoli-Leydig cell tumors 0.05 %, and others 0.05 % [1].

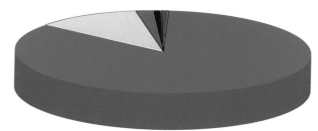

■ 87,0%: Thecoma-fibroma
□ 12,0%: Granulosa cell tumors
■ 1,00%: Steroid cell tumors
■ 0,05%: Sertoli-Leydig cell tumors
■ 0,05%: Others

Fig. 11.1 Repartition of sex cord and stromal tumors of the ovary

11.5 Biology of the Normal Ovary

See Chap. 3.

11.6 Classification and General Features

The World Health Organization (WHO) histological classification is reported in Table 11.1 [3].

A simplified classification is reported in Table 11.2.

Their clinical and biological characteristics are summarized in Table 11.3.

Table 11.1 WHO histological classification of sex cord-stroma cell tumors

1. Granulosa-stromal cell tumors
   1.1. Granulosa cell tumor
       1.1.1. Adult
       1.1.2. Juvenile
   1.2. Tumors in thecoma-fibroma group
       1.2.1. Thecoma
           – Typical
           – Luteinized
       1.2.2. Fibroma
       1.2.3. Cellular fibroma
       1.2.4. Fibrosarcoma
       1.2.5. Stromal tumor with mixed sex cord elements
       1.2.6. Sclerosing stromal tumor
       1.2.7. Unclassified
       1.2.8. Others
2. Sertoli-stromal cell tumors: androblastomas
   2.1. Well differentiated
       2.1.1. Sertoli cell tumor (tubular androblastoma)
       2.1.2. Sertoli-Leydig cell tumor
       2.1.3. Leydig cell tumor
   2.2. Sertoli-Leydig cell tumor of intermediate differentiation
       2.2.1. Variant-with heterologous elements (specific type)
   2.3. Sertoli-Leydig cell tumor, poorly differentiated (sarcomatoid)
       2.3.1. Variant-with heterologous elements (specific type)
   2.4. Retiform
       2.4.1. Variant-with heterologous elements (specific type)
3. Sex cord tumor with annular tubules (SCTAT)
4. Gynandroblastoma
5. Unclassified
6. Steroid (lipid) cell tumors
   6.1. Stromal luteoma
   6.2. Leydig cell tumor
       6.2.1. Hilus cell tumor
       6.2.2. Leydig cell tumor, non-hilar type

Table 11.2 Simplified classification of sex cord-stromal cell tumors

1. Tumors in the thecoma-fibroma group
   1.1. Thecoma (B), fibroma (B), fibrothecoma (B)
   1.2. Sclerosing stromal tumor (B)
   1.3. Cellular fibroma
   1.4. Fibrosarcoma (M)
2. Granulosa cell tumor (Bo)
3. Sertoli-Leydig cell tumors (M)
4. Sex cord Tumor with annular tubules (M)
5. Steroid (lipid) cell tumors
   Leydig cell tumor (B)
   Luteoma
   Not otherwise specified
6. Gynandroblastoma (M)

B benign, *Bo* borderline, *M* malignant

Table 11.3 Clinical and biological characteristics

Normal precursor cell	Tumor	Biology	Age
Stroma cells	Fibroma	NF	PM
Internal theca cells	Thecoma	O, a (rare)	M
Granulosa	Granulosa cell tumors	O, a (rare)	M
	Sertoli-Leydig cell tumors	NF (50 %)	Y
		A (1/3), o (rare)	
	Gynandroblastoma	A, O	
	SCTAT	A, O	
Stroma cells	Stromal luteoma	O (60 %), a (rare)	M
Hilar cells	Leydig cell tumors	A (75 %), o (rare)	M
	Nonclassified sex cord tumor	A (50 %), o (rare)	PM

SCTAT sex cord tumor with annular tubules, *A* androgen secretion most common, *a* androgen secretion uncommon, *O* estrogen secretion most common, *o* estrogen secretion uncommon, *NF* nonfunctioning, *Y* young, *M* menopause, *PM* perimenopause

11.7 Radiologic Findings

11.7.1 Tumors in the Thecoma-Fibroma Group

11.7.1.1 Fibromas-Fibrothecomas

Thecomas and fibromas form a spectrum of benign tumors extending from thecomas in which the tumor is mainly composed of cells containing abundant cytoplasm with large amounts of lipid to fibromas composed entirely or almost entirely of spindle cells producing variable amounts of collagen. Both populations of cells can be mixed in the same tumor. According to the predominant cell component at pathology, the tumor is designated as a thecoma, a fibroma, or a fibrothecoma. Because of the overlap between them, some authors use the designation of fibrothecomas [3].

In fibromas, the average patient age is 48 years; in thecomas, 84 % are postmenopausal; in both types, 10 % are under 30 years of age [4, 5].

Fibroma is usually nonfunctional; it is exceptionally associated with steroid hormone production. It is usually discovered during a routine ultrasound examination.

Thecomas are usually estrogenic; 60 % of the postmenopausal women present with uterine bleeding [4]. In luteinized thecomas, half of them are estrogenic, 39 % are nonfunctioning, and 11 % are androgenic [6].

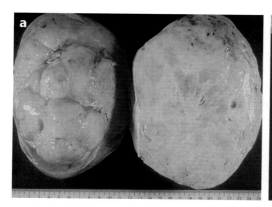

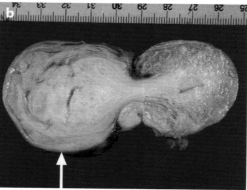

Fig. 11.2 (**a**) **Section of an ovarian fibroma.**
(**b**) Section of a subserous pedunculated leiomyoma (*arrow*)

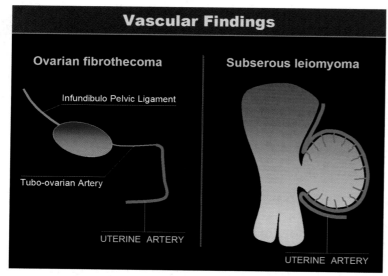

Fig. 11.3 Vascularization of ovarian fibrothecoma versus vascularization of subserous leiomyoma. Vascularization of a fibrothecoma is produced by the ovarian artery and the tubo-ovarian artery of the uterine artery which are of small caliber so that vascularization is poor and mainly central. On the opposite, vascularization of a subserous leiomyoma is produced by the marginal segment of the uterine artery and its branches (the arcuate arteries and the perforating arteries) with a characteristic peripheral vascularization more or less associated with a central vascularization

Macroscopy

Thecomas and fibromas are unilateral in 97 % [3] and in 92 % [5], respectively; they range in size from small to large solid masses; most are 5–10 cm in diameter.

In fibromas, sectioning typically reveals hard, flat, chalky white surfaces, resembling a uterine leiomyoma (Fig. 11.2). In thecomas, sectioning typically discloses a solid yellow mass, but in some cases, the tumor is white with only focal tinges of yellow.

In both tumors, areas of edema, occasionally with cyst formation are present. Hemorrhage is occasionally seen. Focal or diffuse calcifications are observed in fewer than 10 % of cases in fibromas [3]. Foci of calcification may be present in thecomas; extensive calcified thecomas tend to occur in young women [7].

Vascular Findings

While the macroscopic aspect of ovarian fibrothecoma and uterine subserous leiomyoma and their degenerative changes can look very similar, their vascular findings are quite different (Fig. 11.3).

Imaging Modalities

The main findings are summarized in Table 11.4.

Table 11.4 Radiologic findings in fibroma-fibrothecomas

Small fibrothecoma (<5 cm)
Ultrasound
2D: similar to subserous leiomyoma
– Smooth or lobulated contour
– Echogenicity close to myometrium
Characteristic sound attenuation without calcification related to **fibrous** tissue
Doppler findings: different from subserous leiomyoma
Fibrothecoma:
– **Very rare tiny vessels**; can be perpendicular to the wall
– Absence of peripheral vessels like in a subserous leiomyoma
– Vascularization can be absent; in this case differential diagnosis with a cystic echogenic mass
Subserous leiomyoma:
– **Characteristic circumscribed peripheral vessels**
CT/MR
CT without injection
Density close to myometrium, noncharacteristic; cannot be visible especially when small
MR on T2
Characteristic **hypointense signal**
DCT, DMR
– Without injection: density on CT and signal on T1 close to myometrium
– Arterial phase: **absence or slight regular vessel**
– Venous phase: **slight or absence of contrast uptake**
– Delayed phase: slight contrast uptake
Differential diagnosis
Brenner tumor
– Identical morphologic and vascular findings
– Psammoma like calcifications
– Association with another tumor: mucinous cystadenoma
Nonneoplastic ovarian processes
(a) Massive edema
(b) Fibromatosis: encompasses follicles and their derivates
(c) Stromal hyperplasia: bilateral, nodular, or diffuse
Large fibrothecoma (≥5 cm)
Radiologic findings
Degenerative changes identical to subserous leiomyoma
– Edema
– Cystic changes
– Calcification
– Hemorrhage
Morphologic changes related to fibrous tissue +++
Differential diagnosis
Subserous leiomyoma
– **Circumscribed peripheral vascularization** (+++) more or less associated with central vascularization
Carcinoma
Morphologic findings
– Can be identical
DCT or DMR
– Arterial phase: **tumoral vessels are central**, can be peripheral but never circumscribed as in subserous leiomyoma
– Venous phase: high contrast uptake, quite different from fibrothecoma but can be identical to subserous leiomyoma

Typical Form Without or with Few Degenerative Changes

Ultrasound

On TAS, the mass is echogenic with or without acoustic shadowing (Fig. 11.4).

On EVS (Figs. 11.5 and 11.6), the mass has a relatively homogeneous echogenicity slightly inferior or equal to myometrium with a very particular ultrasonic finding, a large area or multiple areas of acoustic shadowing in the absence of any hyperechogenic focus related to calcification [8–12]. Such a pattern on US is well displayed on in vivo and in vitro study (Fig. 11.6) and is typical of fibrous tissue (Table 11.4). It can be observed in other diagnosis (Table 11.5) mainly and subserous leiomyomas and Brenner tumors [10].

For subserous leiomyoma, visualization of the normal ipsilateral ovary separated from the mass can make the differential diagnosis, while presence of follicles around the mass can exclude this diagnosis.

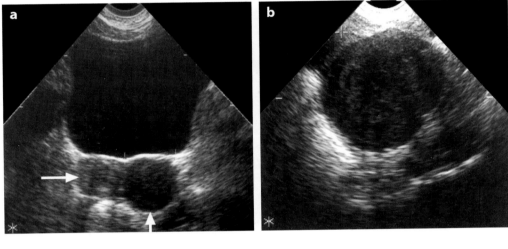

Fig. 11.4 Fibroma: typical form on ultrasound.
(**a**) Left ovarian mass (*vertical arrow*) with an echogenicity lower than myometrium (*horizontal arrow*) without acoustic shadowing on TAS. (**b**) Areas of acoustic shadowing are displayed on EVS

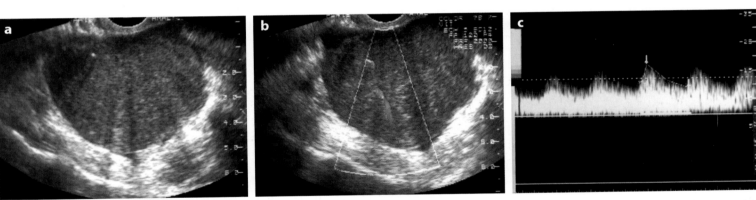

Fig. 11.5 Fibrothecoma: typical aspect on US and color doppler. Seventy-four years old woman with right ovarian mass discovered at a routine gynecologic examination. (**a**) US: 4.8 cm right ovarian mass, with an echogenicity close to myometrium containing multiple acoustic shadowings without hyperechogenic foci (except for one) very likely related to fibrous tissue. (**b**) Color Doppler displays very few vessels in the mass without any peripheral vascularization, which is very suggestive of ovarian fibroma. (**c**) Spectral Doppler: the resistivity index is of 0.50, which is of no help in the diagnosis. At pathology a fibrothecoma was confirmed

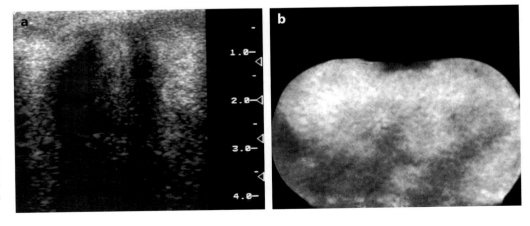

Fig. 11.6 In vitro imaging of fibrothecoma.
(**a**) In vitro ultrasound shows multiple acoustic shadowing without any hyperechogenic focus suggestive of calcification. (**b**) In vitro CT confirms the absence of calcification

Table 11.5 Ultrasound attenuation in the differential diagnosis of adnexal tumors

Structure	Histology	US attenuation
Normal ovary		
Normal ovarian stroma	– Spindle-shaped stromal cells that resemble fibroblasts – Dense reticulum network – A variable amount of collagen which is most abundant in the superficial cortex	Absent
Nonneoplastic ovarian lesions		
PCOD	The superficial cortex is fibrotic and hypocellular	Absent
Fibromatosis	Proliferation of collagen-producing spindle cells	Present
Stromal hyperplasia	Proliferation of ovarian stromal cells	Absent
Ovarian tumors		
Epithelial tumors		
Cystadenofibroma	The stroma can resemble normal ovarian stroma but is generally more fibrous	Absent
Brenner tumor	Stroma varies from closely resembling ovarian cortical stroma to densely fibrous	Present
Sex cord-stromal tumors		
Fibroma	Intersecting bundles of spindle cells and production of abundant dense collagen	Present
Sclerosing stromal tumor	Nodules spindle cells with sclerosis (fibers) separated by densely collagen or edematous tissue	Present
Sertoli-Leydig	Nodular architecture with fibrous bands separating nodules	Present
Metastases		
Carcinoid metastases	– Extensive stromal proliferation that closely resembles an ovarian fibroma – Occasionally the stroma is extensively hyalinized	Present
Krukenberg	– Cellular ovarian stroma – Occasionally, the stroma has a storiform pattern – In large masses, abundant collagen formation, marked stromal edema	Present
Non-ovarian masses		
Leiomyoma	– Whorled anastomosing fascicles of spindle cells (smooth muscle cells) – Hyaline fibrosis in 60 % of cases	Present

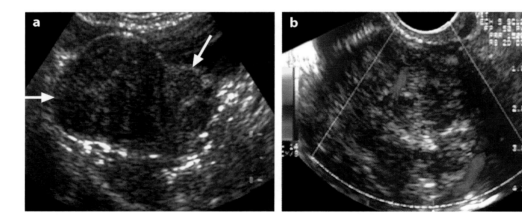

Fig. 11.7 Uterine subserous leiomyoma: ultrasound features. (**a**) TAS shows an echogenic mass (*horizontal arrow*) containing multiple acoustic shadowing, on the right side of the uterus (*oblique arrow*). (**b**) EVS with Doppler demonstrates a peripheral vascularization typical of a uterine subserous leiomyoma

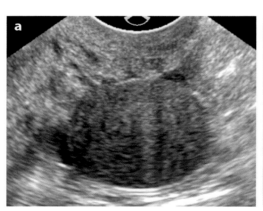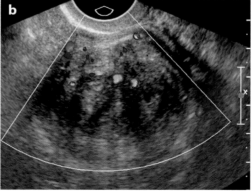

Fig. 11.8 Subserous leiomyoma: ultrasound pattern. (**a**) Round echogenic mass against the posterior wall of the isthmus of the uterus, containing multiple acoustic shadowing without any calcification, very suggestive of fibrous tissue. As the ipsilateral ovary was not visualized, differential diagnosis between a subserous leiomyoma and an ovarian fibroma could not be made. (**b**) On color Doppler, a typical peripheral vascularization, with some central vessels, allowed to make the diagnosis of a subserous leiomyoma. At coelioscopy, this diagnosis was confirmed

Color Doppler allows in most cases to distinguish ovarian fibroma and Brenner tumor from subserous leiomyoma. In ovarian fibromas, the vascularization is very poor, made of small, sparse vessels in the center of the mass (Fig. 11.5), sometimes at the periphery, while a peripheral ring vascularization is typical for a subserous leiomyoma (Figs. 11.7 and 11.8) and is not observed in ovarian fibroma [11]. However, this finding can be observed in the uncommon sclerosing stromal tumor (see later on) and cellular fibroma.

MR and CT Findings
On MR (Fig. 11.9)

On T2W images, the tumors are predominantly of low signal intensity (like pelvic muscle, lower than normal ovarian tissue) [13, 14] so that even when the tumor is small, it can be easily detected. This low signal is very suggestive of the presence of fibrous tissue. This low signal can be homogeneous particularly in case of small tumor [14].

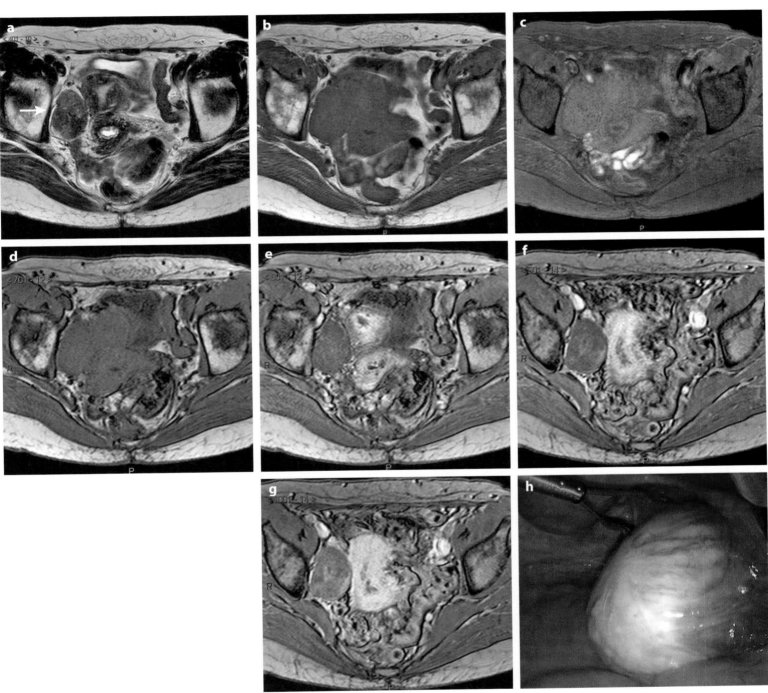

Fig. 11.9 Typical fibrothecoma at MR. Sixty-six years old woman with hormonal replacement and metrorrhagia. A right ovarian mass is discovered on US. MR axial T2 (**a**), axial T1 (**b**), axial T1 fat suppression (**c**), DMR without injection (**d**), at the arterial phase (**e**), at the venous phase (**f**), and on the delayed phase (**g**). On T2 (**a**), the right ovarian mass (*arrow*) appears with overall low signal intensity very suggestive of fibrous tissue. On T1 and T1 fat suppression, the mass is of low signal intensity. On DMR, at the arterial phase, no tumoral vessel is visualized; a slight contrast uptake is displayed at the venous phase, which slightly increases on the delayed phase remaining very low typical for benign fibrous tissue. Preoperative diagnosis: the low signal on T2 and this type of contrast enhancement are typical for fibrothecoma. At surgery (**h**), a tumor suggestive of fibrothecoma was removed. Pathology: histology confirmed the diagnosis of fibrothecoma

OnT1W images, the signal intensity is low, close to pelvic muscles [14].

On DWI (Fig. 11.10), the tumor appears with low signal intensity.

On CT without contrast, the mass has a density equal or slightly inferior to the myometrium [8] (Fig. 11.11).

On DCT (Fig. 11.11) *and DMR* (Fig. 11.9)

At the arterial phase, no arterial vessel is visualized.

At the parenchymal, no contrast uptake is visualized.

On the delayed phase, a slight contrast uptake is displayed.

These findings: (1) absence of arterial vessel at the arterial phase, (2) absence of early contrast uptake, and (3) delayed contrast uptake are typical for a benign convective tissue. They are really different from the malignant tumors where irregular tumoral vessels can be observed at the arterial phase with an early intense contrast uptake. They are also very different from a uterine subserous leiomyoma (Fig. 11.12) [13–15] where multiple more or less regular vessels are present at the arterial phase at the periphery and in the center of the mass, with an intense contrast uptake at the parenchymal phase.

Demonstration of a pedicle to the uterus or of two normal ovaries excludes the diagnosis of an ovarian mass.

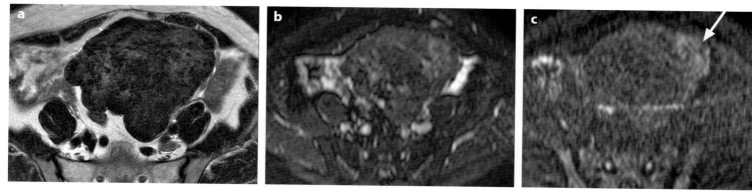

Fig. 11.10 Fibrothecoma on DWI. Sixty-six years old woman. Hormonal replacement for 10 years. Metrorrhagia related to hyperplasia of the endometrium on ultrasound. CA 125: 73 IU/ml. (**a**) MR axial T2 shows a large bosselated mass with overall low signal intensity. (**b, c**) DWI at b0 (**b**) and b1000 (**c**) shows overall low signal intensity in the mass except for some areas of slighter higher intensity related to slight degenerative changes, the most prominent one on the left (*arrow* in **c**). These areas are also slightly hyperintense on the T2WI

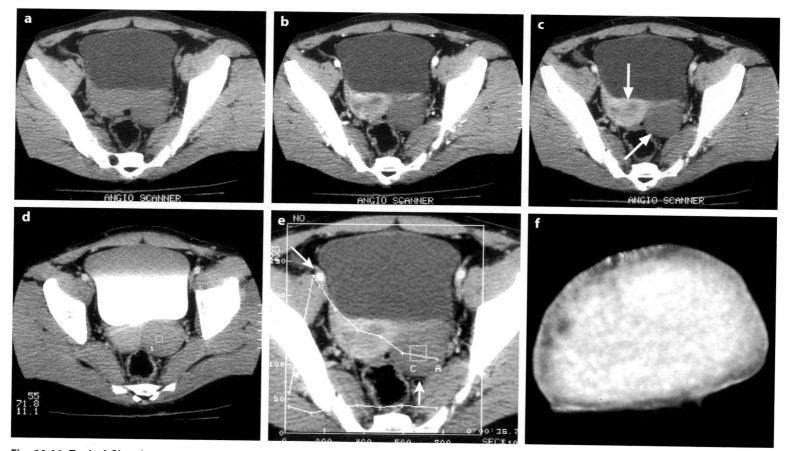

Fig. 11.11 Typical fibrothecoma on CT. (**a–d**) Dynamic CT scan without contrast (**a**), at the arterial phase (**b**), at the parenchymal phase (**c**), and delayed CT (**d**) shows low enhancement of the tumor (*oblique* in **c**) compared to myometrium (*vertical arrow* in **c**). (**e**). Time-intensity curves of the right external iliac artery and the mass show typical low enhancement of the ovarian tumor (*vertical arrow*) compared to the iliac artery (*oblique arrows*), typical for an ovarian fibroma. (**f**) In vitro CT displays a relatively homogeneous fibrous mass (Figures from Author's personal publication: Bazot et al. [8])

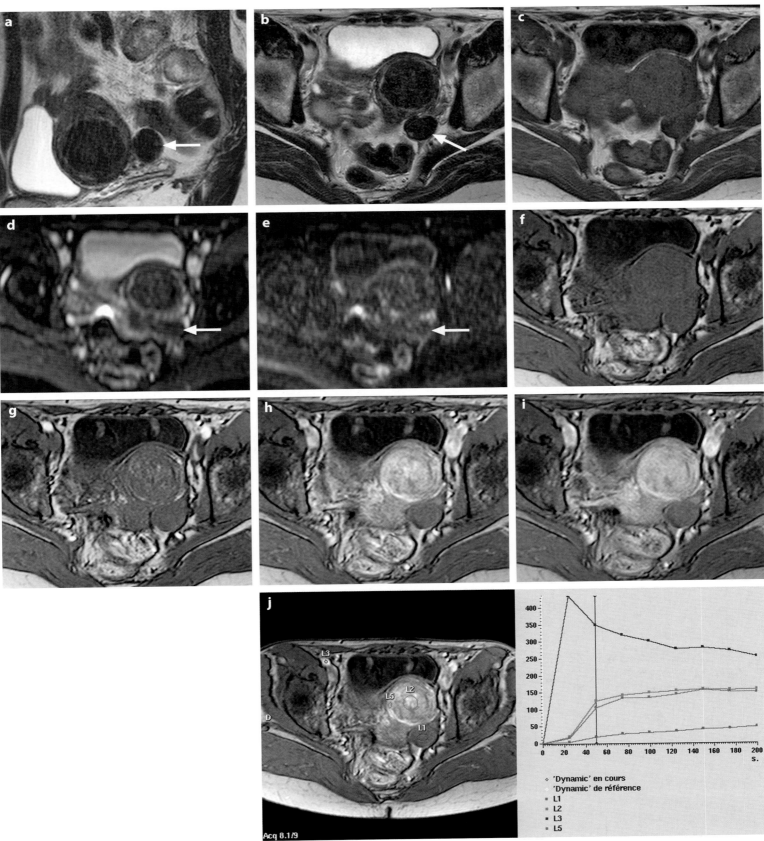

Fig. 11.12 Fibrothecoma without degenerative changes versus subserous leiomyoma. (**a, b**) Sagittal T2 (**a**) and axial T2 (**b**) display a left ovarian mass (*arrows*) with homogeneous low level intensity behind the uterus that contains a leiomyoma. (**c**) Axial T1: the ovarian mass has a low intensity identical to the subserous leiomyoma. (**d, e**) Diffusion b0 (**d**) and b1000 (**e**) show low intensity in both masses (ovarian tumor = *arrows*). (**f–i**) DMR without injection (**f**), at the arterial phase (**g**), at the venous phase (**h**) and on the delayed (**i**) displays: At the arterial phase, no vessel is displayed in the ovarian mass while peripheral and some central vessels are seen in the leiomyoma. At the venous phase, an absence of contrast uptake in the ovarian mass, a peripheral, and central contrast uptake in the leiomyoma. On the delayed a slight contrast uptake in the ovarian mass. (**j**) Time-intensity curves in the mass (*L1*), the center of the leiomyoma (*L2*), the periphery of the leiomyoma (*L5*), and the right external iliac artery (*L3*) show slow a low contrast uptake in the ovarian mass compared to the leiomyoma and the artery

Form with Degenerative Changes

The aspect of these tumors is variable, mainly because of the degenerative changes.

- Edema, Cystic Degeneration

On US, ill-defined anechoic spaces can be related to edema [6] (Fig. 11.13), while clearly anechoic delineated spaces can be related to cystic degeneration (Fig. 11.14) [16, 17].

On MR, distinction between both is easier. While both types of degeneration appear on MR with a high signal on T2 and on CT as low-density areas, after contrast injection, cystic spaces do not enhance while contrast diffuses progressively in edema areas (Figs. 11.13 and 11.14).

- Hemorrhage can be visualized on CT or MR (Fig. 11.15).
- Calcifications

On US, strong echoes can be present. They are usually better detected and characterized on CT and are hardly depicted on MR (Fig. 11.16) [8, 16]. However, when these calcifications are coarse, they can be detected on MR (Fig. 11.17).

- Myxoid degeneration (Fig. 11.18)

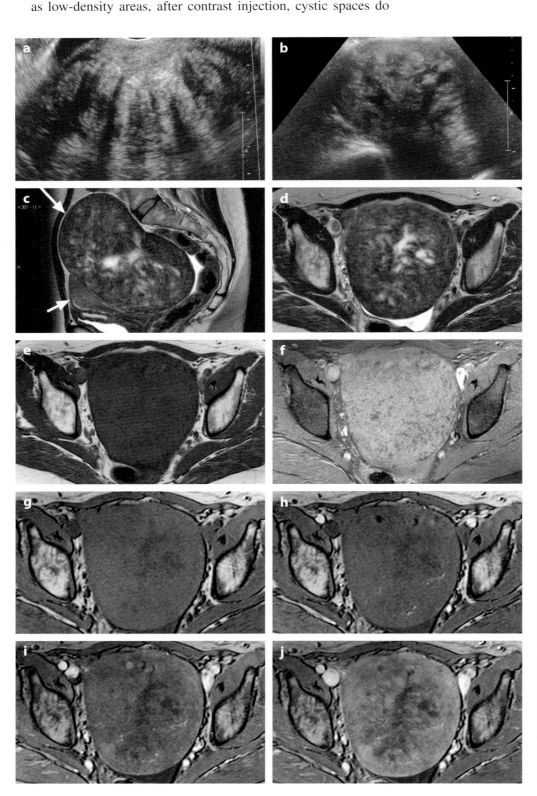

Fig. 11.13 Fibrothecoma with edematous and cystic changes. Fifty-seven years old woman without hormonal replacement. Pollakiuria. CA 125 normal. (**a**) EVS demonstrates an ovarian mass with a pattern very suggestive of an ovarian fibroma. (**b**) TAS displays well-delineated anechoic structures related to edema or cystic changes. (**c**, **d**) On sagittal (**c**) and axial (**d**) T2WI, the mass (*long arrow* in **c**) contains areas of high signal intensity and is posterior to the uterus (*short arrow* in **c**). (**e**, **f**) Axial T1 (**e**) and T1 fat suppression (**f**) show absence of hemorrhage. (**g**–**j**) DMR before injection (**g**), at the arterial phase (**h**), venous (**i**) and parenchymal phase (**j**) show the areas of edema to fill slowly with contrast medium, while no contrast enhancement can be seen in the cystic changes

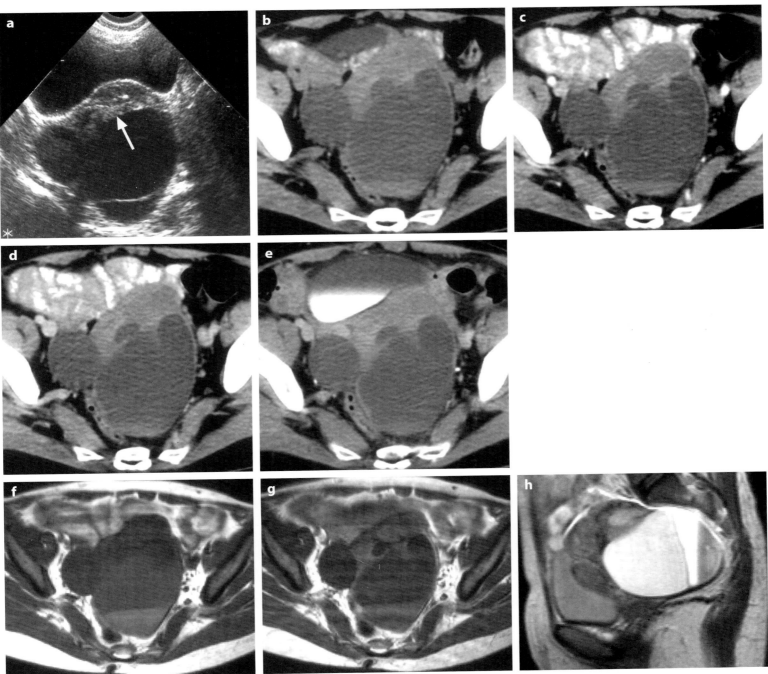

Fig. 11.14 Fibrothecoma of the ovary with cystic degeneration. The mass is mainly cystic multilocular with a tissular potion, very unusual presentation for a fibrothecoma. Sixty-three years old woman with pelvic mass at physical examination. (**a**) TAS: bilateral or biloculated mainly cystic ovarian mass: a small echogenic portion (*arrow*) is visualized anteriorly. No definite diagnosis was suggested. (**b–e**) Dynamic CT without contrast (**b**), at the arterial phase (**c**), at the parenchymal phase (**d**), and on the delayed CT (**e**). Absence of tumoral vessel in the tissular portion at the arterial phase rules out a carcinoma. A slight contrast uptake on the delayed CT (**e**) highly suggests the presence of benign connective tissue. A preoperative diagnosis of benign tumor was established; a diagnosis of cystadenofibroma was suggested. (**f–h**) Axial MR T1W without (**f**) and after injection (**g**), and sagittal T2W images (**h**). Slight contrast uptake is visualized in the tissular portion (**g**). Two fluid-fluid levels with a high signal intensity band are visualized in the dependent portion of the mass. Because of the age of the patient, a total hysterectomy with bilateral adnexectomy was performed. At pathology, a left ovarian fibrothecoma with a multiloculated cystic component containing only clear fluid was diagnosed

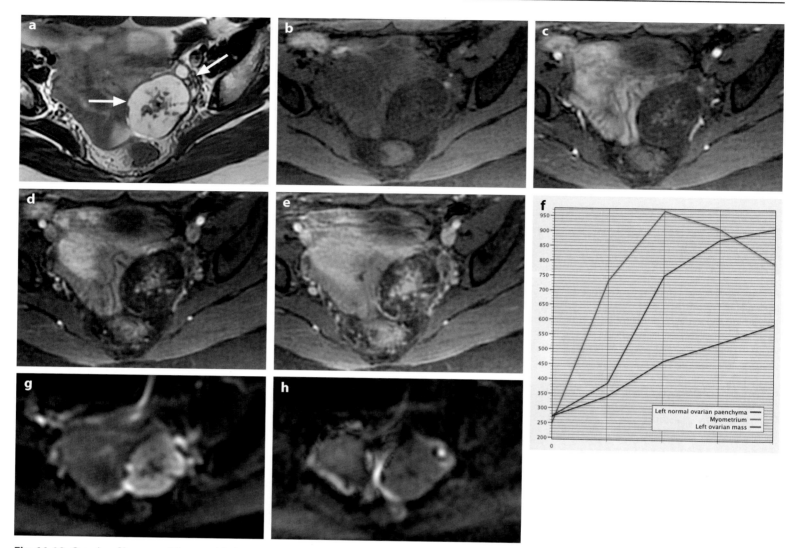

Fig. 11.18 Ovarian fibroma with myxoid changes and cellular areas in a 24 years old woman discovered during routine ultrasound examination. (a) T2W image shows a left ovarian mass (*horizontal arrow*) with a hypointense irregular cellular center and hyperintense periphery with myxoid changes. Normal ovarian left parenchyma is seen anterolaterally (*oblique arrow*). (b–f) Dynamic MRI before injection (b), at the arterial (c), venous (d), and late (e) phases, with corresponding time-intensity curves (f), shows rapid and high contrast uptake in the central portion, close to that of the myometrium and much higher than the normal ovarian parenchyma. Uptake in the other parts of the tumor was absent or low. The left ovarian parenchyma contains also some hyperintense endometriotic spots. (g, h) Diffusion weighted images b0 (g) and b1000 (h) show low signal in the central solid hypervascularized portion with an ADC value of 1.82×10^{-3} mm^2/s. In the myxoid hyperintense portion on T2 and b0, the signal was low on b1000 with an ADC of 2.2×10^{-3} mm^2/s

Particular Patterns

A hyperechogenic aspect has been observed in a series in 3/22 cases [8].

Exceptionally:
- The fibroma is related to the ovary by a small pedicle (Fig. 11.19).
- The fibroma can be included in an ovarian cyst simulating an endocystic papillary projection of an epithelial ovarian tumor (Fig. 11.20).

Associated Findings: Ascites

Thirty percent of the tumors are associated with ascites. Isolated pelvic ascites which is not dependant but in contact with the mass [8, 14] is very particular to this type of benign tumor.

Differential Diagnosis

Unilateral
1. Subserous leiomyoma
2. Brenner tumor
3. Fibromatosis (80 % of cases are unilateral)
4. Carcinoma

Bilateral
5. Stromal hyperplasia: it is almost always bilateral
6. Metastases: mainly Carcinoid and Krukenberg (Table 11.5)

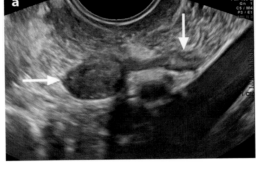
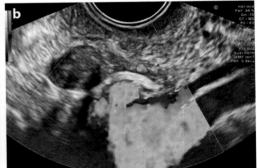

Fig. 11.19 Pedunculated ovarian fibroma. Menopausal woman without hormonal treatment; an ovarian mass is discovered during a routine examination. (**a**) EVS displays an 8 mm in diameter echogenic adnexal mass (*horizontal arrow*) with acoustic shadowing suggestive of a fibrothecoma. It is related to the left ovary (*vertical arrow*) by a narrow band. (**b**) Color Doppler displays a vascularization in the narrow band suggesting the diagnosis of a pedunculated ovarian fibroma. Pathology confirmed this diagnosis

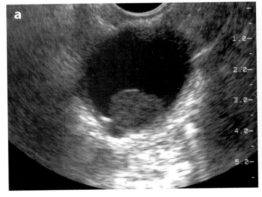
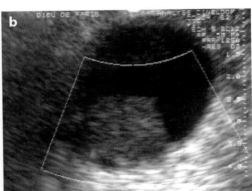

Fig. 11.20 Fibrothecoma of the ovary: unusual aspect in a cyst. (**a, b**) TVS (**a**) and color Doppler (**b**) demonstrate an echogenic round 2 cm mass without acoustic shadowing with a tiny vessel at the periphery, within a cyst. A papillary projection in an epithelial ovarian cyst was suggested. At pathology: a small ovarian fibroma was present in an inclusion cyst

Complications

- *Common*: *Torsion*

  Torsion in this type of tumor is not uncommon (Fig. 11.21) [18].

- *Uncommon*: *Demons-Meigs Syndrome* (Figs. 11.22 and 11.23)

  This syndrome complicates 1–3 % of ovarian fibromas [19]. In 1954, after its initial report, Meigs [20] redefined the syndrome that bears his name as an association of an ovarian fibroma or a predominantly fibrous tumor (including thecoma, granulosa cell tumor, and Brenner tumor) with ascites and pleural effusion (most often unilateral right-sided), with disappearance of the ascitic fluid and effusion(s) after removal of the ovarian tumor [20, 21].

The ascites has been ascribed to the irritation of the peritoneum by the hard tumor mass [20]. The pleural effusion is thought to develop secondary to lymphatic flow across the diaphragm.

On CT, an ovarian cellular fibroma associated with ascites and a right pleural effusion has been reported [22]. Although malignancy is statistically more likely when ascites and pleural effusion are associated with an ovarian tumor, the accumulation of fluid may also been the result of a Meigs syndrome or other benign process.

CA 125 can be increased as in the case reported by Massoni [23]. This syndrome must be distinguished from the pseudo-Meigs' syndrome in which the features of the syndrome are associated with a primary or a secondary ovarian cancer and in which the fluid has not been shown to contain malignant cells [6].

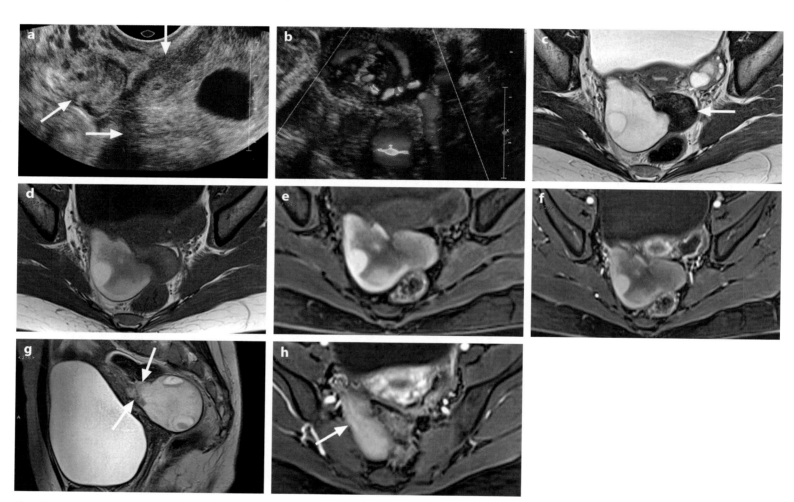

Fig. 11.21 Fibrothecoma complicated with torsion. Thirty-six years old woman with acute pelvic pain, increased leucocytes, increased sedimentation rate and at CRP 73 mg/l. (**a**) EVS displays an echogenic right ovarian mass (*horizontal arrow*) suggestive of an ovarian fibroma or Brenner tumor, containing a cystic portion. The ovarian parenchyma (*vertical arrow*) looks hypoechoic surrounding follicle structures containing echogenic material. A vascular thick pedicle running laterally is seen (*oblique arrow*). (**b**) Color Doppler displays tortuous vessels in the pedicle. Torsion is suspected and an MR performed. (**c–f**) MR axial T2WI (**c**), T1WI (**d**), and T1WI-FS before (**e**) and after injection (**f**). On T2WI, the ovarian mass comprises two components. A hypointense medial component (*arrow*) that was related to fibrous tissue complicated with necrosis at pathology. A lateral solid component that is hyperintense (related to edema) and that contains a cystic portion. On T1 and T1 fat suppression, hyperintense hemorrhage is seen at the periphery of the mass, in the cyst, and in some central areas. After injection, nonobvious contrast uptake is detected. (**g, h**) Sagittal T2 (**g**) and axial T1FS after injection (**h**) demonstrate a thickened hyperintense vascularized pedicle (*arrows*). At surgery, torsion of the ovary around the lombo-ovarian ligament with four turns, without tubal torsion, was found. A right ovariectomy was performed. At pathology, a tumor of the fibrothecal group comprising a cystic and a solid component complicated with necrosis and hemorrhage was diagnosed

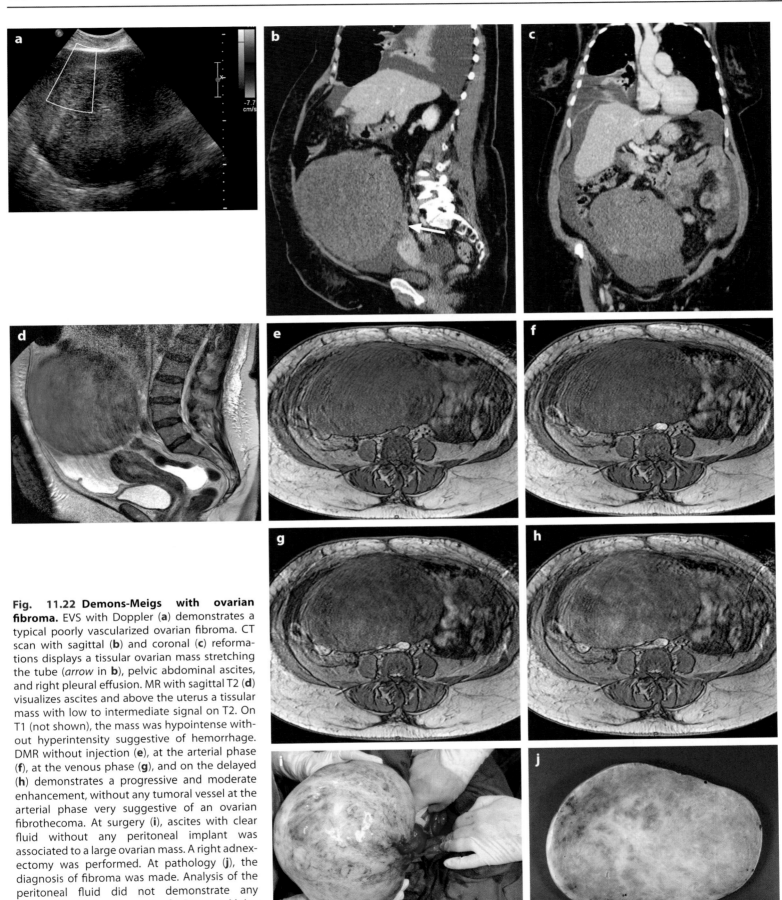

Fig. 11.22 Demons-Meigs with ovarian fibroma. EVS with Doppler (**a**) demonstrates a typical poorly vascularized ovarian fibroma. CT scan with sagittal (**b**) and coronal (**c**) reformations displays a tissular ovarian mass stretching the tube (*arrow* in **b**), pelvic abdominal ascites, and right pleural effusion. MR with sagittal T2 (**d**) visualizes ascites and above the uterus a tissular mass with low to intermediate signal on T2. On T1 (not shown), the mass was hypointense without hyperintensity suggestive of hemorrhage. DMR without injection (**e**), at the arterial phase (**f**), at the venous phase (**g**), and on the delayed (**h**) demonstrates a progressive and moderate enhancement, without any tumoral vessel at the arterial phase very suggestive of an ovarian fibrothecoma. At surgery (**i**), ascites with clear fluid without any peritoneal implant was associated to a large ovarian mass. A right adnexectomy was performed. At pathology (**j**), the diagnosis of fibroma was made. Analysis of the peritoneal fluid did not demonstrate any abnormal cell. The diagnosis of a Demons-Meigs syndrome complicating an ovarian fibroma was retained

The Solid or Mainly Solid Form

The tumor can be mainly solid (Fig. 11.36) or entirely solid (Fig. 11.37) [52, 54].

On US, the mass can be homogenously isoechoic or slightly hypoechoic to the uterus.

On DCT and DMR, a vascularization of endocrine type is displayed with at the arterial phase, regular vessels, and contrast uptake. This contrast uptake is higher than myometrium at the arterial phase but can become less on the following phases (Fig. 11.36) or entirely solid (Fig. 11.37). No significant washout is observed.

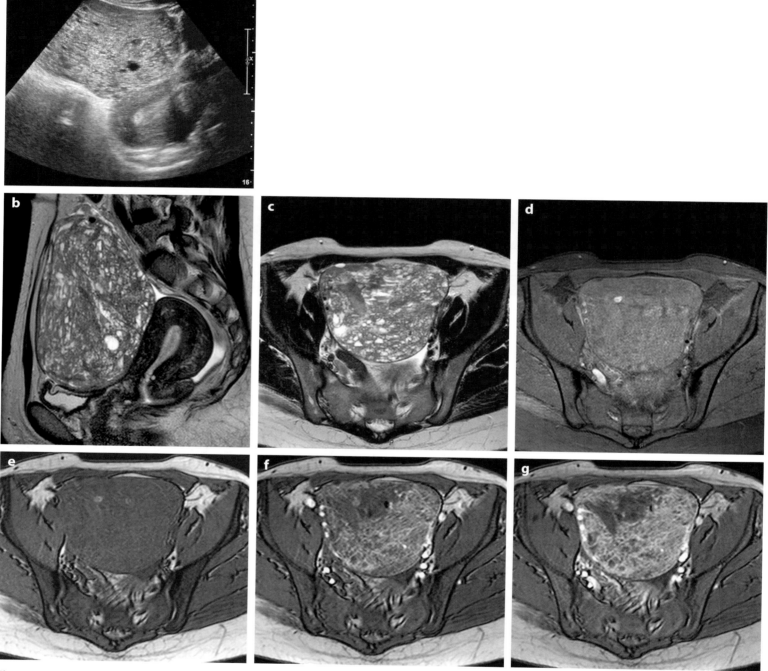

Fig. 11.36 Granulosa cell tumor. (a) TAS displays a mainly solid mass with some cystic spaces. The endometrium is thickened. (b–d) MR sagittal T2 (b), axial T2 (c), and axial T1 with fat suppression (d) show a large mainly solid mass with some cystic spaces and some small hemorrhagic components hyperintense on T1 and T1FS. (e–i) DMR without injection (e), at the arterial phase (f), at the venous phase (g),

The Cystic Mass

The mass can be entirely multicystic [55] resembling a mucinous cystadenoma.

On rare occasions, the mass can be unilocular and cystic mimicking a cystadenoma [55].

Particular Form: Granulosa Cell Tumor

It is a very rare pattern (Fig. 11.38).

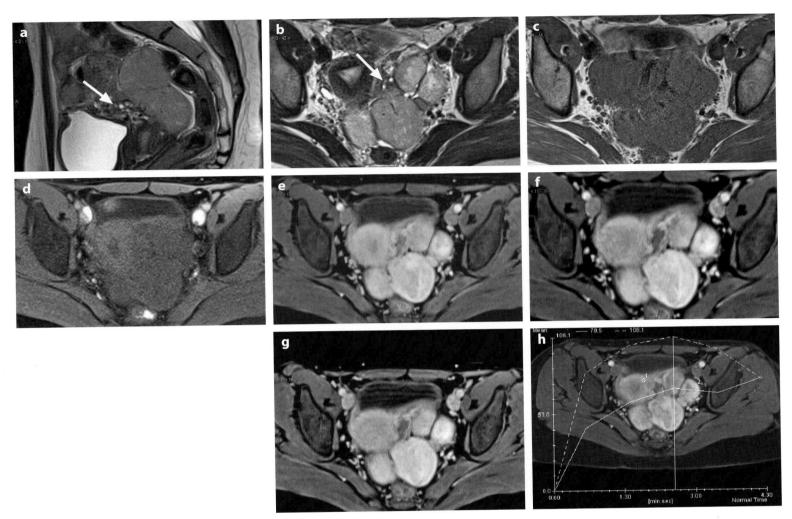

Fig. 11.38 Surface granulosa cell tumor: very unusual pattern. (**a–c**) MR sagittal T2 (**a**), axial T2 (**b**), and axial T1(**c**) display a multilobulated left and middle pelvic mass arising from the left ovary (*arrow* in **a**, **b**) and extending outside the ovary, of intermediate signal on both sequences. (**d–g**) DMR without injection (**d**) at the arterial phase (**e**) allows to precise that this mass is mainly solid and displays within the solid tissue regular vessels associated with a high contrast uptake in the peripheral part of the masses, while the contrast uptake diffuses in the central part on the following sequences (**f**, **g**). (**h**) Time-intensity curve: Peak of contrast enhancement in the tumor is at 2 min after injection. The tumor (ROI 1) enhances more than the myometrium (ROI 2)

The Uterus

Endometrial hyperplasia (related to the estrogen-producing tumor). Thickening of the endometrium sometimes containing small cysts can be depicted (Fig. 11.31).

An endometrial polyp can be observed (Fig. 11.33).

Associated Findings

Peritumoral fluid or a small amount of ascites can be present [52].

A peritumoral hematoma can be rarely discovered [52].

Complication

Rare cases of rupture have been reported with hemoperitoneum [56] (Fig. 11.39).

Laboratory Test

Inhibin in the plasma is significantly increased.

Epithelial tumoral makers CA 125 and CA199 are negative.

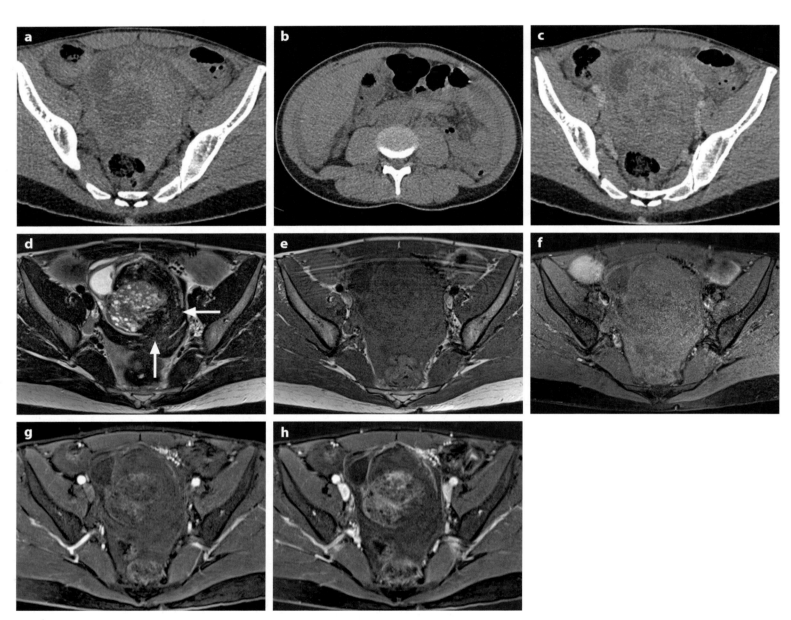

Fig. 11.39 Rupture granulosa cell tumor. CT scan without contrast of the pelvis (**a**) and of the right subhepatic space (**b**) demonstrates a pelvic mass with a high suspicion of hemorrhage and hemoperitoneum. After injection (**c**), the left border of the mass is ill defined. MR axial T2 (**d**) displays a solid mass containing multiple follicle-like spaces very suggestive of a granulosa cell tumor; the left and posterior part of the mass is ruptured (*arrows*). On T1 (**e**) and T1 fat suppression (**f**), the overall same signal intensity of the mass and of the peritoneal fluid suggests the possibility of hemorrhage. DMR at the arterial phase (**g**) makes the diagnosis of a tumor of endocrine type and of rupture that is confirmed at the venous phase (**h**)

Differential Diagnosis

1. Mixed cystic and solid form
   – Carcinoma
2. Multilocular and unilocular (see Table 11.5)

Spread and Recurrence

1. Granulosa cell tumors have a malignant potential with a capacity to extend beyond the ovary. Unlike epithelial carcinomas, 78–91 % of tumors are stage 1 [45, 46, 57, 58] at presentation; most of the remainder are stage 2. The pathway to metastatic spread appears to be similar to that seen in epithelial carcinomas [59]. CT scan is the more appropriate method at the time of presentation to define the extent of the disease.

2. Recurrence can occur late, even decades after resection [46]. CT is a good modality to evaluate the staging of the relapses and the disease progression. Recurrences occur commonly in the pelvis. Lomboaortic and pelvic lymph nodes, and peritoneal extension can be displayed (Figs. 11.40 and 11.41).

3. Metastases
   Hepatic metastases occur in 5–6 % of cases.
   Metastases can be observed on the surface of the spleen (Fig. 11.42). Spleen metastases can be depicted [60]. Exceptionally, these locations can lead to splenic rupture [61].
   The pattern of these metastases can closely recall the aspect of the original tumor.

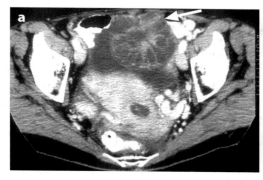
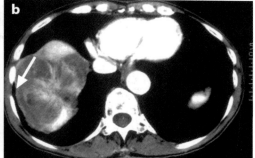

Fig. 11.40 Recurrent granulosa cell tumor (same patient as Fig. 11.33). CT scan 2 years after surgery for granulosa cell tumor recurrence is displayed in the pelvis (*arrow* in **a**) and the right subphrenic space (*arrow* in **b**). It is striking to notice how the pattern of the recurrent mass is very similar to the primary tumor (see Fig. 11.33)

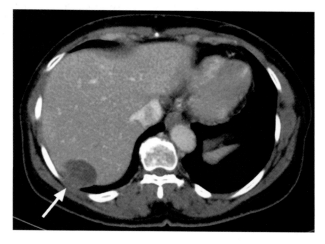

Fig. 11.41 Granulosa cell tumor: recurrence in the subhepatic space. Granulosa cell tumor of the left ovary operated 10 years before with total hysterectomy and bilateral adnexectomy. CT scan discovers a nodule (*arrow*) in the right subphrenic space. Biopsy confirms the diagnosis of recurrence of the granulose cell tumor

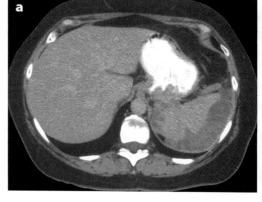
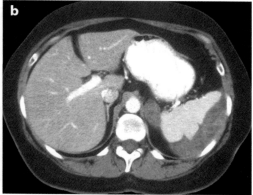

Fig. 11.42 Granulosa cell tumor: recurence on the surface of the spleen. (**a**, **b**). CT scan before (**a**) and after contrast (**b**): peritoneal left subphrenic mass encasing the spleen and creating a scalloping of its surface. The mass is multiloculated and has a pattern which reminds the initial tumor

11.7.3 Androgen-Secreting Tumors

11.7.3.1 Sertoli-Leydig Cell Tumor

Definition

This group comprises the rare Sertoli cell tumor and the more common Sertoli-Leydig cell tumors.

Sertoli Cell Tumor

This tumor is characterized by hollow or solid tubules separated by a stroma that contains only rare or no Leydig cells [62].

The tumors form typically lobulated solid yellow or brown masses.

They may be seen at any age with an average of 30 years. They are usually nonfunctioning.

Sertoli-Leydig Cell Tumor

These tumors are composed of Sertoli cells and cells of stromal derivation, including Leydig cells. There may be a prominent component of cells resembling rete epithelial cells growing in patterns similar to those of the rete testis.

General Features

These tumors account for less than 0.5 % of all ovarian tumors [63].

Seventy-five percent of the patients are 30 years of age or younger.

Sertoli-Leydig cell tumor is the most common virilizing tumor in premenopausal women [64]. However, 50 % of patients have no endocrine manifestations and complain of abdominal swelling or pain.

A hyperandrogenism occurs in about one-third of cases:

- Hirsutism
- Findings of virilization: acne temporal balding, deepening of the voice, atrophy of the breast, clitoromegaly
- During the reproductive age years oligomenorrhea followed by amenorrhea
- In the plasma, the testosterone is markedly increased. The androstenedione can be elevated. In contrast with virilizing adrenal tumors, the urinary 17-ketosteroids are normal.

Occasional tumors have been associated with estrogenic manifestations.

Rare associations with sarcoma botryoides of the cervix and thyroid disease have been reported [65].

Twenty percent of these tumors are associated with elevated serum levels of alpha-fetoprotein [66], but values as high as those accompanying yolk sac tumors are rare [67].

Microscopic Findings

1. *Well-differentiated* forms have a predominant tubular pattern [68]. On low-power examination, fibrous bands are conspicuous, separating lobules composed of hollow or less often solid tubules and Leydig cells. The tubules contain cells with moderate to large amounts of cytoplasm that may be dense or vacuolated and lipid-rich. The stromal component consists of bands of mature fibrous tissue in which variable but usually conspicuous numbers of Leydig cells are present.

2. *Poorly differentiated* forms either lack the lobulation or orderly arrangement of cells with a high mitotic rate. Intermediate forms can be observed.

3. *Retiform component* are present in 15 % of tumors. Microscopic examination shows a network of irregularity branching tubules and cysts into which polypoid structures or papillae may project.

4. *Heterologous components* occur in approximately 20 % of cases. Most commonly, glands and cysts lined by moderately to well-differentiated gastric-type or intestinal-type mucinous epithelium are seen [69, 70]. Stromal heterologous elements encountered in 5 % of cases [71] include islands of cartilage arising on a sarcomatous background, embryonal rhabdomyosarcoma, or both .

Gross Findings

Over 98 % are unilateral. The tumors are stage 1a in 80 % of cases. Rupture or involvement of the external surface occurs in 12 % of cases.

They are often solid, lobulated yellow masses.

Poorly differentiated tumors including those with the heterologous elements tend to be larger and contain areas of hemorrhage and necrosis more frequently.

Tumors with a large heterologous mucinous component may be mistaken for a mucinous tumor.

Tumors with a retiform component are mainly cystic. The cysts may contain numerous papillae and polypoid excrescences that vary from small to large and edematous, simulating serous papillary cystic tumors or a hydatidiform mole [72].

Imaging Findings

1. When the mass is mainly solid, US can display a well-defined hypoechoic mass [30]. The mass can be isoechoic and can be overlooked on conventional US. The mass can detected on color Doppler which can display vessels appearing to arc around a spherical mass. Spectral Doppler showed resistive indices from 0.39 to 0.51

   CT shows an enhancing solid mass. At MR, their signal intensity on T2W images reflects their extent of fibrous stroma.

2. A minority can be indistinguishable from granulosa cell tumors [30].

3. Solid masses with well-demarcated cystic lesions have been reported [73] (Figs. 11.43 and 11.44). This pattern is very similar to that observed in most of the Krukenberg tumors [73]. This aspect has also been reported in granulosa cell tumor, bilateral endometrioid carcinoma, and dysgerminoma.

11.7.4 Sex Cord Tumors with Annular Tubules (SCTAT)

This tumor is characterized by simple and complex ring-tubules, often exhibiting focal differentiation into typical Sertoli cell tumor, granulosa cell tumor, or both [74] (Fig. 11.45).

Doppler

Doppler ultrasound combined with the morphologic findings seems fundamental to delineate the tumor in displaying a peripheral vascularization of the mass, sometimes with a curvilinear aspect more or less associated with a central vascularization (Figs. 11.46 and 11.47).

This hypervascularization may be confused with that of the hormonally active corpus luteum; correlation to the day of the menstrual cycle and to the clinical presentation is needed.

Doppler studies can demonstrate low-impedance flows with RI <0.40 [78].

MR

On T2W images, the mass has heterogeneous intermediate signal.

After injection, vascularization is of endocrine type (Figs. 11.47, 11.48, and 11.49)

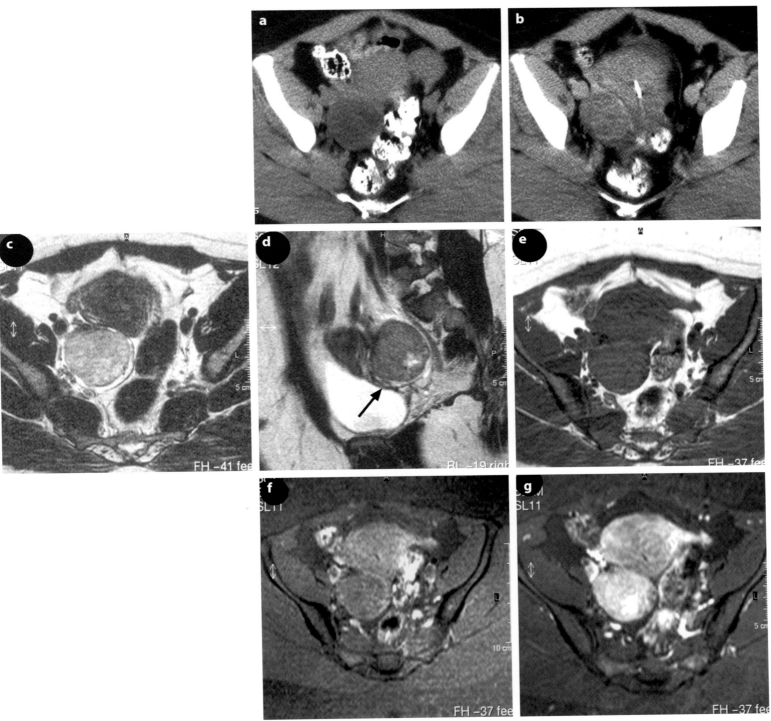

Fig. 11.48 Not otherwise specified steroid cell tumor. Obesity, hirsutism, testosterone ten times the upper normal level. (**a, b**) CT without (**a**) and after early IV contrast (**b**): 5.5 cm right ovarian mass, well limited, with an early intense relatively homogeneous contrast uptake. (**c, d**) MR axial (**c**) and sagittal (**d**) T2. The mass is well delineated from the normal (*arrow* in **d**) ovarian parenchyma. It has an intermediate signal, with some hyperintense foci. (**e**) MR axial T1. The mass has a homogeneous low signal close to myometrium. (**f, g**) MR axial T1 fat suppressed image without (**f**) and after IV injection (**g**). High contrast uptake in the ovarian mass like in the myometrium. At microscopy, a steroid cell tumor is diagnosed which did not contain any Reinke crystal. A non classified steroid cell tumor was finally diagnosed

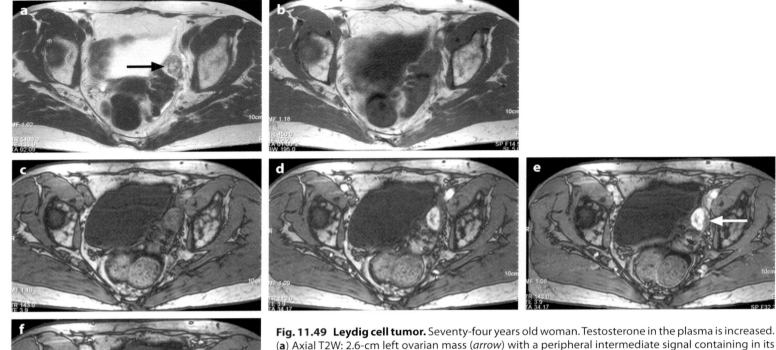

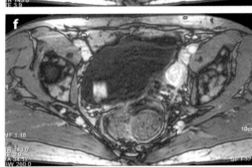

Fig. 11.49 Leydig cell tumor. Seventy-four years old woman. Testosterone in the plasma is increased. (**a**) Axial T2W: 2.6-cm left ovarian mass (*arrow*) with a peripheral intermediate signal containing in its center hyperintense areas. (**b**) Axial T1W images. The mass is hypointense. (**c–f**) Dynamic MR without contrast (**c**), at the arterial phase (**d**), at the venous phase (**e**), and on the delayed MR (**f**). At the arterial phase (**d**), no tumoral vessel is displayed; a significant high contrast uptake is visualized at the periphery of the mass, which increases at the venous phase (**e**) and diffuses centripetally on the delayed MR (**f**). Differentiation from normal ovarian parenchyma (*arrow* in **e**) is best at the venous phase. The absence of tumoral vessel at the arterial phase and the early high contrast uptake without washout of contrast medium highly suggest the diagnosis of endocrine tumor. Association with a high level of testosterone in a woman at that age suggested the diagnosis of a Leydig cell tumor, which was confirmed at pathology

Abdominal Pelvic CT

Abdominal CT has the main interest to rule out an adrenal tumor. Otherwise, the tumor enhance as an endocrine tumor (Figs. 11.48 and 11.50).

Selective Venous Bilateral Ovarian and Adrenal Catheterization

It is used when imaging is negative in case of androgenic and estrogenic disorders to rule out an endocrine ovarian or adrenal tumor.

11.7.6 Gynandroblastoma

This tumor is characterized by the presence of clearly recognizable well-differentiated ovarian and testicular cells [79–81]. Each of these components should account for at least 10 % of a mixed tumor [82].

They usually occur in young women.

They may have androgenic or estrogenic manifestations.

Almost all are stage 1.

Imaging features have not been reported.

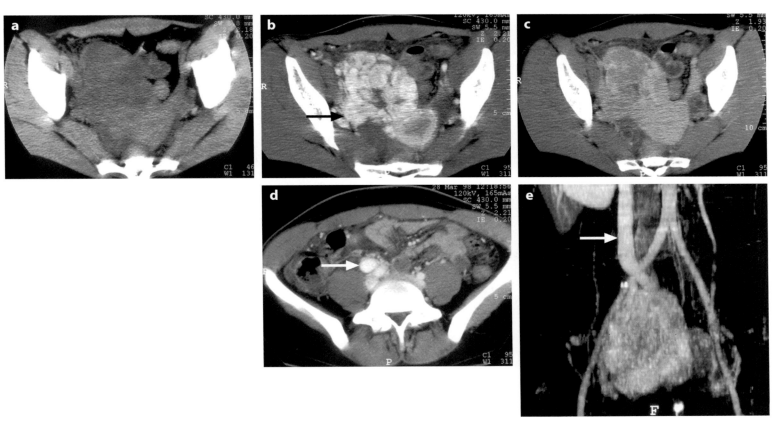

Fig. 11.50 Hilus cell tumor. Acute right lower quadrant pain suggesting appendicitis. No findings of hyperandrogenism. (**a–c**) Incremental dynamic CT scan without injection (**a**), at the arterial phase (**b**), and on the delayed CT (**c**). Right adnexal mass that seems to be developed in the hilus of the right ovary (*arrow* in **b** = right ovary). At the arterial phase, the tumor is highly vascularized (**b**). Contrast uptake is not as high on the delayed CT (**c**). (**d, e**) Axial CT (**d**) with MIP reformation (**e**) displays a huge right ovarian vein (*arrow* in **d, e**) draining the tumor. At surgery, a normal appendix is visualized. The right adnexal mass was in the hilus of the ovary. At pathology, a tumor arising from cortical adrenal rests or a Leydig cell tumor was diagnosed

References

1. Gee DC, Russel P (1981) The pathological assessment of ovarian neoplasms. IV. The sex cord stromal tumors. Pathology 13:235–255
2. Young RH, Scully RE (1994) Sex cord-stromal, steroid cell and other ovarian tumors with endocrine, paraendocrine and paraneoplastic manifestations. In: Kurman RJ (ed) Blaustein's pathology of the female genital tract, 4th edn. Springer, New York, pp 783–847
3. Scully RE, Young RH, Clement PB (1998) Tumors of the ovary, maldeveloped gonads, fallopian tube, and broad ligament, 3rd edn. Armed Force Institute of Pathology, Washington, DC, pp 169–188
4. Bjorkholm E, Silfversward C (1980) Theca-cell tumors. Clinical features and prognosis. Acta Radiol Oncol 19:241–244
5. Dockerty MB, Masson JC (1944) Ovarian fibromas: a clinical and pathologic study of two hundred and eighty-three cases. Am J Obstet Gynecol 47:741–752
6. Zhang J, Young RH, Arseneau J, Scully RE (1982) Ovarian stromal tumors containing lutein or Leydig cells (luteinized thecomas and stromal Leydig cell tumors). A clinicopathological analysis of fifty cases. Int J Gynecol Pathol 1:270–285
7. Young RH, Clement PB, Scully RE (1988) Calcified thecomas in young women. A report of four cases. Int J Gynecol Pathol 7:343–350
8. Bazot M, Ghossain MA, Buy JN et al (1993) Fibrothecomas of the ovary: CT and US findings. J Comput Assist Tomogr 17:754–759
9. Atri M, Nazarnia S, Bret PM, Aldis AE, Kintzen G, Reinhold CE (1994) Endovaginal sonographic appearance of benign ovarian masses. Radiographics 14:747–760
10. Stephenson WM, Laing FC (1985) Sonography of ovarian fibromas. AJR 144:1239–1240
11. Buy JN, Ghossain MA, Hugol D et al (1996) Characterization of adnexal masses: combination of color doppler and conventional sonography compared with spectral Doppler analysis alone and conventional sonography alone. AJR 166:385–393
12. Conte M, Guariglia L, Benedetti Panici P et al (1991) Ovarian fibrothecomas: sonographic and histologic findings. Gynecol Obstet Invest 32:51–54
13. Weinreb JC, Barkoff ND, Megibow A, Demopoulos R (1990) The value of MR imaging in distinguishing leiomyomas from other solid pelvic masses when sonography is indeterminate. AJR 154:295–299
14. Troiano RN, Lazzarini KM, Scoutt LM et al (1997) Fibroma and fibrothecoma of the ovary: MR imaging findings. Radiology 204:795–798
15. Scoutt L, Mc Carthy S, Lange R, Bourque A, Schwartz P (1994) MR evaluation of clinically suspected adnexal masses. J Comput Assist Tomogr 18:609–618
16. Athey PA, Malone RS (1987) Sonography of ovarian fibromas/thecomas. J Ultrasound Med 6:431–436
17. Chechia A, Koubaa A, Makhlouf T et al (2001) Ovarian fibrothecal tumors. A propos of 12 cases. Gynecol Obstet Fertil 29:349–353
18. Jones HW, Jones GS (eds) (1981) Novak's textbook of gynecology. Williams and Wilkins, Baltimore, pp 582–584
19. Droegemueller W, Herbst AL, Mishell DR, Stterchever MA (eds) (1987) Comprehensive gynecology. CV Mosby, St. Louis, pp 479–482
20. Meigs JV (1954) Fibromas of the ovary with ascites and hydrothorax-Meig's syndrome. Am J Obstet Gynecol 67:962–987
21. Meigs JV, Cass JW (1937) Fibroma of the ovary with ascites and hydrothorax: with a report of seven cases. Am J Obstet Gynecol 33:249–267
22. Bierman SM, Reuter KL, Hunter RE (1990) Meigs syndrome and ovarian fibroma: CT findings. J Comput Assist Tomog 14:833–834
23. Massoni F, Carbillon L, Azria E, Uzan M (2001) Demons-Meigs syndrome: a propos of one case. Gynecol Obstet Fertil 29:905–907
24. Laufer L, Barki Y, Mordechai Y, Maor E, Mares A (1996) Ovarian fibroma in a prepubertal girl. Pediatr Radiol 26:40–42
25. Tytle T, Rosin D (1984) Bilateral calcified ovarian fibromas. South Med J 77:1178–1180
26. Diakoumatis E, Vieux U, Seife B (1984) Sonographic demonstration of thecoma: report of two cases. Am J Obstet Gynecol 150:787–788
27. Yaghoobian J, Pinck RL (1983) Ultrasound findings in thecoma of the ovary. J Clin Ultrasound 11:91–93
28. Williams LL, Fleisher AC, Jones HW 3rd (1992) Transvaginal color Doppler sonography and CA-125 elevation in a patient with ovarian thecoma and ascites. Gynecol Oncol 46:115–118
29. Togashi K (1993) MRI of the female pelvis. Igaku-Shoin, Tokyo, pp 227–279
30. Outwater EK, Wagner BJ, Mannion C, McLarney JK, Kim B (1998) Sex cord-stromal and steroid cell tumors of the ovary. Radiographics 18:1523–1546
31. Takemori M, Nishimura R, Hasegawa K (2000) Ovarian thecoma with ascites and high serum levels of CA125. Arch Gynecol Obstet 264:42–44
32. Clement PB, Young RH, Hanna W, Scully RE (1994) Sclerosing peritonitis associated with luteinized thecomas of the ovary. A clinicopathological analysis of six cases. Am J Surg Pathol 18:1–13
33. Khan EM, Pandey R (1994) Sarcoma-like ovarian nodules associated with retractile mesenteritis and retroperitoneal fibrosis. Histopathology 24:276–278
34. Reginella RF, Sumkin JH (1996) Sclerosing peritonitis associated with luteinized thecomas. AJR 167:512–513
35. Chalvardjian A, Scully RE (1973) Sclerosing stromal tumors of the ovary. Cancer 31:664–670
36. Ihara N, Togashi K, Todo G et al (1999) Sclerosing stromal tumor of the ovary: MRI. J Comput Assist Tomogr 23:555–557
37. Joja I, Okuno K, Tsunoda M et al (2001) Sclerosing stromal tumor of the ovary: US, MR, and dynamic MR findings. J Comput Assist Tomogr 25:201–206
38. Kawauchi S, Tsuji T, Kaku T et al (1998) Sclerosing stromal tumor of the ovary: a clinicopathologic, immunohistochemical, ultrastructural, and cytogenetic analysis with special reference to its vasculature. Am J Surg Pathol 22:83–92
39. Tang MY, Liu TH (1982) Ovarian sclerosing stromal tumors. Clinicopathologic study of 10 cases. Clin Med J 95:186–190
40. Lee MS, Cho HC, Lee YH, Hong SR (2001) Ovarian sclerosing stromal tumors: gray scale and color Doppler sonographic findings. J Ultrasound Med 20:413–417
41. Torricelli P, Caruso Lombardi A, Boselli F, Rossi G (2002) Sclerosing stromal tumor of the ovary: US, CT, and MRI findings. Abdom Imaging 27:588–591
42. Matsubayashi R, Matsuo Y, Doi J, Kudo S, Matsuguchi K, Sugimori H (1999) Sclerosing stromal tumor of the ovary: radiologic findings. Eur Radiol 9:1335–1338
43. Prat J, Scully RE (1981) Cellular fibromas and fibrosarcomas of the ovary: a comparative clinico-pathologic analysis of seventeen cases. Cancer 47:2663–2670
44. Outwater EK, Seligman ES, Talerman A, Dunton C (1997) Ovarian fibromas and cystadenofibromas: MRI features of fibrous component. JMRI 7:465–471
45. Bjorkholm E (1980) Granulosa cell tumors: a comparison of survival in patients and matched controls. Am J Obstet Gynecol 138:329–331
46. Stenwig JT, Hazekamp JT, Beecham JB (1979) Granulosa cell tumors of the ovary. A clinicopathological study of 118 cases with long-term follow-up. Gynecol Oncol 7:135–152
47. Nakashima N, Young RH, Scully RE (1984) Androgenic granulosa cell tumors of the ovary. A clinicopathological analysis of seventeen cases and review of the literature. Arch Path Lab Med 108:786–791
48. Norris HJ, Taylor HB (1968) Prognosis of granulosa-theca tumors of the ovary. Cancer 21:255–263
49. Gusberg SB, Kardon P (1967) Proliferative endometrial response to theca-granulosa cell tumors. Am J Obstet Gynecol 111:633–643
50. Young RH, Dickersin GR, Scully RE (1984) Juvenile granulosa cell tumor of the ovary. A clinicopathologic analysis of 125 cases. Am J Surg Pathol 8:575–596
51. Zaloudek C, Norris HJ (1982) Granulosa tumors of the ovary in children. A clinical and pathological study of 32 cases. Am J Surg Pathol 6:503–512
52. Kim SH, Kim SH (2002) Granulosa cell tumor of the ovary: common findings and unusual appearances on CT and MR. J Comput Assist Tomogr 26:756–761
53. Sugimura K (1993) MRI diagnosis of the ovary (Japanese). In: Sugimura K (ed) MRI diagnosis of pelvis. Igaku-Shoin, Tokyo, pp 88–132
54. Jabra AA, Fishman EK, Taylor GA (1993) Primary ovarian tumors in the pediatric patient: CT evaluation. Clin Imaging 17:199–203
55. Ko SF, Wan YL, Ng SH, Lee TY, Lin JW, Chen WJ, Kung FT, Tsai CC (1999) Adult ovarian granulosa cell tumors: spectrum of sonographic and CT findings with pathologic correlation. AJR 172:1227–1233

56. Melemed A, Desouky S, Allen DB, Gilbert-Barness E (1993) Juvenile granulosa cell tumor. Am J Dis Child 147:209–210
57. Bjorkholm E, Pettersson F (1980) Granulosa-cell and theca cell tumors. The clinical picture and long term outcome for the Radiumhemmet series. Acta Obstet Gynecol Scand 59:361–365
58. Bjorkholm E, Silversward C (1981) Prognostic factors in granulosa cell tumors. Gynecol Oncol 11:261–274
59. Thorvinger B, Samuelsson S, Skyaerris J (1987) CT of malignant ovarian disease. Acta Radiol 28:739–742
60. Margolin KA, Pak HY, Esensten ML, Doroshow JH (1985) Hepatic metastases in granulosa cell tumor of the ovary. Cancer 56:691–695
61. Chew DKW, Schutzer RW, Domer G, Jaloudi MA, Rogers AM (2003) Splenic rupture from metastatic granulosa cell tumor 29 years after curative resection: case report and review of the literature. Am Surg 69: 106–108
62. Scully RE, Young RH, Clement PB (1998) Tumors of the ovary, maldeveloped gonads, fallopian tube, and broad ligament, 3rd edn. Armed Force Institute of Pathology, Washington, DC, pp 227–238
63. Novak ER, Long JH (1965) Arrhenoblastoma of the ovary. A review of the ovarian tumor registry. Am J Obstet Gynecol 92:1082–1093
64. Wong IL, Lobo RA (1996) Reproductive endocrinology, surgery, and technology, 1st edn. Lippincott-Raven, Philadelphia, pp 1571–1598
65. Young RH, Scully RE (1985) Ovarian sertoli-leydig cell tumors. A clinicopathological analysis of 207 cases. Am J Surg Pathol 9:543–569
66. Gagnon S, Tetu B, Silva EG, McCaughey WT (1989) Frequency of alpha-fetoprotein production by Sertoli-Leydig cell tumors of the ovary: an immunohistochemical study of eight cases. Mod Pathol 2:63–67
67. Young RH, Perez-Atayde AR, Scully RE (1984) Ovarian Sertoli-Leydig cell tumor with retiform and heterologous components. Report of a case with hepatocytic differentiation and elevated serum alpha-fetoprotein. Am J Surg Pathol 8:709–718
68. Young RH, Welch WR, Dickersin GR, Scully RE (1982) Ovarian sex cord tumor with annular tubules: review of 74 cases including 27 with Peutz-Jeghers syndrome and 4 with adenoma malignum of the cervix. Cancer 50:1384–1402
69. Aguirre P, Scully RE, Delellis RA (1986) Ovarian heterologous Sertoli-Leydig cell tumors with gastrointestinal-type epithelium. An immunohistochemical analysis. Arch Pathol Lab Med 110:528–533
70. Young RH, Prat J, Scully RE (1982) Ovarian Sertoli-Leydig cell tumors with heterologous elements. (i) Gastrointestinal epithelium and carcinoid: a clinicopathologic analysis of thirty-six cases. Cancer 50:2448–2456
71. Prat J, Young RH, Scully RE (1982) Ovarian Sertoli-Leydig cell tumors with heterologous elements. (ii) Cartilage and skeletal muscle: a clinicopathologic analysis of twelve cases. Cancer 50:2465–2475
72. Young RH, Scully RE (1983) Ovarian Sertoli-Leydig cell tumors with a retiform pattern: a problem in histopathologic diagnosis. A report of 25 cases. Am J Surg Pathol 77:755–771
73. Kim SH, Kim WH, Park KJ, Lee JK, Kim JS (1996) CT and MR findings of Krukenberg tumors: comparison with primary ovarian tumors. J Comput Assist Tomogr 20:393–398
74. Scully RE, Young RH, Clement PB (1998) Tumors of the ovary, maldeveloped gonads, fallopian tube and broad ligament, 3rd edn. Armed Force Institute of Pathology, Washington, DC, pp 189–202
75. McGowan L, Young RH, Scully RE (1980) Peutz-Jeghers syndrome with "adenoma malignum" of the cervix. A report of two cases. Gynecol Oncol 10:125–133
76. Srivatsa PJ, Keeney GL, Podratz KC (1994) Disseminated cervical adenoma malignum and bilateral ovarian sex cord tumors with annular tubules associated with Peutz-Jeghers syndrome. Gynecol Oncol 53:256–264
77. Cserepes E, Szücs N, Patkos P et al (2002) Ovarian steroid cell tumor and a contralateral ovarian thecoma in a postmenopausal woman with severe hyperandrogenism. Gynecol Endocrinol 16:213–216
78. Wang PH, Chao HT, Lee RC et al (1998) Steroid cell tumors of the ovary: clinical, ultrasonic, and MRI diagnosis—a case report. Eur J Radiol 26:269
79. Anderson MC, Rees DA (1975) Gynandroblastoma of the ovary. Br J Obstet Gynaecol 82:68–73
80. Chalvardjian A, Derzko C (1982) Gynandroblastoma: its ultrastructure. Cancer 50:710–721
81. Neubecker RD, Breen JL (1962) Gynandroblastoma. A report of five cases with a discussion of the histogenesis and classification of ovarian tumors. Am J Clin Pathol 38:60–69
82. Scully RE, Young RH, Clement PB (1998) Tumors of the ovary, maldeveloped gonads, fallopian tube, and broad ligament, 3rd edn. Armed Force Institute of Pathology, Washington, DC, pp 203–226
83. Deval B, Raffi A, Darai E, Hugol D, Buy JN (2003) Slerosing stromal tumor of the ovary. Ultasound Obstet Gynecol 22:531–534

Metastatic Tumors of the Ovary and Lymphomas

12

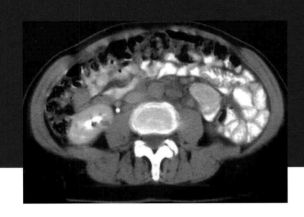

Contents

12.1 General Features

When an ovarian mass suspicious for malignancy is identified at an imaging examination, primary ovarian cancer is generally the main concern [1]. However, malignant tumors of the ovary are metastatic in 5–7% of cases [2]. While metastases are uncommon in daily practice, metastatic neoplasms may be misdiagnosed as primary ovarian neoplasms [3, 4], potentially leading to inappropriate management [1].

Breast cancer, colon cancer, gastric cancer, and lymphoma are the most frequent secondary neoplasms of the ovary [2, 5–7].

The average age of patients with ovarian involvement for each of the most common forms of cancer that spread to the ovary (intestinal, gastric, and mammary) is significantly lower than that of patients without ovarian spread, presumably because of the greater vascularity in younger women [8]. The non-ovarian primary neoplasm is often diagnosed before an ovarian mass is found [3, 6, 9–11]. Occasionally, a primary tumor may not be discovered until several years after removal of the metastatic ovarian tumor [8].

Metastases can be predominantly solid, solid-containing small cysts, or more rarely, multicystic. The solid component of the mass contains tumoral vessels. Although their pattern can resemble a primary ovarian, knowledge of the main etiologies, most commonly of a previous history of an extra-ovarian cancer, of the routes of dissemination, and of particular radiologic findings must draw the attention to the possibility of metastasis.

The main findings of ovarian metastases are summarized in Table 12.1.

J.N. Buy, M. Ghossain, *Gynecological Imaging*,
DOI 10.1007/978-3-642-31012-6_12, © Springer-Verlag Berlin Heidelberg 2013

Table 12.1 Main findings of ovarian metastases

1. Etiologies
  1. Breast
  2. Female genital tract
  3. GI tract
     Carcinoma of the stomach, most often Krukenberg tumor
     Intestinal carcinoma
     Tumors of the appendix
     Carcinoid tumors
     Pancreas, bile ducts, liver
  4. Renal, urinary tract (ureter, bladder, urethra) and adrenal tumors
  5. Melanoma
  6. Pulmonary and mediastinal tumors
  7. Extragenital sarcomas
  8. Ovarian involvement by peritoneal tumors
2. Most common previous history of one of these tumors
  More rarely discovering of ovarian and a malignant extra-ovarian tumor
  at the same time
3. Routes of dissemination
  Direct spread (uterus tube mesothelium)
  Through the lumen of the fallopian tube and onto the surface of the
  ovary
  From more distant sites via blood vessels and lymphatics
4. Bilateral topography in 2/3 to 3/4 of cases [12]
  While serous carcinomas and undifferentiated carcinomas are also
  bilateral in 2/3 of cases, primary mucinous and endometrioids are
  bilateral in 7% and in 13% of cases, respectively [13]
5. Morphologic characters
  Peripheral capsule with a regular lateral border
  Multiple nodules
  Location of the nodules on the surface of the ovary
  Presence of cysts which often are large and thin-walled despite the
  absence of cysts in the primary neoplasm
  Follicle-like spaces:
     Gastric, intestinal, appendix
     Small cell
     Malignant melanomas
6. Vascular findings
  Usual findings of malignancy
  A peripheral vascularization at the arterial phase with a significant
  contrast uptake at the venous phase (related to a capsule) when present is
  very suggestive
7. Very suggestive patterns
  Krukenberg tumor
  Cystic form of metastasis from intestinal carcinoma
  Melanoma (melanocytic type)

Table 12.2 Imaging findings of ovarian metastases from breast carcinoma

Common findings
Bilateral two-thirds of cases
Size <5 cm (85% of cases) [11]
Solid mass made up of nodules of different sizes [12]
Containing cysts (20%)
Surface:
  1. Nodular surface
  2. Smooth-surfaced or bosselated (when the ovary is replaced by tumor)
Usually accompanied by other intra-abdominal metastases [11]
Uncommon
Entirely cystic
Papillae on gross examination

Roughly 75% of ovarian metastases of breast cancer are of the ductal type.

Lobular carcinomas spread to the ovary more often than ductal carcinomas. However, because of the higher frequency of ductal carcinomas, metastases from ductal carcinomas are more common.

Rarely, ovarian metastases of breast carcinoma is a typical Krukenberg; in a series [7] about 1.8% of Krukenberg tumors were of breast origin.

Radiologic Findings are summarized in Table 12.2.

Imaging findings are illustrated on the following figures (Figs. 12.1, 12.2, and 12.3).

12.2.2 Female Genital Tract

12.2.2.1 Endometrial Carcinoma and Endometrial Stromal Sarcomas

Metastases of endometrial carcinoma to the ovary are present in 5–10% of hysterectomies.

Criteria of diagnosis [12]:
1. Extension of endometrial carcinoma deeply into the myometrium
2. Tumor present in the fallopian tube
3. Tumor on the ovarian surface

Metastases of endometrial stromal sarcomas are much more uncommon; metastases from leiomyosarcomas are even more exceptional.

12.2.2.2 Cervical Carcinoma

Ovarian metastases are rare. Ovarian metastasis of adenocarcinoma is a little higher than squamous carcinoma. In a series from the Armed Forces Institute of Pathology, 10% of mucinous adenocarcinomas of the cervix were reported to metastasize to the ovary.

A case of ovarian metastases from invasive verrucous carcinoma (a variant of squamous cell carcinoma) is illustrated (Fig. 12.4).

12.2 Metastatic Tumors

12.2.1 Breast

Usually, breast metastases are discovered in the follow up of breast cancer with a median interval of 11.5 months and are related to the stage of cancer [11].

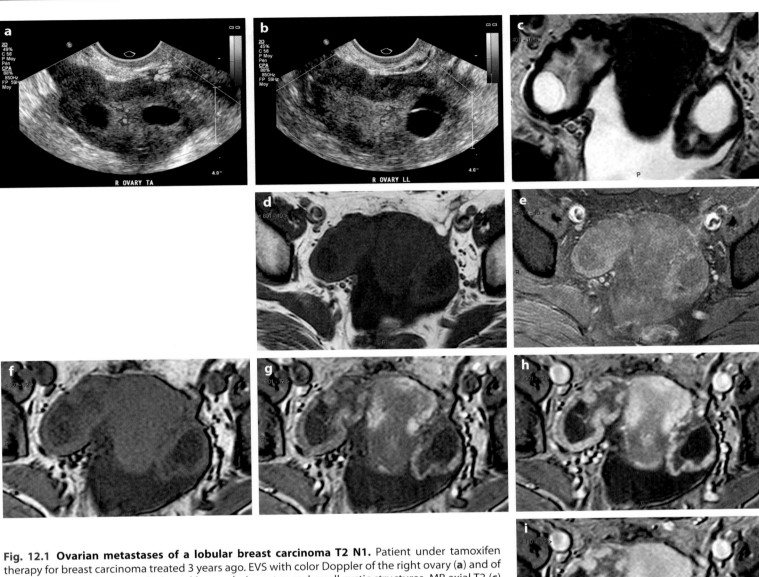

Fig. 12.1 Ovarian metastases of a lobular breast carcinoma T2 N1. Patient under tamoxifen therapy for breast carcinoma treated 3 years ago. EVS with color Doppler of the right ovary (**a**) and of the left ovary (**b**) displays a thickened hypoechoic cortex and small cystic structures. MR axial T2 (**c**) displays a bilateral ovarian mass with a lobulated contour and regular thickening of the cortex that appears with low signal intensity. On T1 (**d**) and T1 fat suppression (**e**), signal intensity is more marked in the cortex especially after fat suppression. DMR without injection (**f**), at the arterial phase (**g**), at the venous phase (**h**) and on the delayed (**i**) show more marked contrast uptake in the cortex. Surgery: Cerebriform ovaries; bilateral adnexectomy was performed. Pathology: (1) Thickening of the ovarian cortex with important fibrosis containing numerous tumoral cells. (2) In the center of the ovaries, the medulla is loose with some tumoral cells

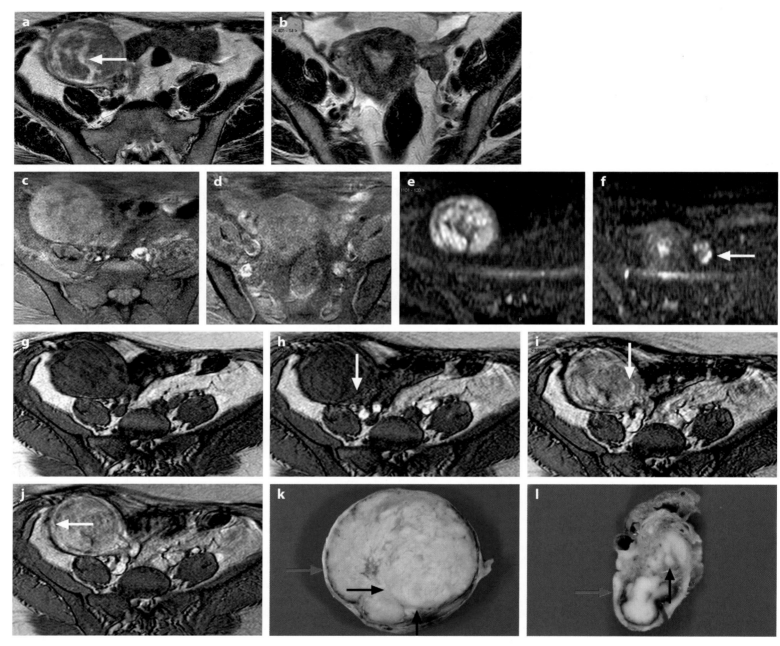

Fig. 12.2 Bilateral ovarian metastasis from breast carcinoma. A 58-year-old woman, 3-cm periareolar lobular invasive carcinoma of the left breast with extension to six axillary lymph nodes operated 4 years ago. Left mastectomy with axillary lymph node dissection, radiotherapy chemotherapy, Arimidex. Left pelvic pain and metrorrhagia for 3 months. CA15-3, CA125 normal. MR axial T2 of the right ovary (**a**) displays an ovarian mass with a thick peripheral rim corresponding to a capsule of intermediate signal with a well delineated regular lateral border and an irregular medial border, containing some edematous changes (*arrow*), and on the left ovary (**b**) a signal close to pelvic muscle. On axial fat suppression of the right ovary (**c**) and of the left ovary (**d**), the masses have an overall signal close to pelvic muscles. Diffusion b1000 of the right ovary (**e**) depicts an overall high signal related to a low ADC. In the left ovary (**f**) nodules of high signal are displayed on DWI (*arrow*), which were not visualized in the previous sequences, which highlights the importance of this sequence in the detection of these nodules. DMR of the right ovary without injection (**g**) at the arterial phase (**h**) displays arterial vessels at the periphery (*arrow*). At the venous phase (**i**), arterial vessels and contrast uptake draw the periphery of nodules like one of these (*arrow*) very suggestive of metastasis. On the delayed (**j**), a regular rim of contrast is visualized at the periphery of the ovary (*arrow*), which is not usually seen in an ovarian carcinoma. CT performed did not demonstrate any extra-ovarian extension. Surgery: bilateral adnexectomy with hysterectomy was performed. Absence of abdominal extension was confirmed. Macroscopic specimen of the right ovary (**k**) depicts (1) the presence of a thick capsule (*red arrow*) with a well defined lateral border of variable thickness and (2) separated nodules (*black arrows*). In the left ovary (**l**), a well defined capsule is also present (*red arrow*); white nodules are clearly seen (*black arrow*). Microscopy: bilateral metastasis of lobular breast carcinoma

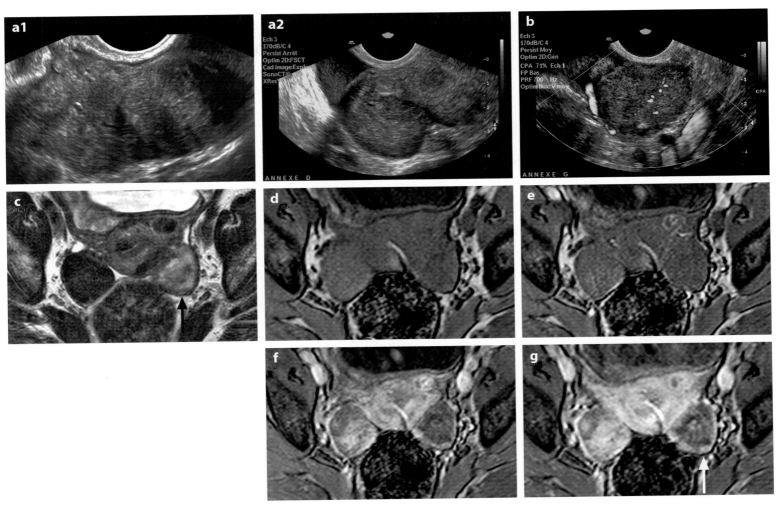

Fig. 12.3 Ovarian metastasis from a breast carcinoma. Association with a subserous leiomyoma; different types of vascularization. A 60-year-old woman, operated 14 years before from a lobular invasive carcinoma of the right breast, treated with tumorectomy, radiotherapy, and chemotherapy. Abdominal pain, CA15-3 increased, ascites. EVS sagittal (**a1**) through the right ovarian mass displays an upper relatively homogeneous echogenic portion (related to the metastasis) and a lower tissular portion with a strong attenuation related to a subserous leiomyoma. Transverse EVS through the right ovarian mass (**a2**) and through the left ovarian mass (**b**) depicts the same type of tumor on both sides. On axial T2 (**c**), (1) the left ovarian mass has an overall intermediate signal with a very particular thick peripheral rim of low signal intensity (*arrow*) corresponding to the capsule with an outer regular border and an inner irregular border, (2) the right subserous leiomyoma is of low signal intensity. DMR without injection (**d**) and at the arterial phase (**e**) depicts (1) in the left ovarian mass large vessels coming from the left ovarian artery with peripheral regular vessels (2) in the right leiomyoma regular peripheral vessel which are very similar. At the venous phase (**f**) (1) in the left ovarian mass, a high contrast uptake is visualized in the thickened wall (*arrow*) which is regular on its lateral border and irregular on its medial border; this finding is very particular to metastases; contrast uptake is much lower in the center. (2) in the right leiomyoma, a peripheral regular rim of contrast uptake associated with a high contrast uptake in the center of the tumor. These differences are even more pronounced on the delayed (**g**). At pathology: bilateral ovarian metastasis; right serous leiomyoma

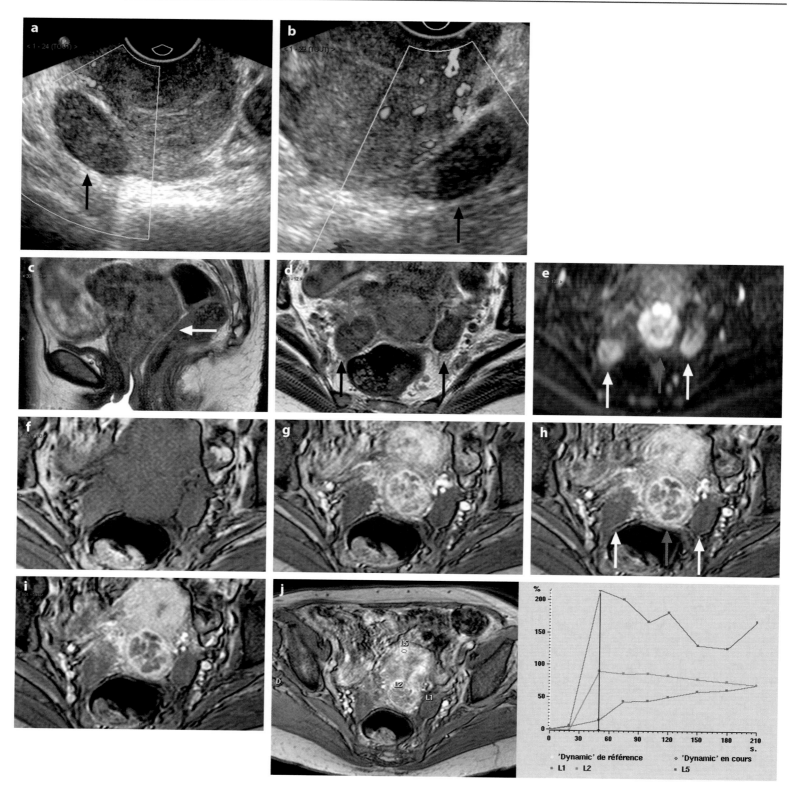

Fig. 12.4 Bilateral ovarian metastasis from carcinoma of the cervix and vagina. A seventy-eight-year-old woman with metrorrhagias. Biopsy of the cervix: well differentiated verucous carcinoma. Transverse EVS with color Doppler (**a, b**) displays (1) a cervical echogenic mass with color flow related to a cervix carcinoma, (2) a bilateral ovarian mass (*arrows*) with a homogeneous echostructure, containing some vessels. MR sagittal T2 (**c**) displays a mass of intermediate signal (*arrow*) involving the cervix and the vagina typical for a carcinoma. Axial T2 (**d**) depicts a bilateral enlarged ovary (*black arrows*) with an overall low signal close to the pelvic muscle, containing in

the right ovarian mass small nodules (*red arrow*). Diffusion using a b1000 sequence (**e**) shows a high signal intensity in the cervix (*red arrow*) while intensity in the ovarian masses (*white arrows*) is much lower. On DMR without injection (**f**) at the arterial phase (**g**), tiny vessels are visualized in the ovarian masses while an intense peripheral and central vascularization appears in the cervix; at the venous phase (**h**) and on the delayed (**i**), contrast uptake in the ovarian masses is low (*white arrows* in **h**), while there is a high contrast uptake in the cervix (*red arrow* in **h**) as it is illustrated on the curve (**j**). PET scan

Fig. 12.4 (*continued*) (**k**) shows a high signal intensity in the cervix with a maximum SUV of 8 units. Bilateral adnexectomy: ovarian metastasis of cervical carcinoma

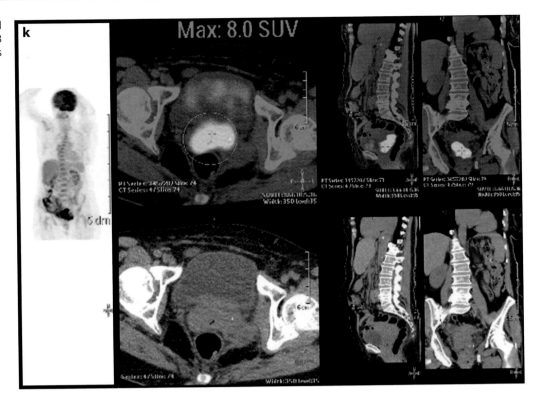

12.2.2.3 Tubal Carcinoma

The ovary is involved secondarily in 13% of tubal carcinomas usually by direct extension, sometimes via tubo-ovarian inflammatory adhesions, or by surface implantation on the ipsilateral or contralateral ovary.

Because most tubal carcinomas closely resemble serous, endometrioid or undifferentiated carcinomas of the ovary, microscopic examination often fails to establish whether a carcinoma involving both organs is primary in one or the other.

12.2.2.4 Vaginal Clear Cell Adenocarcinoma

In this case, there is an extensive pelvic spread.

12.2.2.5 Imaging Findings

No particular morphologic features about these different locations has been reported.

12.2.3 GI Tract

12.2.3.1 Carcinoma of the Stomach Including Krukenberg Tumors

Microscopic Definition [14]

Non-ovarian neoplasm in which:
1. Mucin-filled signet-ring cells account for at least 10% of the neoplasm.
2. Mucin-free epithelial cells, small glands with flattened lining cells and larger glands with flattened lining cells and larger glands of typical intestinal and mucinous type may be present.

3. A fibrous stroma ranging from densely cellular to edematous and extracellular mucin may be prominent.

Frequency

Most ovarian metastases of gastric origin are Krukenberg tumors [12].

Two-thirds of Krukenberg arise from the stomach. Carcinomas of appendix, colon, breast, small intestine, and rectum are then the most common primary tumors [14].

The average age of patients is about 45 years.

Macroscopic and radiologic findings are summarized in Table 12.3.

Microscopic Findings

Multiple nodules separated by normal stroma are seen in small neoplasm and focally in larger ones.

The tumor is often more cellular at the periphery and edematous or gelatinous centrally. It typically reveals mucin-laden, signet-ring cells strewn individually, in small clusters or in aggregates within a cellular ovarian stroma; occasionally, the stroma has a storiform pattern. Frequent variations include mucin-poor tumor cells, abundant collagen formation, and marked stromal edema. Occasionally, small or large cysts form a conspicuous component of the tumor [8].

Extracellular mucin is often conspicuous and, when associated with scant acellular stroma, gives a distinctive appearance referred to as feathery degeneration [14].

Lutein cells are occasionally present in the stroma, particularly if the patient is pregnant [8].

Radiologic Findings

Radiologic findings in US, CT, and MR are reported in Table 12.4.

Table 12.3 Common macroscopic and radiologic findings of Krukenberg tumors

1. Bilateral (80%) usually asymmetrically enlarged [8]
   Involvement of smaller ovary can only be found at microscopic examination [6]
2. Round or reniform [8]
3. Capsular surface smooth, nodular, or bosselated [14] free of peritoneal deposits [15]
4. Typically solid with often ill defined nodules [14]
   Fibrous or edematous gelatinous with focal or diffuse hemorrhage or necrosis
   Containing thin-walled cysts (1/3) filled with mucinous hemorrhage or watery fluid
   Multicystic rarely
5. Blood vessels occasionally striking in the neoplasm [14]
6. Ascites (43%) [14]

Table 12.4 Radiologic findings of Krukenberg tumors

1. US
   Hyperechoic solid pattern (related to intra- and extracellular mucin)
2. MR and CT
   1. Solid component
      On T2: hypointense fibrous periphery:
      After injection: moderate or strong enhancement different from fibrothecoma or Brenner tumor
   2. Mucinous material
      On T2: hyperintense
   3. Cystic component
      After injection: strong enhancement of the cyst wall

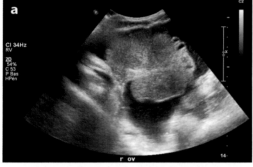
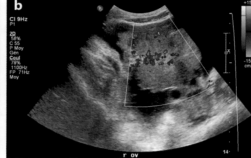
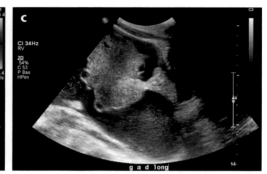
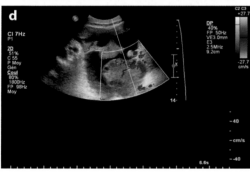

Fig. 12.5 Bilateral Krukenberg tumor. A 26-year-old woman. Epigastric pain and weight loss associated with abdominal swelling. Endoscopy with biopsy diagnoses a mucinous gastric adenocarcinoma (independent cells Her 2-). EVS and color Doppler of the right ovary (**a**, **b**) and of the left ovary (**c**, **d**) depict a bilateral ovarian echogenic mass containing some hyperechoic areas, pushing follicle-like structures at the periphery, with a high degree of vascularization in some parts of the tumor; abundant ascites. Prospective diagnosis: bilateral ovarian metastasis. MR and CT are performed (Fig. 12.7)

US Findings (Figs. 12.5 and 12.6)

The ultrasonic findings of primary ovarian cancer and Krukenberg tumor have been reported initially to be very similar.

In fact, in most of the cases of Krukenberg tumors, the masses have clear tumor margins, a very characteristic irregular hyperechoic solid pattern [16–18] very likely related to the diffuse infiltration of mucin-producing cancer cells [17], and moth-eaten cyst formation.

In contrast, primary ovarian carcinomas have unclear tumor margins, an irregular hypoechoic solid pattern, clear cyst formation, papillary proliferation, and irregular thickness of the septa [17]. However, later in the course of development, Krukenberg tumors become more cystic and necrotic [16] and look like primary ovarian cancers [17].

CT and MR Findings (Figs. 12.6, 12.7, and 12.8)

The masses have sharp margins. The oval configuration is most commonly preserved [19].

On CT and MR, three different patterns have been observed [20].

Solid masses with intramural cysts are the most common pattern.

Solid masses without intratumoral cysts are less frequent.

Predominantly, multilocular cystic masses can rarely be observed.

1. On MR

Various amounts of hypointense solid components on T2W images and isointense components on T1W images, located predominantly in the periphery or randomly distributed can be displayed, like in 57% of cases in HA's series [19]; pathologically, these components corresponded to areas of dense collagenous stroma. Although this finding is very suggestive of fibrous tissue, it is not specific and can be also observed in benign ovarian masses (fibroma or fibrothecoma, Brenner tumor) and subserous leiomyoma. After injection, the solid components were moderately or densely enhanced, which is not usually observed in fibrothecomas and in Brenner tumor.

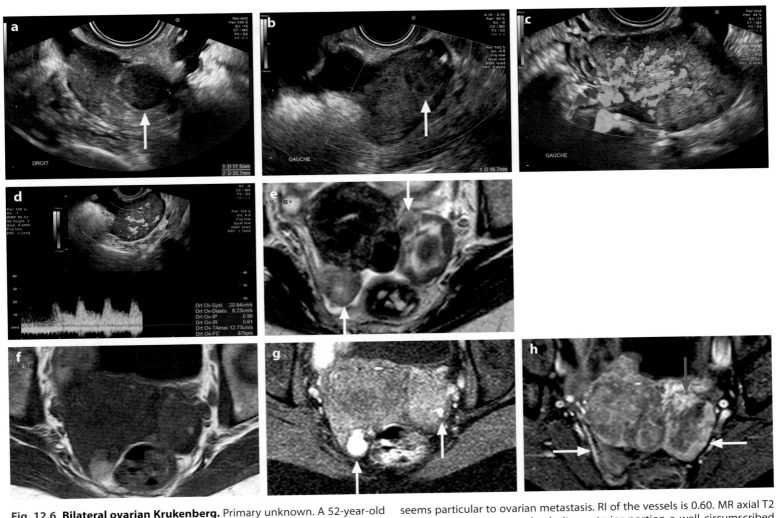

Fig. 12.6 Bilateral ovarian Krukenberg. Primary unknown. A 52-year-old woman. Left latero uterine mass discovered during a routine physical examination. Normal tumoral markers: CA125, CA 19-9, and ACE. EVS depicts a bilateral ovarian mass. Sagittal view of the right ovary contains (**a**) a well delineated hypoechoic nodule in its posterior part (*arrow*); the left ovary (**b**), a hypoechoic nodule of the same nature (*arrow*). Color Doppler of the left ovary (**c**) displays large vessels in the hilum of the ovary, extending in the central part of the mass, with a topography which is not encountered in case of primary carcinoma. On pulsed Doppler (**d**), a regular well delineated hypoechoic capsule is seen at the periphery of the mass (*arrow*), which seems particular to ovarian metastasis. RI of the vessels is 0.60. MR axial T2 (**e**). The right ovary contains in its posterior portion a well circumscribed nodule with an intermediate signal (*arrow*), and the left ovary, a nodule on its medial surface (*arrow*), associated with a thickened peripheral subcapsular band of low signal. On T1 (**f**) and fat suppression (**g**), the cystic content of nodules has a high signal (*arrows*); association of these findings is very suggestive of a mucinous content. DMR at the arterial phase (**h**), arterial vessels are visualized in the capsule of both ovaries (*white arrows*), with a large arterial pedicle in the hilum of the ovary (*red arrow*). Coelioscopy: bilateral adnexectomy. Microscopy: bilateral krukenberg tumor

Because mucinous materials usually show hyperintensity on T2W images, solid components containing a large amount of free or intracellular mucin may exhibit an increase in signal intensity even though stromal overgrowth is present. Indeed, the mucin produced by signet-ring cells may be sometimes so profuse that the cells burst, resulting in dispersion of mucin among stromal cells.

2. On CT and MR

In solid masses with intramural cysts, a very particular strong enhancement of the cyst wall on contrast-enhanced CT scan and on contrast-enhanced T1-weighted MRI has been described by KIM et al. [20] as in 14/22 cases in his series. This enhancement correlated with relatively compact tumor cells in the cyst wall and relatively loose stroma with scanty tumor cells in pericystic areas. Solid masses with well demarcated intratumoral cystic lesions can also been observed in endometrioid carcinomas, Sertoli-Leydig tumors, granulosa cell tumor, and dysgerminoma; but these tumors do not demonstrate relatively strong enhancement of the tumoral cysts [20].

Cystic components within the masses have either well defined or ill defined borders or both [19].

The appearance of entirely cystic masses did not differ from other multiloculated cystic masses such as mucinous tumors [19].

Luteinized fat diagnosed on T1 and fat suppression has been reported [21].

3. CT has two main advantages:

CT can detect the primary tumor particularly a gastric or colonic carcinoma [4, 22].

CT allows to evaluate the extension [3]:

1. Pelvic extension
2. Urinary obstruction
3. Peritoneal metastases
4. Lympadenopathy
5. Hepatic metastases

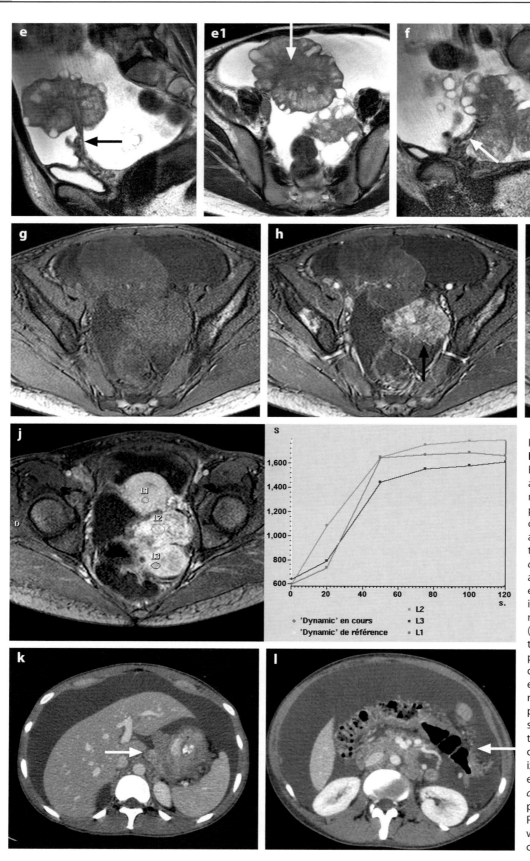

Fig. 12.7 Same patient as Fig. 12.5. Bilateral Krukenberg tumor. Twenty-six-year-old woman. Epigastic pain and weight loss associated with abdominal swelling. Endoscopy with biopsydiagnoses a mucinous gastric adenocarcinoma (independent cells Her 2-). MR Sagittal and axial T2 (**e**, **e1**) of the right ovary and (**f**, **f1**) of the left ovary display a bilateral ovarian mass related by the mesovarium to the posterior part of the broad ligament (*black arrow* in **e** and *white arrow* in **f**), surrounded by ascites. The reniform aspect of the masses, the presence in the right one of central fibrous tissue (*arrow* in **e1**), surrounded by portions of intermediate signal, and the small cystic portions at the periphery (*arrow* in **f1**) are very suggestive of a Krukenberg tumor. DMR without injection (**g**), at the arterial phase (**h**) irregular tumoral vessels (*black arrow*) are displayed particularly in the left ovarian mass with early contrast enhancement (*red arrow*) very likely related to arteriovenous shunts. At the venous phase (**i**) a high contrast uptake is visualized in the solid tissue of the left ovarian mass, illustrated on the dynamic curve (**j**), much more important than on the right side. Multiple cystic portions are visualized at the periphery. CT performed to evaluate extension, depicts carcinoma of the cardia (**k**, *arrow*) and disseminated peritoneal metastases particularly to the greater omentum (**l**, *arrow*). Prospective diagnosis: carcinoma of the stomach with bilateral ovarian Krukenberg tumor. Pathology confirmed the diagnosis

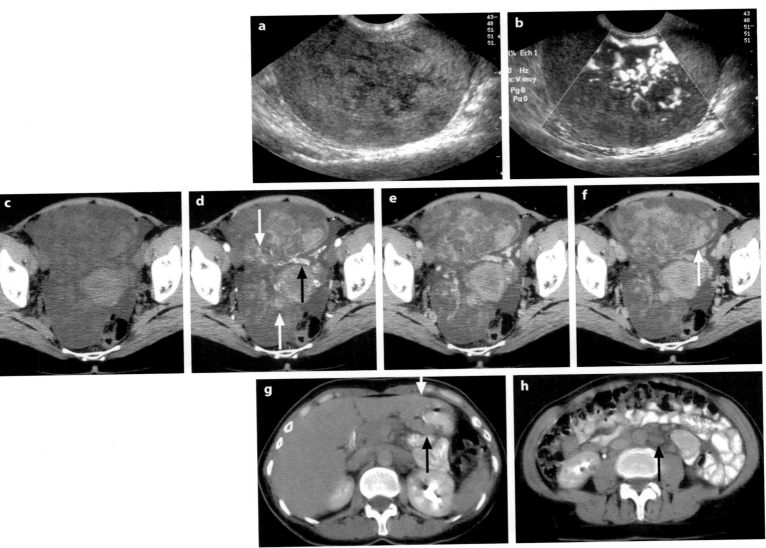

Fig. 12.8 Bilateral ovarian Krukenberg tumor. Forty-eight-year-old woman. EVS of the right ovarian mass (**a**) and with color Doppler (**b**) depict a tissular mass with a high degree of central vascularization. DCT without injection (**c**) at the arterial phase (**d**) display a large left ovarian artery (*black arrow*) and tumoral vessels in both ovarian masses (*white arrows*). At the venous phase (**e**) the masses look very heterogeneous, with contrast uptake in the solid tissues; on the delayed (**f**) some washout is visualized in the tis-sular portions (*arrow*). A bilateral malignant ovarian tumor is diagnosed. CT of the upper abdomen (**g**) shows a circumferential thickening of the antrum (*arrows*) and at a section above the renal pedicles (**h**) left latero aortic lymph node metastasis (*arrow*). Prospective diagnosis: Gastric carcinoma with bilateral ovarian metastases. Pathology: adenocarcinoma of the stomach with bilateral ovarian Krukenberg tumor

Differential Diagnosis

Morphologic and vascular findings of Krukenberg and primary ovarian carcinoma can be very similar (Fig. 12.9). However, the absence of a previous primary malignant tumor and the pathways of dissemination are different; particularly the peritoneal dissemination is much more in favor of a primary.

12.2.3.2 The Predominantly Cystic and Multiloculated Pattern

Intestinal Carcinomas

Most arise from the large intestine occasionally from the small intestine. In one study, 77% were from the rectum or sigmoid colon [23].

Approximately 4% of women with intestinal cancer have ovarian metastases at some time in the course of their disease.

Except for those in the sex cord-stromal tumors, metastatic intestinal carcinomas are among the most common ovarian tumors associated with estrogenic or androgenic manifestations, which result from stimulation of the ovarian stroma by the neoplastic cells.

The common macroscopic and radiological findings are reported in Table 12.5.

Microscopy

The neoplastic cells grow in a pattern similar to those of primary carcinoma.

Mucin containing cells including goblet cells may be scattered among mucin-free cells.

Imaging Findings

The masses are most often large, predominantly cystic, multilocular, with solid masses having morphologic, and vascular findings of

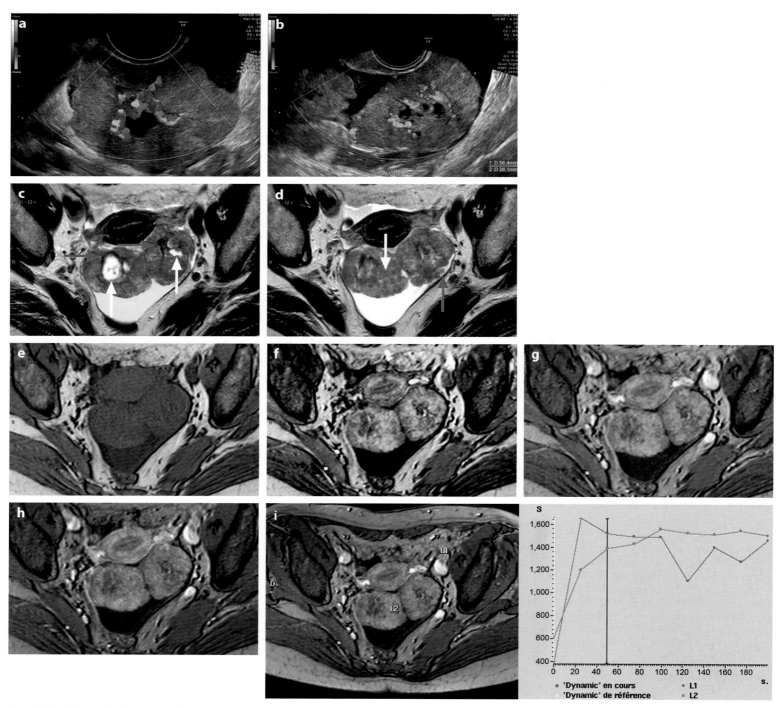

Fig. 12.9 Bilateral primary malignant ovarian tumor resembling a Krukenberg bilateral. A 57-year-old woman. For 6 months, pelvic pain with abdominal swelling. Absence of hormonal treatment. CA 125:140 UI/ml. (1) EVS with Doppler depicts a bilateral ovarian mass. The right ovarian mass (**a**) and the left ovarian mass (**b**) are mainly solid with an echogenicity close to the echogenicity of the myometrium, with lobulated contours, containing in their central portion degenerative changes; the vascularization is made of large vessels with a central distribution in the right one and a mainly central with a slight peripheral distribution in the left one. Slightly echogenic peritoneal fluid is visualized in the pelvis. A bilateral malignant ovarian tumor is diagnosed. Because of the bilaterality and the lobulated contour, a possibility of Krukenberg is suggested. (2) MR axial T2 (**c**, **d**). The ovarian masses displayed have three main morphologic findings: Their overall signal is intermediate on T2 which suggests as a first possibility a malignant tumor. In (**c**), central degenerative changes with a high signal on T2 (*white arrows*) with absence of contrast uptake on the DMR are suggestive of necrosis. Low signal intensity (*red arrows*) around the areas of necrosis are related to fibrosis, which is quite common in Krukenberg tumor. In (**d**), multiple low intensity nodules from 1 to 3 mm are widespread in the masses (*white arrow*) and at their surface (*red arrow*), which are very suggestive of a metastatic process. DMR without injection (**e**), at the arterial phase (**f**), at the venous phase (**g**), and on the delayed (**h**) and curve of contrast enhancement (**I**) depict a bilateral large ovarian artery with tumoral vessels in the masses (**f**), a significant contrast uptake (**g**). Dynamic curve (**i**) displays a rapid intense contrast enhancement with a peak enhancement 100 s after injection. Prospective diagnosis: (1) The morphologic findings of the tumor particularly the multinodular architecture are very suggestive of metastases and as a first possibility a Krukenberg. (2) However, the absence of a primary (on the CT) makes this hypothesis difficult to ascertain, and the much higher frequency of a primary ovarian malignancy and the type of peritoneal dissemination (on the CT) let us discuss the possibility of a primary carcinoma. Definite diagnosis: Bilateral primary serous cystadenocarcinoma of the ovary with peritoneal metastases

Table 12.5 Common macroscopic and radiological findings of metastases from intestinal carcinomas

> 1. Frequently large and commonly rupture
> 2. Findings of mucinous malignant ovarian tumor:
>   Most often predominantly cystic with solid friable tissue and cysts that contain necrotic tumor, mucinous or clear fluid, or blood
>   Multilocular thin-walled cysts filled with clear or mucinous fluid simulating a mucinous cystadenoma or a mucinous cystadenocarcinoma
>   More rarely, solid masses
> 3. Particular findings of metastasis:
>   Bilateral in 60% of cases while primary tumors are bilateral in 6% of cases
>   Different pathways of extension
>   Previous or synchronous tumor mainly of the GI tract

malignancy, indistinguishable from primary mucinous carcinomas (Fig. 12.10).

Uni- or bilateral character is essential to the differential diagnosis. While primary tumors are bilateral in only 6% of cases, metastatic tumors are bilateral in 60% of cases [13] (Fig. 12.11).

Pathways of dissemination can also suggest the diagnosis of metastasis. While primary mucinous carcinomas have GIGO stage 1 in 63% of cases (see Chap. 9), dissemination outside the ovary and some locations of metastasis like liver metastasis can occur in case of mucinous ovarian metastasis while hepatic metastasis are exceptional in case of primary ovarian carcinomas at the time of diagnosis of ovarian tumors.

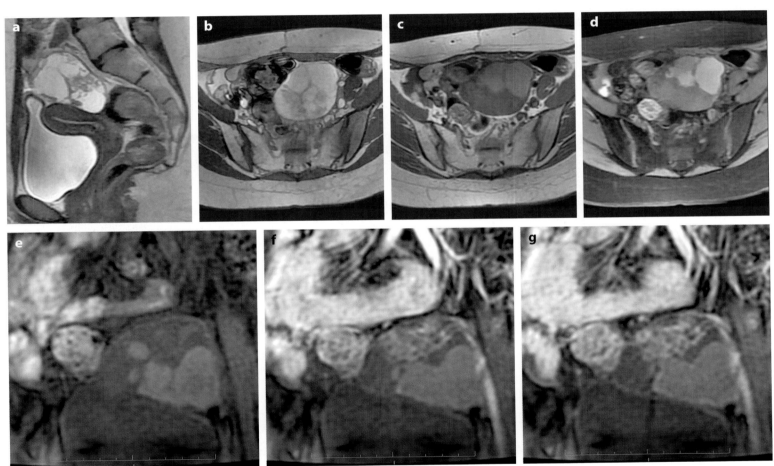

Fig. 12.10 Ovarian metastasis from an adenocarcinoma of the colon.
A 24-year-old woman with previous surgery for colon adenocarcinoma when 19 years old followed 3 years later by right adnexectomy for ovarian metastasis. The left ovary was normal on an MRI done 6 months before. Sagittal T2 (**a**) and Axial T2 (**b**), disclose a 7.5 cm multilocular cystic mass with thickened and irregular septa containing liquids of different signal intensity. On (**b**) is also displayed ascites with thickening of the peritoneum and a small nodule in the right iliac fossa very suggestive of carcinomatosis (which was confirmed at surgery). On axial T1 (**c**) and T1 with fat suppression (**d**) some loculi have a high signal intensity related to hemorrhage. On Coronal DMR before contrast (**e**) and at the arterial phase (**f**) arterial vessels are visualized in the septa. At the venous phase (**g**) contrast uptake is displayed in the irregular wall and septa which increases on the delayed phase

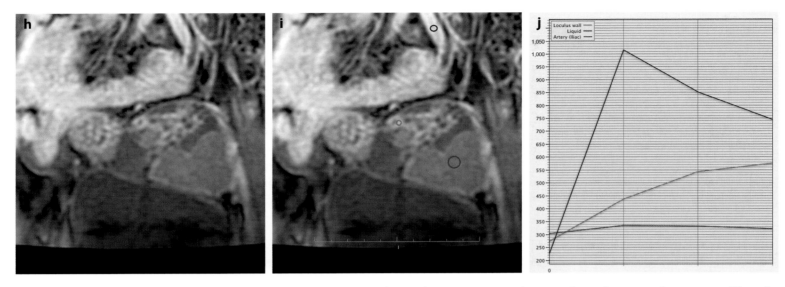

Fig. 12.10 (*continued*) (**h**) Signal-intensity curves are shown in the septa and the loculi (**i, j**). Surgery disclosed left ovarian mass with carcinomatosis. At pathology the mass was a mucinous metastasis from the carcinoma of the colon. *Teaching points*: Ovarian metastasis from mucinous adenocarcinoma may have a similar appearance as primary ovarian malignant mucinous tumors. Bilaterality and history of previous primary adenocarcinoma elsewhere favor the diagnosis of metastatic tumor

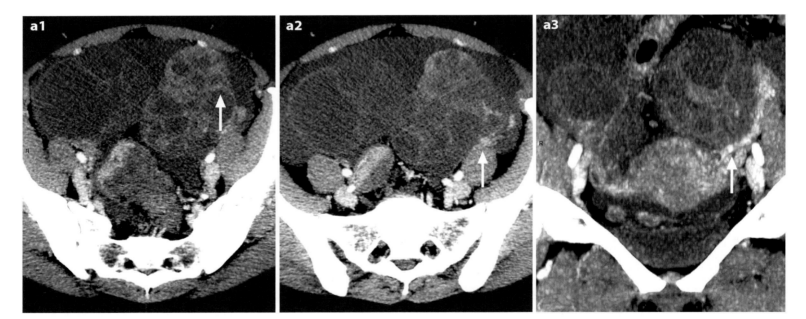

Fig. 12.11 Bilateral mucinous metastasis of sigmoid carcinoma. DCT at the arterial phase (**a1**) depicts: (1) a bilateral multilocular cystic ovarian masses; tumoral arterial vessels (*white arrow*), solid tissue, and thickened and irregular septa reflect findings of malignancy; (2) a sigmoid mass with tumoral arterial vessels highly suggesting a sigmoid carcinoma. At a higher level (**a2**), a large left ovarian artery (*arrow*) and on coronal reformation (**a3**), a large left tubo-ovarian artery (*arrow*) also express findings of malignancy. Transverse view of the omentum

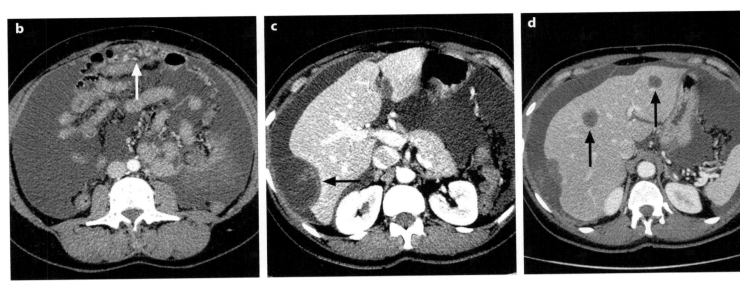

Fig. 12.11 (*continued*) (**b**) displays peritoneal metastases associated with increase of vascularization (*arrow*). On (**c**), peritoneal metastases with a scalloping of a metastasis on the liver capsule and ascites suggest a pseudomyxoma (*arrow*). On (**d**), liver metastases are shown (*arrows*). Prospective diagnosis: Morphologic and vascular findings of the ovarian masses are typical for malignant mucinous tumors. Bilaterality of the masses, extension beyond the ovaries particularly hepatic metastasis, and association with a sigmoid tumor highly suggest bilateral mucinous ovarian metastasis of a sigmoid carcinoma. Laparotomy confirmed the diagnosis of bilateral ovarian masses, sigmoid tumor, with pseudomyxoma. Pathology: Sigmoid mucinous carcinoma. Bilateral ovarian mucinous metastasis of intestinal type

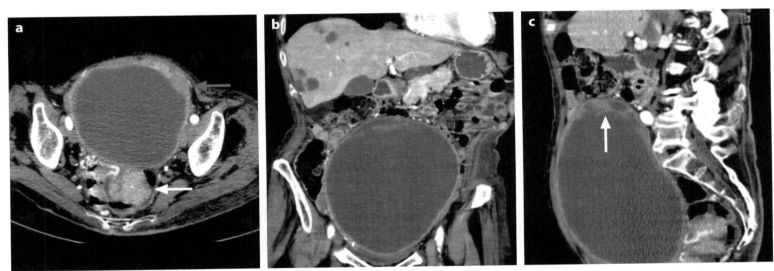

Fig. 12.12 Ovarian metastasis from the rectum. CT at the arterial phase (**a**) displays a carcinoma of the rectum (*white arrow*) and a cystic ovarian mass, with a thickened wall in the anterior part of the mass (*red arrow*). Coronal reformation (**b**) depicts a huge mainly cystic ovarian mass, with hepatic metastases. Sagittal reformation (**c**) shows that the wall of the mass is thick and irregular (*arrow*). No papillary projection is visualized. Prospective diagnosis of ovarian metastasis from a carcinoma of the rectum. Definite diagnosis confirmed this diagnosis

Uncommonly, the mass looks like a multilocular mucinous cystadenoma.

The mass can also be cystic and unilocular. Absence of papillary projection and an irregular thickened wall can suggest the diagnosis (Fig. 12.12).

12.2.3.3 Appendiceal Tumors

Most often, they are borderline mucinous tumors. They typically appear as mucoceles, but can appear grossly normal, associated with similar tumors in one or both ovaries accompanied by pseudomyxoma peritonei (see Sect. 9.4.2.3). Ovarian masses are large frequently bilateral and multilocular.

More rarely the primary tumor is adenocarcinoma, including tumors of typical intestinal, colloid, and signet ring cell types.

12.2.3.4 Pancreas, Gallbladder, and Bile Ducts

Mucinous metastases from the pancreas have been reported for up to 10% of ovarian metastases. Some tumors considered as mucinous carcinomas or borderline tumors of the ovary were in fact ovarian metastases from pancreatic carcinoma.

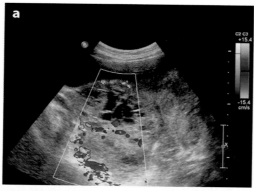
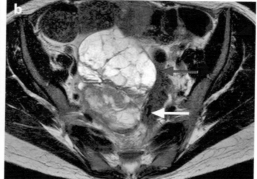
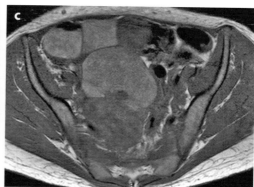
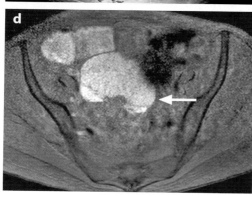

Fig. 12.13 Ovarian metastasis from renal cell carcinoma. A 33-year-old woman. Eight months ago, right nephrectomy for adenocarcinoma. Right pelvic pain. EVS with color Doppler (**a**) displays a right mixed ovarian mass with a multiloculated cystic component and a tissular component, with vessels in the septa and in the solid tissue. MR axial T2 (**b**) depicts a right ovarian mass with an anterior cystic multiloculated portion (*red arrow*) and a posterior solid portion (*white arrow*). On axial T1 (**c**) and fat suppression (**d**), the cystic component is mainly hemorrhagic (*arrow*)

Metastases from gallbladder and bile ducts are much more uncommon; exceptional metastases from hepatocellular carcinomas have been described.

12.2.3.5 Carcinoid Tumors

The primary tumors are mostly in the small intestine [24].
  Extra-ovarian metastases are found in at least 90% of the cases. Most are bilateral.
  They are *predominantly solid*, containing single or confluent nodules, which may resemble ovarian fibromas or thecomas. However unlike ovarian fibromas, carcinoids are usually hypervascularized. Cysts are occasionally present. Necrosis and hemorrhage may occur but are usually focal.

Differential Diagnosis

1. Primary carcinoid tumors
2. Granulosa cell tumor
3. Sertoli or Sertoli-Leydig cell tumor

12.2.4 Urinary Tract

12.2.4.1 Renal

Macroscopy: Solid or mixed
Microscopy:
  The primary is a well differentiated clear cell carcinoma.
  The metastase: A relatively uniform pattern of diffuse sheats of clear cells or tubules lined by similar cells.
  A prominent sinusoidal vascular pattern.

  Radiologic findings: A case of a mixed tumor is reported (Fig. 12.13).

12.2.4.2 Urinary Bladder, Ureter, Urethra

These sites are very uncommon.
  In case of transitional cell carcinoma metastatic to the ovary, it is difficult to distinguish between a metastatic tumor and a borderline or malignant Brenner tumor of the ovary.

12.2.4.3 Adrenal

Neuroblastoma spreads to the ovary more frequently than other tumors of the adrenal gland.

12.2.5 Melanoma

Although some patients have a known primary tumor and evidence of metastases elsewhere, isolated ovarian spread is seen occasionally, sometimes with a negative or remote history of a primary melanoma [25].
  The tumors are bilateral in 45% of cases [25, 26].

12.2.5.1 Gross Examination

1. The tumor is black or brown in 30% of cases.
2. It contains multiple nodules.

12.2.5.2 Microscopy

1. Most commonly: Large cells with abundant eosinophilic cytoplasm.
2. When associated with follicle-like spaces (40% of cases), the tumor may mimic a juvenile granulose cell tumor.
   (a) A helpful diagnostic feature is the presence of rounded aggregates with a nevoid appearance.

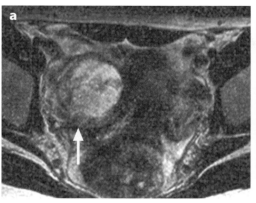
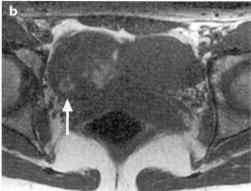
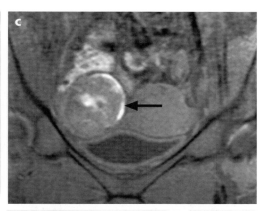
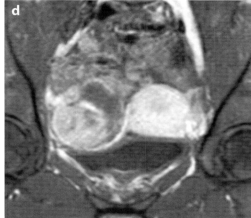

Fig. 12.14 Previous surgery for melanoma of the choroid 7 years before. MR axial T2 (**a**) depicts a right well-delineated ovarian mass. This mass contains mainly a tissular portion of high signal intensity, and its posterior part areas of low signal intensity (*arrow*). These areas of low signal intensity are of high signal intensity on Axial T1 (**b**) (*arrow*) and on coronal fat suppression (**c**) (*arrow*). Association of these characters of signal in a tissular mass are very suggestive of a melanotic type of melanoma. Coronal T1 after contrast (**d**) shows a high contrast uptake in most of the part of the mass. Surgery: right adnexectomy. Pathology: ovarian metastasis of melanoma. Courtesy of Pr Yann Robert

Table 12.6 MR findings of metastatic melanoma

Melanotic type: characters of signal very suggestive
On T1 and fat suppression: mass or areas of high signal intensity (related to hemorrhage and or paramagnetic effects), very suggestive
On T2: low signal intensity
Amelanotic type: characters of signal nonspecific
On T1: low signal intensity
On T2: intermediate high signal intensity

   (b) The presence of melanin is a clue to the nature of the tumor; however, this pigment is inconspicuous or absent in approximately 50% of cases.

3. Immunohistochemistry: In problem cases, demonstration of S-100 protein and HMB-45 are helpful to make the diagnosis.

12.2.5.3 MR Findings (Fig. 12.14)

MR findings are different according to the presence or absence of melanin in the tumor and are reported in Table 12.6.

12.2.5.4 Differential Diagnosis

A primary melanoma can arise in the wall of a dermoid cyst. The cyst may show junctional activity beneath its squamous lining cells. Rarely another teratomatous component such as a struma ovarii accompanies the primary melanoma.

12.2.6 Pulmonary and Mediastinal Tumors (Fig. 12.15)

Usually the pulmonary tumor precedes the discovery of the ovarian metastatic tumor, or both are synchronous. The most common cell type is a small cell carcinoma.

Small cell carcinoma can also originate in the mediastinum, where the primary tumor can be of thymic origin.

12.2.7 Extragenital Sarcomas

Extragenital sarcomas uncommonly metastasize to the ovaries.

There are mainly rhabdomyosarcomas, more rarely leiomyosarcomas, fibrosarcomas, osteosarcomas, chondrosarcomas, and hemangiosarcomas.

12.2.8 Ovarian Involvement by Peritoneal Tumors

Ovarian involvement in cases of malignant mesothelioma and malignant serous tumors of the peritoneum is secondary in most of the cases.

The differential diagnosis in these cases is primarily with an ovarian surface epithelial carcinoma, particularly serous carcinoma, with peritoneal metastases.

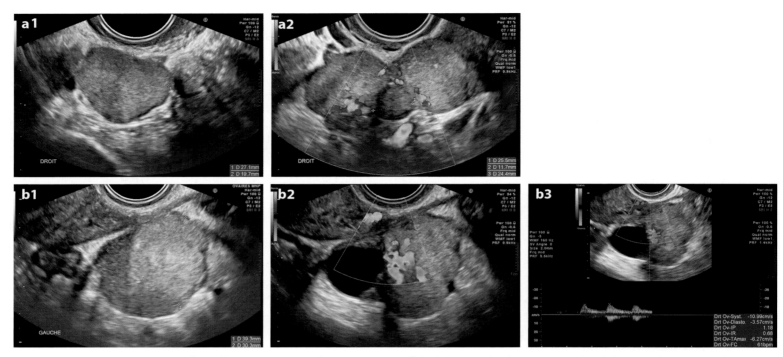

Fig. 12.15 Ovarian metastases of a pulmonary neuroendocrine carcinoma. A 51-year-old woman. Neuroendocrine pulmonary tumor operated 3 years before. Metrorrhagias. EVS transversal (**a1**), longitudinal with color Doppler (**a2**) of the right ovary depicts a multinodular mass, relatively homogeneous, with an echogenicity like myometrium; a rich vascularization is displayed in the mass. EVS longitudinal (**b1**) with color Doppler (**b2**) of the left ovary displays a mass with solid tissue of the same echogenicity as in the right ovarian mass, associated with a small cystic component. On spectral Doppler, the systolic velocity is of 10 cm/s (**b3**). Prospective diagnosis: A bilateral ovarian malignant tumor is suggested. Because of the rarity of ovarian metastatic tumor of the lung, the preoperative diagnosis was not suspected

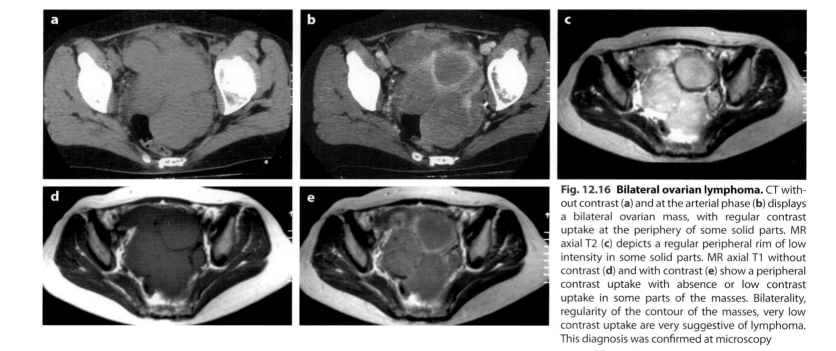

Fig. 12.16 Bilateral ovarian lymphoma. CT without contrast (**a**) and at the arterial phase (**b**) displays a bilateral ovarian mass, with regular contrast uptake at the periphery of some solid parts. MR axial T2 (**c**) depicts a regular peripheral rim of low intensity in some solid parts. MR axial T1 without contrast (**d**) and with contrast (**e**) show a peripheral contrast uptake with absence or low contrast uptake in some parts of the masses. Bilaterality, regularity of the contour of the masses, very low contrast uptake are very suggestive of lymphoma. This diagnosis was confirmed at microscopy

12.3 Malignant Lymphomas (Figs. 12.16 and 12.17)

1. There are three main types:
   (a) The most common: Disseminated being either the first manifestation or occurring during the course of a disseminated disease. The peak incidence is from 20 to 50 years.
   (b) Very uncommonly, a primary extranodal (the presence of lymph node as well as blood and bone marrow being excluded).
   (c) Burkitt's lymphoma is a poorly differentiated malignant lymphoma, which typically appears in endemic areas, but also can

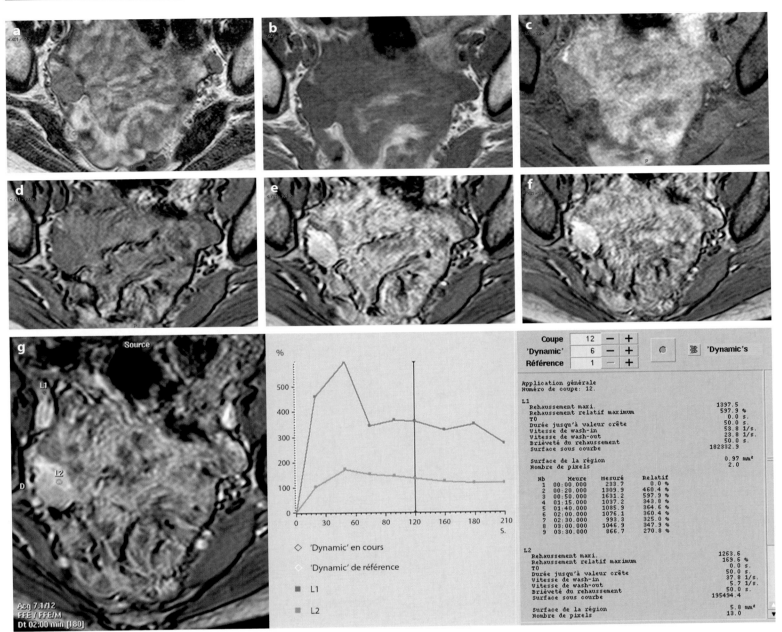

Fig. 12.17 Bilateral ovarian B lymphoma. A 63-year-old woman. Left breast carcinoma treated with tumorectomy and radiotherapy 1 year before. During a routine US examination, a right ovarian mass is discovered. On MR axial T2 (**a**) a bilateral ovarian mass with an overall intermediate signal, containing multiple small nodules is displayed; the masses appear with a low signal on T1 (**b**) and T1-FS (**c**). On DMR focused on the right ovarian mass without injection (**d**) and at the arterial phase (**e**), vessels are displayed at the periphery and in the central part of the mass. At the venous phase (**f**) a peak of contrast enhancement is visualized with a slight wash out on the delayed (**g**) the overall contrast enhancement in the mass (*green curve*) is relatively low compared to the peak of enhancement in the iliac artery (*red curve*). A prospective diagnosis of bilateral metastases was suggested. Surgery: a bilateral adnexectomy was performed. At microscopy, confirmed with immunomarquage, a bilateral follicular small cell type B lymphoma was diagnosed

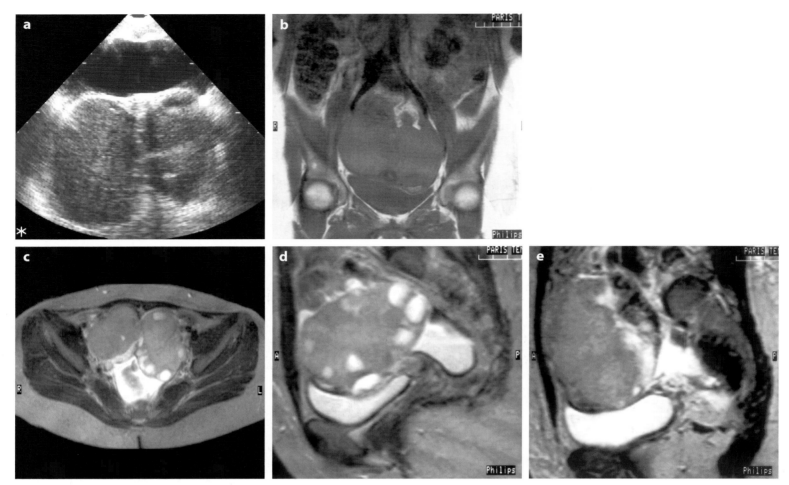

Fig. 12.18 Bilateral Burkitt lymphoma. TAS (**a**) depicts a bilateral ovarian mass with regular contours and an overall low echogenicity. MR coronal T1 (**b**): the masses have a signal intensity close to pelvic muscles; a small area at the lower part of the left ovarian mass has a high signal intensity suggestive of hemorrhage. Axial T2 (**c**) and sagittal T2 through the right (**d**) and left (**e**) ovarian masses display a bilateral ovarian mass with an intermediate signal containing at the periphery multiple cystic spaces

be observed outside these zones. It mainly involves young adults and children (Fig. 12.18).

2. The common macroscopic and radiologic findings in US, CT, and MR are summarized in Table 12.7.

Table 12.7 Imaging findings of ovarian lymphomas in US, CT, and MR

1. Common findings
   Bilateral 50% of cases
   Surface smooth, nodular, or bosselated
   Most often homogeneous
   May spare ovarian follicles
   Uncommonly cystic degeneration, hemorrhage, and necrosis
2. EVS
   Homogeneous and hypoechoic
3. CT
   Without contrast: density close to pelvic muscles
4. MR
   T2: Intermediate signal
   T1: Signal close to pelvic muscles
5. Vascular findings on US, CT, MR
   Mild vascularization
   Mild homogeneous contrast uptake

References

1. Brown DL et al (2001) Primary versus secondary ovarian malignancy: imaging findings of adnexal masses in the Radiology Diagnostic Oncology Group Study. Radiology 219(1):213–218
2. Ulbright TM, Roth LM, Stehman FB (1984) Secondary ovarian neoplasia. A clinicopathologic study of 35 cases. Cancer 53(5):1164–1174
3. Megibow A, Hulnick D, Bosniak M (1985) Ovarian metastases: computed tomographic appearance. Radiology 156:161–164
4. Cho KC, Gold BM (1985) Computed tomography of Krukenberg tumors. AJR Am J Roentgenol 145(2):285–288
5. Demopoulos RI, Touger L, Dubin N (1987) Secondary ovarian carcinoma: a clinical and pathological evaluation. Int J Gynecol Pathol 6(2):166–175
6. Holtz F, Hart WR (1982) Krukenberg tumors of the ovary: a clinicopathologic analysis of 27 cases. Cancer 50(11):2438–2447
7. Yakushiji M et al (1987) Krukenberg tumors of the ovary: a clinicopathologic analysis of 112 cases. Nippon Sanka Fujinka Gakkai Zasshi 39(3):479–485
8. Scully RE, Young RH, Clement PB (1998) Tumors of the ovary, maldeveloped gonads, fallopian tubes and broad ligament. In: Rosai J, Sobin LH (eds) Atlas of tumor pathology, vol 3. Armed Force Institute of Pathology, Washington, DC, pp 335–372
9. Kuhlman JE, Hruban RH, Fishman EK (1989) Krukenberg tumors: CT features and growth characteristics. South Med J 82(10):1215–1219

10. Choi HJ et al (2006) Contrast-enhanced CT for differentiation of ovarian metastasis from gastrointestinal tract cancer: stomach cancer versus colon cancer. AJR Am J Roentgenol 187(3):741–745

11. Gagnon Y, Tetu B (1989) Ovarian metastases of breast carcinoma. A clinicopathologic study of 59 cases. Cancer 64(4):892–898

12. Young RH, Scully RE (2002) Metastatic tumors of the ovary. In: Kurman RJ (ed) Blaustein's pathology of the female genital tract. Springer, New-York, pp 1063–1101

13. Seidman JD, Kurman RJ, Ronnett BM (2003) Primary and metastatic mucinous adenocarcinomas in the ovaries: incidence in routine practice with a new approach to improve intraoperative diagnosis. Am J Surg Pathol 27(7): 985–993

14. Kiyokawa T, Young RH, Scully RE (2006) Krukenberg tumors of the ovary: a clinicopathologic analysis of 120 cases with emphasis on their variable pathologic manifestations. Am J Surg Pathol 30(3):277–299

15. Al-Agha OM, Nicastri AD (2006) An in-depth look at Krukenberg tumor: an overview. Arch Pathol Lab Med 130(11):1725–1730

16. Athey PA, Butters HE (1984) Sonographic and CT appearance of Krukenberg tumors. J Clin Ultrasound 12(4):205–210

17. Shimizu H et al (1990) Characteristic ultrasonographic appearance of Krukenberg tumor. J Clin Ultrasound 18:697–703

18. Choi BI et al (1988) Sonographic appearance of Krukenberg tumor from gastric carcinoma. Gastrointest Radiol 13(1):15–18

19. Ha HK et al (1995) Krukenberg's tumor of the ovary: MR imaging features. AJR Am J Roentgenol 164(6):1435–1439

20. Kim SH et al (1996) CT and MR findings of Krukenberg tumors: comparison with primary ovarian tumors. J Comput Assist Tomogr 20(3):393–398

21. Jeong YY et al (2002) Luteinized fat in Krukenberg tumor: MR findings. Eur Radiol 12(Suppl 3):S130–S132

22. Mata JM et al (1988) CT findings in metastatic ovarian tumors from gastrointestinal tract neoplasms (Krukenberg tumors). Gastrointest Radiol 13(3): 242–246

23. Lash RH, Hart WR (1987) Intestinal adenocarcinomas metastatic to the ovaries. A clinicopathologic evaluation of 22 cases. Am J Surg Pathol 11(2): 114–121

24. Robboy SJ, Scully RE, Norris HJ (1974) Carcinoid metastatic to the ovary. A clinocopathologic analysis of 35 cases. Cancer 33(3):798–811

25. Young RH, Scully RE (1991) Malignant melanoma metastatic to the ovary. A clinicopathologic analysis of 20 cases. Am J Surg Pathol 15(9):849–860

26. Fitzgibbons PL, Martin SE, Simmons TJ (1987) Malignant melanoma metastatic to the ovary. Am J Surg Pathol 11(12):959–964

Tumors with Functioning Stroma

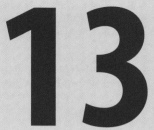

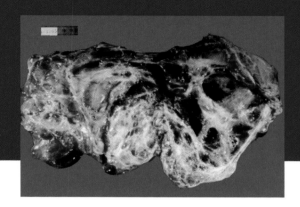

Contents

13.1 Definition

These are tumors other than those in the sex cord-stromal and steroid cell categories that are characterized [1] by (1) a stroma that is morphologically compatible with steroid hormone secretion and (2) clinical biochemical or pathologic incidence of endocrine abnormalities [2] of estrogenic androgenic or rarely progestogenic type, or a combination of them.

In 1958, Hughesdon [3] described serous, mucinous, clear cell, and endometrioid tumors associated with what he termed a "thecal reaction" of the stroma. In four of six cases in which the uterus was available, the endometrium showed cystic hyperplasia.

Such observations, as well as frequency of vaginal bleeding and the association of endometrioid hyperplastic conditions in patients with ovarian epithelial tumors, suggest some of these nonfunctioning tumors do demonstrate endocrine activity, which in most instances is of the estrogenic type.

13.2 Frequency and Distribution

Ovarian tumors with functioning stroma (OTFSs) are common at least at a laboratory level [4]. Approximately, 50% of postmenopausal women with benign and malignant surface epithelial-stromal tumors or carcinomas metastatic to the ovary have elevated urinary estrogen levels (5). Endocrine manifestations are much rarer. Few if any estrogenic tumors of this type have been reported in women in the reproductive age group because of the difficulty in establishing a cause-and-effect relationship between an ovarian tumor and estrogenic manifestations in that age category. There are over 60 reported examples of virilizing ovarian tumors with functioning stroma, slightly over one third of which occurred in pregnant women. Some of these women had virilized offspring as well [1]. Rare tumors are associated with progestational changes manifested by a decidual reaction [6, 7] or an Arias-Stella change in the endometrium.

13.3 Mechanism of Hormone Secretion

The explanation for the stromal stimulation is not clear. The high level of circulating luteinizing hormone in postmenopausal women could be responsible for stromal stimulation. Progressive expansion of aggregates of tumor cells could exert mechanical pressure on the stroma, stimulating it to transform into homono-producing tissue. Carcinoma cells may have aromatase activity and therefore a capacity to convert androgens to estrogens [8].

13.4 Microscopy Findings and Histochemical Investigations

The functioning stroma of the tumor may be its intrinsic stroma which is derived from the ovarian stroma, the stroma adjacent to the tumor, or a combination of the two [9]. The stromal cells transform into plump spindle cells resembling theca externa cells, theca lutein cells, stromal lutein cells, or a combination of these cell types, or rarely into Leydig cells [9].

Histochemical investigation of the luteinized stromal cells demonstrated that, in addition to their lipid content, these cells contained different oxidative enzymes as G6P-dehydrogenase or lactic acid dehydrogenase. Scully and Cohen [10] called them enzymatically active stromal cells (EASC).

EASC are present in 37% of ovarian tumors described by Pfleiderer and Teufel [11]. Since the ovarian stroma is generally considered a primarily androgen component of the ovary, it is not surprising that in some of the estrogenic OFTSs the neoplasm itself produces androgens, which are converted peripherally in estrogens [12].

13.5 Types of Tumors with Functioning Stroma

Tumors accompanied by *estrogenic manifestations* (proliferative or hyperplastic endometrium, swelling or tenderness of the breast) are reported in Table 13.1.

The most common ones are the surface epithelial-stromal tumors, particularly those of the mucinous and endometrioid categories and metastatic carcinomas, especially from the large intestine [5]. Almost

Table 13.1 Tumors accompanied by estrogenic manifestations

1. **Surface epithelial-stromal tumors mucinous and endometrioid**
2. **Metastatic carcinomas especially from the large intestine**
3. **Brenner tumors**

Table 13.2 Tumors accompanied with androgenic manifestations

Common
1. **Krukenberg tumor (gastric origin)**
2. **Primary mucinous cystic tumors (mostly benign)**
Less common
1. **Rete cystadenoma**
2. **Metastatic carcinoma (large intestine)**
3. **Dermoid cysts**
4. **Stromal carcinoid tumors**

50% of patients with Brenner tumors [13] have either endometrioid hyperplasia, polyps or carcinoma, all indicating hyperestrogenism.

Tumors accompanied with *androgenic manifestations* are reported in Table 13.2.

A few cases were reported to display androgenic activity and clinical masculization [14]. Of the over 60 reported ovarian tumors with an androgenic stroma, one third had Krukenberg tumors mostly of gastric origin, one fifth had primary mucinous cystic tumors mostly benign, less common have been rete cystadenomas, metastatic carcinomas from the large intestine, dermoid cysts, stromal carcinoid tumors, and miscellaneous others [1].

Of all epithelial tumors, the levels of androstenedione and testosterone in peripheral and ovarian venous blood are highest in women with mucinous ovarian tumors [15].

13.6 Imaging Findings

13.6.1 On MR

Two cases of OTFS have been reported [16]: one case of carcinoid with androgen manifestations and one case of mucinous cystadenoma with elevated serum level of estrogen. Both tumors looked multiloculated. The imaging feature mimicked those of Sertoli-Leydig tumor and granulosa tumor.

13.6.1.1 Differential Diagnosis

It is important not to be misled by the presence of endocrine manifestations into making an erroneous diagnosis of a sex cord-stromal tumor. Mucinous cysts may be a prominent feature of Sertoli-Leydig cell tumors; therefore, any virilizing tumor with a mucinous component must be searched carefully for Sertoli-Leydig cell elements before making a diagnosis of a virilizing mucinous cystic tumor.

References

1. Scully RE (1995) Ovarian tumors with functioning stroma. In: Fox H (ed) Haines and Taylor obstetrical and gynaecological pathology. Churchill Livingstone, Edinburgh
2. Morris JM, Scully RE (1958) Endocrine pathology of the ovary. Mosby, St Louis
3. Hughesdon PE (1958) Thecal and allied reactions in epithelial ovarian tumors. J Obstet Gynaecol Br Commonw 65:702
4. Scully RE, Young RH, Clement PB (1998) Tumors of the ovary, maldeveloped gonads, fallopian tubes and broad ligament. In: Rosai J, Sobin LH (eds). Atlas of tumor pathology, 3rd edn. Armed Force Institute of Pathology, Washington, DC, pp 373–378
5. Rome RM et al (1981) Functioning ovarian tumors in postmenopausal women. Obstet Gynecol 57(6):705–710
6. Bruno G et al (1988) A case of giant serous cystadenoma of the ovary. Minerva Chir 43(12):1095–1097
7. Ober WB et al (1959) Krukenberg tumor with androgenic and progestational activity. Am J Obstet Gynecol 84:739–744
8. Thompson MA et al (1988) Aromatization of testosterone by epithelial tumor cells cultured from patients with ovarian carcinoma. Cancer Res 48(22):6491–6497
9. Hameed K (1972) Brenner tumor of the ovary with Leydig cell hyperplasia. A histologic and ultrastructural study. Cancer 30(4):945–952
10. Scully RE, Cohen RB (1964) Oxidative-enzyme activities in normal and pathologic human ovaries. Obstet Gynecol 24:667
11. Pfleiderer A Jr, Teufel G (1968) Incidence and histochemical investigation of enzymatically active cells in stroma of ovarian tumors. Am J Obstet Gynecol 102(7):997–1003
12. MacDonald PC et al (1976) Origin of estrogen in a postmenopausal woman with a nonendocrine tumor of the ovary and endometrial hyperplasia. Obstet Gynecol 47(6):644–650
13. Ming S, Goldman H (1962) Hormonal activities of Brenner tumors in postmenopausal women. Am J Obstet Gynecol 83:666–673
14. De Lima GR et al (1989) Virilizing Brenner tumor of the ovary: case report. Obstet Gynecol 73(5 Pt 2):895–898
15. Heinonen PK (1991) Androgen production by epithelial ovarian tumours in post-menopausal women. Maturitas 13(2):117–122
16. Tanaka YO et al (2002) Ovarian tumor with functioning stroma. Comput Med Imaging Graph 26(3):193–197

Hyperandrogenism

14

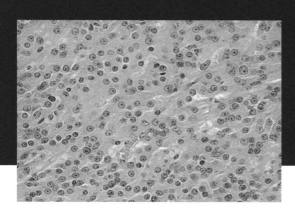

Contents

Hyperandrogenism is a clinical and biological syndrome secondary to an increase of secretion of androgens. The androgens can be produced by the cortex of the adrenal gland in its inner layer, the reticularis; by the ovary in the theca of the ovarian follicle, the stroma or the hilus Leydig cells; and in some cases, as in the PCOD, both in the ovary and in the adrenal gland.

This hyperandrogenism has particular clinical and biological findings which can be isolated. Or it can be associated with clinical and biological findings of virilization.

In clinical practice:

1. The adrenal or ovarian origin of these syndromes can be difficult to determine, leading sometimes to venous catheterization of the adrenal and the ovarian veins.
2. The etiology, functional or tumoral, can be difficult to assess.
3. As the ovarian etiologies are discussed in three different chapters of the book (Chaps. 7, 11, and 13), it seemed to us interesting to report in a chapter of synthesis the main clinical and biological findings of these syndromes, the site of secretion and the biochemistry of the synthesis in the different compartments of the ovary, and the overview of the most frequent etiologies.

14.1 Biosynthesis of Adrenal and Ovarian Androgens

Biosynthesis of adrenal and ovarian androgens is reported in the biochemistry chapter (Chap. 3).

J.N. Buy, M. Ghossain, *Gynecological Imaging*,
DOI 10.1007/978-3-642-31012-6_14, © Springer-Verlag Berlin Heidelberg 2013

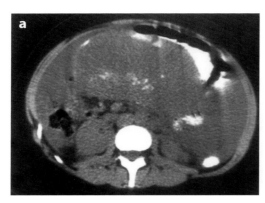
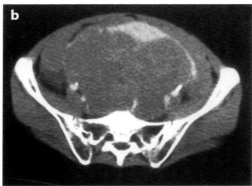

Fig. 14.7 Gonadoblastoma with dysgerminoma developed on a gonadal dysgenesis in a 26-year-old woman with left pelvic pain, constipation, and fever. (a) CT scan without contrast displays a pelvic abdominal mass containing multiple tiny calcifications and high-density ascites. (b) CT scan after contrast shows that the mass pushes the uterus and tubes forward and the rectum backward. Vessels inside the tumor are displayed

14.7 Ovarian Gonadoblastoma

See Chap. 10 (Fig. 14.7)

14.8 Tumors with Functioning Stroma

See Chap. 13

Reference

1. Ghossain MA, Buy JN, Ruiz A, Jacob D, Sciot C, Hugol D, Vadrot D (1998) Hyperreactio luteinalis in a normal pregnancy: sonographic and MRI findings. J Magn Reson Imaging 8(6):1203–1206

15.2.3 Rhabdomyosarcoma

Macroscopic findings are identical to leiomyosarcomas.

15.3 Tumors of Vascular and Lymphatic Origin

15.3.1 Hemangioma

The lesions are small, measuring from few millimeters to 1.5 cm in diameter.

The medulla and the hilar region are the most common sites.

It is of the cavernous or mixed capillary-cavernous type. It consists of collections of vascular spaces lined by endothelial cells.

Hemangioma can be confused with proliferation of dilated blood vessels, frequently seen in the hilar region of the ovary.

15.3.2 Lymphangioma

At macroscopy, it is composed of numerous cystic spaces.

Microscopically the tumor is composed of small thin-walled vascular spaces lined by flattened endothelial cells.

15.3.3 Hemangioendothelial Sarcoma

Hemangioendothelial has a vascularization composed of vascular spaces lined by endothelial cells which are large, with atypical appearance, bizarre nuclei, and mitotic activity.

15.4 Tumors of Cartilage Origin

At pathology, only a few reports of chondromas of the ovary have been reported. According to Talerman [1], it is most likely that most ovarian tumors described as chondromas were either fibromas showing cartilaginous metaplasia or teratomas having a prominent cartilaginous component.

A single case of chondrosarcoma has been reported [1].

15.5 Tumors of Bone Origin

15.5.1 Osteoma

Although an origin from ovarian stroma is possible, most such lesions reported probably were metaplasia occurring in fibromas or leiomyomas.

15.5.2 Osteosarcoma

Histologically, the tumors show typical appearance osteosarcoma occurring in the skeleton.

Although it is believed that these tumors originate directly from ovarian stroma, their histogenesis is uncertain.

These tumors are different from osteosarcomas originating in ovarian teratomas and from MMMTs with a prominent osteosarcomatous component.

15.6 Tumors of Neural Tissue Origin

15.6.1 Neurofibroma, Neurofibrosarcoma, Ganglioneuroma, and Pheochromocytoma

Neurofibromas and one case of neurofibrosarcoma have been reported by Talerman (1) in patients with Recklinghausen's disease. Their macroscopic findings were reported to be identical to these types of tumors occuring elsewhere.

Neurinofibromas are usually well delineated masses, with or without degenerative changes as in the example of a presacral neurinoma displayed in chap 2 (Fig 2.30) These tumors are usually hypervascularized.

A single case of ganglioneuroma, and a single case of pheochromocytoma have been reported at pathology (1).

15.6.2 Primitive Neuroectodermal Tumor (Figs. 10.128 and 10.129)

See Chap. 10.4.3.3.

15.7 Tumors of Adipose Tissue Origin

Lipomas of the ovary have been reported. A single personal case on CT (unfortunately lost) was a regular and homogeneous mass with a typical low-density content.

Benign adipose tissue seen in the ovary may be part of a teratoma.

Malignant adipose tissue may be part of MMMT.

15.8 Tumors of Mesothelial Origin

15.8.1 Adenomatoid Tumor

Their origin is presumed to be from the cells of the serosal mesothelium.

Microscopically, they are composed of multiple small, slitlike, or ovoid spaces lined by a single layer of low cuboidal or flattened epithelia-like cells.

They are usually found where there is the mesovarium in the hilus of the ovary.

They are usually solid 1–2 cm in diameter. Rarely, the cystic spaces are sufficiently large to give a macroscopic pattern of cystic or multilocular mass.

Lesions of this type can be found in the tube, the uterus, and cul-de-sac (see Chap. 20).

15.8.2 Peritoneal Mesothelioma

Peritoneal mesothelioma may involve the ovary. The involvement can be very extensive, and the presentation is that of a primary ovarian neoplasm (see Chap. 16).

15.9 Ovarian Tumors of Probable Wolffian Origin

15.9.1 Embryologic Definition of Wolffian Remnants [2], (See Chap. 1)

Late in the fourth week of embryogenesis, caudal to the pronephroi, the mesonephroi develop, which consist of mesonephric ducts and tubules. The mesonephric ducts open into bilateral mesonephric ducts, which open into the cloaca.

The mesonephric tubules will give rise in males to efferent ductules of testis and paradidymis; in females, to remnants epoophoron and paroophoron.

The mesonephric ducts will give rise in males to appendix of epididymis duct of epididymis and ductus efferens; in females, to remnants appendix vesiculosa duct of epoophoron and Gartner duct.

15.9.2 Pathological Definition of Tumors of Probable Wolffian Origin

The tumor is composed of relatively uniform epithelial cells that line cysts and tubules, associated with connective tissue.

15.9.3 Gross Findings

They are mainly located between the leaves of the broad ligament (see Chap. 31).

The tumors are unilateral, from 2 to 20 cm. They have regular contours, sometimes bosselated.

They are either solid or solid and cystic.

15.10 Rete Cysts and Tumors

15.10.1 Embryological Definition of Rete Ovary [2], (See Chap. 1)

At the stage of the indifferent gonad, gonadal cords extend into the medulla, where they branch into the medulla.

In males, the rete testis becomes continuous with 15–20 mesonephric tubules that become efferent ductules. These ductules are connected with the mesonephric duct, which becomes the duct of epididymis.

In females, gonadal cords do not become prominent, but they extend into the medulla and form a rudimentary rete ovarii.

15.10.2 Pathological Definition of Rete Cysts and Tumors

Rete cysts and tumors are located in the ovarian hilus.

They are lined by nonciliated epithelium and characterized by crevices along their inner surface and smooth muscle in their walls.

15.10.3 Gross Findings

They are usually unilocular, but may be multilocular, with a thin wall.

The content is clear fluid or more rarely mucoid.

15.11 Hamartomas

While hamartomas have been described in testes in androgen insensitivity syndrome [3], no case of ovarian hamartoma has been reported in the textbooks of Scully et al. [3] and Talerman [1].

A single personal case of ovarian hamartoma on US and MR is reported (Fig. 15.3). This hamartoma contained a high proportion of smooth muscle, a vascular component mainly of capillary type, and a thecal component. Should this case be classified as a variety of teratoma?

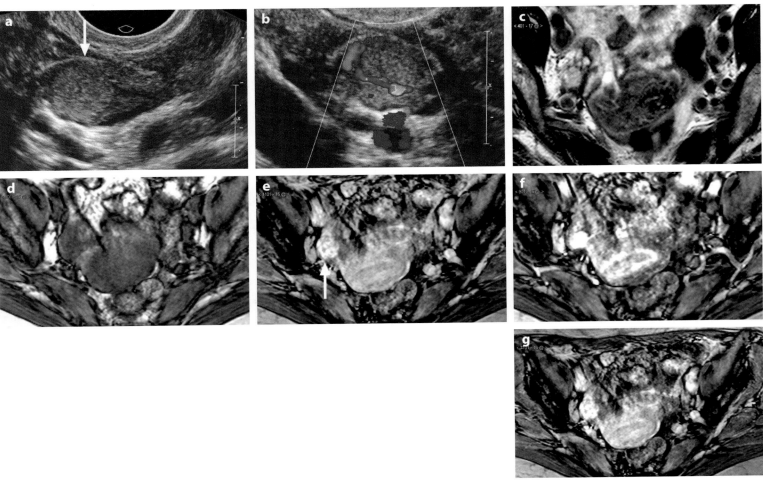

Fig. 15.3 Hamartoma of the right ovary. Sixty-year-old woman. Colic resection 14 years ago for carcinoma. Right pelvic pain. EVS of the right ovary (**a**) depicts a round mass (*arrow*) of 1.5 cm in diameter; the mass has an echogenicity slightly superior to normal ovarian parenchyma. On color Doppler (**b**) a peripheral and central vascularization is depicted. On MR axial T2 (**c**) the mass has a homogeneous signal more intense than the normal ovary. On DMR without injection (**d**) and at the arterial phase (**e**) no vessel is visualized but a high contrast uptake (*arrow*) suggesting the possibility of an endocrine tumor, with an increase in contrast uptake at the venous phase (**f**) and on the delayed (**g**). Prospective diagnosis: endocrine tumor. Pathology: hamartoma containing a high proportion **f** smooth muscle, a vascular component mainly of capillary type, and a thecal component

References

1. Talerman A (2002) Nonspecific tumors of the ovary, including mesenchymal tumors, and malignant lymphomas. In: Blaustein's pathology of the female genital tract, 15th edn. Springer, New York, pp 1035–1061, Chap 21
2. More KL, Persaud TVN (2008) The developing human; clinically oriented embryology, 8th edn. Saunders, Philadelphia, pp 243–284, Chap 12
3. Scully RE, Young RH, Clement PB (1998) Miscellaneous primary tumors. In: Tumors of the ovary, maldeveloped gonad, fallopian tube, and broad ligament. Armed Forces Institute of Pathology, Washington, DC, pp 313–334, Chap 17

Peritoneum

Part 3

Diseases of the Peritoneum

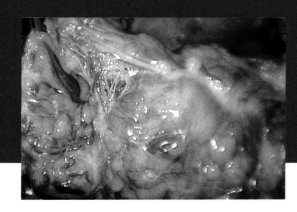

Contents

16.1 Inflammatory Lesions

16.1.1 Acute Peritonitis

Acute diffuse peritonitis is characterized by serosal fibrinopurulent exudates. It is most commonly associated with a perforated viscus. Rare infectious causes include candida and actinomycetes.

Localized acute peritonitis may be secondary to appendicitis (Fig. 16.1), sigmoiditis (Figs. 16.2 and 16.3), or can be associated with PID (Fig. 16.4).

16.1.2 Granulomatous Peritonitis

16.1.2.1 Tuberculous Peritonitis

Tuberculous peritonitis, which is increasing in incidence, particularly among immunosuppressed patients, may be secondary to spread from a focus within the abdominopelvic cavity or be a manifestation of miliary spread.

The granulomas are characterized by caseous necrosis and Langhans giant cells; mycobacteria may be demonstrated by acid-fast stains or immunofluorescence methods.

There are several reports that point out to uncertainty in the preoperative diagnosis of peritoneal tuberculosis and advanced ovarian cancer [1–6]:

(a) Clinical findings: PT presents with nonspecific findings and symptoms such as ascites and pelvic and abdominal pain and mass, and hence mimic ovarian cancer. Progression of PT often takes months or even years.

(b) CA125 is elevated with a median of 331 IU/ml (41–560) in BILGIN's series [1].

J.N. Buy, M. Ghossain, *Gynecological Imaging*,
DOI 10.1007/978-3-642-31012-6_16, © Springer-Verlag Berlin Heidelberg 2013

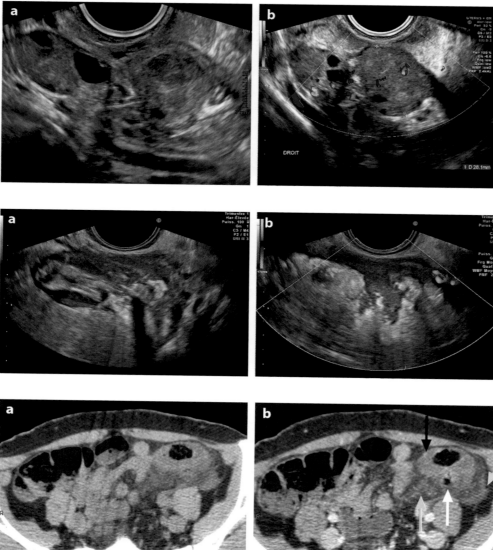

Fig. 16.1 Appendicular perforation complicated with localized peritonitis. EVS (**a**) and color Doppler (**b**) display a normal right ovary and medially a localized peritonitis

Fig. 16.2 Perforation of a sigmoid diverticulum complicated with sigmoiditis. (**a**) Sigmoid diverticulum. (**b**) Thickening of the mesosigmoid associated with echogenic peritoneal fluid, related to a localized peritonitis

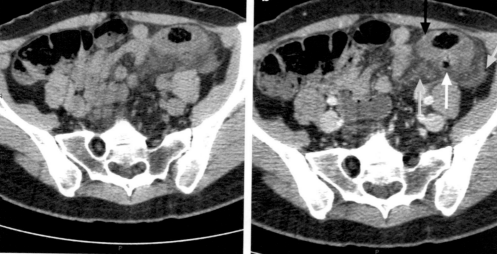

Fig. 16.3 Sigmoid diverticulum perforation complicated with sigmoiditis and peritoneal inflammatory reaction. Forty-three-year-old woman. Acute left pelvic pain. Increased white cell count 12,000/ml, CRP 113. CT without (**a**) and with IV contrast (**b**) displays (1) a thickening of the sigmoid wall (*black arrow*), (2) a perforated diverticulum (*white arrow*), and (3) an inflammatory reaction of the mesosigmoid (*yellow arrows*)

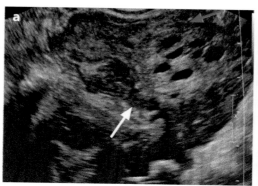
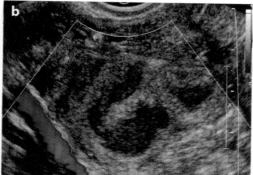

Fig. 16.4 Peritonitis complicated with left pyosalpinx following an appendicitis with peritonitis operated 10 days before (with right salpingectomy). Recurrence of fever, right pelvic pain, white cell count 19,000/ml CRP 48. EVS (**a**) depicts an inflammatory involvement of the right iliac fossa around the lateral face of the right ovary (*red arrow*) with peritoneal fluid related to a recurrence of peritonitis (*white arrow*). Transverse view of the left iliac fossa (**b**) displays a left pyosalpinx.

Fig. 16.4 (*continued*) CT without (**c**) and with injection (**d**) depicts a huge abscess of the right iliac fossa (*black arrow*), extending to the anterior abdominal wall (*yellow arrow*), encasing small bowel loops, a left pyosalpinx (*white arrow*), an abscess in the Douglas (*red arrow*) with pelvic peritonitis

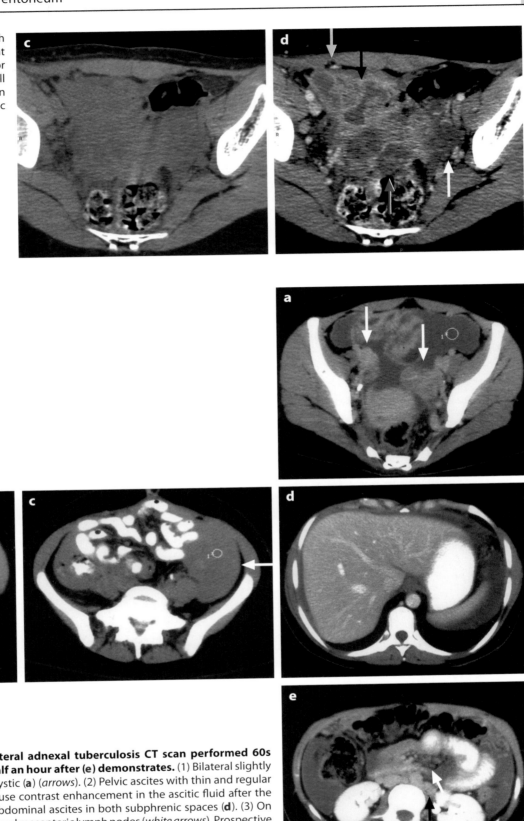

Fig. 16.5 Peritoneal tuberculosis with bilateral adnexal tuberculosis CT scan performed 60s after contrast (a), 4 min after (b, c, d), and half an hour after (e) demonstrates. (1) Bilateral slightly enlarged ovaries which look on the left multicystic (**a**) (*arrows*). (2) Pelvic ascites with thin and regular thickening of the peritoneum (**b**) (*arrow*). Diffuse contrast enhancement in the ascitic fluid after the delayed sequence is remarkable (**c**) (*arrow*). Abdominal ascites in both subphrenic spaces (**d**). (3) On (**e**), slightly enlarged lomboaortic (*black arrow*) and mesenteric lymph nodes (*white arrows*). Prospective diagnosis: Association of these different findings raised preoperatively the diagnosis of bilateral ovarian tumors with peritoneal metastases. Definite diagnosis: bilateral TB of the adnexae with peritonitis. The smooth pattern of the peritoneum without any focus or nodule or plaque and the pattern of the ovaries should have suggested the possibility of peritoneal tuberculosis

(c) US of PT with female genital tract tuberculosis: adnexal masses, adhesions, and septate or particulate ascites. Omental and peritoneal thickening can also be seen.

(d) CT (Figs. 16.5 and 16.6): smooth peritoneum with minimal thickening and pronounced enhancement suggests peritoneal tuberculosis, whereas nodular implants and irregular thickening

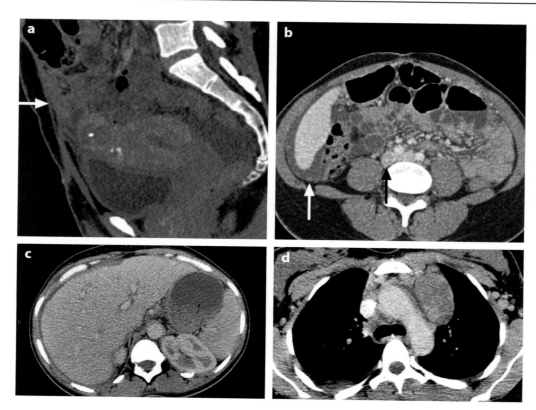

Fig. 16.6 Peritoneal tuberculosis. Thirty-year-old woman VIH+. CT after injection displays: (**a**) ascites in the Douglas and thickening of the greater omentum (*arrow*); (**b**) ascites of the subhepatic space, with thickening of the peritoneum (*white arrow*), lomboaortic lymph nodes, one of these with a necrotic center (*black arrow*); (**c**) ascites in the right subphrenic space; (**d**) the mediastinum: huge adenopathies. Prospective diagnosis: Association of the peritoneal lesions with the necrotic lomboaortic mediastinal lymph node suggested the diagnosis of TB. Fine-needle aspiration of the ascetic fluid confirmed the diagnosis of tuberculosis

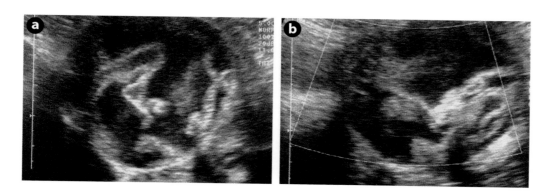

Fig. 16.7 Retained surgical sponge with abscess. Fifty-two-year-old woman, operated from perforation of the splenic flexure during colonoscopy a year before. Pelvic pain and dysuria. US without (**a**) and with color Doppler (**b**) depicts in the vesicouterine pouch a 6-cm round cystic mass with adhesion to the sigmoid containing an echogenic structure suggesting a retained sponge. Around the mass, thickening of the peritoneum suggests an abscess. Surgery confirms the diagnosis of abscess around the sponge, associated with adhesion to small bowel loops and localized inflammation of the peritoneum

suggest peritoneal carcinomatosis; however, peritoneal implants have also been observed in tuberculosis [1]. Omental and mesenteric thickening were demonstrated in all patients in BILGIN's series [1]. Extensive adhesions can cause bowel obstruction. Para-aortic lymph nodes can be present.

(e) MR: usually, the peritoneum is regular and thin, with a miliary diffusion.

(f) Laparotomy is usually performed in the preoperative presumptive diagnosis of adnexal ovarian cancer. A rather pathognomonic picture of miliary tuberculosis with peritoneal thickening, omental cake formation, and adhesions are discovered throughout the peritoneal cavity.

16.1.2.2 Noninfectious

Foreign material (Fig. 16.7), sebaceous material, and keratin from ruptured dermoid cyst, spillage of amniotic fluid at caesarean section can produce a granulomatous peritonitis.

16.2 Tumor-Like Lesions

16.2.1 Peritoneal Inclusion Cysts

Peritoneal pseudocyst occurs in different circumstances, all of them related to peritoneal adhesions: (1) after pelvic surgery, (2) after PID, and (3) after endometriosis.

Definition [7].

It is defined histologically by an inner sheet of peritoneal flat cells of mesothelial type.

These cells usually secrete clear fluid responsible for the development of the cyst. But in some circumstances, different kinds of fluid may be encountered.

Table 16.1 Surgical and radiologic findings of peritoneal inclusion cysts

Common
Size: usually between 4 and 10 cm
Mainly or exclusively cystic
Wall and septa thin and regular (loose fibrovascular connective tissue)
Solid tissue can be present(related to inflammatory tissue)
Usually not round, conforming to surrounding structures
Lying against the peritoneum
Most commonly multilocular, may be unilocular
Adhesions to surrounding structures vey common(bladder, sigmoid)
Uncommon
May resemble simple free peritoneal fluid
Small papillae present(exceptionally)

The surgical and radiologic findings are reported in Table 16.1.

16.2.1.1 US, CT, and MR Findings

1. Unilocular cystic mass

   The wall is thin and regular, without papillary projection. Its shape can be round or oval. Content of the cyst is usually clear fluid, anechoic, of a density close to 0 UH, with a signal close to urine on T1 and T2. Close relationship with the peritoneum can suggest the diagnosis.

   However, differential diagnosis may include other differential diagnosis of unilocular cystic masses, particularly functional ovarian cyst, ovarian serous cystadenoma, paraovarian cyst, and hydrosalpinx.

2. Multilocular pattern: the multilocular peritoneal inclusion cyst (MPICs) (Figs. 16.8 and 16.9).

   (a) The characteristic overall shape of the mass is not round, conforming to the surrounding structures, encasing the ovary (which either looks normal or may contain large follicles related to some degree of ovaritis), and in direct relationship with the parietal and visceral.

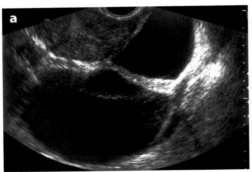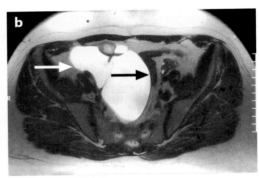

Fig. 16.8 Inclusion peritoneal cyst: multilocular form. Forty-year-old woman; right adnexectomy 3 years before. EVS (**a**) displays a multilocular collection, with a regular wall and septa. MR axial T2 (**b**) depicts and confirms the data concerning the shape and the structure of the collection and visualizes in its anterior part some tissue (which was inflammatory at pathology); MR precisely defined the topography of the mass, which follows the posterior, lateral (*white arrow*), anterior parietal peritoneum, and medially the sigmoid (*black arrow*). These relationships with the peritoneum are characteristic for inclusion peritoneal cyst

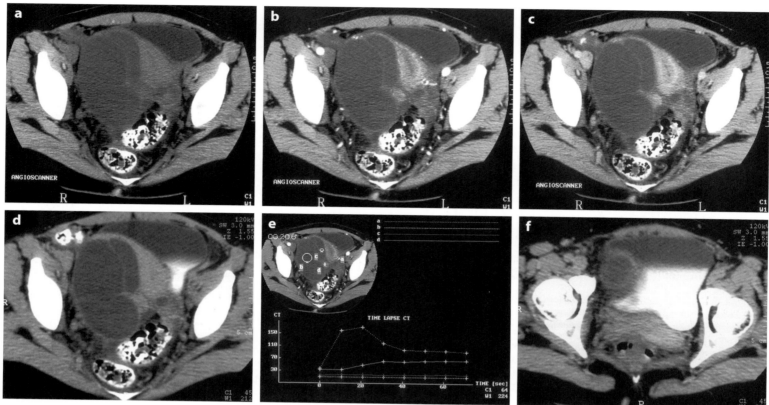

Fig. 16.9 Forty-year-old women. Right ovariectomy 2 years ago. A right pelvic collection is found at physical examination, which is confirmed on ultrasound. DCT without injection (**a**) at the arterial phase (**b**) at the venous phase (**c**) and on the delayed (**d**) display a right multiloculated cystic pelvic mass. The wall and the septa are thin and regular without any papillary projection. The mass is in contact with the parietal peritoneum, pushes forward the right tube and the uterus to the left seems adherent to the mesosig- moid. On the ROC curve (**e**) no contrast uptake is visualized in the center of the mass, while a slight contrast uptake is visualized in the wall. At a lower level (**f**) adhesion to the bladder wall is displayed; a previous surgery, the morphologic findings of the collection, adhesions to the neighbouring organs are very suggestive of peritoneal inclusion cyst, which was confirmed at surgery

   (b) The different loculi can be of the same or of different natures, separated by thin and regular septae. Regular vessels in the wall and in the septa can be displayed.

   When a tissular portion is present, it looks regular with absence of tumoral vessel.

   (c) Although definite diagnosis of adhesions is difficult to assess, asymmetrical deformation of a full bladder and a close and identical relationship to contiguous organs according to different positions of the patient are very suggestive.

   (d) The pelvic ureter may be surrounded by fibrosis, resulting in a partial obstruction.

3. Collection resembling simple free peritoneal fluid (Fig. 16.10). The only way to make the diagnosis is for the patient to change from position and to display exactly the same topography of the fluid in the peritoneal cavity (Fig. 16.11).

4. Uncommon particular form containing small papillae (Figs. 16.12 and 16.13).

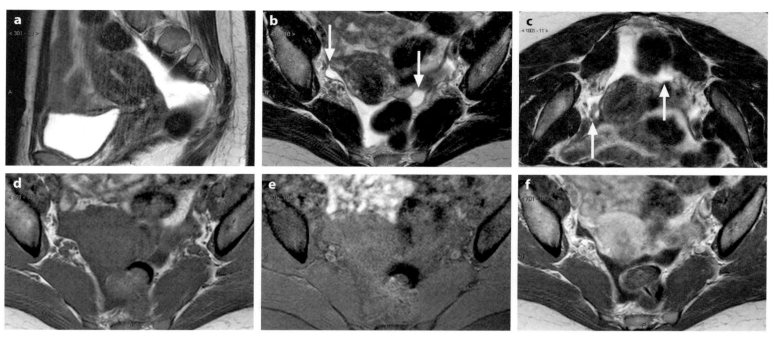

Fig. 16.10 Peritoneal inclusion cyst: interest of the prone position. Forty-year-old woman operated from appendicular peritonitis 4 years ago. Two months ago, an abscess in contact to the anterior border of the right ovary was drained, but a posterior collection was left. MR with sagittal T2 (**a**) and Axial T2 in supine position (**b**) posterior peritoneal collection between the rectum and the posterior part of the uterus and the broad ligaments (*arrows*), which resembles free peritoneal fluid. Because of the previous clinical history, a prone position is performed. Axial T2 in prone position (**c**) The relationships of the peritoneal effusion with the pelvic structures do not change (*arrows*), allowing to make the diagnosis of a peritoneal inclusion cyst. Axial T1 (**d**) and fat suppression (**e**). Content of the collection is watery. After injection (**f**). This collection has a very thin wall with no contrast uptake

Fig. 16.11 Peritoneal inclusion cyst secondary to PID. Thirty seven years old woman. Left pyosalpinx diagnosed at coeliscopy 4 years before. Infertility. EVS (**a**) displays a right pelvic multiloculated cystic extraovarian mass, which is not of round shape, containing anechoic fluid, with regular and thin septa. Transversal EVS (**b**) shows that the mass encases the normal right ovary (*arrow*) and extends along the pelvic wall anteriorly and posteriorly

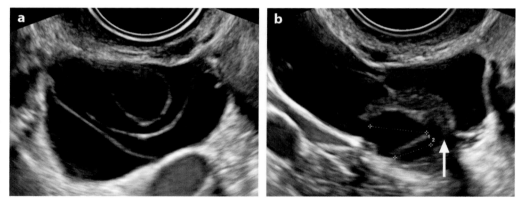

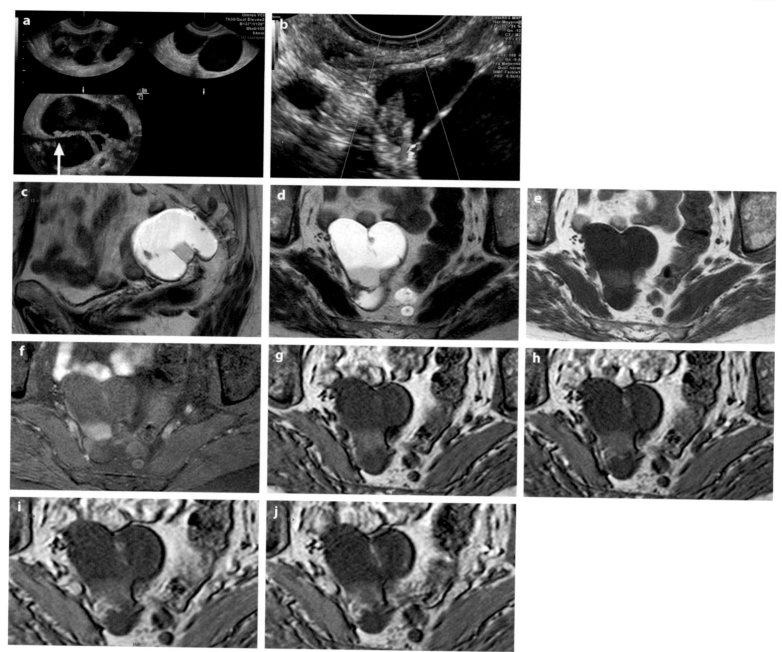

Fig. 16.12 Multilocular peritoneal pseudocyst with papillary projections. Seventy-one-year-old woman operated 50 years ago from left unilateral ovariectomy and 1 year before from endometrial carcinoma. During the follow-up, a routine EVS examination is performed. EVS with 3D reformation (**a**) displays a multiloculated right and posterior pelvic mass which is not round in close relationship with the parietal peritoneum, suggesting an extraovarian mass. Multiple endocystic papillary projections (*arrow*), some of them with color flow, are displayed (**b**). A preoperative diagnosis of hydrosalpinx was proposed. On MR examination, on sagittal T2 (**c**) and axial T2 (**d**), the shape of the mass confirms the impression of an extraovarian origin.

Liquids of different signals with a posterior one containing a high signal on t1 (**e**) and fat suppression (**f**) are displayed. DMR without injection (**g**) at the arterial phase (**h**) at the venous phase (**i**) and on the delayed (**j**) is performed. At the arterial phase, contrast uptake is visualized in papillary projection which slightly increases at the venous phase and persists on the delayed. These findings wrongly suggest the possibility of either papillary projections in a hydrosalpinx or in an ovarian mass. At surgery, a subperitoneal collection was resected. At pathology, a peritoneal inclusion cyst containing multiple papillary projections was diagnosed

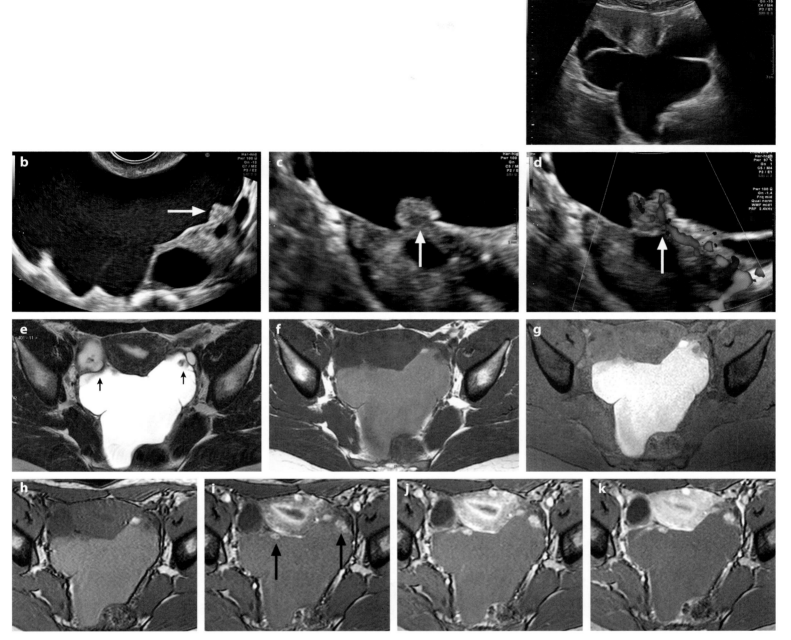

Fig. 16.13 Peritoneal inclusion cyst with papillary projections. Simulating a papillary surface serous tumor. Forty-four-year-old woman. Previous polymyomectomy 4 years ago. For some months, abdominal swelling. Pelvic mass at clinical examination. Transverse TAS (**a**) displays a collection in the Douglas, which follows the lateral walls of the pelvis. Transverse EVS (**b**) shows an echogenic collection, with papillary projection (*white arrow*) at the surface of the left ovary. Transverse EVS (**c**) of the right ovary also displays a papillary projection (*arrow*), forming an obtuse angle with the surface of the ovary; on color Doppler (**d**), a large vessel penetrates at its base (*arrow*). MR axial T2 (**e**) depicts a large posterior collection, with

papillary projections at the surface of both ovaries (*arrows*) and against the posterior face of the uterus. On MR axial T1 (**f**) and on fat suppression (**g**) the liquid has a high signal suggesting either hemorrhage of a high protein content. On DMR without injection (**h**) and at the arterial phase (**i**) depict vessels in the papillary projections (*arrows*), with a high contrast uptake at the venous phase (**j**) and on the delayed (**k**), associated with a high contrast uptake on the right parietal peritoneum. Prospective diagnosis: surface borderline tumor. Surgery: A subperitoneal inclusion peritoneal cyst encasing and hiding both adnexae is displayed. Resection of the collection and bilateral adnexectomy. Microscopy: benign peritoneal inclusion cyst

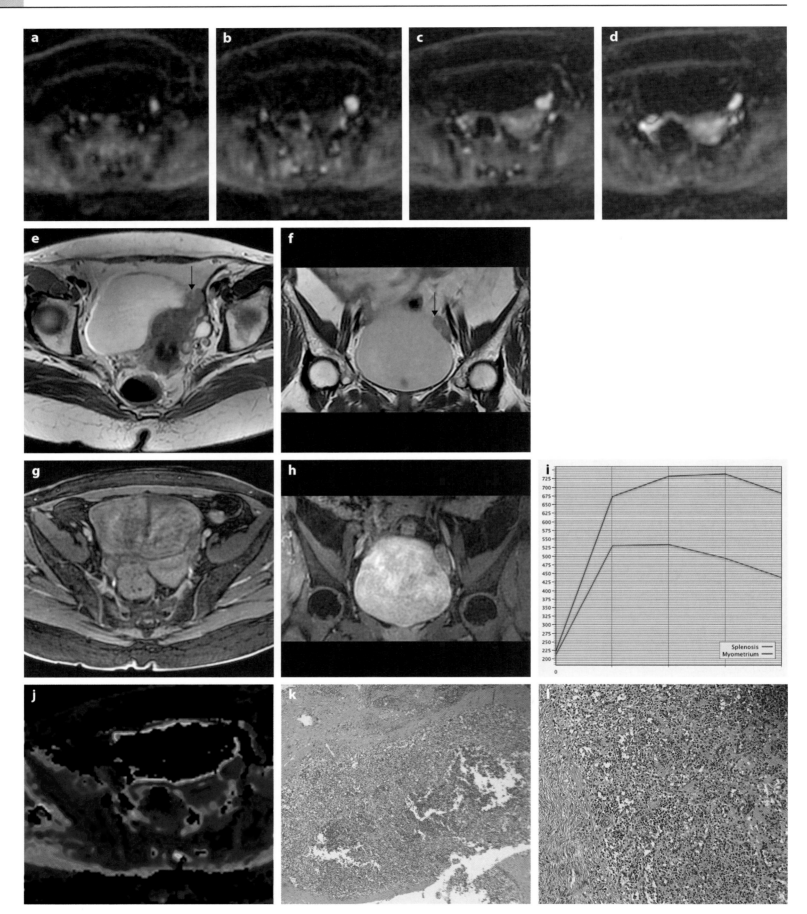

Fig. 16.14 Splenosis of the mesosalpinx (a–d). DW images at b1000 nicely display several adjacent hyperintense lesions of the fallopian tube. (**e**, **f**) On T2W axial and coronal images these lesions (arrows) are seen with an intermediate signal between pelvic mucles and adipose tissue. (**g–i**) Axial DMR at the late phase followed by similar coronal sequence, with time intensity curves, show the lesion to have a contrast uptake lower than that of myometrium and very close to that of endometrium. (**j**) ADC map at b1000 showed an ADC of 0.76×10^{-3} mm²/s. A fallopian tube tumor or malignant peritoneal implants were suspected. (**k**, **l**) Laparotomy and histology revealed splenosis of the mesosalpinx. Anamnesis revealed past splenectomy for trauma

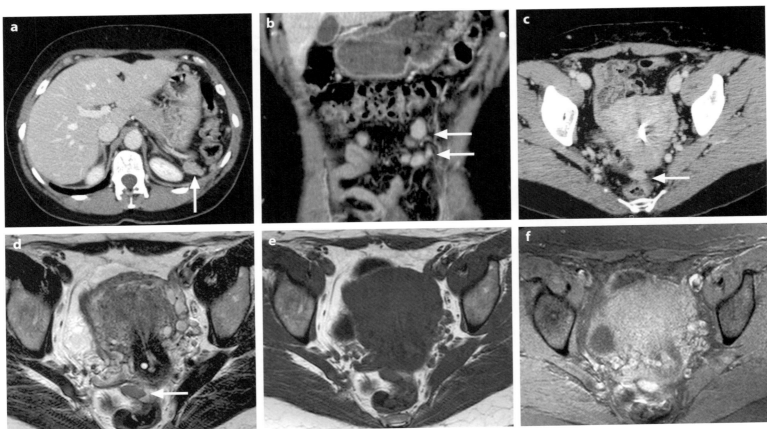

Fig. 16.15 Splenosis. Forty-nine-year-old woman. Splenectomy after trauma with rupture of the spleen 20 years ago. During a routine US examination, splenic nodules in the peritoneum particularly in the Douglas and on the greater omentum have been seen. CT after contrast (**a**) a round nodule is visualized in the posterior part of the lodge of splenectomy (*arrow*). On coronal reformation (**b**), multiple nodules with the same density are depicted in the omentum (*arrows*). A nodule of the same type is depicted in the Douglas (**c**) (*arrow*). On MR axial T2 (**d**) axial T1 (**e**) and fat suppression (**f**) the nodule in the Douglas (*arrow* in **d**) appears with a signal intensity close to myometrium on T2 and on the other sequences

16.2.2 Splenosis (Figs. 16.14 and 16.15)

Definition: Implantation of splenic tissue on the peritoneum after splenectomy.

A few to innumerable peritoneal nodules, ranging from punctuate to 7 cm in diameter, are scattered widely throughout the abdominal and less the peritoneal cavity [7].

The intraoperative appearance may mimic endometriosis, benign or malignant vascular tumors, or metastatic cancer [7].

Accessory spleen uncommonly in the pelvis can be displayed (Fig. 16.16).

16.3 Mesothelial Neoplasms

The classification of mesothelial neoplasms is reported in Table 16.2.

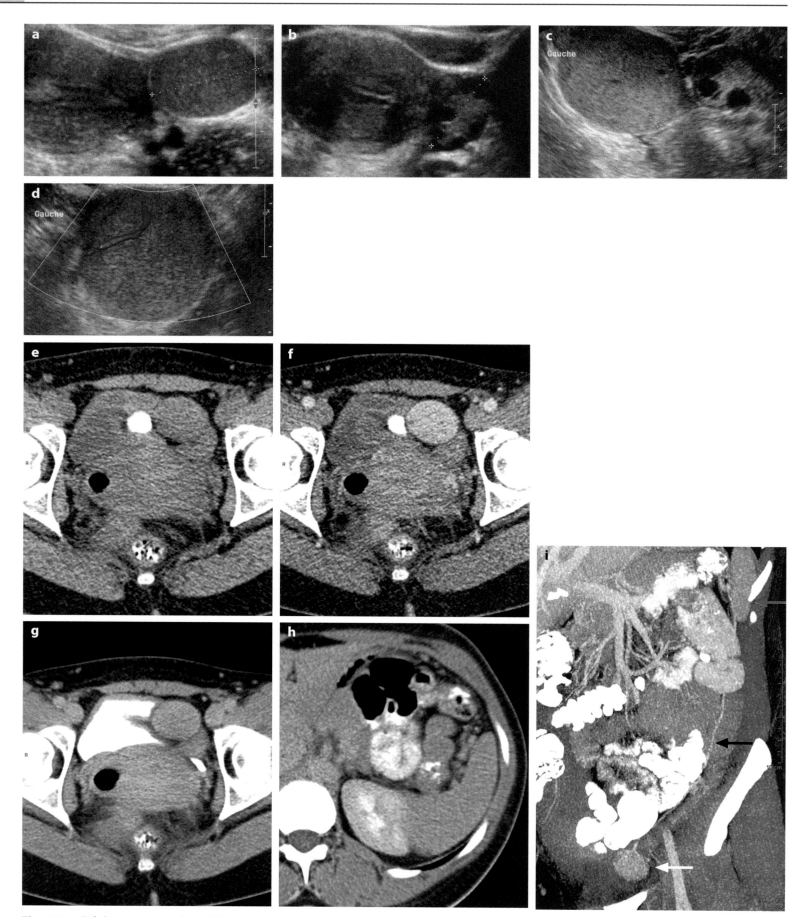

Fig. 16.16 Pelvic accessory spleen. EVS (**a–c**) displays a round echogenic homogeneous mass, separated from the uterus in (**a**) and from the ovary in (**b, c**) containing vessels on color Doppler (**d**). DCT without injection (**e**) and at the arterial phase (**f**) display a round mass with an early and homogeneous contrast uptake; on the delayed (**g**), contrast uptake is identical to the spleen (**h**). CT with oblique coronal reformation and MIP (**i**) depicts the accessory spleen (*white arrow*) related by a cord (*black arrow*) to the lower pole of the spleen (*red arrow*). Prospective diagnosis: pelvic accessory spleen. Coelioscopy confirmed the diagnosis

Table 16.2 Classification of mesothelial neoplasms

Type	Macroscopy	Microscopy
Localized		
1. Solitary fibrous tumor	Localized mass	Submesothelial Fibroblast proliferation
2. Adenomatoid tumor	Localized mass	Mesothelial proliferation
Diffuse		
1. Well-differentiated papillary mesothelioma	Papillary or nodular, less than 2 cm	A single layer of flattened or cuboidal mesothelial cells
2. Low-grade cystic mesothelioma	Multicystic	Atypical mesothelial cells
3. Diffuse malignant mesothelioma	Nodules and plaques on the parietal and visceral peritoneum; viscera often encased, may be invaded	Tubulopapillary and solid patterns Invasion of subperitoneal tissues Mild degrees of nuclear atypicality, mitotic figures

16.3.1 Localized Neoplasms

16.3.1.1 Solitary Fibrous Tumor

Definition: Proliferation of submesothelial fibroblasts.
Macroscopic findings are the usual findings of a fibroma.

16.3.1.2 Adenomatoid Tumors

Their origin is presumed to be from the cells of the serosal mesothelium. Microscopically, they are composed of multiple small slitlike or ovoid spaces lined by a single layer of low cuboidal or flattened epithelia-like cells [7].

The tumor can resemble a leiomyoma. Continuity with the overlying mesothelium is occasionally seen.

The main findings are reported in Table 16.3.

Immunostaining is positive for mesothelial markers as cytokeratine, vimentine, and calretinin.

Table 16.3 Findings in adenomatoid tumors

1. **Location**:
   Subserous cornual myometrium
   Tube
   Ovary (hilum)
   Peritoneum
2. **Size**
   – Usually small, 1–2 cm
   – May be larger
3. **Pathology**
   – Collagen, elastic tissue, smooth muscle surround the epithelial elements
   – Smooth muscle can be so predominant that the tumor can resemble a leiomyoma
   – Rarely the cystic spaces are sufficiently large to give a macroscopic pattern of cystic or multilocular mass

16.3.2 Diffuse Neoplasms

16.3.2.1 Well-Differentiated Mesothelioma

Eighty per cent occur in women during reproductive age year.
History of asbestos exposure is possible.
Definition [7]:
1. The fibrous papillae are covered by a single layer of flattened to cuboidal cells.
2. The nuclear features are bland, and mitotic figures absent.
3. The stroma can be extensively fibrotic.
   The main findings are reported in Table 16.4.

Table 16.4 Well-differentiated papillary mesothelioma

1. Aspect: solid nodules less than 2 cm; psammoma bodies uncommon
   Number: usually multiple
2. Location: mainly pelvic peritoneum and omentum
3. Ascites uncommon
4. Pleura and pericardium involvement possible

Table 16.5 Low-grade cystic mesothelioma

1. Aspect: commonly often multicystic, grapelike clusters, serous fluid
   Septa of variable thickness
   Uncommonly unilocular
2. Location: cul-de-sac, in contact with uterus, ovary, and rectum
   May extend in the abdominal cavity
   Multifocality possible
3. Ascites absent
4. Pleura and pericardium: absence of involvement
5. Follow-up
   50 % of recurrences 1–27 years after diagnosis
   Malignant transformation possible

16.3.2.2 Low-Grade Cystic Mesothelioma [7, 8]

Definition: In contrast to MPICs, cysts are lined, at least focally by markedly atypical mesothelial cells with hyperchromatic, pleomorphic nuclei.

The main findings are reported in Table 16.5.

A case of low-grade cystic mesothelioma is reported (Fig. 16.17).

16.3.2.3 Diffuse Malignant Mesothelioma [9]

Diffuse malignant mesotheliomas of the peritoneum are much less common than those of the pleura and account for 10–20 % of all mesotheliomas.

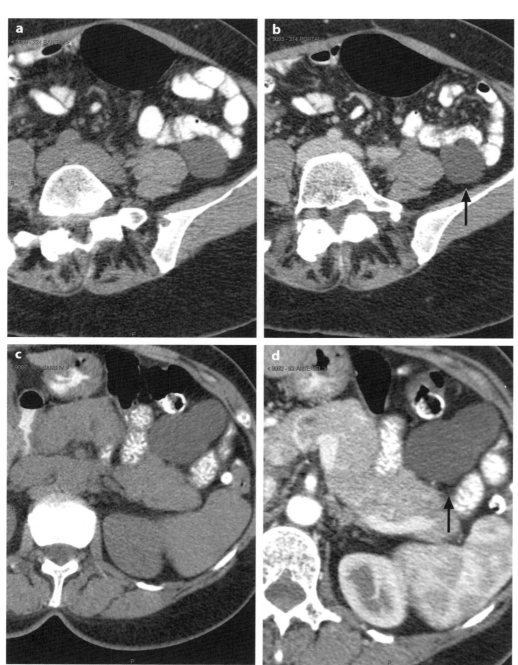

Fig. 16.17 Recurrence of low-grade cystic mesothelioma. Fifty-year-old woman operated 4 years ago from a low-grade cystic mesothelioma. During the follow-up, US examination discovers peritoneal collections. CT without (**a**) and after injection at the venous phase (**b**) shows a peritoneal collection (*arrow*) with a thin wall at the level of the left iliac crest. CT without (**c**) and at the arterial phase (**d**) shows in the left subphrenic space the same type of collection (*arrow*)

One third of patients are women.

Eighty per cent of patients have a history of asbestos exposure.

Definition [7]:

Epithelial cells are arranged in tubulopapillary and solid patterns.

The tumor cells retain some resemblance with mesothelial cells with a cuboidal shape and eosinophilic cytoplasm; mild to moderate nuclear atypicality, variably prominent nucleoli, and mitotic figures are present.

Sarcomatoid and biphasic may occur.

Immunochemistry: positivity for cytokeratins 5 and 7, calretinin.

The main findings are reported in Table 16.6.

Table 16.6 Diffuse malignant mesothelioma

1. Aspect:
Pattern:
Diffuse: plaques and nodules
Localized: focal masses
Homogeneous or with necrotic or cystic changes
Striking desmoplastic reaction in some cases
Invasion of subperitoneal tissues
Calcification rare
2. Location: visceral and parietal peritoneum
3. Viscera: often encased by the tumor
May be invaded
4. Ascites: generalized or localized
5. Pleura: calcified pleural plaques, thickening and masses can be present

Malignant mesothelioma may

1. Infiltrate the small bowel mesentery, thickening the leaves of the mesentery and producing a pleated or stellate appearance; tumor infiltration fixates the small bowel, straightening the course of the mesenteric vessels.
2. Extend to the visceral peritoneum of the small bowel, giving to the small bowel wall a thickened appearance [10].

Nodal metastases are rare. Therefore, the presence of lymph node enlargement in a patient with diffuse peritoneal disease suggests another etiology, such as peritoneal carcinomatosis, lymphomatosis, or tuberculous peritonitis.

Differential Diagnosis

1. Adenocarcinoma with diffuse peritoneal involvement.
2. Primary peritoneal adenocarcinoma with secondary ovarian involvement.

16.4 Metastatic Tumors

16.4.1 Metastatic Tumors of Ovarian Tumors

See Chap. 9.

16.4.2 Metastatic Tumors of Extraovarian Tumors
(Figs. 16.18 and 16.19)

Tumors other than ovarian tumors, particularly of the gastrointestinal tract, may spread to the peritoneum.

16.4.3 Pseudomyxoma Peritonei

See Chap. 9 Sect. 9.4.2.3.

16.5 Other Diseases of the Peritoneum

16.5.1 Lesions of the Secondary Mullerian System

Endometriosis, endosalpingiosis, endocervicosis, mullerianosis
They are developed from the pelvic peritoneum and the subjacent mesenchyma (see Chap. 17).

16.5.2 Primary Serous Carcinoma of the Peritoneum (PSCP)

Definition: Widespread peritoneal tumor associated with ovaries of normal size and shape, with normal surface or involved in many cases by small surface implants.

Microscopic examination reveals no tumor of the ovaries or tumor confined to the surface epithelium of the ovaries or invading the underlying cortical stroma but less than 5×5 mm [11].

PSCP is also called by Feuer et al. [12] the "normal size ovary carcinoma syndrome.

The main differential diagnosis is the primary small ovarian carcinoma with peritoneal metastases (Fig. 9.63). In PSCP, on US, ovaries of normal size associated with ascites and peritoneal metastases can be displayed. Echogenic foci at the surface of the ovaries can be displayed which are very difficult to characterize as lesions on the peritoneum, lesions on the ovaries, or adjacent bowel loops. On CT and on MR, diffuse peritoneal disease with normal size ovaries is most commonly observed. Exceptionally, nodularities along the surface of normal-sized ovaries can be demonstrated.

Thoracic findings may be associated; they include cardiophrenic nodes and pleural effusion.

CA125 is elevated in all cases.

16.5.3 Extraovarian Abdominal Tumors Resembling Ovarian Tumors

A variety of extraovarian neoplasms resemble histologically and often clinically tumors of ovarian origin. These tumors include those that arise from the secondary Mullerian system, that is, the pelvic and lower abdominal mesothelium and subjacent mesenchyma.

Among these tumors, tumors of epithelial origin are the most frequent. Although the different subtypes can be encountered, the serous tumors are the most common.

Serous tumors may have two different presentations:

– Diffuse peritoneal involvement called the primary serous carcinoma of the peritoneum.
– Localized cystic mass.

16.5.3.1 Rare Extraovarian Serous Tumors

Rare extraovarian serous tumors occur as localized typically cystic masses usually within the broad ligament (see Chap. 31). These tumors can be benign, borderline, or malignant [11].

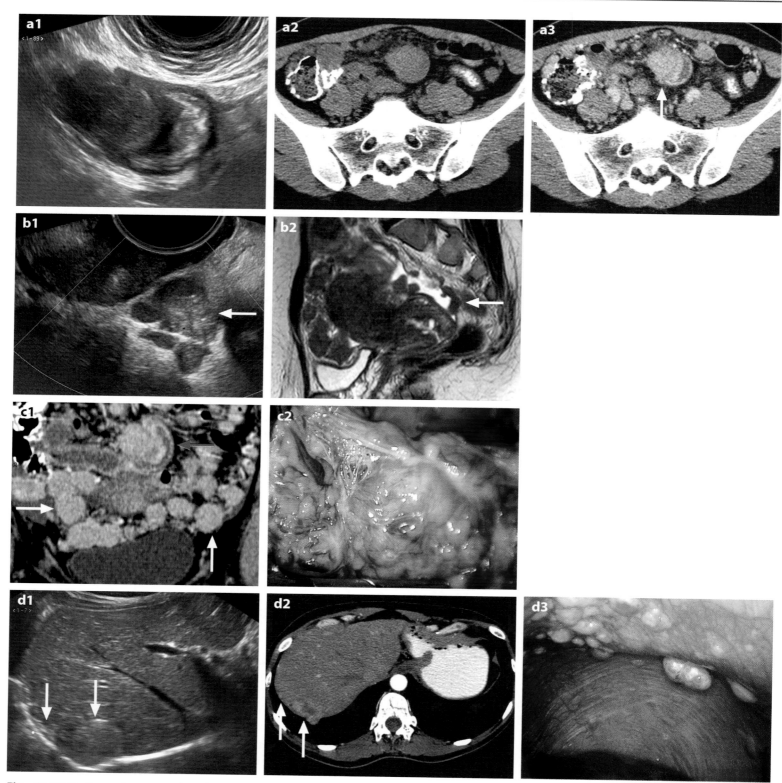

Fig. 16.18 Peritoneal metastasis of carcinoid tumor. Fifty-year-old woman. (1) Tumor of the small bowel US (**a1**) displays a round low echogenic mass in the anterior part of the small bowel. DCT without injection (**a2**) and at the arterial phase (**a3**) confirms the presence of a tumor in the small bowel with an early and high contrast uptake, very suggestive of a tumor of endocrine type (*arrow*). (2) Implants in the Douglas are shown on US in (**b1**) (*arrow*) and confirmed on MR on sagittal T2 (**b2**). (3) Peritoneal metastasis. On CT with coronal reformation (**c1**) multiple hypervascularized nodules of the omentum (*white arrows*) with the tumor of small bowel (*red arrow*) are visualized and confirmed at coelioscopy (**c2**). (4) Liver metastasis is depicted on US (**d1**) (*arrow*). CT (**d2**) precise that the peritoneal metastasis involve the liver (*arrow*); one of them extends to the diaphragm (**d3**)

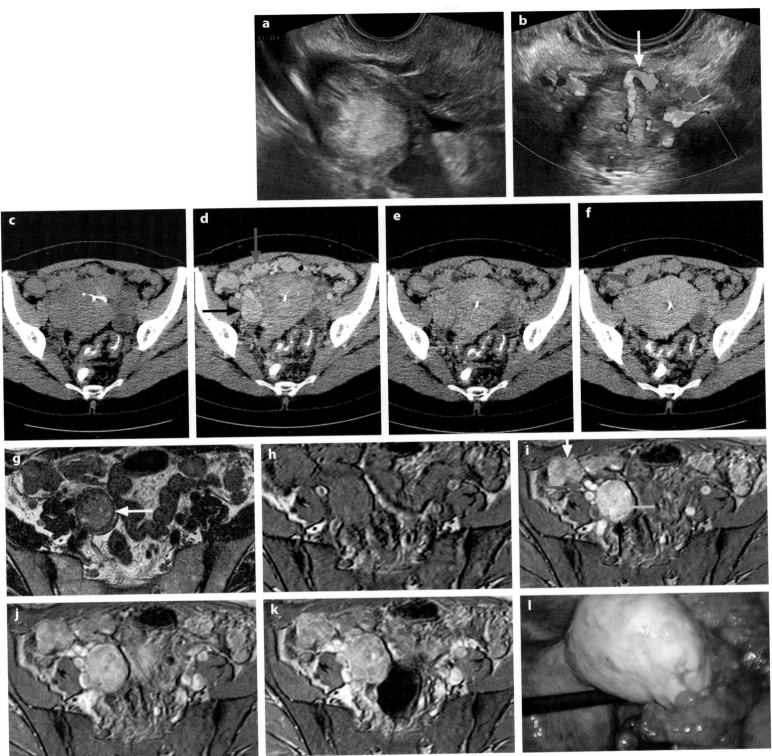

Fig. 16.19 Ovarian metastasis of carcinoid tumor. Fifty-year-old woman. Abdominal pain. EVS (**a**) displays a round well-delineated ovarian mass with an overall hyperechogenicity. On color Doppler (**b**), a large vascular pedicle (*arrow*) with central vessels is seen. DCT without injection (**c**) at the arterial phase (**d**) displays some vessels and overall an intense and homogeneous contrast uptake very suggestive of a tumor with a vascularization of endocrine type (*black arrow*); metastases in the omentum are shown (*red arrow*). At the venous phase (**e**) a washout is observed in the tumor which increases on the delayed (**f**). MR axial T2 (**g**) depicts a well-circumscribed ovarian mass with an intermediate signal surrounded by a low-intensity peripheral rim (*arrow*) pushing the normal ovarian parenchyma to the periphery. DMR without injection (**h**) and at the arterial phase (**i**) depicts large arterial pedicle (*red arrow*) regular arterial vessels mainly at the periphery of the mass (suggestive of ovarian metastasis) (*black arrow*) associated with an early and intense and relatively homogeneous contrast uptake very suggestive of an endocrine tumor (*yellow arrow*); metastasis to the omentum is seen (*white arrow*). As on DCT, an early washout is visualized at the venous phase (**j**), which increases on the delayed (**k**). Coelioscopy visualized (1) diffuse abdominopelvic peritoneal metastases, (2) a slightly enlarged right ovary (**l**), and (3) an ileal tumor (*arrow*). Peritoneal biopsies: microscopy and immunochemistry – peritoneal metastases of a carcinoid tumor (chromogranin positive), very likely of a small bowel tumor

16.5.3.2 Mucinous Tumors (Fig. 16.20)

Ovarian-type mucinous neoplasms, in the absence of a primary tumor within the ovary, have been described in extraovarian sites, typically in the retroperitoneum [11].

These tumors form large cystic masses that on histologic examination resemble ovarian mucinous tumors (benign, borderline, or malignant).

Although it is possible that some of these tumors originate within a supernumerary ovary, the great rarity of the latter, the absence of follicules or their derivatives within the ovarian-like stroma, and the rare occurrence of similar tumors in males strongly support a peritoneal origin.

An example of retroperitoneal sero-mucinous tumor is reported (Fig. 16.21).

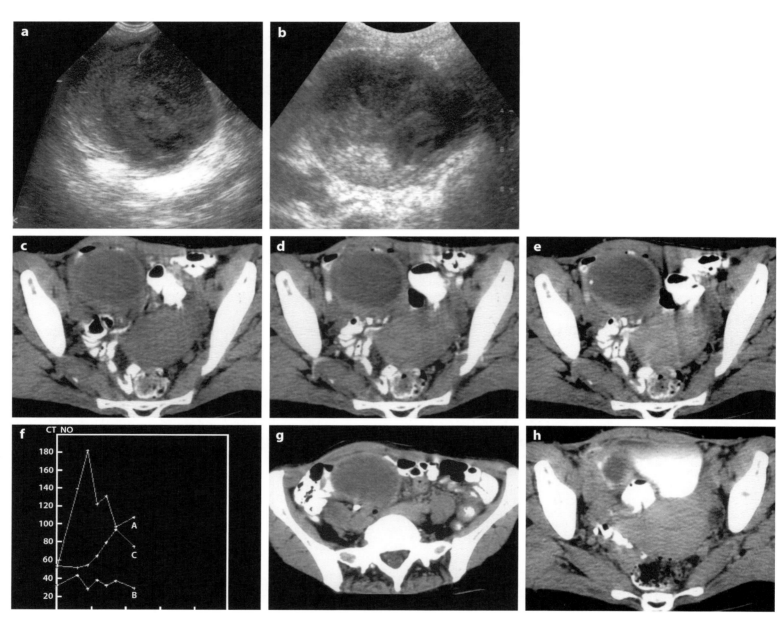

Fig. 16.20 Extraovarian mucinous tumor. Forty-nine-year-old woman with urinary incontinence and irregular menstrual cycle. EVS (**a, b**) right laterouterine pelvic mass, with a mixed echogenic pattern and a good ultrasound transmission: An ovarian mass of indeterminate nature is diagnosed. DCT: (**c**) (without contrast), (**d**) (arterial phase), (**e**) (1 mn after injection), (**f**) (dynamic curve) demonstrate a mass anterior to the right broad ligament, mainly cystic with a mass density of 30 HU and a thickened wall with a significant contrast uptake. Delayed CT (**g, h**) precise the topography of the mass lying in contact to the cecum (**g**), independent of the right ovary (**h**). At laparotomy: The mass is extraovarian, seems to be cecal in origin, developed independently from the appendix. Right hemicolectomy was performed. Pathology: cystic mass with a mucinous content. Primary borderline peritoneal mucinous tumor. Normal appendix

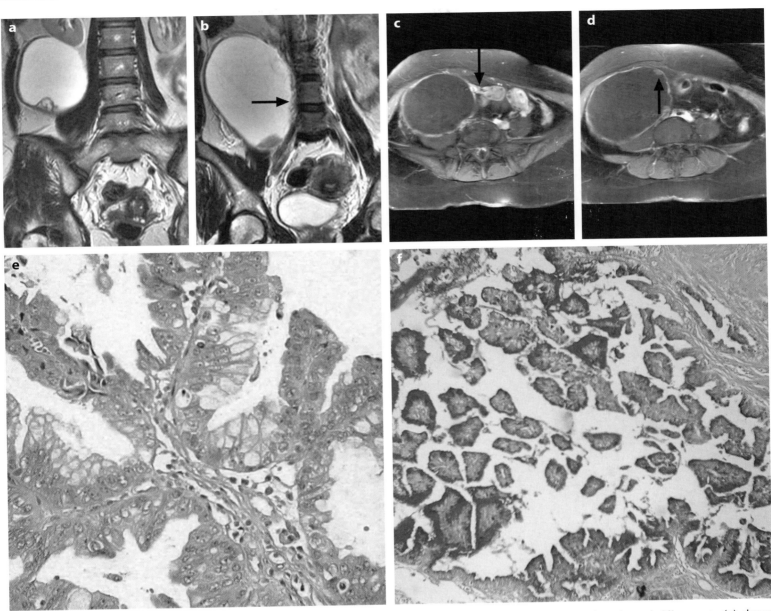

Fig. 16.21 Retroperitoneal sero-mucinous borderline cystadenoma. MR coronal T2 (**a**, **b**) display in (**a**) above the right iliac crest a cystic mass with little loculi at its lower pole and in (**b**) along its inner border small papillary projections (*arrow*). Axial T1 after injection (**c**, **d**) depicts in (**c**) that the mass is separated from the right ovary (*arrow*) and in (**d**) shows contrast enhancement in the papillary projections (*arrow*). Microscopy (**e**) shows papillary projections ;the cellular proliferation is pluristratified with a serous and a mucinous component. Coloration with PAS (**f**) depicts the mucinous epithelial cells

16.5.3.3 Extraovarian Brenner Tumors

Exceptional extraovarian Brenner tumors have been reported.

16.5.4 Leiomyomatosis

See Chap. 24.

References

1. Bilgin T et al (2001) Peritoneal tuberculosis with pelvic abdominal mass, ascites and elevated CA 125 mimicking advanced ovarian carcinoma: a series of 10 cases. Int J Gynecol Cancer 11(4):290–294

2. Yoshimura T, Okamura H (1987) Peritoneal tuberculosis with elevated serum CA 125 levels: a case report. Gynecol Oncol 28(3):342–344

3. Sheth SS (1996) Elevated CA 125 in advanced abdominal or pelvic tuberculosis. Int J Gynaecol Obstet 52(2):167–171

4. Rao GJ et al (1996) Abdominal tuberculosis or ovarian carcinoma: management dilemma associated with an elevated CA-125 level. Medscape Womens Health 1(4):2

5. Gurgan T et al (1993) Pelvic-peritoneal tuberculosis with elevated serum and peritoneal fluid Ca-125 levels. A report of two cases. Gynecol Obstet Invest 35(1):60–61

6. Groutz A, Carmon E, Gat A (1998) Peritoneal tuberculosis versus advanced ovarian cancer: a diagnostic dilemma. Obstet Gynecol 91(5 Pt 2):868

7. Clement PB (2002) Disease of the peritoneum, chapter 17. In: Blaustein's pathology of the female genital tract. Springer, New York, pp 729–789

8. Levy AD, Arnaiz J, Shaw JC et al (2008) Primary peritoneal tumors: imaging features with pathologic correlation. Radiographics 28: 583–607

9. Goldblum J, Hart WR (1995) Localized and diffuse mesotheliomas of the genital tract and peritoneum in women. A clinicopathologic study of nineteen true mesothelial neoplasms, other than adenomatoid tumors, multicystic mesotheliomas, and localized fibrous tumors. Am J Surg Pathol 19(10):1124–1137

10. Whitley NO, Brenner DE, Antman KH et al (1982) CT of peritoneal mesothelioma: analysis of eight cases. Am J Roentgenol 138:531–535

11. Scully RE, Young RH, Clement PB (1998) Tumors of the ovary, maldeveloped gonads, fallopian tubes and broad ligament, vol 3. Armed Forces Institute of Pathology, Washington, DC, pp 451–456, Chap 23

12. Feuer GA, Shevchuk M, Calanog A (1989) Normal -sized ovary carcinoma syndrome. Obstet Gynecol 73:786–792

Secondary Mullerian System

Part 4

Secondary Mullerian System

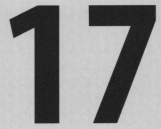

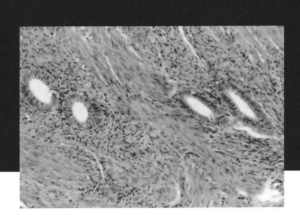

Contents

Anatomical definition: The secondary mullerian system is the pelvic and lower abdominal mesothelium and the subjacent mesenchyma [1, 2]. The mullerian potential of this layer is consistent with its close embryonic relation to the mullerian ducts that arise by invagination of the coelomic epithelium.

Pathological definition: The peritoneal lesions of the secondary mullerian system are characterized by:

1. Epithelial differentiation in serous, endometrioid, and mucinous epithelium, simulating normal or neoplastic tubal, endometrial, endocervical epithelium; (rarely differentiation in urothelial epithelium exemplified by Walthard nests).

2. Proliferation of the subjacent mesenchyme may accompany epithelial differentiation in endometrial stromal-type cells, decidua, or smooth muscle.

Lesions

Endometriosis

Endosalpingiosis

Endocervicosis

Extra-ovarian serous and mucinoustumors (see Chap. 16)

Leiomyomatosis (see Chap. 24)

17.1 Endometriosis

17.1.1 Microscopic Definition

Presence of endometrial epithelium and stroma in an ectopic site excluding the myometrium. Usually both epithelium and stroma are seen, but occasionally, the diagnosis can be made when only one component is present [3].

J.N. Buy, M. Ghossain, *Gynecological Imaging*,
DOI 10.1007/978-3-642-31012-6_17, © Springer-Verlag Berlin Heidelberg 2013

17.1.2 Introduction

1. Pelvic endometriosis is a common disease associated with a variety of symptoms principally pain and infertility. It is estimated to occur in 10 % of women of reproductive age [4]. This prevalence may be as high as 24.5 and 19.6 %, respectively, in patients undergoing laparoscopy for pelvic pain and infertility [5].
2. Endometriosis affects in more than 80 % of cases women in the reproductive age group, typically between 25 and 40 years of age [3]. Almost 10 % (8.5 %) of patients are adolescents [6] and less than 5 % postmenopausal [7].
3. Although classically this disease uses to have mainly gynecologic sites of implantations mainly ovaries, tubes, and peritoneum covering these organs, presentations have significantly changed these past years with tremendous increase in subperitoneal locations particularly GI tract locations mainly the rectum and sigmoid, so that this disease leads the patient to consult not only the gynecologist but also the gastroenterologist.
4. Considered classically as a benign disease, it can be very painful and disabling for the patient, can cause difficulties of dissection for the surgeon because of extensive adhesions, and in some cases, especially in cases of low rectal lesions, can lead to aggressive surgery [8, 9].

17.1.3 Pathology

17.1.3.1 Microscopic Findings

Typical

In reproductive-age woman, the typical appearance is one or more glands lined by endometrial epithelium, surrounded by a mantle of dense packed small fusiform cells with scanty cytoplasm and bland cytology, typical of nonneoplastic endometrial stromal cells.

Small blood vessels may be engorged. When seen in the ovary, endometriosis varies from microscopically dilated glands to grossly recognizable cysts, while in extra-ovarian sites cysts are less common to rare.

Unusual

1. Metaplastic glandular changes: These changes include ciliated, eosinophilic, hobnail, and rarely squamous and mucinous metaplasia (see Chap. 22.3.3).
2. Hyperplastic glandular changes: Hyperplastic changes similar to those occurring in the endometrium have been described in endometrial glands, sometimes related to an endogenous or exogenous estrogenic stimulus, or tamoxifen therapy. Hyperplastic changes are particularly common in cases of polypoid endometriosis. Such atypical changes have a malignant potential.
3. Stromal changes: The endometriotic stroma may undergo metaplasia, typically smooth muscle metaplasia, which is most often encountered in the wall of ovarian endometriotic cysts but occasionally elsewhere. Extensive amounts of smooth muscle within the endometriotic stroma can result in endomyometriosis.

17.1.3.2 The Appearance of Endometriotic Tissue Varies with Hormonal Changes and with the Location of the Disease

With Hormonal Changes

In reproductive age woman:

In approximately 80 % of patients, the endometriotic lesions show cyclic changes although considerable variability in glandular and epithelial cell morphology may be observed [10, 11].

Periodic menstrual changes within the endometriotic focus will result in histologic evidence of recent and remote hemorrhage within the endometriotic stroma and glandular lumens and a secondary inflammatory response consisting predominantly of a diffuse infiltration of histiocytes [3]. The histiocytes convert the extravasated red blood cells into glycolipid and granular brown pigment, becoming so-called pseudoxanthoma cells, that can replace most or all the endometriotic stroma. Most of the pigment is hemofuscin and hemosiderin is typically present to a much lesser extent. The amount of pigment in an endometriotic lesion appears to increase with its age, and early lesions are frequently nonpigmented [12]. Variable numbers of lymphocytes and smaller numbers of other inflammatory cells may be present. Large numbers of neutrophils with microabscess formation should raise the possibility of secondary bacterial infection.

During pregnancy or progestin therapy:
1. The endometriosis glands become atrophic, which are small and lined by cuboidal or flattened epithelial cells.
2. The stroma exhibits marked decidual transformation (see Chap. 21.3.2).

In postmenopausal women:

The aspect is similar to a simple or cystic atrophy of the endometrium.
1. The endometriotic glands become atrophic, which occasionally are cystic lined by flattened epithelial cells.
2. The stroma is dense fibrotic with sometimes a barely perceptible tendency for the stroma to be more cellular close to the gland.

With the Location of the Disease

1. In the *ovary*, the predominant pattern is a small hemorrhagic focus or a larger cyst containing menstrual debris and lined by endometrial epithelium associated by endometrial stroma. However, the epithelial and stromal lining of an endometriotic cyst frequently becomes attenuated and difficult to recognize. Commonly, this cyst lining is totally lost and is replaced by granulation tissue, dense fibrous tissue, and numerous pigmented macrophages. In this case, a definitive diagnosis of endometriosis cannot be made because a similar appearance can be seen in an old corpus luteum cyst [3].
2. In the *peritoneum*, the endometrial lesions are constituted by implants and adhesions secondary to the inflammatory process. Implants can have different patterns and are classically divided in red, black, and white lesions [13].
3. When endometriotic lesions are located in *tissues containing smooth* muscle such as the uterine ligaments or the muscular wall of the bladder, rectum, and abdomen, or connective tissue,

the predominant pattern is that of a nodule constituted of smooth muscle hyperplasia and fibrosis surrounding or not tiny endometrial foci or cavities [3, 14]. The appearance is similar to that of adenomyosis with secondary striking myometrial hypertrophy, and the term adenomyoma was used by some authors to describe these lesions [3, 14, 15].

17.1.4 Etiology and Pathogenesis

The pathogenesis of endometriosis remains controversial. The two principal histogenetic theories are (a) metastasis of endometrial tissue to its ectopic location (metastatic theory) and (b) metaplastic development of endometrial tissue at the ectopic site (metaplastic theory). The two theories are not mutually exclusive, and it is likely that both are valid [3].

17.1.4.1 Metastatic Theory

Several ways of dissemination have been suggested:

Retrograde menstruation, that is, reflux of endometrial tissue through the fallopian tubes during menstruation, with subsequent implantation and growth on peritoneal surfaces, has been proposed by Sampson [16] to explain endometriosis. An experiment in human [17] has demonstrated that the shed endometrium is viable and may be implanted within the host. Retrograde menstruation is a common physiologic process occurring in approximately 90 % of menstruating women with patent tubes [18, 19]. Why only some of these women will develop endometriosis is not clear. Different factors have been incriminated including genetic factor, hormonal factor, menstrual factor, and immune factor [20]. Observations supporting the theory of retrograde menstruation are numerous and include the distribution of endometriotic lesions which are most common on the surfaces of the ovaries and fallopian tubes and the high frequency of endometriosis in females with congenital obstruction to menstrual flow [21–23].

Intraoperative implantation has been proposed to explain the presence of endometriosis in abdominal scars after uterine surgery [24, 25].

Hematogenous spread has been proposed to explain endometriosis in distant sites such as lungs, skeletal muscle, subarachnoid space, and kidneys, while endometriosis in lymph nodes is most easily explained by *lymphatic spread* [26].

17.1.4.2 Metaplastic Theory

The development of peritoneal endometriosis by a process of metaplasia of coelomic epithelium is consistent with the putative Müllerian potential of the pelvic peritoneum, which has been referred to as the secondary Müllerian system [1, 3]. Metaplasia of Müllerian remnants was also advocated as the cause of endometriosis [14]. Observations supporting the metaplastic theory include the demonstration of endometriosis in patients with Turner's syndrome and pure gonadal dysgenesis who are amenorrheic and have hypoplastic uteri [27–30] and in males with endometriosis of the prostate, bladder, abdominal wall, and scrotum [31–33].

17.1.5 Distribution

Endometriosis can involve almost any part of the body with a notary exception, the spleen [34, 35]. However, by far, the most common locations are the ovaries and the pelvic peritoneum followed in order of frequency by the GI system and the urinary system (Table 17.1).

1. Ovarian lesions may be constituted of small implants inferior to 1 cm or larger endometriotic cysts.
2. Peritoneal implants are subdivided in superficial and deep implants.
3. Deep infiltration is defined as the presence of endometrial tissue 5 mm or more under the peritoneum [36]. Deep infiltration leads to invasion of the subperitoneal space. The two major involved sites are (a) the anterior vesicouterine pouch with infiltration of the bladder wall and (b) the posterior cul-de-sac of Douglas with infiltration of the rectal wall, the posterior fornix of the vagina, the uterosacral ligaments, and the rectovaginal septum. The pelvic ureters are also frequently involved.

Another common manifestation of endometriosis is peritoneal adhesions that may lead to fimbriae agglutination and cul-de-sacs obliteration.

Distribution and type of endometriotic lesions are reported in Table 17.1.

Table 17.1 Distribution and type of endometriotic lesions

Common lesions
Ovaries:
– Ovarian **implant** (<1 cm)
– Endometrial *cyst*
Pelvic peritoneum:
– **Implants** covering the uterus, the tubes, the uterine ligaments, the anterior and posterior cul-de-sacs, the rectosigmoid, and the bladder
Peritoneal cavity:
– **Adhesions**
Subperitoneal space:
– **Anterior** with involvement of the bladder
– **Posterior** with involvement of the torus, the uterosacral ligaments, the posterior fornix of the vagina, the anterior wall of the rectosigmoid junction, and the rectovaginal septum
– **Lateral** involvement of the ureter (extrinsic location)
Other GI tract locations:
– Lower rectum and sigmoid
Less common lesions
Intratubal implants
Peritoneal endometriotic pseudocysts
Other GI tract locations: appendix, caecum, small bowel, and transverse colon
Cutaneous: scars, umbilicus, and inguinal region
Rare lesions
Diaphragm
Thoracic cavity: pleural and lung
Other urinary tract locations: kidneys and ureters (intrinsic location)
Other GI tract locations: gallbladder, liver, and pancreas
Nervous system: CNS and peripheral nerves locations
Lymphatic system: pelvic lymph nodes
Others

17.1.6 Classification

1. Criteria

   The classification of endometriosis [37] is based on a scoring system with extensive evaluation of the site and the size of the following:

   – Implants of endometriosis (superficial or deep) on the ovary. Ovarian endometriotic cyst should be confirmed by histology or by the presence of the following features: (a) cyst diameter <12 cm, (b) adhesion to pelvic side wall, (c) endometriosis on the surface of the ovary, and (d) tarry thick chocolate-colored fluid content.

   – Implants of endometriosis on the peritoneum (superficial or deep).

   – Cul-de-sac obliteration is considered if endometriosis or adhesions have obliterated part of the cul-de-sac: partial, some normal peritoneum is visible below the uterosacral ligaments and complete, no peritoneum is visible below the uterosacral ligaments.

   – Adhesions filmy or dense of the ovary and the tube.

   According to the amount of the different scores, the disease is classified as stage I (score 1–5), stage II (score 6–15), stage III (score 16–40), and stage IV (score >40).

   Furthermore, this classification suggests to include information on the morphologic appearance of the implants categorized as:
   1. Red-red red-pink, and clear lesions.
   2. White-white yellow-brown, and peritoneal defects.
   3. Black-black and blue lesions.

2. Critics

   Deep endometriosis is confirmed to be poorly reflected in the revised AFS classification.

   The most severe type III lesion is most frequently scored in revised AFS class I. This lends further support to Koninckx's previous considerations for including deep endometriosis in a revision of the revised AFS classification or in a new functional classification.

17.1.7 Clinical Findings

Clinical findings are reported in Table 17.2.

Table 17.2 Clinical findings

Symptoms
Mainly catamenial
Common
1. Infertility
2. Dysmenorrhea with abdominal swelling; vomiting; and sacral, lower back pain
3. Deep dyspareunia
4. GI tract findings: dyschesia, diarrhea
5. Urinary findings: dysuria, urgenturia
Uncommon
1. Rectorrhagia
2. Hematuria
3. Sciatica
4. Right shoulder pain, pneumothorax
Physical examination
1. Diffuse or focal abdominal tenderness
2. A retroverted uterus, an adnexal mass
3. Decreased motility and/or tenderness of the uterus and ovaries
4. Nodules or tenderness in the cul-de-sac, the rectovaginal septum, the uterosacral ligaments, and the abdominal wall

Table 17.3 Elevation of CA-125

1. Ovarian disease
Epithelial ovarian tumors (borderline and carcinomas)
Non epithelial ovarian malignant tumors
Germ cell tumors
Sex cord-stromal cell tumors
2. PID
3. Uterine disorders
Leiomyomas
Adenomyosis
4. Peritoneal disorders
Primary peritoneal carcinoma
Peritoneal metastases
Tuberculosis

17.1.8 Laboratory Tests

CA-125 (normal value <35 UI/ml) is commonly increased in endometriosis. It increases with the stage of the disease [38, 39]. However, this marker is also increased in many other gynecologic disorders (Table 17.3).

Serum levels of CA-125 are usually higher with ovarian cancer [40], but occasionally very high levels may be found with endometriomas [41, 42].

17.1.9 Laparoscopy

1. Definite diagnosis of endometriosis and evaluation of its extension are usually done through laparoscopy preferably with histologic examination [43]. Laparoscopic techniques allow also surgical resection of lesions in most instances without the need to perform a laparotomy [44].

   Imaging modalities are an alternative to the diagnosis and precede generally laparoscopy.

2. Difficulties of Correlation

   While the gold standard in the diagnosis of endometriosis is the presence at pathology of endometrium in an ectopic location, in routine clinical practice, difficulties in surgical pathological and radiological correlations are underestimated.

   – At laparoscopy, diagnosis of endometriosis can be established because the aspect of the lesion and its location are very suggestive of endometriosis (a thickening of a uterosacral ligament for instance), while no biopsy is performed. In other cases, biopsy of a suspected lesion only demonstrates fibrosis without endometrium, while the macroscopic aspect is characteristic enough to suggest endometriosis.

   – At laparoscopy or laparotomy, involvement of a posterior subperitoneal lesion can be overlooked because the lesion is exclusively subperitoneal in location, or can be hidden by dense adhesions, or because the lesions are so extensive that the surgeon gives up dissection, preventing to evaluate accurately the lesions which are clearly demonstrated on US or MR. Should these lesions depicted on US or MR be considered as false positives or rather as lesions impossible to classify as endometriotic?

17.1.10 Imaging Modalities

17.1.10.1 Methods

Two methods are essential: ultrasound and MR.

1. *Ultrasound (US)* is usually performed first.

   A transabdominal and a transvaginal approach must be used systematically whenever possible.

   Rectal endoscopic ultrasonography can be performed in case of suspicion of GI tract involvement [45, 46].

2. *MR* is a complementary imaging modality in evaluating endometriosis.

   Vaginal opacification is performed whenever possible. Some authors join opacification of the rectum.

   The following protocol is performed:

   Sagittal and axial T2 sequences.

   Axial T1.

   Sagittal and axial fat suppression.

   Sagittal and axial T1 after injection of gadolinium.

   Other methods:

- *CT*, with IV contrast followed by opacification of the large bowel, can be performed.

  1. To make the differential between adhesion and invasion of the rectosigmoid wall and determine the extension and to look for another location.

  2. To precise the relationship of the pelvic ureters with the endometriotic lesions or adhesions and eventually to diagnose a bladder or a ureteral location.

- *HSG*

  Although less and less performed, in patients with infertility, HSG allows to evaluate the permeability of the tubes, can detect adenomyosis or tubal endometriosis.

17.1.10.2 Ovary

Macroscopy (Fig. 17.1) (Table 17.4)

1. *Hemorrhagic content.* Endometriotic lesions of the ovary vary from a small focus on the surface of the ovary to a large mass. Because the ectopic endometrium bleeds, it produces a small hematoma at the surface of the ovary. Later on, this hematoma increases in size and produces an hemorrhagic cyst which progressively invaginates into the ovary pushing the ovarian parenchyma at the periphery [47] (Fig. 17.2).

   The content of the hemorrhagic cyst consists of semifluid or inspissated chocolate-colored material [3, 48]. It may contain *clots* that are typically peripheral but more rarely central.

2. *Thickened wall.* Endometriotic cysts have typically a fibrotic wall of variable thickness, comprised between 1 and 3 mm. Its inner wall is smooth or granular [3].

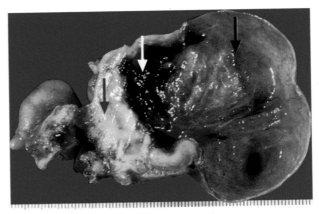

Fig. 17.1 (1) Ovarian cyst (*black arrow*), (2) clots (*white arrow*), and (3) normal ovarian parenchyma (*blue arrow*)

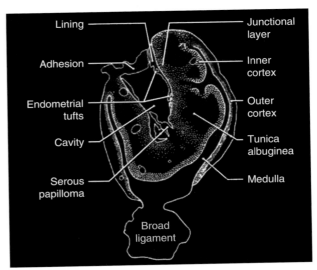

Fig. 17.2 Endometriotic cyst [47]. Endometrial tufts penetrating from outside to inside into the ovary. Tunica albuginea pushed at the periphery. Adhesion created at the surface of the endometriotic cyst

Table 17.4 Macroscopic features and pathological surgery

Hemorrhagic content: chocolate cyst, clots
Thickened wall
Size <9 cm
Shape not rounded
Normal ovarian parenchyma pushed at the periphery
Uni- or bilateral 1/3 to 1/2 cases
Unique or multiple lesions
Location backward and inward
Adhesions to the neighboring structures or peritoneum

3. *Size* is usually between 2 and 7 cm exceptionally superior to 9 cm [49]. The smaller cysts consist of only one cavity. The larger ones can appear uni- or multilocular.

4. The other findings will be described with the different imaging modalities.

US

US Findings

The main findings of endometrial cyst are reported in Table 17.5.

Table 17.5 Ultrasound findings of endometriomas and functional hemorrhagic cysts

	Endometrioma	Functional hemorrhagic cyst
Size	<8 cm	<8 cm
Shape	Not round with protrusion	Round
Bilateral	1/2 to 1/3 of cases	Exceptional
Multiple cysts in the same ovary	Possible	Exceptional
Location	– Ovarian fossa – Displaced inward and backward	Ovarian fossa
Internal echo pattern	– Ground-glass pattern	– Fishnet pattern – Whirled pattern – Heterogeneous pattern
Clots	– Echogenic foci – Peripheral – Round or curvilinear	– Large hyperechoic central portion
Wall	Thick	Thick
Layering	Possible	Possible
Acoustic enhancement	Very common	Very common
Follow-up ultrasound	No modification in size and echo pattern	Modification in size and echo pattern
Normal parenchyma pushed toward the periphery	Common finding	Common finding
Adhesions	Possible	Absence

As far as hemorrhagic functional cyst is the main differential diagnosis, its findings are also reported in the same table.

Typical Form

1. *Hemorrhagic content:* On transvaginal ultrasound, the hemorrhagic content of an endometrioma appears most commonly and typically as a *homogeneous low-level echo pattern* of lesser echogenicity than myometrium [50–52], defined by some authors as a ground-glass pattern (Figs. 17.3 and 17.4). Using this finding as the only criterion to diagnose ovarian endometriosis, it has a sensitivity of 84–95 % [53] and a specificity of 81–90 % [54]. This pattern is very suggestive of the diagnosis but can also be found in other adnexal masses (Table 17.6).

2. *Clots:* They appear as echogenic foci usually with a more intense echogenicity than myometrium but can have more rarely the same echogenicity.

   (a) *Shape:* They can be round, oval (Fig. 17.5), or curvilinear (Fig. 17.6). When curvilinear, they are very typical for endometriosis [55].

Table 17.6 Etiology of ground-glass pattern

Common
Hemorrhagic cyst of small size or in a portion of a larger cyst
Mucinous cystadenoma
Abscess
Cystic forms of epithelial tumors with papillary projection
Uncommon
Dermoid cyst (a portion)
Ovarian lymphoma

   (b) *Acoustic shadowing:* These clots can present without or with acoustic shadowing.

   (c) *Border:* Their border can be sharp or ill defined.

   (d) *Size:* Size is variable from some millimeters to 1 or 2 cm, rarely more.

    When there are punctiform, with or without acoustic shadowing, they look like calcifications (Figs. 17.7 and 17.8); in this case, absence of vessel in the mass on color Doppler rules out a solid mass containing calcifications.

   (e) *Location:* Usually they lie against the inner wall [55] and commonly in the dependent portion but can be located more centrally.

Association of these echogenic foci to a ground-glass pattern is pathognomonic of ovarian endometriosis.

When the clot is round or oval and lies against the inner wall, it can simulate a papillary projection (BUY AJR); however, in some cases, a section in another plan can demonstrate a typical clot (Fig. 17.9). More rarely it can confused with a calcification or a tooth in a Rokitansky protuberance [56].

3. *Wall:* The wall of endometriomas is relatively thick (1–3 mm) compared to functional cysts and epithelial cystadenomas [52].

   Acoustic enhancement can be present.

   Fissure of the wall can occur (Fig. 17.10).

4. *Color Doppler findings:* Color Doppler can show vessels in the wall of the endometrioma and in the septa. However, no vessel is seen inside the endometrioma confirming its cystic nature [50].

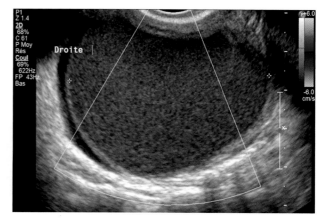

Fig. 17.3 Forty-three-year-old woman, dysmenorrhea, homogeneous low-level echo, and pushing the normal ovarian parenchyma toward the periphery. Color Doppler does not display any vessel in the wall

Fig. 17.4 Typical echogenic pattern of endometriotic cyst on EVS. Twenty-seven-year-old woman with dysmenorrhea and CA-125 at 80 IU/ml. (**a**) TVS shows a 4-cm right ovarian mass with homogeneous echogenicity and an intensity lower than myometrium. Normal ovarian parenchyma (*arrow*) is pushed toward the periphery. (**b**) Color Doppler shows no vascularization in the mass proving its cystic nature. A small vessel is visualized in the wall

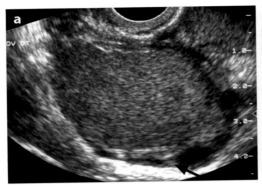
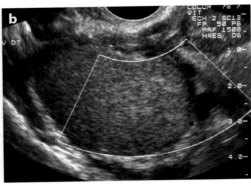

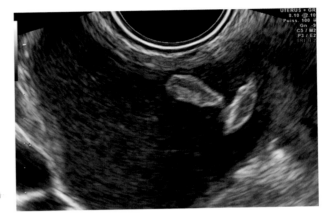

Fig. 17.5 Clots in endometrioma. Clots are situated at the periphery of the cyst oval in shape, echogenic with a central lower echogenicity

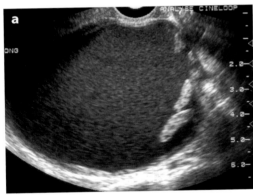
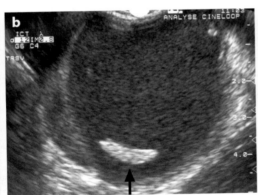
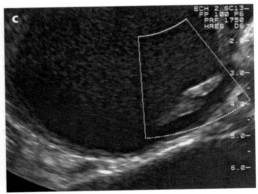

Fig. 17.6 Ovarian endometrioma on US with clots. EVS Sagittal (**a**) and transverse, (**b**) show a left 8-cm cystic ovarian mass with a homogeneous low-level echoes containing semilunar clots typical of endometriomas (*arrow*), and with absence of vessel in the mass on color Doppler (**c**)

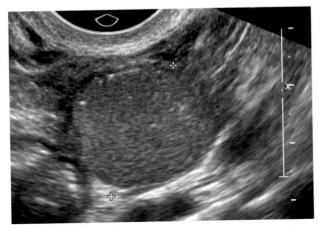
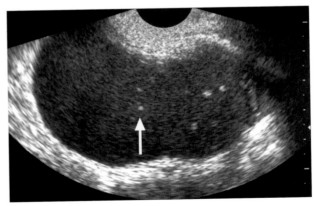

Fig. 17.7 Typical ground-glass pattern containing echogenic foci without acoustic shadowing and looking like tiny calcifications

Fig. 17.8 Anterior endometriotic cyst with clots resembling calcifications. Fifty-three-year-old woman. EVS Sagittal (**a**): Cystic low echogenic ovarian mass containing small hyperechoic clots (*arrow*) without acoustic shadowing which could have been confused with dots or lines of hair in a dermoid cyst

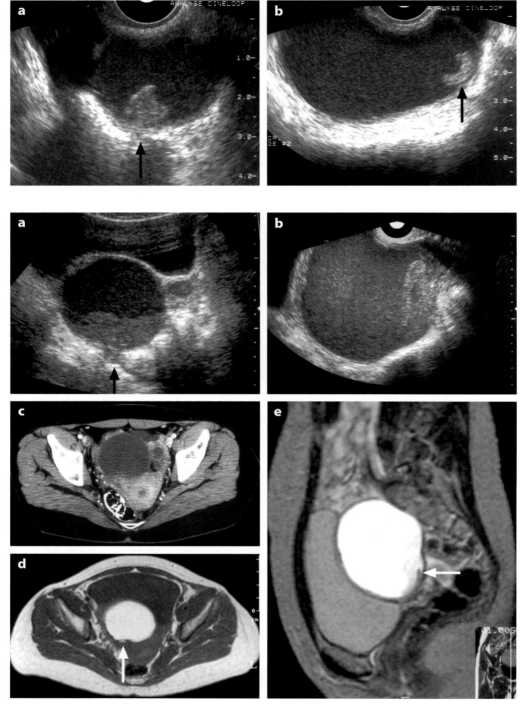

Fig. 17.9 Clot simulating a papillary projection. Thirty-one-year-old woman with primary infertility and CA-125 at 117 IU/ml. (**a**) Coronal TVS: low echogenic ovarian cyst containing against its inner wall an echogenic focus resembling a papillary projection (*arrow*). (**b**) Longitudinal TVS: the echogenic focus appears as a semilunar echogenic clot (*arrow*) in the dependant portion of the mass is characteristic for endometrioma

Fig. 17.10 Right cystic ovarian mass with clots and an irregularity of the ontour due to posterior rupture and adhesions. Twenty-eight years old woman with pelvic mass and pelvic pain. Transverse TAS (**a**) (*arrow*) and sagittal EVS, (**b**) display in the posterior wall of the cyst an interruption of the wall suggesting a focal rupture. CT after injection (**c**) and on MR axial T1 (**d**) (*arrow*) and sagittal T2 (**e**) (*arrow*) confirm this impression

The Other Forms

1. *Mixed echogenic pattern* (Fig. 17.11). Usually, Doppler allows to prove its cystic nature. However, in uncommon cases, the pattern is very atypical, while MR allows to make the diagnosis.
2. *Layering* (Fig. 17.12). A layering or a fluid-fluid level is an uncommon finding. It was found in 2 of 38 (5 %) endometriomas in the series of Kupfer et al. [52]. When a layering is present in a hemorrhagic cyst, a functional hemorrhagic cyst is discussed.
3. *Atypical forms of clots and hemorrhagic contents* (Fig. 17.13).
4. *Exceptionally with attenuation of the US beam simulating an ovarian fibroma* (Fig. 17.14). In this case, other imaging modalities may suggest the diagnosis.

Other US Findings Common to the Different Imaging Modalities

1. *Shape*: Cysts are commonly covered by fibrous adhesions which can result in fixation to adjacent structures [3]. This is the reason why the shape of these ovarian masses, at the opposite of most primary ovarian tumors, is not rounded. The cyst conforms to the shape of the adjacent structures. In some cases, localized outward protrusions of the cyst and/or sharp inward invaginations of the cyst wall simulating incisures are very characteristic.
2. The *normal ovarian parenchyma* is often seen pushed to the periphery of the lesion.
3. *Unilateral or bilateral lesions:* Bilateral lesions happen from 1/3 to 1/2 cases [3, 49].

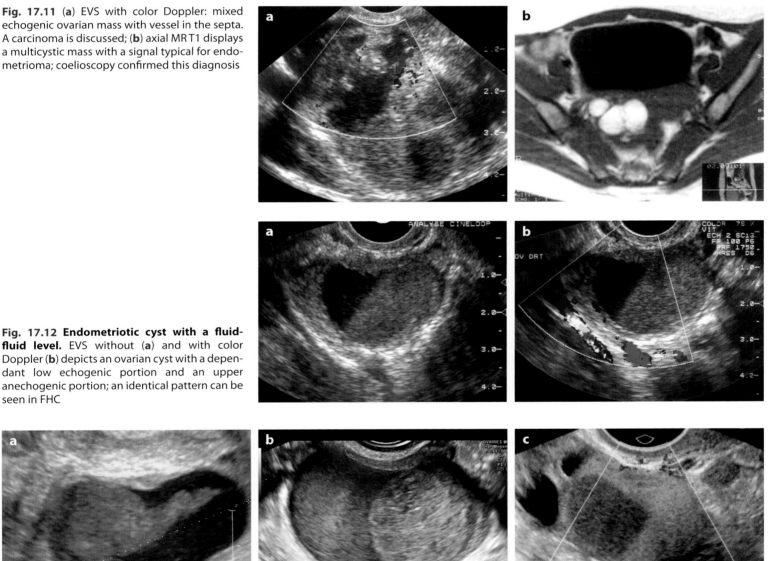

Fig. 17.11 (**a**) EVS with color Doppler: mixed echogenic ovarian mass with vessel in the septa. A carcinoma is discussed; (**b**) axial MR T1 displays a multicystic mass with a signal typical for endometrioma; coelioscopy confirmed this diagnosis

Fig. 17.12 Endometriotic cyst with a fluid-fluid level. EVS without (**a**) and with color Doppler (**b**) depicts an ovarian cyst with a dependant low echogenic portion and an upper anechogenic portion; an identical pattern can be seen in FHC

Fig. 17.13 (**a**) Elongated clot; (**b**) ground-glass pattern with a round clot; and (**c**) endometriotic cyst with two components, one with a ground-glass pattern and the other one with a more echogenic and homogeneous pattern

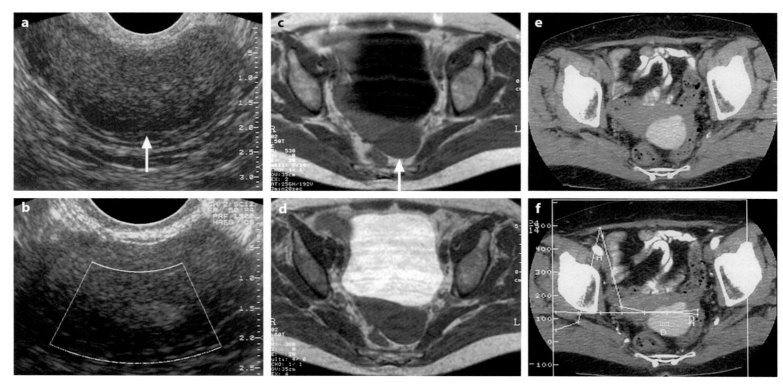

Fig. 17.14 Endometriotic cyst with unusual pattern on US and on MR (low signal on T1 and T2). EVS (**a**) and color Doppler (**b**), a low echogenic mass containing a more echogenic focus is depicted. There is an overall strong posterior attenuation (*arrow*) in (**a**), suggesting an ovarian fibroma. No vessel is seen on color Doppler inside the mass. MR Axial T1 (**c**): left adnexal mass with signal intensity slightly superior to pelvic muscles is displayed (*arrow*). On T2 (**d**), the signal intensity of the mass is close to pelvic muscles. No definite diagnosis is proposed. CT without contrast (**e**) and DCT (**f**): cystic mass with a density of 110 HU is visualized corresponding to a hemorrhagic content. A small anterior protrusion is depicted. Prospective diagnosis: an ovarian hematoma is diagnosed on CT. The very high density excludes a functional hemorrhagic cyst. Laparoscopy: ovarian hemorrhagic cyst. Pathology: endometriotic cyst

4. *Unique or multiple lesions:* The lesion can be unique or multiple in the same ovary and in this last case can simulate a multilocular mass (Fig. 17.15). Invaginations or localized protrusions related to adhesions give to the mass a shape which is not round. The different loculi in the same ovary or ovarian cysts in both ovaries can appear with different echogenicities (Fig. 17.16).

5. *Location* is variable. The mass can be in the ovarian fossa. However, because of the retraction inflammatory in origin and adhesions, the mass has a tendency to be situated more backward and inward. When the mass is in such a situation and bilateral, cysts are opposed to each other tethering the rectosigmoid. This topography is very characteristic; however, one can also see it in case of bilateral carcinomas of the ovary. Exceptionally, the mass is anterior to the broad ligament.

6. *Adhesion* to the neighboring structures or to the peritoneum is very common (Fig. 17.17).

7. *Stability of the internal echo pattern*: Endometriomas do not resolve or diminish in size during a short period of time, and their internal echo pattern is stable.

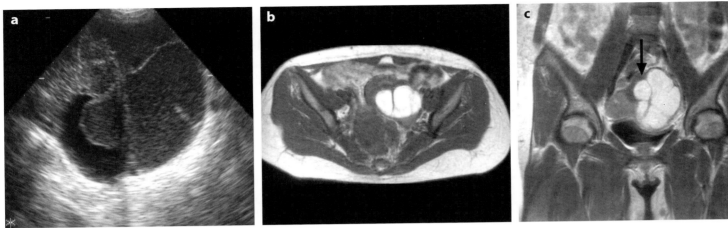

Fig. 17.15 Multiloculated endometriotic cyst with sharp inward invaginations of the cyst wall simulating incisures. (a) Coronal TVS: multicystic left hypoechoic mass with a sharp incisure that looks like an incomplete septum. (b) Axial MR T1 and coronal T2 (c) definitely confirm the deep longitudinal incisure (*arrow* in c) in the anterior part of the mass. This incisure is related to adhesions, which are very characteristic of endometriomas

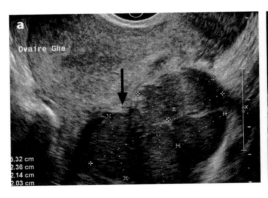

Fig. 17.16 Bilateral endometriotic cyst with different echogenicities. Right (*black arrow*) and left ovarian (*red arrow*) cysts have different echogenicities

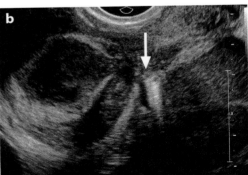

Fig. 17.17 Adhesion. Longitudinal EVS (a) displays adhesion of a left ovarian endometriotic cyst to the posterior wall of the uterus (*black arrow*). Axial EVS (b) depicts a right multilocular and a left unilocular ovarian endometriotic cyst with adhesion to the torus (*arrow*)

Differential Diagnosis

The main differential diagnosis is reported in Table 17.7.

Table 17.7 Differential diagnosis

Common
The other adnexal cystic echogenic masses
Functional hemorrhagic cyst
Dermoid cyst
Mucinous cystadenoma
Tuboovarian abscess
Cystic epithelial ovarian tumor with papillary projection
The echogenic solid ovarian masses
Ovarian fibrothecoma
Subserous leiomyoma
Uncommon
Lymphoma and metastases

The Other Adnexal Cystic Echogenic Masses

1. Functional hemorrhagic cyst (Table 17.5):

   (a) The patterns of FHC are very variable.

   Some echogenic patterns are typical for functional hemorrhagic cysts: Fishnet appearance, a central clot related to the periphery with thin echogenic lines, and a small echo-free area in an echogenic cysts [50, 51, 57] (Fig. 17.18).

   However, in some cases, differentiation with endometrioma can be very difficult. Some aspects of echogenic cysts suggestive of FHC are very uncommonly related to endometriosis (Fig. 17.19). Very similar small echogenic cysts can be related to FHC and endometriosis (Fig. 17.20). Not exceptionally, FHC and endometriotic cyst can be associated in the same ovary or in the contralateral ovary (Fig. 17.21).

   (b) On ultrasound follow-up, functional hemorrhagic cysts not only have a tendency to resolve or diminish in size but their internal echo pattern is modified. In Okai et al. series [57], 7 of 24 functional hemorrhagic cysts (29 %) disappeared within 2 weeks, and the remaining had different sonographic appearance with time until they disappeared finally within 8 weeks.

2. *Dermoid cyst:* While some echogenic patterns like a highly echogenic focus with broad acoustic shadowing, a hair ball, or an entirely hyperechoic mass are very suggestive of the diagnosis, the echogenic pattern can be less characteristic especially when the mass is relatively uniformly echogenic; in this case, dermoid cyst can mimic an endometrioma (Fig. 17.22).

3. *Mucinous cystadenoma* when unilocular can be difficult to differentiate from endometrioma. Accumulation of mucin can resemble clots (Fig. 17.23).

4. *Ovarian abscess* can look like exactly like an ovarian endometrioma (Fig. 17.24). However, usually a significant peripheral vascularization is present.

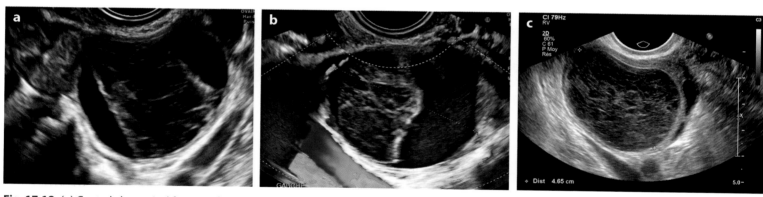

Fig. 17.18 (**a**) Central clot typical for FHC, (**b**) color Doppler does not display any vessel in the clot, and (**c**) characteristic fishnet appearance

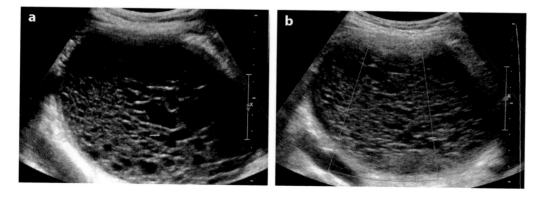

Fig. 17.19 (**a**) Endometriotic cyst with absence of vessel on color Doppler (**b**)

Fig. 17.20 EVS (**a**) Endometrioma, (**b**) functional hemorrhagic cyst with a ground-glass pattern

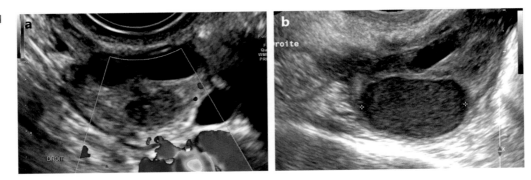

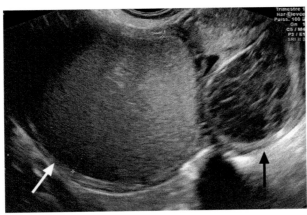

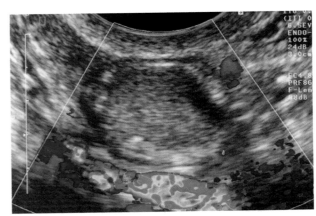

Fig. 17.21 Association of a FHC and an edometriotic cyst in the same ovary. Association of a FHC with a characteristic fishnet appearance (*black arrow*) and endometriotic cyst with a typical ground-glass (*white arrow*) pattern in the same left ovary

Fig. 17.22 Atypical dermoid cyst looking like endometriosis. The cyst with a ground-glass pattern considered as an endometriotic cyst was in fact a dermoid cyst

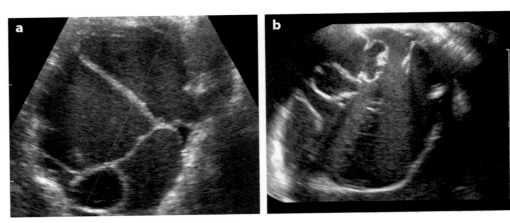

Fig. 17.23 (**a**) Multilocular endometriotic cyst and (**b**) multilocular mucinous cystadenoma

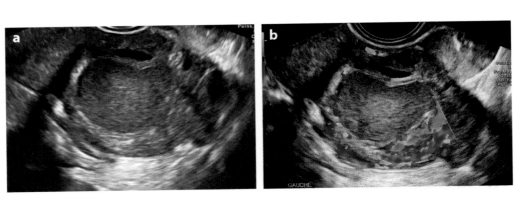

Fig. 17.24 EVS without (**a**) displays a low-level echogenic mass. Color Doppler (**b**) depicts a peripheral hypervascularization, very suggestive of an abscess

The Echogenic Solid Ovarian Masses

1. *Ovarian fibroma.* When small, without degenerative changes, ovarian fibromas can present relatively uniform echogenic pattern (Fig. 17.25). Two main findings allow to make the differential: (1) numerous discrete acoustic shadowing not related to calcifications but to fibrous tissue and (2) color Doppler usually demonstrates vessels in the mass which typically are scarce and central, but in some cases, vessels are barely seen. DMR makes the diagnosis.

2. *Pedunculated subserous leiomyoma* can also appear as a homogeneous echogenic mass. As ovarian fibroma, it may present numerous discrete shadowing.

   Its vascularization is richer than that of ovarian fibroma often realizing a peripheral hypervascular rim. Other findings that allow to differentiate uterine subserous leiomyoma from ovarian fibroma and ovarian endometrioma are (a) visualization of a normal ipsilateral ovary and (b) a vascular pedicle linking the mass to the uterus.

3. Less commonly, the *epithelial cystic tumors* with papillary projections particularly the borderline and malignant forms (Fig. 17.26).

   When a clot lies against the inner wall of a cyst, it can resemble in some cases to a papillary projection. When this echogenic focus is superior to 1 cm in diameter, color doppler usually demonstrates color flow in the papillary projection while color flow is absent in the clot. On the opposite, when the echogenic focus is inferior to 1 cm in diameter, differential diagnosis may be impossible as far as color flow is absent in both. In these cases, injection of IV contrast on MR usually depicts contrast uptake in the papillary projection.

MR

After US examination, MR is advocated:

1. For the diagnosis, (a) when the clinical findings are very suggestive of endometriosis while the US is normal, (b) when the cysts are of small size, and when the pattern of the ovarian cyst is not sufficiently characteristic to diagnose endometriosis.

2. To evaluate extension particularly to look for or to confirm subperitoneal locations.

3. For the follow-up under medical treatment or to diagnose a recurrence.

MR Findings

It is practical to distinguish small intraovarian implants (<1 cm) and larger endometrioma (>1 cm).

Endometrioma

1. *The wall:* The wall is hypointense on T1 but mainly on T2 related to fibrosis with hemosiderin [58]. After gadolinium injection, the wall slightly enhances [59].

2. *Hemorrhagic content*:
   The main findings are reported in Table 17.8.

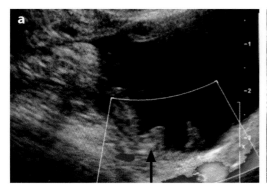

Fig. 17.25 Low-level echogenic ovarian mass; although a slight attenuation is displayed, the diagnosis of ovarian fibroma cannot be ascertained

Table 17.8 Signal intensity of endometriomas on T1, T1 with fat suppression, and T2

T1	T1 with fat suppression	T2
Signal ≥ adipose tissue	High signal in 100 %	Intermediate signal , between pelvic muscle and adipose tissue Signal ≥ urine[a]
Muscle < signal < adipose tissue	High signal Low signal	Signal ≥ urine Signal < adipose tissue
Signal = muscle	Low signal	Signal = pelvic muscle

[a]Uncommonly

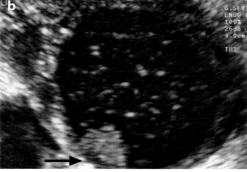

Fig. 17.26 (**a**) EVS with color Doppler: endometriotic cyst, containing multiple clots lying against the inner wall of the cyst (*arrow*). These clots can simulate papillary projections like in this case of mucinous cystadenofibroma (*arrow* in **b**). Color flow (in **a**) is absent in the clots

1. The most common form of presentation present in 80/86 (93 %) [60] and the most characteristic (Figs. 17.27 and 17.28).

On T1W images, a predominantly high-signal intensity ≥ adipose tissue. The cyst can be homogeneously hyperintense or heterogeneous because the blood products are in various stages of degradation from multiple episodes of bleeding.

On fat suppression, a high-signal intensity is maintained in 100 % of cases [59, 61], allowing to rule out fatty content present in dermoid cyst or immature cystic teratoma.

On T2W images:

(a) In the characteristic form, the overall signal becomes lower, intermediate between adipose tissue and pelvic muscle. While the signal in almost all ovarian cysts increases on T2, this decrease in signal on T2 is very particular to endometrioma. This decrease in signal is homogeneous (Fig. 17.27) or heterogeneous (Fig. 17.28).

This T2 shortening has been designated the shading sign [58]. Shading is a focal [58] or diffuse [62] or appears as a loss

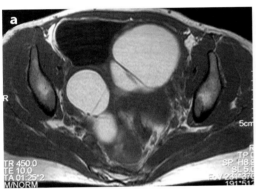
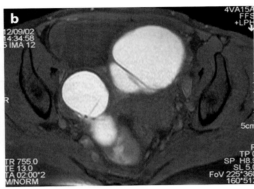
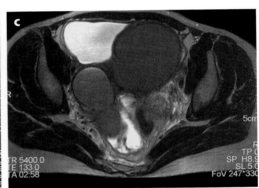
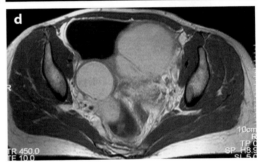

Fig. 17.27 MR characteristic pattern bilateral multicystic ovarian endometriotic cyst. MR axial T1 (**a**) fat suppression (**b**), T2, and (**c**) after injection (**d**). The content of the cysts has a signal identical to fatty tissue on T1 (**a**) with a high signal on fat suppression (**b**) and a decrease of the signal on T2 with an intermediate signal between adipose tissue and pelvic muscle. Association of these findings is specific for endometriosis; after injection there is a slight contrast uptake in the wall of the cysts. Bilaterality and presence of multiple cysts in the ovaries are characteristic additional findings

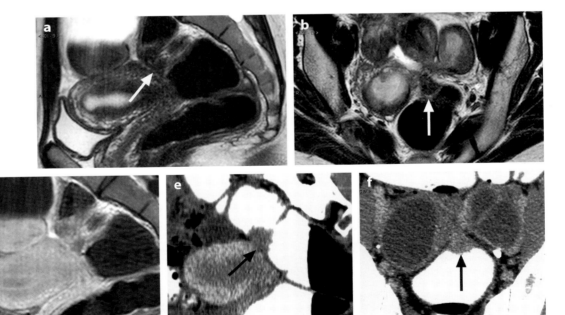
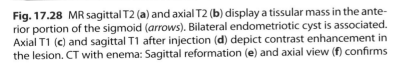

Fig. 17.28 MR sagittal T2 (**a**) and axial T2 (**b**) display a tissular mass in the anterior portion of the sigmoid (*arrows*). Bilateral endometriotic cyst is associated. Axial T1 (**c**) and sagittal T1 after injection (**d**) depict contrast enhancement in the lesion. CT with enema: Sagittal reformation (**e**) and axial view (**f**) confirms the presence of an endometriotic location in the anterior portion of the sigmoid (*arrows* in **e** and **f**); the irregular aspect of the mucosa precises that the lesion extends deeply at least into the muscular layer. Enema also allowed to precise that this location was unique, which was confirmed at operation

of signal in the dependant layering with a hypointense fluid level [60]. When it is focal, it can be located peripherally or centrally with a relatively sharp margin from the high-signal intensity loculize content or marge imperceptibly with it [58]. It can be attributable to the highly viscous content of the cyst or to the extremely high concentration of methemoglobin or a high protein concentration [60] or iron products.

In a cystic mass, association of an overall signal equal to adipose tissue on T1, a high signal on fat suppression, and a decrease signal on T2 comprised between adipose tissue and pelvic muscle is almost pathognomonic for diagnosis of endometrial cyst+++.

(b) On T2W images, a hyperintense signal can be present like in a chronic stage hematoma and in this case, is considered not definite but very suggestive of endometriosis [60, 63] (Fig. 17.29).

After injection, a slight contrast uptake is visualized in the wall.

2. Uncommonly, on T1W images, the signal is intermediate comprised between muscle and adipose tissue (Fig. 17.30).

   On fat suppression, the cysts may have a high or a low signal [63].

   On T2W images, signal can be > urine [64] or < adipose tissue [59].

3. Exceptionally, on T1W images, in 6–7 % of cases [60, 61] the signal is equal to pelvic muscle (Fig. 17.14).

   On fat suppression, the signal remains low [61].

   On T2W images, the signal remains low [60].

3. *Clots:* The morphologic findings are the same as those mentioned on ultrasound (paragraph ultrasound) (Fig. 17.31).

   Signal intensity of the clots is either equal to muscle [55] or comprised between muscle and adipose tissue on both T1- and T2-weighted images. Absence of contrast uptake allows to distinguish a clot from a papillary projection.

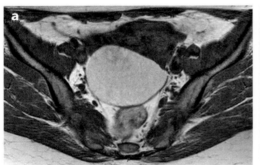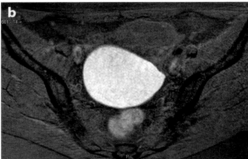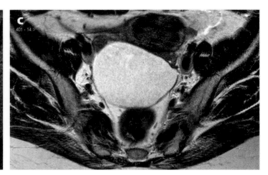

Fig. 17.29 Endometriotic cyst with a high signal on T1 and T2. Forty-three-year-old woman with dysmenorrhea. MR axial sequences: right ovarian cyst with a signal comprised close to adipose tissue on T1 (**a**) with a high signal on fat suppression (**b**) and a high signal close to urine on T2 (**c**)

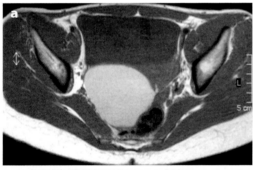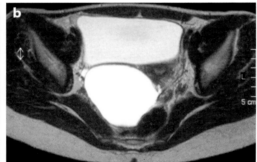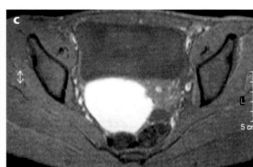

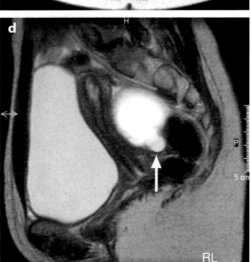

Fig. 17.30 Ovarian cyst with an intermediate signal on T1. MR axial T1 (**a**) fat suppression (**b**) and axial T2 (**c**): content of the cyst has an intermediate signal on T1, a high signal on fat suppression and a signal close to urine on T2. On sagittal T2 (**d**): protrusion of the lower part of the cyst, an additional characteristic finding of endometriosis, is displayed (*arrow*)

4. While *layering* can be observed in functional hemorrhagic cyst [65], exceptionally this finding can be observed in endometrioma [58, 60, 66] (Fig. 17.32). The dependent portion had a low signal in 2/12 endometriomas on T1-weighted images and in 10/12 endometriomas on T2-weighted images in Zawin et al. series [66].

In very common cases, signal intensity of the FHC can be the same as endometriosis; only the follow-up with US can make the differential diagnosis (Fig. 17.32).

5. Other MR findings common to the different imaging modalities.

The *shape*: Inward invaginations of the wall simulating incisures, localized outward protrusions, and irregularity of the external wall are related to peripheral adhesions and are typical for endometriomas.

Bilateral topography is very suggestive.

Multiple lesions considered by Togashi et al. [58, 60] as typical for endometriomas and are better visualized on MR (Fig. 17.33).

Precise *location* of the mass is also better depicted on MR than on ultrasound.

Adhesions can be highly suspected when (1) obliteration of Douglas outlined by an incompletely declive peritoneal effusion is present; (2) the cysts are posteromedially situated, due to retraction of the posterior leaf of the broad ligament, giving in case of bilateral lesion(s) a typical tethered aspect of the rectosigmoid; and (3) when a plane separating two contiguous anatomic structures is obliterated on T2 and after injection, mainly when there is an associated attraction; however, this last finding can be over or underestimated.

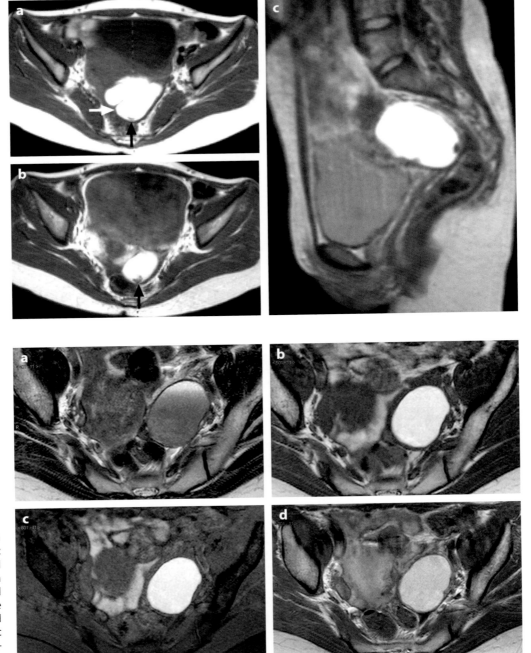

Fig. 17.31 Characteristic semi-lunar clot in an endometrial cyst. Thirty-one-year-old woman with primary infertility and CA-125 at 117 IU/ml. (**a**) MR axial T1: the mass appears with a irregular contour and a characteristic indentation (*white arrow*). Signal intensity is equal to adipose tissue. A semi-lunar clot is visualized in the dependant portion of the cyst with a signal slightly superior to pelvic muscles (*black arrow*). (**b**) MR axial T1 after contrast injection. No contrast uptake is depicted in the semi-lunar focus confirming it is related to a clot (*arrow*). (**c**), sagittal T2. The cystic content has a signal intensity superior to urine. The clot has a signal equal to pelvic muscles (). Marked irregular contour are related to adhesions

Fig. 17.32 Differential diagnosis between endometrioma and functional hemorrhagic cyst. *Endometriotic cyst in one patient*: MR axial on T1 (**a**) displays a 5.5 cm left ovarian cyst with an intensity close to adipose tissue a high-signal intensity on fat suppression (**b**) with a decrease of signal which is intermediate with a fluid level on T2 (**c**) which is typical for an endometriotic cyst; a slight contrast uptake in the wall is displayed after injection (**d**).

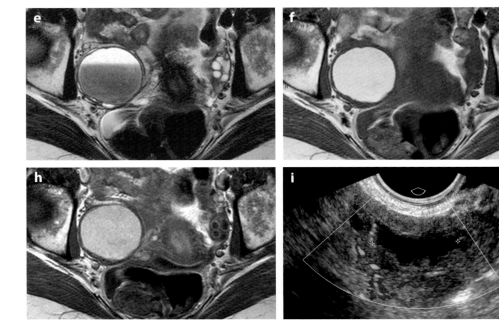

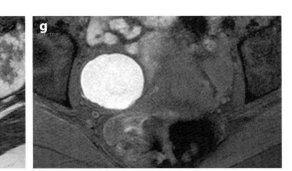

Fig. 17.32 (continued) Functional hemorrhagic cyst in an other patient: MR axial T1 (**e**) Fat suppression (**f**) T2 (**g**) and after injection (**h**) display a 5 cm right ovarian cyst which has exactly the same features of signal, suggesting an endometriotic cyst; because of the rapid increase in size (this cyst measured 3 cm on a US performed 2 months earlier), a functional hemorrhagic cyst could not be excluded. EVS (**i**) performed at the beginning of the next cycle demonstrated a significant decrease in size of the cyst associated with a flattened pattern proving the functional nature of the cyst. This pattern in MR is quite unusual, but outlines in some cases the necessity to perform an ultrasound examination after the next period to make the differential diagnosis

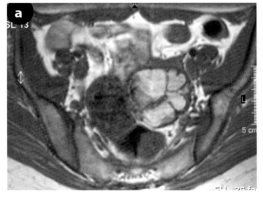
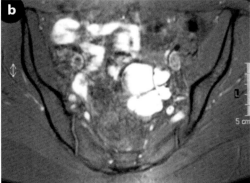
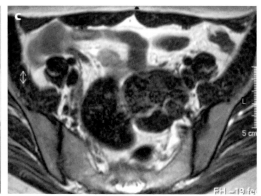

Fig. 17.33 Multicystic left endometioma. Thirty-four-year-old woman with dysmenorrhea. (**a**), MR axial T1: a 5-cm left ovarian multicystic mass with an overall signal close to adipose tissue. (**b**) axial T1 with fat suppression: an overall bright signal is seen in the mass confirming its hemorrhagic nature. (**c**) axial T2: the signal in the mass is significantly decreased. Multiplicity of hemorrhagic cysts allows the definite diagnosis of endometriosis. Diffuse superficial peritoneal implants in the sub-diaphragmatic spaces and the paracolic gutters not evaluated by MR, were discovered at surgery

Intraovarian Implants (Endometriomas <1 cm)

Impossible to detect and especially to characterize on ultrasound, they can be visualized as hyperintense foci on T1-weighted images coupled with fat suppression [67]. They have variable intensity on T2-weighted images. Even, when they are tiny, they can be detected because of the high contrast between them and the ovarian parenchyma. They can be totally overlooked by laparoscopy.

When these implants are unique and unilateral, they lack of specificity and can correspond to a corpus luteum cyst or small hemorrhagic follicles. That is why, MR should be performed in the first part of the cycle when possible.

Differential Diagnosis

1. *Functional hemorrhagic cyst.* Three main aspects can be observed.
   (1) In the most common and characteristic form of FHC (Table 17.9):

Table 17.9 Differential diagnosis endometrioma versus FHC

	T1	Fat suppression	T2
Endometrioma	= Adipose tissue	Elevated	Decrease between adipose tissue and muscle
FHC	= Muscle	Low	High signal ≥ urine heterogeneous

(2) Uncommonly, signal intensity is comprised between muscle and adipose tissue on T1-weighted images, with high signal on T1-weighted fat suppression images and a signal superior or equal to urine on T2-weighted images [68]. This pattern can be observed occasionally in endometrioma.

(3) An uncommon pattern of subacute hematoma first reported by Gomori et al. [69] in the brain and later on by Hahn et al. [70] in the duodenum has been also observed by Togashi [60] in the ovary, while this aspect has never been observed in case of endometrioma.

Layering is more frequent in functional hemorrhagic cysts than in endometriomas.

Endometrial cyst is not exceptionally associated with FHC in the same (Fig. 17.34) or in the contralateral ovary.

Dermoid cyst. This differential does not include the regular dermoid with signal ≥ adipose tissue on T1 with low signal on T1 fat-suppression sequences but dermoids with signal inferior to adipose tissue on T1-weighted images. CT can be very helpful in this last case in demonstrating small areas of low density of fat or a Rokitansky protuberance.

Mucinous cystadenoma, which can be a problem on US, has usually a different patten on MR. In case of the most frequent multiloculated form, on T1-weighted, the loculation with the highest signal is comprised between muscle and adipose tissue. On fat suppression, the signal is intermediate. On T2, the different loculi are of different signals.

In case of the unilocular form on T1, the signal is comprised between muscle and adipose tissue. On T2, the signal is ≥ urine.

Ovarian abscess. On T1, signal is intermediate between pelvic muscles and adipose tissue.

On fat suppression, a very high signal can be confused with the signal of an endometrioma.

On T2, the signal is high as urine.

After injection, there is a characteristic high-contrast uptake in the wall on the delayed phase associated with a blurring at the periphery of the lesion (see Chap. 33).

Ovarian fibroma. This differential diagnosis is only discussed in the exceptional cases of endometriomas with signal equal to muscle on T1. Delayed contrast uptake is displayed in a fibroma [71].

Epithelial cystic mass with papillary projection. When an endometrioma contains a clot lying against its wall, an epithelial cystic mass with papillary projections is a differential diagnosis. However, (1) the cystic content in case of borderline or carcinoma has a signal usually comprised between pelvic muscle and adipose tissue and (2) injection of gadolinium always demonstrates a contrast uptake in the papillary projections.

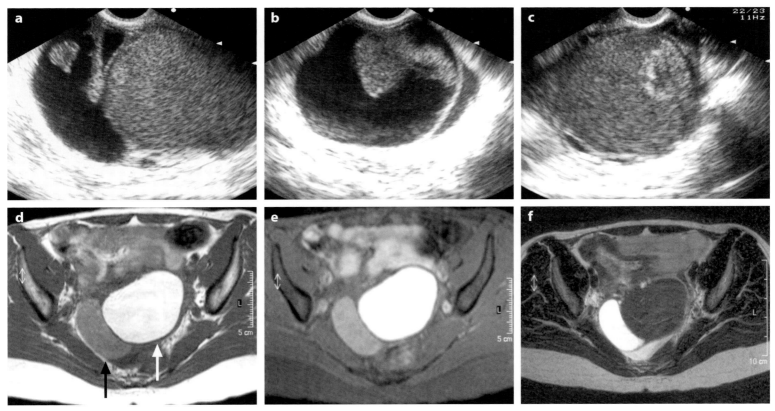

Fig. 17.34 Association of a FHC and an endometrioma in the same ovary. EVS transverse of the right ovary (**a**) and sagittal through the lateral cyst (**b**) and through the medial cyst (**c**) displays a lateral cyst I with typical findings of a hemorrhagic functional and a typical medial endometrioma. MR axial T1 (**d**), fat suppression (**e**) and T2 (**f**) depict: (1) a lateral cyst with an intermediate signal on T1 and fat suppression and a signal close to urine on T2; these findings are typical for a FHC (*black arrow*). (2) In the medial part of the ovary a cyst with a signal close to adipose tissue on T1 (*white arrow*), with a high-signal intensity on fat suppression, and an intermediate signal between adipose tissue and pelvic muscle (decrease of the signal) on T2; these findings are typical for an endometrioma

CT Pattern

CT has no place in the current diagnosis of endometrioma. However, because endometriosis can be discovered by chance on a CT examination and because endometrioma can be a differential diagnosis with other adnexal masses where CT has major indications, the aspect and the main findings of endometrioma on CT must be known.

The wall: Without injection, the wall can be dense; the external surface may have a blurred appearance due to adhesions, while the inner wall may have a shaggy appearance due to small clots against its inner wall (Fig. 17.35). After contrast injection, contrast uptake is visualized in the inner wall, external wall remains blurred at the arterial phase of a dynamic CT injection, and regular vessels are usually visualized giving the wall a double contour aspect.

The hemorrhagic content: Without contrast, density of the cyst is usually higher than that of urine and close to myometrium (Fig. 17.36). After contrast, absence of contrast uptake in the cyst easily allows to prove its cystic nature.

Exceptionally, the overall density of the cysts is very high, around 100 HU (Fig. 17.14). These cases are also correlated with very peculiar aspects on ultrasound and MR.

Clots: They appear with the different shapes described above. They can resemble to calcifications; however, their density is usually comprised between 90 and 140 HU [55] which is much lower than regular calcifications. Their exact location, separate from the wall, can clearly be seen and a particular semilunar shape is specific for endometrioma (Fig. 17.37).

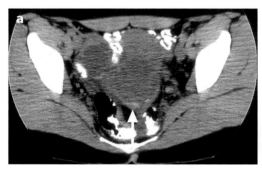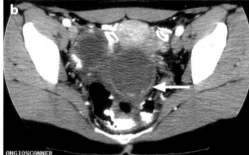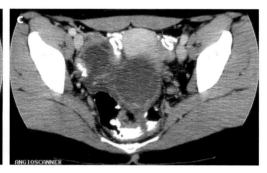

Fig. 17.35 Bilateral ovarian endometrioma typical aspect on DCT. CT without contrast (**a**): the walls of the cysts are slightly denser than the cystic content. Hyperdense foci (*arrow*) related to clots lie in the dependent portion of the left cyst. At the arterial phase (**b**): tiny vessels (*arrow*) are visualized in the inner walls. At the parenchymal phase (**c**): contrast uptake in the walls is depicted

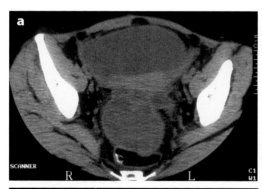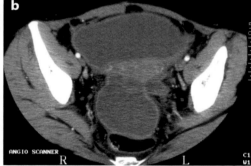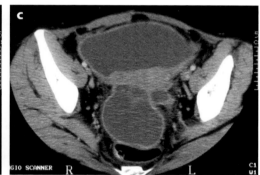

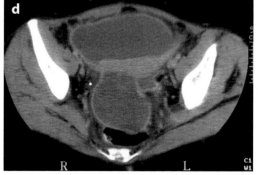

Fig. 17.36 CT findings of hemorrhagic content in endometrioma. DCT without injection (**a**): the cyst is not round; its wall is thick; and density of the content is 20 HU, related to the hemorrhagic content. At the arterial phase (**b**), a regular vessel is seen in the wall, with a contrast uptake at the venous phase (**c**) which is more pronounced on the delayed (**d**)

Fig. 17.37 **Characteristic curvilinear clot on CT.** (a) In vivo CT scan: a characteristic declive curvilinear clot in the dependent portion of an ovarian endometriotic cyst is displayed (*arrow*). (b) In vitro CT scan: density of the clot measures 90 HU (*arrow*)

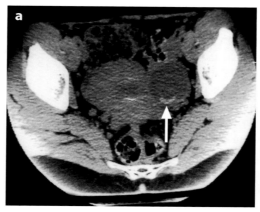 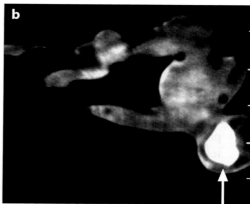

Differential diagnosis: Except in the case where a typical clot is found or where secondary findings such as bilateral and multiple lesions, localized protrusions, and incisures are seen (Table 17.2), the diagnosis can hardly be made on CT.

17.1.10.3 Subperitoneal Endometriosis

Deep endometriosis is defined by some authors as an infiltration of the implant penetrating ≥5 mm under the surface of the peritoneum [36]. In fact, any type of endometriotic lesion under the peritoneum is considered as a subperitoneal location.

The depth of an endometriotic lesion cannot be anticipated at coelioscopy. A small pelvic lesion can hide a deep and larger endometriotic lesion, especially in types II and III [72]. Deep endometriosis is poorly reflected in the AFS classification.

As it has been already mentioned, the pattern of endometriotic lesions is quite different according to the tissue in which endometriosis develops. Indeed in the subperitoneal space, endometriotic implants grow in conjunctive tissue, which is quite different from stroma of the ovary.

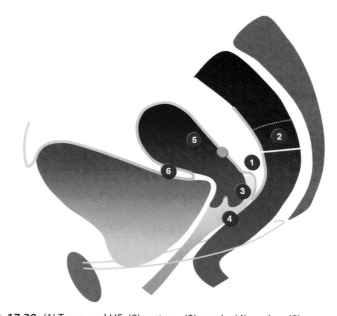

Fig. 17.38 (1) Torus and US, (2) rectum, (3) cervix, (4) vagina, (5) uterus, and (6) vesicouterine pouch

Macroscopy and Imaging Findings

They are reported in Table 17.10.

Table 17.10 Macroscopic and imaging findings

1. US
1. Fibromuscular component echogenic or hypoechoic
2. Endometriotic foci: may appear hyperechoic or anechoic

2. MR
1. Fibromuscular component:
   T1, fat suppression, and T2. Overall signal close to pelvic muscle or of intermediate signal
   After injection, fibrotic component slightly enhances
2. Endometriotic foci:
   Hemorrhagic foci: high signal on T1, after fat suppression, and variable signal on T2
   Cavities containing a clear fluid: low signal on T1 and a high signal on T2

The pattern of the lesion is mainly related to the fibromuscular hyperplasia surrounding the endometriotic foci that can contain small cavities [36].

Subperitoneal endometriosis (Fig. 17.38) can involve:

1. The posterior subperitoneal space, most often secondary to peritoneal implants in the pouch of Douglas that extends into the vaginal fornix; the anterior wall of the rectum; the rectovaginal wall; and laterally, the uterosacral ligaments.
2. The anterior subperitoneal space, mainly the bladder wall secondary to implants in the vesicouterine pouch Sampson.
3. The lateral subperitoneal space.

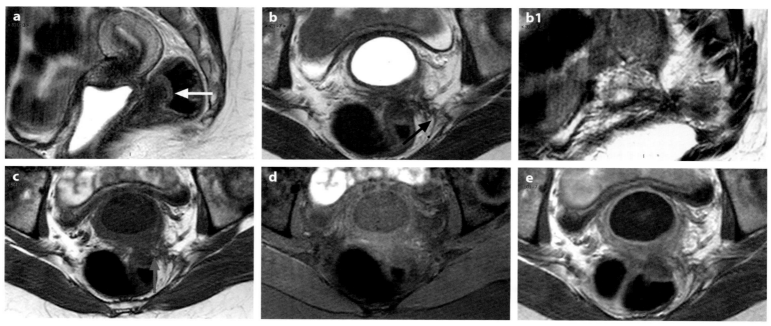

Fig. 17.53 Endometriosis of the low rectum, USL and sacrorectogenital septum. MR sagittal T2 (**a**) depicts a tissular mass in the posterior wall of the cervix and the upper vagina infiltrating the upper part of the rectovaginal septum and extending to the anterior wall of the low rectum (*white arrow*); the inferior pole of the lesion is 4 cm above the anorectal junction. On axial T2 (**b**), the lesion involves the anterior rectal wall from 10 to 2 o'clock, extending laterally the left US ligament; deep extension of the lesion of the US to the sacrorectogenital septum is visualized on **b1** and to the pelvic fascia (*black arrow*). On axial T1 (**c**) and fat suppression (**d**), a small hemorrhagic focus (*red arrow*) is present in the tissular mass of the rectum, while multiple foci are displayed in the left US ligament. After injection (**e**), a slight contrast uptake in the rectal mass is visualized

4. Extension (Fig. 17.38). Involvement of the torus, of the terminal portion of the US ligaments, may extend through continuity.

   (a) Downward medially to the posterior wall of the cervix and the posterior wall of the vagina and laterally to the sacrorectogenital septum following a backward direction with spicules joining the posterior deep pelvic fascia and or a downward direction into the thickness of the septum with a possible extension into the inferior hypogastric plexus (Figs. 17.49, 17.53, and 17.54); as far as branches of this inferior hypogastric plexus are connected with the inferior branches of the sacral plexus ,these abnormalities may explain the possibility of a sciatica or pain in the territory of the obturator nerve;

   (b) Upward to the serosa of the uterus body and through contiguity to the posterior myometrium, creating lesions of external adenomyosis;

   (c) Backward to the rectosigmoid junction;

   (d) Uncommonly anteriorly, to the parametrium and the ureter. In this location, MR or CT with injection seems more accurate in the diagnosis than US.

Posterior Part of the Cervix and the Vagina

1. Involvement of the posterior part of the cervix and vagina is most often secondary to a lesion of the torus or of the USL. More rarely, involvement of the cervix or the vagina is primary [75].

2. On US, echogenicity of the lesion is usually a little lower than echogenicity of the uterus. Several implants can be present (Fig. 17.55). More rarely, the nodule is roughly of the same echogenicity (Fig. 17.56).

   Contours are regular (Fig. 17.57) or spiculated (Fig. 17.58). Echogenic foci related to clots typical for endometriosis can be visualized in the nodule. The lesion can extend posteriorly to the rectum.

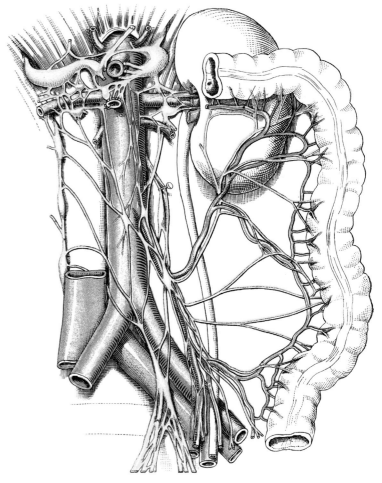

Fig. 17.54 Abdominal aortic plexus, superior mesenteric plexus, inferior mesenteric plexus, superior hypogastric plexus. Presacral nerve in front of the bifurcation the abdominal aorta, with its bifucation (*upper dotted line*). Hypogastric nerve (*inferior dotted line*)

Fig. 17.55 Endometriosis of the posterior fornix. Longitudinal EVS (**a**) and axial (**b**) visualize two low echogenic nodules protruding under the mucosa of the posterior wall of the fornix (*arrows*)

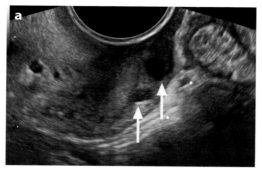
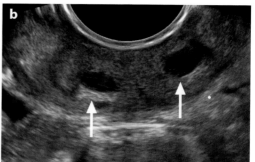

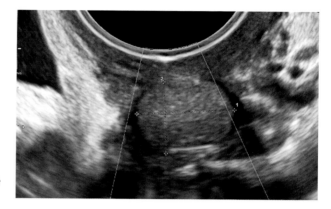

Fig. 17.56 Endometriosis of the posterior fornix. Longitudinal EVS depicts in the posterior fornix a nodule of the same echogenicity as the wall of the vagina

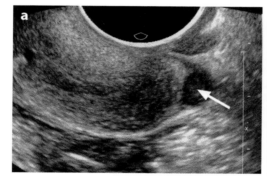
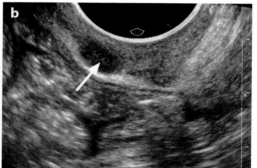

Fig. 17.57 Endometriosis of the posterior fornix. Forty-eight-year-old woman with dysmenorrhea and dyspareunia. Longitudinal EVS (**a**) and transverse EVS (**b**) display a round hypoechoic nodule (*arrow*) with regular border in the right portion of the posterior fornix

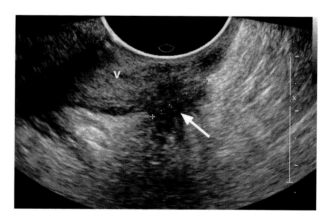

Fig. 17.58 Twenty-year-old-woman with deep dyspareunia. Longitudinal EV displays a hypoechogenic nodule (*arrow*) with spiculated contours invading the vaginal wall anteriorly (*V*)

Douglas (Figs. 17.63, 17.64, and 17.65)

On US, some hyperechogenic foci can be visualized. These foci can be even better displayed when they are outlined by some fluid in the cul-de-sac. Infiltration through contiguity in the underlying structures can be seen.

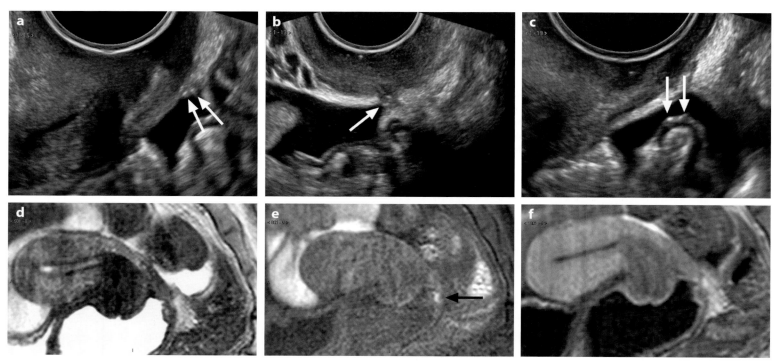

Fig. 17.63 Endometriosis of the Douglas. Twenty-five-year-old woman with dysmenorrhea and deep dyspareunia. At physical examination, painful nodule in the posterior fornix. EVS sagittal (**a**) displays echogenic foci (*arrows*) in the *bottom* of the Douglas, very likely related to hemorrhagic endometriotic implants; axial view (**b**) depicts a stellated endometriotic lesion in the posterior fornix of the vagina (*arrow*); sagittal view (**c**) endometriotic foci are present in the Douglas on the anterior serosa of the rectum (*arrows*). MR sagittal T2 (**d**) depicts (1) an endometriotic mass in the posterior fornix with hemorrhagic foci on fat suppression (**e**) (*arrow*) and contrast uptake in the mass after contrast (**f**); (2) tiny peritoneal implants in the Douglas outlined by the peritoneal fluid on (**d**)

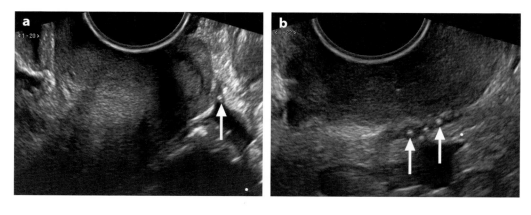

Fig. 17.64 (**a**) Longitudinal and axial (**b**) EVS display hyperechogenic foci (*arrows*) related to hemorrhagic implants in the bottom of the Douglas

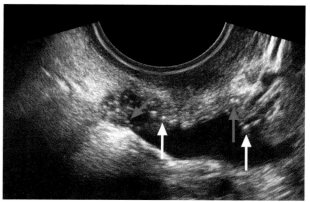

Fig. 17.65 Peritoneal implants in the Douglas. Axial EVS (**a**) displays multiple echogenic foci (*white arrows*) in the anterior portion of the Douglas extending in the right fornix (*red arrow*)

External Adenomyosis

External Adenomyosis (posterior wall) [76]. From the torus, the endometriotic lesions extend centrifugally to the posterior wall of the uterus on the serosa, extending into the external myometrium where they create external adenomyosis (Fig. 17.66).

Rectosigmoid Wall: Other GI Tract Locations

Rectosigmoid Involvement

Involvement of the anterior wall of the rectum or the inferior wall of the sigmoid is usually continuous with involvement of the posterior wall of the uterus body, the cervix most often the torus, the US, and the posterior wall of the vagina.

Clinical Findings

Most commonly, as far as endometriosis of the wall involves the serosa and the muscular layer protruding under the submucosa, patients complain of dyschesia and in some cases of findings of the rectal syndrome.

In uncommon cases, the lesion extends beyond the submucosa until the mucosa and is responsible for catamenial rectorrhagia.

Common Macroscopic and Radiologic Findings Are Reported in Table 17.12.

Imaging Findings

(a) *On EVS or on endorectal sonography* [77], the different layers of the normal rectosigmoid wall can be displayed (Fig. 17.67).

Table 17.12 Common macroscopic and radiologic findings

1. Site:
    Most commonly rectosigmoid junction
    Less commonly rectum above or at the level of the rectovaginal septum
    Sigmoid
    Double location possible

2. Pattern:
    Tissular mainly fibrotic
    Containing sometimes foci of endometriosis
    Surface regular or irregular.
    Homogeneous or slightly inhomogeneous

3. Morphology:
    Sagittal plane : obtuse angles with the rectum wall
    Axial plane: From 10 to 2 h
    Triangular aspect with anterior tip, posterior base

4. Associated findings:
    Rectum attracted forward, separated from the normal concavity of the sacrum, and converging toward the torus
    Ascitic fluid behind the rectum can be present

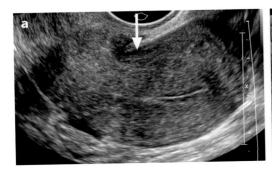
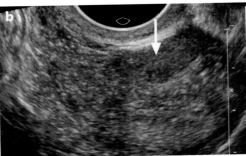
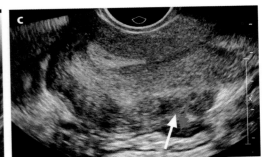
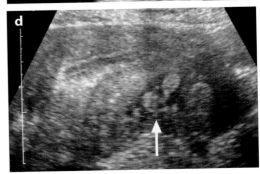

Fig. 17.66 Longitudinal EVS (**a**): low echogenic involvement of the torus extending upward on the posterior wall of the uterus (*arrow*). Longitudinal EVS (**b**): involvement of the posterior wall extends until the fundus (*arrow*). Longitudinal EVS (**c**): involvement of the torus extends posteriorly to the anterior wall of the rectosigmoid junction (*red arrow*) and upward all along the posterior wall of the uterus (*white arrow*). Longitudinal TAS (**d**): very extensive on both sides of the torus infiltrating deeply the posterior myometrium, with a retroflexion of the uterus (*arrow*)

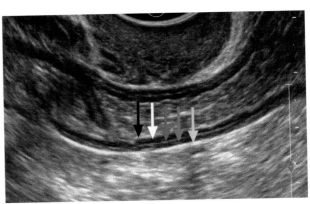

Fig. 17.67 (1) Mucosa (superficial layer) hyper echogenic (*black arrow*). (2) Muscularis mucosae hypoechoic (*white arrow*). (3) Submucosa echogenic (*red arrow*). (4) Muscularis propria hypoechoic (*green arrow*). (5) Serosa hyperechoic (*yellow arrow*)

The tissular lesion has an echogenicity equal or slightly inferior to the rectal wall; it is poorly or not vascularized on color Doppler. The degree of extension through the different layers of the wall can be displayed. Extension to the muscular wall is commonly associated with an edema of the submucous layer; clear delineation of both layers indicates absence of invasion of the submucosa, while irregularity of the interface corresponds to invasion of the submucosa. Involvement of the rectal mucosa can be depicted (Fig. 17.68). The height of extension can be measured (Fig. 17.69).

While involvement of a higher location is more difficult to detect, involvement of the sigmoid can be displayed.

Thickening of the hypoechoic muscular layer outlined by a hyperechoic thickening of the submucosa on its innerside, associated with a retraction, and a hyperechoic thickening of the serosa and very likely of the mesosigmoid are characteristic (Fig. 17.70). On color Doppler, vessels at the base probably in the mesosigmoid can be depicted.

(b) *On MR*, the main fibrotic component of the mass looks hypointense (like pelvic muscles) on T2 and T1. In some cases, hemorrhagic foci, hyperintense on T1 and on fat suppression, can be displayed (Fig. 17.53). After injection of gadolinium, this component has a contrast uptake lower than the normal wall and is clearly delineated from the normal rectal wall (Fig. 17.71).

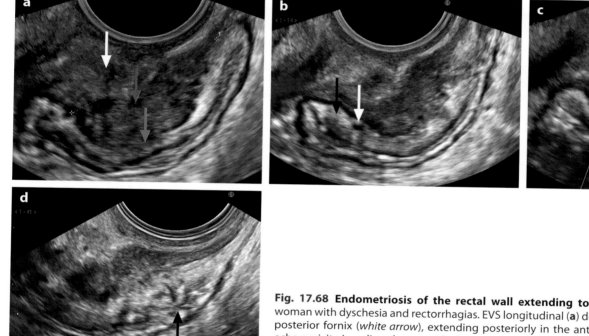

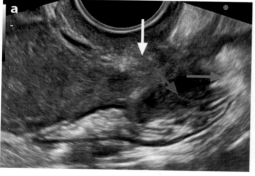

Fig. 17.68 Endometriosis of the rectal wall extending to the mucosa. Twenty-nine-year-old woman with dyschesia and rectorrhagias. EVS longitudinal (**a**) displays an endometriotic lesion of the posterior fornix (*white arrow*), extending posteriorly in the anterior rectal wall; the mass has a low echogenicity invading the muscular layer (*red arrow*); there is a focal interruption of the submucosa (*green arrow*). The submucosa is thickened (*black arrow*), containing tiny cystic cavities (*white arrow*) related to endometriotic implants (**b**) with vessels on color Doppler (**c**). A focal extension into the mucosa (*black arrow*) is visualized (**d**)

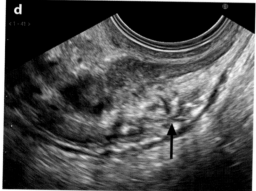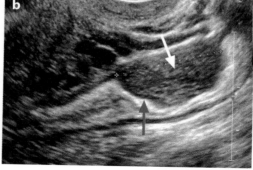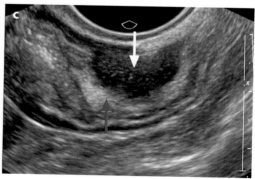

Fig. 17.69 Involvement of the rectum and the rectosigmoid junction. (**a**) Thirty-eight-year-old woman with dyschesia and catamenial rectorrhagias. Endometriosis of the posterior cervix and the posterior fornix (*white arrow*) obliterating the hypoechoic layer corresponding to the muscularis propria (*red arrow*) and obliterating the submucosa (*green arrow*) of the anterior rectal wall, making the hypothesis of involvement of the mucosa very likely. (**b**) Nodule of 2-cm length involving the muscular layer (*white arrow*) protruding under the submucosa which is normal (*red arrow*). (**c**) Involvement of the muscularis (*white arrow*) of the anterior wall of the rectosigmoid junction associated with an edema of the submucosa (*red arrow*) and a ill-defined limit of its deepest portion related to an infiltration of this layer.

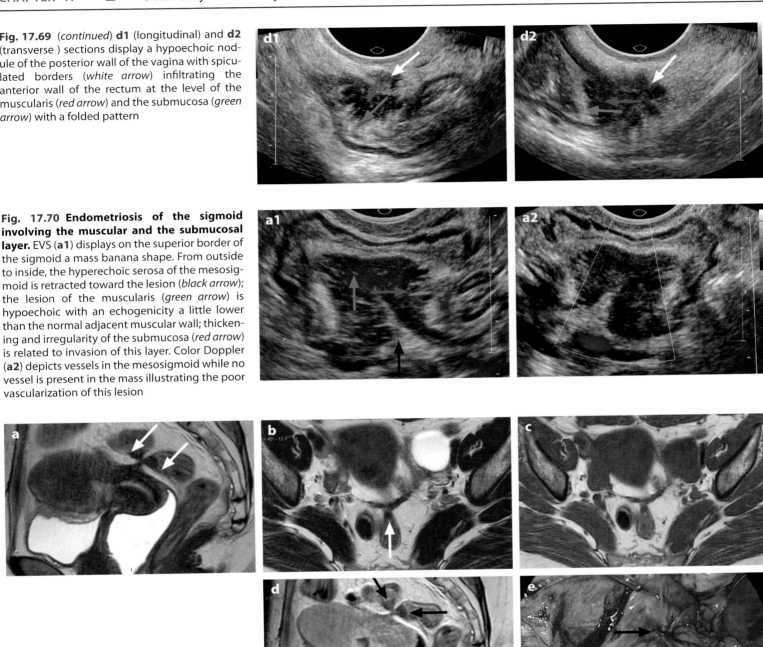

Fig. 17.69 (*continued*) **d1** (longitudinal) and **d2** (transverse) sections display a hypoechoic nodule of the posterior wall of the vagina with spiculated borders (*white arrow*) infiltrating the anterior wall of the rectum at the level of the muscularis (*red arrow*) and the submucosa (*green arrow*) with a folded pattern

Fig. 17.70 Endometriosis of the sigmoid involving the muscular and the submucosal layer. EVS (**a1**) displays on the superior border of the sigmoid a mass banana shape. From outside to inside, the hyperechoic serosa of the mesosigmoid is retracted toward the lesion (*black arrow*); the lesion of the muscularis (*green arrow*) is hypoechoic with an echogenicity a little lower than the normal adjacent muscular wall; thickening and irregularity of the submucosa (*red arrow*) is related to invasion of this layer. Color Doppler (**a2**) depicts vessels in the mesosigmoid while no vessel is present in the mass illustrating the poor vascularization of this lesion

Fig. 17.71 Rectal involvement of endometriosis. Forty-five-year-old woman with dysmenorrhea and deep dyspareunia. Treated with progesterone. MR sagittal T2 (**a**) and axial T2 (**b**) display at the rectosigmoid junction a tissular fibrotic mass 3-cm length, contiguous with an involvement of the torus with an attraction (*arrow*). This pattern is typical for an endometriotic location of the rectosigmoid junction. On axial T1 (**c**), no hemorrhagic focus in the lesion is visualized. Sagittal after IV injection of gadolinium (**d**) depicts a slight contrast uptake of the fibrotic tissue (*arrow*). At coelioscopy (**e**), rectosigmoid junction (*blue arrow*) has an adhesion to the torus (*black arrow*) situated just immediately below the inferior part of the uterus body (*green arrow*). Adhesiolysis with shaving of the rectosigmoid junction was performed which confirmed the diagnosis and the extension of the lesion

Extension through the wall can be precised. Involvement can be limited to the serosa and in this case, cannot be distinguished from a simple adhesion (Fig. 17.72). Interruption of the muscular layer with extension to the submucosa can be displayed (Fig. 17.73); in this case, a higher-contrast uptake than in the muscular layer can be visualized (Fig. 17.74). When there is a contrast uptake in the mucosa, an extension until this layer can be suspected (Fig. 17.75).

While a location at the rectosigmoid junction (Fig. 17.73) or lower on the rectum (Fig. 17.53) is usually easily diagnosed, difficulties of diagnosis on the sigmoid are variable; low location on the sigmoid (Fig. 17.28) can be easily recognized,

while higher or small locations can be overlooked (Fig. 17.76).

Extension in height is usually clearly established; the relationship of the inferior border of the lesion with the anorectal junction (which is essential to know preoperatively) is usually clearly established.

In some cases, diagnosis of a double location particularly of another location on the sigmoid at some distance from the rectosigmoid junction can be performed.

Although MR can be sufficient to diagnose involvement of the rectum or the rectosigmoid location, when surgery is considered, CT with enema is advocated.

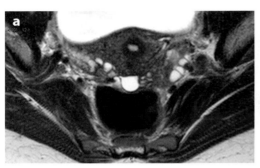
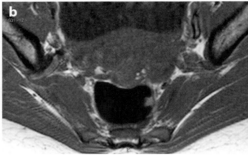
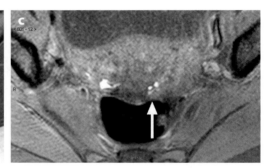

Fig. 17.72 Endometriosis of the left US ligament extending to the serosa of the rectum without involvement of the muscularis. MR axial T2 (**a**) shows involvement of the left US ligament in contact with the serosa of the anterior wall of the rectum at 1 o'clock. On T1 (**b**) and on fat suppression (**c**) at the same location, the signal of the serosa is interrupted (*arrow*). Prospective diagnosis: Endometriosis or simple adhesion at this level, without invasion of the muscularis propria, was suggested. Surgery: endometriosis of the serosa

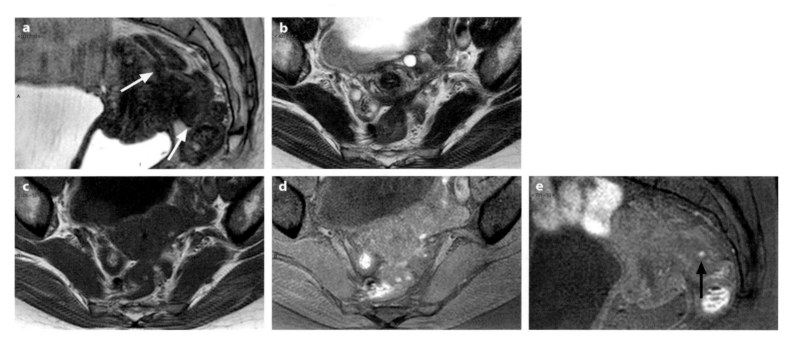

Fig. 17.73 Rectosigmoid lesion with extension to the mucosa. Thirty-seven-year-old woman with dyschesia and rectorrhagias. MR sagittal T2 (**a**) and axial T2 (**b**) display in continuity with endometriosis of the cervix a low-intensity mass involving the posterior wall of the high rectum and the rectosigmoid junction, making obtuse angles with the normal rectal wall (*two white arrows*). On axial T1 (**c**), axial and sagittal fat suppression (**d** and **e**) and multiple hemorrhagic foci are visualized in the lesion (*arrow*).

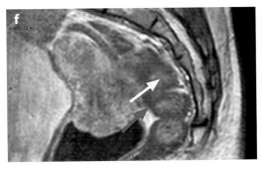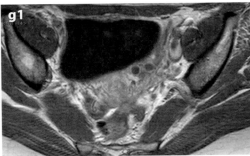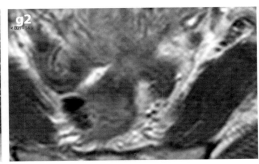

Fig. 17.73 (continued) On sagittal after injection (**f**), the overall intensity of the mass is higher than the normal muscular wall which is pushed backward at the inferior pole of the mass. Complete interruption of this layer is visualized (*white arrow*), related to invasion of the submucosa. Normal muscular wall is indicated (*red arrow*). On axial after injection (**g1**) and with magnification (**g2**), the lesion is in contact with the mucosa. Prospective diagnosis: endometriosis of the rectal wall extending to the mucosa. Surgery: resection rectosigmoid through coelioscopy with colorectal anastomose. Macroscopy: The mass is 5-cm length; at the section, the mass is fibrous with hemorrhage. Microscopy: involvement of (1) the serosa and the subserosa, (2) the muscular layer with hyperplasia and dissociation of the muscular fascicles, and (3) the submucosa

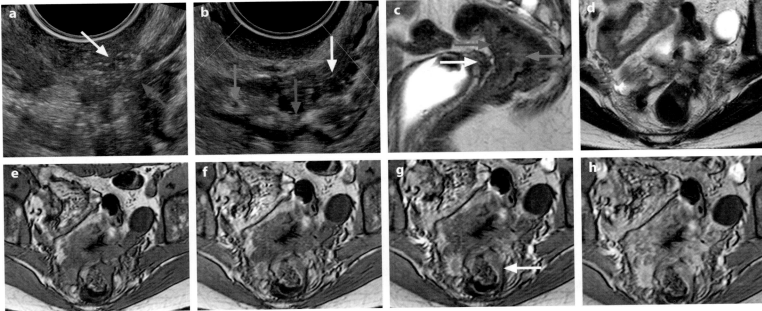

Fig. 17.74 Endometriosis of the rectal wall involving the submucosa. Forty-nine-year-old woman. Total hysterectomy for adenomyosis. Dyschesia. (**a**) Longitudinal EVS displays an endometriotic lesion of the posterior fornix (*white arrow*) extending to the anterior wall of the rectum (*red arrow*). Longitudinal EVS through the rectal wall (**b**) depicts a low echogenic tissular mass involving the muscularis (*white arrow*) containing some echogenic foci; interruption of the normal muscular wall and submucous irregular thickening indicate invasion of the submucosa (*red arrow*). A small cystic lesion in the submucosa (*green arrow*) is displayed. (**c**) MR sagittal (**c**) and axial T2 (**d**) confirm endometriosis of the posterior fornix (*white arrow*) and of the anterior rectal wall. Extension in the muscularis (*red arrow*) appears as a mass of low signal intensity close to pelvic muscle, while invasion of the submucosa (*green arrow*) appears with a high signal intensity. DMR without injection (**e**), and at the arterial phase (**f**) visualize vessels in the lesion (in **f**), with a slight contrast uptake at the venous phase (**g**) (*arrow*) which increases on the the delayed (**h**)

Fig. 17.75 Twenty-nine-years-old woman with catamenial rectorrhagias. MR sagittal T2 (**a1** and **a2**) displays a 4–5-cm lesion in the inferior and anterior portion of the terminal segment of the sigmoid. On **a1**, the mainly fibrous component of the mass of low signal is underlined by a thin layer of high-signal intensity which corresponds to an edema of the submucosa (*arrow*). On **a2**, small cystic cavities with a high-signal intensity are visualized in the upper part of the mass (*arrow*).

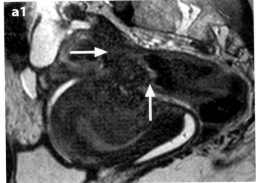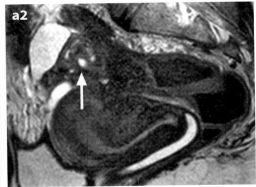

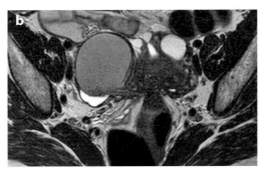
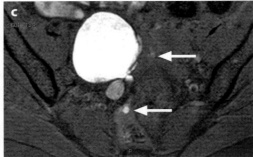
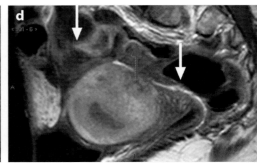

Fig. 17.75 (*continued*) On axial T2 (**b**), multiple high-signal spots are present in the mass, which appear with a characteristic high signal on axial T1 with fat suppression (**c**) (*arrows*) related to their hemorrhagic content. Sagittal T1 after contrast injection (**d**) better delineates the mass (*white arrows*) and shows an overall low contrast of the mass with a high-contrast uptake in the mucosa (*red arrow*). Coelioscopy: partial resection of the sigmoid was performed. Pathology: endometriotic lesion of the sigmoid involving the wall until the mucosa

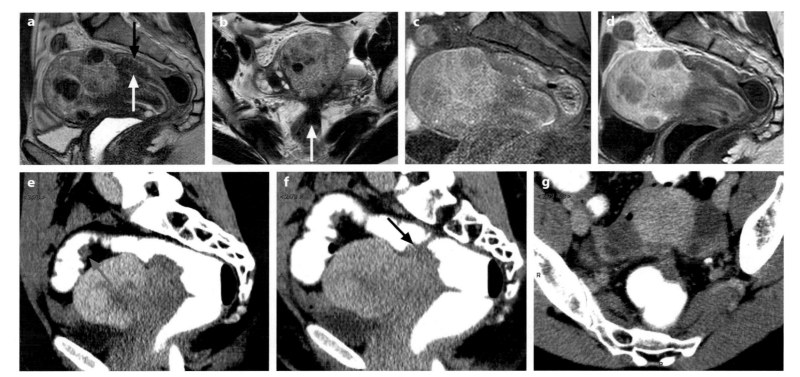

Fig. 17.76 Rectosigmoid endometriosis with a second sigmoid location. MR sagittal T2 (**a**) and axial T2 (**b**) display involvement of the torus extending to the anterior wall of the rectosigmoid junction, between 10 and 2 o'clock, on both sides to the lower sigmoid and the upper rectum over a length of 5 cm. The mass has a low-signal intensity (*white arrow*). Its shape with obtuse angles with the normal wall is characteristic. Invasion of the muscular wall until the deep part of the submucosa (*black arrow*) which appears with a high-signal intensity is displayed. On sagittal T1 with fat suppression (**c**), the mass contains hemorrhagic implants. On sagittal T1 after injection (**d**), the mass has a low-contrast uptake with a signal inferior to myometrium. CT with enema with sagittal reformation (**e, f**) and transverse view (**g**) performed after MR (**e**) (1) confirms the diagnosis with a very particular crenelated pattern of the mucosa (*black arrow*) reflecting involvement of the muscularis, and extension of the lesion of the rectosigmoid (2) displays a little second location (*green arrow*) on the inferior part of the sigmoid, overlooked on MR

(c) *CT with enema.* CT is performed in prone position (which allows a perfect opacification of the anterior and inferior wall of the rectosigmoid), with IV contrast which better displays the lesion but overall allows in the same time to study the ureters and the bladder.

The mass has a tissular density. A slight IV contrast enhancement is displayed. In case of involvement of at least the muscular layer, the mucosa has a flattened or a crenelated aspect.

1. CT is very accurate to make the diagnosis of involvement of the rectum and the sigmoid; this last location can be overlooked on MR (Fig. 17.77). It allows to differentiate extension to the serosa from extension to the wall.

2. It allows to precise the height of extension (Fig. 17.78) and the position of the lower pole compare to the anorectal junction.

3. CT with enema is the best method to detect another location on the colon. About 15 % of patients have a double location (Figs. 17.76 and 17.79) and in very uncommon cases more than two locations.

(d) With the different imaging modalities, when the posterior endometriotic lesion arrives just in contact with the serosa of the rectum, it can be difficult to diagnose the presence or absence of adhesion. EVS, because of the dynamic aspect, can be helpful to diagnose adhesions.

When the rectum is attracted toward the posterior wall of the uterus or vagina, it can be difficult to differentiate a simple adhesion from a true invasion of the rectal wall.

Fig. 17.77 Sigmoid involvement better displayed on CT than on MR. MR Sagittal T2 (**a**) and T1 after injection (**b**) barely display an endometriotic involvement of the lower part of the sigmoid (*arrow*); CT with enema on sagittal reformation (**c**) and on axial view (**d**) depicts a typical location on the anterior portion of the sigmoid (*arrow*) with a pattern of partial obstruction on the axial view (*arrow*)

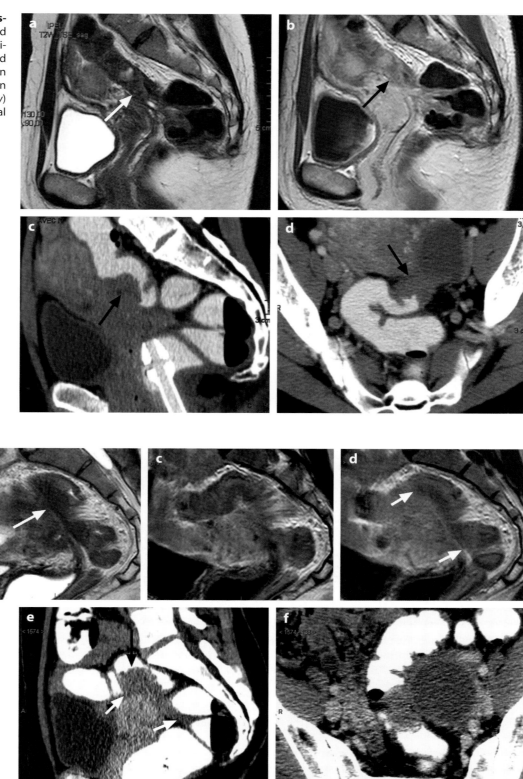

Fig. 17.78 Rectal and sigmoid endometriosis. MR sagittal T2 (**a**, **b**) (two contiguous sections) shows an involvement of the torus with an attraction and involvement of the rectosigmoid junction extending to the upper portion of the rectum and the inferior portion of the sigmoid; the lesion appears as a low-intensity infiltration of the wall with obtuse angles with the normal wall (*arrow*). After injection (**c**, **d**) (two contiguous sections), contrast uptake delineates accurately extension of the lesion (*two small arrows*). CT enema sagittal (**e**) axial (**f**) displays involvement of the wall with a crenelated aspect of the mucosa (*black arrow*) which indicates involvement of the wall extends at least into the muscle layer; the length of extension and the distance of the lower part to the anorectal junction are well documented (*two small white arrows*). Pathology: endometriosis involvement of the serosa, the muscular layer, and the submucosa except the mucosa

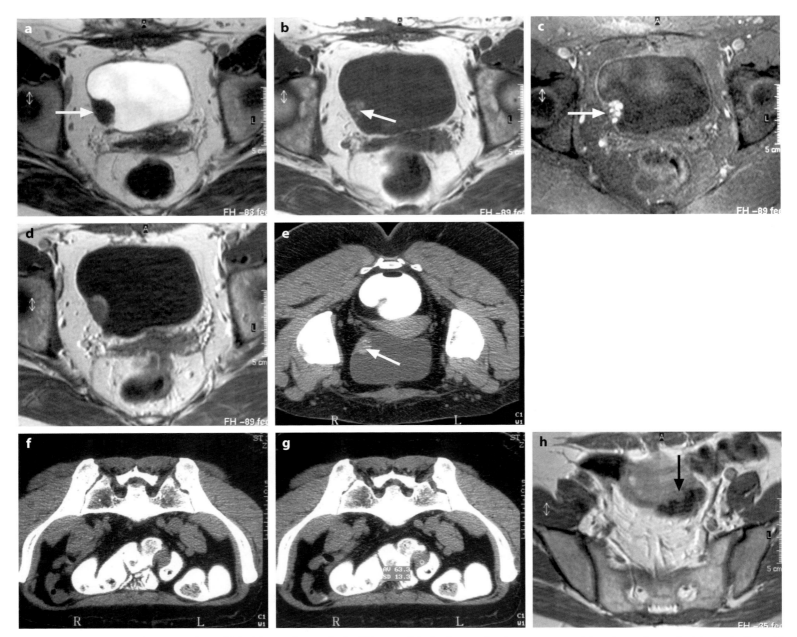

Fig. 17.79 Sigmoid endometriosis and bladder endometriosis. Thirty-five-year-old woman with menometrorrhagia and dyspareunia. At colonoscopy, there was a regular narrowing of the sigmoid with an intact mucosa. *Bladder endometriosis.* MR axial T2 (**a**): the mass with an overall signal close to pelvic muscles is clearly seen (*arrow*). Axial T1 (**b**) and with fat suppression (**c**): mass contains hyperintense foci (*arrow*). Axial T1 after injection (**d**) demonstrates contrast enhancement in the mass. CT without injection (**e**) displays a tissular mass containing hyperdense foci (*arrow*). *Sigmoid endometriosis.* CT with enema (**f, g**) visualizes a smooth mass of 63 HU in the lower part of the sigmoid (*small ROI in g*), very suggestive of an endometrial location, which was confirmed at surgery. This lesion was missed on a prospective evaluation on MR (**h**) and was very difficult to diagnose (*arrow*) even on a retrospective study

Other Gastrointestinal Tract Locations

They can involve more rarely the caecum (Fig. 17.80), the appendix, and the small bowel. These locations can be isolated or associated with other GI tract locations. They can be associated with other endometriotic locations and particularly subperitoneal locations.

Rectovaginal Septum (Fig. 17.81)

RVS is often diagnosed at vaginal examination.

There are mainly two types of involvement:

Rectovaginal septum (RVS) lesion is caused by invasion of Douglas pouch or by a subperitoneal location (USL, sacrorectovaginal septum, anterior mesorectum, anterior wall of the rectum, cervix, vagina (Fig. 17.82)).

Rarely endometriosis of the RVS can originate in the RVS tissue and looks like a circumscribed nodular aggregate of smooth muscle containing active endometrial glands and scanty stroma, so that Donnez [78] suggests to call this form rectovaginal adenomyosis.

Association of Subperitoneal Lesions (Fig. 17.53)

While in some patients endometriosis can be located only to one subperitoneal location (USL for example), in other patients, different locations can be involved most often contiguous more rarely distinct from each other (nodule on USL and a separated rectal location, a double GI tract location for example).

Fig. 17.80 Endometriosis of the caecum. Forty-one-year-old had appendicectomy 30 years ago and catamenial right pelvic pain since the interruption of oral contraceptive. EVS (**a**) displays a thickening of the wall of the caecum, containing some echogenic fluid, with a localized pain at the pressure of the probe (*arrow*). On color Doppler (**b**), vessels are visualized in the wall. Association with the clinical findings suggested the possibility of an endometriotic location to the caecum. CT without injection (**c**) and after injection (**d**) confirms the impression of the EVS examination. The wall of the caecum is thickened (*arrow*). Fibrotic tissue around the caecum is visualized (*arrow*). Surgery: 3-cm nodule situated at the junction of the terminal ileum and the caecum. Ilecolic resection. Pathology: endometriosis on the serosa infiltrating the wall until the mucosa

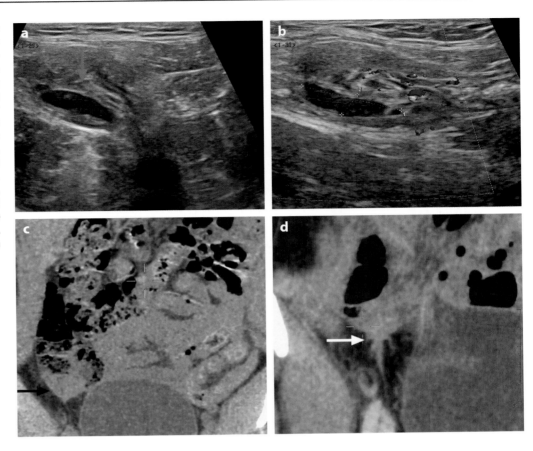

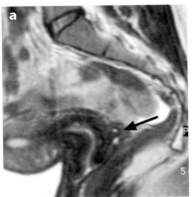
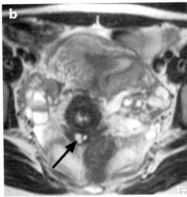
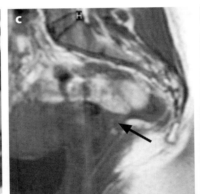
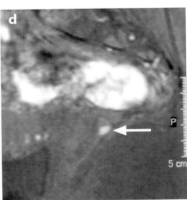

Fig. 17.81 Small endometriotic nodule of the upper part of the rectovaginal septum. Twenty-six-year-old woman with dyspareunia and dysmenorrhea. (**a** and **b**) Sagittal and axial T2: 2-cm nodule (*arrow*) with hyperintense foci involves the Douglas pouch, the posterior wall of the vagina, and the top of the rectovaginal septum. (**c** and **d**) Sagittal T1 without and with fat suppression confirms the presence of hyperintense hemorrhagic foci (*arrows*)

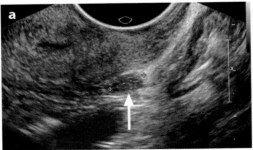
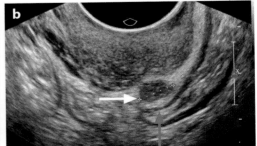

Fig. 17.82 Nodule of the Douglas pouch. Longitudinal (**a**) and transverse (**b**) EVS display an oval low echogenic nodule (*white arrow*) in the bottom of the Douglas infiltrating the top of the rectovaginal septum. The nodule is clearly separated from the anterior wall of the rectum (*red arrow*)

Anterior Subperitoneal Space

Anatomy

Anteriorly peritoneum covers the anterior wall of the uterus and reflects in front of the isthmus over the superior wall of the bladder to form the vesicouterine pouch.

Locations

Locations are reported in Table 17.13 (Fig. 17.83).

Table 17.13 Anterior subperitoneal lesions

1. Vesicouterine pouch
2. Anterior adenomyosis
3. Bladder wall
4. Vesicovaginal septum

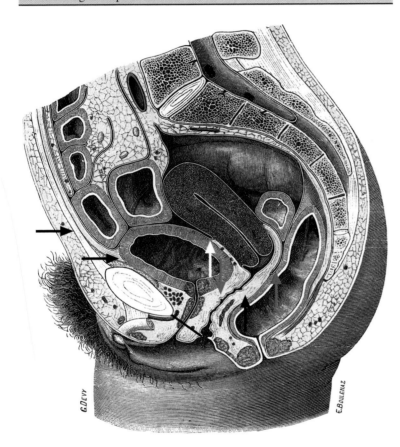

Fig. 17.83 Intraperitoneal space (indicated in front of the *superior horizontal black arrow*), anterior subperitoneal space (*Inferior horizontal black arrow*), perineal space (*below the black bar*), vesicouterine pouch (*white arrow*), vesicouterine septum (*green arrow*), Douglas (a little above the tip of the *red arrow*), and rectovaginal septum (vertical *black arrow*)

Vesicouterine Pouch Involvement

Findings are the same as for the Douglas.

Anterior Adenomyosis

Findings are the same as posterior external adenomyosis (Fig. 17.84).

Bladder Wall Involvement

Bladder endometriosis is relatively rare, representing 2 % of all endometriosis cases [79].

Age: The majority of cases occurs between the ages of 25 and 40 [79].

Some cases have been reported after menopauses [80].
Pathogeny:
Three different opinions have been suggested:

- Koninckx and Martin [72] and Vercellini [81] suggested that peritoneal lesions are able to penetrate under the peritoneum and develop into deeply infiltrating endometriosis.
- Donnez [82] suggests that bladder endometriosis is a consequence of metaplasia of Müllerian remnants which can be found in the rectovaginal septum as well as in the vesicovaginal septum [13].
- According to Fedele [83], detrusor endometriosis could result from the extension of adenomyotic lesions from the anterior uterine wall to the bladder.

Clinical Findings

At least 50 % of patients have a history of previous pelvic surgery [79] and particularly a cesarian.

Painful micturition with straining and increased pain at the close of voiding has been first reported by JUDD [84]. Some patients experience a sense of pressure, a heaviness most frequently in the suprapubic region, usually relieved by voiding [79]. Associate symptoms suggestive of cystitis are frequent: urinary urgency, frequency, and burning [79]. Hematuria is present in only one-fourth of the cases [79]. The symptoms are classically cyclic [79]. However, absence of cyclic symptoms should not preclude a diagnosis of endometriosis [80].

At physical examination, a tender nodule can be palpated on the anterior fornix of the vagina [82].

Improvement of bladder symptoms during pregnancy has been reported [85].

Macroscopic and Radiological Findings Are Reported in Table 17.14

Imaging Findings

1. Ultrasound
   - Technical aspect:
   Transabdominal ultrasound with a full bladder can detect the lesion that appears as a mural mass that can extend both inside

Table 17.14 Common macroscopic and radiologic findings

1. Site:
   Most commonly superior face of the bladder in the vesicouterine cul-de-sac
   Less commonly trigone or floor of the bladder, the lateral walls, the dome, or the uterovesical junction [86]
   Double location possible
2. Pattern:
   Tissular mainly fibrotic
   Containing cystic cavities and endometriotic foci (more commonly than in subperitoneal posterior locations)
   Surface regular or irregular
3. Morphology:
   Size usually comprised between 2 and 3 cm [82][a]
   Extension from the vesicouterine pouch into the bladder wall, protruding into the lumen of the bladder common and very suggestive
4. Associated findings:
   Anterior adenomyosis (uncommonly inter-uterovesical block)
   Posterior subperitoneal location

[a]May range from several millimeters to 14 cm in diameter [86]

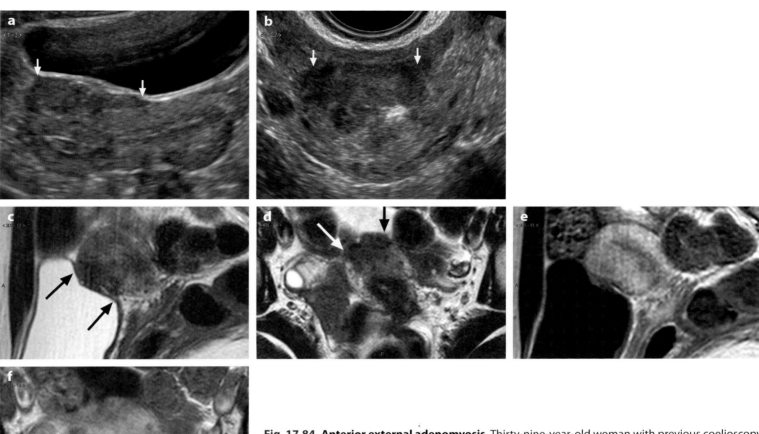

Fig. 17.84 Anterior external adenomyosis. Thirty-nine-year-old woman with previous coelioscopy for endometriosis. EVS sagittal (**a**) and axial (**b**) display a tissular infiltration between the uterus body and the bladder wall, less echoic than normal myometrium (*two small arrows*). MR sagittal T2 (**c**) and axial T2 (**d**) depict a lesion from the fundus to the *bottom* of the of the vesicouterine pouch, with a signal inferior to normal myometrium, extending to the outer layer of the anterior wall of the uterus body (*black arrows* in **c** and *black* and *white arrows* in **d**). On sagittal (**e**) and axial T1 (**f**) after injection, this tissular infiltration enhances less than normal myometrium

the bladder lumen and outside [87]. However, EVS allows a better depiction of the lesion [88].

Findings: (Figs. 17.85, 17.86, and 17.87)

– Location of the mass is variable. However, the mass is most often in the vesicouterine pouch, by its size is usually comprised between 2 and 3 cm.

The mass is oblong, conforming to the bladder wall with obtuse angles. It looks echogenic roughly like myometrium, with regular borders.

Two different findings can strongly suggest the diagnosis of endometriosis:

• The mass is usually surrounded by a very particular regular echogenic line, especially against the lumen of the bladder [89, 90]. This aspect has not been mentioned in cases of carcinoma.

• The mass may contain small cystic cavities surrounded by an echogenic line, like in adenomyosis.

Color Doppler may demonstrate some vessels in the mass. Bladder endometriotic lesions can be continuous with adenomyosis in the anterior uterine wall [91].

2. MR (Fig. 17.88)

– On MR, the mass looks with an overall signal close to pelvic muscle or of intermediate signal on T1-weighted images, on fat suppression, and T2W images [89]. Inside tiny cavities with high signal on T1W images, especially after fat suppres-

sion and variable signal on T2W images can be seen. Some cavities may show a low signal on T1W images and a high signal on T2W images. After injection of gadolinium, the fibrotic component enhances.

MR can delineate contiguous lesions of adenomyosis in the anterior uterine wall and can clearly depict abnormalities in the uterine cesarian scar in continuity with the bladder lesion (Fig. 17.89).

– In some rare cases, a complete block between the uterus and the bladder wall extending from the vesicouterine pouch to the anterior parietal peritoneum can be displayed (Fig. 17.90). These extensive endometriotic lesions can even involve posteriorly the vesicouterine septum.

3. CT (Fig. 17.79)

CT is not performed in usual practice to diagnose vesical endometriosis. However, the lesion can be discovered by chance, during an abdominopelvic examination. The lesion appears with a soft tissue density, which may contain hyperdense foci.

The main interest of CT is to display after IV injection on the delayed CT the relationships of the bladder lesion with the ureters. The choice of treatment depends on the patient's age, desire for pregnancy, extent of the vesicle lesion, severity of urinary symptoms or menstrual disorders, and associated pelvic pathologic conditions [92]. The preferred treatment is surgical excision. Unfortunately, in young women, recurrences are not

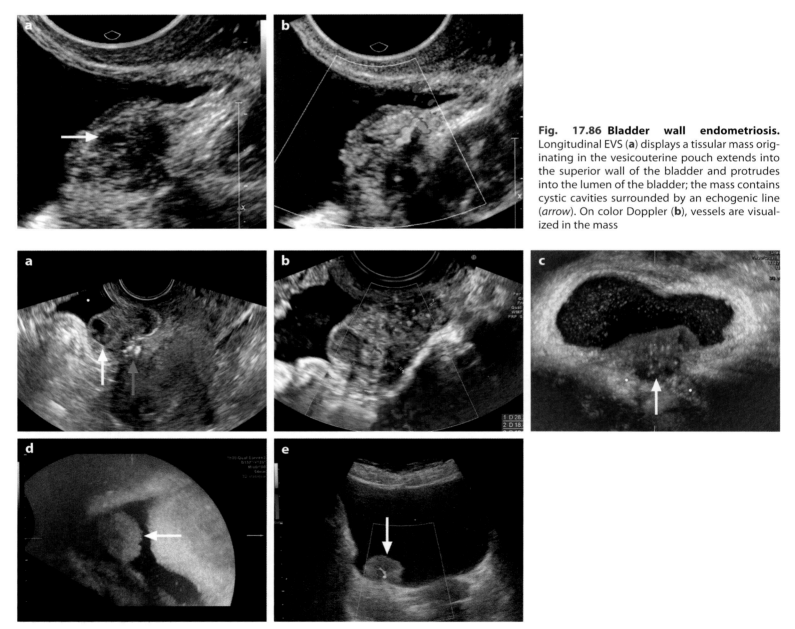

Fig. 17.85 *Vesical endometriosis.* Thirty-three-year-old woman with vesical pain at the end of micturition without hematuria. Sagittal TAS (**a**) and EVS (**b**): in front of the vesicouterine pouch, there is a 2.5-cm echogenic mass with regular border that ends smoothly with the bladder wall. It contains tiny anechoic cavities with an echogenic border typical of endometriotic cavities (*arrow*). EVS with Doppler (**c**) shows arterial vessels in the lesion

Fig. 17.86 Bladder wall endometriosis. Longitudinal EVS (**a**) displays a tissular mass originating in the vesicouterine pouch extends into the superior wall of the bladder and protrudes into the lumen of the bladder; the mass contains cystic cavities surrounded by an echogenic line (*arrow*). On color Doppler (**b**), vessels are visualized in the mass

Fig. 17.87 Vesicouterine pouch involvement associated with extension into the bladder wall. (1) Thirty year-old-woman with previous history of endometriosis and catamenial pollakiuria. Sagittal EVS (**a**) displays in the vesicouterine pouch an oval echogenic mass protruding into the bladder wall (*white arrow*) with adhesion to the anterior wall of the uterus. Echogenic foci related to clots (*red arrow*) are visualized at the level of the adhesions. On color Doppler (**b**), some vessels are visualized in the mass. On 3D reformation with 2D reconstruction (**c**), the topography of the mass outside the bladder wall protruding into the bladder (*arrow*) is depicted. Coelioscopy: endometriosis of the vesicouterine pouch with adhesions. Cystoscopy: mass protruding into the bladder wall with normal mucosa. (2) Differential diagnosis: polyp of the bladder. EVS with 3D reformation (**d**): a mass originating in the bladder wall protrudes into the lumen of the bladder (*arrow*). On color Doppler (**e**), a vascular pedicle (*arrow*) lies in the center of the mass. These findings are typical for a polyp

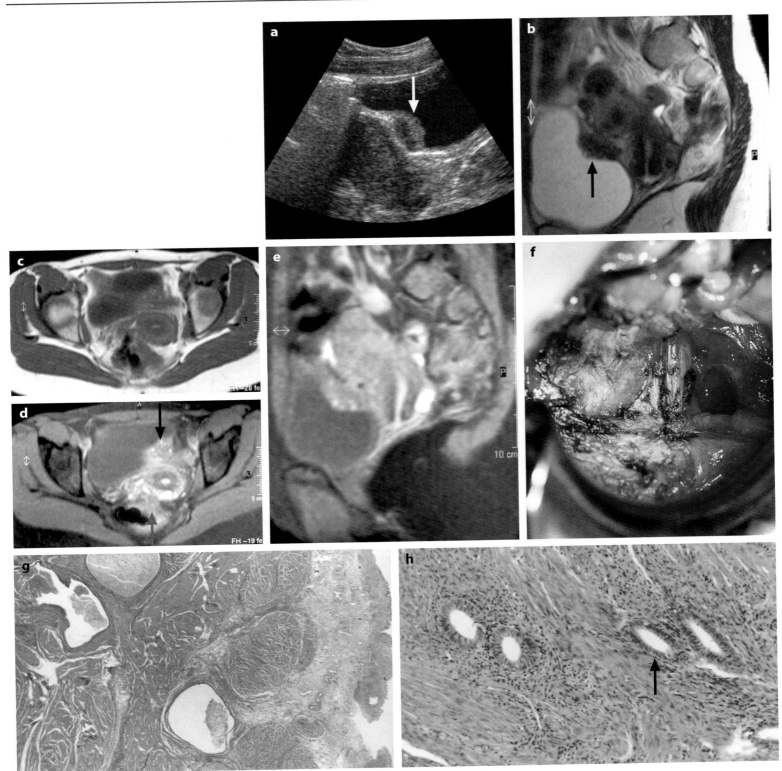

Fig. 17.88 Vesical endometriosis. Association with Douglas and rectal wall endometriosis. Thirty-year-old woman with pelvic pain. (1) Vesical endometriosis. Sagittal TAS (**a**) shows a 3-cm mass in the bladder wall in the front of the vesicouterine pouch (*arrow*). It is surrounded by an echogenic line. Its margins form an obtuse angle with the bladder wall. This pattern is very suggestive of bladder endometriosis. MR Sagittal T2 (**b**): the hypointense bladder wall is interrupted by the mass that has a signal close to pelvic muscle and contains small hyperintense foci (*arrow*). Axial T1 (**c**): the vesical mass has an overall signal intensity equal to pelvic muscles containing tiny hyperintense foci. Hyperintense foci are barely seen between the cervix and the rectum. Axial and sagittal T1 with fat suppression (**d, e**) highlight the endometriotic foci in the bladder wall (*black arrow* in **d**), in the Douglas (*gray arrow* in **d**). At operation (**f**), the normal vesical serosa is displayed on the right of the image. On the *left*, the bladder wall is *thickened*, *white*, and *fibrotic*. A partial bladder resection is performed. Histologic specimen from the bladder wall (**g**) displays the serosa and the muscularis layer and small endometriotic tubes. At a higher magnification (**h**), endometriotic tubes (*arrow*) are visualized in the muscular layer.

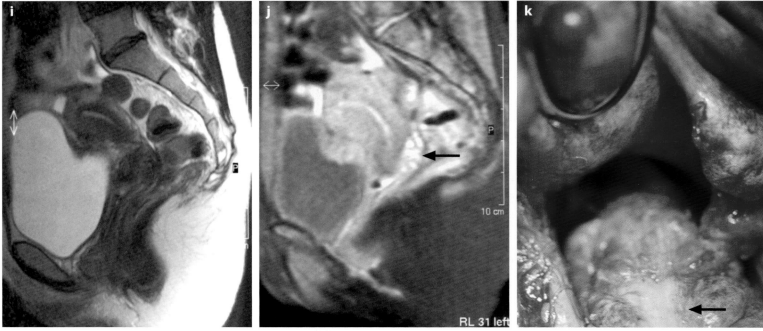

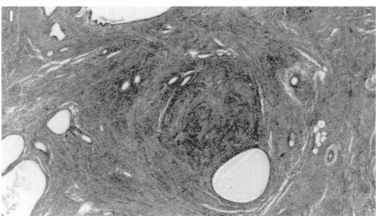

Fig. 17.88 (*continued*) (2) Rectal endometriosis. Sagittal T2 (**i**) and sagittal T1 with fat suppression (**j**) visualize the endometriotic lesion of the Douglas pouch and the anterior wall of the rectum (*arrow* in **j**). Surgical view showing the anterior wall of the rectum (**k**): the uterus is reclined forward. White fibrotic serosa (*arrow*) is displayed. At microscopy (**l**) endometrial tubes are visualized in the specimen

uncommon, and further surgery may be necessary to effect a permanent cure [93]. Hormonal treatment has proved effective in the treatment of some patients of endometriosis [92].

Other Methods

- Cystoscopy
  - Bladder endometriosis varies both cystoscopically and histologically during the menstrual cycle.
    Cystoscopy can be normal. Vesical endometriosis appears as a lobulated mass beneath an intact urothelium [94]. The most diagnostic appearance is the presence of translucent blue, blue-black, or red-brown cysts [95].
    The size of the mass, size of the cysts, and coloring of the cysts increase preceding and during menstruations, and even actual bleeding and sloughing may be observed.
    Biopsy is recommended but seldom provides the diagnosis [79].
  - The main use of this procedure is to exclude an epithelial tumor of the bladder mucosa and more uncommonly mesenchymal tumors such as hemangioma fibroma and leiomyoma [83], although in rare cases, a nonspecific appearance may mimic other bladder lesions ranging from cystitis to carci-

noma [95]. It demonstrates the relationship of the lesion with the ureteral meatuses [83].

- *IVP and Cystography*:
  These procedures are less and less performed and are replaced by CT.
  Cystography may reveal a filling defect that cannot be differentiated from a bladder neoplasm. However, urinary opacification may not detect lesions involving only the serous or muscular layers of the bladder [96].

Vesicovaginal Septum

Involvement of the vesicovaginal septum is exceptional.

Lateral Subperitoneal Space

Parametrium with Ureter (Including Intrinsic Location)

Visualization of the topography of the ureter (Fig. 17.91) is essential for the surgeon. CT with IV contrast is the most appropriate method to visualize the relationship of the lesion with the ureters.

Ureteral involvement is less frequent than bladder endometriosis [97]. Nonspecific flank pain, hematuria sometimes exaggerated

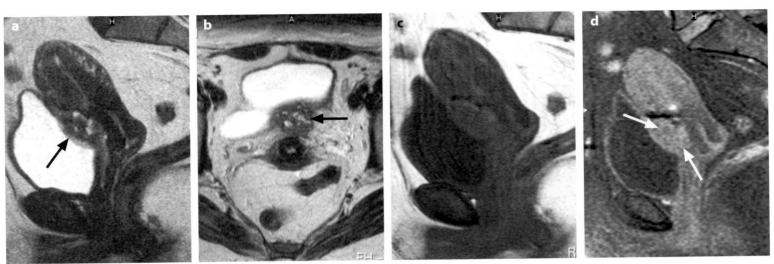

Fig. 17.89 Vesical endometriosis secondary to endometriosis in a cesarian scar. Dysmenorrhea, vesical burning at the end of micturition, and previous history of three cesarians. MR sagittal T2 (**a**) and axial T2 (**b**): a 3-cm ovoid mass is visualized in front of the cesarian scar in the vesicouterine pouch (*arrow*), extending in front of the cervix. The mass involves the bladder wall. The mass has an overall signal close to pelvic muscles and contains multiple hyperintense foci. Sagittal T1 without (**c**) and with fat suppression (**d**), displays the mass with a signal equal to pelvic muscles. A hyperintense endometriotic focus is visualized at the level of the cesarian scar while no hyperintense signal is visualized in the mass (*white arrows*)

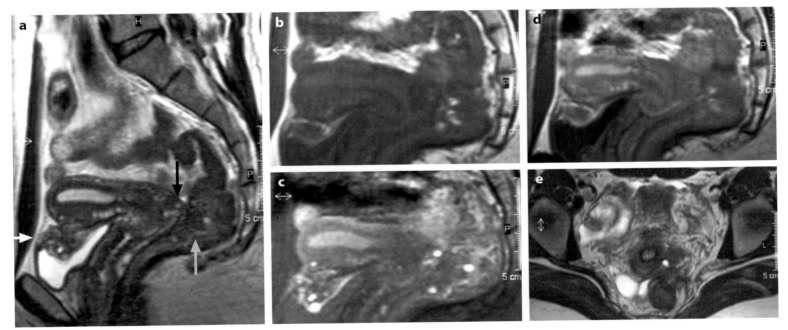

Fig. 17.90 Posterior and anterior subperitoneal endometriosis. Twenty-five-year-old woman with (1) dysuria and pain at the end of micturition, (2) dyspareunia, (3) pain at defecation, and (4) left sciatica. At endorectal sonography, rectal wall invasion was present. MR sagittal T2 (**a**): (1) Anterior subperitoneal space: A mass (*white arrow*) with identical morphologic findings involves the anterior wall of the uterus, the vesicouterine pouch, and the superior bladder wall. (2) Posterior subperitoneal space: a mass with an overall signal close to pelvic muscles, containing small hyperintense foci, involves the anterior rectal wall (*gray arrow*), the posterior wall of the vagina (*black arrow*), the Douglas, the rectovaginal septum (*arrow*), and the torus uterinus. Its lower part is approximately 5-cm above the levator anus. On sagittal T1 (**b**) and with fat suppression (**c**), hyperintense foci (*arrows*) are visualized in both masses (*arrows*). On sagittal T1 after injection (**d**), contrast enhancement is displayed in both subperitoneal masses. On axial T2 (**e**), the posterior subperitoneal lesion involves the left uterosacral ligament and extends laterally to the paracervical region and posteriorly to the anterior wall of the rectum and to the pelvic wall. *Pathology:* (1) In the bladder, endometriosis involved the serosa and the muscularis layers. (2) In the rectum, endometriosis involved the serosa, the muscularis layers, and the submucosa

at the time of menstruation [96], a pelvic mass [98], previous pelvic or abdominal surgery can be observed, or patients can be asymptomatic.

1. *Most commonly, in 75–85 % of cases* [97], *involvement of the ureter is extrinsic compression.* The pelvic ureter is surrounded by adjacent endometriosis and its attendant inflammation and fibrosis [99] making ureterolysis by the surgeon necessary. Radiologic Findings:

IVP: radiologic findings include hydro-uretero-hydronephrosis above a pelvic ureteral stricture [100], or rarely an intraluminal mass [101].

The strictures are short (0.5–2.2 cm), mainly located in that portion of the pelvic ureter projected within 3 cm of the inferior margin of the sacroiliac joint, which corresponds to the cross with the uterosacral ligaments [102]. The ureteral structures show smooth, often abrupt tapering.

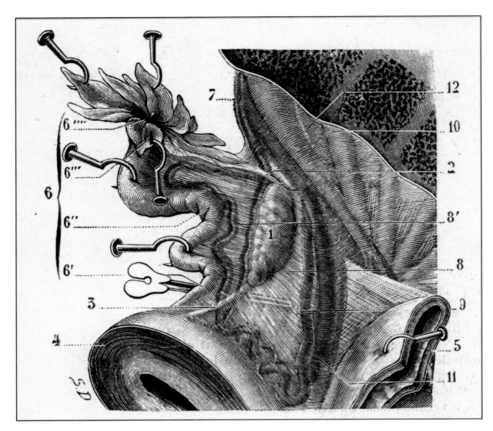

Fig. 17.91 Pelvic ureter and its relationships with the uterine artery and the other surrounding structures. *1* Ovary; *2* Tuboovarian ligament; *3* Ovarian ligament; *4* Uterus; *5* Rectum; *6* Tube with *6'* isthmus, *6"* ampulla, *6'''* infundibulum; *7* Suspensory or Infundibulopelvic ligament containing in its thickness the ovarian artery and vein and lymphatics; *8* Mesometrium; *8'* Mesosalpinx; *9* Uterine artery; *10* Sacral plexus; *11* Ureter in its extraperitoneal portion behind the uterine artery; *12* Internal iliac vein

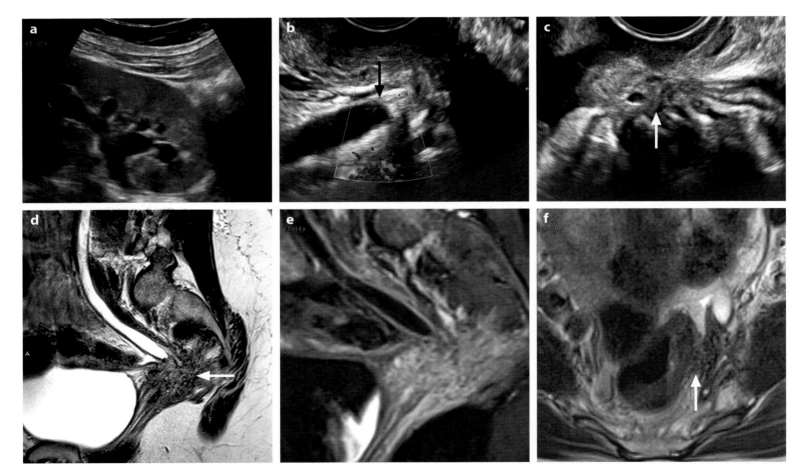

Fig. 17.92 Obstruction of the left ureter by an endometriosis of the left US ligament and parametrium. Forty-two-year-old woman with dysmenorrhea, dyspareunia, and left catamenial sciatalgy. Transabdominal ultrasound (**a**) and EVS (**b**) depict an obstruction of the left pelvic ureter (*black arrow*). On EVS (**c**), the obstruction is related to a hypoechoic infiltrating lesion which involves the lateral wall of the fornix, the USL, and the parametrium (*white arrow*). MR sagittal T2 (**d**) displays the obstruction of the left pelvic ureter by an endometriotic subperitoneal mass involving the left US ligament, extending into the sacrorectogenital septum (*arrow*), with a high-contrast uptake on sagittal T1 after injection (**e**). On axial T2 (**f**), this lesion involves the left lateral wall of the rectum, the left mesorectum, and anteriorly the left parietal peritoneum (*arrow*)

Fig. 17.93 Thirty-year-old woman operated from endometriosis; left pelvic pain. CT after IV contrast (**a**) displays an obstruction of the left pelvic ureter secondary to an involvement of the left uterosacral ligament. On the MIP coronal reformation (**b**), at the level of obstruction, the ureter is tapering progressively without any intrinsic abnormality

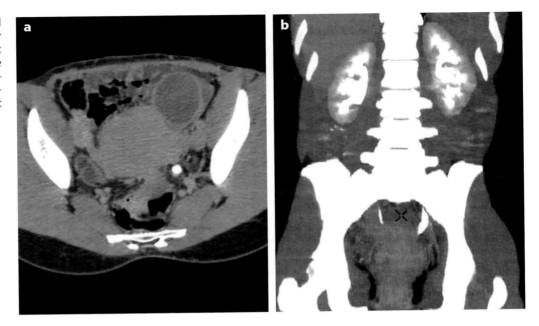

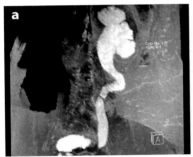
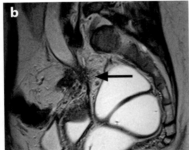
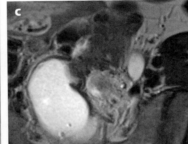
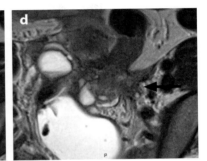

Fig. 17.94 Extrinsec compression of the ureter by the left USL. MR coronal T2 (**a**) and sagittal T2 (**b**) depict an obstruction of the left ureter at the level S1–S2 by a characteristic stellate fibrotic endometriotic lesion (*arrow*). On axial T2 immediately above (**c**) and at the level of the obstruction (**d**), the endometriotic lesion lies in the USL, extending anteriorly into the parametrium (*arrow*)

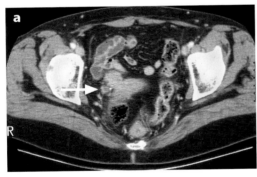
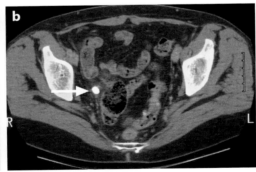
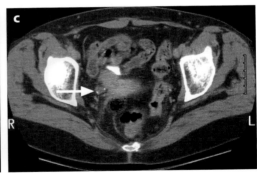

Fig. 17.95 Intra-ureteral endometriosis. Sixty-three-year-old woman with pelvic pain and hematuria. Previous subtotal hysterectomy and bilateral ovariectomy for pelvic endometriosis. CT at the arterial phase (**a**) displays a round nodule (*arrow*) protruding in the lower portion of the right pelvic ureter; tiny dense foci are visualized at the periphery of the lesion. CT performed 4 mn after injection: dilatation of the ureter (**b**) (*arrow*) above the intrinsic lesion (**c**) (*arrow*). Surgery and pathology: intrinsic endometriotic location in the ureter

Medial angulation of the ureter in the region of the narrowed segment may be due to displacement by an extrinsic mass of endometrial tissue or retraction by fibrosis, which is usually present (Figs. 17.92, 17.93, and 17.94).

2. *Uncommonly, involvement is intrinsic invasion.* Thickening of the wall, or a polyp-like lesion or both can be observed [93]. This form has been often mistaken for a primary ureteral neoplasm [99] (Fig. 17.95).

On CT, the mass has a tissular density [103]. Dynamic CT scan can depict an intense contrast enhancement, while an urothelial tumor is poorly vascularized.

On MR (Fig. 17.95), fibrotic linear lesions encasing the pelvic ureter along the lateral pelvic wall can be displayed.

Only one case of endoluminal mass with a low signal on T1W images and an intermediate signal on T2W images has been reported [103].

Other Urinary Locations

Kidney

Endometriosis of the kidney is extremely rare [104].

On gross examination, a typically solitary well-circumscribed, hemorrhagic, solid, and cystic mass focally replaces the renal parenchyma [86]. The cysts contain bloody serous fluid and small clots [104].

Polypoid masses may project in the renal pelvis [104].

Urethra

Only two cases of urethral endometriosis have been described [86], one case of a nodule projecting from the urethral orifice and the other in the wall of a large urethral diverticulum.

Anterior and Posterior Subperitoneal Space Involvement Can Be Associated

Figure 17.79 very extensive endometriotic lesions associated with adhesions can create a frozen pelvis (Fig. 17.96).

17.1.10.4 Peritoneal Endometriosis

Laparoscopic Findings

Laparoscopy remains the best modality to detect peritoneal implants. The most common locations are the cul-de-sac and the broad ligament [105]. Most of the implant measure from 1 to 10 mm. Diagnosis may be only made by direct visualization of the lesions or may require biopsy.

The classical pigmented lesions appear as brownish, bluish, or purplish hemorrhagic areas often associated with stellate scaring. However, lesions associated with old sutures, epithelial inclusions, residual carbon from previous laser surgery, and inflammatory cysts may be mistaken for endometriosis [44].

Multiple nonpigmented lesions can be observed. The most common are scarred white lesions, polyps, peritoneal pockets, petechial peritoneum, areas with peritoneal hypervascularization, clear vesicular lesions, and sub-ovarian adhesions [12, 13, 106]. These lesions are usually less specific than the classical pigmented lesions. Indeed, scarred white lesions may be confused with fibrotic tissue from previous inflammatory disease or postoperative scarring. Moreover,

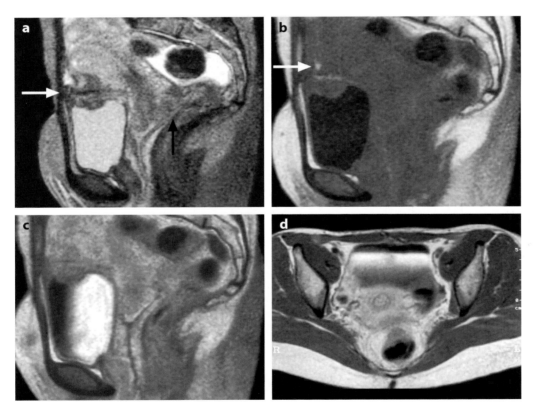

Fig. 17.96 Posterior and anterior subperitoneal endometriosis. Twenty-nine-year-old woman with pelvic pain and dyspareunia. MR sagittal T2 (**a**): (1) posterior subperitoneal space: large lesion (*black arrow*) involving the inter-uterorectal space with invasion of the posterior wall of the vagina, the anterior wall of the rectum, and the rectovaginal septum obliterating the Douglas pouch; some peritoneal fluid is seen just above. (2) Anterior subperitoneal space: Large lesion (*white arrow*) in the inter-vesicouterine space invading the anterior wall of the uterus and the superior wall of the bladder obliterating completely the vesicouterine pouch. Sagittal T1 (**b**): a hyperintense focus (*arrow*) is visualized in the anterior lesion. Sagittal T1 after injection (**c**): Both lesions enhance. Axial T1 after gadolinium (**d**): fibrotic thickening of the torus uterinus and the left uterosacral ligament were confirmed at surgery. *At pathology,* the muscular layers of the rectal and bladder walls were invaded, but their mucosa was spared

many patients have clear vesicular lesion which can be difficult for even the most experienced laparoscopist to visualize [106].

Pigmented and nonpigmented lesions may be present in the same patient [12]. Changes of coloration of endometriosis can occur during the menstrual cycle, and progression from nonpigmented to pigmented lesions has also been observed.

Endometriosis can also be deeply infiltrating, while the lesion can appear just superficial to the untrained eye.

US Findings

Peritoneal implants appear as hyperechogenic foci (Figs. 17.63 and 17.64).

MR Findings

1. *Implants*:
   (a) *Pelvic*
      When the implant has an hemorrhagic content, association of T1-weighted spin-echo and fat-suppressed T1-weighted images displays a hyperintense foci without mass formation [61, 107, 108]. Their signal on T2-weighted images may be hyperintense or hypointense (Fig. 17.63). The detection rate of endometrial implants depends on the size of the implants,

that is, superior to 4 mm, on their location and on their morphology. Moreover, these hyperintense foci are sometimes very difficult to distinguish from vessels and GI tract.

When the implants correspond to clear vesicles, they look hypointense on T1 and hyperintense on T2.

Scarred lesions are difficult to visualize. Injection of gadolinium can depict a localized area of contrast enhancement with stellate contour.

Other lesions such as petechial lesions and peritoneal hypervascularization that are very suggestive of endometriosis at laparoscopy are impossible to detect on MR, so that a normal examination does not exclude peritoneal endometriosis.

Detection rate as high as 61 % has been reported in the literature using T1-weighted fat suppression [109], but in our own experience, detection rate is much lower.
   (b) Very uncommonly abdominal implants can be visualized (Fig. 17.97).
2. Exceptionally, *a peritoneal endometrioma* can develop (Fig. 17.98).
3. *Adhesions*:
   Adhesions can be secondary to endometriosis or develop after surgery. During the life of the cysts, material escapes from them into the peritoneal cavity which was irritating and gives rise to

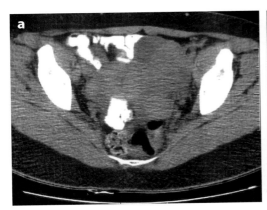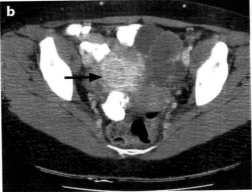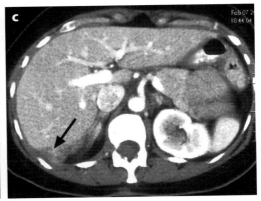

Fig. 17.97 Pseudometastatic abdominal peritoneal endometriotic implants. Pelvic CT. (**a** and **b**) Axial CT of the pelvis before and after IV contrast: Left multiloculated cystic mass with one of the loculi containing a liquid as dense as myometrium before injection (*arrow*). Abdominal CT. (**c**) Axial CT after injection at the level of the subphrenic space: Peritoneal implants (*arrows*) are visualized in the posterior part of the right subphrenic space which wrongly suggested metastatic peritoneal implants from an ovarian carcinoma, although no morphologic findings of carcinoma of the left ovary were present. *At surgery and pathology*, a left endometrioma with abdominal endometriotic peritoneal implants was diagnosed

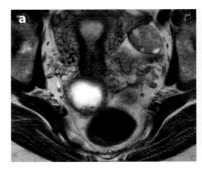
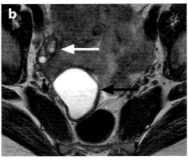
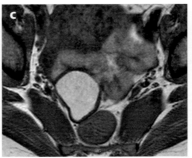
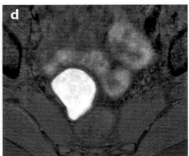

Fig. 17.98 Extra-ovarian endometriotic cyst. Forty-one-year-old woman with prior appendicectomy. After a misabortion, a US discovers a hemorrhagic cystic mass in the right portion of the Douglas pouch. MR axial T2 (**a**) displays a cystic mass (*black arrow*) separated from the right ovary (*white arrow*) in the right portion of the Douglas pouch in contact with the serosa of the rectum. Its signal intensity is superior to adipose tissue. On axial T2 (**b**) at another level, left ovary is normal. On axial T1 (**c**) and fat suppression (**d**), the cystic mass has a signal equal to adipose tissue which is very suggestive of an endometriotic cyst. Diagnosis of an endometrioma in a peritoneal location is suggested. At surgery, the mass is intraperitoneal, adherent to the rectum. Pathology confirms the diagnosis of endometriosis

adhesions. Adhesions vary in extent, density, and location. They may be slight , as those resulting from a mild pelvic peritonitis or extensive and dense causing the most part involved to become fused with one another and thus making their separation very difficult [76].

On EVS, three morphologic findings allow to suspect adhesions (Fig. 17.99): (1) a hypoechoic cord between to structures; (2) attraction and convergence of a wall of an organ or an anatomical structure toward a neighboring structure, for instance, a lesion of the rectosigmoid junction with a folded appearance, and the torus, or the bladder and the anterior wall of the uterus (Fig. 17.100); (3) low echogenic structure related to fibrosis. Moreover, EVS allows to perform a dynamic evaluation and to suspect adhesions in case of inability to separate two contiguous anatomical structures sometimes associated with pain, mainly when a localized pressure of the probe is performed.

Adhesions may sometimes be identified as:

1. Low-signal intensity cords (Fig. 17.101).
2. Obliteration of the contour of an organ in contact with another one or with the peritoneum particularly on T2 images and after contrast injection (Fig. 17.102).
3. Distortion or displacement of an organ: posterior displacement of the uterus and ovaries, angulation of bowel loops, elevation of the posterior vaginal fornix, loculated fluid collections, hydrosalpinx; and displacement with retraction of the peritoneum.

Although the extent and severity of adhesions can be difficult to determine with imaging [110] and laparoscopy is required for definite diagnosis, preoperative diagnosis or at least high suspicion allows to alert the surgeon of the difficulties of adhesiolysis.

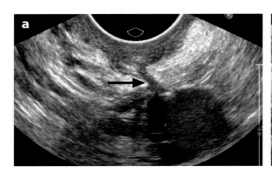
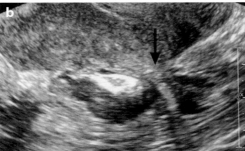
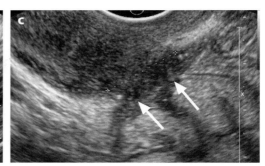

Fig. 17.99 (**a**) Cord between the torus and a left ovarian endometrioma (*arrow*). (**b**) Attraction and convergence of the anterior wall of the layers of rectosigmoid junction with a folded appearance and the torus (*arrow*). Which is not documented on this figure was the pain and the inability during the examination to separate both anatomical structures. (**c**) Low echogenic structure related to fibrosis with symphysis of the posterior wall of the cervix and the vagina and the anterior wall of the rectum, obliterating the Douglas (*two arrows*)

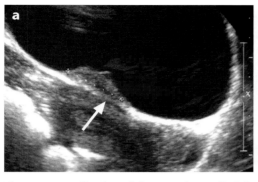
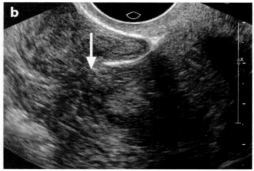
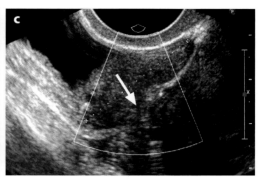

Fig. 17.100 Adhesion of the anterior wall of the uterus to the bladder. (a) Longitudinal TAS displays an interruption of the bladder wall and an echogenic mass protruding into the lumen of the bladder. (b) EVS shows external adenomyosis with an interruption of the echogenic line, corresponding to an adhesion between the uterus and the bladder at the level of the vesicouterine pouch. (c) EVS displays extension to the bladder wall with an echogenic mass corresponding to an endometriotic involvement of the bladder

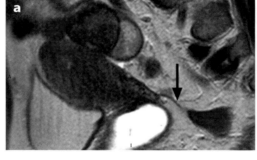
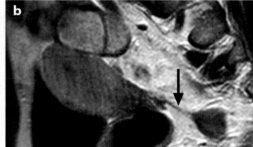

Fig. 17.101 Fourty-eight-year-old woman with pelvic pain. Adhesion between rectum and uterus. MR sagittal T2 (a) and after injection (b) display a cord (*arrows*) between the anterior wall of the rectum and the posterior wall of the cervix obliterating the Douglas pouch. This was confirmed at surgery

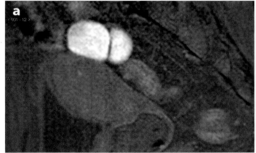
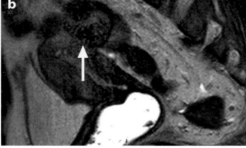
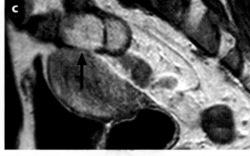

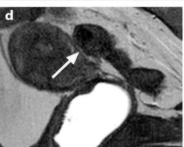
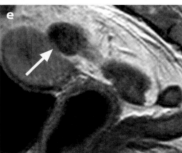
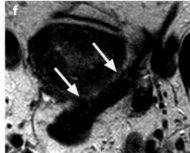
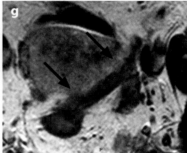

Fig. 17.102 Fourty-eight-year-old woman with pelvic pain. (1) Adhesion between right ovary and uterus (a–c). MR sagittal fat suppression (a): right bilobulated endometrioma; on sagittal T2 (b) (*arrow*), the right ovarian cysts and the uterus are close in contact; after injection (c), absence of contrast uptake at this level is very suggestive of adhesion (*arrow*). (2) Sagittal T2 (d) (*arrow*) and after injection (e) (*arrow*) demonstrate adhesion between rectum and uterus according to the same findings. (3) Axial T2 (f) and after injection (g) (*arrows*) display adhesion between the medial and anterior border of the sigmoid with the uterus according to the same findings. These three locations of adhesions were confirmed at surgery

17.1.10.5 Other Locations

- Uterus
- Tubes
- Peritoneal Pseudocysts
- Abdominal Wall
- Diaphragm and Thorax
- Miscellaneous

Uterus

(a) *Adenomyosis*

Definition:

Adenomyosis: Implantation of endometrium into the myometrium.

Endometriosis: Implantation of endometrium outside the myometrium.

Pathology:

Two different types of adenomyosis must be distinguished:

1. *The internal adenomyosis* (see Chap. "Benign and Malignant Mesenchyma").
2. *The external adenomyosis*, secondary to involvement of uterine serosa by endometriotic implants extending from outside to inside into the external myometrium (see Section 17.1.10.3).

(b) *Endometriosis on Cesarian Scar*

Endometriosis on *cesarian scar* can develop after surgery (Fig. 17.103). The lesions of endometriosis progress steadily on to the vesicouterine pouch and later on can involve the bladder wall.

(c) *Endometriosis of the Cervix*

Endometriosis of the cervix can be superficial or deep:

1. Superficial endometriosis

   This condition may be asymptomatic or be associated with premenstrual or postcoital bleeding. Before menses, the lesions typically enlarge and change of color from bright red to blue.

   The solitary or multiple lesions typically involve the ectocervix, rarely the endocervix. The endometriotic foci appear as streaks, nodules, or cysts measuring from 1 mm to 2 cm. Although usually superficial endometriosis of the cervix is not associated with deep pelvic endometriosis, occasionally, this association can be encountered (Fig. 17.104).

   On US, content of the cyst is low echogenic. On MR, the usual characteristics of signal of endometriosis allow to differentiate them from Nabothian's cysts.

2. Deep endometriosis is usually an extension of a subperitoneal location of the cul-de-sac or from the torus extending down to the cervix.

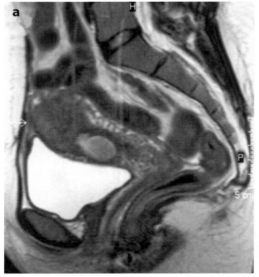 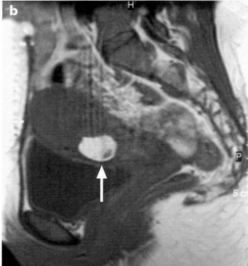 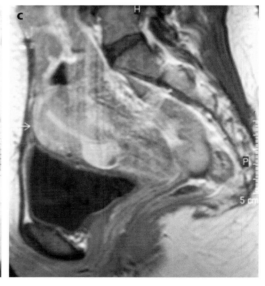

Fig. 17.103 Endometriosis in a cesarian scar. Forty-year-old woman. Previous cesarian 5 years. Secondary dysmenorrhea. MR is performed at days 10 of the menstrual cycle. Sagittal T2 (**a**) shows a pouch of intermediate signal at the level of the cesarian scar communicating with the endometrial cavity. On sagittal T1 (**b**), content of the pouch has a signal close to adipose tissue, suggestive of endometriosis (*arrow*). On sagittal after injection (**c**), a contrast uptake in the wall of the pouch and a curvilinear clot in the bottom of the pouch are visualized

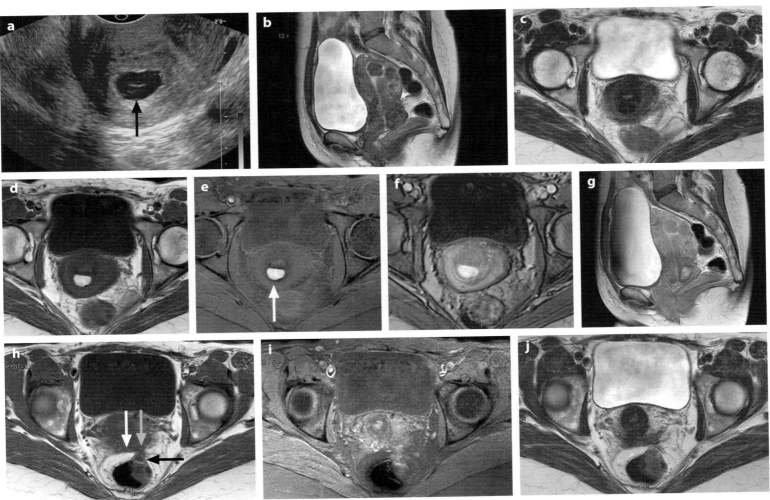

Fig. 17.104 Endometriosis of the cervix. Forty-two-year-old woman with deep dyspareunia. EVS transverse (**a**) depicts in the posterior portion of the cervix a low echogenic nodule (*arrow*). MR sagittal T2 (**b**) and axial T2 (**c**) depict in the posterior lip of the cervix a cyst with a signal slightly lower than the normal stroma. On T1 (**d**) and fat suppression (**e**), the cyst has a signal intensity close to adipose tissue, which is very suggestive of endometriosis (*arrow*). On axial T1 (**f**) after injection and on the delayed sagittal T1 (**g**), the wall of the cyst has a lower signal than the cervical stroma. On axial T1 (**h**), fat suppression (**i**) and after injection (**j**) endometriosis of the torus (*white arrow*) extending to the left USL (*yellow arrow*) and to the anterior wall of the rectum (*black arrow*) are displayed

Tubes

There are three different types:

1. By far, the most common lesions of endometriosis are implants on the serosa of the tubes, associated to endometriosis elsewhere in the pelvis. The myosalpinx is typically not involved [86].

2. Endometrial tissue may extend directly from the uterine cornu and replace the mucosa of the interstitial and isthmic portions of the tube. In some cases, it may give rise to intratubal polyps.

3. The third type occurs typically 1 to 4 years after tubal ligation, in the tip of the proximal tubal stump. Endometrium extends from the endosalpinx to the myosalpinx and frequently to the serosal surface. It may be associated to salpingitis isthmic nodosa (outpouching of tubal epithelium into the surrounding tubal muscularis; see Chap. 20.2.4).

In fact, the most common internal lesions observed in patients operated from endometriosis are diagnosed as nonspecific chronic salpingitis.

HSG realized in the checkup of infertility can be normal, can demonstrate obstruction of the tubes, or rarely opacified small cavities lying against the lumen of the tube. MR and US miss the great majority of these lesions.

Approximately, 30 % of women with endometriosis have associated tubal abnormalities present at laparoscopy [111].

Hydrosalpinges have a tubular, often folded configuration.

On EVS, content of the tube is echogenic. The wall is thickened (Fig. 17.105).

On MR, (Figs. 17.105 and 17.106) the content has a high-signal intensity on T1 and on fat suppression. The fallopian tubes do not always show T2 shortening typical of endometrial cysts. In addition, debris can be present within the dependent portions of the tube [112].

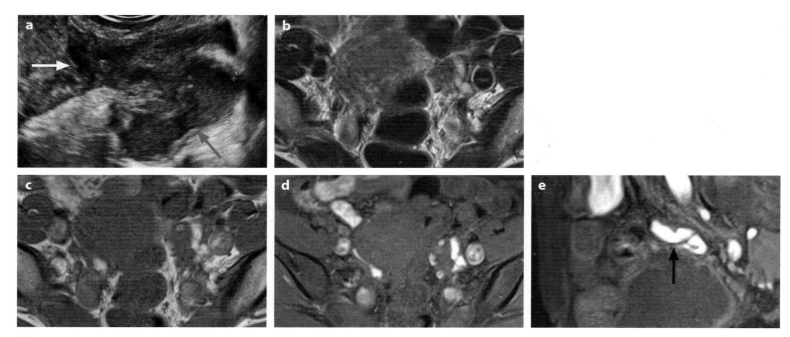

Fig. 17.105 Tubal endometriosis. Thirty-five-year-old woman. Endometriosis with left ovarian cystectomy performed 6 years before. Left pelvic pain. EVS transverse (**a**) depicts lateral to the left ovary (*white arrow*) dilatation of the tube with an echogenic content and a thickened wall (*red arrow*). Endometriosis of the tube is suspected. A small endometriotic cyst in the left ovary is visualized. MR axial T2 (**b**) displays dilatation of the left tube. Content of the tube has an intermediate signal. On axial T1 (**c**) with fat suppression (**d**) and sagittal with fat suppression (**e**), content of the tube has a high-signal characteristic of endometriosis (*arrow*)

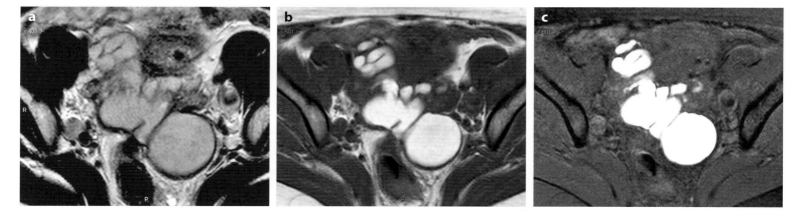

Fig. 17.106 Tubal endometriosis. Thirty-five-year-old woman with sub-peritoneal and bilateral adnexal endometriosis known for 3 years and treated with progesterone. Six months after interruption of the hormonal treatment, right pelvic pain. MR axial T2 (**a**) displays an extra-ovarian elongated cystic mass with multiple plicae and an intermediate signal content. On T1 (**b**), the mass has a signal intensity close to adipose tissue and a high-signal intensity on fat suppression (**c**). Sagittal oblique reformation on fat suppression (**d**) displays clearly the elongated shape of the mass with multiple plicae. Prospective diagnosis: endometriosis of the right tube with hematosalpinx. Coelioscopy confirmed the diagnosis

Peritoneal Pseudocysts (Fig. 17.107)

Non endometriotic peritoneal pseudocysts are not exceptional after surgery for pelvic endometriosis because of the development of adhesions that are particularly common in this condition. However, peritoneal pseudocysts presenting authentic endometriotic lesions in the border of the collection have been reported. As usual pseudocysts, they conform to the shape of the surrounding structures. They are often multilocular. They can lie on both side of the broad ligament. Their cystic content is hemorrhagic. On US, their cystic content is echogenic with different loculi separated by regular septa. On CT scan, the cystic content is denser than urine. The wall and the septa enhance after contrast injection. On MR, signal intensity is intermediate to muscle or adipose tissue on T1 and hyperintense on T2 in our three cases.

These entities are quite difficult to manage because the patients usually have a history of previous surgeries. Percutaneous drainage can be proposed in these patients with the usual limits of success.

Abdominal Wall

They involve usually a scar after abdominal surgery or the umbilicus (Fig. 17.108).

Usually, clinical findings are very suggestive. A painful blue nodule increases in size during the menstrual cycle.

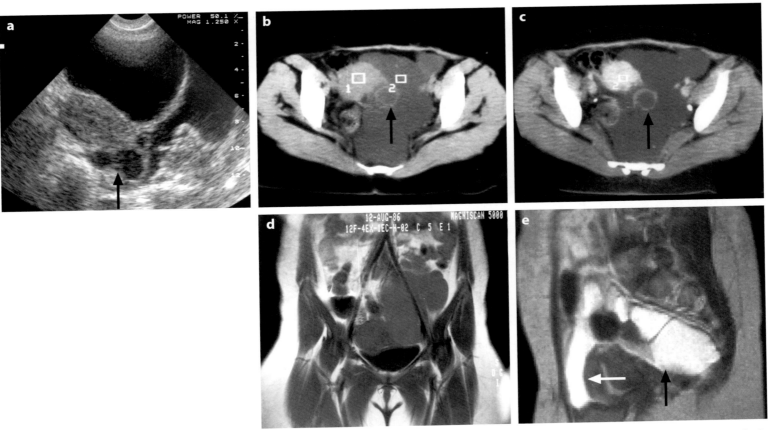

Fig. 17.107 Peritoneal endometriotic pseudocysts. Thirty-two-year-old woman with pelvic pain and previous right adnexectomy for endometriosis. *Ultrasound*: Transverse TAS (**a**): the uterus is pushed forward and to the right by a multicystic mass with echogenic septa that lies posterior and anterior to the broad ligament (*arrow*). *CT*: CT before (**b**) and after IV injection (**c**): the mass conforms to the surrounding structures. Septa of loculi (*arrow*) appear slightly denser than the liquid on non contrast CT. After injection, a significant contrast uptake is visualized in the septa (*arrow*). MR. On coronal T1 (**d**), the collection appears with a signal comprised between pelvic muscles and adipose tissue and conforms to the adjacent structures. On sagittal T2 (**e**), the collection appears anterior and posterior to the broad ligament and has a high signal (*arrows*). *At surgery*, numerous pelvic adhesions were associated with a periadnexal collection containing a chocolate liquid. Pathologic examination of the septa confirmed the diagnosis of endometriotic pseudocysts

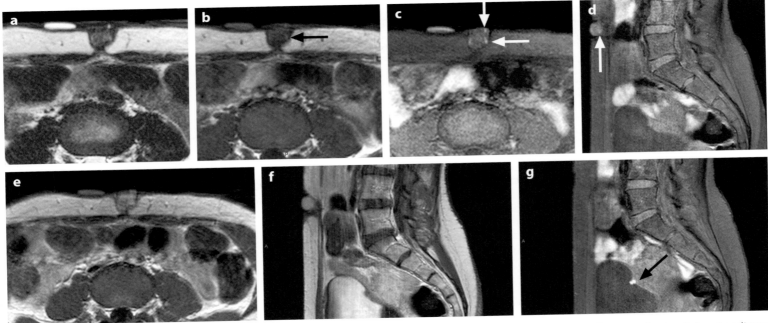

Fig. 17.108 Endometriosis of the umbilicus. Thirty-five-year-old woman operated 2 years before from an umbilical hernia. Three months later, catamenial hematuria. For 6 months, catamenial swelling of the umbilicus. MR axial T2 (**a**) displays a nodule 17-mm width at the umbilicus with a regular hypointense wall and a content of intermediate signal. On axial T1 (**b**) and axial and sagittal fat suppression (**c** and **d**), spots of a signal close to adipose tissue in the mass allow to characterize the mass as an endometriotic location (*arrows*). On axial and sagittal T1 after injection (**e** and **f**), contrast uptake is displayed in the nodule. Sagittal T1 with fat suppression (**g**) displays endometriosis in superior wall of the bladder (*arrow*)

At macroscopy (Fig. 17.109), the mass is mainly tissular, containing some cystic cavities usually less than 3 mm in diameter, filled with clear or hemorrhagic fluid, and sometimes with clots. At microscopy, the tissular component is fibromuscular.

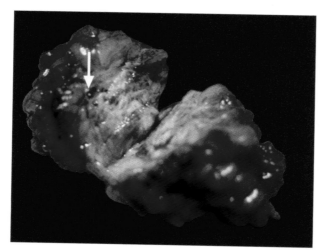

Fig. 17.109 Endometriosis of the abdominal wall. Fibromuscular mass containing tiny cavities filled with clear fluid or hemorrhage or clots (*arrow*). At microscopy the cystic cavities were limited by endometrium

On US (Fig. 17.110), the mass is usually oval in shape, lying in the subcutaneous tissue and/or the muscle of the abdominal wall. Its limits are irregular. It is usually low echogenic of lower echogenicity than the echogenicity of the muscle (Fig. 17.111). While in most of the cases an echogenic areas in the mass are displayed (which may contain echogenic foci), the diagnosis of cystic spaces related to endometriosis can be impossible. On color Doppler, few vessels can be depicted in the mass. Exceptionally, vascularization is more pronounced (Fig. 17.112). Differential diagnosis with tumors of the abdominal wall as desmoids tumor can be difficult.

On MR (Figs. 17.110, 17.111, and 17.113), on T2, the fibromuscular component has a signal close to the muscle of the abdominal wall; well-delineated small cystic cavities surrounded by a line of intermediate signal related to endometrium are usually displayed. On T1. hemorrhagic foci of a signal close to adipose tissue mass, with a high signal on fat suppression typical for endometriosis, are usually displayed.

Exceptionally, location to the extra pelvic portion of *the round ligament* can be encountered (Fig. 17.114).

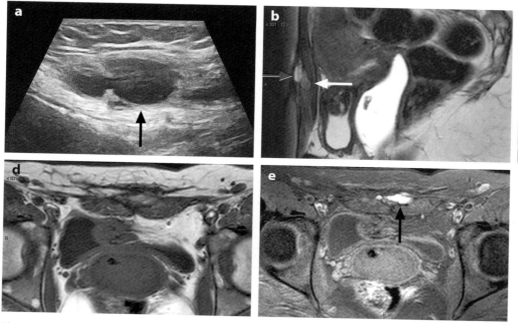

Fig. 17.110 Parietal endometriosis of the recti abdomini adenomyoma of the vesicouterine pouch. Thirty-three-year-old woman with previous endometriotic lesions on the bladder wall operated 2 years before, a cesarian 1 year before, and dysmenorrhea. TAS of the abdominal wall (**a**) depicts on the midline a cystic mass, between the aponevrosis of the recti abdominis and the recti abdomini muscle backward (*arrow*). MR with sagittal (**b**) axial T2 (**c**) displays on the midline, 5 cm above the pubic symphysis an oval mass lying in the subcutaneous tissue, invading the anterior wall of the left rectus abdominis (*white arrows*); a small collection in the subcutaneous tissue is associated (*red arrow*). Axial T1 (**d**) and fat suppression (**e**) display multiple hemorrhagic foci in the mass (*arrow*) allowing to definitely diagnose a parietal endometriosis. Moreover sagittal MR T2 (**b**) and the axial MR sequences (**c–e**) show in the vesicouterine pouch an adenomyoma containing hemorrhagic implants associated with adhesion to the uterus, the bladder wall, and the anterior abdominal wall

Fig. 17.111 Endometriosis of the abdominal wall. Thirty-one-year-old woman three cesarians. For a year, nodule of the abdominal wall above the pubic symphysis with cyclic pain. TAS (**a**) displays an oval mass in the rectis abdominis; color Doppler (**b**) displays few vessels in the mass

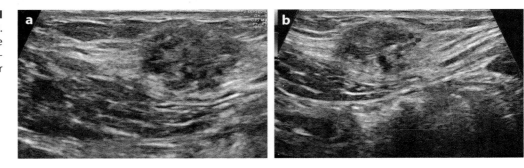

Fig. 17.112 Parietal endometriosis. Thirty-nine-year-old woman. Previous cesarian. Cyclic pelvic pain of a nodule palpated in the abdominal wall. TAS (**a**) displays an echogenic oval parietal mass, containing anechoic areas with irregular infiltrating margins lying in the recti abdominis pushing anteriorly the aponevrosis (*arrows*). On color Doppler (**b**), large vessels are shown in the mass

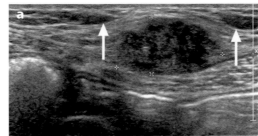
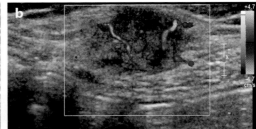

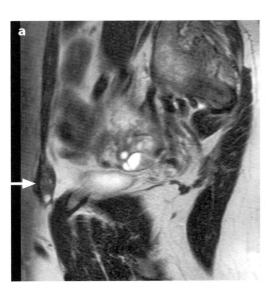
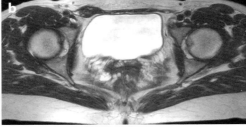
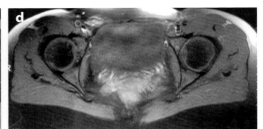
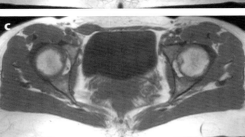

Fig. 17.113 Sagittal T2 (**a**) and axial T2 (**b**) display a mass in the right anterior abdominal wall between in front aponevrosis of the external oblique and the fascia transversalis backward 3 cm above the pubic symphysis. The mass has an overall signal close to pelvic muscle, containing some cystic cavities (*arrow*). Axial T1 (**c**) and fat suppression (**d**) display hyperintense foci in the mass (*arrow*) allowing to definitely diagnose a parietal endometriosis. Surgery: The tissular mass was removed. Microscopy: parietal endometriosis

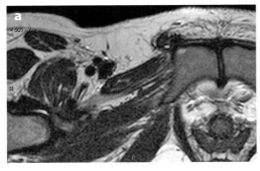
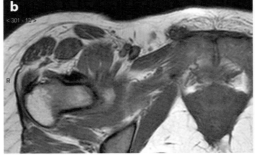
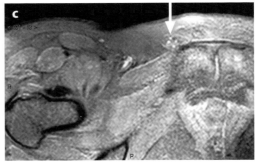

Fig. 17.114 Endometriosis of the round ligament. Thirty-one-year-old woman catamenial pelvic pain close to the mons pubis. Axial T2 (**a**) displays close to the external orifice of the right inguinal canal a low-intensity tissular mass with irregular limits containing a small cystic cavity. On axial T1 (**b**) and fat suppression (**c**) hyperintense hemorrhagic foci are typical for endometriosis (*arrow* in **c**)

Diaphragmatic and Pleuropulmonary Endometriosis

Clinical Findings (Table 17.15)

Generally associated with coexistent endometriosis and usually occurs 5 years after the diagnosis of pelvic endometriosis.

Macroscopic and Radiological Findings

1. Diaphragmatic lesions and pleural nodules.
   They are most commonly right sided; they can be bilateral, exceptionally only on the left hemidiaphragm.

Table 17.15 Clinical findings

1. Common
Catamenial pneumothorax[a]
Hemothorax
Hemoptysia
Pulmonary nodules
2. Uncommon
Non catamenial pneumothorax
Catamenial thoracic pain

[a]Right sided

They lie most commonly in the fibrous center of the diaphragm, usually 2 to 3 cm laterally and posteriorly to the entrance of the IVC into the diaphragm. Small nodules from 1 to some millimeters can be seen. On MR these nodules are difficult to demonstrate; they can appear with a high signal on T1 and fat suppression (Fig. 17.116). At surgery holes in the diaphragm can be displayed (Fig. 17.115).

A pneumothorax without or with pleural effusion can be associated.

2. Uncommonly, perforation of the diaphragm can occur (Fig. 17.117).
   These lesions are not necessarily associated with gynecological locations.

Miscellaneous

Almost any organ in the body can be involved with the exception of the spleen, but these sites are quite uncommon (Table 17.1). Lymph node involvement has been described as well as sciatic nerve involvement, subarachnoid involvement, and breast involvement [86].

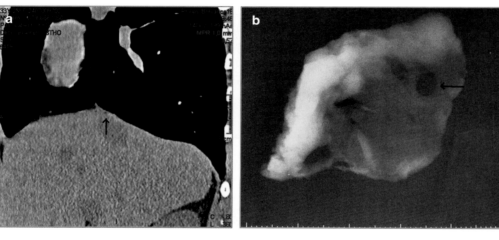

Fig. 17.115 Pleural endometriosis. Thirty years old woman with catamenial right pneumothorax. CT of the right thoracoabdominal junction with sagittal reformation (**a**), displays a small hyperdense focus on the diaphragm with low density nodules (*arrow*). Radiography of the resection of this part of the right hemidiaphragm (**b**) displays holes of 2 to 3 mm in the diaphragm. (*arrow*)

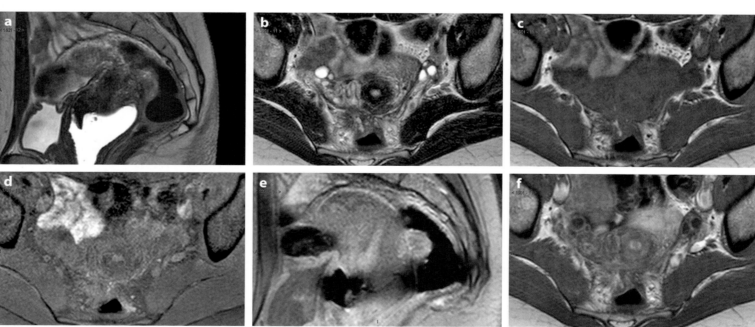

Fig. 17.116 Twenty-seven-year-old woman with right recurrent catamenial pneumothorax. Sagittal T2 (**a**), axial T2 (**b**) axial T1 (**c**) and axial T1 fat suppression (**d**) and sagittal fat suppression (**e**) depict a important posterior subperitoneal endometriosis with involvement of the rectal wall, containing hemorrhagic implants. Sagittal (**f**) and axial T1

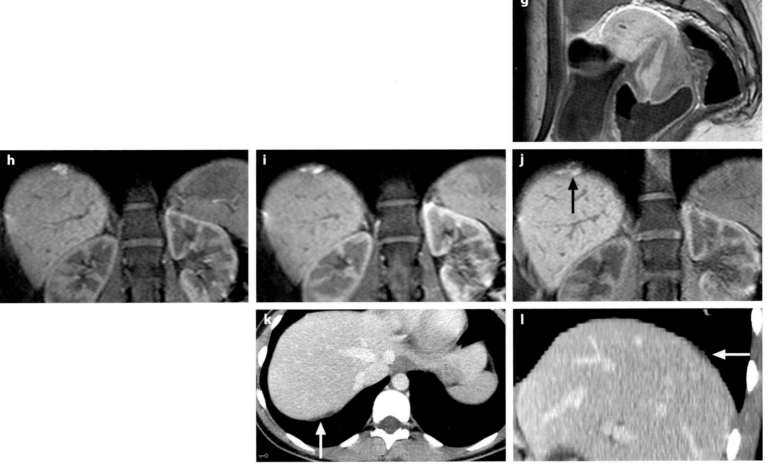

Fig. 17.116 (*continued*) (**g**) after injection display contrast uptake in the lesions. Coronal T1 (**h** and **i**) and fat suppression (**j**) visualize hemorrhagic implants over the right hemidiaphragm (*arrow*), situated roughly 2 cm lateral and posterior to the entrance of the IVC into the right hemidiaphragm. This pattern and that location are very suggestive of endometriosis. CT after injection on axial view (**k**) and sagittal after reformation (**l**) display the endometriotic implants at the same level (*arrows*)

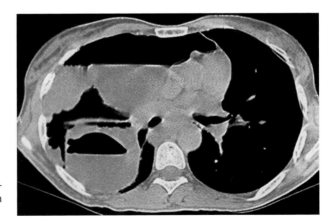

Fig. 17.117 Diaphragmatic rupture with pneumothorax. CT at the level of the thoracoabdominal junction depicts a right pneumothorax with a posterior cystic mass with an air fluid level

17.1.10.6 Association with Mullerian Congenital Abnormalities

Endometriosis can be associated with septated uterus, bicornis uterus (Fig. 17.118) or agenesis of the uterus.

17.1.10.7 Complications

1. Focal leaks with inflammation, fibrosis, and adhesion formation are characteristics of endometriosis, whereas acute cystic rupture is a relatively uncommon complication. It has been reported in pregnancy and likely occurs because of softening of the lesion from stromal decidualization combined with pressure from the expanding uterus. Patients with a rupture cyst present with symptoms of an acute abdomen.
2. Torsion: Endometriosis may predispose to twist less than ovarian masses possibly because of the surrounding adhesions.
3. Ascites: Massive, sometimes serosanguineous, ascites occurs in patients with endometriosis; a right pleural effusion is also present in one-third of cases. If one or both ovaries are involved, the operative findings may simulate those of an ovarian carcinoma. The pathogenesis of ascites is not clear. Possible sources include production by endometriotic cysts, irritated peritoneal mesothelial cells, or the ovarian serosa (Meigs-like syndrome).

17.1.10.8 Neoplasms Arising from Endometriosis

Malignant Tumor

According to Sampson [113], the criteria for malignant change in endometriosis are (1) endometriosis and carcinoma coexisting in the same ovary, (2) carcinoma in the region of endometriosis that is not metastatic, and (3) transitional lesion between the carcinoma focus and the endometriosis lesion. Transitional lesions are atypical changes seen in endometriosis, which on occasion, displays the full morphologic spectrum of neoplastic progression, that is, endometriosis without atypia, with atypical hyperplasia, and well-differentiated endometrioid adenocarcinoma (Fig. 17.119).

Malignant tumors arising in a focus of endometriosis have been documented in 0.3–0.8 % of cases [86]. But the exact incidence is unknown because in many cases, tumor arising in endometriosis may obliterate the latter or the endometriosis may not be sampled microscopically.

Approximately, 75 % of tumors complicating endometriosis arise within the ovary. The most common extra-ovarian site is the rectovaginal septum, less frequent sites include the vagina, colon, rectum, urinary bladder, and other sites in the pelvis and abdomen [86]. In patients with endometriosis who develop ovarian cancer, endometrioid carcinoma is the most common reported malignant tumor, after clear carcinoma, when the primary site is the ovary [114]. Extragonadal lesions are reported to be mostly endometrioid tumors and sarcomas [114]. This disease is seen in women who are 10–20 years younger than those who develop endometrial or ovarian cancer [114].

Findings of ovarian carcinoma in patients with endometriosis have been reported on MR [115, 116, 117]. The mean diameter of endometrioma with malignant transformation is higher than in usual endometrioma, measuring 9.4 and 5 cm, respectively. The cysts were unilocular or multilocular. On T1W images, the signal of the cystic content was slightly higher than that of myometrium, but not as high as adipose tissue, like it is most often the case in a regular endometrioma. Low-signal intensity on T2W images was only observed in two of ten endometrial cysts in Tanaka's series [115]. One or several nodules were observed in all cases in Tanaka's series. Size of the nodules ranged from 2 to 6.5 cm; the mural nodules showed low-signal intensity on T2W images compared with that of myometrium. When the maximum diameter of the mural nodules surrounded by hyperintense fluid is smaller than 3 cm, it may be difficult to evaluate whether the nodules enhance after administration of meglumine gadopentate. Dynamic images or even better dynamic substraction images can be advocated [115].

Imaging findings of malignant transformation in extra-ovarian endometriosis have already been reported [118, 119].

Rare epithelial tumors of other types arising from endometriosis include ovarian serous cystadenoma of low malignant (Fig. 17.120), benign and malignant mucinous tumors, and squamous cell carcinomas. Endometrioid stroma sarcomas, MMMT, and adenosarcomas account for approximately 10 and 20 % of tumors arising in ovarian and extra-ovarian endometriosis, respectively.

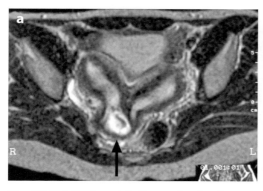 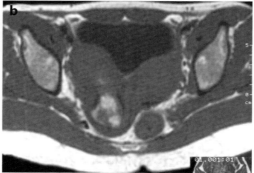 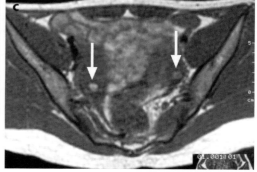

Fig. 17.118 Endometriotic ovarian implants associated to congenital abnormality of the Mullerian system. Twenty-year-old woman with congenital abnormality of the uterus. Axial T2 (**a**) and T1(**b**): Bicorne uterus with hemorrhagic pouch (*arrow*) communicating with the right hemi-uterus. On axial T1 (**c**), bilateral endometriotic ovarian impants are visualized with hyperintense signal on T1 (*arrows*)

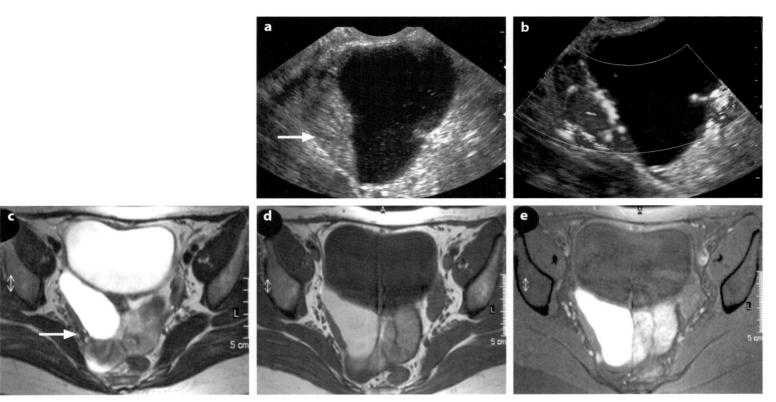

Fig. 17.119 Right peritoneal non-endometriotic pseudo-cyst. Thirty-year-old woman operated a year before from a bilateral endometrioma. Non-catamenial pelvic pain for some months. (1) EVS: Transverse and color Doppler (**a** and **b**): a fluid collection which conforms to the shape of adjacent structures is visualized in contact with the medial face of the right ovary (*arrow*). (2) MR: On axial T2 (**c**) the fluid collection conforms to the shape and seems to share adhesions with the medial face of the right ovary (*arrow*), the parietal peritoneum, the bladder and behind with small bowel. Signal intensity of the fluid is high on T2 (**c**) and intermediate on T1 (**d**). These characters of signal are usual in case of peritoneal pseudocyst and are different from those of an endometriotic collection. However signal intensity is high on T1 with fat suppression (**e**)

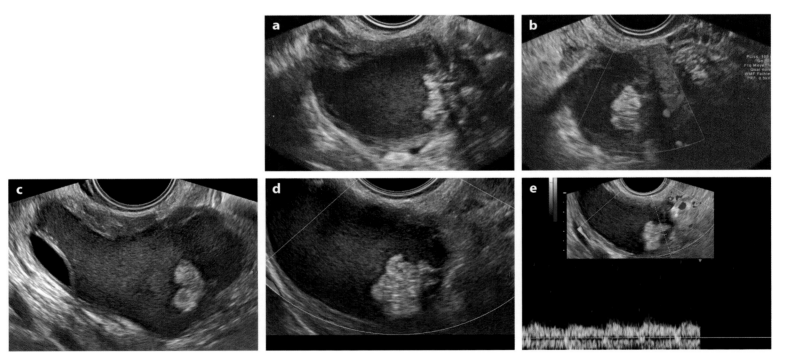

Fig. 17.120 Papillary projections in a cyst considered as an endometriotic cyst. Forty-three-year-old woman operated in 2008: (1) left adnexectomy for endometriotic cyst proved at pathology (2) aspiration of a right chocolate ovarian cyst considered as an endometriotic cyst. EVS in 2009 longitudinal (**a**) and transverse with color Doppler (**b**) display a right 5-cm ovarian cyst with a ground-glass pattern; close to the inner wall of the cyst an echogenic foci, without color flow, is considered as a clot. EVS in 2011 longitudinal (**c**), transverse (**d**), and with color Doppler (**e**) show that the echogenic focus (1) has a broad base of implantation with obtuse angles on the inner wall, (2) an increase in size, and (3) contains vessels, proving that it is a papillary projection.

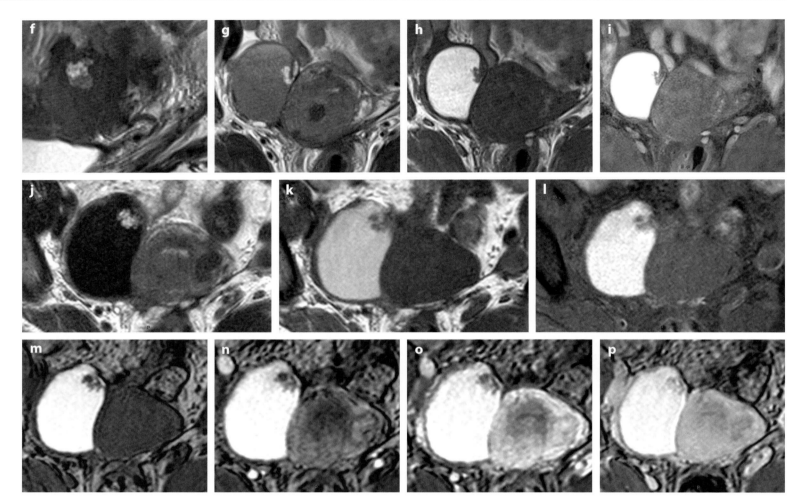

Fig. 17.120 (*continued*) In 2009, MR sagittal T2 (**f**), axial T2 (**g**), axial T1 (**h**), and fat suppression (**i**) depict a right ovarian cyst with a content of low signal on T2, a signal close to adipose tissue on T1 and a high signal on fat suppression typical for an endometriotic cyst. Against the inner wall of the cyst, a focus has a low signal on T1 and fat suppression and a high signal on T2 which is unusual for a clot. In 2011 MR axial T2 (**j**), T1 (**k**), and fat suppression (**l**) depict (1) a slight increase in size of the cyst; (2) a modification of the signal intensity of the cyst on T2, which is close to pelvic muscles; a significant increase in size of the focus lying against the inner wall of the cyst; and a modifications of its morphologic findings which first suggest that it is related to papillary projections. DMR without injection (**m**), at the arterial phase (**n**), show a slight contrast uptake in the papillary projection, which progressively increase at the venous phase and on the delayed at the venous phase (**o**), and on the delayed (**p**). Prospective diagnosis: endocystic papillary projections developed in an endometriotic cyst. Two possibilities are discussed: a cystadenoma and a borderline tumor. Because of the poor vascularization of the papillary projection and its low progression over 2 years, a carcinoma is excluded. Definite diagnosis: at present this patient declined the operation

17.1.10.9 Evaluation of Lesions Under Hormonal Treatment

Different conception of treatment is actually proposed which can be gathered in two mains groups:
- Association of estrogen and progesterone like regular pill or isolated progesterone.
- More specific medication which is LH-RH analogs.

Size of the lesions has been for a long time considered as an important factor of success in the medical treatment as well as the stage.

In fact, the response is mainly related to the location of the lesions. Ovarian cysts decrease significantly in size or even disappear, while endometriotic implants encased in fibromuscular tissue, particularly in subperitoneal locations, do not respond to medical treatment as well.

Comparative studies on ultrasound or MR, associated with clinical findings and CA125, allow to evaluate correctly the response under treatment.

It must be mentioned particularly in young women, that oral contraceptive can hide endometriosis. Indeed, after stopping intake of oral contraceptive, patients complain of symptoms of endometriosis.

17.2 Endosalpingiosis

Endosalpingiosis occurs during reproductive age years with a mean age of 30 years [120].

17.2.1 Microscopic Definition [86]

Epithelium: Presence of benign glands often cystically dilated lined by a single layer (focal cellular pseudostratification may be present) of tubal-type epithelium (with its three cells: ciliated cells, secretory cells, peg cells) involving the peritoneum and subperitoneal tissues.

The glands may exhibit irregular contours, crowding, and intraluminal stromal papillae.

Stroma: Glands are commonly surrounded by a loose or dense stroma.

17.2.2 Locations

The main locations of endosalpingiosis are reported in Table 17.16.

Table 17.16 Locations of endosalpingiosis

Locations of endosalpingiosis
Most commonly
Peritoneum covering
Uterus
Fallopian tubes
Ovaries
Cul-de-sac
Less commonly
Pelvic parietal peritoneum
Omentum
Bladder and bowel serosa
Para-aortic area
Skin including laparotomy scars

17.2.3 Aspect

1. Usually inapparent at operation.
2. May be visible.

Multiple cysts 1–2 mm, rarely larger, and rarely grossly apparent transmural uterine cysts.

Psammoma bodies frequently present within the lumen or the adjacent stroma.

17.2.4 Association

Chronic salpingitis.
Atypical proliferative serous tumors.

17.2.5 Imaging Findings

Peritoneal endosalpingiosis can sometimes be detected as multiple peritoneal calcified nodules, without ascites which are well displayed on CT.

Mass like is rare. On US and CT, solid or cystic adnexal masses can be displayed and can mimic tumors [4, 86, 120–123].

17.3 Endocervicosis

17.3.1 Microscopic Definition

Benign glands of endocervical type involving the peritoneum.

17.3.2 Location

The main locations are reported in Table 17.17.

17.3.3 Aspect

In the bladder, the lesions usually form tumor-like masses that involve the posterior wall or posterior dome in women of reproductive age year.

Table 17.17 Main locations

Posterior uterine serosa
Cul-de-sac
Vaginal apex
Outer wall of the uterine cervix
Urinary bladder

At microscopy, these lesions can simulate a well-differentiated adenocarcinoma.

17.3.4 Clinical Findings

Commonly asymptomatic, pelvic pain, and a palpable mass.

17.3.5 Imaging Findings [121]

They commonly manifest as cystic structures which range from 1 to 5 cm.

On MR, the cystic content is of low intensity on T1 and high intensity on T2.

The findings of paracervical endocervicosis are indistinguishable from those of primary mucinous minimal-deviation adenocarcinoma.

17.4 Extra-Ovarian Serous and Mucinous Tumors

See Chap. 16.

17.5 Leiomyomatosis

See Chap. 24.

References

1. Lauchlan SC (1972) The secondary mullerian system. Obstet Gynecol Surv 27:133–146
2. Lauchlan SC (1994) The secondary mullerian system revisited. Int J Gynecol Pathol 13(1):73–79
3. Clement PB (1987) Endometriosis, lesions of the secondary mullerian system, and pelvic mesothelial proliferations. In: Kurman RJ (ed) Blaustein's pathology of the female genital tract. Springer, New-York, pp 516–559
4. Wheeler JM (1989) Epidemiology of endometriosis-associated infertility. J Reprod Med 34(1):41–46
5. Eskenazi B, Warner ML (1997) Epidemiology of endometriosis. Obstet Gynecol Clin North Am 24(2):235–258
6. Chatman DL, Ward AB (1982) Endometriosis in adolescents. J Reprod Med 27(3):156–160
7. Kempers RD et al (1960) Significant postmenopausal endometriosis. Surg Gynecol Obstet 111:348–356
8. Bailey HR, Ott MT, Hartendorp P (1994) Aggressive surgical management for advanced colorectal endometriosis. Dis Colon Rectum 37(8):747–753
9. Bromberg SH et al (1999) Surgical treatment for colorectal endometriosis. Int J Surg 84(3):234–238
10. Bergqvist A, Ljungberg O, Myhre E (1984) Human endometrium and endometriotic tissue obtained simultaneously: a comparative histological study. Int J Gynecol Pathol 3(2):135–145
11. Roddick JW, Conkey G, Jacobs EJ (1960) The hormonal response of endometrium in endometriotic implants and its relationship to symptomatology. Am J Obstet Gynecol 79:1173–1177
12. Jansen RP, Russell P (1986) Nonpigmented endometriosis: clinical, laparoscopic, and pathologic definition. Am J Obstet Gynecol 155(6):1154–1159
13. Nisolle M et al (1989) Peritoneal endometriosis: typical aspect and subtle appearance. In: Donnez J (ed) Laser operative laparoscopy and hysteroscopy. Nauwelaerts Printing, Leuven, p 25
14. Nisolle M, Donnez J (1997) Peritoneal endometriosis, ovarian endometriosis, and adenomyotic nodules of the rectovaginal septum are three different entities [see comments]. Fertil Steril 68(4):585–596
15. Cullen TS (1920) The distribution of adenomyomas containing uterine mucosa. Arch Surg 1:215–283
16. Sampson JA (1940) The development of the implantation theory for the origin of peritoneal endometriosis. Am J Obstet Gynecol 40:549–557
17. Ridley JH, Edwards IK (1958) Experimental endometriosis in the human. Am J Obstet Gynecol 76:783–790
18. Blumenkrantz MJ et al (1981) Retrograde menstruation in women undergoing chronic peritoneal dialysis. Obstet Gynecol 57:667–670
19. Halme J et al (1984) Retrograde menstruation in healthy women and in patients with endometriosis. Obstet Gynecol 64(2):151–154
20. Oral E, Arici A (1997) Pathogenesis of endometriosis. Obstet Gynecol Clin North Am 24(2):219–233
21. Henriksen E (1955) Endometriosis. Am J Surg 90:331–337
22. Schifrin BS, Erez S, Moore JG (1973) Teen-age endometriosis. Am J Obstet Gynecol 116:973–980
23. Hanton EM et al (1966) Endometriosis associated with complete or partial obstruction of menstrual egress. Report of 7 cases. Obstet Gynecol 28(5):626–629
24. Chatterjee SK (1980) Scar endometriosis: a clinicopathologic study of 17 cases. Obstet Gynecol 56(1):81–84
25. Steck WD, Helwig EB (1966) Cutaneous endometriosis. Clin Obstet Gynecol 9:373–383
26. Javert CT (1951) Observations on the pathology and spread of endometriosis based on the theory of benign metastasis. Am J Obstet Gynecol 62:477–487
27. Binns BA, Banerjee R (1983) Endometriosis with Turner syndrome treated with cyclical oestrogen/progesterone. Br J Obstet Gynaecol 90:581–582
28. Doty DW et al (1980) 46, XY pure gonadal dysgenesis: report of 2 unusual cases. Obstet Gynecol 55(3 Suppl):61S–65S
29. El-Mahgoub S, Yassen S (1980) A positive proof for the theory of coelomic metaplasia. Am J Obstet Gynecol 137:137–140
30. Peress MR et al (1982) Pelvic endometriosis and Turner's syndrome. Am J Obstet Gynecol 144:474–476
31. Beckman EN et al (1985) Endometriosis of the prostate. Am J Surg Pathol 9(5):374–379
32. Schrodt GR, Alcorn MO, Ibanez J (1980) Endometriosis of the male urinary system: a case report. J Urol 124:722–723
33. Scully RE (1981) Smooth-muscle differentiation in genital tract disorders (editorial). Arch Pathol Lab Med 105:505–507
34. Jubanyik KJ, Comite F (1997) Extrapelvic endometriosis. Obstet Gynecol Clin North Am 24(2):411–440
35. Markham SM, Carpenter SE, Rock JA (1989) Extrapelvic endometriosis. Obstet Gynecol Clin North Am 16(1):193–219
36. Cornillie FJ et al (1990) Deeply infiltrating pelvic endometriosis: histology and clinical significance. Fertil Steril 53:978–983
37. (1997) Revised American Society for Reproductive Medicine classification of endometriosis: 1996. Fertil Steril 67(5):817–821
38. Chen FP et al (1998) The use of serum CA-125 as a marker for endometriosis in patients with dysmenorrhea for monitoring therapy and for recurrence of endometriosis. Acta Obstet Gynecol Scand 77(6):665–670
39. Mol BW et al (1998) The performance of CA-125 measurement in the detection of endometriosis: a meta-analysis. Fertil Steril 70(6):1101–1108
40. Eltabbakh GH et al (1997) Serum CA-125 measurements >65 U/mL. Clinical value [see comments]. J Reprod Med 42(10):617–624
41. Kashyap RJ (1999) Extremely elevated serum CA125 due to endometriosis. Aust N Z J Obstet Gynaecol 39(2):269–270
42. Johansson J, Santala M, Kauppila A (1998) Explosive rise of serum CA 125 following the rupture of ovarian endometrioma. Hum Reprod 13(12):3503–3504
43. Duleba AJ (1997) Diagnosis of endometriosis. Obstet Gynecol Clin North Am 24:331–346
44. Adamson GD, Nelson HP (1997) Surgical treatment of endometriosis. Obstet Gynecol Clin North Am 24(2):375–409
45. Schroder J et al (1997) Endoluminal ultrasound diagnosis and operative management of rectal endometriosis. Dis Colon Rectum 40(5):614–617
46. Chapron C et al (1998) Results and role of rectal endoscopic ultrasonography for patients with deep pelvic endometriosis. Hum Reprod 13(8):2266–2270
47. Hughesdon PE (1957) The structure of endometrial cysts of the ovary. J Obstet Gynaecol Br Emp 64:481–487
48. Fox H, Buckley CH (1984) Current concepts of endometriosis. Clin Obstet Gynaecol 11(1):279–287
49. Sampson JA (1922) The life history of ovarian hematomas (hemorrhagic cysts) of endometrial (Mullerian) type. Am J Obstet Gynecol 4:451–512
50. Buy JN et al (1996) Characterization of adnexal masses: combination of color Doppler and conventional sonography compared with spectral Doppler analysis alone and conventional sonography alone. AJR Am J Roentgenol 166(2):385–393
51. Jain KA et al (1993) Adnexal masses: comparison of specificity of endovaginal US and pelvic MR imaging. Radiology 186(3):697–704
52. Kupfer MC, Schwimer SR, Lebovic J (1992) Transvaginal sonographic appearance of endometriomata: spectrum of findings. J Ultrasound Med 11:129–133
53. Mais V et al (1993) The efficiency of transvaginal ultrasonography in the diagnosis of endometrioma. Fertil Steril 60(5):776–780
54. Patel MD et al (1999) Endometriomas: diagnostic performance of US. Radiology 210(3):739–745
55. Buy JN et al (1992) Focal hyperdense areas in endometriomas: a characteristic finding on CT. Am J Roentgenol 159:769–771
56. Laing FC (1994) US analysis of adnexal masses: the art of making the correct diagnosis. Radiology 191(1):21–22
57. Okai T et al (1994) Transvaginal sonographic appearance of hemorrhagic functional ovarian cysts and their spontaneous regression. Int J Gynaecol Obstet 44(1):47–52
58. Nishimura K et al (1987) Endometrial cysts of the ovary: MR imaging. Radiology 162(2):315–318
59. Ascher SM et al (1995) Endometriosis: appearance and detection with conventional and contrast-enhanced fat-suppressed spin-echo techniques. J Magn Reson Imaging 5:251–257
60. Togashi K (1993) Endometriosis. In: MRI of the female pelvis. Igaku-Shoin, Tokyo, pp 203–226
61. Sugimura K et al (1993) Pelvic endometriosis: detection and diagnosis with chemical shift MR imaging. Radiology 188:435–438
62. Glastonbury CM (2002) The shading sign. Radiology 224(1):199–201

63. Sugimura K, Imaoka I, Okizuka H (1996) Pelvic endometriosis: impact of magnetic resonance imaging on treatment decisions and costs. Acad Radiol 3 Suppl 1:S66–S68

64. Stevens SK, Hricak H, Campos Z (1993) Teratomas versus cystic hemorrhagic adnexal lesions: differentiation with proton-selective fat-saturation MR imaging. Radiology 186(2):481–488

65. Nyberg DA et al (1987) MR imaging of hemorrhagic adnexal masses. J Comput Assist Tomogr 11(4):664–669

66. Zawin M et al (1989) Endometriosis: appearance and detection at MR imaging. Radiology 171(3):693–696

67. Bis KG et al (1997) Pelvic endometriosis: MR imaging spectrum with laparoscopic correlation and diagnostic pitfalls. Radiographics 17:639–655

68. Outwater EK, Dunton CJ (1995) Imaging of the ovary and adnexa: clinical issues and applications of MR imaging. Radiology 194(1):1–18

69. Gomori JM et al (1985) Intracranial hematomas: imaging by high-field MR. Radiology 157(1):87–93

70. Hahn PF et al (1986) Duodenal hematoma: the ring sign in MR imaging. Radiology 159:379–382

71. Bazot M et al (1993) Fibrothecomas of the ovary: CT and US findings. J Comput Assist Tomogr 17:754–759

72. Koninckx PR, Martin DC (1992) Deep endometriosis: a consequence of infiltration or retraction or possibly adenomyosis externa? [see comments]. Fertil Steril 58:924–928

73. Uhlenhuth E, Wolfe WM, Middleton EB (1948) The rectovaginal septum. Surg Gynecol Obstet 76:148–163

74. Sampson JA (1927) Peritoneal endometriosis due to the menstrual dissemination of endometrial tissue into the peritoneal cavity. Am J Obstet Gynecol 14:422–469

75. Nguyen BD et al (1994) Primary cervicovaginal endometriosis: sonographic findings with MR imaging correlation. J Ultrasound Med 13:809–811

76. Sampson JA (1921) Perforating hemorrhagic (chocolate) cysts of the ovary. Arch Surg 3:245

77. Fedele L et al (1998) Transrectal ultrasonography in the assessment of rectovaginal endometriosis. Obstet Gynecol 91(3):444–448

78. Donnez J et al (1995) Rectovaginal septum, endometriosis or adenomyosis: laparoscopic management in a series of 231 patients. Hum Reprod 10(3):630–635

79. Fein RL, Horton BF (1966) Vesical endometriosis: a case report and review of the literature. J Urol 95(1):45–50

80. Skor AB, Warren MM, Mueller EO (1977) Endometriosis of bladder. Urology 9:689–692

81. Vercellini P et al (1996) Bladder detrusor endometriosis: clinical and pathogenetic implications. J Urol 155(1):84–86

82. Donnez J et al (2000) Bladder endometriosis must be considered as bladder adenomyosis. Fertil Steril 74(6):1175–1181

83. Fedele L et al (1998) Bladder endometriosis: deep infiltrating endometriosis or adenomyosis? Fertil Steril 69(5):972–975

84. Judd ES (1921) Adenomyomata presenting as a tumor of the bladder. Surg Clin North Am 1:1271–1278

85. Moore TD, Herring AL, McCannel DA (1943) Some urologic aspects of endometriosis. J Urol 40:171

86. Clement PB (2002) Diseases of the peritoneum. In: Kurman RJ (ed) Blaustein's pathology of the female genital tract. Springer, New-York, pp 729–789

87. Bree RL, Silver TM (1981) Sonography of bladder and perivesical abnormalities. AJR Am J Roentgenol 136(6):1101–1104

88. Damani N, Wilson SR (1999) Nongynecologic applications of transvaginal US. Radiographics 19 Spec No:S179–S200

89. Buy JN (2001) Pelvic endometriosis. J Radiol 82(12 Pt 2):1867–1879

90. Deval B et al (2000) Bladder endometriosis. Apropos of 4 cases and review of the literature. Gynecol Obstet Fertil 28(5):385–390

91. Fedele L et al (1997) Pre-operative assessment of bladder endometriosis. Hum Reprod 12(11):2519–2522

92. Buka NJ (1988) Vesical endometriosis after cesarean section. Am J Obstet Gynecol 158:1117–1118

93. O'Conor VJ, Greenhill JP (1945) Endometriosis of the bladder and ureter. Surgery 80:113–119

94. Sircus SI, Sant GR, Ucci AA Jr (1988) Bladder detrusor endometriosis mimicking interstitial cystitis. Urology 32(4):339–342

95. Young RH (1988) Pseudoneoplastic lesions of the urinary bladder. Pathol Annu 23(Pt 1):67–104

96. Fagan C (1974) Endometriosis: clinical and roentgenographic manifestations. Radiol Clin North Am 12:109–125

97. Sepich CA et al (1997) Urinary tract endometriosis: report of 2 cases and a review of the literature. Int Urol Nephrol 29(4):433–436

98. Yates-Bell AJ, Molland EA, Pryor JP (1972) Endometriosis of the ureter. Br J Urol 44(1):58–67

99. Klein RS, Cattolica EV (1979) Ureteral endometriosis. Urology 13(5):477–482

100. Berlin L et al (1964) Endometriosis of the ureter. AJR Am J Roentgenol 92:351–354

101. Kaplan JH, Kudish HG (1974) Endometrial obstruction of ureter. Urology 3(3):327–329

102. Pollack HM, Wills JS (1978) Radiographic features of ureteral endometriosis. AJR Am J Roentgenol 131(4):627–631

103. Roy C et al (1993) Ureteral endometriosis. Role of medical imaging. J Radiol 74(3):165–169

104. Miles HB, Falconer KW (1969) Renal endometriosis associated with hematuria. J Urol 102(3):291–293

105. Redwine DB, Koning M, Sharpe DR (1996) Laparoscopically assisted transvaginal segmental resection of the rectosigmoid colon for endometriosis [see comments]. Fertil Steril 65:193–197

106. Adamson GD (1990) Diagnosis and clinical presentation of endometriosis. Am J Obstet Gynecol 162:568–569

107. Ha HK et al (1994) Diagnosis of pelvic endometriosis: fat-suppressed T1-weighted vs conventional MR images. Am J Roentgenol 163:127–131

108. Takahashi K et al (1994) Diagnosis of pelvic endometriosis by magnetic resonance imaging using "fat-saturation" technique. Fertil Steril 62(5):973–977

109. Ha HK et al (1994) Diagnosis of pelvic endometriosis: fat-suppressed T1-weighted vs conventional MR images. AJR Am J Roentgenol 163(1):127–131

110. Woodward PJ, Sohaey R, Mezzetti TP Jr (2001) Endometriosis: radiologic-pathologic correlation. Radiographics 21(1):193–216

111. Ott DJ, Fayez JA (1991) Tubal and adnexal abnormalities. In: Ott DJ, Fayez JA (eds) Hysterosalpingography: a text and atlas. Urban and Schwartzenberg, Baltimore, pp 103–125

112. Gougoutas CA et al (2000) Pelvic endometriosis: various manifestations and MR imaging findings. AJR Am J Roentgenol 175(2):353–358

113. Sampson JA (1924) Benign and malignant endometrial implants in the peritoneal cavity, and their relation to certain ovarian tumors. Surg Gynecol Obstet 38:287–311

114. Heaps JM, Nieberg RK, Berek JS (1990) Malignant neoplasms arising in endometriosis. Obstet Gynecol 75(6):1023–1028

115. Tanaka YO et al (2010) MRI of endometriotic cysts in association with ovarian carcinoma. AJR Am J Roentgenol 194(2):355–361

116. Fujiwara T et al (1994) MR findings of two cases of endometrial carcinoma accompanied with endometrial cysts. Jpn J Clin Radiol 39:983–986

117. Nobusawa H et al (1995) MR imaging of malignant tumor arised from the wall of endometrial cysts: report of two cases. Jpn J Clin Radiol 40:745–748

118. Weinfeld RM et al (1998) CT diagnosis of perihepatic endometriosis complicated by malignant transformation. Abdom Imaging 23(2):183–184

119. Stringfellow JM, Hawnaur JM (1998) CT and MRI appearances of sarcomatous change in chronic pelvic endometriosis. Br J Radiol 71(841):90–93

120. Zinsser KR, Wheeler JE (1982) Endosalpingiosis in the omentum: a study of autopsy and surgical material. Am J Surg Pathol 6(2):109–117

121. Katre R et al (2010) Tumors and pseudotumors of the secondary mullerian system: review with emphasis on cross-sectional imaging findings. AJR Am J Roentgenol 195(6):1452–1459

122. Bazot M, Vacher Lavenu MC, Bigot JM (1999) Imaging of endosalpingiosis. Clin Radiol 54(7):482–485

123. Katre R, Morani AK, Prasad SR et al (2010) Tumors and pseudotumors of the secondary mullerian system: with emphasis on cross-sectional imaging findings. AJR Am J Roentgenol 195:1452–1459

Muller Duct

Part 5

Introduction

18

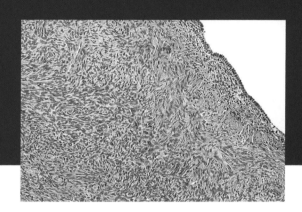

Contents

18.1 Embryology [1, 2]

18.1.1 Development of the Female Genital Ducts and Glands

1. During the fifth and sixth weeks, the genital system is in an indifferent state. Two pairs of genital ducts are present, the mesonephric ducts (or Wolffian ducts) and paramesonephric ducts (or mullerian ducts).

2. The paramesonephric ducts develop lateral to the gonads and to mesonephric ducts on each side from longitudinal invaginations of the mesothelium on the lateral aspects of the mesonephroi. The edges of these paramesonephric grooves approach each other and fuse to form the paramesonephric ducts. The funnel-shaped cranial ends of these ducts open into the peritoneal cavity. Caudally, the paramesonephric ducts run parallel to the mesonephric ducts until they reach the future pelvic region of the embryo. Here they cross ventral the mesonephric ducts, approach each other in the median plane, and fuse to form a Y-shaped uterovaginal primordium.

3. This tubular structure projects in the dorsal wall of the *urogenital sinus*[1] and produces an elevation the sinus tubercle which defines the site of the future hymenal membrane.

---

[1]At fifth week, a septum divides the cloaca into rectum and urogenital sinus that later on will give rise to bladder, urethra, and phallus.

J.N. Buy, M. Ghossain, *Gynecological Imaging*,
DOI 10.1007/978-3-642-31012-6_18, © Springer-Verlag Berlin Heidelberg 2013

4. Contact of the uterovaginal primordium with the urogenital sinus induces the formation of paired endodermal outgrowths – the sinovaginal bulbs. They extend from the urogenital sinus to the caudal end of the uterovaginal primordium. The sinovaginal bulbs fuse to form a vaginal plate. Later the central cells of this plate break down, forming the lumen of the vagina. The epithelium of the vagina is derived from the peripheral cells of the vaginal plate.

Until fetal life, the lumen of the vagina is separated from the cavity of the urogenital sinus by a membrane – the hymen. The membrane is formed by invagination of the posterior wall of the urogenital sinus, resulting from expansion of the caudal end of the vagina. The hymen usually ruptures during the perinatal period.

The unfused portion of the ducts gives rise to the tubes, the fused portions of the ducts to the uterovaginal primordium. The uterovaginal primordium gives rise to the body and cervix of the uterus and superior part of the vagina.

The anatomical origin of tubes, uterus, and vagina are summarized in Table 18.1.

Table 18.1 Anatomical origin of tubes, uterus, and vagina

Muller ducts	
Unfused part	Tubes
Uterovaginal primordium (fused part)	Uterus body and cervix
	Upper vagina
Urogenital sinus	Lower vagina

At tenth week, the mullerian ducts are completely fused (entire septum gone).

Fusion of the paramesonephric ducts also brings together a peritoneal fold that forms the broad ligament and two peritoneal compartments – the rectouterine pouch and the vesicouterine pouch. Along the sides of the uterus, between the layers of the broad ligament, the mesenchyme proliferates and differentiates into cellular tissue the parametrium, which is composed of loose connective tissue and smooth muscle.

The histological origin of epithelium and connective tissue of tubes, uterus, and vagina is summarized in Table 18.2.

Table 18.2 Histological origin of tubes, uterus, and vagina

Embryology	Histology
1. Mullerian duct (of mesodermal origin)	Epithelial component Subepithelial stroma of the mucosa (uterine corpus, endocervix) Muscularis (tube, myometrium, vagina) and Fibrous stroma of the ectocervix
2. Vaginal plate (fusion of uterovaginal primordium with urogenital sinus)	Peripheral cells of the vaginal plate: Epithelium of the vagina Mesenchyme: Fibromuscular wall of the vaginal

The urogenital sinus in which the vagina opens enlarges as the embryo grows, so that it becomes the vestibule of the adult external genitalia.

18.1.2 Mesonephric Ducts Remnants

In female embryos, the mesonephric ducts regress because of the absence of testosterone and only a few nonfunctional remnants persist (Table 18.3).

The mesonephric ducts remnants and their location are reported in Table 18.3.

Table 18.3 Mesonephric ducts remnants, embryological origin and location

Mesonephric ducts remnants	Embryological origin	Location
Appendix vesiculosa	Cranial end of the mesonephric duct	Lateral to ovary
Epoophoron	Corresponding to Efferent ductules and duct of the epididymis in male	Mesovarium
Paroophoron	Corresponding to Rudimentary tubules	Mesosalpinx
Gartner's duct cyst	Corresponding to Ductus deferens and ejaculatory duct in males	Mesometrium Lateral wall of the uterus and vagina

18.1.3 Development of the Male Genital Ducts and Glands

In the presence of fetal testes:
(a) Sertoli cells begin to produce MIS at 7 weeks. MIS causes the paramesonephric ducts to disappear by epithelial-mesenchymal transformation.
(b) Interstitial cells produce testosterone in the eighth week. Testosterone stimulates:
  • The mesonephric ducts which will give rise to the epididymis and the ductus efferens
  • Glands development:
    – Seminal glands (from lateral outgrowths of the caudal end of each mesonephric duct)
    – Prostate (from the prostatic part of the urethra)
    – Bulbourethral glands (from the spongy part of the urethra)
The paramesonephric ducts remnants are reported in Table 18.4.

Table 18.4 Paramesonephric ducts remnants and location

Hydatid of Morgagni	Cranial end of the paramesonephric duct	Lateral to infundibulum

18.2 Different Types of Lesions Along the Mullerian Duct According to Histology

Insofar as the Mullerian ducts will produce the tubes, the uterine corpus, the endocervix, the exocervix, and the upper vagina, one can understand that the histology of these different segments have many points in common but with differences that are very likely related to adaptation of the functions of the different organs (i.e., ciliated cells in the tube, glands in the uterine corpus and endocervix, squamous pluristratified epithelium in the cervix and vagina to protect against infection and trauma).

According to the histologic structure of the different layers of the wall at each level, one can observe different pathologies that can be benign or malignant, epithelial, mesenchymal, or mixed in origin. Moreover, because most of histologic structures are in common, most of these different segments share at least for some of them the same pathological entities.

References

1. Moore KL, Persaud TVN (2008) The developing human clinically oriented embryology, 8th edn. Saunders-Elsevier, Philadelphia, pp 243–284
2. Robboy SJ, Bently RC, Russell P (2002) Embryology of the female genital tract and disorders of abnormal sexual development. In: Kurman RJ (ed) Blaustein's pathology of the female genital tract. Springer, New York, pp 3–36

Congenital Abnormalities of the Mullerian Ducts

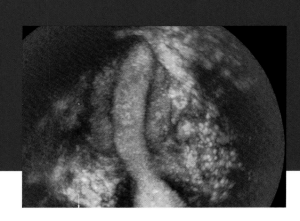

Contents

19.1 Three Main Types

The three main types of müllerian duct abnormalities (congenital abnormality of the paramesonephric duct) are agenesis, bicornuate uterus, and septated uterus.

19.1.1 Agenesis

19.1.1.1 Bilateral: Mayer-Rokitansky-Kuster-Hauser Syndrome (Fig. 19.1)

Definition

The main features and associated findings of Mayer-Rokitansky-Kuster-Hauser syndrome are summarized in Table 19.1.

Table 19.1 Mayer-Rokitansky-Kuster-Hauser syndrome

Main features
– 46XX chromosome
– Normal ovaries
– Hypoplasia of the tubes, aplasia of uterus and vagina until the hymen
– Normal external female genitalia
Associated abnormalities
– Renal anomalies (40–50 % of cases)
– Associated skeletal or spinal anomalies in 10–12 % of cases
– Hearing loss in 10–25 % of cases

J.N. Buy, M. Ghossain, *Gynecological Imaging*,
DOI 10.1007/978-3-642-31012-6_19, © Springer-Verlag Berlin Heidelberg 2013

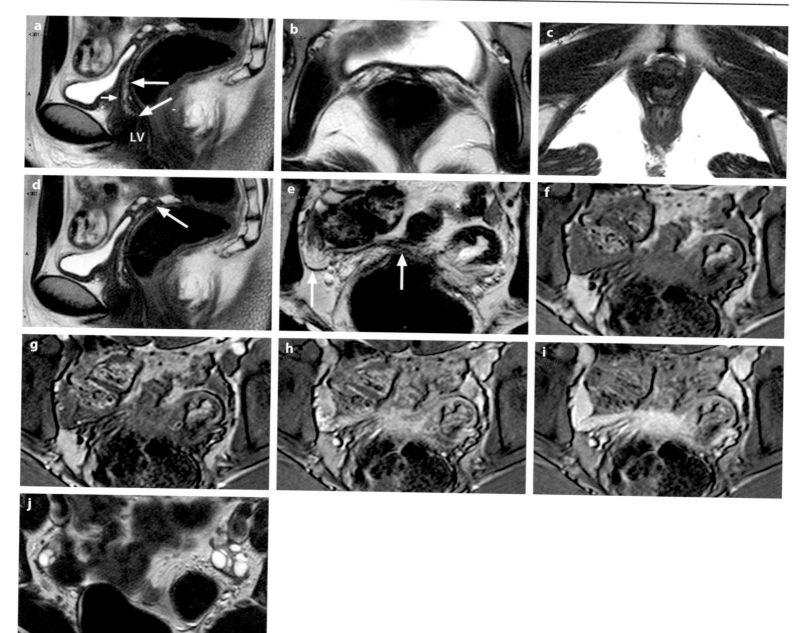

Fig. 19.1 Mayer-Rokitansky-Kuster-Hauser syndrome. Twenty-year-old woman with amenorrhea. (1) *Absence of vagina.* (**a**) MR sagittal T2 on the midline displays absence of vagina almost until the introitus, with adipose tissue between two hypointense lines very likely representing the rectovaginal septum (*long horizontal arrow*) and the vesicovaginal septum (*short horizontal arrow*). The lower vagina (*LV*) is present with a cone shape and an apex (*oblique arrow*) representing the junction with the remnant upper two-thirds vagina. (**b–c**). Axial T2 at two levels. Through the middle part of the posterior wall of the bladder (**b**) allows to definitely confirming the absence of vagina until the introitus; At the level of the posterior and inferior part of the pubis (**c**) displays a normal vestibular vagina. (2) Uterine and tubal remnants. (**d, e**). Sagittal T2 through the midline (**d**) displays between the upper part of the bladder and rectum low intensity tissue (*arrow*). Axial T2 through this tissular mass (**e**) shows a central mass (*central arrow*) with irregular borders related to a remnant of the uterus and laterally two tubular structures with a hyperintense to intermediate signal related to tubal remnants (*lateral arrow*). (**f, i**). DMR without injection (**f**) at the arterial (**g**), venous (**h**), and late (**i**) phases. At the arterial phase (**g**), tubal arterial vessels are displayed in the tubal remnants. At the venous phase (**h**) and even better on the delayed (**i**), a significant contrast uptake is visualized in the uterus and tubes remnants, with a characteristic fold appearance in the right tube at the venous phase. (3) *Normal ovaries* are visualized on axial T2 (**j**)

Differential Diagnosis

The main differential diagnosis is androgen insensitivity syndrome (AIS). AIS findings are displayed in Table 19.2 (Fig. 19.2).

Persons with partial AIS exhibit some masculinization at birth, such as ambiguous external genitalia and may have an enlarged clitoris.

Table 19.2 Findings of androgen insensitivity syndrome (AIS)

– 46XY chromosome
– Testis in the abdomen or in the inguinal canals
– Aplasia of tubes, uterus, and vagina until the hymen due to secretion of müllerian-inhibiting substance (MIS) also called anti-mullerian hormone (AMH) by the Sertoli cells of the testis
– Normal external female genitalia (insensitivity to androgens secreted by the interstitial cells of the testis)

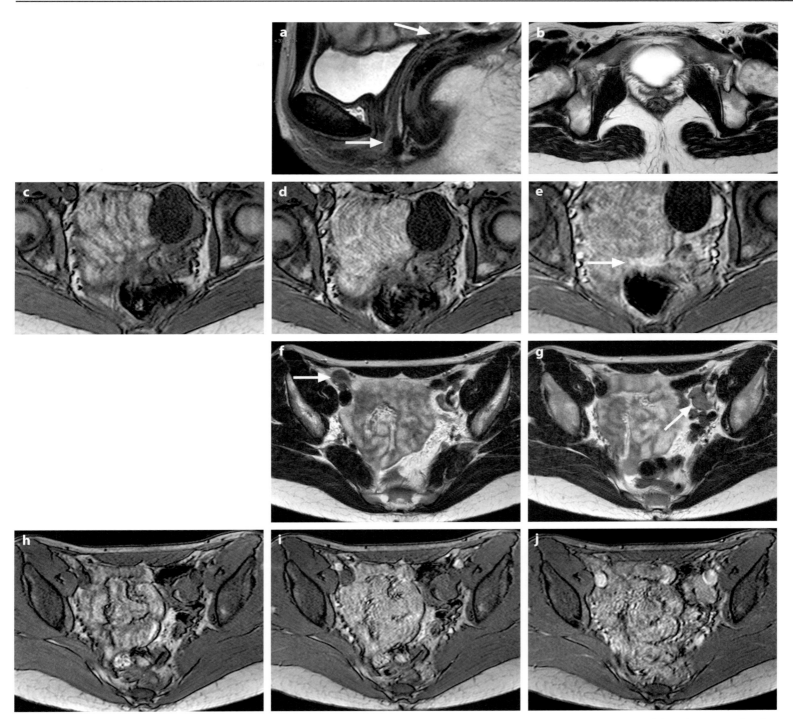

Fig. 19.2 Androgen insensitivity syndrome (AIS). Sixteen-year-old girl with primary amenorrhea. (1) Absence of vagina. (**a, b**) Sagittal T2W image (**a**) and axial T2W image at the level of the middle third of the vagina (**b**) show absence of uterus and collapsed walls of the upper two-thirds of the vagina with no vaginal mucosa seen at this level. *Horizontal arrow* in (**a**) points to mucosa of the lower third of the vagina, which is hypoplastic compared to the corresponding part in the Rokitansky syndrome (see Fig. 19.1). (2) Absence of tubal remnants. On sagittal T2 (**a**), a hypointense tissue (*oblique arrow*) is displayed in front of the anterior part of the rectum. (**c–e**) DMR at the level of this tissue before injection (**c**), at the arterial (**d**), and late (**e**) phases. At the arterial phase, no tubal arteries are displayed. Contrast uptake at the venous phase and especially on the delayed (**e**) is visualized in this little solid tissue (*arrow*), which is smaller and less well delineated than in Rokitansky syndrome. An associated anterior left cyst is visualized in contact at a higher level with the medial border of the testis, probably related to a cyst of the epididymis. (3) Testis. (**f, g**) Axial T2W images at the level of the right gonad (*arrow* in **f**) and the left gonad (*arrow* in **g**), show absence of follicle with a pattern more suggestive of testicles than ovaries. (**h–j**) DMR at the level of (**g**), before injection (**h**), at the arterial (**i**), and late (**j**) phases confirms absence of follicles or nodular enhancement in the left gonad. Similar findings were found in the right gonad

19.1.1.2 Unilateral Agenesis

Complete: Unicornis (Figs. 19.3 and 19.4)

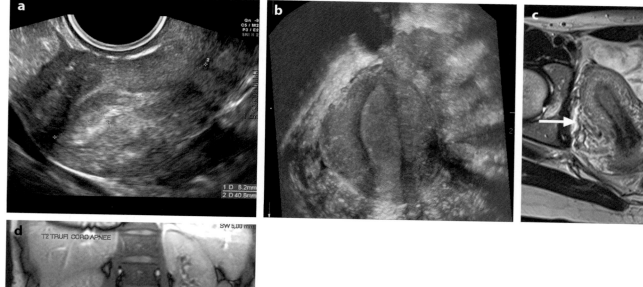

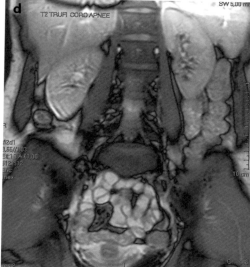

Fig. 19.3 Unicornuate uterus. (**a**) Sagittal EVS displays a uterus that is deviated to the right (*cursors = endometrium*). (**b**) 3D reformation with 2D coronal reconstruction confirms the presence of only one cavity. (**c**) MR axial T2 confirms the US impression and better displays a banana-like uterus very suggestive of a unicornuate uterus. The mesometrium is well displayed on the right (*horizontal arrow*), while on the left, it is absent with presence only of the Mackenrodt (paracervix) ligament (*oblique arrow*). The left round ligament (which originate from the gubernaculums) is visualized in the inguinal canal (*vertical arrow*). (**d**) Coronal T2 shows the presence of two normal kidneys. Coelioscopy confirmed the diagnosis

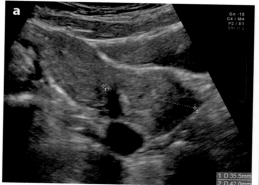

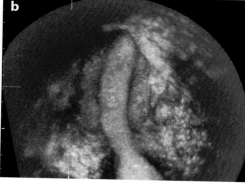

Fig. 19.4 Unicornis right hemiuterus. (**a**) Transabdominal sonography displays a *right banana shaped* unicornis hemiuterus measured using two distances. (**b**) 3D with 2D reformation well displayed the *banana shaped* endometrium. Coelioscopy confirmed the diagnosis

Definition

Small elliptical uterus deviated on one side of the pelvis with single cornu, with an elliptic endometrial cavity well displayed on US with 3D reformation.

On the side of the absent hemiuterus, the round ligament seems to start directly from the ovary (Fig. 19.5).

Differentiation from a normal uterus deviated to one side is made on the following findings:

1. Shape of the uterine fundus is normal with a triangular aspect of the endometrial cavity.
2. Both round ligaments start from the uterine cornua.

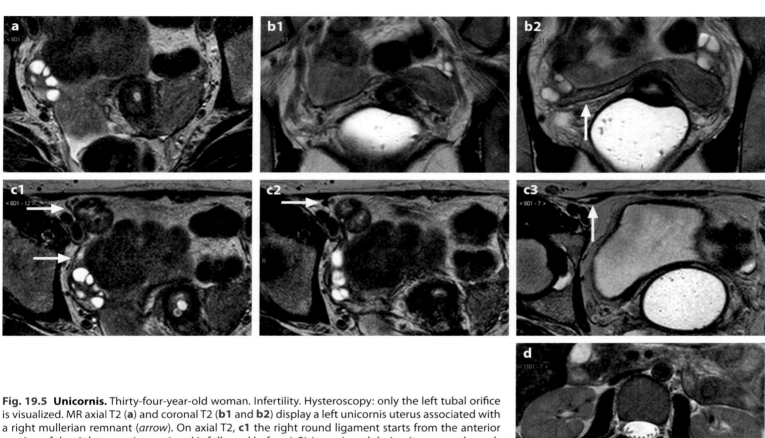

Fig. 19.5 Unicornis. Thirty-four-year-old woman. Infertility. Hysteroscopy: only the left tubal orifice is visualized. MR axial T2 (**a**) and coronal T2 (**b1** and **b2**) display a left unicornis uterus associated with a right mullerian remnant (*arrow*). On axial T2, **c1** the right round ligament starts from the anterior portion of the right ovary (*arrows*) and is followed before (**c2**) (*arrow*), and during its course through the inguinal canal (**c3**) (*arrow*). Although coelioscopy has not yet been performed, this relationship of the round ligament suggests the possibility that in the absence of one uterus cornua, the gubernaculum on the same side (because of the absence of utero-ovarian ligament) starts directly from the ovary. Axial T2 shows (**d**) two normal kidneys in normal situation

Incomplete: Pseudounicornis

Definition

Unicornis with contralateral rudimentary uterus:

- Contralateral rudimentary uterus with endometrium (Fig. 19.6) or without a cavity covered by endometrium.

- Contralateral rudimentary uterus communicating or not communicating (Figs. 19.6 and 19.7) with the normal uterus.
- Bilateral kidneys (Fig. 19.8) or unilateral renal aplasia (Fig. 19.6) can be present.

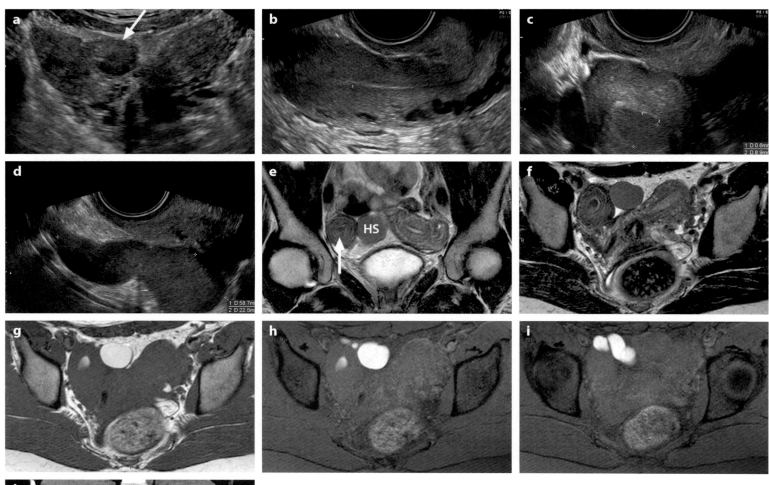

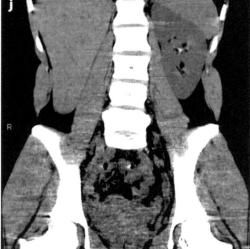

Fig. 19.6 Noncommunicating pseudounicornis uterus with menstrual retention subperitoneal endometriosis and agenesis of the right kidney. Twenty-three-year-old woman with dysmenorrhea. (**a**) TAS, transverse section, displays a left hemiuterus and a smaller right hemiuterus with medial to it an echogenic collection (*arrow*). (**b**) EVS, longitudinal section, depicts a normal left uterus with a thin endometrium. (**c**) EVS longitudinal section on the right shows a right uterus not communicating with the cervix; a hematic collection of 9 mm thickness is displayed in the endometrial cavity. The endometrium is thin. (**d**) EVS, through the right collection identified it as a 59 × 23 mm hematosalpinx (*cursors*). A diagnosis of pseudounicornis uterus is diagnosed. Abdominal ultrasound (not shown) demonstrates absence of the right kidney and normal left kidney. (**e**, **f**) MR coronal T2 (**e**) and axial T2 (**f**): left hemiuterus and tube are normal. On the right side, a small right hemiuterus is present, with hypointense blood in the endometrial cavity (*arrow*), without any communication with the left hemiuterus associated with a right hematosalpinx (letters *HS*). Hypointense thickening of the torus and uterosacral ligament is seen related to endometriosis. Vagina and cervix are unique. (**g–i**) Axial T1 (**g**) and T1 fat suppression (**h**, **i**) show blood in the endometrial cavity of the right hemiuterus and in the right tube. (**j**) CT with coronal reformation confirms absence of right kidney

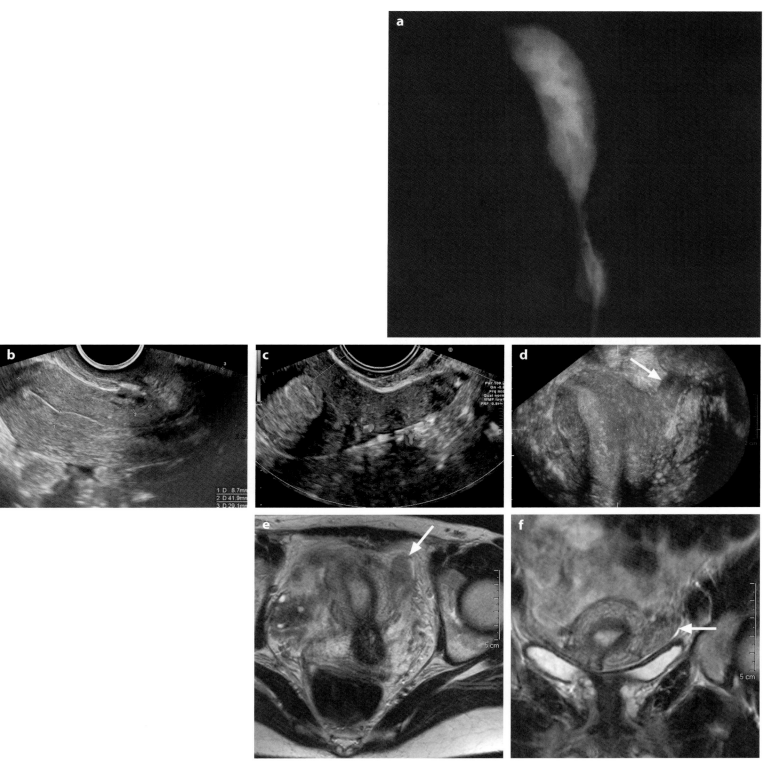

Fig. 19.7 Pseudounicornis with rudimentary noncommunicating horn and without endometrium. Thirty-three-year-old woman with primary infertility. (**a**) HSG: uterus with a right lateral orientation and opacification of the right tube with a little phimosis of the infundibulum, without opacification of the left tube. A unicorn uterus is suggested. Endometrium has a polypoid aspect. (**b–d**) EVS, longitudinal scan (**b**), falsely gives the impression of a normal uterus. Transverse scan with Doppler (**c**) displays against the left wall of the uterus a mass of the same echogenicity as myometrium. 3D with 2D reformation (**d**) allows to precise that the left mass (*arrow*) is in continuity with the myometrium and to diagnose a left pseudou-

nicornis uterus without endometrium. Abdominal US (not shown) displayed two normal kidneys in their lumbar fossa. (**e, f**) MR axial T2 (**e**) and coronal T2 (**f**) confirm the diagnosis made with US (*arrows* = rudimentary left uterus). Hysteroscopy: an endometrial cavity with a tube shape and a hypertrophic endometrium was demonstrated. Right ostium was present with absence of left ostium. Coelioscopy: The distal portion of the left tube was present, but blue injection in this tube did not opacify its proximal part. A diagnosis of noncommunicating pseudounicornis uterus is thus confirmed. EVS and MR allowed to precise the absence of endometrium in the left rudimentary uterine horn

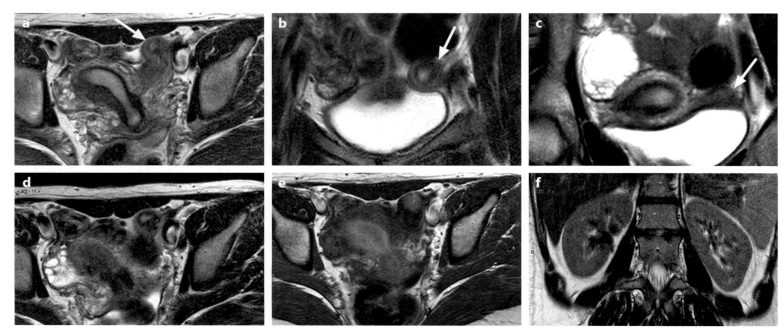

Fig. 19.8 Pseudounicornis uterus. (a–c) MR axial T2W (a) and coronal T2W (b, c) show: right hemiuterus. Left uterine horn (*arrows*) connected to the right hemiuterus with a bridge. A left broad ligament is present. (d) Axial T2 shows a left round ligament going to the inguinal canal. (e) On axial T1 after injection, contrast uptake in the left uterine horn is similar to that of the right uterus. (f) Coronal T2 of the lumbar fossae does not display any abnormality of the kidneys

19.1.2 Incomplete Fusion of Normally Developed Mullerian Ducts

19.1.2.1 Definition

Two types are cited in the American Fertility Society classification (AFS), bicornuate and didelphys [1].

Bicornuate Uterus (Fig. 19.9) [2]

Definition

The distance between the serosa of the middle part of the fundus and the line joining the external portion of the horns is superior to 1 cm.

Anatomical and Imaging Findings

They are displayed in Table 19.3.

Didelphys

Definition

Complete duplication of uterine horns and cervices

Anatomical and Imaging Findings

They are displayed in Table 19.4.

Table 19.3 Bicornis or bicornuate uterus

Uterine horns symmetric in size and appearance Different degrees of fusion between horns: – **Incomplete**: The intervening cleft is of variable length but above the internal os. – **Complete**: The intervening cleft extends at least until the internal cervical os (bicornuate unicollis) or further to form two cervices (bicornuate bicollis), but a degree of communication is maintained between the two horns, the feature that differentiates it from didelphys uterus.

Table 19.4 Uterus didelphys

– Complete duplication of uterine horns and cervices – No communication between the two horns – Longitudinal vaginal septum in 75 % of cases – Occasionally complicated by transverse vaginal septum causing obstruction

Fig. 19.9 Complete bicornis bicervical with complete vaginal septum. Twenty-year-old woman with deep dyspareunia. MR T2W axial (**a**) and coronal (**b**) images through the bodies display a bicornis uterus. The endometrium is present in each uterine body, but it is difficult to assess as far as the patient has her period at the time of examination. Both ovaries are present (*arrows* in **a**). The right vagina is opacified (*arrow* in **b**). T2W axial (**c**) and coronal (**d**) images through the cervix depict two cervices which are in contact of each other. T2W axial (**e**) and coronal (**f**) images through the vaginas demonstrate (1) a unique vulvar portion of the vagina, (2) an opacified upper right vagina, and (3) a collapsed left upper vagina. Duplication starts just at the level of the hymen upon the vestibular bulbs (*arrow* points to left vestibular bulb). Axial T2 (**g**) at the level of the torus and uterosacral ligaments suggests the possibility of endometriosis (*arrow* points to left uterosacral ligament). Coronal view (**h**) of the kidneys depicts two normal kidneys in their lumbar fossae

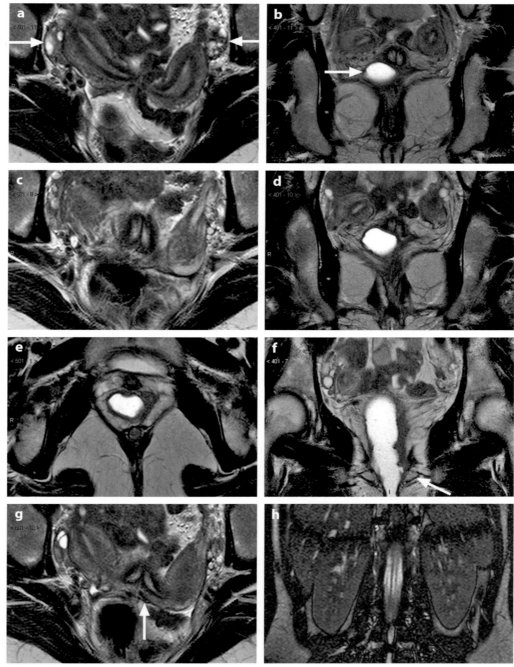

19.1.3 Septated Uterus

It is the most common congenital mullerian abnormality.

19.1.3.1 Definition

Incomplete resorption of medial uterovaginal septum.

The distance between the serosa of the middle part of the fundus and the line joining the external portion of the horns is inferior to 1 cm.

It can be partial or total.

19.1.3.2 Partial

Septum ends proximal to the cervical os (Fig. 19.10).

19.1.3.3 Total

Septum extends to the cervical os (Fig. 19.11). A vaginal septum of variable length can be associated (Fig. 19.12). Opacification of the vagina can confirm the presence of a vaginal septum and precise its extension (Fig. 19.13).

19.2 Associated Lesions

19.2.1 Congenital Abnormalities of the Urinary Tract

Renal aplasia (Fig. 19.6)
   Pelvic kidney

19.2.2 Endometriosis (Fig. 19.6)

Endometriosis is more frequent in females with congenital obstruction to menstrual flow. The implants may involve the the different locations of endometriosis (see Sect. 17.10.1.6, Fig. 17.118) but mainly the ovaries, the peritoneum and the subperitoneal spaces.

19.2.3 Endometrial Hyperplasia (Fig. 19.7)

Endometrial hyperplasia can be associated wih congenital anomaies of the Muller duct, mainly uterus bicornis.

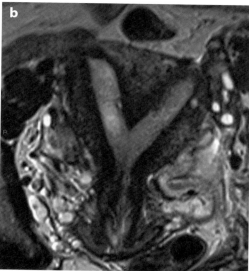

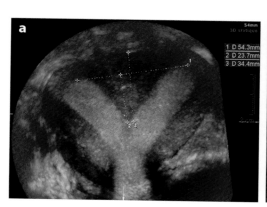

Fig. 19.10 Septated uterus. (a) US with 3D and 2D coronal reformation depicts a septated uterus. The surface of the serosa of the fundus is almost flat, eliminating a bicornuate uterus. Two endometrial cavities are present in the upper part of the uterus. The distance between the apices of the two cavities is 54 mm. The distance between the point of junction of the two cavities and the line joining the apices of the two cavities is 24 mm. The ratio of these two distances is 24/54 = 44 %, definitely classifying this uterus as septated and not arcuate (ratio less than 10 %). **(b)** MR T2W image through the body of the uterus shows approximately the same findings as 3D US and confirms the absence of endometrial abnormality and endometriosis

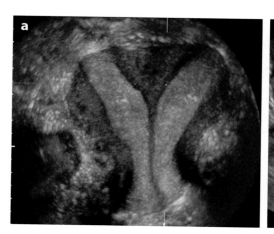

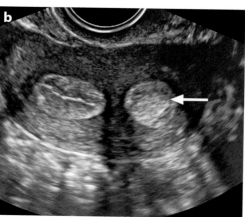

Fig. 19.11 Complete septated uterus. (a) 3D EVS with 2D reformation clearly depicts a complete septated uterus. **(b)** EVS transverse view shows a normal right endometrium with a well-delineated hyperechogenic midline corresponding to an empty cavity. On the *left*, this line is blurred by a hyperechoic structure (*arrow*) related to a polyp

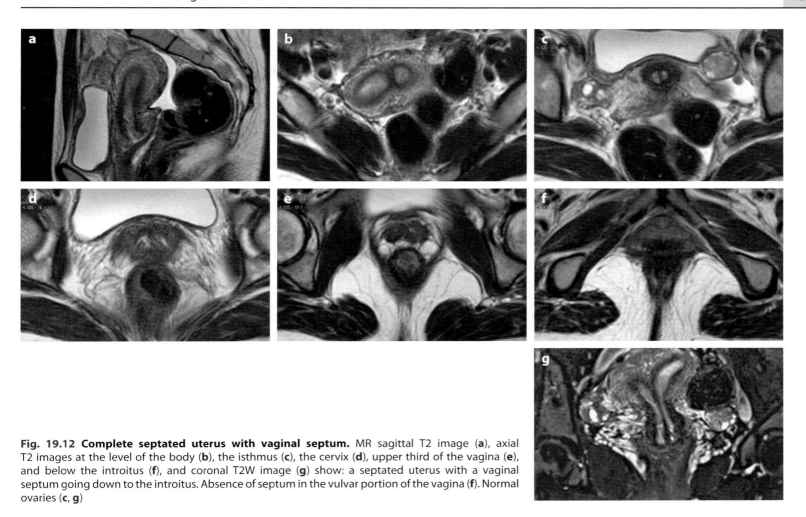

Fig. 19.12 Complete septated uterus with vaginal septum. MR sagittal T2 image (**a**), axial T2 images at the level of the body (**b**), the isthmus (**c**), the cervix (**d**), upper third of the vagina (**e**), and below the introitus (**f**), and coronal T2W image (**g**) show: a septated uterus with a vaginal septum going down to the introitus. Absence of septum in the vulvar portion of the vagina (**f**). Normal ovaries (**c**, **g**)

Fig. 19.13 Completed septated uterus with incomplete vaginal septum. (**a**) MR coronal T2 with vaginal opacification displays a complete septated uterus. The lower part of the vaginal septum starts above the introitus. Transverse T2 (**b**) at the level of the base of the bladder well depicts the sagittal septum

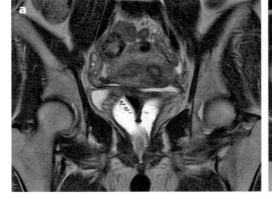
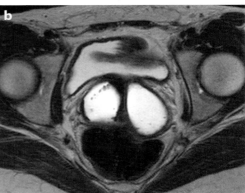

19.3 Other Abnormalities

19.3.1 Uterus-Like Mass (Figs. 19.14 and 19.15)

19.3.1.1 Definition

The pelvic uterus-like mass is a well-delineated mass composed of smooth muscle and a central cavity lined by endometrium [3], or tubal type mucosa [4], or both [5]. It can be a differential diagnosis of adenomyoma (Table 19.5). It is a very uncommon phenomenon.

It could be related to the primary or secondary mullerian system (see Chap. 17). The mass can lie in the following locations (Table 19.6):

Such a mass has even been reported following total hysterectomy and bilateral salpingo-oophorectomy [10].

19.3.2 DES-Related Disorders [11]

19.3.2.1 General Features

Diethylstilbestrol (DES) is a synthetic estrogen prescribed for women with recurrent spontaneous abortions and poor reproductive outcome, between 1940 and 1980. It was responsible for several abnormalities in children (male and female) of pregnant women who received this drug during their pregnancy.

These abnormalities also depend on the amount of DES given to the pregnant mother. Similar changes reported without history of DES exposure suggest that this may represent a müllerian abnormality expressed following in utero exposure to DES.

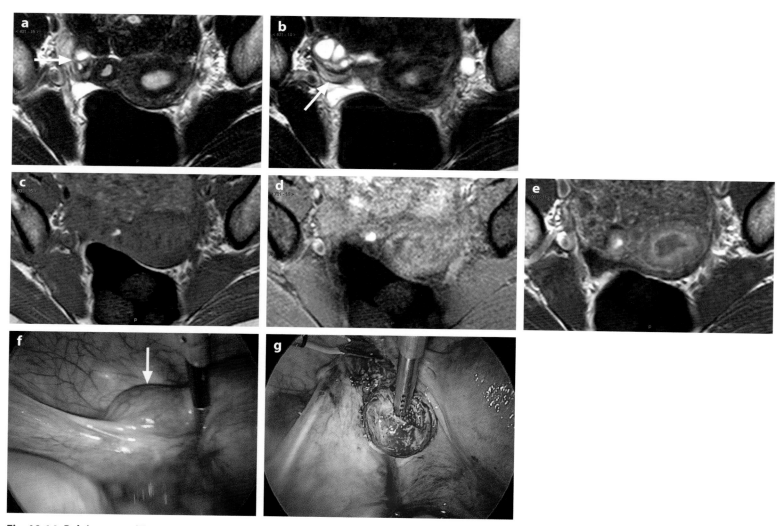

Fig. 19.14 Pelvic uterus-like mass. MR. (**a**) Axial T2 displays in contact with the upper right lateral border of the uterus body a mass with the same structure as the uterus with central endometrium and peripheral myometrium, surrounded by serosa in continuity with serosa of the uterus. It is just medial to the right ovary (*arrow*). Axial T2 (**b**) at a level just above the previous section depicts a normal right tube (*arrow*) starting from the right horn of the uterus joining the posterior border of the right ovary. This finding allows ruling out a pseudounicornis uterus and allows diagnosing a uterus-like mass. (**c, d**) Axial T1 (**c**) and T1W fat suppression (**d**) demonstrate blood in the endometrial cavity of the mass. (**e**) On axial T1 after injection, contrast enhancement in the myometrium and the mass is similar. On US, both normal kidneys were visualized. Coelioscopy. (**f, g**) Coelioscopy (**f**) demonstrates a mass (*arrow*) independent of the right ovary enclosed in the uterus with a tube encompassing the mass and going normally into the uterine horn. At opening (**g**), the mass has a peripheral portion with a central cavity filled with blood. At pathology, diagnosis of a uterus-like mass is confirmed

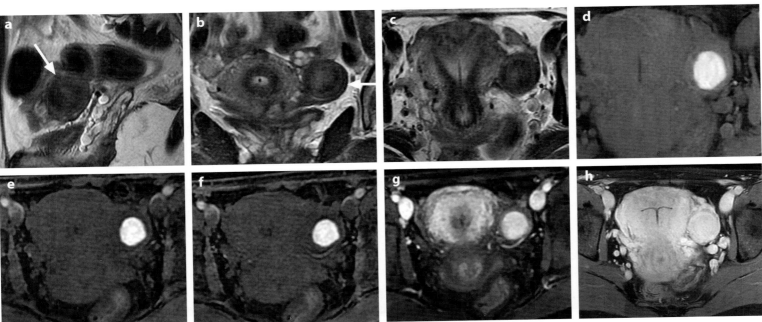

Fig. 19.15 Uterus-like mass. (a–c) MR sagittal (a), coronal (b), and axial (c) images display a well-delineated extraovarian mass (*arrow* in a, b) in contact with the inferior border of the left ovary, surrounded by the uterine serosa. (d) On T1 fat suppression, the central part of the mass contains a hyperintense cystic hemorrhagic portion. (e–h) On DMR without injection (e), at the arterial phase (f), at the venous phase (g), and on the delayed phase (h), contrast uptake in the peripheral tissular portion is identical to peripheral myometrium. An IUD is well depicted. Prospective diagnosis: The intrauterine topography of the mass and its hemorrhagic content suggest either an adenomyoma or a uterus-like mass; its regular contour is more in favor of a uterus-like mass. Surgery: resection of the mass was performed. Pathology: uterus-like mass

Table 19.5 Macroscopic and microscopic findings of adenomyoma and uterus-like mass

Adenomyoma	Uterus-like mass
Circumscribed mass with ill-defined borders	Circumscribed mass with well-delineated borders
Containing: 1. Smooth muscle 2. Endometrial glands and usually endometrial stroma [6]	Containing: 1. Smooth muscle 2. Central cavity lined by endometrium, tubal type mucosa, or both

Table 19.6 Locations of uterus-like mass versus adenomyoma

Adenomyoma	Uterus-like mass
Body of the uterus [7]	Uterine wall
Endocervix [8]	Adjacent to the uterine horn [3]
Tube [9]	Ovary Vaginal cuff At a site of a previous removed ovary [3] Pelvis (broad ligament, small bowel mesentery, uterosacral ligament)

19.3.2.2 Clinical Findings

Clinical findings of women exposed to DES area mainly infertility, ectopic pregnancy, and spontaneous abortion.

19.3.2.3 Imaging and Pathological Findings (Fig. 19.16)

They are summarized in Table 19.7.

Pseudopolyp

The pseudopolyp is caused by a peripheral concentric cervical band, which gives the portio vaginalis (central to it) the appearance of a protruding polyp. However, the presence of an external os at its center differentiates it from a true polyp.

The cervix may be hypoplastic.

The vaginal fornices can be obliterated. A ridge consisting of fibrous tissue covered by squamous epithelium can traverse the vagina.

Adenosis

Definition

The epithelium of the vagina is replaced by mucinous columnar cells lining glands resembling those of the normal endocervical mucosa. This epithelium not only lines the surface of the vagina but also is found in the lamina propria. Vaginal mucosa contains red granular spots or patches and does not stain with an iodine solution.

Location

Most frequently the anterior wall
- Upper third of the vagina: 34 % of patients exposed to DES
- Middle third: 9 %
- Lower third: 2 %

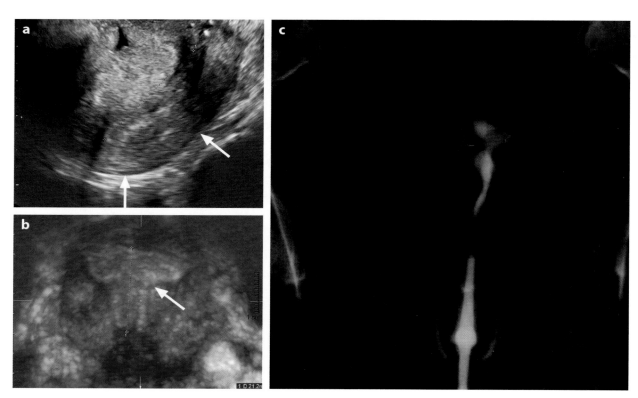

Fig. 19.16 DES-related uterus. Sagittal EVS (**a**) depicts a small uterus (*arrows*). (**b**) 3D with coronal T2 reformation displays a T-shaped uterus with two constriction bands at the junction of the vertical portion of the body and the transverse endometrial cavity of the fundus. *Arrow* points to left constriction band. *Cursors* = height of the endometrial cavity. (**c**) Hysterosalpingography confirms a small uterus with a small endometrial cavity, a T shape, and constrictions bands

Table 19.7 DES-related abnormalities in women

Body of the uterus   Hypoplastic with: – T-shaped endometrial cavity due to constriction bands   – Narrowed fundal segment of the endometrium   – Irregular endometrial margins
Uterine cervix   – Hypoplasia or stenosis   – Pseudopolyp
Fallopian tubes   – Short with irregular contours
Associated abnormalities   – Vaginal adenosis in 67 % of cases   – Clear cell carcinoma of the vagina in 0.14–1.4 per 1,000

19.3.3 Localized Atresia

- Cervical atresia (Fig. 19.17)
- Vaginal agenesis

Complete vaginal agenesis is rare. It results from incomplete caudal development and fusion of the lower part of the müllerian ducts. The defect is often associated with the absence of the uterus and fallopian tubes and with anomalies of the urinary tract.

The commonest cause is Mayer-Rokitansky-Kuster-Hauser syndrome. Other causes for agenesis or hypoplasia of the uterus and vagina include gonadal dysgenesis, Turner syndrome (45 XO), pseudohermaphroditism, and testicular feminization syndrome, which are conditions associated with ambiguous genitalia. MRI is helpful to demonstrate absence of vagina, uterus, and ovaries and assist in surgical planning.

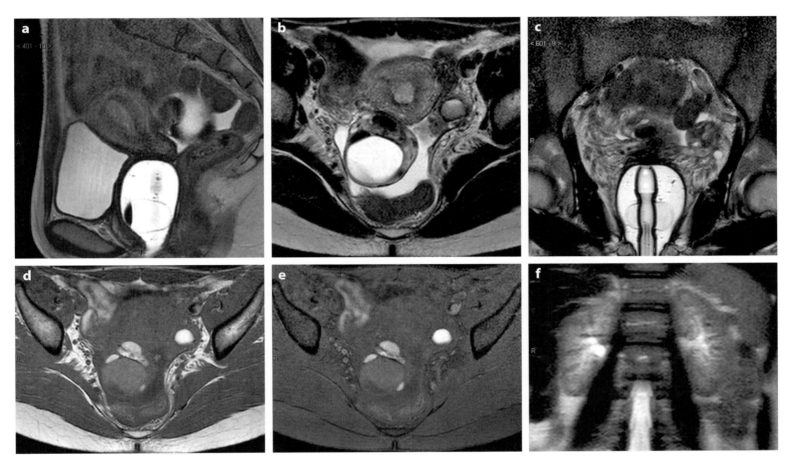

Fig. 19.17 Atresia of the cervix and the vaginal fornices. Twenty-nine-year-old woman with primary amenorrhea and periodic pain suggesting primary dysmenorrhea. MR T2W sagittal (**a**), axial (**b**), and coronal (**c**) depict atresia of the cervix, particularly the anterior lip with absence of endocervical mucosa and external cervical os. Atresia of the lateral and posterior for-nices gives to the superior portion of the opacified vagina a circular form. Axial T1 (**d**) and T1 with fat suppression (**e**) display several associated lesions of endometriosis on the torus and one in the left ovary. Coronal T2 (**f**) depicts both kidneys. Vaginoscopy confirmed atresia of the cervix with hypoplasia of the fornices of the vagina

19.3.4 Vaginal Septum

Vaginal septum can be transversal and longitudinal. Both may occur either isolated or with other müllerian duct abnormalities.

Transversal vaginal septum is uncommon (of about 1 in 50,000 women). It may occur anywhere within the vagina and most frequently at the junction of the cranial and middle thirds. It results from incomplete migration or excavation of the vaginal plate.

Longitudinal vaginal septa arise either as a failure of lateral fusion of the müllerian ducts or due to incomplete resorption of the vaginal septum. They occur in 75 % of cases of uterine didelphys. Renal agenesis often occurs on the side of the obstructed vagina.

On MRI, these septa appear as thin, low signal intensity structures best delineated on T2-weighted sequences on the coronal and axial plane (Fig. 19.18).

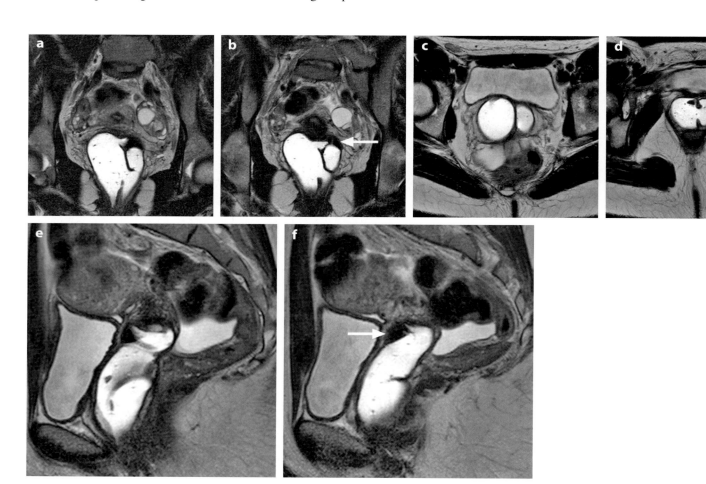

Fig. 19.18 Vaginal septum with rudimentary left cervix and normal right uterus (**a–d**). T2W images with vaginal opacification in the coronal (**a, b**) and axial (**c, d**) planes disclose vaginal septum in the upper vagina with a normal right uterus and a rudimentary left cervix (*arrow*). The right ovary is normal. The left one contains a dominant follicle. (**e, f**). T2W sagittal views show the normal right uterus (**e**) and the left rudimentary cervix (**f**) (*arrow*) and the vaginal septum (in **e** and **f**).

19.3.5 Imperforated Hymen

Imperforated hymen is the most common congenital anomaly of the vagina. Any obstruction of the vaginal tract during the prenatal, perinatal, or adolescent period results in the entrapment of vagina and uterine secretions, and menstrual blood. The obstruction is at the level of introitus. The presence of a thick mucoid secretion that distends the vagina may provide a clue to diagnosis in neonatal.

Abdominal and pelvic ultrasonography provides means for rapidly diagnosing for hematocolpos or hematometrocolpos. If a complex anomaly is suspected or a detailed description of the abnormality is needed, MRI can give full details (Fig. 19.19).

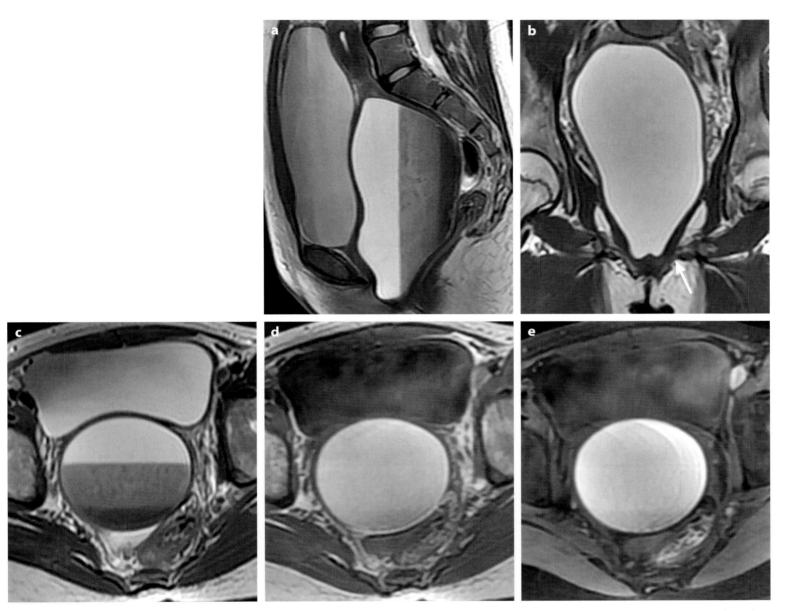

Fig. 19.19 Imperforated hymen. Premenarchal 12-year-old girl with periodic pain. MR sagittal T2 (**a**) displays an important collection distending the vagina from the fornix to its lower part without any retention in the uterus. Coronal T2 (**b**) shows that the lower portion is at the level of the deep transverse muscle (*arrow*) which indicates the level of the introitus. The vulvar portion of the vagina is normal. Axial T2 (**c**) displays two fluid-fluid levels in this collection. Axial T1 without (**d**) and with fat suppression (**e**) demonstrates the hemorrhagic nature of the fluid

19.3.6 Arcuate Uterus

It is a mild indentation of the fundal cavity with no real septum (differentiation from septated uterus). It is most often considered as a normal variant with no real effect on pregnancy. That is why the American Fertility Society classification (AFS) classified it in a different category that septated uterus [1].

However, the AFS did not define the limit between them. A ratio of less than 10 % between the height of the fundal indentation and the distance between the lateral apices of the cavities may be indicative of arcuate uterus [2]. Indeed on the basis of HSG findings, an adverse reproductive outcome is not anticipated in these cases [2].

References

1. The American Fertility Society (1988) Classifications of adnexal adhesions, distal tubal occlusion, tubal occlusion secondary to tubal ligation, tubal pregnancies, mullerian anomalies and intrauterine adhesions. Fertil Steril 49(6):944–955
2. Troiano RN et al (2004) Mullerian duct anomalies: imaging and clinical issues. Radiology 233(1):19–34
3. Kaufman Y, Lam A (2008) The pelvic uterus-like mass. A primary or secondary mullerian system anomaly? J Minim Invasive Gynecol 15(4): 494–497
4. Gurel D, Tuna B, Yorukoglu K (2007) Uterus-like mass of the ovary. Turkish J Pathol 23(2):103–106
5. Cozzutto C (1981) Uterus-like mass replacing ovary: a report of a new entity. Arch Pathol Lab Med 105:508–511
6. Zaloudek C (2002) Mesenchymal tumors of the uterus. In: Kurman RJ (ed) Blaustein's pathology of the female genital tract. Springer, New York, pp 561–615
7. Clement PB (2002) Nonneoplastic lesions of the ovary. In: Kurman RJ (ed) Blaustein's pathology of the female genital tract. Springer, New York, pp 675–727
8. Wright CT, Ferenczy A (2002) Benign diseases of the cervix. In: Kurman RJ (ed) Blaustein's pathology of the female genital tract. Springer, New York, pp 225–252
9. Wheeler JE (1987) Diseases of the fallopian tube. In: Kurman RJ (ed) Blaustein's pathology of the female genital tract. Springer, New York, pp 409–413
10. Redman RWEJ, Massol NA (2005) Uterus-like mass with features of an extrauterine adenomyoma presenting 22 years after total abdominal hysterectomy-bilateral salpingo-oophorectomy: a case report and review of the literature. Arch Pathol Lab Med 129(8):1041–1043
11. Hricak H (2007) Diagnostic imaging gynecology, Section 2: uterus. Amirsys, Salt Lake City, Utah, pp 1–247

Diseases of the Fallopian Tube

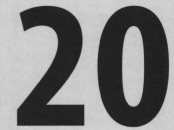

20

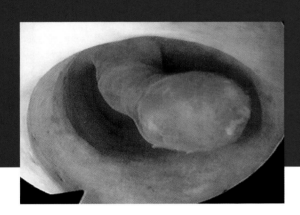

Contents

20.1 Anatomy and Histology

20.1.1 Anatomy (Fig. 20.1) [1]

20.1.1.1 Location

The tube is situated in the upper part of the broad ligament.
The broad ligament comprises:
- The mesosalpinx
- The mesovarium
- The mesometrium

The mesosalpinx is a fold of peritoneum attached:
- Above to the uterine tube
- Below and posteriorly to the mesovarium
- Laterally to the suspensory ligament of the ovary
- Medially to the ovarian ligament

20.1.1.2 Description

The tube comprises four different parts from medial to lateral:
- The intramural part (1 cm length): It lies within the wall of the uterus. It opens into the uterine cavity, near the cornu, through the uterine os.
- The isthmus (2 cm length): It forms its medial third. Its lumen is narrow.
- The ampulla (6 cm length).
- The infundibulum (1 cm length): Its circumference is prolonged into a variable number of finger-like processes, the fimbriae. One of these, the ovarian fimbria, is longer than the others (2–3 cm). It goes from the posterior part of the infundibulum, follows the upper border of the tubo-ovarian ligament.

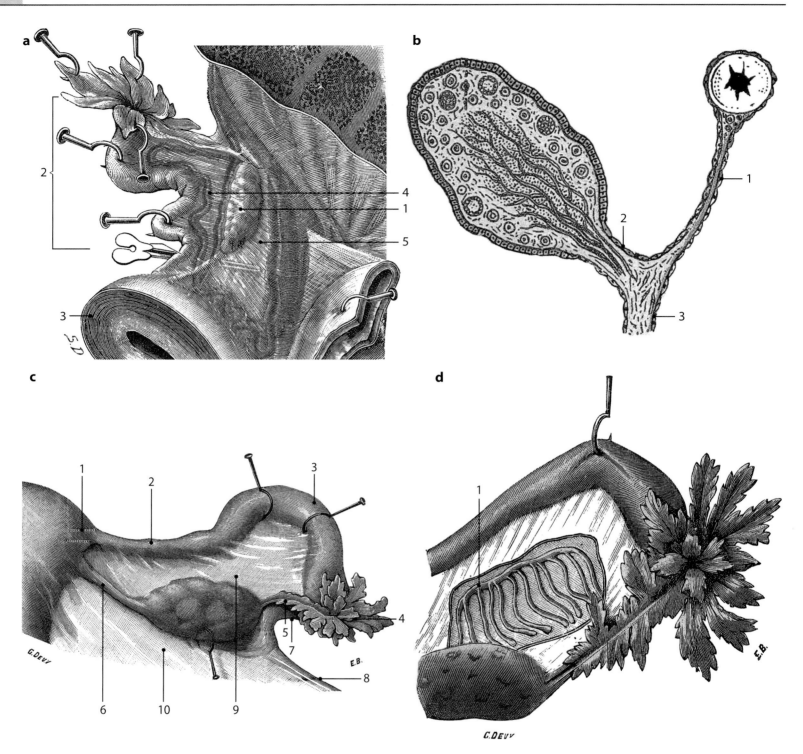

Fig. 20.1 (**a**) Ovary (*1*), Tube (*2*), Uterus (*3*), Mesosalpinx (*4*), Mesometrium (*5*). (**b**) Mesosalpinx (*1*), Mesovarium (*2*), Mesometrium (*3*). (**c**) Tube: Intramural (*1*), isthmus (*2*), ampulla (*3*), infundibulum, fimbriae (*4*), and ovarian fimbria (*5*) Ovarian ligament (*6*), Tuboovarian ligament (*7*), Lomboovarian ligament (*8*), Mesosalpinx (*9*), Mesometrium (*10*). (**d**) Mesonephric duct remnants (*1*) (From Testut [1])

20.1.2 Histology (Fig. 20.2) [2]

20.1.2.1 Mucosa

The mucosal layer consists of a luminal epithelial lining and a scanty lamina propria.

(a) The epithelium is composed of:
  - Columnar secretory cells (55–65 %).
  - Ciliated cells (20–30 %).
  - Intercalary or peg cells: Columnar cells occupied by a thin dark staining nuclei.
  - Scattered lymphocytes may be seen located above the basement membrane.

(b) The lamina propria contains spindly or angular cells and vessels.

The mucosa increases in its gross structural complexity as the lumen enlarges from the uterine to the ovarian end.

The interstitial and intramural portions each contain about five or six blunt plicae or folds. In the isthmus, the plicae increase in height to more nearly occupy the larger lumen. A dozen or more plicae, some with secondary folds, are present.

In the ampulla, the plicae are frond-like and delicate, and both secondary and tertiary branches are visualized.

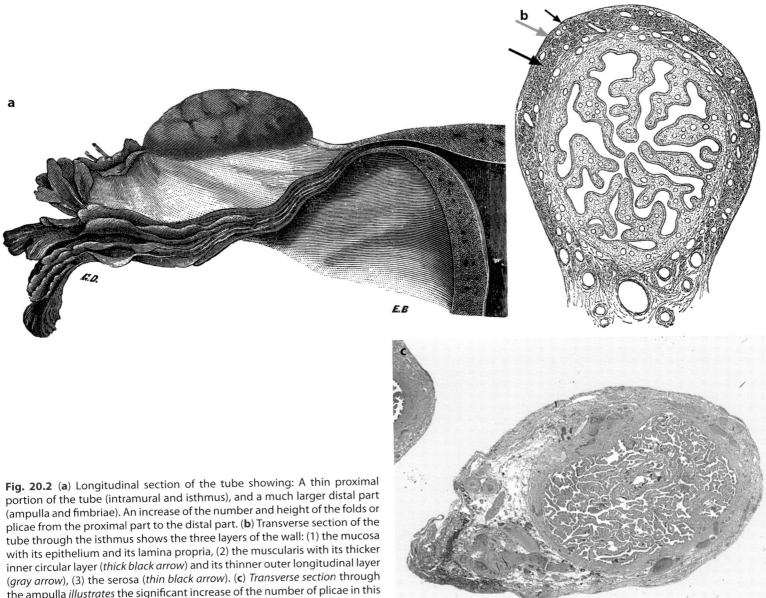

Fig. 20.2 (**a**) Longitudinal section of the tube showing: A thin proximal portion of the tube (intramural and isthmus), and a much larger distal part (ampulla and fimbriae). An increase of the number and height of the folds or plicae from the proximal part to the distal part. (**b**) Transverse section of the tube through the isthmus shows the three layers of the wall: (1) the mucosa with its epithelium and its lamina propria, (2) the muscularis with its thicker inner circular layer (*thick black arrow*) and its thinner outer longitudinal layer (*gray arrow*), (3) the serosa (*thin black arrow*). (**c**) *Transverse section* through the ampulla *illustrates* the significant increase of the number of plicae in this portion of the tube (Fig. 20.2a, b from Testut [1])

20.1.2.2 Muscularis

The muscularis has two layers, mainly an inner circular layer that has a variable thickness, being about 0.5 mm in the isthmus and 0.1 mm in the ampulla, and an outer longitudinal layer.

At the uterine end, beginning in the intramural tube and extending laterally about 2 cm, there is in addition an inner longitudinal layer.

20.1.2.3 Serosa

The serosa is lined by flattened mesothelial cells. Beneath the mesothelium, there is a small amount of collagen and blood vessels.

20.2 Non-Tumoral Tubal Lesions

(a) Metaplasia
(b) Endometriosis (see Chap. 17.1.10) and endosalpingiosis (see Chap. 17.2.4)
(c) Salpingitis (see Chap. 33)
(d) Salpingitis isthmica nodosa
(e) Tubal infertility

20.2.1 Metaplasia [2]

The metaplastic cells are squamous, transitional, or mucinous resembling the endocervical epithelium. Mucinous metaplasia may be associated with Peutz-Jeghers syndrome or chronic inflammation.

20.2.2 Endometriosis and Endosalpingiosis

See Chap. 17.

20.2.3 Salpingitis

See Chap. 33.

20.2.4 Salpingitis Isthmica Nodosa [2]

20.2.4.1 Definition

One or more outpouchings or diverticula of the epithelium, surrounded by nodular hyperplasia of the muscularis, are located in the isthmic portion of the tube (Table 20.1).

Table 20.1 Clinical and imaging findings in salpingitis isthmica nodosa

– 30 years
– Isthmic portion of the tube
– Often bilateral
– Nodules of 1–2 cm in diameter centered by a diverticulum
– Serosa smooth
– Complications: infertility, ectopic pregnancy, and exceptionally rupture

20.2.4.2 Etiology

The etiology is unknown. Salpingitis or adenomyosis-like process has been suggested.

20.2.4.3 Clinical and Imaging Findings

They are reported in Table 20.1.

At hysterosalpingography, the pattern of diverticles of the isthmic portion is very characteristic (Fig. 20.3).

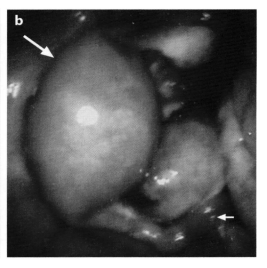

Fig. 20.3 Hysterosalpingography (a) displays multiple diverticles on the isthmic portion of the right fallopian tube (*arrow*) (Courtesy of Professor Antoine Maubon). Coelioscopy (b) depicts small outpouchings under the serosa (*small arrow*) of the isthmic portion and a hydrosalpinx of the ampulla (*large arrow*)

20.2.5 Tubal Infertility

Infertility may be due to tubal patency or dysfunction (Table 20.2). Tubal patency is commonly assessed by hysterosalpingography.

Table 20.2 Etiology of tubal infertility

Patency
– Peri-tubal adhesions (endometriosis, PID, surgery)
– Obliterative fibrosis possibly secondary to inflammation within the uterus
– Polyp formation at the uterotubal junction
Dysfunction
– Dysfunction in the immotile cilia of Kartagener's syndrome

20.3 Benign Tubal Neoplasms

(a) Inclusion cysts and Walthard nests
(b) Epithelial papilloma
(c) Leiomyoma and adenomyoma
(d) Adenomatoid tumor
(e) Other benign mesenchymal and mixed epithelial mesenchymal tumors
(f) Teratoma

20.3.1 Inclusion Cysts and Walthard Nests [2]

20.3.1.1 Pathology

Inclusion Cyst

The tubal serosa, by invagination, may give rise to an inclusion cyst. The cyst is unilocular, lined by one or more layers of mesothelial cells. It lies directly beneath the serosal surface.

Walthard Nest

A process of metaplasia can fill the inclusion cyst, partially or completely, with polygonal epithelia-like cells. The cavity can be completely filled with a central groove giving a coffee-bean appearance. On gross examination, they appear as yellowish subserosal nodules.

20.3.1.2 Imaging

Both inclusion cysts and Walthard nests are frequent incidental findings at pathology of 1–2 mm in size, often not seen on imaging modalities.

20.3.2 Epithelial Papilloma or Polyp

They are composed of a single layer of nonciliated columnar or oncocytic cells that line a delicate, branched papillary core [3].

They appear as a filling defect or obstructive lesions on hysterosalpingography (Fig. 20.4).

20.3.3 Leiomyoma and Adenomyoma

Tumors of the smooth muscle chiefly leiomyoma (Fig. 20.5) and rarely adenomyoma can arise in the tube.

They look microscopically and radiologically as their uterine counterparts that are much more common.

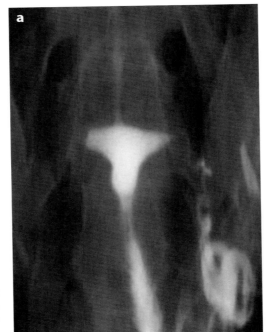
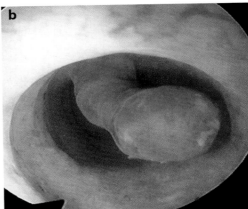

Fig. 20.4 Hysterosalpingography (**a**) displays a filling defect with a regular border in the right cornu. At hysteroscopy (**b**), a tubal polyp protruding into the uterine cavity is seen (Courtesy of Professor Antoine Maubon)

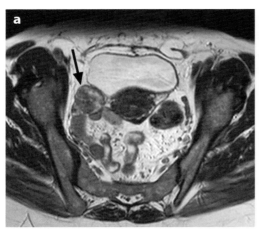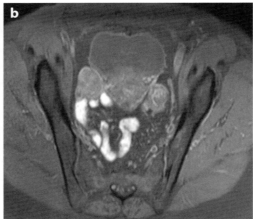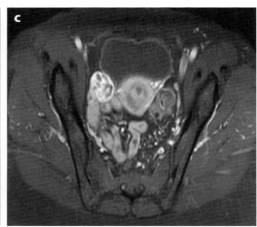

Fig. 20.5 MR axial T2 (**a**) displays an extraovarian mass (*arrow*) close to the right horn of the uterus. The mass is round, of 2 cm in diameter, and heterogeneous with an overall intermediate signal. On T1 with fat suppression before injection (**b**), the mass has an overall signal close to myometrium. After contrast (**c**), at the arterial phase, peripheral arterial vessels associated with central vessels are typical for a leiomyoma. Prospective diagnosis: leiomyoma of the broad ligament. Coelioscopy: leiomyoma of the tube (Courtesy of Professor Antoine Maubon)

20.3.4 Adenomatoid Tumor (Benign Mesothelioma) (See Fig. 24.22)

Their origin is presumed to be from the cells of the serosal mesothelium.

It is the most frequent type of benign tubal tumor.

Microscopically they are composed of multiple small slit-like or ovoid spaces lined by a single layer of low cuboidal or flattened epithelia-like cells. Immunostaining is positive for mesothelial markers as cytokeratin, vimentin, calretinin.

Macroscopically they appear as nodular swelling under the tubal serosa and can resemble a leiomyoma. Continuity with the overlying mesothelium is occasionally seen.

Lesions of this type can be found in the uterus, cul-de-sac, ovary, and elsewhere in the body. They are usually solid 1–2 cm in diameter. Rarely the cystic spaces are sufficiently large to give a macroscopic pattern of cystic or multilocular mass [4, 5].

The main findings are reported in Table 20.3.

Table 20.3 Findings in adenomatoid tumors

1. Location: Subserous
– Cornual myometrium
– Tube
– Ovary(hilum)
– Peritoneum
2. Size
– Usually small 1–2 cm
– May be larger
3. Pathology
– Collagen, elastic tissue, and smooth muscle surround the epithelial elements
– Smooth muscle can be so predominant that the tumor can resemble a leiomyoma
– Rarely the cystic spaces are sufficiently large to give a macroscopic pattern of cystic or multilocular mass

20.3.5 Other Benign Mesenchymal and Mixed Epithelial-Mesenchymal Tumors

Other tumors of mesenchymal origin are rare (hemangioma, lipoma [6], chondroma, angiomyolipoma, adenofibroma, cystadenofibroma, and neural tumors have been reported) [2]. Their pathologic and radiologic pattern is the same as elsewhere in the body.

20.3.6 Teratoma

Tubal teratomas are rare [7]. They have the same pathologic and radiologic characteristics of their more frequent ovarian counterparts.

20.4 Malignant Tubal Neoplasms

(a) Carcinoma *in situ*
(b) Invasive adenocarcinoma
(c, d) Sarcomas and mixed epithelial mesenchymal tumors
(e) Metastatic tumors
(f) Lymphomas

20.4.1 Carcinoma *In Situ*

Radiological findings are negative.

20.4.2 Invasive Adenocarcinoma

It constitutes 0.2–0.5 % of primary female malignancies (Table 20.4).

Table 20.4 Tubal invasive adenocarcinoma

The lumen is filled and dilated by papillary or solid and necrotic tumor
The fimbriated end is closed in about half of the cases

20.4.2.1 Clinical Findings

It is usually found in the sixth or seventh decade. Thirty percent are in nulliparous women.

The most common clinical findings are vaginal bleeding, clear or serosanguinous vaginal discharge, pelvic pain, or pelvic mass.

20.4.2.2 Microscopy [2]

Serous (70 %): They are similar to serous carcinomas of the ovary (Fig. 20.6).

They are composed of fine branching papillae covered by one or more layers of epithelium with enlarged pleomorphic hyperchromatic nuclei with both increased and abnormal mitoses.

In poorly differentiated areas, the tumor may grow in solid sheets and cells with small or large foci of necrosis.

Endometrioid (10 %) and transitional cell (10 %) types are next in frequencies.

Others, 10 % are mucinous, clear cell, squamous, and undifferentiated. Mucinous carcinomas may be of borderline histology or in situ. Synchronous mucinous primaries have been reported in the tube and endocervix [8].

20.4.2.3 Common Macroscopic and Imaging Findings

They are reported in Table 20.4.

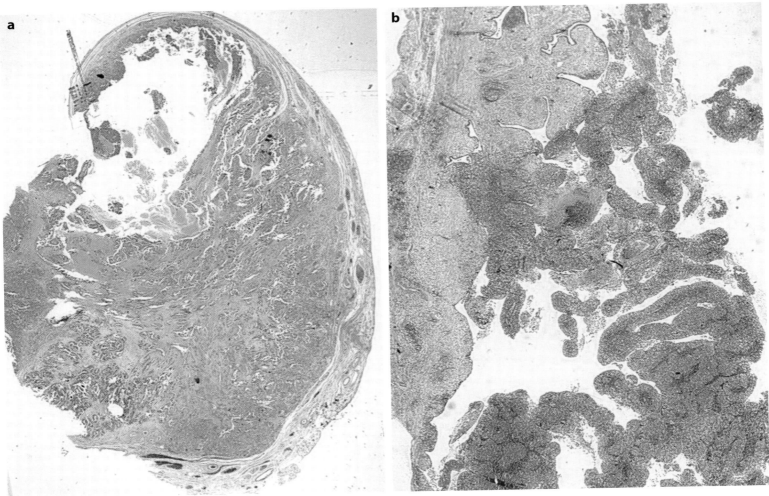

Fig. 20.6 Carcinoma of the tube. At low magnification (**a**), a tumor of the ampulla is displayed. At higher magnification (**b**), papillary projections are visualized related to a serous carcinoma

20.4.2.4 Imaging Findings

They have the usual vascular findings of malignancy.

On US, the mass is echogenic with irregular borders. On color Doppler, arterial tumoral vessels can be displayed (Fig. 20.7).

On MR, the mass has an intermediate signal on T2. On DMR, at the arterial phase, arterial tumoral vessels can be displayed. At the venous phase, a high contrast uptake is depicted. Necrosis can be present (Figs. 20.7 and 20.8). Also not necessary for characterization of the mass, DW images allow however easy detection of the lesion and appraisal of its shape (Fig. 20.8).

On CT, the tumor is solid, with malignant vessels. As for other malignant processes, CT is appropriate to evaluate extension (Fig. 20.9).

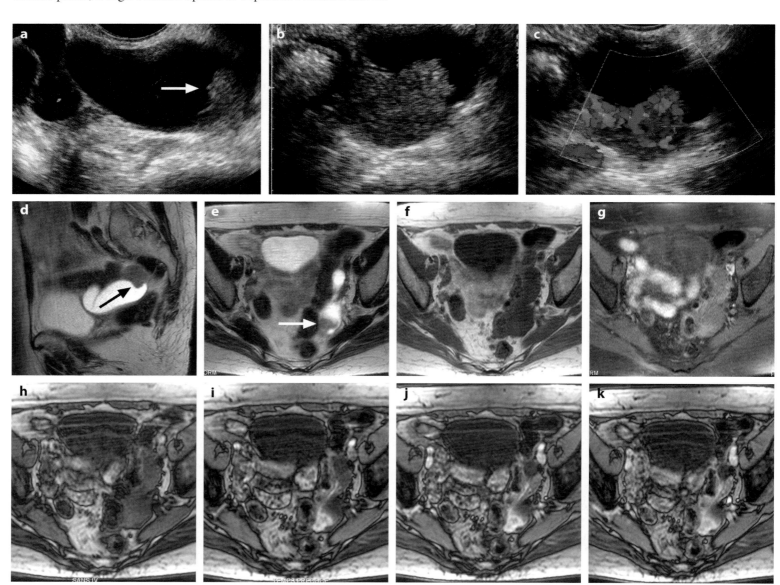

Fig. 20.7 Invasive carcinoma of the left tube. Seventy-two-year-old woman with metrorrhagias. EVS (**a**, **b**) displays, in the distal part of the distended left fallopian tube, a solid mass (*arrow* on **a**) with irregular borders. On color Doppler (**c**), the mass is hypervascularized. On MR sagittal T2 (**d**) and axial T2 (**e**), the mass (*arrow*) situated in the distal part of the tube has an intermediate signal. On T1 (**f**) and on fat suppression (**g**) no hyperintensity related to hemorrhage is seen in the tumor. DMR without injection (**h**) at the arterial (**i**), venous (**j**), and delayed (**k**) phases. At the arterial phase (**i**), tumoral vessels in the tumor and along the medial border of the ampulla are visualized. At the venous phase (**j**) and on the delayed (**k**) phases, a significant contrast uptake in the tumor is depicted, with central necrosis. Prospective diagnosis: carcinoma of the tube. Surgery: total hysterectomy, with bilateral adnexectomy. Microscopy: serous carcinoma of the ovary

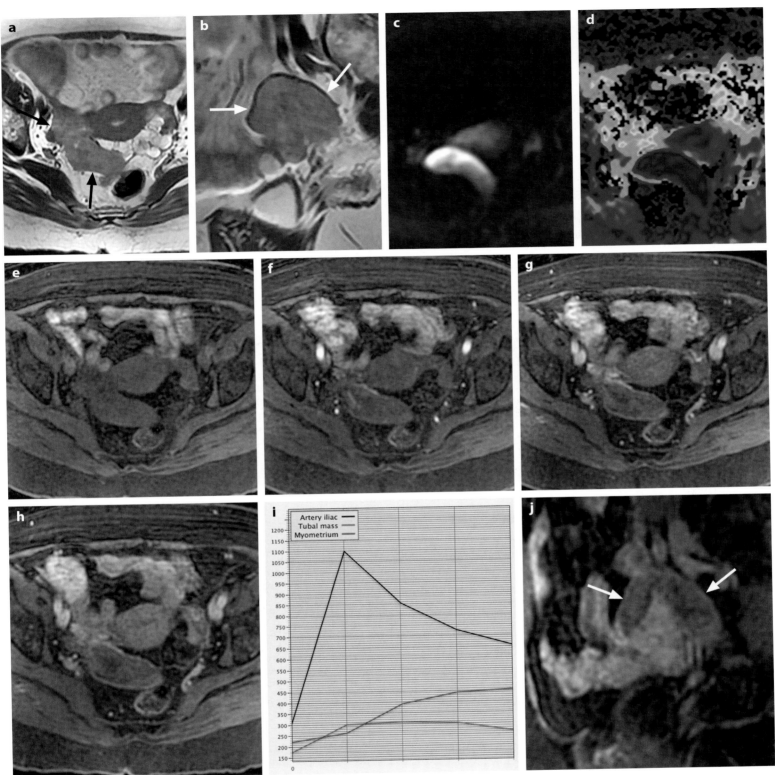

Fig. 20.8 Tubal adenocarcinoma (serous). Metrorrhagia in a 68-year-old woman. Hysteroscopy done before imaging was negative. (**a** and **b**) Axial (**a**) and sagittal (**b**) T2W images show a tubular right adnexal structure of intermediate signal intensity (*arrows*). The right ovary was not identified. (**c**) On consecutive DW images at b1000, the tubal structure was very clearly depicted and easy to follow due to its hyperintensity. (**d**) ADC map shows a low ADC (mean 0.5×10^{-3} mm²/s). (**e–i**) DMR before (**e**) and 25 (**f**), 70 (**g**), 125 and 240 (**h**) seconds after injection with corresponding time-intensity curves (**i**) show early uptake in the tumor with a peak starting at the arterial phase. Some parts of the tumors were not enhancing related to necrosis or blood. The wall of the fallopian tube was more enhancing than the endoluminal tumor. (**j**) On delayed sagittal T1FS image, the tubular shape is well depicted (*arrows*)

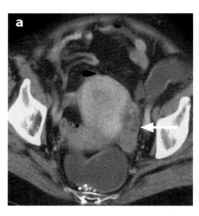
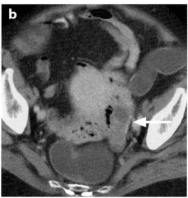
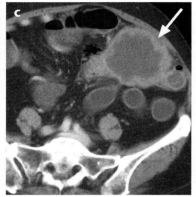
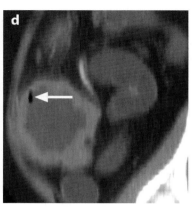

Fig. 20.9 Carcinoma of the tube with peritoneal metastases. Seventy-five-year-old woman with metrorrhagias. CT at the venous phase (**a**, **b**) displays a tumoral mass (*arrows*) occupying the ampulla, with areas of necrosis. CT at a higher level (**c**) and with sagittal reformation (**d**) depicts a necrotic peritoneal metastases of the omentum (*arrow* in **c**) with a small air-fluid level (*arrow* in **d**). A fistula into the transverse colon was displayed at surgery. Histology: serous carcinoma of the left tube with peritoneal metastases

20.4.2.5 Extension

FIGO classification is reported in Table 20.5 [2].

Bilaterality is observed in 7 % of stage 0–II and in 30 % of stage III and IV.

20.4.2.6 Recurrence

Same findings as other recurrent gynecologic malignancies are depicted (Fig. 20.10).

20.4.3 Sarcomas and Mixed Epithelial-Mesenchymal Tumors

They can be pure or mixed with epithelial element. They are called adenosarcoma if mixed with benign epithelial elements and malignant mesenchymal mixed tumors (MMMT) if mixed with malignant epithelial tumors.

The most common pure sarcoma is leiomyosarcoma.

20.4.4 Metastatic Tumors

They are secondary to spread from the ovary or endometrium.

20.4.5 Lymphomas

Tubal lymphoma is rare and is usually associated with lymphoma of the ovary.

Table 20.5 FIGO classification of fallopian tube tumor

Stage 0: Carcinoma in situ
Stage I: Growth limited to fallopian tubes
IA. Growth limited to one fallopian tube
With extension into submucosa and/or muscularis but not penetrating serosal surface; no ascites
IB. Growth limited to both tubes
With extension into submucosa and/or muscularis but not penetrating serosal surface; no ascites
IC. Tumor either stage IA or IB with
– Extension through or onto tubal serosa
– Or with ascites containing malignant cells or with positive peritoneal washings
Stage II: Growth involving one or both fallopian tubes with pelvic extension
IIA. Extension and/or metastases to uterus and/or ovaries
IIB. Extension to other pelvic tissues
IIC. Tumor either stage IIA or IIB with:
Ascites containing malignant cells or with positive peritoneal washings
Stage III: Tumors involving one or both fallopian tubes with peritoneal implants outside pelvis and/or positive retroperitoneal or inguinal lymph nodes
Superficial liver metastases equal stage III
Tumor appears limited to true pelvis but with histologically proved malignant extension to small bowel or omentum
IIIA. Tumor grossly limited to the true pelvis with:
Negative nodes but with histologically confirmed microscopic seeding of abdominal peritoneal surfaces
IIIB. Tumors involving one or both fallopian tubes with histologically confirmed implants of abdominal peritoneal surfaces, none exceeding 2 cm in diameter
Lymph nodes are negative
IIIC. Abdominal implants >2 cm in diameter
And/or positive retroperitoneal or inguinal nodes
Stage IV: Growth involving one or both fallopian tubes with distant metastases
If pleural effusion is present, there must be positive cytology to allot a case of stage IV
Parenchymal liver metastasis equals stage IV

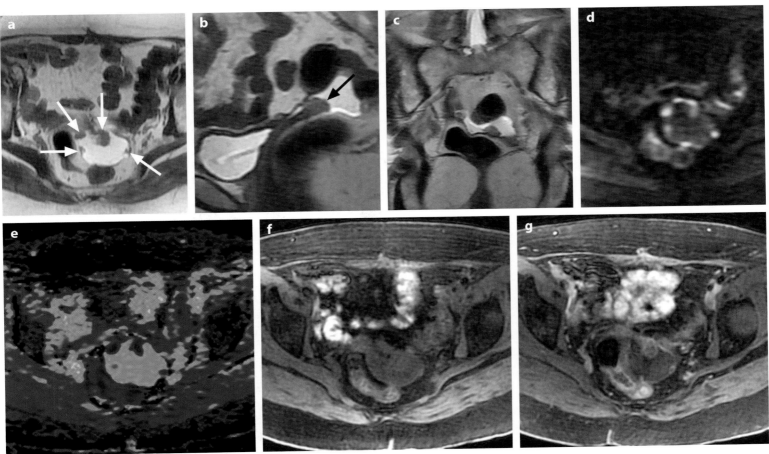

Fig. 20.10 Peritoneal metastasis following surgery for serous tubal carcinoma (same patient as Fig. 20.8). (**a**–**c**) Axial, sagittal, and coronal T2W images, 1 year and a half after hysterectomy and bilateral adnexectomy for tubal serous adenocarcinoma, show ascites and hypointense peritoneal implants (*arrows*) in the pouch of Douglas. (**d**) Axial DW b1000 image shows the peritoneal implants to be hyperintense. (**e**) Corresponding ADC map discloses sharply the implants that have a low ADC (0.9×10^{-3} mm²/s) compared to the ascites (2.7×10^{-3} mm²/s). (**f, g**) Axial T1W FS images, before and after gadolinium injection, confirm enhancement in the peritoneal implants

References

1. Testut L (1931) Appareil urogenital, peritoine. In: Latarget A Traité d'anatomie humaine. 8th edn. revue par. G Doin et Cie Editeurs, Paris, pp 1–595
2. Wheeler JE (1987) Diseases of the fallopian tube. In: Kurman RJ (ed) Blaustein's pathology of the female genital tract. Springer, New York, pp 409–413
3. David MP, Ben-Zwi D, Langer L (1981) Tubal intramural polyps and their relationship to infertility. Fertil Steril 35(5):526–531
4. Hong R et al (2009) Multicentric infarcted leiomyoadenomatoid tumor: a case report. Int J Clin Exp Pathol 2(1):99–103
5. Kim JY et al (2002) Cystic adenomatoid tumor of the uterus. AJR Am J Roentgenol 179(4):1068–1070
6. Baeyens K et al (2004) CT features of a tubal lipoma associated with an ipsilateral dermoid cyst (2004:6b). Eur Radiol 14(9):1720–1722
7. Yoshioka T, Tanaka T (2000) Mature solid teratoma of the fallopian tube: case report. Eur J Obstet Gynecol Reprod Biol 89(2):205–206
8. Jackson-York GL, Ramzy I (1992) Synchronous papillary mucinous adenocarcinoma of the endocervix and fallopian tubes. Int J Gynecol Pathol 11(1):63–67

Anatomy, Histology, and Normal Imaging of the Endometrium

21

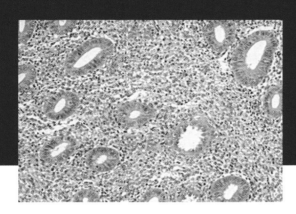

Contents

21.1 Vascular Anatomy

The endometrial arteries originate from the arcuate arteries of the myometrium and are drained by corresponding veins (Fig. 21.1). Their pattern changes during the menstrual cycle [1].

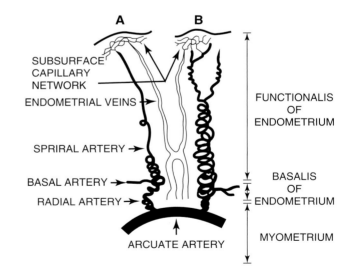

Fig. 21.1 The coiled endometrial spiral arteries originate from the myometrial arcuate arteries and have connections with the subsurface capillary network, which in turn is drained by dilated veins. Arborization and coiling of spiral arteries are amplified in the postovulatory period (**B**) compared with the preovulatory phase (**A**) of the menstrual cycle (From Mutter and Ferenczy [1])

J.N. Buy, M. Ghossain, *Gynecological Imaging*,
DOI 10.1007/978-3-642-31012-6_21, © Springer-Verlag Berlin Heidelberg 2013

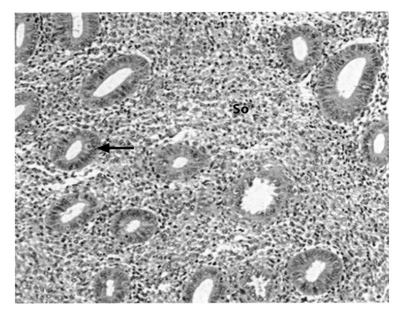

Fig. 21.2 Mid-proliferative phase endometrium (day 10) showing glands with columnar cells (*arrow*) and stromal edema (letters *So*)

21.2 Morphology and Physiology of the Normal Endometrium [1]

At birth the endometrial surface and glands are lined by a low columnar or cuboidal epithelium, which is devoid of either proliferative or secretory changes.

21.2.1 Proliferative Phase

The preovulatory endometrium is characterized by proliferation of gland cells, stromal cells, and vascular endothelial cells (Fig. 21.2).

21.2.1.1 Gland Cells

The straight glands in the early proliferative phase become progressively more voluminous and tortuous during the mid- and late phases of proliferation. Glands are lined by columnar cells with pseudostratified pencil-shaped nuclei.

21.2.1.2 Stroma

The somewhat edematous stroma of the functionalis layer contrasts with the dense stroma of the basalis layer.

The endometrium demonstrates zonal variations in response to hormonal stimuli. This geographic variation correlates with different biologic functions; the upper functional layer serves as the implantation site. The lower functionalis provides the integrity of the endometrial mucosa.

21.2.2 Secretory Phase

21.2.2.1 Postovulation Days 1–3

In the functional layer, subnuclear glycogen vacuoles appear in the base of the gland cells. As a result, the nuclei are pushed to the center of the cells producing nuclear palisading.

21.2.2.2 Postovulation Days 4–6

Supranuclear vacuolization is established.

21.2.2.3 Postovulation Days 7–10

The glands show dilated lumen with secretions; the lining epithelium is low columnar.

Then intraluminal epithelial projections appear (glandular ferning).

The stroma shows edema and increased vascularization.

Edema

These alterations are mediated by prostaglandin F2 (PGF2) and PGE2. The elevated concentrations of midluteal phase E on cycle day 22 increase the synthesis of the enzyme cyclooxygenase, responsible for PG production. PGE2 in turn promotes capillary permeability, leading to maximal stroma edema on day 22.

Coiling of the Spiral Arteries

PGE presumably also promotes vascular endothelial mitotic activity. Endothelial proliferation leads to coiling of the arterial system of the endometrium, a phenomenon that produces vascular clusters in the upper functionalis layer.

Vascular permeability and edema of the stroma are the essential prerequisites for the predecidual transformation. Perivascular *predecidualization of the stroma* around the spiral arteries is characterized by the conversion of uncommitted spindle-shaped stromal cells into plump epithelia-like cells with enlarged nuclei and increased cytoplasm.

21.2.2.4 Postovulation Days 11–13

Predecidual transformation of the stromal cells under the surface epithelium is achieved by day 25 producing the compacta layer.

21.2.3 Menstrual Phase

The upper two-thirds of the endometrium on cycle days 28–2 contain fissures and degenerative predecidual cells admixed with epithelial glandular cells as well as acute and chronic inflammatory cells.

21.3 Morphology of the Gestational Endometrium [1]

21.3.1 Glandular Epithelium

1. The gestational endometrium becomes distinctive by the fourth week of gestation.
   Many gestational glands display intraluminal epithelial projections (glandular ferning), and often they are lined with large cells with clear or eosinophilic cytoplasm and nuclei of varying size.
2. Exaggeration of these cytonuclear alterations produces the *Arias-Stella reaction (ASR)*, which is characterized at microscopy by voluminous glandular cells with:
   - Large hyperchromatic nuclei and irregular nuclear membranes.
   - Large cytoplasm often clear and vacuolated.
   - Normal nuclear/cytoplasm ratio; both the cytoplasm and nucleus being enlarged (cytonucleomegaly).

ASR results from hyperstimulation by chorionic gonadotropin, estrogen, and progesterone. ASR is associated with intra- or extrauterine pregnancy or trophoblastic disease.

21.3.1.1 Differential Diagnosis: Clear Cell Carcinoma

Unlike clear cell carcinoma, ASR is focal, and the adjacent endometrium shows normal gestational changes, that is, a prominent decidual reaction.

Malignant clear cells have a high nucleocytoplasmic ratio.

21.3.2 Stroma

The predecidual cells are transformed into larger epithelioid decidual cells termed decidua vera. The cells are particularly prominent in the upper one-third of the endometrium and produce the compact layer.

Ultrastructurally, predecidual cells lack the typical features of epithelial cells such as glandular lumens, bundles of tonofilaments, or desmosal connections. Gestational decidual cells contain more organelles than their predecidual nongestational counterparts.

Histochemically, the predecidual cells contain glycogen and PAS positive mucosubstances.

These cells have phagocytic properties and digest extracellular collagen matrix by removing the collagen; this may facilitate the development of the decidual reaction. If conception does not occur, predecidual cells by removing the collagen may contribute to menstrual breakdown of the endometrial stroma.

The gestational decidual reaction can be seen not only in intrauterine pregnancy but also in ectopic pregnancy or as a result of exogenous progestational therapy.

On MR, at 5 weeks of amenorrhea, the endometrium in the upper half of the body is very thick containing a gestational sac (Fig. 21.3). This pattern must be recognized immediately to stop the examination.

21.4 Morphology of Inactive and Atrophic Endometrium

It is as thick as early to mid-proliferative-phase endometrium but devoid of morphologic features of either active proliferation or

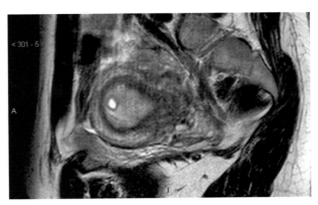

Fig. 21.3 Morphology of the gestational endometrium. Twenty-five-year-old woman with dysmenorrheal and infertility. MRI performed at 33 days of amenorrhea with negative B-HCG the day before. MR sagittal T2 displays in the upper half of the endometrial cavity a gestational sac associated with marked thickened endometrium. The examination was stopped immediately

secretion. The glands and stroma resemble proliferative endometrium, but the glands are usually oriented parallel rather than perpendicular to the surface epithelium. It is about 0.5 mm in thickness or 1 mm for the two layers [1].

At US, using a 5-mm threshold (for two layers) to define abnormal endometrial thickening [2], in a meta-analysis of 5,892 postmenopausal women with vaginal bleeding, with or without hormone replacement found:
- Ninety-six percent of women with cancer, and 92 % with an endometrial disease had an abnormal thickening.
- Conversely 23 % using hormone replacement therapy and 8 % without using hormone replacement had normal histology.

21.5 Normal Imaging

21.5.1 Ultrasound

Just after the menses, the endometrium is thin and often reduced to a thin echogenic line corresponding to the interface between the two layers of the endometrium. Prepubertal, postmenopausal, and atrophic endometrium of any reason has the same pattern.

Then during the proliferative phase, the endometrium becomes progressively thicker and composed of:
- A thin median echogenic line corresponding to the interface between the two endometrial layers
- On each side of this median line, a hypoechoic band corresponding to the functional endometrium
- A peripheral thin hyperechoic line corresponding to the basal endometrium

The thickness of the endometrium is usually measured on a longitudinal view from one peripheral line to the opposite one, perpendicularly to the median line, including the two layers of the endometrium (Fig. 21.4). Exceptionally, it could be useful to measure one layer as in the presence of liquid in the endometrial cavity.

During the periovulatory phase, the endometrium has the same architecture as in the proliferative phase but is thicker, and the peripheral hyperechoic line becomes thicker and a little bit convoluted (Fig. 21.5).

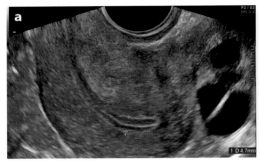
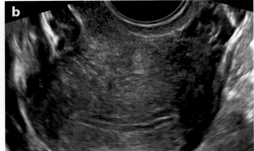

Fig. 21.4 Endometrium at day 5 of the menstrual cycle. (**a**, **b**) Endovaginal ultrasound, longitudinal (**a**) and transverse (**b**) views, displays a retroverted uterus with a typical endometrium of proliferative phase measuring 5 mm in thickness (*cursors* in **a**). The echogenic middle and peripheral lines are well visualized. The junctional zone is not well individualized in this patient

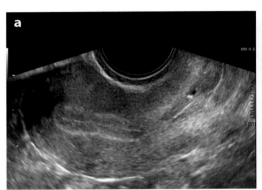
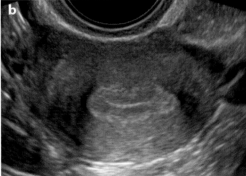
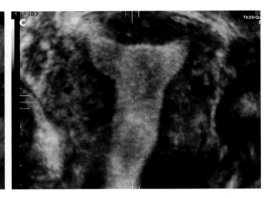

Fig. 21.5 Endometrium at day 14 of the menstrual cycle. (**a**, **b**) Endovaginal ultrasound, longitudinal (**a**) and transverse (**b**) views, displays an anteverted uterus with an endometrium of periovulatory phase measuring 9.4 mm in thickness. The echogenic middle and peripheral lines are still visualized, but the hypoechoic bands start to be more echoic especially in periphery. (**c**) On coronal 3D reformation, the junctional zone of the myometrium, not seen on 2D views, is identifiable

During the secretory phase, the hypoechoic band becomes progressively hyperechoic, and it is often impossible to identify the median line corresponding to the interface between the two layers of the endometrium; this is the reason why thickness of the endometrium is routinely expressed from peripheral border to the opposite one including the two layers (Fig. 21.6).

The junctional zone of the myometrium corresponds to the inner part of the myometrium that is in contact with the basalis of the endometrium. It appears as a hypoechoic band compared to the outer myometrium and is not always seen. It is well depicted in Fig. 21.6 and less well delineated in Figs. 21.4 and 21.5. When the endometrium is reduced to a thin echoic line, as just after the menses or in prepubertal, postmenopausal, and atrophic endometrium, care must be taken not to include the junctional zone in the measurement of the thickness of the endometrium, confusing it with an endometrium of proliferative type. This may happen when the technical conditions are not optimal. The junctional zone, unlike the endometrium in the proliferative phase, is not bordered by a peripheral hyperechoic line.

21.5.2 MR

On MR, the endometrium appears hyperintense on T2 and is usually measured on this sequence using the sagittal plane (Figs. 21.7 and 21.8). As on ultrasound, thickness includes the two layers of the endometrium. A pitfall is the presence of liquid in the uterine cavity that appears hyperintense like the endometrium and indistinguishable from it. This results in majoring the thickness of the endometrium by including the liquid. A good habit is the to compare the sagittal T2 sequence to a sagittal post-contrast T1 sequence, allowing identification of liquid in the cavity and assessing the true thickness of the endometrium. As on ultrasound, the hypointense junctional zone must not be included in the measurement (Fig. 21.8).

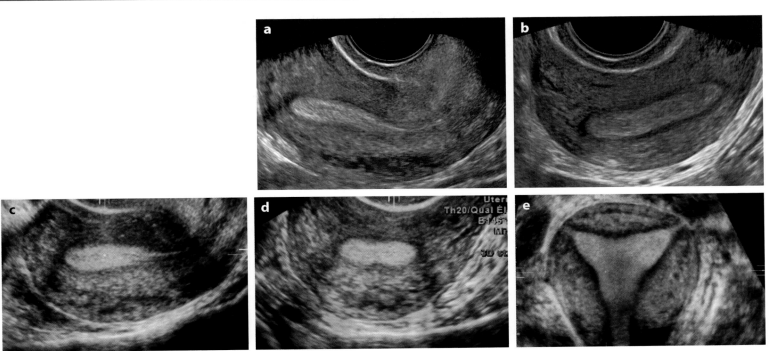

Fig. 21.6 Endometrium at day 18 of the menstrual cycle. (**a, b**) Endovaginal ultrasound, longitudinal (**a**) and transverse (**b**) views, display an anteverted uterus with a typical endometrium of the secretory phase. The endometrium is entirely hyperechoic and the interface between the two layers is not depicted. (**c–e**) 3D with sagittal (**c**) transverse (**d**) and coronal reformation (**e**) well display the hyperechoic endometrium and the hypoechoic junctional zone mainly on (**e**)

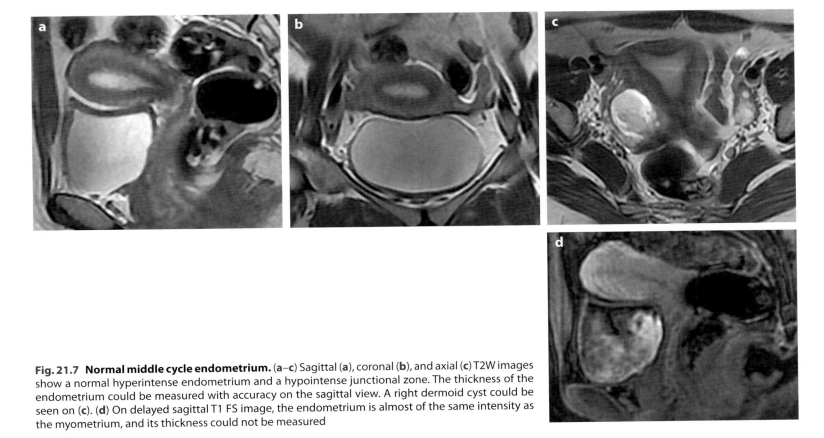

Fig. 21.7 Normal middle cycle endometrium. (**a–c**) Sagittal (**a**), coronal (**b**), and axial (**c**) T2W images show a normal hyperintense endometrium and a hypointense junctional zone. The thickness of the endometrium could be measured with accuracy on the sagittal view. A right dermoid cyst could be seen on (**c**). (**d**) On delayed sagittal T1 FS image, the endometrium is almost of the same intensity as the myometrium, and its thickness could not be measured

On DW images, the endometrium appears hyperintense, and the junctional zone hypointense compared to endometrium and outer myometrium (Fig. 21.9).

On DMR, the endometrium enhances less rapidly than the myometrium but usually becomes isointense to it on the late phase (Fig. 23.9). On delayed phase, the endometrium may or may not be differentiate from the myometrium (Figs. 21.7 and 23.10).

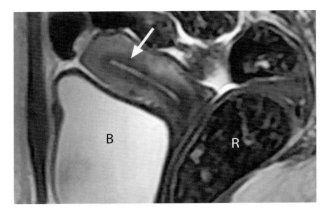

Fig. 21.8 Thin endometrium at third day of the menstrual cycle. A Sagittal T2W images depict a thin hyperintense endometrium and a well-delineated hypointense junctional zone (*arrow*) of the myometrium. *B* bladder, *R* rectum

21.5.3 CT

CT is not the preferred modality to visualize the myometrium. Before injection, it could not be individualized and is seen after injection because it enhances less than the myometrium especially at early phases (Fig. 21.10).

References

1. Mutter GL, Ferenczy A (2002) Anatomy and histology of the uterine corpus. In: Kurman RJ (ed) Blaustein's pathology of the female genital tract. Springer, New-York, pp 383–418
2. Smith-Bindman R et al (1998) Endovaginal ultrasound to exclude endometrial cancer and other endometrial abnormalities. JAMA 280(17): 1510–1517

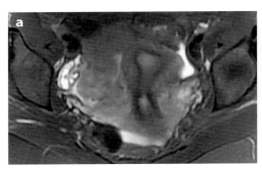
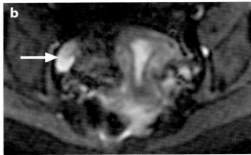
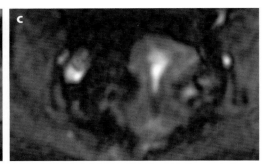

Fig. 21.9 Endometrium on DWI. (**a–c**) Axial T2 FS (**a**) and DW at b500 (**b**) and b1000 (**c**) images show a normal endometrium, hyperintense on T2 and on DW images. The junctional zone of the myometrium is well delineated, appearing hypointense on all three sequences. Note that the normal ovary appears hyperintense on DW image (*arrow* in **b**)

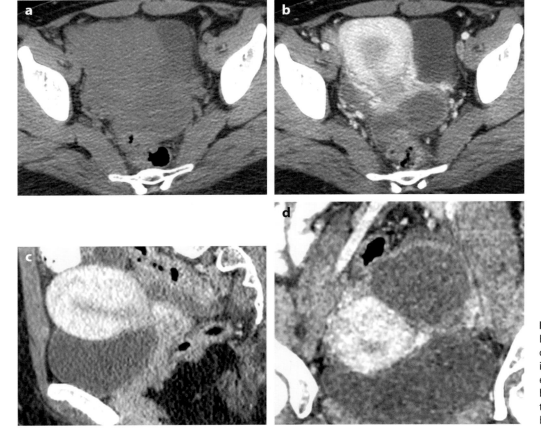

Fig. 21.10 Normal endometrium on CT. (**a**) Before injection, the endometrium has the same density as the myometrium and could not be identified. (**b**) After injection, the endometrium enhances less than the myometrium and could be identified. (**c**, **d**) 2D reformations in the sagittal (**c**) and coronal (**d**) planes could be obtained but with lesser definition than MR and US

Benign and Malignant Endometrium

22

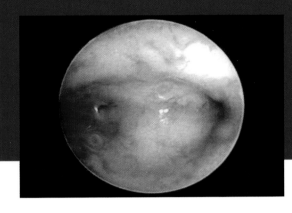

Contents

22.1 Atrophy

22.1.1 Definition

22.1.1.1 Microscopy

Glands are lined by a single layer of flattened or cuboidal epithelial cells containing bland nuclei without mitoses. Mucus is scant. Glands may be fragmented.

Stroma is markedly reduced.

22.1.1.2 Macroscopy

The endometrium is thin (0.5 mm for one layer). The glands are often cystic [1].

J.N. Buy, M. Ghossain, *Gynecological Imaging*,
DOI 10.1007/978-3-642-31012-6_22, © Springer-Verlag Berlin Heidelberg 2013

22.1.2 Etiology

Atrophy is related to insufficient estrogen stimulation in:
1. In premenopausal women
   - Women taking oral contraceptives
   - Drugs:
     - Oral contraceptive
     - GnRH agonists
     - Progestin
   - Premature ovarian failure
   - Radiation
   - Functional hypothalamic amenorrhea
2. In postmenopausal women without hormonal treatment

22.1.3 Clinical Findings

In premenopausal women, atrophy of the endometrium may be responsible of amenorrhea or vaginal bleeding.

In postmenopausal women, atrophy may account for up to 82 % of vaginal spotting or bleeding [2, 3] (Fig. 22.1).

22.1.4 Ultrasound

The endometrium is thin (Fig. 22.2). Cystic spaces may be present.

22.2 Polyps

22.2.1 Generalities

22.2.1.1 Definition

Endometrial polyps are benign localized overgrowths of endometrial glands and stroma that are covered by epithelium and project above the adjacent surface epithelium.

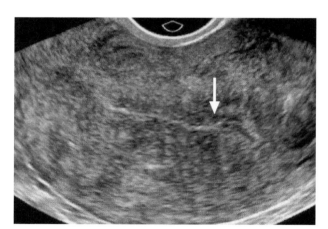

Fig. 22.1 Atrophy of the endometrium. Postmenopausal women without hormonal replacement. Longitudinal EVs displays an endometrium of 3 mm thickness (*arrow*)

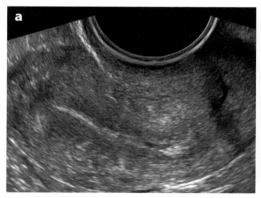
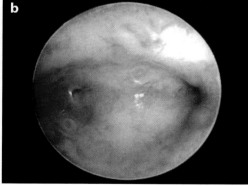

Fig. 22.2 Atrophy of the endometrium. Thirty-eight-year-old woman. Secondary amenorrhea with a low anti-Mullerian hormone (AMH) related to premature ovarian failure. Longitudinal EVS (**a**) displays a thin endometrium, related to atrophy. Because of a desire of pregnancy, a hysteroscopy is performed. Hysteroscopy (**b**) confirms a marked atrophy with a pale mucosa

22.2.1.2 Pathology

Macroscopic and Radiologic Findings

They are reported in Table 22.1 [4] (Fig. 22.3).

Table 22.1 Macroscopic and radiologic findings of endometrial polyps

– Broad base or pedunculated or attached to the endometrium by a slender stalk
– May contain small cystic spaces
– Size: from 1 mm to a large mass filling the entire cavity
– Site: anywhere in the uterine cavity but most common in the fundus
– Surface: glistening or hemorrhagic
– Multiple in 20 % of cases

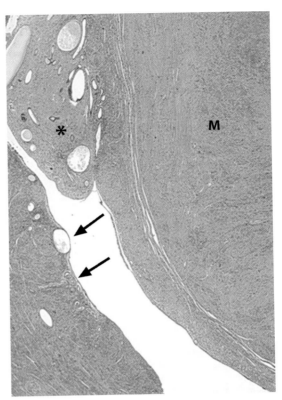

Fig. 22.4 Endometrial polyp with cystic atrophy. Histology of a polyp in a menopausal woman displays: an atrophic endometrium (*lower oblique arrow*) with a thin epithelium and cystic glands (*upper oblique arrow*). Small polyp (*asterisk*) with cystic atrophy. Adjacent leiomyoma (*M*)

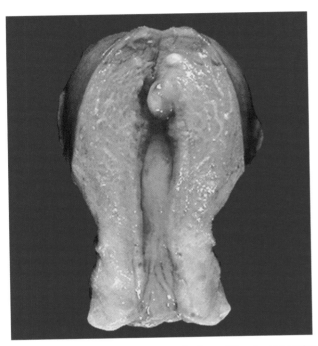

Fig. 22.3 Endometrial polyp. Macroscopic view of the uterine cavity shows a well-delineated pedunculated polyp of the fundus

Microscopy

Stroma

May contain endometrial stroma, fibrous tissue, or smooth muscle, but generally the stroma appears more fibrous than normal fundic endometrium.

Vessels

Thick-walled vessels are seen at the base.

Epithelium and Glands

Secretory changes in the endometrial glands may be weak or absent, or the glands may appear dilated and inactive. Most are categorized as hyperplastic, functional, or atrophic.

- Hyperplastic polyps contain proliferating irregularly shaped glands resembling diffuse hyperplasia.
- Atrophic polyps consist of low columnar or cuboidal cells lining cystic dilated glands; they are typically found in postmenopausal women (Fig. 22.4).
- Functional polyps containing glands resembling normal cycling endometrium are relatively uncommon.

Hyperplasia, carcinoma (any type), and carcinosarcoma may involve or be entirely confined to a polyp [4].

22.2.1.3 Clinical Findings

It is common in women over 40 years.

During reproductive age years, the most common presentations are metrorrhagia or menometrorrhagia. It may be a cause of infertility.

After menopause, postmenopausal bleeding is the common finding.

A polyp should always been considered after curettage (if not associate to hysteroscopy), because polyps that contain a delicate stalk may elude the curette.

22.2.2 Imaging Findings

22.2.2.1 Ultrasound

Endovaginal US with eventually hysterosonography is the best method to detect small polyps that can be missed or misdiagnosed with MR. Endometrial polyp usually appears as a round or elongated mass. In premenopausal woman, it is usually well depicted during the first part of the endometrial cycle. Indeed, at this phase, the polyp, which echogenicity is high and identical to the basalis layer of the endometrium, is clearly distinguished from the low echogenicity of the functionalis layer of the endometrium. On the opposite, an endometrial polyp can be difficult to visualize during the second part of the cycle because the deep and superficial layers of the endometrium and the polyp have the same echogenicity. In some cases, it is covered by a thin layer of superficial endometrium (Fig. 22.5).

In some cases, endometrial polyp can appear only as an endometrial thickening (Fig. 22.6) mainly when associated to a premenopausal or postmenopausal atrophic endometrium. In these difficult cases, a vascular pedicle or hysterosonography may be very useful to diagnose them.

The morphologic and vascular findings are reported in Table 22.2 (Figs. 22.7 and 22.8).

Cystic spaces: Small cystic spaces usually from 2–3 mm in diameter, with a regular border typically surrounded with a hyperechoic line, when present are typical for a benign polyp. Cystic spaces have also been reported in some cases of carcinomas, although they are much more uncommon [5] and do not have the same morphologic features, i.e., are not as regular and particularly are not surrounded by a hyperechoic line.

2D [6] and 3D hysterosalpingo sonography [7] have been demonstrated valuable in the diagnosis of endometrial polyps and particularly to demonstrate the pedicle and the peripheral hyperechoic line.

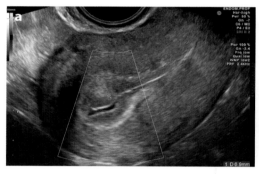
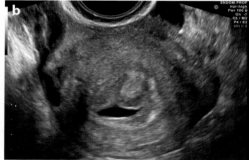
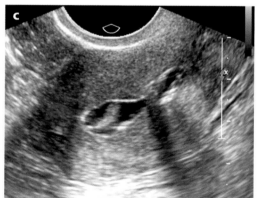

Fig. 22.5 Endometrial polyp in a 39-year-old woman with menometrorrhagia. (a, b) Sagittal (a) and transverse (b) endovaginal ultrasound during the first part of the menstrual cycle discloses a 9 mm hyperechoic polyp (*cursors*) of the anterior endometrium with no vascular pedicle on color Doppler. The hyperechoic polyp is in contact with the basal endometrium and covered by a normal hypoechoic superficial endometrium. Some liquid is present in the endometrial cavity. (c) Hyteroscopy confirmed the presence of an anterior polyp (*arrow*)

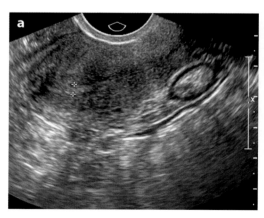
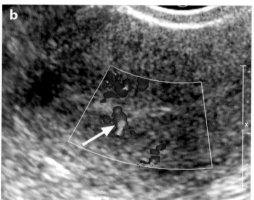
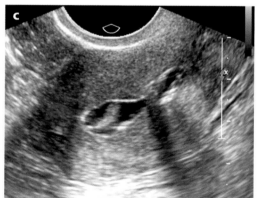

Fig. 22.6 Endometrial polyp appearing as a localized endometrial thickening. Forty-year-old woman with menometrorrhagia. (a) EVS, very early in the menstrual cycle, displays a thin endometrium in the lower part of the corpus and a localized thickening (*cursors*) of about 3 mm in the fundus. (b) Doppler demonstrates a posterior pedicle (*arrow*) entering the endometrial thickening, very suggestive of an endometrial polyp. (c) Hysterosonography definitely confirms the diagnosis of an endometrial polyp

Table 22.2 Morphologic and Doppler findings of endometrial polyps

– Round or elongated echogenic mass; sometime localized thickening of the endometrium
– Hyperechoic; may contain cystic spaces
– Regular limit; sometimes peripheral hyperechoic line
– Narrow or broad base attachment
– Vascular pedicle

Hyperechoic line: A peripheral hyperechoic line has been demonstrated as a valuable finding of focal process (polyp or submucous leiomyoma) (Fig. 22.9). This finding is usually not present in endometrial hyperplasia and carcinoma.

Vascular pedicle: Visualization of a central vascular pedicle usually with a single regular vessel is a fundamental finding of a polyp (Fig. 22.10).

However, no arterial flow was detected in 30 % of nonfunctional polyps, 0 % of proliferative polyps, 11 % of secretory polyps, 25 % of hyperplastic polyps, and 33 % of malignant polyps in a series [8]; mean resistive index and mean pulsatility index were not different in the different categories.

3D reformation has the main interest to give a more precise location of the endometrial polyp than 2D (Fig. 22.11).

22.2.2.2 Differential Diagnosis

Localized Lesions

1. Submucous leiomyoma
   - Acoustic shadowing
   - Peripheral vascularization
2. Clots
3. Polypoid adenocarcinoma
4. Polypoid adenofibroma and adenosarcoma

Diffuse Lesion

1. Endometrial hyperplasia [9]

22.2.2.3 MR

Detection

Small polyps detected on EVS can be difficult to visualize or even can be overlooked on MR. It is the combination of a low intensity on T2W images and a higher uptake than endometrium on early DMR that best allows to detect them.

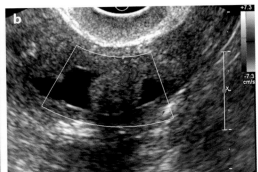
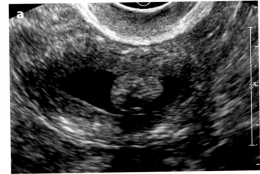

Fig. 22.7 Endometrial polyp. Seventy-nine-year-old woman with genital prolapse. EVS (**a**), transverse view, displays a mass protruding into the endometrial cavity, well delineated by hydrometria. Its echogenicity superior to myometrium and cystic spaces contained within the mass are very suggestive of an endometrial polyp. Doppler (**b**), longitudinal view, demonstrates an anterior vascular pedicle typical for an endometrial polyp

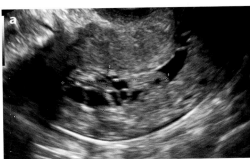
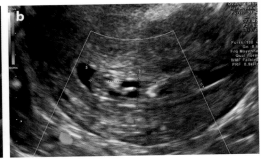

Fig. 22.8 Endometrial polyp. Forty-year-old woman with menometrorrhagia. EVS (**a**) displays a 2.5-cm elongated mass protruding in the endometrial cavity with a smooth regular limit. The mass is echogenic containing multiple cystic spaces with regular limits typical for an endometrial polyp. Doppler (**b**) does not display any pedicle or any vessel in the polyp

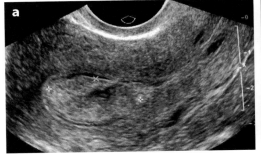
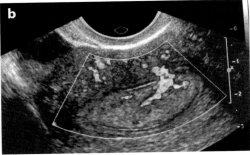

Fig. 22.9 Endometrial polyp in a 58-year-old postmenopausal woman with metrorrhagia. (**a**) Sagittal endovaginal ultrasound discloses a hyperechoic endometrial polyp (*cursors*). A thin layer of anechoic liquid separates the hyperechoic line corresponding to the atrophic endometrium from the hyperechoic line covering the polyp. (**b**) Color Doppler clearly displays a vascular pedicle. Hysterectomy confirmed the presence of a fibro-glandular not-proliferative polyp

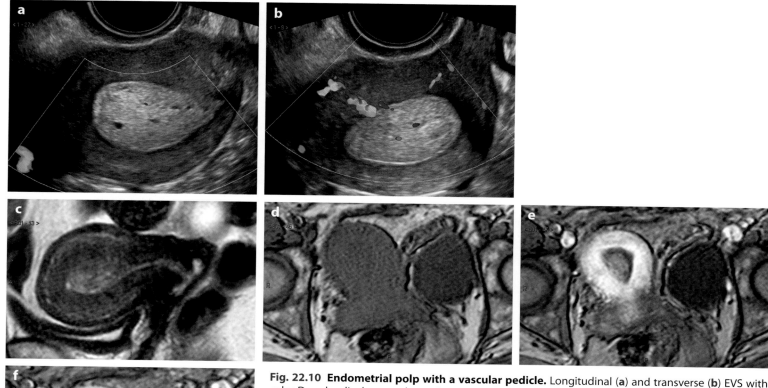

Fig. 22.10 Endometrial polp with a vascular pedicle. Longitudinal (**a**) and transverse (**b**) EVS with color Doppler display an echogenic mass (with an echogenicity superior to myometrium), occupying most of the endometrial cavity. A peripheral hyperechoic line indicating a focal process allows to differentiate this mass from endometrial hyperplasia. This mass contains small cystic cavities underlined at their periphery by hyperechoic lines, which are typical for a benign process. Transverse view with color Doppler in (**b**) shows a vascular pedicle which definitely confirms the diagnosis of endometrial polyp. On MR sagittal T2 (**c**), the polyp has an overall intermediate signal, with some cystic spaces not as well demonstrated as on ultrasound. The limits of the mass are regular and the interface between the endometrium and the myometrium is well defined. On axial T1 (**d**) signal intensity of the polyp is slightly lower than myometrium. On DMR at the venous phase (**e**) cystic cavities are surrounded by a contrast uptake more intense than in the rest of the polyp. Thirty seconds later (**f**), the endometrial mass is clear defined with a contrast uptake inferior to myometrium and superior to normal endometrium

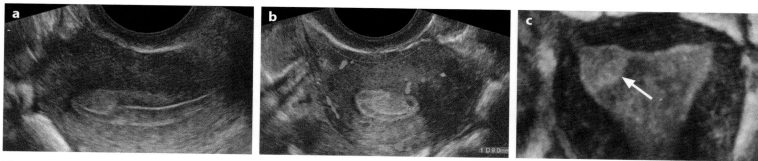

Fig. 22.11 Endometrial polyp in a 44-year-old asymptomatic woman. (**a, b**) Sagittal (**a**) and transverse (**b**) endovaginal ultrasound during the second part of the menstrual cycle discloses a 9 mm endometrial polyp (*cursors* in **b**), arising in the anterior endometrium at the level of the fundus, pushing the echogenic endometrial line posteriorly. The polyp is slightly more hyperechoic than the normal endometrium. (**c**) 3D reconstruction clearly shows the precise location of the polyp (*arrow*) in the right cornual endometrium that was not as clearly localized on the 2D views

Morphologic Findings [10]

Small polyps (<1 cm), because of their signal intensity identical to the signal intensity of normal endometrium on T1 and identical or slightly less intense than endometrium on T2 are very difficult to detect, while they are much better displayed on endovaginal ultrasound (where they look more echogenic than normal endometrium). They can be only or better detected on DMR (Fig. 22.12). However, they can be also overlooked on DMR.

Larger polyps (>1 cm) are usually displayed. While on T1 they have roughly the same signal intensity as endometrium, on T2 they appear clearly as a well delineated endometrial masses, with a regular interface with the junctional zone, usually localized, containing sometimes a central fibrous core of lower signal intensity than endometrium and cystic cavities with regular borders of high signal intensity (Figs. 22.10 and 22.13).

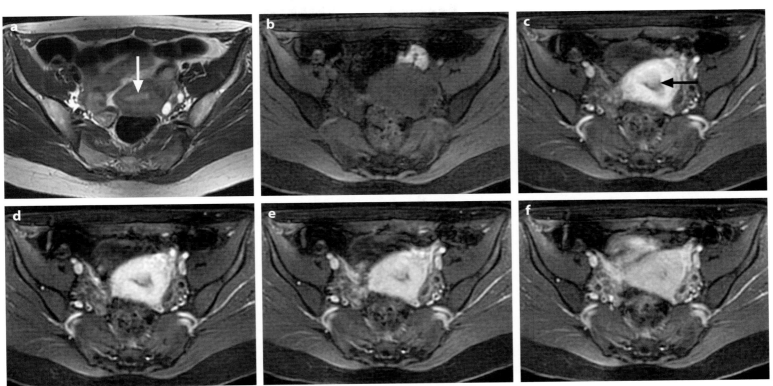

Fig. 22.12 Endometrial polyp hardly seen on T2 images and well depicted on DMR. (a) On T2, a small hypointense zone (*arrow*) is seen in the endometrium that could correspond to blood or partial volume effect. (**b–f**) On DMR before (**b**), at the arterial (**c**), venous (**d**), parenchymal (**e**), and late (**f**) phases, a well-delineated structure is seen at the early phases (*arrow* in **c**) contrasting with the less-enhancing normal endometrium. At the late phase, the polyp becomes isointense and indistinguishable from the normal endometrium

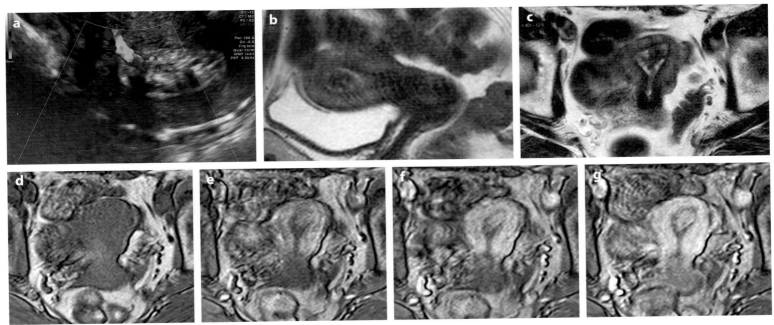

Fig. 22.13 Typical endometrial polyp containing small cystic cavities. A 65-year-old woman with hormonal treatment; absence of metrorrhagia. (**a**) Transvaginal ultrasound displays a typical endometrial polyp, hyperechoic with small glandulocystic cavities, surrounded by a hyperechoic line and associated to a clear vascular pedicle on color Doppler. (**b, c**) Sagittal (**b**) and axial (**c**) T2W images display the polyp as a hypointense intracavitary mass containing small cystic cavities and surrounded by a hyperintense endometrium. (**d–g**). DMR before (**d**) and after gadolinium injection (**e–g**) shows the polyp to enhance more rapidly than the normal endometrium with maximum contrast between the two structures at the early phase (**e**); however, the polyp is better delimited on the last phase (**g**)

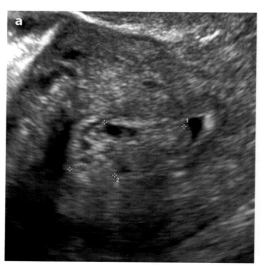
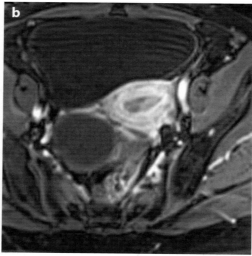

Fig. 22.14 Endometrial polyp with glandulo-cystic cavities. A 61-year-old woman with right ovarian cyst, without hormonal treatment, absence of menometrorrhagia. (**a**) Transvaginal ultrasound, transverse view, discloses a 2.5 cm endometrial polyp (*cursors*) with small glandulocystic cavities. Otherwise the endometrium is thin with a small quantity of intracavitary fluid. (**b**) On axial T1W-FS MR after injection, the polyp appears as a well-delineated endocavitary mass containing small cystic cavities. Right cystadenoma is also displayed

22.2.2.4 Vascular Findings (Fig. 22.15)

1. Right from the arterial phase, a significant contrast uptake is seen superior to the endometrium.
2. The peak enhancement is at 2–3 min (Fig. 22.15 and Table 22.3).
3. The overall contrast uptake is superior to normal endometrium.
4. In some cases, the center of the polyp (around the vascular pedicle) enhances earlier than the periphery (Fig. 22.13). This allows to differentiate a polyp from an endocavitary leiomyoma where contrast uptake is more prominent at the periphery at the early phase.

These morphologic and vascular findings are illustrated in the following figures (Figs. 22.10, 22.12, and 22.16).

As it has been reported by Park et al. [11], if these findings are close to those of endometrial hyperplasia, they are different from those of endometrial carcinomas (Table 22.3).

Endometrial carcinoma shows usually earlier (1 min) mild peak enhancement and late gradual washout.

Sarcomas demonstrate early (1 min) more intense enhancement and late peak enhancement.

22.2.2.5 CT

Polyps are usually not visualized or visualized with difficult on CT. They can appear as a thickening of the endometrium. Hydrometry may help to detect them.

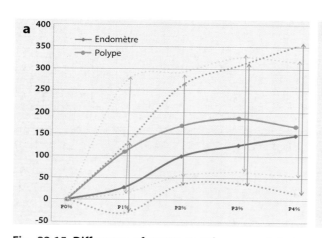
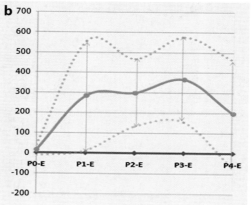

Fig. 22.15 Difference of contrast enhancement between polyp and endometrium. DMR, with sequences performed before and 25, 70, 125, and 240 s after injection (Materials: ten patients, Author's personal series). (**a**) Right from the arterial phase, contrast in the polyp is superior to the endometrium. Peak enhancement in the polyp is at 2 min. The overall contrast enhancement in the polyp is superior to normal endometrium. (**b**) The *plain orange line* illustrates the mean difference of contrast enhancement between the polyp and the endometrium with the most marked difference at 70 and 125 s. *Dots orange lines* correspond to minimal and maximal difference in contrast uptake

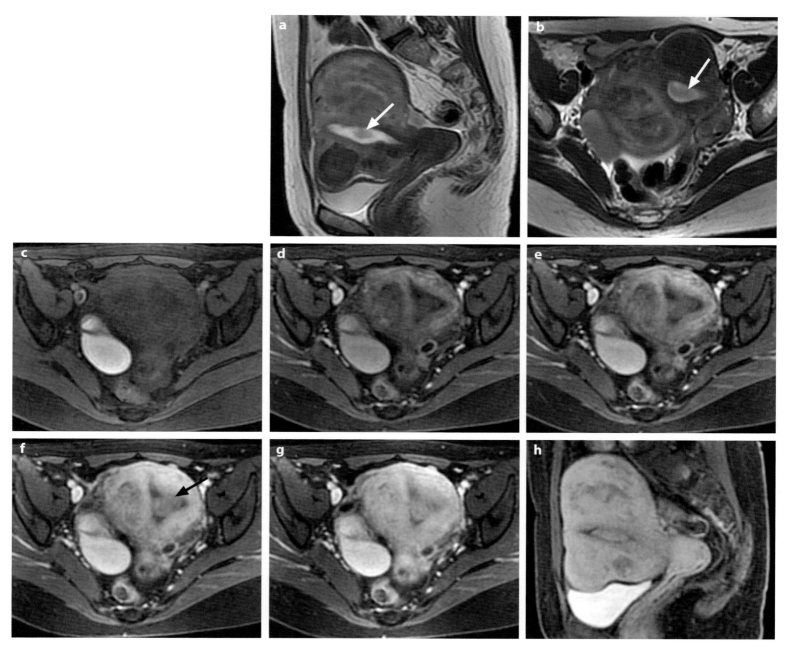

Fig. 22.16 Endometrial polyp well delineated on T2, DMR, and late post-contrast sequences. (**a, b**) Sagittal (**a**) and Axial (**b**) T2W images show in the posterior middle part of the endometrium an ovoid shape mass (*arrows*) with an intermediate signal intensity less than endometrium. Uterine leiomyomas and right endometrioma are also present. (**c–g**) On DMR before (**c**), at the arterial phase (**d**), the venous phase (**e**) and on the following phase (**f**), a significant contrast uptake in the mass superior to that of the endometrium is typical for endometrial polyp (*arrow* in **f**). On the delayed phase (**g**), signal intensity of the polyp is identical to endometrium. (**h**) Sagittal delayed T1FS sequence shows that the polyp, which has now the same intensity as the myometrium and the normal endometrium, is still visible because surrounded by some liquid

Table 22.3 Vascular findings

	DMR					
	Peak enhancement (time)					
	≤1 min	**2 min**	**3 min**	**PE/WA (degree)**	**Late contrast enhancement/outer M**	**Enhancement pattern**
Polyp (9)	0	4	5	Intense PE		Homogeneous (6/9)
Hyperplasia (3)	0	2	1			Homogeneous (2/3)
End Carc (32)	23	9	0	Mild gradual WA	Gradual WA<M	Homogeneous (29/32)

According to Park et al. [11]

End Carc endometrial carcinoma, *PE* persistent enhancement, *WA* washout, *M* myometrium

22.2.3 Atypical Polypoid Adenomyoma (APA)

22.2.3.1 Pathology

It is a benign condition [4] although APA associated with adenocarcinomas have been rarely reported [12].

Histology

It is composed of
- Irregularly shaped hyperplastic glands arranged haphazardly
- Stroma containing abundant smooth muscle [13]. In fact, the stroma usually contains also a mixture of fibrous tissue and endometrial stroma which has suggested some authors [14] to designate this entity atypical polypoid adenomyofibroma to emphasize their stromal heterogeneity.
- Extensive morular squamous metaplasia sometimes showing central necrosis may exaggerate the appearance of glandular crowding and raises concern regarding the possibility of a carcinoma.

Macroscopy [4]

It resembles a typical endometrial polyp.
It often involves the lower uterine segment.

22.2.3.2 Clinical Findings

- During the reproductive and perimenopause period
- Abnormal uterine bleeding

22.2.3.3 Follow-Up

Longacre et al. [14] reported that 45 % of the lesions treated conservatively recurred clinically, although none progressed to invasive carcinoma.

22.2.3.4 Radiologic Findings

MR Findings

The polypoid mass was [15]
- On T1, isointense to myometrium
- On T2, slightly hyperintense to myometrium containing markedly hyperintense foci

- After contrast irregular enhancement
- PET/MR fused images 18 F-FDG localized the abnormality to the endometrial cavity and showed focal intense accumulation with a SUV of 5.8.

22.3 Endometrial Hyperplasia

22.3.1 Generalities

22.3.1.1 Definition

Proliferation of glands of irregular size and shape with an increase in the gland/stroma ratio compared with proliferative endometrium. Generally diffuse but may be focal.

22.3.1.2 Pathology [16]

Macroscopy

Endometrium has a velvety knobby surface with spongy tissue and vague borders.

Diffuse thickening is usually present, but focal overgrowth may occur and simulate a polyp.

Histology

The lesions are classified in:
1. Typical or atypical hyperplasia: according to the cytologic findings
   - Typical hyperplasia: absence of cytologic atypia
   - Atypical hyperplasia: presence of cytologic atypia: (a) stratified cells (b) loss of polarity (c) increase in the nuclear/cytoplasmic ratio
2. Simple or complex hyperplasia according to the architectural features (Fig. 22.17):
   - Simple hyperplasia: the glands are cystically dilated with occasional outpouchings surrounded by an abundant cellular stroma. Occasionally the glands are minimally dilated.
   - Complex hyperplasia: crowded glands with little intervening stroma.

Fewer than 2 % of hyperplasias without cytologic atypia progress to carcinomas whereas 23 % of atypical hyperplasias progress to carcinomas [16].

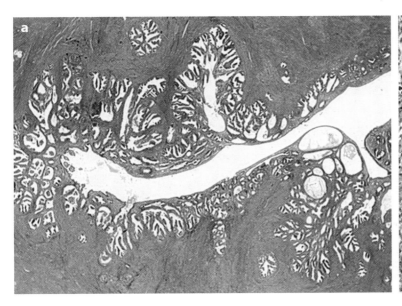

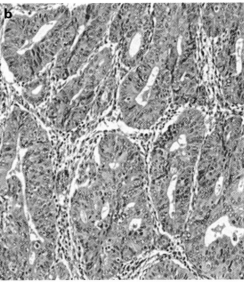

Fig. 22.17 (a) Simple hyperplasia. (b) Complex hyperplasia

22.3.1.3 Clinical Features

Hyperplasia develops as a result of exogenous unopposed estrogenic stimulation or a history of persistent anovulation. It is most common in perimenopausal and menopausal women and uncommon during the reproductive years. Bleeding may be moderate, heavy, or absent (hyperplasia being fortuitously discovered during biopsy).

It can be associated to some special clinical conditions:
- Obesity associated with PCOD
- Estrogen secreting ovarian tumors (see Chap. 11)

22.3.2 Imaging Findings

22.3.2.1 Ultrasound

Ultrasound findings are reported in Table 22.4 (Figs. 22.18 and 22.19).

In a series of 23 patients with hyperplasia of the endometrium, metaplasia, or both studied by transvaginal sonography and saline hysterosonography, Jorizzo et al. [9] found endometrial thickness to increase with atypia, complexity of hyperplasia and associated metaplasia, but with a lot of overlap. Lobular contours were present in 9 % patients. Cysts were contained in the thickened endometrium in 57 % of patients. Concomitant polyps were present in 26 %.

Table 22.4 Ultrasound findings of endometrial hyperplasia

1. Morphological findings
Thickness (diffuse or more rarely focal thickening of the endometrium)
Postmenopausal woman
- Without hormonal treatment >5 mm
- With hormonal treatment >8 mm
Reproductive age years
- No clear cutoff (depending on the time of study during the menstrual cycle)
Pattern
- Regular interface with myometrium
- Echogenicity as normal endometrium
- Homogeneous (non-suggestive) or contain cystic spaces (very suggestive)
2. Doppler findings:
Regular vessels when seen
3. Hysterosonography [9]
Better evaluates the thickness and detects or rules out associated polyps

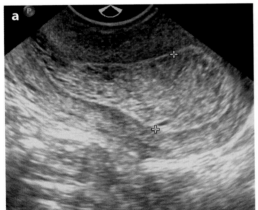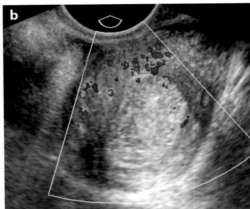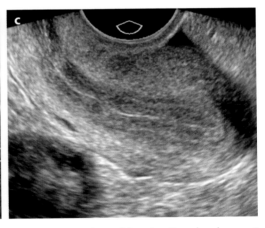

Fig. 22.18 Endometrial hyperplasia. A 39-year-old woman with PCOS and secondary amenorrhea. (**a**) Transvaginal sagittal ultrasound discloses a retroverted uterus with a diffuse echogenic and homogeneous thickened endometrium (18 mm for two layers) from the fundus to the isthmus. This pattern is suggestive of endometrial hyperplasia. The peripheral basal endo-metrial line is well seen. (**b**) Transverse view with color Doppler does not show a vascular pedicle. (**c**) Ultrasound performed after treatment with Duphaston shows a normal 7 mm endometrium (for two layers) with a well-delineated endocavitary line

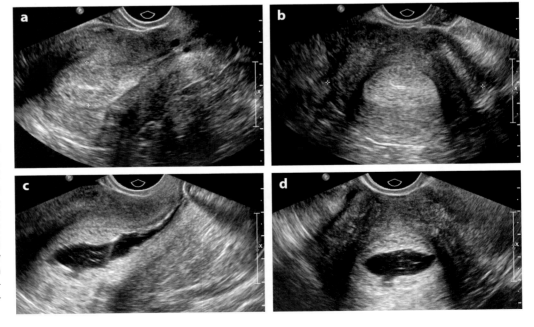

Fig. 22.19 Endometrial hyperplasia in a 45 years old woman with menometrorrhagia. (**a**, **b**) Sagittal (**a**) and transverse (**b**) transvaginal ultrasound display a thickened endometrium (20 mm for two layers) containing small cystic cavities. The endocavitary line is well displayed on both views, well centered. The peripheral basal endometrium appears as a peripheral hyperechoic line. (**c**, **d**) Hysterosonography confirms absence of focal endometrial growth and a thickened regular hyperechoic endometrium. Echoic lines in the endocavitary liquid correspond to blood and/or air

22.3.2.2 MR

Simple and Typical Hyperplasia

Simple and atypical hyperplasia presents as a diffuse or less commonly localized endometrial thickening sometimes containing cystic spaces (Fig. 22.20). The interface with the myometrium is well defined.

1. The thickened endometrium
   On T2, hyperplasia is isointense or slightly hypointense relative to the normal endometrium.

On DMR, during the early post-contrast images, hyperplasia like the normal endometrium is hypointense relative to the myometrium.

On the delayed, it becomes isointense or hyperintense or sometimes slightly hypointense relative to the adjacent myometrium.

2. Small hyperintense foci on T2, hypointense after injection representing cystic glandular dilatations may be seen [17].

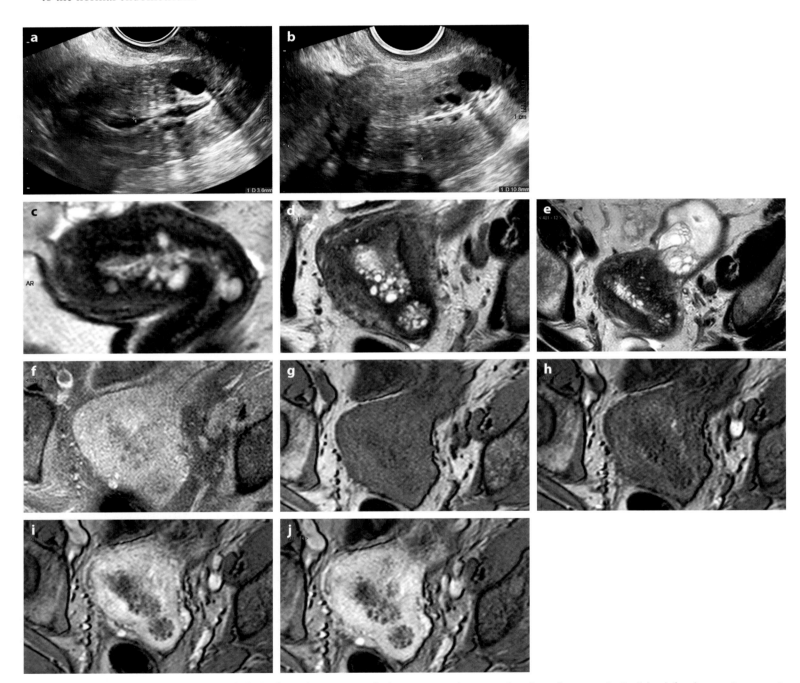

Fig. 22.20 Endometrial hyperplasia with foci of mucinous metaplasia and associated adenomyosis. Association with a mucinous ovarian borderline cystadenoma. Seventy-five-year-old woman with metrorrhagias and hydrorrhea. (**a**, **b**) Longitudinal EVS (**a**) and (**b**) display some fluid in the endometrial cavity, a thickening of the endometrium at 7 mm, containing small cystic cavities. Cystic spaces are also visualized in the inner myometrium related to adenomyosis. (**c–e**) MR T2W sagittal (**c**) axial (**d**, **e**) depict a thickening of the endometrium containing unusual numerous small cystic cavities suggesting endometrial hyperplasia. Large and small endometrial cysts in the myometrium are related to adenomyosis. On (**e**), a left tubo-ovarian mass is seen that was related to a mucinous borderline tumor with tubal intussusception at pathology. (**f**) On axial T1 fat suppression, no hemorrhage is displayed in the endometrium. (**g–j**) On DMR without injection (**g**), at the arterial phase (**h**), few vessels are visualized in the endometrium, with unusual tortuous vessels at the endometrial myometrial junction. At the venous phase (**i**) and on the delayed (**j**), a slight contrast uptake is depicted. Prospective diagnosis: endometrial hyperplasia with adenomyosis. Microscopy: confirmed the diagnosis and showed association to mucinous metaplasia of the endometrium

Atypical and Complex Hyperplasia

Although Jorrizo et al. [9] have reported that the thickness of endometrium in atypical and complex hyperplasia is significantly higher than in simple and typical hyperplasia, the pattern of this last entity has not been reported. In our case (Fig. 22.21), the endometrium does not contain any cystic spaces; the overall signal of endometrium is not as hyperintense as in simple and typical hyperplasia, limitation with the junctional zone is not as clearly demarcated. However, at present, the final diagnosis is histological.

22.3.2.3 CT

As for polyps, hyperplasia in not well characterized on CT. It could appear as thickening of the endometrium. Cystic spaces are hard to see.

22.3.3 Endometrial Cellular Changes: Metaplasia, Cellular Differentiation [16]

22.3.3.1 Definition

Metaplasia is the replacement of one type of adult tissue by another type that is not normally found in that location.

In contrast to hyperplasia that is a proliferative response to estrogenic stimulation, metaplasia is a cytoplasmic differentiation secondary most commonly to estrogenic and progestational stimulation.

22.3.3.2 Histology

Eosinophilic changes are the most common, among them several types of eosinophilic cytoplasmic transformation: ciliated cells, squamous cells, oncocytes, and papillary and surface syncytial changes.

Other types are:
- Squamous cells, round or polygonal, may be spindle shaped forming a circumscribed nest (squamous morule)
- Ciliated cells (tubal metaplasia)
- Secretory cells: columnar cells with sub- or supranuclear vacuoles
- Clear cells: polygonal cells with clear cytoplasm containing glycogen
- Hobnail changes, reminiscent of the Arias-Stella reaction
- Mucinous

The various forms of cellular differentiation are typically focal when unaccompanied by hyperplasia but can be diffuse when hyperplasia is present.

22.3.3.3 Clinical Features

Metaplasias develop most commonly in response to estrogenic and progestational stimulation.

The frequent association of the various cytoplasmic changes with hyperplasia is probably because both result from a hyperestrogenic state.

More than 70 % of perimenopausal and postmenopausal women with metaplasia have received exogen estrogen [18]. Most young women with metaplasia have clinical manifestations of anovulation and primary infertility.

Metaplasia also may occur in benign conditions as polyps, endometritis, trauma, and vitamin A deficiency.

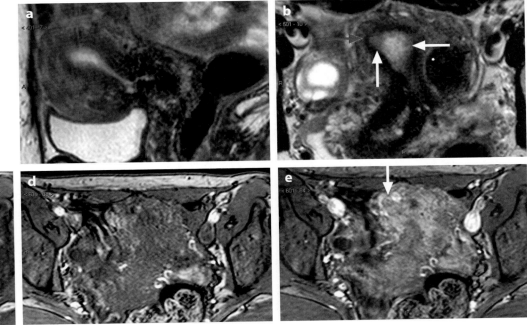

Fig. 22.21 Atypical and complex hyperplasia. Fifty-year-old woman. Absence of clinical finding. During a routine EVS examination, an endometrial polyp is discovered. At pathologic examination, atypical and complex endometrial hyperplasia is diagnosed. MR sagittal (**a**) and axial T2 (**b**) displays a diffuse thickening of the endometrium of 13 mm (measured in the upper third). No cystic space is visualized in the endometrium, signal intensity of the endometrium is not as hyperintense as usually, and signal intensity is not homogeneous, with some areas of intermediate signal (*white arrows*). In the right and upper portion of the endometrium, the limit between the outer part of the endometrium and the junctional zone is not clearly demarcated, and the junctional zone at this point is thinner (*red arrow*). On DMR without injection (**c**) and at the arterial phase (**d**), a slight increase of arterial vascularization is displayed at the same level, with at the venous phase (**e**), a slightly increase of the venous vascularization (*arrow*)

22.3.3.4 Imaging

Jorizzo et al. [9] have reported thickening of the endometrium in metaplasia, isolated (5–12 mm) or associated with hyperplasia (10–20 mm) (Fig. 22.20).

Differentiation with hyperplasia is based on histology.

22.4 Primitive Malignant Tumors

22.4.1 Endometrial Carcinoma

22.4.1.1 Endometrial Intraepithelial Carcinoma (EIC) [16]

Definition

Markedly atypical nuclei identical to those of invasive serous carcinomas, lining the surfaces and glands of an atrophic endometrium.

Serous carcinoma is the prototypic endometrial carcinoma that is not related to estrogenic stimulation and typically occurs in the setting of endometrial atrophy.

Macroscopy

The surface often demonstrates a slightly papillary contour.

EIC can be found on the surface of a polyp in an atrophic endometrium.

22.4.1.2 Endometrial Invasive Carcinoma

Different Pathologic Types

Endometrioid Carcinoma

The most common form accounting for more than three quarters of cases.

Definition

(a) This tumor is so-called because it resembles proliferative phase of the endometrium.

(b) It does not contain more than 10 % of squamous, serous, mucinous, or clear cell differentiation (if these components are more than 10 %, it is called mixed type carcinomas).

Pathology

Gross findings are reported in Table 22.5 [16] (Fig. 22.22).

Table 22.5 Macroscopic findings of endometrioid carcinoma

1. Morphologic findings
– Focal or diffuse
– Endometrial surface shaggy, glistening and tan, and may be focally hemorrhagic
– Almost uniformly exophytic even when deeply invasive
– At times separated polypoid masses
– Necrosis usually not evident macroscopically in well-differentiated carcinoma may be seen in poorly differentiated carcinoma
2. Extension
(a) Myometrial invasion
– Well-demarcated gray white tissue with linear extensions beneath an exophytic mass
– Multiple white nodules with yellow areas of necrosis within the uterine wall
(b) In the lower uterine segment: common
(c) In the cervix in 20 % of cases

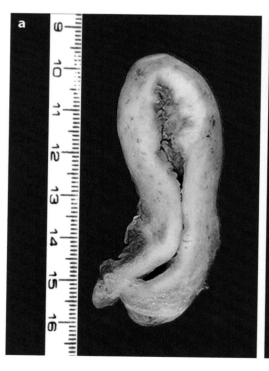 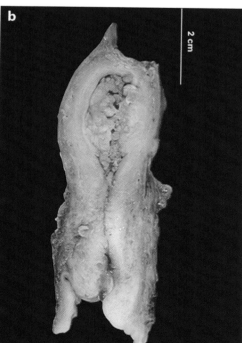

Fig. 22.22 Endometrial carcinoma: macroscopic specimen. (**a**, **b**) Exophytic mass occupying the entire endometrial uterine cavity extending to the posterior wall into the inner half of the myometrium. The isthmus and the cervix are not invaded

Microscopic Findings

Grading [16]

Grade is based on cytologic and architectural features:

1. Cytologic features (Nuclear features)
   - Grade 1. Nuclei oval, mildly enlarged, evenly dispersed chromatin.
   - Grade 2. Features intermediate between 1 and 2.
   - Grade 3. Nuclei markedly enlarged and pleomorphic, irregular coarse chromatin, prominent eosinophilic nucleoli.
2. Architectural features are determined by the extent to which the tumor is composed of solid masses of cells as compared with well-defined glands:
   - Grade 1. No more than 5 % of the tumor is composed of solid masses.
   - Grade 2. 6–50 % of the tumor is composed of solid masses.
   - Grade 3. More than 50 % of the tumor is composed of solid masses.

   The tumors are graded primarily by their architecture, with the overall grade modified by the nuclear grade when there is discordance.

Other Types of Endometrioid Carcinoma

- *Villoglandular* (Latin: villous= hair):
  Displays a papillary (Latin: papilla=nipple) architecture with thin delicate fronds.
  Covered by stratified columnar epithelial cells.
  The main differential diagnosis is serous carcinoma.
  They have thick densely fibrotic papillary fronds with papillary clusters detached from the papillary fronds.
  The cells tend to be rounder.
- *Secretory*
  Well-differentiated glandular pattern.
  Columnar cells with sub- or supranuclear vacuolization closely resembling days 17–22 secretory endometrium.
- *Ciliated*
  Well differentiated often cribriform pattern
  Cells with prominent eosinophilic cytoplasm and cilia
- *With squamous differentiation*
  Low Grade
  - The nests of squamous epithelium are confined to gland lumens.
  - The squamous cells resemble metaplastic squamous cells of the cervical transformation zone.
  - Frequently nests of cells with a prominent oval to spindle appearance referred to as morules are observed.
  High Grade
  - The squamous cells may not be in direct continuity with the glandular epithelium, appearing in isolated nests within the myometrium.
  - Keratinization and pearl formation occur to varying degrees.

- The most common problem is atypical hyperplasia with squamous metaplasia.

Other Types of Endometrial Carcinomas

- *Mucinous*
  Has an appearance similar to mucinous carcinoma of the endocervix
- *Serous*
- *Clear cell*
- *Squamous*
- *Mixed types*
- *Undifferentiated*

Clinical Findings

Most women are postmenopausal with a mean age of 59 years.
   Only 1–8 % occur in women under 40 years.
   A small number have been reported in women under 30 years; in these cases, the tumor is usually low grade, and the majority of patients have had polycystic ovary disease.
   Rarely, it occurs during pregnancy.
   The initial manifestation is abnormal vaginal bleeding.
   Rarely the diagnosis is made fortuitously.

Imaging Findings

US

Tumor
Endometrial carcinoma may be detected first on US.
   On conventional US, carcinoma of the endometrium usually appears as an echogenic mass homogeneous or heterogeneous with an overall echogenicity close to endometrium and superior to myometrium (Fig. 22.23).
   3D reformation can be helpful to precise clearly the location of the tumor and its extension.
   Color Doppler can display few vessels, while in other cases vascularization is intense (Fig. 22.24).

Myometrial Involvement [19]

- If limited to the endometrium: subendometrial halo is preserved [20].
- If invasion <50 %: segmental or complete interruption of the subendometrial halo.
  On 3D US, virtual navigation through three orthogonal planes to identify the shortest myometrial tumor-free distance to serosa was shown to be reliable to assess myometrial infiltration using subjective impression of the examiner [21].

MR

MR is the preferred modality to evaluate the tumor. MR findings are reported in Table 22.6.

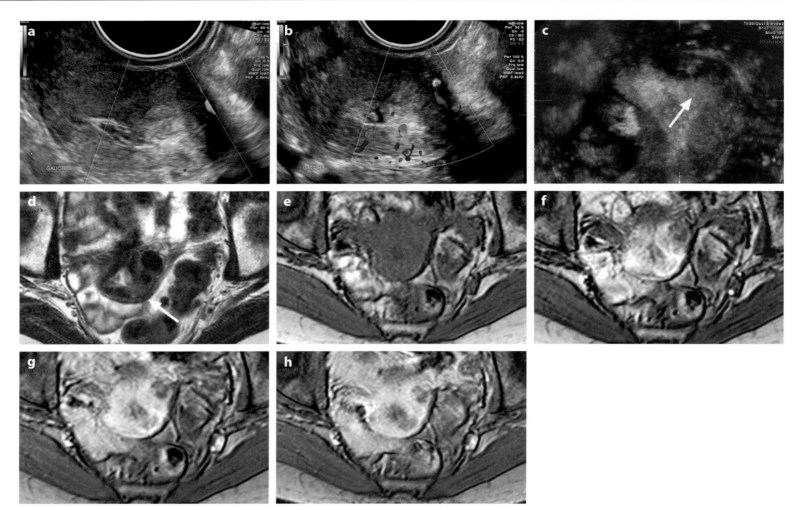

Fig. 22.23 Stage 1B endometrial carcinoma. Sixty-seven-year-old woman; metrorrhagia. EVS with color Doppler (**a**, **b**): an echogenic mass in the left part of the fundus containing some vessels extends into the myometrium. EVS with 3D reformation (**c**) better localizes the mass in the left uterine horn (*arrow*). MR axial T2 (**d**) displays better than US the degree of extension into the outer myometrium (*arrow*). Two left hypointense uterine leiomyomas are seen, the smallest one close to the carcinoma. DMR without contrast (**e**) at the arterial phase (**f**) at the venous phase (**g**) and on the delayed (**h**) confirms that the extension involves the outer myometrium almost until the serosa

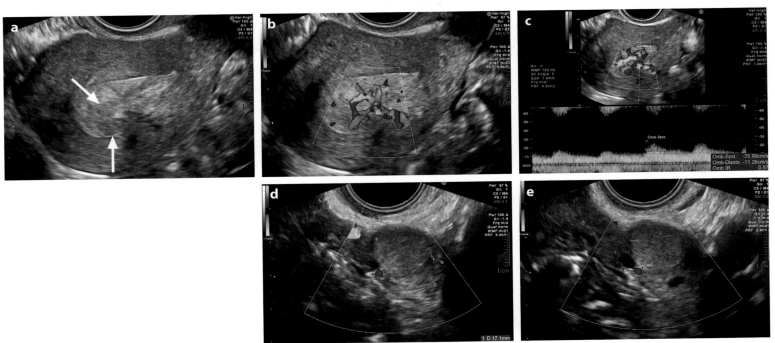

Fig. 22.24 Endometrioid carcinoma of the endometrium stage IIIA. EVS (**a**) with color Doppler (**b**) and spectral Doppler (**c**) display an endometrial mass at the junction between the left border and the posterior wall of the uterus of an echogenicity lower than normal endometrium (*arrows* in **a**). On color Doppler, the tumor is highly vascularized. On spectral Doppler, the maximum systolic velocity is high 25 cm/s and the resistive index 0.57. Color Doppler (**d**, **e**) depicts an ovarian mass (*cursors* in **d**) of intermediate signal containing few vessels; a metastasis was diagnosed at pathology

Table 22.6 Endometrial carcinoma: MR findings

1. Location
Endometrial lesion expanding the endometrial cavity
2. Morphologic findings
– Focal or diffuse
– Endometrial surface may be focally hemorrhagic
– Almost uniformly endocavitary even when deeply invasive
– At times separated polypoid masses
– Necrosis usually not evident in well-differentiated cases
T1: lesion isointense to the adjacent myometrium
T2: heterogeneous mass of intermediate signal between myometrium and adipose tissue
3. Diffusion
• On DW images, all endometrial cancers appear hyperintense [22]
• ADC values less than 1.15×10^{-3} mm²/s [23]
4. Vascular findings
– Arterial phase: arterial vessels can be seen in the tumor
– Peak enhancement within 1 min and 2 min but never later. This peak enhancement is of mild intensity, much less than inner myometrium [24]
– Late (3 min) gradual washout [11]
– Maximum of contrast between tumor and inner myometrium is between 50 s and 3 min [24, 25]
5. Extension
Myometrial invasion
– Disruption of the junctional zone
– Well-demarcated tissue with linear extensions beneath an endocavitary mass
– Multiple nodules with areas of necrosis within the uterine wall
Intracavitary extension
– In the lower uterine segment: common
– In the cervix: 20 % of cases

The Tumor

Morphologic Findings

- On T1, the lesion is isointense to the adjacent myometrium.
- On T2, the mass is heterogeneous of intermediate signal between muscle and adipose tissue (Figs. 22.25, 22.26, and 22.27).

Compared with the adjacent myometrium, in 86 % of cases hyperintense, it is rarely isointense exceptionally hypointense [26].

Compared to endometrium, it is usually slightly hypointense [27].

Vascular Findings

Endometrial carcinomas contain a peripheral vascularized solid tissue with usually a large central component of necrosis. These two parts are usually clearly distinguished right on the early phases of the DMR.

(a) In the solid tissue

- At the arterial phase, irregular tumoral vessels can be visualized (Fig. 22.27).
- Peak enhancement within 1 min (Fig. 22.26) and at 2 min (Fig. 22.25) but was never present later Table 22.7 [11], of mild intensity, much less than inner myometrium [26].
- Late (3 min) gradual washout [11]
- Maximum contrast between tumor and inner myometrium has been reported to be at 3 min in Manfredi series [26], while in JOJA's series [25], it was at approximately at 50 s. In general, endometrial cancer enhances earlier than normal endometrium but later than adjacent myometrium [28], allowing identification of small tumors.

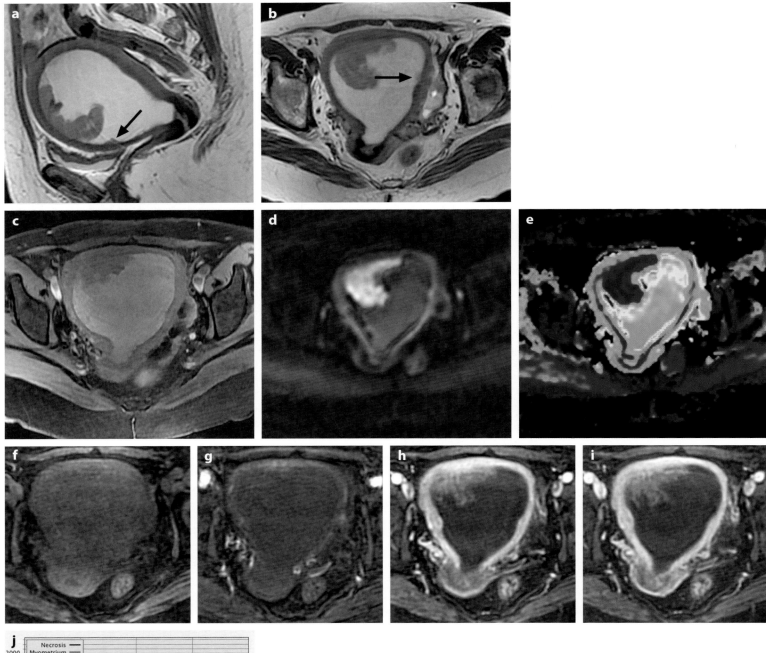

Fig. 22.25 Endometrial serous adenocarcinoma stage 1A. (a, b) T2W images shows an intracavitary mass occupying the entire endometrial cavity which has two components: (1) a cauliflower mass of the fundus with an inner irregular border associated with other small nodules (*arrows*) with a regular junctional zone (2) a large component extending until the upper part of the endocervix with a high signal on T2. (c) T1W image with fat suppression show this large portion is related to necrotico-hemorrhagic material. (d–e) DWI b1000 (d) and ADC map (e) at b1000 show the solid part of the lesion to be hyperintense on DW images with a low ADC of 0.75×10^{-3} mm^2/s. (f–j) DMR without injection (f), at 25 s (g), 70 s (h), 125 s (i), 240 s and time-intensity curves (j) displays: (1) in the solid tissue a slight contrast uptake at the arterial phase (g) with a peak of enhancement at 2 min after injection (i) clearly inferior to contrast enhancement in the normal myometrium, followed by a slight washout on the delayed time (j). (2) Absence of contrast uptake in the large necrotico-hemorrhagic portion. These findings are typical for an endometrial carcinoma. On the MR, the carcinoma was assessed to be limited to the endometrium. Macroscopy confirmed these data, while at microscopy a slight invasion of the inner myometrium was diagnosed

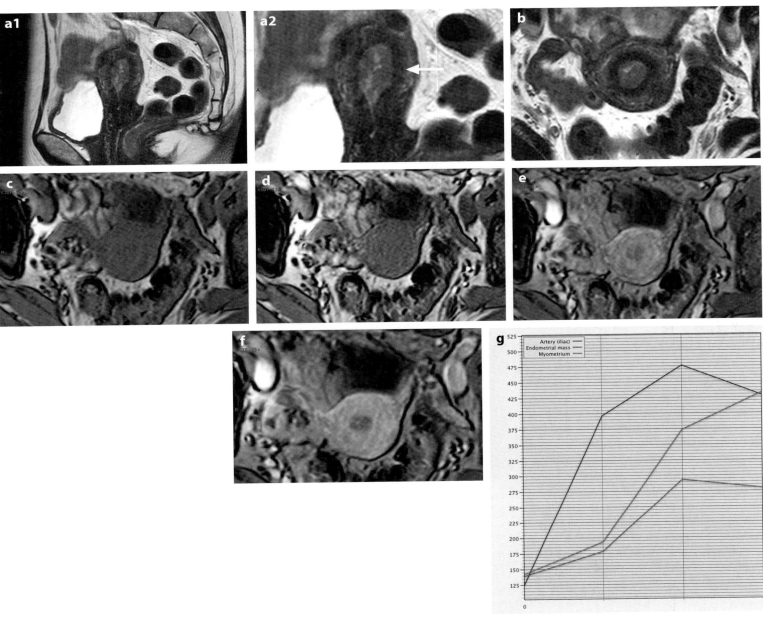

Fig. 22.26 Stage 1A endometrioid carcinoma. Fifty-nine-year-old woman; hormonal treatment stopped 3 month before; red blood metrorrhagia. Sagittal T2 (**a1** and localized view **a2**) and axial T2 (**b**) display an endometrial mass with an overall intermediate signal occupying the entire endometrial cavity, very suggestive of endometrial carcinoma. On the magnified view, on the posterior wall, a localized rupture of the junctional zone with exten-sion to the inner myometrium (*arrow*) could be visualized (3 out of 15 mm at pathology). DMR performed without injection (**c**), 25 sec after injection (**d**), 1 min after injection (**e**), and 4 min after injection (**f**). At the arterial phase (25 s), absence of tumoral vessels. At 1 min, there is a typical peak contrast enhancement and a slight wash out on the delayed phase (**f**), as it is shown on the curve of contrast enhancement (**g**)

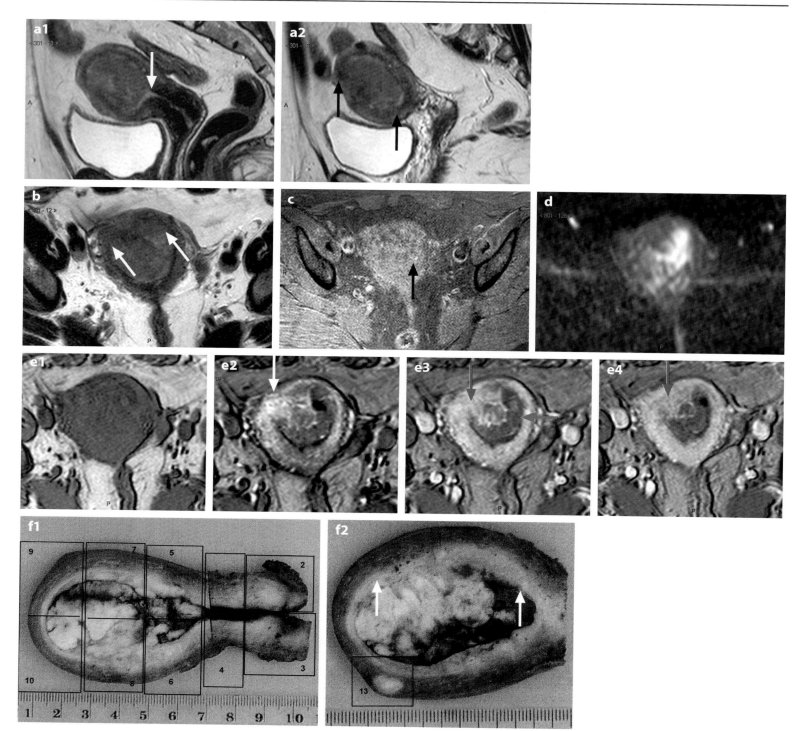

Fig. 22.27 Endometrioid carcinoma extending to the outer half of the myometrium stage 1B. Sixty-year-old woman. Postmenopausal metrorrhagias. MR sagittal T2 (**a1**, **a2**) displays an endometrial mass occupying the entire endometrial cavity of intermediate signal, respecting the isthmus (*arrow* in **a1**), invading the outer half of the myometrium of the anterior wall (*arrows* in **a2**). On axial T2 (**b**), extension in the outer myometrium is depicted (*arrows*). On T1 with fat suppression (**c**), areas of high signal intensity related to hemorrhage are displayed (*arrow*). Diffusion using a b1000 (**d**) shows a maximum hyperintense signal in the necrotic portion. On DMR without injection (**e1**), and at the arterial phase (**e2**), depicts irregular tumoral arterial vessels in the sold tissue (*arrow*) typical for a malignant process of the endometrium. At the venous phase (**e3**), a significant contrast uptake is visualized in the solid tissue (*red arrow*), while the necrotic portion (*green arrow*) does not enhance. On the delayed sequence (**e4**), a typical washout is demonstrated in the solid tissue (*arrow*). No extrauterine extension was displayed. Macroscopy (**f1** and **f2**): the tumor occupies the entire endometrial cavity, contains necrotic changes, and infiltrates the outer half of the myometrium (*arrows*). Microscopy: well-differentiated endometrioid carcinoma stage 1B

Table 22.7 Vascular findings of polyps, hyperplasia, and endometrial carcinomas according to Park

| | DMR | | | | | |
| | Peak enhancement (time) | | | | | |
	≤1 min	2 min	3 min	PE/WA (degree)	Late contrast enhancement /outer M	Enhancement pattern
Polyp (9)	0	4	5	Intense PE		Homogeneous (6/9)
Hyperplasia (3)	0	2	1			Homogeneous (2/3)
End Carc (32)	23	9	0	Mild gradual WA	Gradual WA<M	Homogeneous (29/32)

According to Park et al. [11]

End Carc endometrial carcinoma, *PE* persistent enhancement, *WA* washout, *M* myometrium

(b) In the portion with necrotic changes, according to the degrees of necrosis (Fig. 22.27), there is an absence or a slight contrast uptake. The limits with the solid tissue are clearly depicted on the delayed views.

Diffusion

On DW images, solid tissue as well as degenerative changes can appear hyperintense (Figs. 22.25 and 22.27) [22].

The mean ADC of endometrial carcinoma has been reported to be 0.864×10^{-3} mm²/s to 0.98 [22, 23, 29] and that of benign endometrial lesions 1.277×10^{-3} mm²/s [29].

ADC value less than 1.15×10^{-3} mm²/s was defined as the best cutoff to differentiate malignant from benign endometrial lesions [23].

Extension

Extension is evaluated according to the FIGO classification (Table 22.8)

Table 22.8 Extension: FIGO staging [30]

Stage I: Tumor confined to the corpus uteri
IA: No or less than half myometrial invasion
IB: Invasion equal to or more than half of the myometrium
Stage II: Tumor invades cervical stroma (ᵃ) but does not extend beyond the uterus
Stage III: Local and/or regional spread of the tumor
IIIA: Tumor invades the serosa of the corpus uteri and/or adnexa
IIIB: Vaginal and/or parametrial involvement
IIIC: Metastases to pelvic and/or para-aortic lymph nodes (ᵇ)
IIIC1: Positive pelvic nodes
IIIC2: Positive para-aortic lymph nodes with or without positive pelvic lymph nodes
Stage IV: Tumor invades bladder and/or bowel mucosa and/or distant metastases
IVA: Tumor invasion of bladder and/or bowel mucosa
IVB: Distant metastases, including intra-abdominal metastases and/or inguinal lymph nodes

All stages either G1, G2, or G3

ᵃEndocervical glandular involvement only should be considered as stage I and no longer as stage II

ᵇPositive cytology has to be reported separately without changing the stage

Myometrial Invasion

Pathology [31]

The myometrium can be invaded

- Along a broad pushing front
- As masses, cords, nodules, or individual glands or diffusely

The maximum depth of invasion is evaluated in millimeters and expressed as a percentage of the myometrial thickness.

It is important to remember that endomyometrial junction is typically irregular, and it is not unusual for endometrial glands to appear to be in the myometrium; this can be confusing in the cornual area, because of tangential sectioning.

It may be difficult to distinguish myometrial invasion from extension of the carcinoma into adenomyosis. This distinction is important because presence of carcinoma in adenomyosis deeper than the true depth of the tumor does not worsen the diagnosis [31].

Morphologic and Vascular Findings

(Figs. 22.27, 22.28, 22.29, and 22.30)

Normal interface between endometrium and myometrium can be evaluated by means of three different limits:

(a) The inner part of the junctional zone on T2 W images.

The junctional zone appears with a low intensity and corresponds roughly to the inner third of the myometrium. However, the junctional zone was only visible in 79 % in the premenopausal women and in only 50 % of postmenopausal women in Seki's et al. series [32].

(b) Myometrial enhancement on DMR at the early phase

- Most often, there is a thin layer of subendometrial enhancement at the early phases that corresponds to the inner myometrium [19, 33]; these findings were present in 60 % of cases in Seki's [32].
- However, it can appear as a thick enhanced layer of the inner myometrium as in 30 % of cases in Seki's series [32], or enhancement of the whole myometrium as in 10 % of cases in Seki's series [32].

(c) Low-intensity zone of the inner myometrium on delayed postcontrast T1W images.

However, it was only found in 35 % of patients in Seki's series [32].

Morphologic and vascular findings of malignancy are reported in Table 22.9.

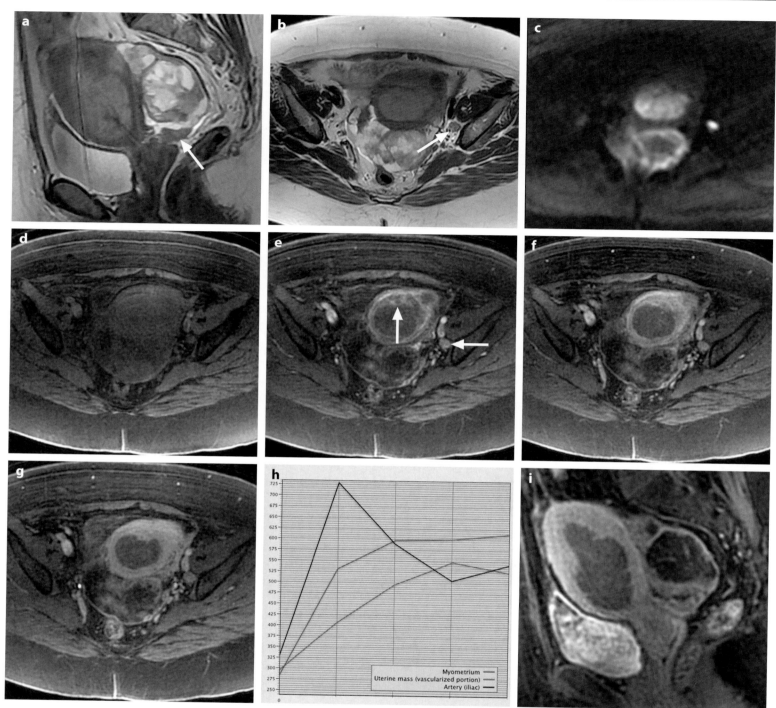

Fig. 22.28 Mixed endometrial adencarcinoma with papillary and neuroendocrine component extending to the ovaries, associated to carcinomatosis and iliac lymph nodes involvement (Stage IIIC1). (a–b) Sagittal (a) and axial (b) T2W images show a large endometrial mass with intermediate signal. On sagittal image, the junctional zone is clearly disrupted especially in its upper and anterior portions. At histology, the myometrium was infiltrated with a depth of 1.5 cm. A 13 × 10 mm left iliac lymph node is seen in (b) (arrow). Another 11 × 8 mm right iliac lymphnode was also seen at higher level. These two lymphnodes were involved at histology. Another left iliac lymphnode was involved at histology but not identified on MR even retrospectively. A mass with cystic and solid components, posterior to the uterus, is seen corresponding to the left ovary involved by metastases. On sagittal image, an implant is seen in the Douglas (arrow in a). (c) DWI at b1000 at the level of the left lymph node shows the lymph node to be hyperintense as well as the endometrial mass and the ovarian nodules. ADC values were 0.50×10^{-3} mm^2/s in the lymph nodes, 0.6×10^{-3} mm^2/s in the uterine mass, and about 1.0×10^{-3} mm^2/s in the ovarian nodules. (d–h) DMR before (d) and 25 (e), 70 (f), 125, and 240 s (g) after injection with corresponding time-intensity curves (h): The peripheral part of the endometrial tumor (vertical arrow in e) enhances more than the central mainly necrotic part. This peripheral part enhances less than the myometrium at the arterial phase, become close to the myometrium on the venous phase, and blend with it at the later phases. Thus the exact size of the tumor is best appreciated at the arterial phase. The ovarian mass contains enhancing and nonenhancing areas, and the enhancing left lymph node is also seen (horizontal arrow). (i) Sagittal delayed view after injection well display absence of extension to the cervix because the cervix is in contact with the poorly vascularized portion of the tumor while extension to the myometrium in the upper uterus is better appreciated on DMR

Fig. 22.28 (*continued*) (**j**) Histology of the ovary shows an endometrial mixed adenocarcinoma with endocrine components

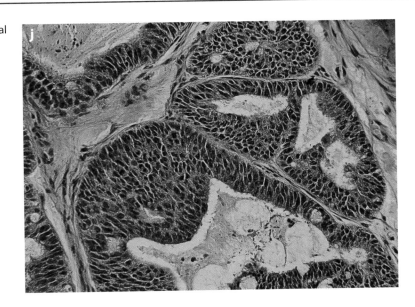

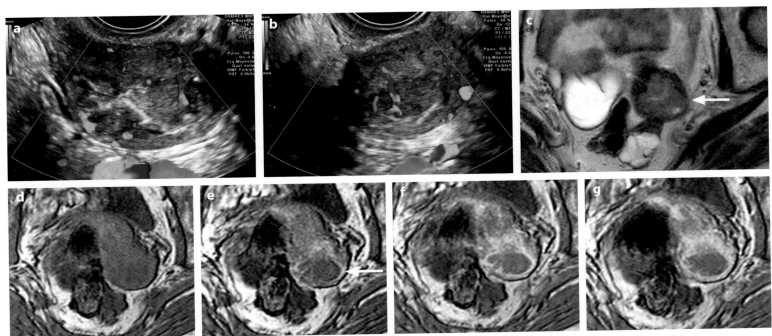

Fig. 22.29 Serous carcinoma of the endometrium stage 1B. (**a**, **b**) EVS with color Doppler, sagittal (**a**), and axial (**b**) views displays an endometrial mass. Delineation from the normal myometrium is ill defined. Large vessels are visualized in the mass. A prospective diagnosis of carcinoma was suggested; however, extension to the myometrium was underestimated. (**c**) MR axial T2 demonstrates an endometrial mass occupying most of the endometrial cavity with an intermediate signal on T2 extending to the half outer part of the myometrium and almost until the serosa in front of the left horn (*arrow*). (**d–g**) DMR without injection (**d**) at 25 s (**e**), 60 s (**f**), and 4 min after injection (**g**) display: At 25 s (the arterial phase), tumoral vessels in the peripheral portion of the tumor particularly a large vessel is depicted on the left side of the tumor (*arrow*). At 60 s, a high contrast uptake in the peripheral portion of the tumor is visualized, while there is poor contrast uptake in the central portion with necrosis. Comparison with T2-weighted image confirms that this ring of enhancement did not correspond to a normal junctional zone but to the periphery of the tumor. The inner limit of this ring, which contains in its left border the large vessel depicted at the arterial phase, clearly shows the landmark between the tumor and its central portion containing necrosis. Its outer limit indicates the separation between the peripheral portion of the tumor and the normal myometrium. At the late phase, contrast between normal myometrium and the periphery of the tumor is almost absent. These morphologic and vascular findings overall display a clear extension to the outer myometrium without extension to the serosa. Absence of extension to the cervix and to the pelvic lymph nodes allowed diagnosing a stage 1B carcinoma

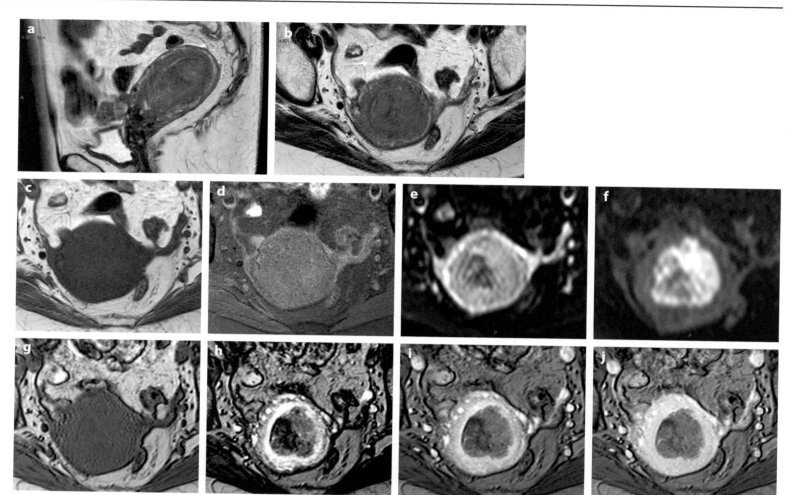

Fig. 22.30 Endometrial carcinoma stage 1B. Eighty-four-year-old woman with metrorrhagias. MR sagittal (**a**) and axial T2 (**b**) display an endometrial mass occupying the entire endometrial cavity, without invasion of the isthmus. In (**b**), from 1 o'clock to 5 o'clock, the myometrium is invaded almost until the serosa. Axial T1 (**c**) and fat suppression (**d**) do not demonstrate any hemorrhage in the tumor. Diffusion at b0 (**e**) and b1000 (**f**) depict a tissular mass with a high signal on the b1000 related to a low ADC. DMR without injection (**g**) and at the arterial phase (**h**) display typical tumoral vessels mainly on the left part of the tumor. At the venous phase (**i**) and on the delayed phase (**j**), a significant contrast uptake in the solid part is depicted, while in the right portion necrosis is suggested. No lymph node in the retrovenous external iliac chains is visualized. Prospective diagnosis: endometrial carcinoma stage 1B. Surgery and pathology confirmed this diagnosis

Table 22.9 MR criteria of extension [32]

Carcinoma limited to the endometrium
– On T2: Junctional zone is intact
– On Dynamic: Subendometrial enhancement (a thin enhanced layer between endometrium and myometrium) is intact
– On delayed contrast-enhanced T1: low-intensity zone of the inner myometrium intact
– When these landmarks are not visible, the inner surface of myometrium is smooth and sharp

Myometrial invasion
Invasion < 50 %
– Disruption or irregularity of the junctional zone, the subendometrial enhancement line, or the low-intensity zone of the inner myometrium.
– When these landmarks are not visible, the inner surface of myometrium is irregular
Invasion > 50 %
– In addition to the previous findings, signal intensity of tumor extends in the outer half of myometrium.
– The outer stripe of the myometrium is preserved

Transmyometrial invasion
– Disruption of the continuity of the residual myometrium is seen

Diffusion

DW Images

1. On high-b value, tumors are defined as masses of high signal intensity in the myometrium with higher signal intensity than the adjacent myometrial parenchyma.
2. ADC map: hypointense areas compared to normal myometrium
3. ADC value: $0.60–1.32 \times 10^{-3}$ mm^2/s [34]

Fused T2W and DW images seem to be better than DMR for assessing the depth of myometrial invasion. Shen et al. [29] report an accuracy of 0.62 using 1.5 T DW images, while Lin et al. [34] reported an accuracy of 0.88 using fused T2W and DW images at 3 T.

Performance and Value of the Different Methods

In atrophic uterus of postmenopausal women, in whom the junctional zone is frequently less conspicuous, DMR images are more useful than T2 images in assessing myometrial invasion [35].

Interest and Limitations

1. Histological grade and myometrial invasion correlate with the prevalence of lymph node metastases. Patients with greater than 50 % myometrial invasion have a six- to sevenfold higher prevalence of pelvic and para-aortic lymph node metastasis than those with less than 50 % myometrial invasion [36].
2. The incidence of early endometrial cancer in patients who want to preserve their childbearing ability has been increasing due to major changes in the lifestyles of women [37]. A good response in well-differentiated carcinoma without myometrial invasion in patients under age 40 by treatment of various doses of progestin has been reported. However, absence of myometrial invasion could only be excluded on MR with a negative predictive value of only 42.2 % of cases in Nakao's series [37].

Reasons for Misinterpretation

Common

- Nonvisualization of a mass after curettage [38]
- Larger tumors tend to diminish myometrial thickness, making difficult to assess myometrial invasion [39]
- Poor tumor/myometrium contrast [19]
- Leiomyoma [39]
- Atrophy of the endometrium [19]

Uncommon

- Endometrial cancer adjacent to adenomyosis [40]. In these cases, DMR seems better than T2 images to assess myometrial invasion because better contrast between tumor and myometrium and good visualization of inner linear enhancement of the myometrium. On the other hand, abnormal myometrial signal on T2 makes this assessment difficult.
- Congenital anomalies [39]
- Small uteri [39]
- Pyometry

Cervical Involvement

Prognosis

Involvement of the cervix is one of the important prognostic factors in addition to histologic tumor grade and depth of myometrial invasion [41–43]. In cases with cervical involvement, radical hysterectomy or preoperative radiotherapy may be necessary because tumor may extend to the parametrium or metastasize to the lymph nodes [44–46].

In the new revised FIGO classification (Table 22.8), involvement localized to the endocervical mucosa does not change the stage. It is invasion of the underlying stroma that changes the staging.

Frequency

In a series, among 154 patients with endometrial cancer operated, prevalence of 17 % for cervical involvement was found at the histology of the hysterectomy specimen [43].

Preoperative Diagnosis

Preoperative pre-hysterectomy curettage for cervical involvement of endometrial carcinoma is less predictive (sensitivity 38 %; specificity 91 %) than the judgment of the intraoperative gross appearance of the cervix (sensitivity 50 %; specificity of 95 %) [43].

Way of Spread

The spread of endometrial carcinoma to the cervix was studied in 19 hysterectomy specimens from patients with stage II disease [47]. None received preoperative irradiation. The tumor was found to spread in continuity from corpus to endocervix where it involved only the surface in five patients, the surface and underlying stroma in 13, and only stroma in one case. Surface only involvement tended to correlate with a lower grade of tumor, less myometrial invasion, and a better prognosis than association with endocervical stromal invasion.

MR Findings

- *On T2W*

  Extension appears as an abnormal signal intensity extending into the cervical canal or into the stroma, or widening of the cervical canal [48–51]. However, false negative can be related to microscopically involvement just beyond the internal cervical os. On the other hand, false positives can be observed related to large tumors widening and protruding into the cervical canal without infiltrating it or associated polyp in the cervical canal [52].

- *On DMR*

  DMR has been proven to be more accurate than T2 sequences in this evaluation [52].

  (a) Cervical epithelium involvement

    In most cases, enhancement of the cervical mucosa (and its subepithelial part) on DMR is greater than that of tumor that is greater than that of cervical stroma especially between 80 sec and 240 sec as shown in Seki et al. [52].

    Disruption of enhancement of the cervical epithelium [50, 51] indicates involvement, while the finding of continuous enhancement of the cervical epithelium rules out a cervical involvement. This finding is fundamental because it allows ruling out extension to the cervix when the cervical canal is widened because a tumor extends near the internal cervical os or is protruding into the cervical canal.

    When the enhanced cervical epithelium is indistinguishable from enhanced cervical stroma, the same criteria as on T2 are used.

    The contrast between the tumor and cervical epithelium is greater on the dynamic MR than on T2W and contrast-enhanced nondynamic T1W images.

On the other hand, contrast between the tumor and cervical stroma is greater on T2 than on the DMR and enhanced T1W.

  (b) Stroma involvement (Fig. 22.31)

    It is characterized by disruption of the enhancing inner line and bulging of the tumor into the stroma. In case the tumor extends directly from the myometrium to the cervical stroma, continuous enhancement of the cervical epithelium may be observed which can lead to a false negative diagnosis.

Local or Regional Spread Including Lymph Nodes (Stage III)

Stage IIIA

Disruption of continuity of the outer myometrium or the presence of nodules on the peritoneal surface or adnexa is indicative of serosal involvement or peritoneal spread of the tumor [35].

The presence of ascites should raise the possibility of peritoneal spread especially in postmenopausal woman [35].

An associated adnexal mass can be metastatic (Figs. 22.28 and 22.32) or can be independent [35].

Metastasis to the ovaries (Stage III A) is suggested when ovarian involement is:

1. Multinodular
2. Bilateral
3. Ovaries are small (<5 cm)
4. When endometrial carcinoma is associated with deep myometrial invasion (stage IB at the level of the uterus)
5. When there is fallopian tube involvement

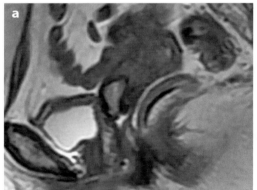
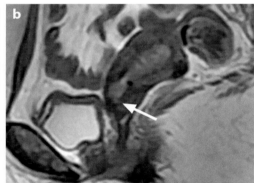
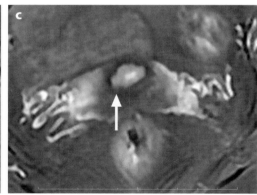
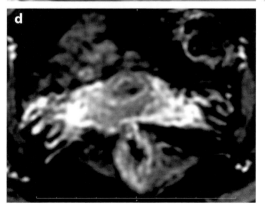

Fig. 22.31 Endometrioid adenocarcinoma of the endometrium invading the inner myometrium and upper cervical stroma (stage II). A 56-year-old woman with metrorrhagia. (**a, b**) Sagittal T2W images show, at the level of the cervix, integrity of the hypointense junctional line in the middle sagittal plane (**a**) while in the right parasagittal plane, this line is interrupted posteriorly (*arrow*). (**c**) Axial T2W FS image at the level of the upper cervix shows the hypointense junctional line to be clearly disrupted posteriorly on the right (*arrow*). (**d**) DMR at 75 s at the same level as (**c**) shows that the peripheral rim enhancement corresponding to the inner stroma is disrupted posteriorly in the right side in the same area

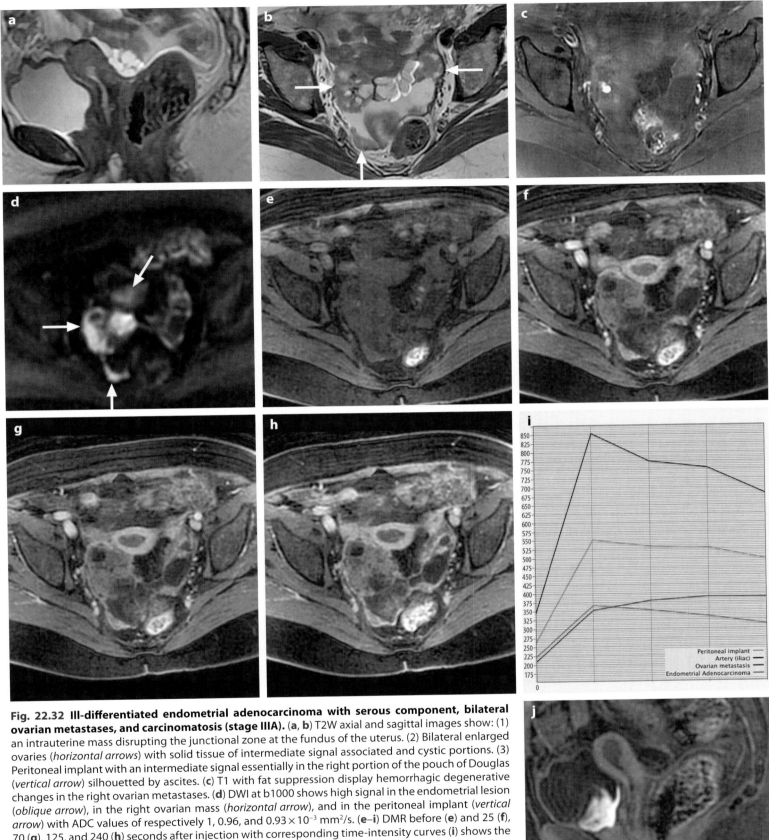

Fig. 22.32 Ill-differentiated endometrial adenocarcinoma with serous component, bilateral ovarian metastases, and carcinomatosis (stage IIIA). (**a**, **b**) T2W axial and sagittal images show: (1) an intrauterine mass disrupting the junctional zone at the fundus of the uterus. (2) Bilateral enlarged ovaries (*horizontal arrows*) with solid tissue of intermediate signal associated and cystic portions. (3) Peritoneal implant with an intermediate signal essentially in the right portion of the pouch of Douglas (*vertical arrow*) silhouetted by ascites. (**c**) T1 with fat suppression display hemorrhagic degenerative changes in the right ovarian metastases. (**d**) DWI at b1000 shows high signal in the endometrial lesion (*oblique arrow*), in the right ovarian mass (*horizontal arrow*), and in the peritoneal implant (*vertical arrow*) with ADC values of respectively 1, 0.96, and 0.93×10^{-3} mm^2/s. (**e–i**) DMR before (**e**) and 25 (**f**), 70 (**g**), 125, and 240 (**h**) seconds after injection with corresponding time-intensity curves (**i**) shows the peritoneal implant to enhance more than the endometrial lesion and the ovarian mass and very close curves of contrast uptake of the primitive endometrial carcinoma and the ovarian metastases. (**j**) Late sagittal T1WFS after injection better delineated the endometrial tumor that enhances less than the myometrium

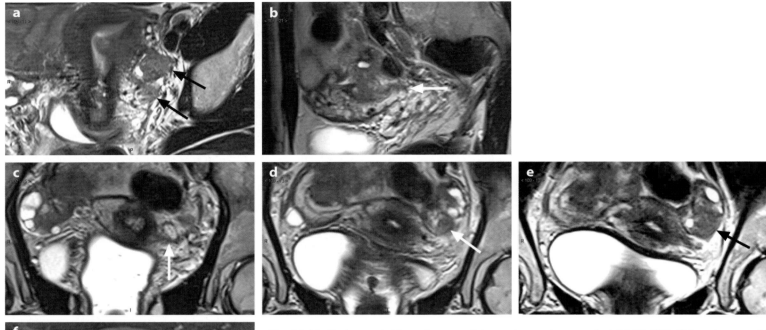

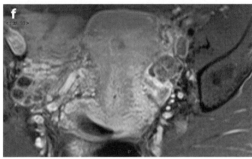

Fig. 22.33 Endometrioid carcinoma of the endometrium grade 3 (FIGO IIIB). Thirty-six-year-old woman. Menometrorrhagias for 3 months. MR axial T2 (**a**) displays: (1) an endometrial carcinoma of left border of the endometrial cavity, extending into the inner half of the myometrium. (2) Lateral to the left border of the uterus, from the isthmus to the fundus two areas of infiltration, one in the broad ligament (*arrow*), the other one immediately in front (*arrow*). Sagittal T2 (**b**) displays an interruption of the posterior leaf of the broad ligament (*arrow*) confirming the invasion of the broad ligament. Coronal T2 with three different sections from the back to the front (**c**–**e**) depict: in (**c**) invasion of the broad ligament (*arrow*), in (**d**) a mass (*arrow*) which corresponded at surgery to invasion of the mesosalpinx and which extended (*arrow* in **e**) through contiguity into the left ovary. Axial T1 after injection (**f**) displays a contrast uptake in the tumoral extension to the broad ligament and into the mesosalpinx and the left ovary

Stage IIIB

Parametrial involvement appears on T2 as a mass of an intermediate signal in the broad ligament; in extensive involvement, extension through the leaf of the ligament can be visualized on MR (Fig. 22.33).

Stage IIIC

A cutoff value of 10 mm for the minimal transverse diameter is used [26]. However, larger lymph node may be benign, and smaller lymph node may be metastatic (Fig. 22.34).

Bladder and Bowel Mucosa (Stage V)

Involvement on MR is assessed using the same findings as for cervical carcinoma.

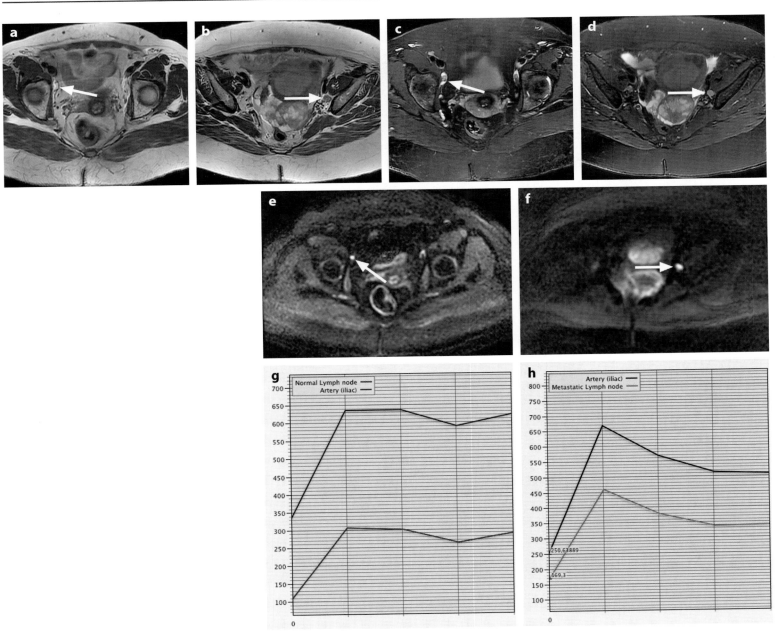

Fig. 22.34 Benign versus malignant lymph node at histology in two patients with pelvic cancer. A right benign lymph node (*arrows*) in a cervical squamous cell carcinoma (**a, c, e, g**) is compared to left malignant lymph node in an endometrial mixed adenocarcinoma (**b, d, f, h**), both lymph nodes confirmed at histology. (**a–d**) On T2WI without (**a, b**) and with (**c, d**) fat suppression, as well as on other sequences, the benign lymph node tends to be oblong (18×10 mm in this case) with fat sinus, while the metastatic lymph node tends to be roundness (12×10 mm in this case) without fat sinus. (**e, f**) On DWI, benign and malignant lymph nodes are hyperintense, perhaps more in malignant with low ADC (0.5×10^{-3} mm²/s in this case) and less in benign with high ADC (1.9×10^{-3} mm²/s in this case). (**g, h**) On DMR, both lymph nodes enhances with a peak at the arterial phase, but enhancement in malignant lymph node is more important

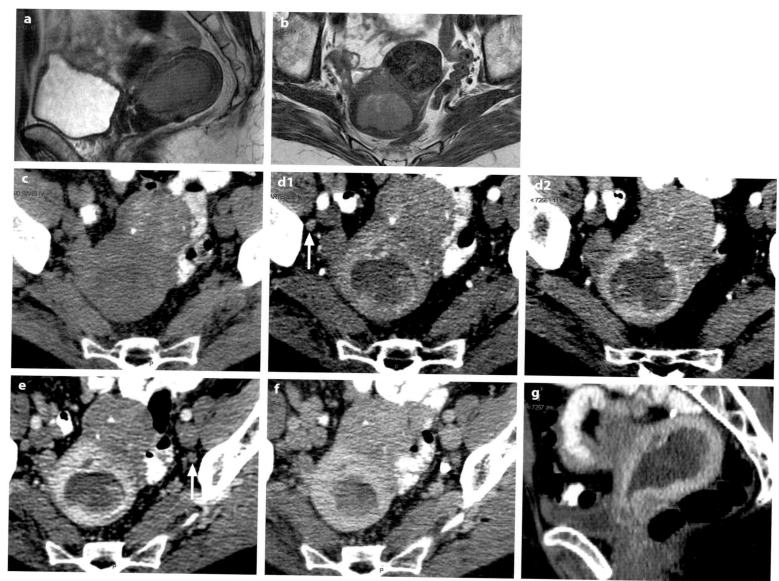

Fig. 22.35 Endometrium carcinoma of the endometrium stage IIIC1. Sixty-two-year-old woman with metrorrhagias. Hysteroscopy with biopsy: endometrioid carcinoma grade 3. (**a**, **b**) MR Sagittal (**a**) and axial (**b**) T2WI: endometrial mass with an intermediate signal occupying the entire uterine cavity typical for an endometrial carcinoma. Extension to the myometrium anteriorly and posteriorly is clearly depicted. However, this extension that has been evaluated to the inner half of the wall on MR involved at pathology the 2/3 of the myometrium. A leiomyoma is displayed anteriorly (with calcification on CT). A thoraco-abdomino-pelvic CT scan has been performed to evaluate the extension. (**c**–**f**) Dynamic CT, at the level of the fundus, without injection (**c**), at the arterial phase (**d1** and **d2** with MIP reformation), at the venous phase (**e**) and 4 min after injection (**f**) displays: (1) in the tumor. (a) At the arterial phase, thin and irregular tumoral vessels that are better displayed on the MIP. Invasion of the myometrium is also better depicted on the MIP. (b) At the venous phase from outside to inside, a high contrast uptake in the solid tissue of the tumor at the periphery; an intermediate zone where contrast uptake is lower; a large portion protruding in the endometrial cavity with few or absence of contrast uptake related to necrosis. (c) On the delayed phase, a slight diffusion in the portion with necrotic changes. (2) In a right iliac lymph node just behind the right external iliac vein, there is a high contrast uptake at the arterial phase (*arrow* in **d1**), while there is no significant contrast uptake until the venous phase in symmetrical left iliac lymph node (*arrow* in **e**). At pathology, the right lymph node was invaded, while the left one was normal. (**g**) Sagittal reformation depicts clearly not only the tumor but also its extension to the myometrium as in MR

CT (Fig. 22.35)

While MR is considered as a good tool to evaluate locoregional extension, thoraco-abdomino-pelvic CT is advocated to evaluate extension in the entire abdominopelvic cavity (particularly to evaluate lomboaortic lymph nodes) and extension to the chest.

Tumor

In fact, CT with DCT can also give information about locoregional extension.

1. DCT of the Tumor

Without injection, the tumor does not appear clearly as far as it has about the same density as normal myometrium.

At the arterial phase (25 s after injection), tumoral vessels are displayed in the solid tissue of the tumor.

At the venous phase (60 s after injection) from the periphery to the inner part of the tumor, three different zoned are displayed:

- A peripheral portion with a high contrast uptake
- A middle zone with an intermediate contrast uptake
- A central zone with a very low or absence of contrast uptake corresponding to necrosis.

On the delayed time, a slight diffusion of contrast uptake can be seen in this last zone.

Myometrial and Cervical Invasion

DCT has been also proved accurate in the evaluation of local extension particularly in evaluating myometrial invasion and cervical infiltration [53].

Extension to the myometrium can be visualized right on the arterial phase and at the venous phase owing to vessels or contrast uptake identical in the tumor and in the invaded myometrium. At the venous phase, an irregular interface between the tumor and the normally enhanced myometrium is seen. However, the degree of extension to the inner or the outer half is difficult to precise.

Cervical involvement is diagnosed when involvement includes widening of the internal cervical os and/or endocervical canal with or without presence of a mass protruding into the cervix [53].

Lymph Nodes

Besides the usual criteria of size, round shape, and necrosis, metastatic lymph nodes can be detected at the arterial phase of the DCT because of a high contrast uptake that is significantly different from a normal lymph node.

Iliac lymph nodes can be detected by MR or CT.

Lomboaortic lymph nodes are better evaluated on CT than on MR. These nodes can be involved through iliac lymph node involvement or directly through a pathway from the uterine fundus to the subrenal lymph nodes via the infundibulopelvic ligament.

Adnexal Metastases

Metastasis to the ovaries can be displayed on CT; however, especially when of small size, MR offers a better contrast to detect them.

Peritoneum

Peritoneal fluid and peritoneal implants are very well depicted on CT.

Liver

Liver metastases are exceptional at time of diagnosis and are usually only displayed during the follow-up.

Thorax

CT has the big advantage during the same rapid examination to evaluate this extension.

Recurrences

CT is a valuable method to detect recurrences [54]. Association with PET scan is appropriate.

22.4.2 Malignant Mesodermal Mixed Tumor (MMMT) or Carcinosarcoma

It is a variant of endometrial carcinoma (see Chap. 25).

22.4.3 Miscellaneous

- Squamous cell
- Choriocarcinoma

22.4.4 Metastasis to the Endometrium

Ovarian carcinoma

Simultaneous carcinomas involving the ovary and the endometrium may represent:

1. Metastasis from the endometrium to the ovary
2. Metastasis from the ovary to the endometrium (which is much less uncommon)
3. Independent primary tumors

Among primary ovarian tumors with extension to the endometrium, ovarian endometrioid carcinoma is the most common. Diagnosis of metastasis to the endometrium based on imaging findings can be difficult. However findings in favour of a primary endometrial carcinoma mentioned above (see Chap. 22.4.1), when present may help to make the differential diagnosis.

Carcinomas from extragenital sites are much more uncommon and usually are a manifestation of obvious dissemination. Among them breast carcinoma and stomach carcinoma are the most common.

22.5 Endometritis

See Chap. 33

22.6 Effects of Therapy

22.6.1 Drugs

Many drugs may have an effect on the endometrium. The most important are:

- Estrogens that induces essentially hyperplasia (see hyperplasia)
- Estrogen and progesterone therapy in postmenopausal women that results in thickness of the endometrium. A threshold of 8 mm is usually used to define normal thickness compared to 5 mm in postmenopausal woman without hormone substitution therapy.
- Tamoxifen (see below)
- Clomiphene citrate (like tamoxifen)

22.6.1.1 Tamoxifen

Pathology

The endometrium shows several benign changes that can be isolated or associated. These changes include glandulocystic atrophy, polyp, adenomyosis and later on hyperplasia. Endometrial carcinoma is exceptional.

1. Glandulocystic atrophy

   At hysteroscopy, the mucosa is smooth, white, hypervascularized, and atrophic, with scattered protuberances [55]. This atrophia differs macroscopically from the atrophic mucosa in postmenopausal women where the mucosa is thin, pale, without protuberances.

   At microscopy, multiple cystic spaces lined by atrophic endometrium are present within a dense fibrous stroma [56].

   Some authors report that the cysts extend to the endometrial-myometrial junction, while others place them in subendometrial location which in this case would correspond to adenomyosis [56–58].

2. Endometrial polyp

   Clinical Findings: Although these polyps may cause abnormal uterine bleeding, most women are asymptomatic.

   Tamoxifen polyps are different from usual polyps:

   • At macroscopy, they are unusually large (mean diameter 5 cm)

   • At microscopy, they have an association of cystic glandular dilatation, epithelial metaplasia, focal periglandular stromal condensation, and extensive fibrosis, which may account for the difficulties in excising them at hysteroscopy

3. Adenomyosis
4. Endometrial hyperplasia (late phase)
5. Endometrial carcinoma (exceptional)

The risk increases with duration of treatment and cumulative tamoxifen dose [59]

Radiology

Ultrasound

• The most common pattern is a thicker endometrium (9–13 mm) as compared with that in control subjects (4–5.4 mm) [60–62]. This endometrium is hyperechoic and contains cystic spaces, which may correspond to glandulocystic atrophy (Fig. 22.36). Other anomalies that can be associated are polyp (Fig. 22.37), adenomyosis (Fig. 22.36), or hyperplasia (Fig. 22.38).

• Hysterosonography can increasingly improve the ability to diagnose the type of pathologic condition.

MR

Glandulocystic atrophy, adenomyosis, polyp, and hyperplasia are well depicted on MR (Figs. 22.39 and 22.40).

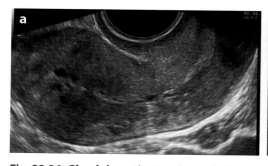
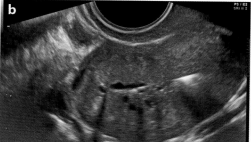
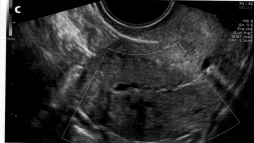

Fig. 22.36 Glandulocystic atrophy and adenomyosis under tamoxifen. Ultrasound in a 41-year-old woman with amenorrhea under tamoxifen therapy since 1 year for breast carcinoma. (**a–c**) Transvaginal ultrasound with Doppler discloses a thin endometrium with small cystic spaces in endometrial and subendometrial locations corresponding to glandulocystic atrophy. Other cystic spaces are seen deeper in the myometrium corresponding to adenomyosis. Color Doppler shows absence of flow in the cystic spaces ruling out vessels

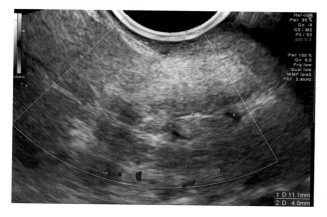

Fig. 22.37 Endometrial polyp under tamoxifen treatment. Routine ultrasound in a 51-year-old woman under tamoxifen since 1 year for breast carcinoma. An 11×5 mm endometrial polyp (*cursors*) is displayed without detectable vascular pedicle. The endometrium is otherwise hyperechoic and thin. The polyp was extracted under hysteroscopy

Fig. 22.38 Glandulocystic hyperplasia under tamoxifen. Routine US follow-up in 80-year-old woman under tamoxifen since 7 years for breast carcinoma. (**a**) Sagittal transvaginal ultrasound discloses a thickness of the entire endometrium with small cystic spaces and hyperechoic endometrium. (**b**) Transvaginal color Doppler shows absence of vascular pedicle but vessels inside the solid part of the endometrium

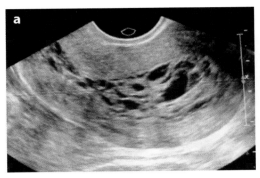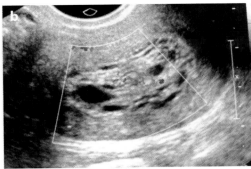

Fig. 22.39 Endometrium with tamoxifen therapy. Sagittal T2W image (**a**) and corresponding delayed T1W-FS image after gadolinium injection (**b**) show hydrometria, thin endometrium and several subendometrial cystic glands related to glandulocystic atrophy or adenomyosis

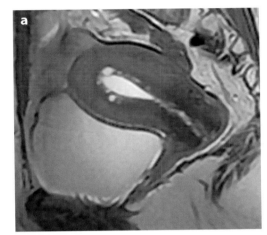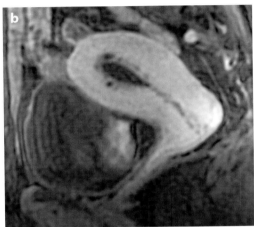

Fig. 22.40 Endometrium with tamoxifen therapy. Sagittal T2W image (**a**) and corresponding delayed T1W-FS image after gadolinium injection (**b**) show an endometrium reaching 8 mm of maximum thickness, several subendometrial cystic glands related to glandulocystic atrophy or adenomyosis, and several other cystic glands deeper in the myometrium related to adenomyosis

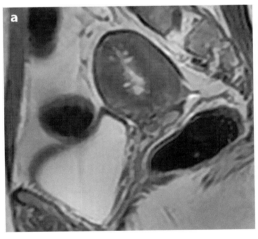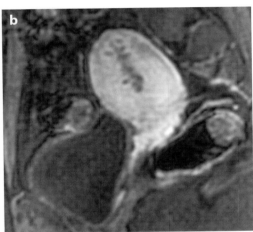

22.6.2 Curettage and Asherman Syndrome

1. *After curettage* transient inflammatory and regenerative changes are seen in the endometrium.
2. *Asherman syndrome*
   Definition: a posttraumatic condition associated with hypomenorrhea or amenorrhea and infertility following endometrial injury.
   Etiology:
   - Postpartum or post-abortal curettage, particularly if infection is present
   - Myomectomy
   - Tuberculous endometritis

Macroscopic and imaging findings are reported in Table 22.10.

Table 22.10 Macroscopic and imaging findings of Asherman syndrome

1. Endometrium Bands of fibrous tissue or smooth muscle traversing or rarely obliterating the endometrial cavity Synechiae (adhesion)
2. Myometrium Retraction (which may extend to the serosa)
3. Associated finding Atrophy and fibrosis of the endometrium

22.6.2.1 Imaging Findings

1. On ultrasound, synechia appears as hyperechoic foci or linear small structures (Fig. 22.41). 3D US reformation and hysterosalpingography may better delineate the lesion (Figs. 22.42 and 22.43).
2. On MR, bands of fibrous tissue appear hypointense on T2. Retraction of the endometrial cavity and deformity of the adjacent endometrium is displayed (Fig. 22.44).

22.6.3 IUD

A significant degree of sharply localized area of decidualization in chronic inflammation is observed in 25–40 % of patients.

Progesterone-impregnated devices release hormones in a slow continuous fashion, producing a sharply localized area of decidualization adjacent to the device.

Complications (PID and Actinomyces) are treated in Chap. 33.

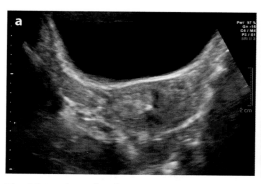
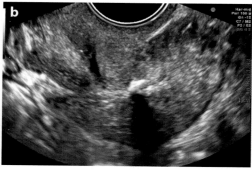
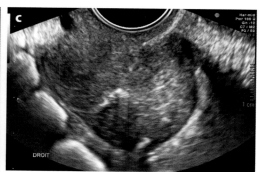

Fig. 22.41 Synechia following myomectomy. A 40-year-old woman with previous embolization for leiomyomas followed by leiomyomas resection through hysteroscopy. (**a**) Transabdominal ultrasound, transverse view, shows a hyperechoic focus with shadowing in the endometrium. (**b, c**) Transvaginal views confirm the presence of a small linear hyperechoic structure with shadowing very suggestive of synechia. Following hysteroscopy confirmed the diagnosis

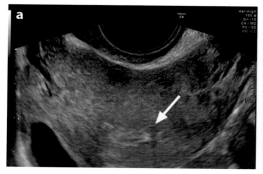
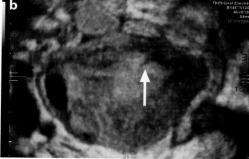
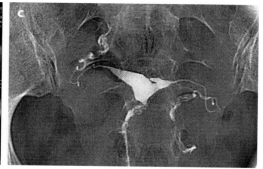

Fig. 22.42 Synechia following sepsis. A 30-year-old woman with previous sepsis following curettage and secondary infertility. (**a**) Transverse transvaginal ultrasound discloses an echogenic 7 mm focus with adjacent shadowing in the left fundus (*arrow*) suggestive of synechia. (**b**) 3D reformation clearly depicts the synechia as an incisure in the left part of the fundus (*arrow*). (**c**) Hysterosalpingography displays clearly the location of the scar going from the fundus to the inferior part of the cornua. The tubes are normally opacified. Hysteroscopy confirms the diagnosis and the location

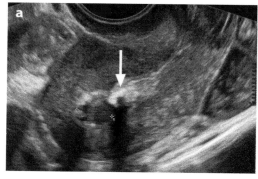
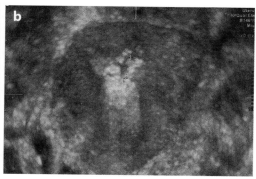

Fig. 22.43 Synechia with residual trophoblastic tissue. A 39-year-old woman with synechia treated by hysteroscopy 2 years ago. Pregnancy occurred 1 year later complicated by placenta accreta treated by embolization. Hysteroscopy showed a residual fibrino-necrotic mass in the left anterolateral fundus with residual trophoblastic tissue and new constituted synechia. Transvaginal ultrasound was done for evaluation and follow-up. (**a**) Sagittal ultrasound view through the left part of the uterus shows a hypoechoic mass (*cursors*) corresponding to the residual fibrino-necrotic mass, a hyperechogenic structure with shadowing (*arrow*) corresponding to the synechia or calcification in the residual trophoblastic tissue. (**b**) 3D reformation clearly demonstrates normal endometrium in the right cornua, the residual trophoblastic tissue centered by a synechia and blurred left cornua

Fig. 22.44 Asherman's syndrome. Sixty-four-year-old woman. Endometrial curettage for polyps of the endometrium 7 years ago. Pelvic pain. MR sagittal T2 (**a**) displays in the upper part of the endometrial cavity fibrous bands (*arrow*), secondary to the curettage. On axial T2 (**b**), retraction of the inner myometrium (*green arrow*) is visualized facing the fibrous bands (*red arrows*). Lesions of adenomyosis with cystic cavities are associated

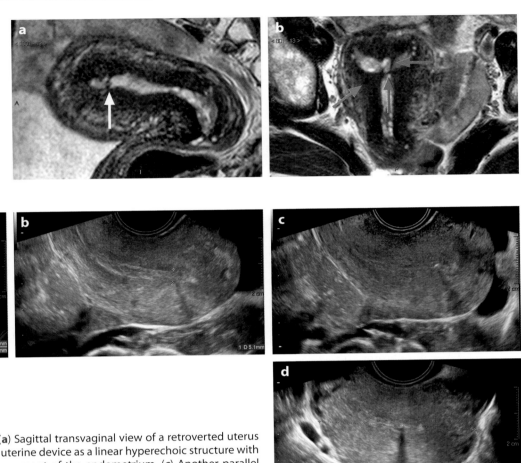

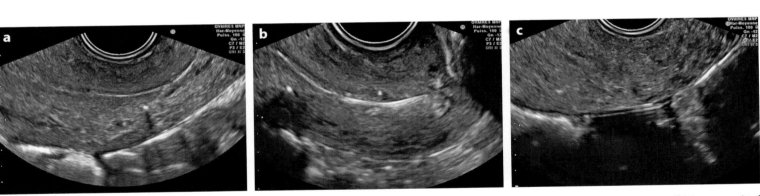

Fig. 22.45 Normal positioned T-shaped IUD. (**a**) Sagittal transvaginal view of a retroverted uterus through the longitudinal part of the T shows the uterine device as a linear hyperechoic structure with shadowing. (**b**) Parallel sagittal view allow measurement of the endometrium. (**c**) Another parallel sagittal view shows a hyperechoic point with shadowing in the fundus due to the horizontal part of the T. (**d**) Transverse view shows the horizontal part of the T in the fundus with a small shadowing in the middle

Fig. 22.46 IUD in ectopic cervicovaginal position. (**a**) Sagittal transvaginal ultrasound shows absence of IUD in the corporeal cavity. (**b**) Lower sagittal view shows part of the IUD in the cervix. (**c**) Another view shows part of the IUD in the vagina

22.6.3.1 US

Ultrasound allows checking for good position of the IUD. The IUD appears as a hyperechoic structures with shadowing (Figs. 22.45 and 22.46). 3D reformation is very useful (Figs. 22.47, 22.48, and 22.49).

22.6.3.2 MR

On MR, the IUD appears hypointense on all sequences (Fig. 22.50).

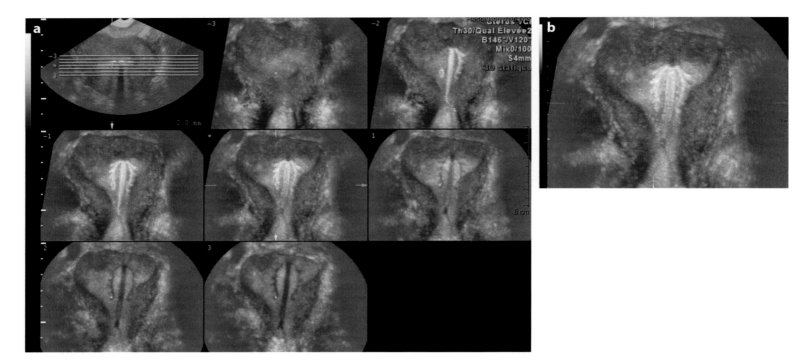

Fig. 22.47 T-shaped IUD with internal bowing of the lateral branches. (**a**) 3D with one axial and several coronal reformations shows the lateral branches of the IUD to be internally bowed. Note that the IUD appears hyperechoic on anterior coronal reformations and hypoechoic on posterior reformations due to shadowing. (**b**) Magnification of one of the anterior coronal reformation showing the IUD

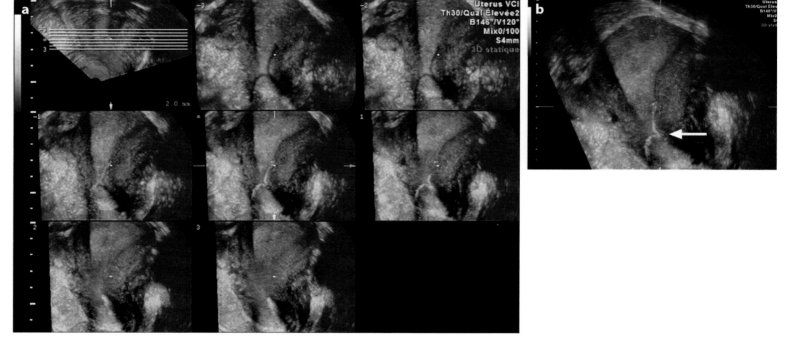

Fig. 22.48 IUD in the isthmic region. (**a**) Transvaginal 3D ultrasound with one axial and several coronal reformations show the T-shaped IUD to be in the isthmic region slightly rotated to the right. (**b**) Magnified view of the most expressive coronal reformation showing the IUD (*arrow*)

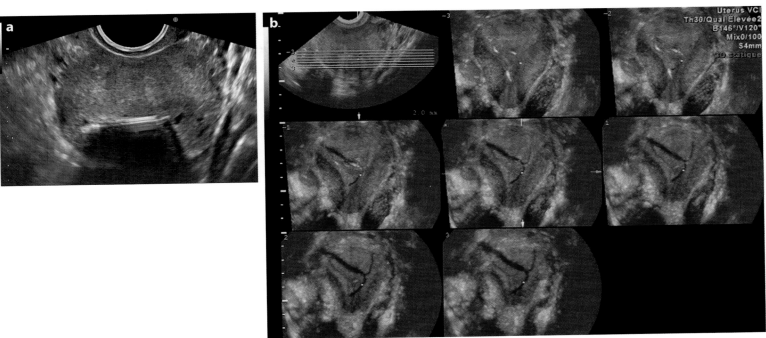

Fig. 22.49 IUD rotated to the left. (a) During transvaginal ultrasound, the IUD is best visualized on the transverse view here shown. **(b)** 3D with one axial reformation and several coronal reformations clearly shows the T-shaped IUD rotated to the left. It is best seen on posterior view where it appears hypoechoic due to shadowing

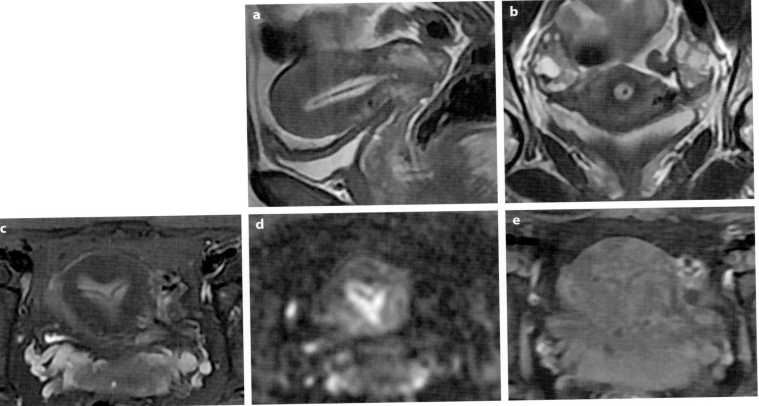

Fig. 22.50 Normal positioned IUD at MR. (a) Sagittal T2W image well delineated the vertical part of the T-shaped IUD as a linear hypointense structure compared to the hyperintense endometrium. **(b)** On coronal T2W image, the IUD appears as a hypointense point in the endometrium that can be followed on consecutives images. **(c, d)** Axial T2W image with fat-saturation and DW b1000 image shows the upper part of the IUD as a truncated T-shaped structure hypointense compared to the hyperintense endometrium. **(e)** Axial T1 FS shows the IUD to be hypointense compared to uterus

22.6.3.3 Essure

A variety of IUD is Essure. It is a permanent contraceptive method. An insert is put in the proximal portion of each tube. Tissue growth related to fibrotic reaction results in complete obliteration of the tube after 3 months. US allows confirmation of the good position of the inserts (Figs. 22.51 and 22.52). Hysterosalpingography is made 3 months later to confirm obliteration of the tubes.

22.6.4 Radiation

The endometrium is thin and easily traumatized; small blood vessels in the stroma are thin walled and ectatic. Some blood vessels form plaques of lipid-filled clear cells in the media [31].

Cells are often enlarged, assume unusual shapes, and display vacuolated cytoplasm. Nuclear changes include enlargement, pleomorphism, and hyperchromasia with poorly preserved chromatin [4].

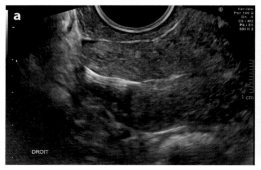 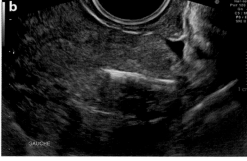 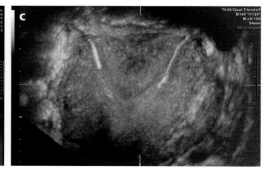

Fig. 22.51 Contraceptive device (Essure). (a) Transvaginal transverse view of the right cornua shows the right insert correctly positioned in the proximal tube. **(b)** On the left, the insert is also correctly positioned but seems extending a little bit more proximal. **(c)** 3D with coronal reformation shows correct positioning of the two inserts although small asymmetry is noted with the left one being a little bit more proximal

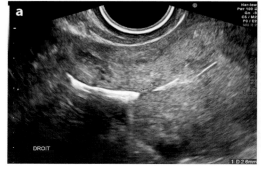 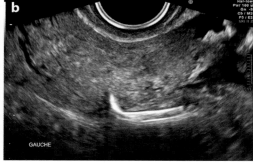 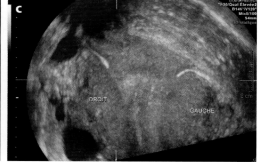

Fig. 22.52 Contraceptive device (Essure) with unusual kinking of the left insert. (a) Transvaginal ultrasound of the right cornua shows the right insert normally positioned in the proximal tube. **(b)** On the left, there is unusual kinking of the proximal extremity of the insert that is probably under the ostium of the tube. **(c)** 3D with corresponding coronal reformation shows on a single view both inserts allowing better comparison

References

1. Smith-Bindman R et al (1998) Endovaginal ultrasound to exclude endometrial cancer and other endometrial abnormalities. JAMA 280(17): 1510–1517

2. Choo YC et al (1985) Postmenopausal uterine bleeding of nonorganic cause. Obstet Gynecol 66(2):225–228

3. Lidor A et al (1986) Histopathological findings in 226 women with post-menopausal uterine bleeding. Acta Obstet Gynecol Scand 65(1):41–43

4. Sherman ME (2002) Benign diseases of the endometrium. In: Kurman RJ (ed) Blaustein's pathology of the female genital tract. Springer, New York, pp 421–466

5. Atri M et al (1994) Transvaginal US appearance of endometrial abnormalities. Radiographics 14:483–492

6. Baldwin MT et al (1999) Focal intracavitary masses recognized with the hyperechoic line sign at endovaginal US and characterized with hysterosonography. Radiographics 19(4):927–935

7. La Torre R et al (1999) Transvaginal sonographic evaluation of endometrial polyps: a comparison with two dimensional and three dimensional contrast sonography. Clin Exp Obstet Gynecol 26(3–4):171–173

8. Goldstein SR et al (2002) Evaluation of endometrial polyps. Am J Obstet Gynecol 186(4):669–674

9. Jorizzo JR, Chen MY, Riccio GJ (2001) Endometrial polyps: sonohystero-graphic evaluation. AJR Am J Roentgenol 176(3):617–621

10. Grasel RP et al (2000) Endometrial polyps: MR imaging features and distinction from endometrial carcinoma. Radiology 214(1):47–52

11. Park BK et al (2006) Differentiation of the various lesions causing an abnormality of the endometrial cavity using MR imaging: emphasis on enhancement patterns on dynamic studies and late contrast-enhanced T1-weighted images. Eur Radiol 16(7):1591–1598

12. Mittal KR et al (1995) Coexistent atypical polypoid adenomyoma and endometrial adenocarcinoma. Hum Pathol 26(5):574–576

13. Mazur MT (1981) Atypical polypoid adenomyomas of the endometrium. Am J Surg Pathol 5(5):473–482

14. Longacre TA et al (1996) Atypical polypoid adenomyofibromas (atypical polypoid adenomyomas) of the uterus. A clinicopathologic study of 55 cases. Am J Surg Pathol 20(1):1–20

15. Maeda T et al (2006) Atypical polypoid adenomyoma of the uterus: appearance on (18)F-FDG PET/MRI fused images. AJR Am J Roentgenol 186(2): 320–323

16. Ronnett BM, Kurman MD (2002) Precursor lesions of endometrial carcinoma. In: Kurman RJ (ed) Blaustein's pathology of the female genital tract. Springer, New York

17. Chaudhry S et al (2003) Benign and malignant diseases of the endometrium. Top Magn Reson Imaging 14(4):339–357

18. Hendrickson MR, Kempson RL (1980) Endometrial epithelial metaplasias: proliferations frequently misdiagnosed as adenocarcinoma. Report of 89 cases and proposed classification. Am J Surg Pathol 4(6):525–542

19. Yamashita Y et al (1993) Assessment of myometrial invasion by endome-trial carcinoma: transvaginal sonography vs contrast-enhanced MR imag-ing. AJR Am J Roentgenol 161(3):595–599

20. Fleischer AC et al (1987) Myometrial invasion by endometrial carcinoma: sonographic assessment. Radiology 162(2):307–310

21. Alcazar JL et al (2009) Assessing myometrial infiltration by endometrial cancer: uterine virtual navigation with three-dimensional US. Radiology 250(3):776–783

22. Tamai K et al (2007) Diffusion-weighted MR imaging of uterine endome-trial cancer. J Magn Reson Imaging 26(3):682–687

23. Fujii S et al (2008) Diagnostic accuracy of the apparent diffusion coefficient in differentiating benign from malignant uterine endometrial cavity lesions: initial results. Eur Radiol 18(2):384–389

24. Manfredi R et al (2005) Endometrial cancer: magnetic resonance imaging. Abdom Imaging 30(5):626–636

25. Joja I et al (1996) Endometrial carcinoma: dynamic MRI with turbo-FLASH technique. J Comput Assist Tomogr 20(6):878–887

26. Manfredi R et al (2004) Local-regional staging of endometrial carcinoma: role of MR imaging in surgical planning. Radiology 231(2):372–378

27. Takeuchi M et al (2005) Pathologies of the uterine endometrial cavity: usual and unusual manifestations and pitfalls on magnetic resonance imag-ing. Eur Radiol 15(11):2244–2255

28. Sala E et al (2007) MRI of malignant neoplasms of the uterine corpus and cervix. AJR Am J Roentgenol 188(6):1577–1587

29. Shen SH et al (2008) Diffusion-weighted single-shot echo-planar imaging with parallel technique in assessment of endometrial cancer. AJR Am J Roentgenol 190(2):481–488

30. Pecorelli S (2009) Revised FIGO staging for carcinoma of the vulva, cervix, and endometrium. Int J Gynaecol Obstet 105(2):103–104

31. Ronnett BM et al (2002) Endometrial carcinoma. In: Kurman RJ (ed) Blaustein's pathology of the female genital tract. Springer, New York, pp 501–559

32. Seki H, Kimura M, Sakai K (1997) Myometrial invasion of endometrial carcinoma: assessment with dynamic MR and contrast-enhanced T1-weighted images. Clin Radiol 52(1):18–23

33. Ito K et al (1994) Assessing myometrial invasion by endometrial carci-noma with dynamic MRI. J Comput Assist Tomogr 18(1):77–86

34. Lin G et al (2009) Myometrial invasion in endometrial cancer: diagnostic accuracy of diffusion-weighted 3.0-T MR imaging – initial experience. Radiology 250(3):784–792

35. Koyama T, Tamai K, Togashi K (2007) Staging of carcinoma of the uterine cervix and endometrium. Eur Radiol 17(8):2009–2019

36. Larson DM et al (1996) Prognostic significance of gross myometrial invasion with endometrial cancer. Obstet Gynecol 88(3):394–398

37. Nakao Y et al (2006) MR imaging in endometrial carcinoma as a diagnos-tic tool for the absence of myometrial invasion. Gynecol Oncol 102(2): 343–347

38. Lee EJ et al (1999) Staging of early endometrial carcinoma: assessment with T2-weighted and gadolinium-enhanced T1-weighted MR imaging. Radiographics 19(4):937–945; discussion 946–947

39. Scoutt LM et al (1995) Clinical stage I endometrial carcinoma: pitfalls in preoperative assessment with MR imaging. Work in progress. Radiology 194(2):567–572

40. Utsunomiya D et al (2004) Endometrial carcinoma in adenomyosis: assess-ment of myometrial invasion on T2-weighted spin-echo and gadolinium-enhanced T1-weighted images. AJR Am J Roentgenol 182(2):399–404

41. Fanning J et al (1991) Prognostic significance of the extent of cervical involvement by endometrial cancer. Gynecol Oncol 40(1):46–47

42. Boente MP et al (1993) Prognostic factors and long-term survival in endo-metrial adenocarcinoma with cervical involvement. Gynecol Oncol 51(3): 316–322

43. Lampe B et al (1997) Accuracy of preoperative histology and macroscopic assessment of cervical involvement in endometrial carcinoma. Eur J Obstet Gynecol Reprod Biol 74(2):205–209

44. Rutledge F (1974) The role of radical hysterectomy in adenocarcinoma of the endometrium. Gynecol Oncol 2(2–3):331–347

45. Rubin SC et al (1992) Management of endometrial adenocarcinoma with cervical involvement. Gynecol Oncol 45(3):294–298

46. Elia G et al (1995) Surgical management of patients with endometrial can-cer and cervical involvement. Eur J Gynaecol Oncol 16(3):169–173

47. Bigelow B, Vekshtein V, Demopoulos RI (1983) Endometrial carcinoma, stage II: route and extent of spread to the cervix. Obstet Gynecol 62(3): 363–366

48. Belloni C et al (1990) Magnetic resonance imaging in endometrial carci-noma staging. Gynecol Oncol 37(2):172–177

49. Chen SS, Rumancik WM, Spiegel G (1990) Magnetic resonance imaging in stage I endometrial carcinoma. Obstet Gynecol 75(2):274–277

50. Murakami T et al (1995) Cervical invasion of endometrial carcinoma – evaluation by parasagittal MR imaging. Acta Radiol 36(3):248–253

51. Takahashi S et al (1998) Preoperative staging of endometrial carcinoma: diagnostic effect of T2-weighted fast spin-echo MR imaging. Radiology 206(2):539–547

52. Seki H, Takano T, Sakai K (2000) Value of dynamic MR imaging in assess-ing endometrial carcinoma involvement of the cervix. AJR Am J Roentgenol 175(1):171–176

53. Tsili AC et al (2008) Local staging of endometrial carcinoma: role of multidetector CT. Eur Radiol 18(5):1043–1048

54. Walsh JW, Goplerud DR (1982) Computed tomography of primary, persis-tent, and recurrent endometrial malignancy. AJR Am J Roentgenol 139(6): 1149–1154

55. Neven P (1993) Tamoxifen and endometrial lesions. Lancet 342(8869): 452

56. McGonigle KF et al (1998) Abnormalities detected on transvaginal ultrasonography in tamoxifen-treated postmenopausal breast cancer patients may represent endometrial cystic atrophy. Am J Obstet Gynecol 178(6): 1145–1150

57. Goldstein SR (1994) Unusual ultrasonographic appearance of the uterus in patients receiving tamoxifen. Am J Obstet Gynecol 170(2):447–451

58. Achiron R et al (1995) Sonohysterography for ultrasonographic evaluation of tamoxifen-associated cystic thickened endometrium. J Ultrasound Med 14(9):685–688

59. van Leeuwen FE et al (1994) Risk of endometrial cancer after tamoxifen treatment of breast cancer. Lancet 343(8895):448–452

60. Lahti E et al (1993) Endometrial changes in postmenopausal breast cancer patients receiving tamoxifen. Obstet Gynecol 81(5 (Pt 1)):660–664

61. Cheng WF et al (1997) Comparison of endometrial changes among symptomatic tamoxifen-treated and nontreated premenopausal and postmenopausal breast cancer patients. Gynecol Oncol 66(2):233–237

62. Kedar RP et al (1994) Effects of tamoxifen on uterus and ovaries of postmenopausal women in a randomised breast cancer prevention trial. Lancet 343(8909):1318–1321

Anatomy and Histology of the Uterus Body

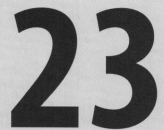

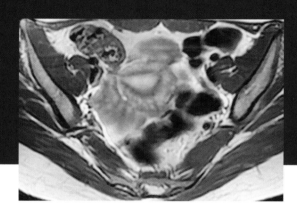

Contents

23.1 Anatomy [1]

The body of the uterus forms the upper two-thirds of the uterus. It is pear shaped, while the cervix is narrower and is cylindrical in shape. The adult nonpregnant uterus is about 7 cm length, 5 cm in breath, and 3 cm thick.

The body of the uterus extends from the fundus at its uppermost part to the cervix inferiorly. Near its upper end, it receives on both sides the uterine tubes. The point of fusion between the uterine tube and body is called the uterine cornu.

Infero-posterior to the cornu is the ovarian ligament. Infero-anterior to the cornu is the round ligament (see Chap. 2). In fact these two structures are in continuity in the embryo and are both derivates from the gubernaculum.

The fundus is covered by peritoneum, which is continuous with that of anterior and posterior surfaces. The lateral margins of the body are convex, and on each side their peritoneum is reflected laterally to form the broad ligament (See Chap. 2).

The peritoneum of the anterior surface is reflected onto the bladder at the uterovesical fold.

The peritoneum of the posterior surface continues down to cover the cervix, and the upper vagina then is reflected back to cover the rectum along the surface of the Douglas.

J.N. Buy, M. Ghossain, *Gynecological Imaging*,
DOI 10.1007/978-3-642-31012-6_23, © Springer-Verlag Berlin Heidelberg 2013

23.2 Structure of the Myometrium [2]

The body of the uterus from outside to inside has three layers (Fig. 23.1):

1. Serosa: it comprises mesothelium and its conjunctive-elastic tissue
2. Muscularis: the myometrium

3. Mucosal layer: the endometrium (see Chap. 21)

The muscularis of the body comprises from outside to inside three different layers (Figs. 23.1 and 23.2).

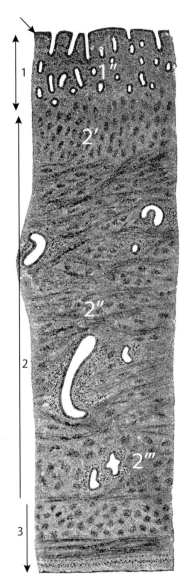

Fig. 23.1 Vertical section of the uterine wall close to the fundus. *1* endometrium: *1″* surface epithelium (*small oblique arrow*), *1″* glands and stroma, *2* muscularis: *2′* inner layer, *2″* middle layer, *2″* outer layer, *3* serosa: mesothelium and its conjunctive layer (From Testut [2])

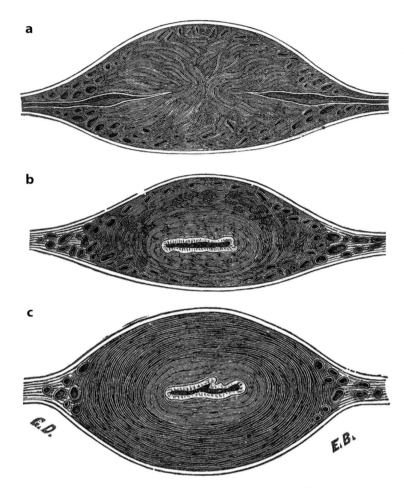

Fig. 23.2 Anatomic constitution of the uterine wall on transverse section of the uterus (the anterior face is at the inferior part of the figure). (**a**) Through the superior portion of the body, at the level of the tubal orifices. (**b**) Through the middle part of the body. (**c**) At the middle part of the cervix (From Testut [2])

23.2.1 The Outer Layer

The outer layer (Fig. 23.3) comprises outer longitudinal fibers and immediately beneath them transverse fibers.

(a) Longitudinal Fibers. They form a flattened fascicle of 10–25 mm width, which occupies the midline of the uterus on its anterior face, on the fundus, and on the posterior face, with a horseshoe shape. This fascicle goes down a little lower on the posterior surface of the uterus until its middle third of the cervix, while on its anterior surface, it stops at the junction of the body and the cervix.

This fascicle is constituted initially on the anterior face as on the posterior face by fibers initially transverse that arise from the lateral parts of the uterus and then straighten up to become vertical.

When they arrive on the fundus of the uterus, the fibers follow a double direction. Some pass directly from the anterior face onto the posterior face and vice versa. The other ones bend outside to become transverse to make one's way to the orifices of the tubes. Among these ones, some cross the midline and draw an elongated Z.

(b) Transverse fibers immediately beneath the previous ones form a regular and continuous plane all over the length of the uterus. On the lateral borders of the uterus:

- Some curve to pass from the anterior face to the posterior face of the uterus; they are crossed by numerous arteries and veins forming around them round or elliptical rings.
- The other go beyond the limits of the organ, disappear in the thickness of the broad ligament, where they constitute the muscular fascicles of the broad ligament, the round ligament, the utero-ovarian ligament, the external layer of the muscularis of the tube.

Transverse fibers go on the cervix. They follow a direction slightly oblique inward and downward. They share some connections in front with bladder fibers. Backward they constitute the uterosacral ligaments. Downward they go on with the muscularis layer of the vagina.

23.2.2 The Middle Layer

The middle layer (Fig. 23.4) is the thickest one, representing half of the thickness of the muscular layer. It is constituted by bundles of muscular fibers that intersect in all the directions and are called for that reason plexiform. What characterizes this layer is the presence in the meshes which circumscribe these bundles of numerous venous channels called uterine sinuses; for that reason, this layer has be called stratum vasculosum. The wall of these sinuses is often reduced to the endothelial layer, which is strongly adherent to the muscular fascicles.

This layer belongs exclusively to the body of the uterus and does not exist in the cervix.

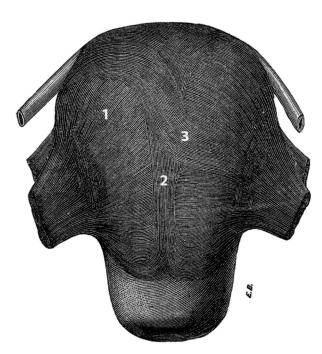

Fig. 23.3 Anterior view of the uterus: muscularis outer layer. *1* transverse fibers, *2* longitudinal fibers, *3* fascicle with a Z shape (From Testut [2])

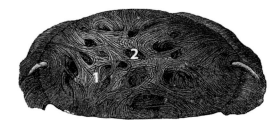

Fig. 23.4 Muscularis middle layer. *1* plexiform bundles, *2* circular or elliptic intervals occupied by uterine sinuses (From Testut [2])

23.2.3 The Inner Layer

The structure of this layer (Fig. 23.5) is very similar to the external layer, except fibers do not go beyond the limits of the organ. It comprises longitudinal fibers immediately beneath the endometrium and outer layer of transverse fibers.

23.2.3.1 Longitudinal Fibers

There are two fascicles of muscular fibers with a longitudinal direction and a triangular shape, the base of which is directed from a tube to the other. As for the external layer, the fibers initially transverse bend close to the midline to become longitudinal some of them bend again to become transversal and join the opposite side of the uterus with a Z shape.

The base of the longitudinal fascicles is the fundus of the uterus. The fibers with a transverse direction very likely constitute the inner longitudinal fibers of the tube.

23.2.3.2 Transverse Fibers

There are two types.
Circular transverse fibers: They pass from one side to the other one and from one face to the other one.
Concentric transverse fibers: At the angles of the body of the uterus, they form concentric rings (Fig. 23.5), the smallest ones surrounding the internal orifice of the tube, while the greatest

ones go until the midline to lean against those of the opposite side. These fibers form at the junction of the body and the cervix a thick ring called the sphincter of the isthmus.

These two types of longitudinal and transverse fibers that constitute the inner muscular layer of the body go on the cervix.

The longitudinal fibers form two median bundles with lateral oblique ramifications, which raise the mucosa and determine the formation of "arbres de vie," which usually stop 6–7 mm above the external cervical os.

The circular fibers form a thick and regular layer that occupies the entire cervix.

23.3 Vascular Supply and Lymphatic Drainage [1, 2]

23.3.1 Arteries

The uterine artery arises as a branch of the anterior division of the internal iliac artery most often of a common trunk with the umbilical artery.

- The artery is lateral to the parietal peritoneum behind the posterior leaf of the broad ligament. The ureter crosses its medial border then goes behind the artery.
- The transverse segment is in the broad ligament roughly at the level of the isthmus. The ureter crosses the inferior border of the artery usually 2 cm lateral to the cervix (Fig. 23.6).
- One major branch ascends tortuously along the lateral border of the body of the uterus within the broad ligament. It gives off the artery to the fundus then goes laterally until it reaches the region of the ovarian hilum where its anastomoses with branches of the ovarian artery. Another branch descends to supply the cervix and anastomoses with branches of the vaginal artery.

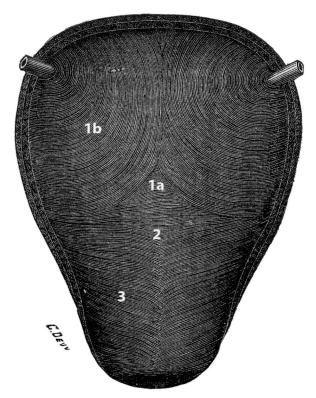

Fig. 23.5 Anterior view of the muscularis inner layer. *1* uterus body: (**a**) transverse circular fibers (**b**) transverse concentric fibers, *2* isthmus: circular bundles, *3* cervix: circular bundles (From Testut [2])

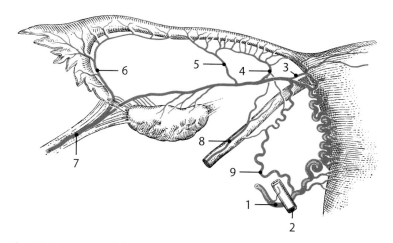

Fig. 23.6 Arteries of the uterus, ovary and tube (Posterior view). *1* uterine artery, *2* ureter, *3* artery of the fundus, *4* medial tubal artery, *5* middle tubal artery, *6* lateral tubal artery, *7* ovarian artery, *8* artery of the round ligament, *9* anastomosis between the uterine artery and its end (From Testut [2])

Each uterine artery gives off numerous branches. These enter the uterine wall, divide and run circumferentially as groups of anterior and posterior actuate arteries. They ramify and narrow as they approach the anterior and posterior midline. The right and left arterial trees anastomose across the midline.

The arcuate arteries supply many tortuous radial branches, which pass through the deeper myomertrial layers. Terminal branches in the myometrium are called helicine arteries, which pass into the endometrium. They also form subendometrual arcuate vessels (see Fig. 21.1).

23.3.2 Veins

The venous drainage is via the uterine veins.

23.3.3 Lymphatic Drainage

- Upper part of the fundus and uterine tubes drain into lateral aortic nodes
- Lower part of the uterus body drains into external iliac nodes

23.4 Histology [3]

The myometrium is composed of smooth muscle cells surrounded by an extracellular matrix of collagen and elastin. The smooth muscle cells are spindled, with blunt-end cigar-shaped elongated nuclei. The volume of the cytoplasm is variable, ranging from 20 μm in nongravid state to 600 μm in the term uterus.

23.5 Radioanatomy of the Myometrium

23.5.1 Ultrasound

On EVS, the landmark between the basal layer of the hyperechoic endometrium and the low echogenic myometrium is clearly displayed. The inner layer of the myometrium, called the junctional zone, is sometimes displayed as a hypointense band compared to the outer myometrium (Fig. 23.7).

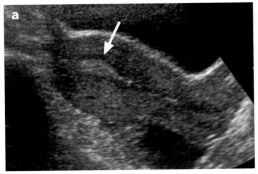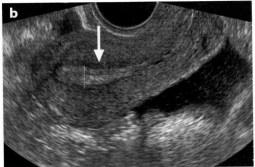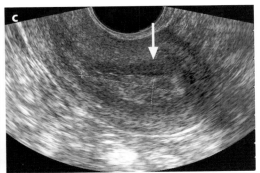

Fig. 23.7 Junctional zone on ultrasound. (**a**, **b**) Trans-abdominal (**a**) and transvaginal (**b**) ultrasound in a patient with otherwise proved ectopic pregnancy show a 7 mm thickness hyperechoic endometrium (*cursors* in **b**) and a well-delineated hypoechoic junctional zone (*arrows*). (**c**) Transvaginal ultrasound in a patient with a proved endometrial polyp (*cursors*) shows a retroverted uterus with a well-delineated hypoechoic junctional zone (*arrow*)

23.5.2 MR

On T2, a clear landmark is displayed between the endometrium which appears with a signal close to urine and the inner part of the myometrium which has a signal close to pelvic muscles.

In the myometrium, the three different layers described by *TESTUT* [2] are clearly depicted (Figs. 23.8 and 23.9).

The inner layer called in MR the junctional zone usually represents roughly the inner third of the myometrium. The middle layer appears with a higher signal comprised between pelvic muscles and urine, the outer layer appears with a low signal as the inner layer but is often more difficult to depict. It has been mentioned that the outer layer becomes of high signal intensity in the mid-secretory phase because of the increased vascularity and prominence of the subserous arcuate vessels.

On DMR at the arterial phase, subendometrial and subserous arteries are visualized (Figs. 23.8 and 23.9).

At the venous phase, high contrast uptake in the venous sinuses of the middle layer is depicted.

On the delayed phase, contrast uptake is about the same in the three different layers and separation between them is no longer established.

The junctional zone on T2 and the inner band on DMR are not always well delineated and sometimes not seen. These anatomical landmarks may help evaluating extension of uterine lesions. The low enhancement of the endometrium on the early phases of DMR is very helpful to detect small endocavitary lesions such as small polyps or submucous leiomyoma.

23.5.3 Contractions

Uterine contractions, frequent in the second part of the cycle, result in hypointense areas than can simulate on MR adenomyosis if irregular or myomas if regular (Fig. 23.10). Bulging may be present.

Diagnosis may be made by comparison to another examination or another sequence during the same examination [4, 5].

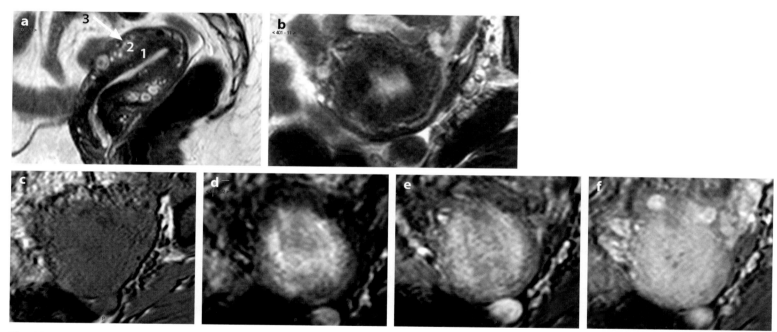

Fig. 23.8 Anatomy of the muscularis of the body of the uterus. (a, b) Sagittal (**a**) and axial T2 (**b**) show the three layer of the myometrium: inner layer (*1*), middle layer (*2*), and outer layer (*3*). (**c, f**) DMR without injection (**c**) and at the arterial phase (**d**) displays subendometrial arterial vessels and some subserous arterial vessels. At the venous phase (**e**), a high contrast uptake is depicted in the venous sinuses of the plexiform muscularis. On the delayed phase (**f**), contrast uptake in the three different layers is about the same so that differentiation between them is no longer possible

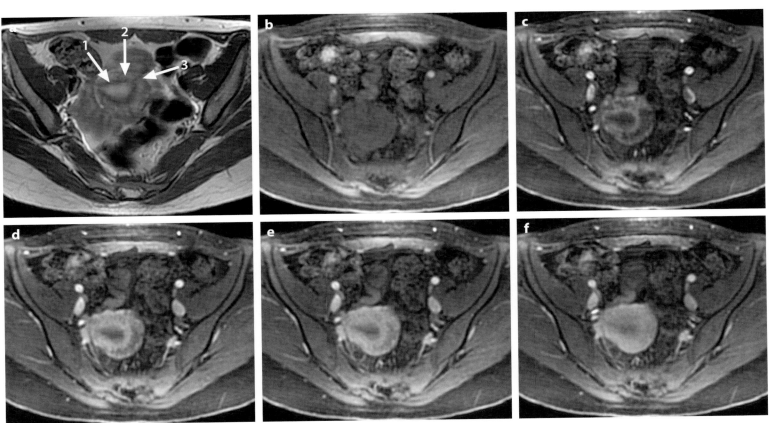

Fig. 23.9 Normal uterine zonal anatomy at T2 and DMR. (a) On axial T2WI, the three layers of the myometrium are depicted. The inner layer or junctional zone (*1*) appears hypointense compared to the middle layer (*2*). The outer hypointense layer (*3*) is more difficult to depict. The endometrium appears hyperintense. (b–f) DMR before (b) and 25 (c), 70 (d), 125 (e) and 240 (f) seconds after injection. At the arterial phase, subendometrial and subserous arcuate vessels enhance delimiting the inner layer (junctional zone) and outer layer of the uterus. The middle layer is mainly hypointense compared to the inner and outer layers. On subsequent phases, the middle layers enhance progressively and heterogeneously to become almost isointense with the remaining of the myometrium on the delayed phase. The endometrium enhances poorly at the early phases to become almost isointense with the myometrium on the late phase

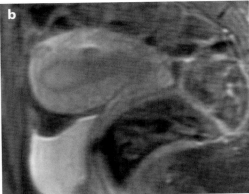

Fig. 23.10 Uterine contraction simulating myoma in a 21-year-old woman in the second part of her menstrual cycle. (a) T2W sagittal image shows a 25×15 mm roughly well-delineated posterior area of the myometrium suggesting a myoma (*arrow*). (b) Sagittal delayed T1FS after injection at the end of the examination shows homogeneous myometrium and disappearance of the bulging in the endometrium confirming it was a contraction. Comparison with a previous MRI performed 3 months earlier showed also that the myometrium was normal

References

1. Standring S (ed) (2005) Gray, anatomy. The anatomical basis of clinical practice, 39th edn. Elsevier/Churchill Livingstone, Edinburgh/New York, pp 1331–1338, Chap. 104
2. Testut L (1931) Appareil urogenital, peritoine. In: Latarget A Traité d'anatomie humaine. 8th edn. revue par. G Doin et Cie Editeurs, Paris, pp 1–595
3. Sternberg SS (1992) Histology for pathologists. Raven, New York
4. Togashi K, Kawakami S, Kimura I, Asato R, Takakura K, Mori T, Konishi J (1993) Sustained uterine contractions: a cause of hypointense myometrial bulging. Radiology 187(3):707–710
5. Togashi K, Kawakami S, Kimura I, Asato R, Okumura R, Fukuoka M, Mori T, Konishi JJ (1993) Uterine contractions: possible diagnostic pitfall at MR imaging. Magn Reson Imaging 3(6):889–893

Benign and Malignant Mesenchymal Tumors of the Uterus

24

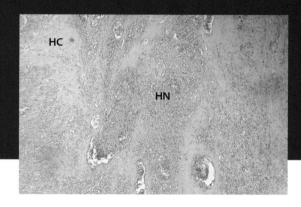

Contents

24.1 Introduction

24.1.1 Embryologic Definition of Mesenchyme

1. At the beginning of the third week, an opacity formed by a thickened linear band of epiblast – the primitive streak – appears caudally in the median plane of the dorsal aspect of the embryonic disc.
2. Shortly after the primitive streak appears, cells leave its deep surface and form mesenchyme, a tissue consisting of loosely arranged cells suspended in a gelatinous matrix. Mesenchymal cells are ameboid and actively phagocytic.
3. Mesenchyme forms the supporting tissues of the embryo, such as most of the connective tissues of the body and connective tissue framework of glands.

Some mesenchyme forms mesoblast (undifferentiated mesoderm) which forms the intraembryonic or embryonic mesoderm.

This chapter considers neoplasms of the uterus in which there is mesenchymal differentiation:

Either pure such as those derived from smooth muscle and endometrial stroma, or associated with epithelial elements such as adenofibroma and adenosarcoma.

The capacity of neoplasms arising in the uterus to form heterologous mesenchymal elements is a reflection of the potentiality of the uterine primordium, which is formed from an anlage of coelomic lining cells and subjacent mesenchymal cells (see Chap. 1).

Within the mesodermal primordium that is to become the uterus, the mesodermal components distinction between duct epithelium and mesenchyme is lost. The Müllerian duct epithelial cells seem to form part of the mesenchyme accompanying the duct before the formation of the uterus. A distinction between the precursors of the endometrium and myometrium is not possible. Neoplasms that subsequently arise in the uterus may express bipotentiality of their ancestry by forming a mixture of epithelial and mesodermal components.

24.2 Classification

Classification of mesenchymal tumors and diseases are presented in Table 24.1.

Table 24.1 Classification of mesenchymal tumors and diseases

1. **Smooth muscle tumors**
   1.1 Leiomyomas
   General features
   Specific subtypes of leiomyomas
   – Mitotically active leiomyoma
   – Cellular leiomyoma
   – Hemorrhagic cellular leiomyoma
   – Epithelioid leiomyoma
   – Myxoid leiomyoma
   – Vascular leiomyoma
   – Lipoleiomyoma
   Leiomyoma versus leiomyosarcoma
   1.2 Smooth muscle tumors of uncertain malignant potential
   1.3 Leiomyosarcoma
   – Usual leiomyosarcoma, epithelioid leiomyosarcoma, myxoid leiomyosarcoma
   1.4 Other smooth muscle tumors
   – Diffuse leiomyomatosis
   – Intravenous leiomyomatosis
   – Metastasizing leiomyoma
   – Disseminated peritoneal leiomyomatosis
   – Parasitic leiomyoma
2. **Endometrial stromal tumors**
   – Endometrial stromal sarcoma
   – Endometrial stromal nodule
3. **Miscellaneous mesenchymal tumors**
   – Homologous and heterologous sarcomas
   – Primitive neuroectodermal tumors (PNET)
   – Vascular tumors
   – Lymphoma
4. **Adenomyosis, adenomyoma, and adenomyotic cyst**

24.3 Smooth Muscle Tumors

24.3.1 Leiomyomas

24.3.1.1 General Features

Clinical Findings

1. Most leiomyomas are detected in middle-aged women.
   They are uncommon in women less than 30 years of age except in black women.

2. Their growth is affected by their hormonal milieu [1] because they contain estrogen and progesterone receptors. They may increase in size during estrogen therapy, and most decrease in size with GnRH agonist.
   Progestins, progesterone, hormonal replacement therapy, and pregnancy occasionally are associated with a rapid increase in size of leiomyomas.
   Some shrink after menopause.

3. Clinical findings depend on their location (body or cervix; interstitial/intramural, submucosal, or subserous) and on their size.
   Most are asymptomatic but may cause pain, a sensation of pressure, or abnormal uterine bleeding.
   Large tumors can produce uterine enlargement or an irregular uterine contour.
   Submucosal leiomyomas, even small ones, can cause uterine bleeding due to compression of the overlying endometrium and compromise of its vascular supply.
   Subserous leiomyomas can be sessile or pedunculated and can be confused with an adnexal mass. Rarely, pedunculated leiomyoma can undergo torsion.

Pathology

Macroscopy

They are multiple in two-thirds of cases [2].

They are spherical bulges above the surrounding myometrium from which they are easily shelled out.

Intramural leiomyomas are the most frequent.

Submucosal leiomyomas are frequently ulcerated and hemorrhagic.

Subserous leiomyomas can be sessile or pedunculated.

Microscopy

Leiomyomas are composed of whorled, anastomosing fascicles of uniform smooth muscle cells. Most are more cellular than the surrounding myometrium.

Degenerative changes are frequent:
- Hyaline fibrosis in more than 60%, particularly in postmenopausal women.
- Edema in 50% of cases.
- Hemorrhage in 10% of cases; zonal and sharply demarcated.
- Cystic in 4% of cases.
- Calcification in 4% of cases.

Most of the leiomyomas are developed in the uterus body. Uncommonly there are leiomyomas of the cervix. Exceptionally, submucosal leiomyomas can extend into the cervix and even protrude into the external cervical os (Fig. 24.1).

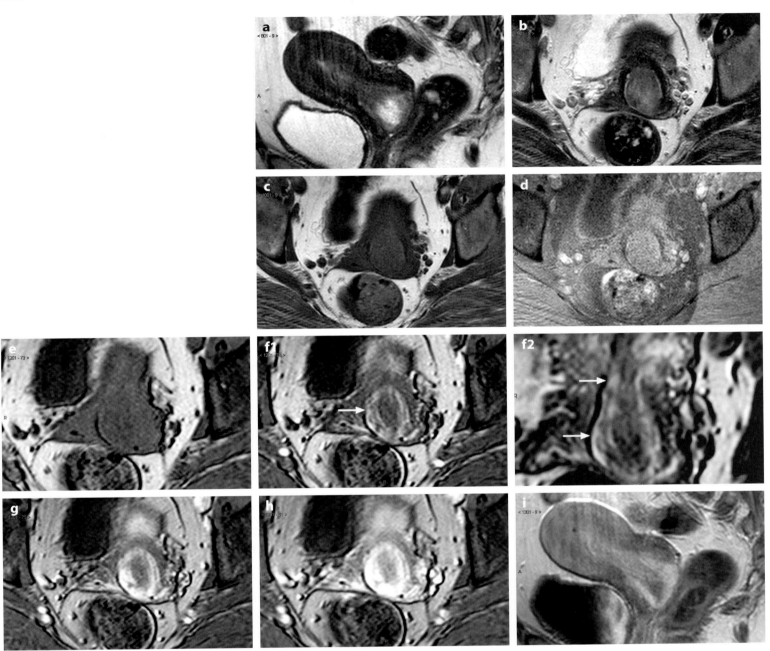

Fig. 24.1 Submucosal leiomyoma of the uterine body protruding into the cervix until the external cervical os. Fifty-year-old woman with metrorrhagias. (**a, b**) MR sagittal (**a**) and axial T2 (**b**) display an endometrial mass with regular contour extending into the internal cervical os and protruding through the external cervical os. The mass is of intermediate signal in its upper two-thirds, while the lower portion is of high signal. (**c, d**) Axial T1 (**c**) and fat suppression (**d**) do not demonstrate any hemorrhage in the mass. (**e–i**) DMR without injection (**e**) and at the arterial phase without (**f1**) and with MIP reconstruction in the coronal plan of the uterus (**f2**) demonstrates peripheral arterial vessels (*arrows*) typical for a submucosal leiomyoma, different from the central arterial vascularization of a polyp. At the venous phase (**g**) and on the delayed (**h**), an intense contrast uptake in the peripheral portion characteristic for a leiomyoma is displayed. (**i**) On sagittal T1 after injection, insertion of the leiomyoma on the posterior wall of the endometrial cavity is depicted. Diagnosis at hysteroscopy: polyp inserted on the left lateral portion of the endometrium. Pathology after resection: submucosal endometrial leiomyoma covered with normal endometrium

Ultrasound

Leiomyoma Without Degenerative Changes

On 2D ultrasound, they are well-circumscribed echogenic masses usually with an echogenicity lower than normal myometrium. They often show acoustic shadowing arising within the substance of the leiomyoma (different from shadowing due to calcification). Pathologic correlation showed that these shadows probably originate from interfaces between the margins of smooth muscle whorls and the margins of fibrous connective tissue, and the edges of whorls and bundles of smooth muscle [3]. Sensitivity of this finding is higher for transvaginal (87%) than for transabdominal (52%) ultrasound [4]. This finding is not specific of uterine leiomyoma and can also be encountered in other entities especially in masses containing fibrous tissue (Table 24.2) [4].

Table 24.2 Differential diagnosis of acoustic shadowing due to fibrous tissue in leiomyomas

Uterine
– Adenomyosis
– Sarcomas
Ovarian
– Fibrothecoma
– Brenner tumor
– Ovarian metastases

On color Doppler, regular peripheral vascularization is usually depicted more or less associated with central vascularization.

Leiomyoma with Degenerative Changes

Echogenicity is variable and is usually heterogeneous.

Locations and Differential Diagnosis

It may be useful for surgeons to classify submucosal leiomyomas into three categories [5]:

- Polypoid.
- <50% contained within myometrium.
- >50% contained within myometrium.

3D saline infusion sonohysterography has been suggested to evaluate the proportion of fibroid contained within the endometrial cavity [6]. The main differential diagnosis of leiomyomas according to their location is listed in Table 24.3.

CT

The main findings are increase is size and bulging of the uterus. Difference in contrast between the leiomyoma and the myometrium may be difficult to appreciate even after contrast injection except in case of necrobiosis. Calcifications are useful for the diagnosis and are better visualized than on US, and especially better than on MR (Fig. 24.2).

Table 24.3 Differential diagnosis of uterine leiomyomas according to their location

Submucosal
Benign
– Polyp
– Atypical polypoid adenomyoma
Malignant
– Endometrial carcinoma
– Sarcomas
Interstitial
– Adenomyoma
– Sarcoma
Subserous
Uterine
– Subserous adenomyoma
Ovarian and extra-ovarian masses
– Ovarian carcinoma
– Ovarian fibrothecoma
– Ovarian Brenner tumor
– Ovarian metastases
– Leiomyoma of the broad ligament

MR

Morphologic Findings

Leiomyoma Without Degenerative Changes

They usually appear as hypointense on T2 compared to the normal myometrium. They are also hypointense or isointense to normal myometrium on DWI. Their contrast uptake is variable, less, like, or more than myometrium (Fig. 24.3). On DMR, endocavitary myomas enhance more than normal endometrium at almost all phases (Fig. 24.4).

Leiomyoma with Degenerative Changes
Hyaline Degeneration

- High-intensity areas on T2, with enhancement on T1 after contrast injection (Figs. 24.5 and 24.6).

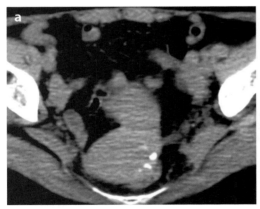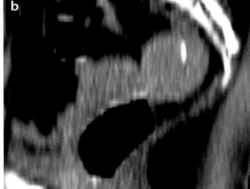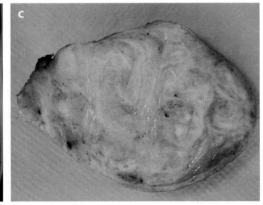

Fig. 24.2 Pedunculated calcified leiomyoma. Pelvic mass in a 75-year-old woman. (**a**) Axial CT view without IV contrast injection shows a calcified mass posterior to the uterus. (**b**) Sagittal reformation clearly shows the mass arising from the uterus typical of a subserous leiomyoma. At surgery, a pedunculated calcified leiomyoma was excised. (**c**) View of the surgical specimen

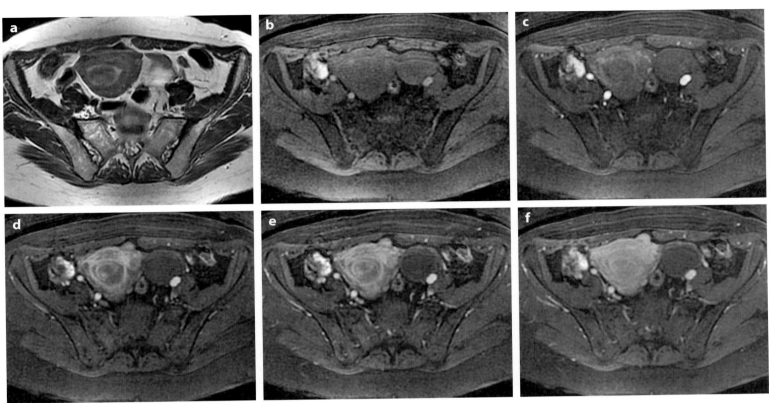

Fig. 24.3 Endocavitary leiomyoma at T2 and DMR. (a) On axial T2W image, an endocavitary lesion, hypointense compared to normal endometrium, with an intensity close to myometrium is seen. **(b–f)**. On DMR before **(b)** and 25, 75, 125, and 240 s after injection, the lesion shows enhancement superior to that of endometrium and close to that of myometrium. At early phases, the center of the tumor enhances heterogeneously with a peripheral enhancing rim like the inner band of the myometrium

Fig. 24.4 Difference of contrast enhancement between endocavitary myomas and normal endometrium. On DMR, with sequences performed before and 25, 70, 125, and 240 s after injection, contrast enhancement in myomas is superior to that of normal endometrium with no overlap at most phases. *Blue line*: signal intensity of normal endometrium minus signal intensity of normal endometrium in the same patient (flat curve = 0). *Mauve lines*: signal intensity of myoma minus signal intensity of normal endometrium in the same patient (mean, minimal and maximal). Materials: 13 patients (author's personal series). *Teaching points*. On DMR, endocavitary myomas enhance more than normal endometrium at almost all phases

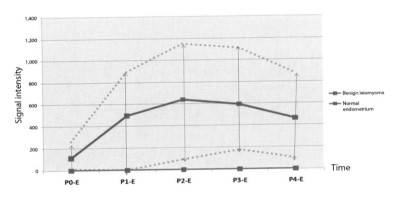

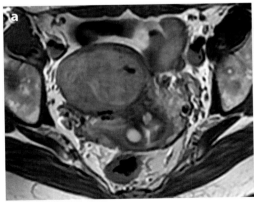
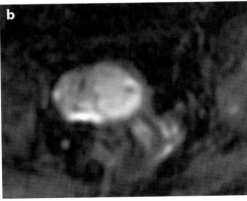
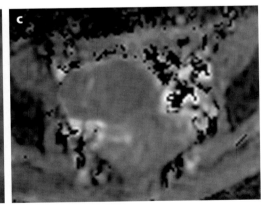

Fig. 24.5 Benign myoma hyperintense on DWI in a 37-year-old woman. (a) Axial T2-weighted image shows a 6.6-cm myoma, hyperintense compared to the normal myometrium, that has increased in size rapidly compared to a previous ultrasound. **(b, c)** DWI b1000 **(b)** with corresponding ADC map **(c)** shows that the myoma is hyperintense on DWI with an ADC of 0.9×10^{-3} mm^2/s in left part of the tumor and 1.1×10^{-3} mm^2/s in the right part of the tumor.

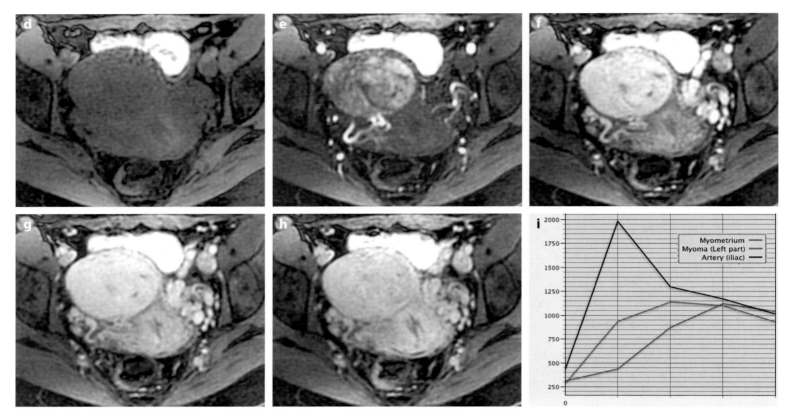

Fig. 24.5 (*continued*) (**d–i**) Dynamic MRI before injection (**d**) and 25, 70, 125, and 240 s (**d–h**) after injection with corresponding time-intensity curves (**i**) shows at the arterial phase areas of rapid contrast uptake in the left part of the leiomyoma superior to that of the myometrium, with equivalent uptake at the late phase. In the right part of the leiomyoma, contrast uptake was close to that of normal myometrium. The association in the left part of the leiomyoma of a higher signal intensity than the myometrium on T2WI, a high signal intensity on DWI, a low ADC value, and a rapid contrast uptake at the arterial phase raised the possibility of a sarcoma or cellular myoma. The patient refused hysterectomy. Transvaginal biopsy in the left part of the tumor showed no malignant tissue. Follow-up was decided

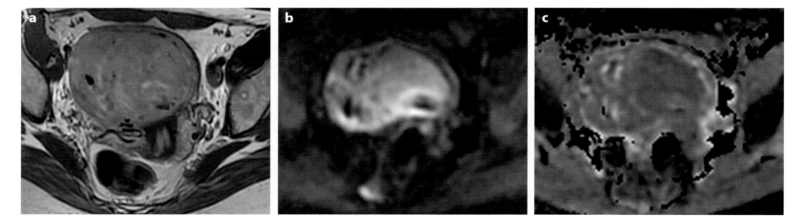

Fig. 24.6 Follow-up of a leiomyoma hyperintense on DWI in a 37-year-old woman (same patient as Fig. 24.5). (**a**) Axial T2-weighted image shows a 9.5-cm myoma, hyperintense compared to the normal myometrium, that has increased in size since the last MRI, 9 months ago, where it measured 6.6 cm. (**b, c**) DWI b1000 (**b**) with corresponding ADC map (**c**) shows that the myoma is still hyperintense on DWI with ADC values that have increased since the last examination: 1.05 (range 0.8–1.0) instead of 0.9×10^{-3} mm²/s in left part of the tumor and 1.5 instead of 1.1×10^{-3} mm²/s in the right part of the tumor

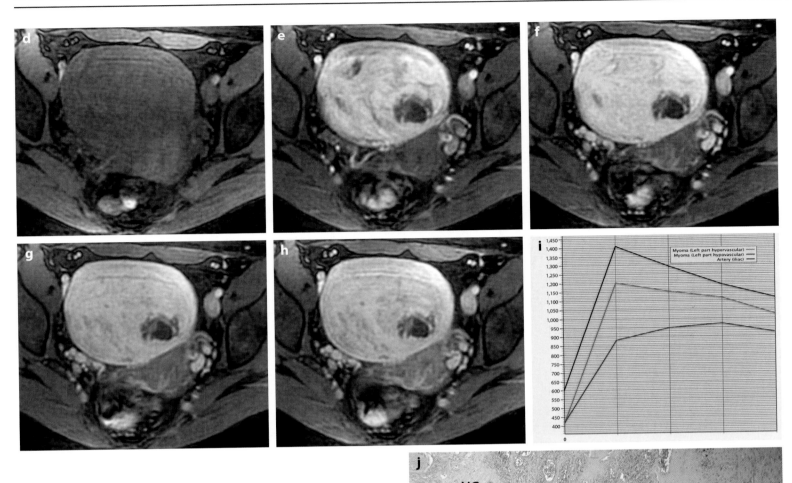

Fig. 24.6 (*continued*) (**d–i**) Dynamic MRI before injection (**d**) and 25, 70, 125, and 240 s (**e–h**) after injection with corresponding time-intensity curves (**i**) still shows rapid contrast uptake at the arterial phase in the left part of the leiomyoma compared to the right part with appearance of areas of necrosis in both parts of the tumor. The patient's wish was conservative surgery. A repeated transvaginal biopsy showed absence of malignant tissue. Myomectomy was then performed. (**j**) Histology showed benign leiomyoma with intermixed hyaline changes (*HC*) and hemorrhagic necrosis (*HN*)

Edema
- Slightly high signal intensity on T2 with enhancement on T1 after contrast injection.

Red Degeneration (Hemorrhagic Necrosis)
- May or may not show high signal intensity on T1 (Fig. 24.6); absence of enhancement in the necrotic areas.
- It is caused by venous thrombosis. Most of them occur during pregnancy.

Cystic Degeneration
- High signal intensity, well-delineated areas on T2 with no enhancement on T1 after injection (Figs. 24.7 and 24.8).
- It may be difficult to differentiate them from pockets of necrotic areas, frequently observed within hemorrhagic degeneration and uterine sarcomas [7].

Necrotic areas are usually but not always less well circumscribed.

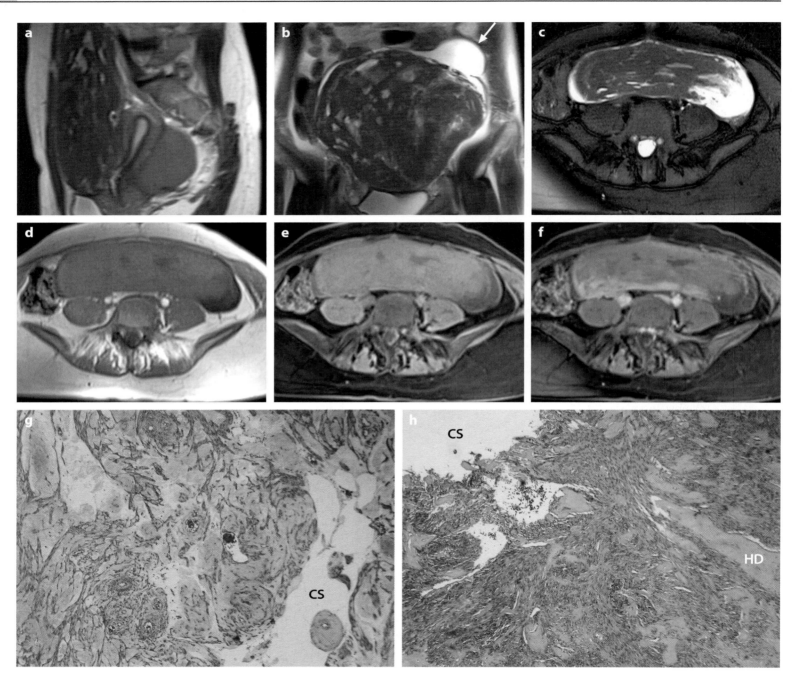

Fig. 24.7 Leiomyoma with cystic degeneration in a 48-year-old woman.
(**a, b**) Sagittal (**a**) and coronal (**b**) T2W images show a huge subserous anterior leiomyoma measuring 17 cm in height, 7 cm anteroposteriorly, and
20 cm transversely. The leiomyoma contains small hyperintense cystic
spaces surrounded by hypointense solid tissue and large peripheral hyperintense spaces abutting against the uterine serosa especially in its upper left
part (*arrow* in **b**). A 10-cm mass of intermediate intensity is seen behind the
uterus on the sagittal view corresponding to an endometrioma of the left
ovary. (**c**) Axial T2WFS image shows that the cystic spaces are sometimes

well delineated and sometimes dissecting the smooth muscle fibers of the
leiomyoma. (**d–f**) Axial T1W image (**d**) and T1WFS images before (**e**) and
after (**f**) gadolinium injection show absence of hyperintensity related to
hemorrhage and absence of contrast uptake in the cystic spaces. (**g, h**)
Histology of the surgical specimen revealed benign leiomyoma with hyaline
degeneration (*HD*) and cystic spaces (*CS*) of different size. The cystic spaces
were in continuity with the smooth muscle fibers of the leiomyoma and in
some locations abutting peripherally against the serosa

**Fig. 24.8 Leiomyoma with cystic degeneration and rapid increase in size.
A 31-year-old woman with metrorrhagia.** (**a**) Axial T2W image shows a well-
circumscribed mass (*arrow*) in the left isthmic region containing small cystic
areas. The solid part of the mass has an intermediate intensity close to that of
peripheral myometrium with a peripheral hypointense rim. Hypointense
rims surround also most of the small cavities. Some of these cavities were
hyperintense on T1 and T1FS images indicating their hemorrhagic nature.
(**b**) On DWI, the mass is hyperintense with an ADC value of 1.6 in the solid
portions (mean values at b500 and b1000). (**c–e**) DMR at early phase before
opacification of the uterus (**c**), at the venous phase (**d**), and following
phases with corresponding time-intensity curves (**e**) shows before uterus

opacification a spontaneous hyperintense hemorrhagic cystic space (*arrow*
in **c**) and after opacification a well-circumscribed mass that enhances slightly
less than myometrium. (**f, g**) Fourteen months later, MRI was performed after
miscarriage. Sagittal T2W (**f**) and corresponding (**g**) T1WFS delayed sequence
after injection showed huge increase of the mass which contains some cystic changes. Transvaginal biopsy was performed and concluded to a benign
leiomyoma. Patient refused hysterectomy, and embolization was performed
in another institution. It was followed by severe metrorrhagia. (**h, i**) Repeated
MRI with sagittal T2W (**h**) and corresponding (**i**) T1WFS showed necrosis of
the majority of the mass. Laparotomy followed by hysterectomy was performed. (**j**) Histology showed areas of necrosis and cystic changes

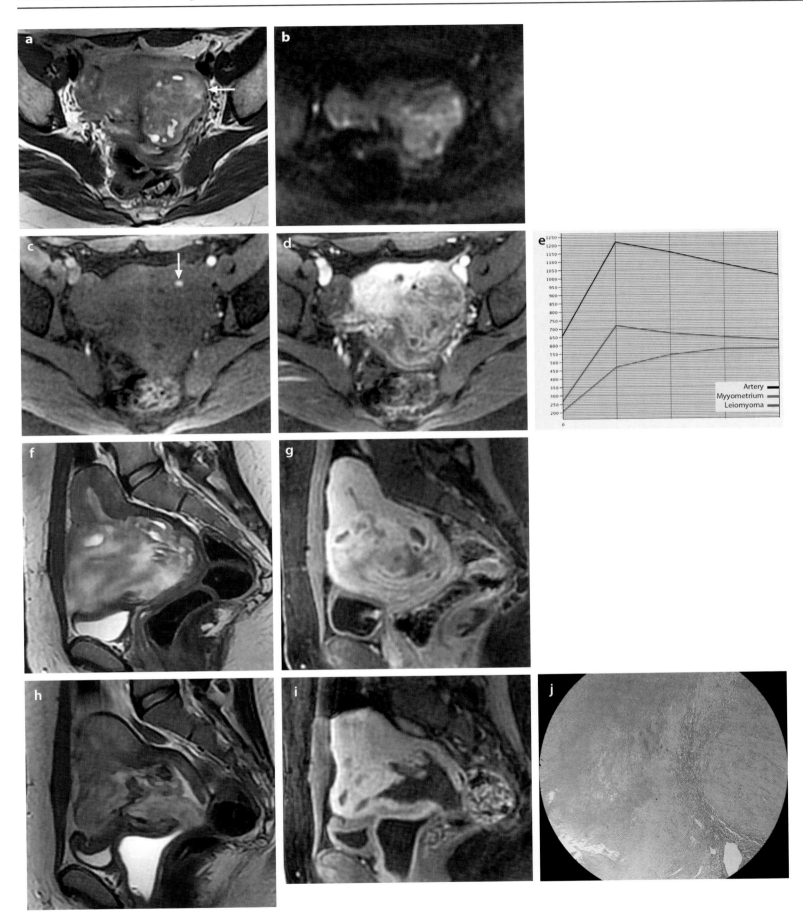

Calcifications

Calcifications are often missed on MR and visualized at best on CT. They appear as hypointense areas on all sequences. If a subserous leiomyoma is calcified, care must be taken not to confuse it with a bowel loop.

Necrobiosis

The diagnosis is made on absence of contrast enhancement in the tumor except for a peripheral rim (Figs. 24.9 and 24.10). On T1 with and without fat suppression, they are entirely or partly hyperintense. On T2, their intensity is variable being hypointense, hyperintense, or heterogeneous.

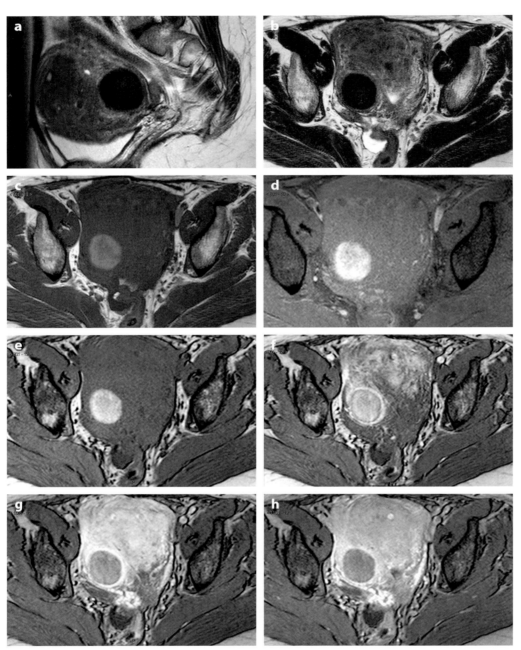

Fig. 24.9 Myoma with hemorrhagic necrosis. (**a, b**) Sagittal and axial T2W images in a patient with leiomyomatosis, and multiple leiomyomas show a well-delineated, right-located interstitial hypointense leiomyoma. (**c, d**) Axial T1W images without (**c**) and with (**d**) fat suppression show the leiomyoma to be hyperintense related to hemorrhage. (**e–h**) DMR before injection (**e**), at the arterial phase (**f**), at the venous phase (**g**), and at the late phase (**h**) shows the wall of the leiomyoma as a peripheral enhancing rim since the arterial phase. Otherwise, no contrast uptake is detected in the hyperintense necrotic and hemorrhagic leiomyoma

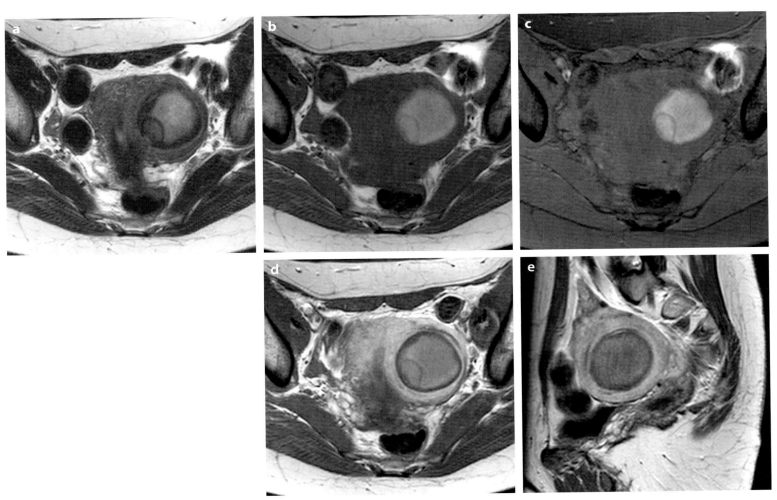

Fig. 24.10 Leiomyoma with necrobiosis. A 44-year-old woman with sudden pelvic pain and contractions. (**a**) Axial T2W image shows a left 5-cm leiomyoma with a central high intensity zone and a hypointense periphery. A pseudoloculation is present in the medial and posterior part of the myoma. (**b**, **c**) Axial T1W (**b**) and T1W-SPIR image (**c**) shows a central large part of the myoma to be hyperintense related to hemorrhagic necrosis. (**d**, **e**) Axial (**d**) and sagittal (**e**) T1W images after gadolinium injection show the myoma to be composed of a central hyperintense nonenhancing portion, a peripheral nonenhancing hypointense rim and a thin peripheral enhancing rim best seen on sagittal view. The wall of the pseudoloculation is not enhancing related to necrotic tissue or fibrin

Vascular Findings

Flow Voids

Flow voids appear as hypointense structures at the interface between the leiomyoma and the myometrium. This sign probably corresponds to dilated feeding arteries with fast flow located outside the capsule of the leiomyoma [8].

In Torashima et al.'s series [8], they were seen more commonly on T1 than on T2, exclusively in leiomyomas >3 cm and in 87% of leiomyomas >7 cm, mainly in leiomyomas with degenerative changes and in the pedicle of subserous leiomyomas [8].

In their series, this finding was not observed in focal adenomyosis, ovarian fibromas, thecomas, ovarian cancer, Krukenberg tumors, and in one case of dysgerminoma [8].

DMR

Main findings at DMR are [9]:

At the arterial phase: regular circumscribed vessels at the periphery.

At the venous phase: high contrast uptake (equal to polyp) at the periphery and less in the center, less than sarcoma.

At the late phase: peak enhancement (less than sarcoma) is usually seen at 3 min but may be present earlier even at the arterial phase (Fig. 24.6).

24.3.1.2 Specific Subtypes of Leiomyomas

Mitotically Active Leiomyoma

Definition: A mitotically active leiomyoma is a typical-appearing leiomyoma in a premenopausal woman with five or more mitotic figures per ten high-power fields [10].

Leiomyomas removed during the secretory phase of the menstrual cycle have a significantly increased mitotic index compared to those removed during the proliferative phase.

Leiomyomas removed from women who are taking progestin have a higher mitotic rate than women who are taking estrogen and progestin or who are not taking any exogenous hormone.

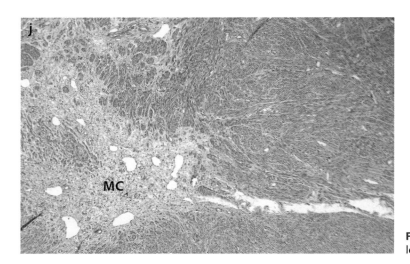

Fig. 24.11 (*continued*) (**j**) Histology showed myxoid changes (*MC*) in both leiomyomas more prominent in the lower one

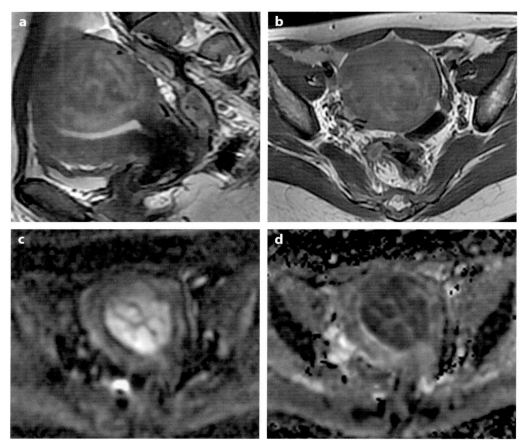

Fig. 24.12 Benign leiomyoma with high intensity on DWI in a 49-year-old woman. (**a, b**) Sagittal T2W image shows a 6-cm posterior myoma slightly more intense than the myometrium. No hyperintensity on T1 (not shown) suggestive of hemorrhage was present. (**c, d**) DWI b1000 (**c**) with corresponding ADC map (**d**) shows that the central part of the myoma is hyperintense on DWI with an ADC of 0.83×10^{-3} mm^2/s.

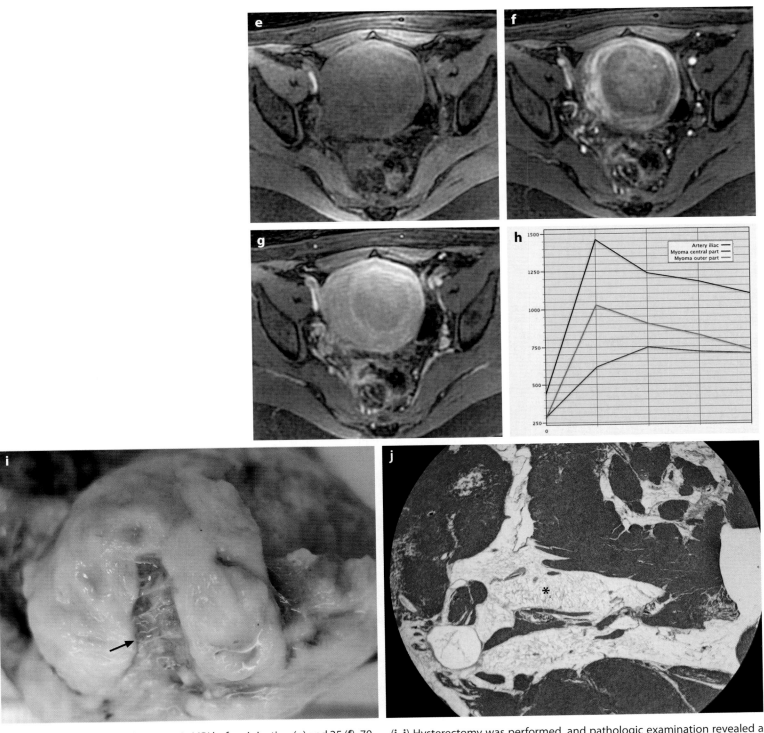

Fig. 24.12 (*continued*) (**e–h**) Dynamic MRI before injection (**e**) and 25 (**f**), 70, 125, and 240 (**g**) seconds after injection with corresponding time-intensity curves (**h**) shows arterial vessels in the outer part of the leiomyoma at the arterial phase with lower contrast uptake in the central part. (**i, j**) Hysterectomy was performed, and pathologic examination revealed a leiomyoma with edematous-myxoid changes (*arrow* in **i** and *asterisk* in **j**) and some hypercellular areas

Vascular Leiomyoma

Definition: It contains numerous large vessels with muscular walls.
Differential diagnosis: Hemangioma, arteriovenous fistula.

Lipoleiomyoma (Fig. 24.13)

Definition: A lipoleiomyoma is a leiomyoma that contains a significant amount of fat.

High signal intensity on T1 with low intensity on fat suppression allows distinguishing fat from blood clot within the tumor.

CT is also diagnostic by easily characterizing fat.

24.3.1.3 Leiomyoma Versus Leiomyosarcoma

One of the most difficult challenges of the radiologists is to differentiate atypical leiomyomas from leiomyosarcomas. If leiomyosarcoma is suspected, hysterectomy is indicated because myomectomy will favor peritoneal spread. This causes an important dilemma in young women seeking pregnancy. Here are presented some examples of these situations.

(a) Intermediate signal leiomyoma, with high signal on diffusion and low ADC (Figs. 24.5 and 24.12).
(b) Leiomyoma with a rapid increase in size (Fig. 24.14).
(c) Leiomyoma with an increase in size, but also with an increase of the ADC (Fig. 24.6).

Some authors found that an intensity superior to myometrium on T2W images associated to an ADC value $<1.05 \times 10^{-3}$ mm^2/s had a sensitivity of 100% and a specificity of 100% in the diagnosis of sarcoma. Some of the above cases show however that such an association can also be present in leiomyomas with myxoid, hyaline, and/or hemorrhagic changes.

Some surgeons have advocated transvaginal biopsy to avoid dissemination, but the efficiency and safety of this method have not been proven (Figs. 24.5 and 24.6).

On the other hand, ADC values $>1.05 \times 10^{-3}$ mm^2/s may be found in leiomyosarcoma (Fig. 24.15).

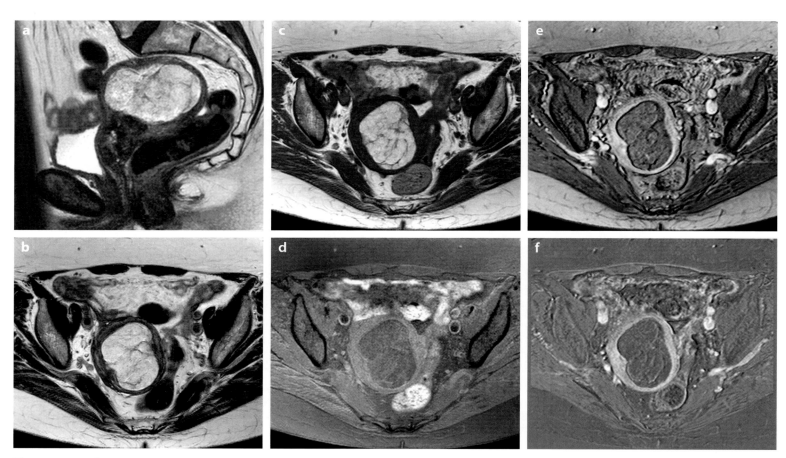

Fig. 24.13 Lipoleiomyoma in a 69-year-old woman. MR sagittal T2 (**a**) and axial T2 (**b**) display a submucosal leiomyoma pushing the endometrium to the right. It has overall high signal intensity, containing septa. On axial T1 (**c**), its signal is identical to adipose tissue and decreases like adipose tissue on fat suppression (**d**). These findings allow making a specific diagnosis of lipoleiomyoma. DMR after injection (**e**) and delayed subtraction (**f**) show small enhancement in the septa without any other significant enhancement ruling out malignancy. Prospective diagnosis: lipoleiomyoma. Pathology confirmed this diagnosis

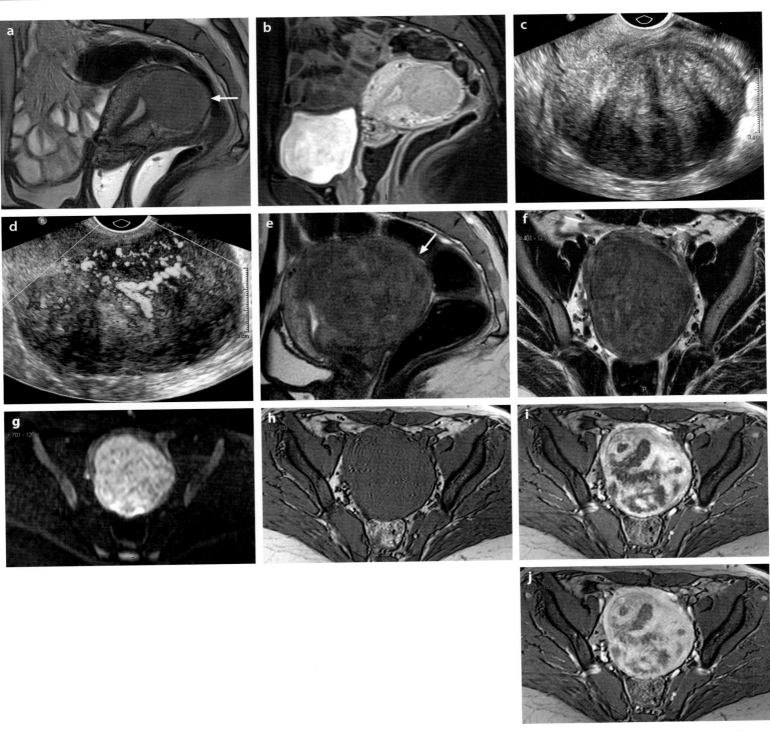

Fig. 24.14 Leiomyoma with rapid and important increase in size versus sarcoma. Thirty-five-year-old woman operated one year before from a posterior leiomyoma through coelioscopy. An incomplete resection was performed. At pathologic examination, the leiomyoma was benign. Five months ago, MR sagittal T2 (**a**) with vaginal and rectal opacification discovers a recurrence of the leiomyoma (*arrow*) that measured 4 cm in diameter. On sagittal T1FS after injection (**b**), homogeneous uptake with no necrosis is visualized. EVS (**c**) displays a unique posterior leiomyoma that has dramatically increased in size with a long axis measuring 9 cm. At Color Doppler (**d**), unusual large vessels are demonstrated in the central part of the mass. On spectral Doppler, the resistive index is 0.60. On MR sagittal T2 (**e**) and axial T2 (**f**), the leiomyoma (*arrow* in **e**) extends from the posterior cervix to the fundus of the uterus; its overall signal is close to pelvic muscle. On T1 and

T1FS (not shown), no hemorrhage is displayed. On b1000 (**g**), signal intensity on the b1000 is superior to normal myometrium; ADC is 1.35×10^{-3} mm²/s. On DMR without injection (**h**), at the arterial phase (**i**), at the venous phase, and on the delayed phase (**j**), a significant contrast uptake is displayed at the arterial phase in some parts of the tumor, while a progressive contrast uptake is seen in portions with degenerative changes. No necrosis was visualized. Prospective diagnosis: while different morphologic and vascular findings were not suggestive of a sarcoma and the value of ADC was not conclusive, the rapid and important increase in size over a short period of time did not allow the ruling out of the possibility of atypical leiomyoma or even a leiomyosarcoma. At pathology, it was in fact a leiomyoma with very few mitoses

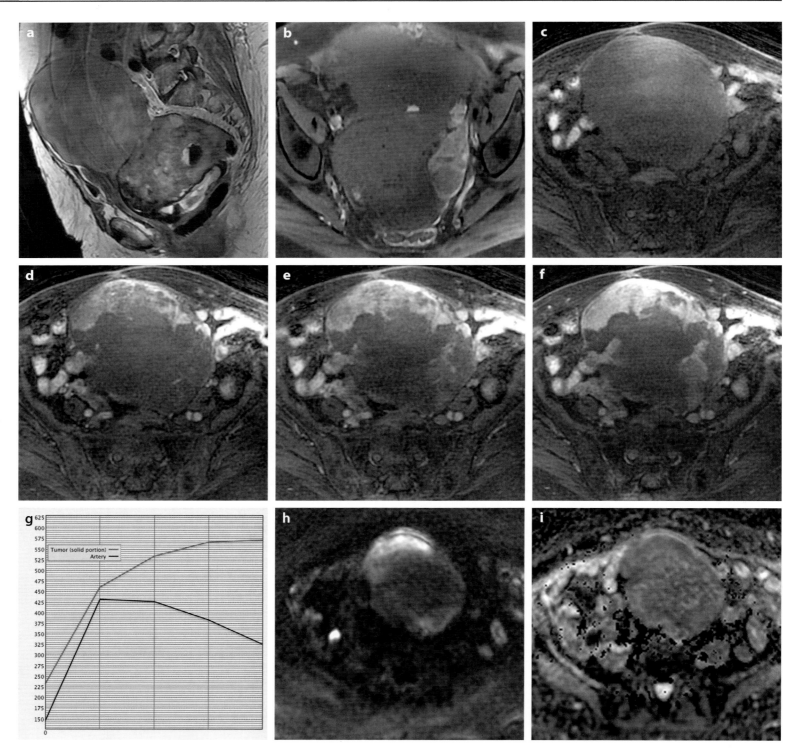

Fig. 24.15 Leiomyosarcoma in a 72-year-old woman. (a) Sagittal T2W image shows an enlarged uterus completely occupied by a huge heterogeneous mass of intermediate intensity containing some cystic structures. (b) Axial T1FSW image through the lower part of the uterus show some hyperintense area related to hemorrhage. Differentiation between solid and necrotic part is not possible in the majority of the tumor on T2- and T1-weighted images. (c–g) DMR before (c), at the arterial phase (d), at the venous phase (e), and at the parenchymal and late phases (f) with corresponding time-intensity curves (g) shows that most of the tumor is necrotic. Uptake in the anterior solid portions is very high since the arterial phase, persisting at the late phases with arterial vessels seen on the arterial phase. (h, i) DWI at b1000 with corresponding ADC map at the same level shows the anterior solid portion to be partially of high intensity on DWI with an ADC value of 1.8×10^{-3} mm²/s (1.3×10^{-3} mm²/s at b500; mean 1.55×10^{-3} mm²/s). At another level, the solid portion was also of high intensity on DWI with an ADC value of 1.3×10^{-3} mm²/s (1.8×10^{-3} mm²/s at b500; mean 1.55×10^{-3} mm²/s). At surgery and pathology, a leiomyosarcoma invading the peritoneum was found. In this case, the morphologic findings of malignancy were obvious, but DWI and ADC values were not helpful for the diagnosis and were even misleading.

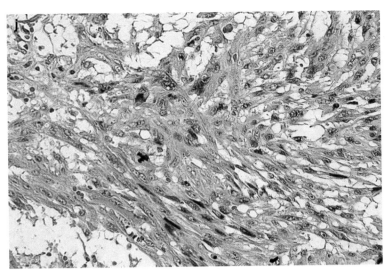

Fig. 24.15 (*continued*) (**j**) Histology of the solid portions showing leiomyosarcomatous cells

24.3.2 Smooth Muscle Tumors of Uncertain Malignant Potential (STUMP) [13]

This denomination is used when there is uncertainty of the diagnosis of malignancy such as:
1. When the clinicopathologic information about a malignant type is scant.
2. When there is uncertainty concerning:
   - The type of smooth muscle differentiation.
   - About the mitotic index in the neighborhood of 10MF/10HPF.
   - About the presence of tumor cell necrosis (distinction with hyaline/infarction necrosis and tumor cell necrosis can be ambiguous).

24.3.2.1 MR Findings

According to Tanaka et al., MR findings favoring the diagnosis of leiomyosarcomas and STUMP are [14]:
1. 50% of the tumor shows high signal on T2.
2. Presence of small area of high signal on T1.
3. Presence of unenhanced pocket-like areas after injection.

24.3.3 Leiomyosarcoma

24.3.3.1 Frequency

They represent about one-third of uterine sarcomas and 1.3% of uterine malignancies [13].

Approximately 1 in 800 smooth muscle tumors of the uterus is a leiomyosarcoma, but less than 1% of women thought to have clinically a leiomyosarcoma prove to have leiomyosarcoma [13].

24.3.3.2 Pathology

Macroscopy is summarized in Table 24.4 [13].

Histological Type

(a) Usual leiomyosarcoma
   Definition: It is composed of fascicles of spindle cells with an abundant eosinophilic cytoplasm.

Table 24.4 Macroscopic differences between leiomyomas and leiomyosarcomas

Leiomyoma	Leiomyosarcoma
No specific location	Intramural
Usually multiple	Usually solitary (50–75%)
Variable size	Large, 6–9 cm and often >10 cm
Firm whorled cut surface	Soft fleshy cut surface
Hemorrhage and necrosis (rare)	Hemorrhage and necrosis (common)
Regular margin	Irregular margin

Modified from Ref. [13]

Cytologic criteria:
Three main findings:
- Nuclear atypia (fusiform nuclei).
- High mitotic index (in excess of 15MF/10HPF).
- Tumor cell necrosis.

Other findings:
- Cellular pleomorphism; multinucleated (50%) or giant cells can be present.

Architectural criteria:
- Myometrial infiltration (common).
- Vascular invasion (10–22%).

(b) Myxoid leiomyosarcoma
   Definition: It is an abundant amorphous myxoid stroma between the smooth muscle cells.
   Macroscopy:
   - Large gelatinous neoplasm.
   Architectural criteria:
   - Myometrial infiltration (common).
   - Vascular invasion (10–22%).

(c) Epithelioid leiomyosarcoma
   Definition: The cells are round or polygonal rather than fusiform.

24.3.3.3 Clinical Findings

The average age is 52 years. The main symptoms are abnormal vaginal bleeding, lower abdominal pain, and a pelvic or an abdominal mass.

A rapidly enlarging leiomyoma should allow the discussion on the possibility of a leiomyosarcoma, although Parker in his series [15] only found 1 in 371 women with this finding to have a leiomyosarcoma.

24.3.3.4 Imaging

Ultrasound and Doppler

In Exacoustos's series [16], they were solitary and had a diameter ≥8 cm.

Degenerative changes were observed in half of the cases.

At color Doppler [16], the peripheral vascularity of leiomyoma is increased compared with that of normal myometrium and to that of the center of the tumor. Leiomyosarcomas have a different vascular distribution with an increased peripheral and central vascularity.

At spectral Doppler analysis [17], the mean resistive index in arterioles of leiomyomas (0.59) was significantly different from MMMTs (0.41) but not significantly different from leiomyosarcomas (0.49).

MR (Figs. 24.15 and 24.16)

T1 and T2 Findings
They often appear as large heterogeneous masses, rarely as endometrial mass [7, 18].

- On T1, a background of low or intermediate low signal intensity with scattered pockets of high signal intensity corresponding to hemorrhage.

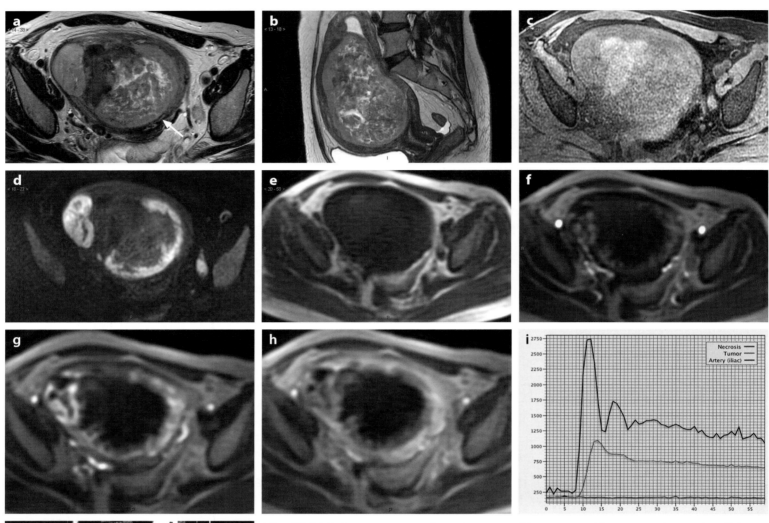

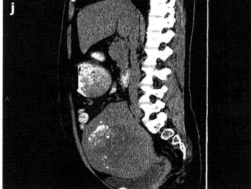

Fig. 24.16 Leiomyosarcoma. Forty-three-year-old woman with menorragias and pollakiuria. Leiomyoma of 9 cm 2 years ago. MR. Axial T2 (**a**) and Sagittal T2 through the endometrial cavity (**b**) display: (1) Significant increase in size of the uterine leiomyoma that correspond now to a 13-cm mass localized to the myometrium, occupying the body of the uterus and pushing the lower endometrium posteriorly and to the left (*arrow* in **a**) without invasion of the cervix.; the endometrium and the cervical mucosa are preserved. (2) On (**a**), a 5-cm right portion of intermediate signal corresponding to a solid portion enhancing after injection. On (**a**), a central portion of heterogeneous intensity related to necrosis not enhancing after injection and a peripheral portion of intermediate signal at the periphery enhancing after injection. Axial T1 fat suppression (**c**) visualizes a large portion of hemorrhage in the right and lower part of the mass. Diffusion b1000 (**d**) shows high signal intensity in the right solid portion and the peripheral solid portion of the mass. DMR without injection (**e**), at the arterial phase 20 s after injection (**f**), at 40 s after injection (**g**), and delayed 150 s after injection (**h**) demonstrates large regular arterial vessels in the solid tissue (**f**). At 40 s after injection (**g**), a high contrast uptake is visualized in the solid portion superior to the myometrium; while the central portion contains a lot of necrosis, only a part of which is hemorrhagic as it is shown in (**c**). A slight washout is displayed on the delayed (**h**) and on the time-intensity curves (**i**). Thoraco-abdomino-pelvic CT scan with sagittal reconstruction (**j**) was performed to evaluate extension. It showed the following: (1) multiple calcifications in the mass. (2) Absence of lymph nodes and metastases. Surgery: colpohysterectomy with bilateral adnexectomy, peritoneal biopsies, and bilateral iliac lymphadenectomy. Microscopy: (1) leiomyosarcoma without extension to the endometrium; (2) absence of extrauterine extension. Immunohistochemistry: smooth muscle actin +, H-Caldesmon slightly +, CD10-; Ki-67 elevated

- On T2, a background of intermediate signal intensity with areas of high signal intensity; the tumor may be of predominantly high signal intensity.

Areas of high T1 and intermediate or high T2 signal intensity correspond to hemorrhagic necrosis.

Areas of low T1 and intermediate or high T2 signal intensity correspond to cystic necrosis (coagulative tumor cell necrosis).

Vascularized solid areas may be of high intensity on T2 due to edema.

DWI

Several studies tried to differentiate leiomyomas from leiomyosarcomas using DWI and ADC values.

In Tamai et al.'s series [19], both uterine sarcomas (5 leiomyosarcomas and 2 endometrial stromal sarcomas) and cellular leiomyomas exhibited high signal intensity on DW images, whereas ordinary leiomyomas and most degenerated leiomyomas showed low signal intensity.

The mean ADC values of sarcomas (1.17×10^{-3} mm^2/s) were lower than those of normal myometrium (1.62×10^{-3} mm^2/s) and degenerated leiomyomas (1.7×10^{-3} mm^2/s) without any overlap; however, they were overlapped with those of ordinary leiomyomas and cellular leiomyomas.

Nanimoto et al. [20] combined T2 and DWI to differentiate sarcomas from leiomyosarcomas. They found that association of a T2 signal superior to that of myometrium and an ADC $<1.05 \times 10^{-3}$ mm^2/s has a sensitivity of 100% and a specificity of 100% for sarcoma.

However, ADC values may be unexpectedly high in solid portions of sarcomas (Fig. 24.15). Even when combining T2 and ADC, differentiation with degenerative benign leiomyomas is not always possible (Figs. 24.5, 24.6, and 24.12).

DMR

In a large series of degenerated leiomyomas ($n = 130$) and leiomyosarcomas ($n = 10$), Goto et al. [18] studied DMR enhancement and LDH isoenzyme values.

Contrast enhancement was seen in the early phase (20–90s) in leiomyosarcomas and was more intense than in leiomyomas with degenerated changes. The myometrium was gradually enhanced in the later phase (120–180s), though differentiation with leiomyosarcomas was at best in the early phase.

LDH isoenzyme type 3 was elevated in LMS with a sensitivity of 90% and specificity of 92%.

With combined use of DMR and LDH, sensitivity and specificity were of 100%, respectively.

24.3.3.5 Differential Diagnosis

(a) When leiomyosarcoma presents as a large mass, which is the most frequent:
- Degenerative leiomyoma [18].
- Cellular leiomyomas.

(b) When leiomyosarcoma presents as an endometrial mass, which is rare [7]:
- Endometrial carcinoma.
- MMMTs.
- Endometrial stromal sarcoma.

(c) Exceptionally an invasive trophoblastic disease (Fig. 24.17). Although usually a history of a recent pregnancy and very high HCG are known, this disease can be revealed as a pelvic mass.

24.3.3.6 Extension

Extension is staged according to FIGO classification [21] (Table 24.5).

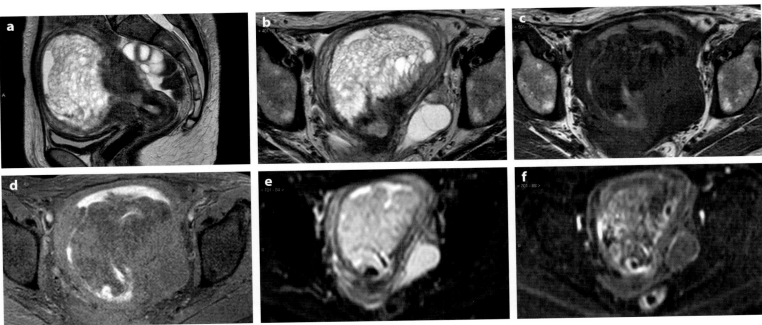

Fig. 24.17 Invasive mole revealed as a pelvic mass. Forty-year-old woman with pelvic pain, abdominal swelling, nausea, and urinary imperiousness since 1 month; absence of metrorrhagia. MR sagittal T2 (**a**) and axial T2 (**b**) display an endometrial mass occupying the entire endometrial cavity, extending into the upper endocervix. The mass is tissular containing multiple cystic cavities. Left ovarian simple cysts are present. Axial T1 without (**c**) and with (**d**) fat suppression display hemorrhage especially at the periphery and in the anterior portion. On diffusion b0 (**e**) and b1000 (**f**), signal intensity is not very high on b1000.

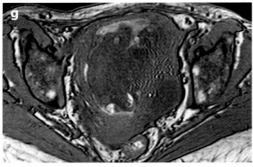
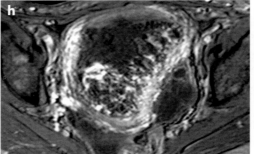
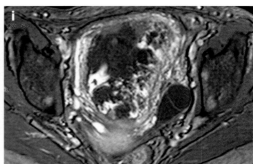
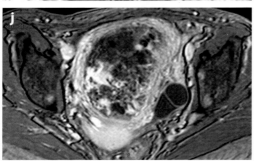

Fig. 24.17 (*continued*) DMR without injection (**g**) and at the arterial phase (**h**) demonstrates large vessels at the periphery invading the myometrium. At the venous (**i**) and on the delayed (**j**) phases, enhancement is seen in the myometrium. Prospective diagnosis: sarcoma or choriocarcinoma. Final diagnosis: invasive mole

Table 24.5 FIGO staging for uterine sarcomas (leiomyosarcomas, endometrial stromal sarcomas, adenosarcomas, and carcinosarcomas)

Leiomyosarcomas and Endometrial stromal sarcomas (ESS)*			**Adenosarcomas**		
I	Tumor limited to uterus		I	Tumor limited to uterus	
	IA	≤5 cm		IA	Tumor limited to endometrium/endocervix with no myometrial invasion
	IB	>5 cm		IB	Less than or equal to half myometrial invasion
II	Tumor extends to the pelvis			IC	More than half myometrial invasion
	IIA	Adnexal involvement	II	Tumor extends to the pelvis	
	IIB	Tumor extends to others pelvic tissue		IIA	Adnexal involvement
III	Tumor invades abdominal tissues (not just protruding into the abdomen).			IIB	Tumor extends to others pelvic tissue
	IIIA	One site	III	Tumor invades abdominal tissues (not just protruding into the abdomen).	
	IIIB	> one site		IIIA	One site
	IIIC	Metastasis to pelvic and/or para-aortic lymph nodes		IIIB	> one site
IV	IVA	Tumor invades bladder and/or rectum		IIIC	Metastasis to pelvic and/or para-aortic lymph nodes
	IVB	Distant metastasis	IV	IVA	Tumor invades bladder and/or rectum
				IVB	Distant metastasis

Carcinosarcomas
Carcinosarcomas should be staged as carcinomas of the endometrium.

* Note: Simultaneous tumors of the uterine corpus and ovary/pelvis in association with ovarian/pelvic endometriosis should be classified as independent primary tumors.

Modified from reference [22]

24.3.4 Other Smooth Muscle Tumors

24.3.4.1 Diffuse Leiomyomatosis (Fig. 24.18)

Definition: Diffuse leiomyomatosis is an unusual condition in which innumerable small smooth muscle nodules produce symmetric enlargement of the uterus.

The nodules range from microscopic to 3 cm in diameter, but most are less than 1 cm.

They are less circumscribed than typical leiomyomas.

24.3.4.2 Intravenous Leiomyomatosis

Definition: Intravenous leiomyomatosis is a very rare condition in which nodular masses of histologically benign smooth muscle cells grow within venous channels.

Pathology

It is a complex coiled or nodular growth within the myometrium with convoluted wormlike extensions that can grow into the uterine veins of the broad ligament or even into other pelvic veins. It reaches the inferior vena cava in more than 10% of patients and in some patients goes as far as the heart.

24.3.4.3 Metastasizing Leiomyoma (Fig. 24.18)

Definition: A nebulous condition in which metastatic smooth muscle tumor deposits in the lung, lymph nodes, or abdomen appear to be derived from a benign leiomyoma of the uterus.

The primary neoplasm, typically removed years before the metastatic deposits are detected, often has been inadequately studied.

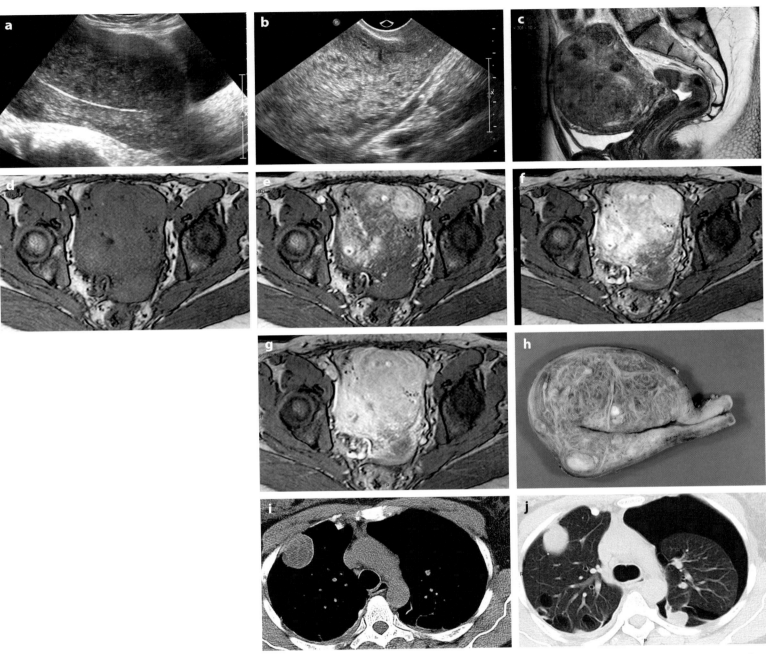

Fig. 24.18 Diffuse leiomyomatosis with benign metastasizing leiomyoma. Metrorragia in a 23-year-old woman with previous myomectomy. TAS (**a**) and EVS (**b**) display diffuse modifications of the echostructure of the myometrium without acoustic shadowing. MR sagittal T2 (**c**) shows nodular, diffuse, ill-defined modification of the structure of the myometrium with signal intensity close to pelvic muscles. On T1 and T1 fat suppression (not shown), the overall signal of the myometrium is also close to pelvic muscles. DMR without injection (**d**), at the arterial phase (**e**), at the venous phase (**f**), and on the delayed phase (**g**) depicts without injection multiple flow voids, at the arterial phase thin regular arteries, and at the venous phase contrast uptake slightly more important in the external part of the myometrium than in the inner myometrium. At macroscopy (**h**), the myometrium is hyperplastic with a fasciculated aspect; inside it, white nodules are disseminated. At microscopy, a diffuse leiomyomatosis was diagnosed. Leiomyomas and adenomyosis were associated. CT scan of the chest (**i**, **j**) displays two subpleural nodules, one in the right upper lobe and one in the apical segment of the left lobe. The right one is of slightly low tissular density containing regular septa; this aspect is very suggestive of metastasizing leiomyoma, which was confirmed at pathology. Parenchymal cysts and pneumothorax are associated

24.3.4.4 Disseminated Peritoneal Leiomyomatosis

Definition: An imprecise condition in which multiple smooth muscle nodules, myofibroblastic and fibroblastic, most of them <1 cm, are found on the peritoneal surfaces of the uterus, adnexa, intestines, omentum, and abdominal cavities in women of reproductive age.

Most cases are associated with pregnancy, an estrinizing granulosa tumor, or oral contraceptive.

24.3.4.5 Parasitic Leiomyoma

Uncommonly, leiomyomas detach from their subserous location and attach to some other pelvic site.

24.4 Endometrial Stromal Tumors

24.4.1 Endometrial Stromal Sarcoma (ESS)

Definition: Endometrial stromal sarcoma is a tumor of endometrial stromal cells that invades the myometrium [23].

ESS is traditionally divided into two categories, low-grade stromal sarcoma and high-grade stromal sarcoma.

24.4.1.1 Pathology [13]

Macroscopy

1. Endometrium
   It usually involves the endometrium sometimes extensively. It forms smooth surface polyps that are occasionally partly infarcted and hemorrhagic.
2. Myometrium
   Myometrial involvement has three main features:
   - Most frequently, tumoral cords or nodules permeate the myometrium.
   - A nodular tumor may be present with soft orange cut surface opposed to the whorled firm surface of a leiomyoma.
   - The myometrium may be diffusely thickened, but a clearly defined tumor is not evident.
   In high-grade tumors:
   - Polypoid tumors bulge into and often fill the endometrial cavity.
   - Multiple masses invade the underlying myometrium.
   - Hemorrhage and necrosis are frequent.

Microscopy

- Endometrial stromal sarcoma cells resemble proliferative phase or hyperplastic endometrial stroma cells.
- (a) *Most are low-grade tumors* with cells of relatively uniform size and shape. The cells have round or oval nuclei with finely dispersed chromatin and small nucleoli. The cytoplasm is amphophilic, and the cell borders are ill defined.
  Rare low-grade tumors consist predominantly of spindle-shaped cells that are fibroblastic in appearance with fusiform nuclei and elongated cell bodies.

Mitotic activity is low in most low-grade tumors usually less than 3MF/HPF.

Proliferation of small vessels and arterioles resembling the endometrial spiral arterioles is a characteristic finding. The arterioles tend to be uniformly distributed among the stroma cells, and capillaries and small veins are often obvious as well.

Low-grade tumors invade the myometrium and may extensively permeate it. Invasion of lymphatic and vascular channels is a characteristic finding.

(b) *High-grade tumors*
   Cytologic features:
   - Larger, more vesicular conspicuous nuclei.
   - Usually more than 10MF/10HPF.
   - Tumor cells tend to be larger.
   Architectural features:
   - A destructive pattern of myometrial invasion with areas of hemorrhage and necrosis.
   - An irregular and pleomorphic vascular pattern.

24.4.1.2 Clinical Findings

The mean age is between 42 and 53 years, and more than 50% of patients are premenopausal.

A few cases have been reported in women treated for breast cancer with Tamoxifen.

The main symptoms are vaginal bleeding, cyclic menorrhagia that gradually becomes more severe, and abdominal pain.

The uterus is enlarged with an irregular contour. A few women have bulky polypoid tumors that protrude from the cervical os.

The usual clinical impression is that the patient has a uterine leiomyoma that is causing an exceptional degree of bleeding.

Occasionally, patients present with abdominal or pulmonary metastases.

24.4.1.3 Imaging Findings

MR findings are reported in Table 24.6 [13, 19, 20, 24, 26] (Fig. 24.19).

The whole tumor may be seen as multiple confluent nodules. The tumor margins are usually irregular [26].

On T1, the tumor is usually isointense to myometrium, sometimes higher than myometrium [24].

On T2, all lesions exhibit higher signal intensity than myometrium [24, 26].

24.4.1.4 Location

1. Tumor predominantly within the endometrial cavity
   - Sharply demarcated polypoid tumor or voluminous polypoid masses with an expanded endometrial cavity. In most cases, obscured endometrial border (sometimes only on a short distance), thinning, or focal disruption of the functional zone is seen [7, 26, 27]. Rarely, the tumor is confined to the endometrium [7, 26].

Table 24.6 MR findings of endometrial stromal cell sarcoma

Location [24]
- Endometrial, protruding predominantly into the endometrial cavity
- Endometrial, protruding into the endometrial cavity with extensive involvement of the myometrium
- Bulky polypoid tumors protruding from the cervical os (rare)

Morphologic findings

(a) In low-grade tumors (the most common)

Endometrium:
- Usually involved by smooth surfaced polyps that are occasionally partly infarcted and hemorrhagic

Myometrium:
- Most frequently permeated by cords or nodules of tumors
- Nodular tumor looking as a leiomyoma
- Myometrium diffusely thickened

(b) In high-grade tumors
- Polypoid tumors bulge into and often fill the endometrial cavity.
- Multiple masses invade the underlying endometrium.
- Hemorrhage and necrosis are frequent.

Signal intensity

T2 images
- Hyperintense to myometrium
- Slightly lower or isointense to endometrium
- Numerous bands of low signal throughout the areas of myometrial involvement
- High signal intensity areas corresponding to hemorrhage or necrosis [25]

T1 images
- Isointense to myometrium [24]
- High signal intensity corresponding to hemorrhage or necrosis

Signal voids
  Prominent in areas of extensive myometrial involvement

DW images
  Reported ADC ranges in the literature: 0.8–1.2 $10^{-3} \times mm^2/s$

DMR and after regular contrast
  Contrast enhancement higher or lower than myometrium

2. Tumor that extensively involves the myometrium
   - Sharply or ill demarcated lesions [24].
   - Mainly located in the myometrium with protrusion in the endometrial cavity.
   - Mainly located in the myometrium mimicking leiomyoma with cystic degenerative changes or leiomyosarcomas.
   - Diffuse myometrial thickening misinterpreted as adenomyosis in one patient [24].
   - Rarely tumor located in the cervix and invading the vagina [26].
   - A case of high-grade ESS completely replacing the uterus has been reported.

24.4.1.5 Myometrial Invasions

Marked myometrial invasion can give one of the following features:
- Bands of low signal intensity on T2 within the area of myometrial invasion [24]. This unique finding is considered to represent bundles of preserved myometrial fibers separated by wormlike plugs of tumor permeating the myometrium, as it has been described at pathology by [13, 28].
- Intramyometrial nodular lesions (related to intralymphatic or intravascular extension). On contrast T1, these lesions do not enhance as much as normal myometrium [26].

24.4.1.6 Extension

Extension is staged according to FIGO classification (Table 24.5).

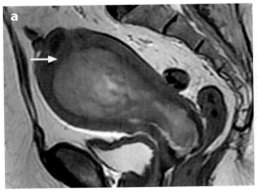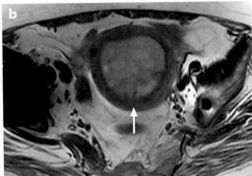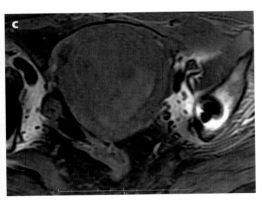

Fig. 24.19 Endometrial stromal sarcoma protruding into the endocervical canal. (**a**) Sagittal T2W images show a mass of intermediate signal intensity distending the uterine cavity and protruding into the endocervical canal. The hypointense junctional line appears disrupted in some places as here at the level of the fundus (*arrow*). At the level of the cervical canal, the tumor appears surrounded by a normal mucosa. Some leiomyomas are present. (**b**) Axial T2W images confirm that the hypointense junctional zone is disrupted in some places as posteriorly on this section (*arrow*). (**c**) Axial T1W image with fat suppression shows some hyperintense areas very suggestive of hemorrhage confirmed at pathology.

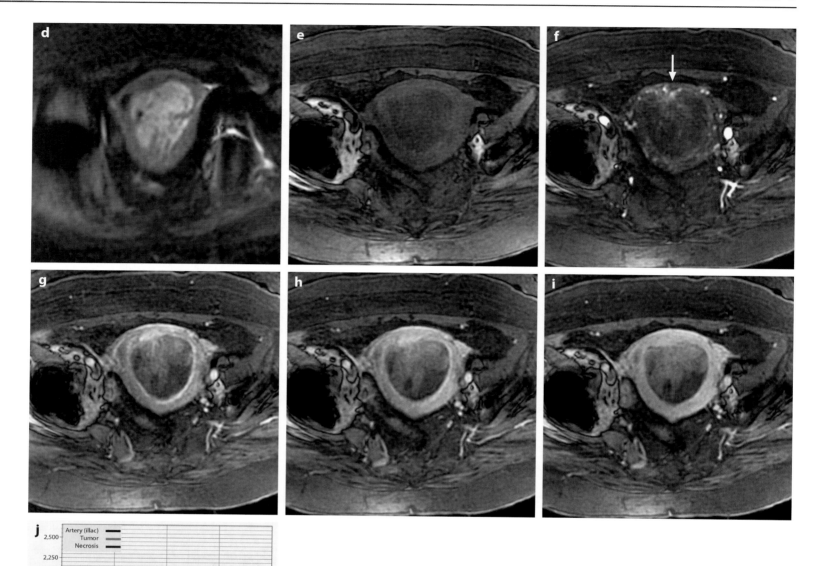

Fig. 24.19 (*continued*) (**d**) DWI at b500 (**d**) and corresponding ADC map (not shown) are unable to differentiate the necrotic from the non-necrotic part of the tumor with ADC values $\geq 1.1 \times 10^{-3}$ mm^2/s (range 1.1–1.4; mean 1.2). (**e–j**) DMR before (**e**) and 25 (**f**), 70 (**g**), 125 (**h**), and 240 (**i**) seconds after injection with time-intensity curves (**j**): at the arterial phase (25 s), tumoral vessels arising from the arcuate arteries of the inner myometrium penetrating into the tumor anteriorly (*arrow*) are typical for a malignant tumor. At the venous (70 s) and following phase (125 s), the peripheral enhancing rim corresponding to the inner myometrium is better seen appearing disrupted posteriorly and anteriorly. Starting at the venous phase, differentiation between the necrotic and non-necrotic part of the tumor is easy. Peak enhancement in the vascularized part is at 125 s

24.4.2 Endometrial Stromal Nodule (Fig. 24.20)

Definition: Endometrial stromal nodules consist of cells that closely resemble normal proliferative-phase endometrial stromal cells. They do not invade the adjacent myometrium.

24.4.2.1 Clinical Findings

They are rare and represent less than a quarter of endometrial stromal tumor.

The median age is 47 years, and 75% of women are premenopausal.

The main symptoms are abnormal vaginal bleeding and menorrhagia.

24.4.2.2 Macroscopy

They have a circumscribed contour.
   The average diameter is 4–5 cm.
- Nearly half of them grow entirely within the myometrium, with no apparent connection with the endometrium.
- Many of them are polypoid and protrude into the uterine cavity.
- Occasionally, tumors are cystic. Foci of hemorrhage and necrosis are rare.

Fig. 24.20 Endometrial stromal nodule versus leiomyoma. EVS longitudinal (**a**) and 3D ultrasound with 2D reformation (**b**) display a 35-mm-long, 14-mm-thick anterior bilobulated mass (*cursors*) of the body extending into the endocervix, protruding into the endometrial cavity. The tumor has an echogenicity close to myometrium without any acoustic shadowing, which is quite unusual for a leiomyoma of this size. At Color Doppler (**c**), peripheral vascularization is absent (which is quite unusual for a leiomyoma) while a central hypervascularization crossing the tumor is present. On pulsed Doppler (**d**), resistivity index is high. Radiological diagnosis: a leiomyoma is unlikely. Diagnosis at surgery performed through hysteroscopy: right leiomyoma occupying the entire endometrial cavity. At pathology: monomorph proliferation of fusiform cells. Immunohistochemistry: CD10, smooth muscle actin minutely expressed. Desmin and H-caldesmon negative. Two diagnoses are discussed: endometrial stromal nodule and cellular leiomyoma

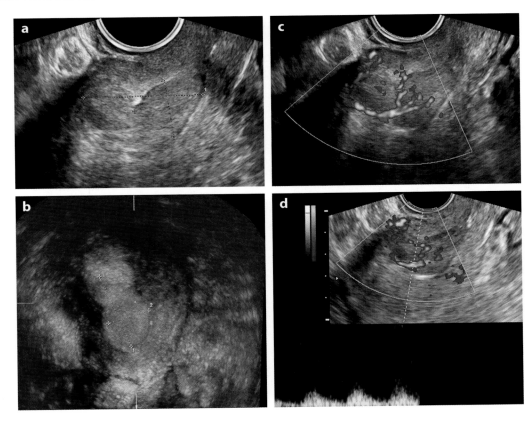

24.4.2.3 Microscopy

Stromal nodules compress the surrounding endometrium and myometrium, without invasion. Gland-like structures are present in some nodules.

Minor irregularities of the margin can be seen.

They are highly vascular with small arterioles distributed throughout.

Minor foci of smooth muscle differentiation are present in 10% of cases. If extensive smooth muscle differentiation is present (>30%), the tumor should be classified as a combined stromal-smooth muscle tumor. In this case, it should be differentiated from a cellular leiomyoma; at immunohistochemistry, stromal nodule staining is weak for smooth muscle actin and negative for desmin.

24.4.2.4 Imaging

Rare cases have been reported [29]. The tumor may be entirely solid or contains large cystic part [29]. It is well demarcated.

On US, the solid part has an echogenicity close to that of myometrium (Fig. 24.20).

On MR, the solid portion is slightly hyperintense than myometrium and enhances slightly more than myometrium [29] (Table 24.7).

Table 24.7 Macroscopic and imaging findings of endometrial stromal nodule

Location
– Intramyometrial
– Protrudes into the cavity
Macroscopic findings
– Solid
– Occasionally cystic component
– Rarely foci of hemorrhage and necrosis
Imaging
– Solid homogeneous or with cystic component
– On US, echogenicity of solid portion close to that of myometrium
– On MR, solid portion slightly hyperintense to myometrium on T2, enhancing more than myometrium

24.5 Miscellaneous Mesenchymal Tumors

24.5.1 Homologous and Heterologous Sarcomas (Fig. 24.21)

Most tumors of this group are high-grade sarcomas.

They consist of round or spindle cells with variable amounts of cytoplasm and pleomorphic atypical nuclei. Mitotic figures are numerous.

24.5.2 Adenomatoid Tumors (Benign Mesotheliomas) (Fig. 24.22)

Their origin is presumed to be from the cells of the serosal mesothelium. Microscopically they are composed of multiple small slit-like or ovoid spaces lined by a single layer of low cuboidal or flattened epithelia-like cells.

The tumor can resemble a leiomyoma. Continuity with the overlying mesothelium is occasionally seen.

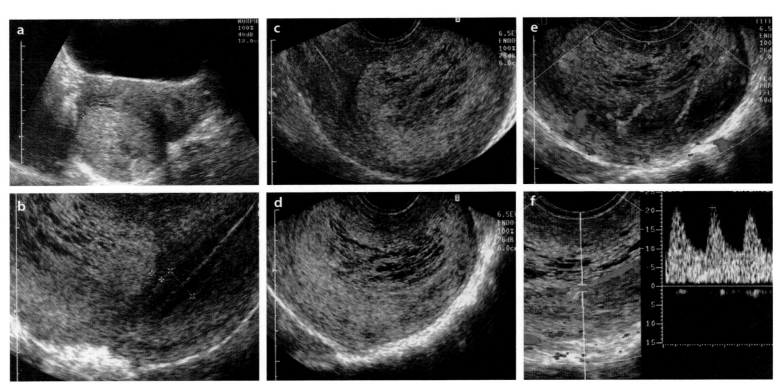

Fig. 24.21 Synovial sarcoma. Fifty-seven-year-old woman with metrorrhagias and normal hysteroscopy. TAS (**a**) displays in the right and posterior region of the body and in the uterine fundus a round, 65-mm well-limited mass situated in contact with the serosa. On EVS (**b**), its deep portion is situated at 3 mm of the deep portion of the endometrium. On longitudinal (**c**) and transverse (**d**) EVS, the structure of the mass is quite unusual for a leiomyoma. The mass is heterogeneous with a fibrillar aspect associated with anechoic spaces. Color Doppler (**e**) displays a quite unusual vascularization for a leiomyoma, peripheral and overall central with a vascular axis crossing the tumor. On Pulsed Doppler (**f**), the PSV is high at 22 cm/s. Surgery: a total hysterectomy with bilateral adnexectomy was performed. Pathology: a synovial sarcoma was diagnosed

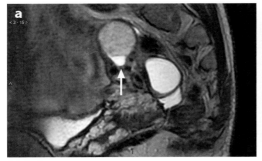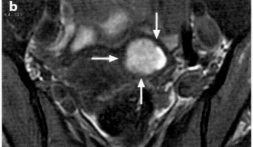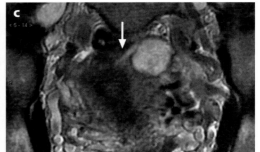

Fig. 24.22 Forty-year-old woman. MR sagittal T2 (**a**), axial T2 (**b**), and coronal T2 (**c**) display a round mass 2.9 cm in size in the left uterine cornua, involving the interstitial segment of the left tube, extending in the proximal portion of the mesosalpinx (*red arrow* in **a**). It has two components: a major component of intermediate signal and a portion particularly at its lower pole of high signal intensity (*white arrow* in **a**). The mass has ill-defined borders (*arrow* in **b**). At its upper pole, the mass presents a linear structure which is linked to the serosa of the fundus of the uterus (*arrow* in **c**).

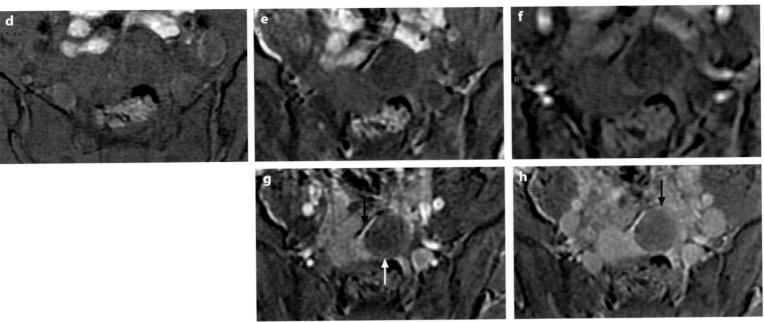

Fig. 24.22 (*continued*) On axial T1 with fat suppression (**d**), the mass has an overall signal close to that of myometrium. On DMR without injection (**e**), the mass has a signal intensity a little lower than that of the myometrium. At the arterial phase (**f**), a peripheral arterial vascularization is not displayed like it usually is in a subserous leiomyoma. At the venous phase (**g**), a slight peripheral contrast uptake is visualized a little inside the outer limit of the mass (*white arrow*), which is not seen in subserous leiomyoma. A particular linear high contrast uptake is shown in the linear structure (*black arrow*) which is depicted in (**c**). A moderate contrast uptake lower than that of myometrium is displayed in the mass, which slightly increases on the sequence performed 4 min after injection (**h**) (*arrow*). Macroscopy: benign mesothelial tumor; some vascular clefts realizing cystic cavities. Immunochemistry: positive for cytokeratins AE1–AE3, and overall for calretinin

Table 24.8 Findings in adenomatoid tumors

1. **Location: subserous** – Cornual myometrium – Tube – Ovary (hilum) – Peritoneum
2. **Size** – Usually small, 1–2 cm – May be larger
3. **Pathology** – Collagen, elastic tissue, and smooth muscle surround the epithelial elements. – Smooth muscle can be so predominant that the tumor can resemble a leiomyoma. – Rarely the cystic spaces are sufficiently large to give a macroscopic pattern of cystic or multilocular mass.

The main findings are reported in Table 24.8.

Immunostaining is positive for mesothelial markers such as cytokeratin, vimentin, and calretinin.

24.5.3 Primitive Neuroectodermal Tumor (PNET)

Rarely, PNET develops in the uterus.

It occurs most commonly in postmenopausal women. Abnormal vaginal bleeding is the usual clinical finding.

24.5.3.1 Macroscopy

A polypoid mass that originates in the endometrium and invades the myometrium.

24.5.3.2 Microscopy

- The tumor is composed of small cells with round to oval hyperchromatic nuclei and scanty cytoplasm.
- Fibrillary foci of glial differentiation.
- Rosettes, Homer-Wright pseudorosettes, and perivascular, ependymal-type rosettes may be present.

Immunostaining is positive for neuron-specific enolase (NSE), glial fibrillary acidic protein (GFAP), chromogranin, or S-100 protein.

24.5.4 Vascular Tumors

Hemangioma, vascular malformations, and more rarely angiosarcomas can occur in the myometrium.

24.5.5 Lymphomas

The uterus is rarely the initial site of uterine lymphoma. When it occurs, the cervix is three times more involved than the uterus body [13].

24.6 Adenomyosis, Adenomyoma, and Adenomyotic Cyst

24.6.1 Adenomyosis

Definition: *Adenomyosis*: Implantation of endometrium into the myometrium.
   Endometriosis: Implantation of endometrium outside the uterus.

24.6.1.1 Pathology

Microscopy

The ectopic endometrium is responsible for two main lesions:
- Small endometriotic foci: They usually appear as round cystic cavities from 1 to 3 mm in diameter but can be larger. They contain clear or hemorrhagic fluid or clots, limited by a regular rim of endometrium. Sometimes direct channels, more or less perpendicular to the deep portion of the endometrium, extending into the myometrium are seen.
- Secondary muscular hyperplasia around the foci.

Macroscopy

There are two main types of adenomyosis:
- The most common one is non-circumscribed adenomyosis.
- Very uncommonly adenomyosis is circumscribed with two different patterns: adenomyoma and adenomyotic cyst.
- A particular form, external adenomyosis, is secondary to involvement of uterine serosa by endometriotic implants extending from outside to inside into the external myometrium (see chapter endometriosis).

24.6.1.2 Clinical Findings

They are essential for the diagnosis. Age is usually comprised between 35 and 45 years old. The most suggestive findings are menorrhagia with clots and dysmenorrhea for several months or years.
   CA-125 can be increased.

24.6.1.3 Non-circumscribed Adenomyosis

US (Figs. 24.23, 24.24, and 24.25)

The main findings [30] are reported in Table 24.9.

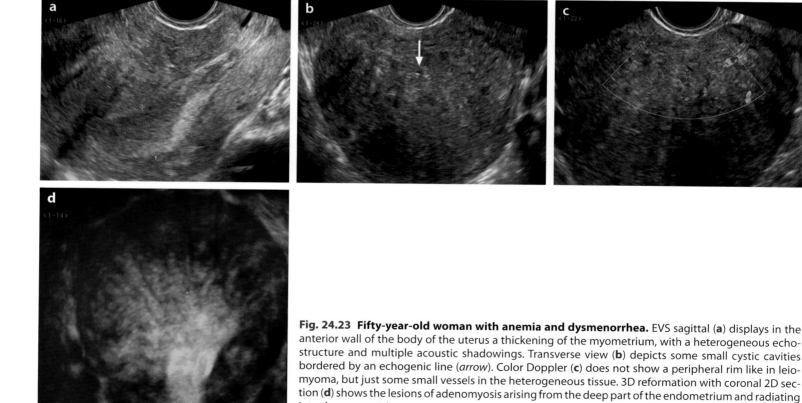

Fig. 24.23 Fifty-year-old woman with anemia and dysmenorrhea. EVS sagittal (**a**) displays in the anterior wall of the body of the uterus a thickening of the myometrium, with a heterogeneous echostructure and multiple acoustic shadowings. Transverse view (**b**) depicts some small cystic cavities bordered by an echogenic line (*arrow*). Color Doppler (**c**) does not show a peripheral rim like in leiomyoma, but just some small vessels in the heterogeneous tissue. 3D reformation with coronal 2D section (**d**) shows the lesions of adenomyosis arising from the deep part of the endometrium and radiating into the myometrium

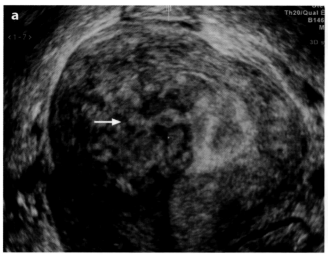
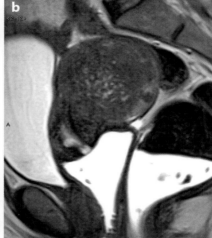
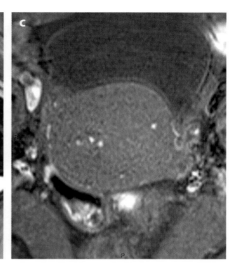

Fig. 24.24 Forty-year-old woman with menorrhagias, clots, and dysmenorrhea. CA 125: 105 UI/ml. EVS with 3D (**a**) reformation displays a diffuse thickening of the anterior wall of the uterus with direct visualization of fragments of endometrium going from the deep part of the endometrium directly into the myometrium (*arrow*). MR sagittal T2 (**b**) displays multiple cystic cavities of adenomyosis, some containing on axial T1 with fat suppression (**c**) hemorrhage

Fig. 24.25 Forty-nine-year-old woman with menorrhagias. EVS longitudinal (**a**) displays a thickening of the endometrium containing cystic cavities related to endometrial hyperplasia. The outer limits of these abnormalities are indistinct. Coronal 2D obtained after 3D reformation (**b**) displays more clearly at the periphery of the myometrium cystic cavities lying in the inner myometrium related to adenomyosis

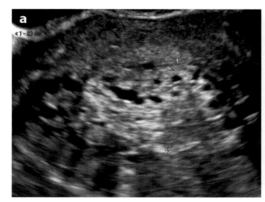
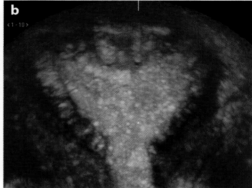

Table 24.9 Findings of internal adenomyosis on US

1. Topography
– Extends from the deep portion of the endometrium into the myometrium
– Classically most frequent on the posterior wall and the cornua, but can lie anywhere in the myometrium
– Usually the inner third; may be localized or diffuse
– May confer a diffuse globulous aspect to the body of the uterus
2. Morphologic findings
(a) Direct findings: small cysts in the myometrium (characteristic for adenomyosis)
– Surrounded by an echogenic line
– Nonhemorrhagic: anechoic
– Hemorrhagic: contain echogenic foci
(b) Findings of secondary hyperplasia of the myometrium:
– Most often heterogeneous myometrium or myometrial areas, with mixed echogenicity and acoustic shadowing (without calcifications)
– More rarely, areas of less echogenicity than normal myometrium
3. Shape of the area of adenomyosis
– Not round as for a leiomyoma
– Poor limitation between the foci of adenomyosis and the external myometrium
4. Color Doppler in the area of adenomyosis
– Absence of peripheral vascularization as in a leiomyoma
– May contain some central vessels

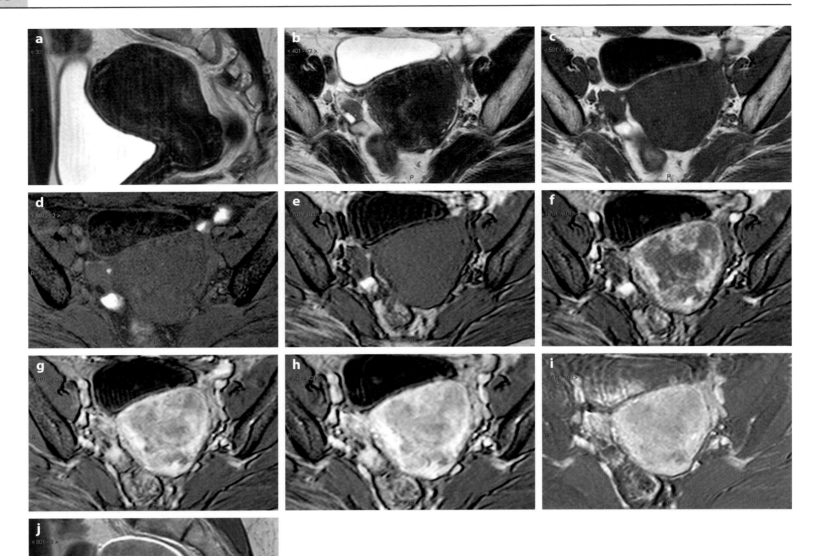

Fig. 24.26 Adenomyosis. Forty-three-year-old woman with dysmenorrhea and menorrhagia with clots. (1) MR sagittal T2 (**a**) and axial T2 (**b**) display a diffuse muscular hyperplasia involving the anterior and posterior walls and the fundus. (2) Hyperintense foci are displayed on the T2 sequences; some of them are better visualized as hyperintense spots on axial T1 (**c**) and T1 fat suppression (**d**). (3) DMR without injection (**e**), at the arterial phase (**f**), at the venous phase (**g**), on the parenchymal phase (**h**), and on the delayed phase (**i**) followed by sagittal delayed (**j**) shows heterogeneous uptake more marked on early phases

24.6.1.4 MR

Morphologic Findings

1. Most often adenomyosis is depicted only with findings related to hyperplasia of the myometrium (Fig. 24.26).

   On T2, hyperplasia is displayed by a low intensity area at the inner part of the myometrium starting at the endometrial myometrial junction, extending outside with a lateral irregular limit with the normal myometrium. As far as signal intensity of this hyperplasia is identical to the signal of the junctional zone, it has been described as a thickening of this junctional zone.

2. The direct findings of cystic cavities are much more uncommon. According to the nature of their content, these cavities appear with high signal intensity on T2 (watery content), or with high signal intensity on T1 and fat suppression (hemorrhagic content) (Figs. 24.27 and 24.28).

DMR is very helpful in some cases to differentiate adenomyosis from leiomyoma (Fig. 24.26; Table 24.10).

DWI

Kilickesmez [31] found an ADC value of $1.24 \pm 0.20 \times 10^{-3}$ mm²/s in adenomyosis and $1.76 \pm 0.19 \times 10^{-3}$ mm²/s in the myometrium. Absolute values differ however between apparatus and patients (Fig. 24.27).

The main findings are reported in Table 24.10.

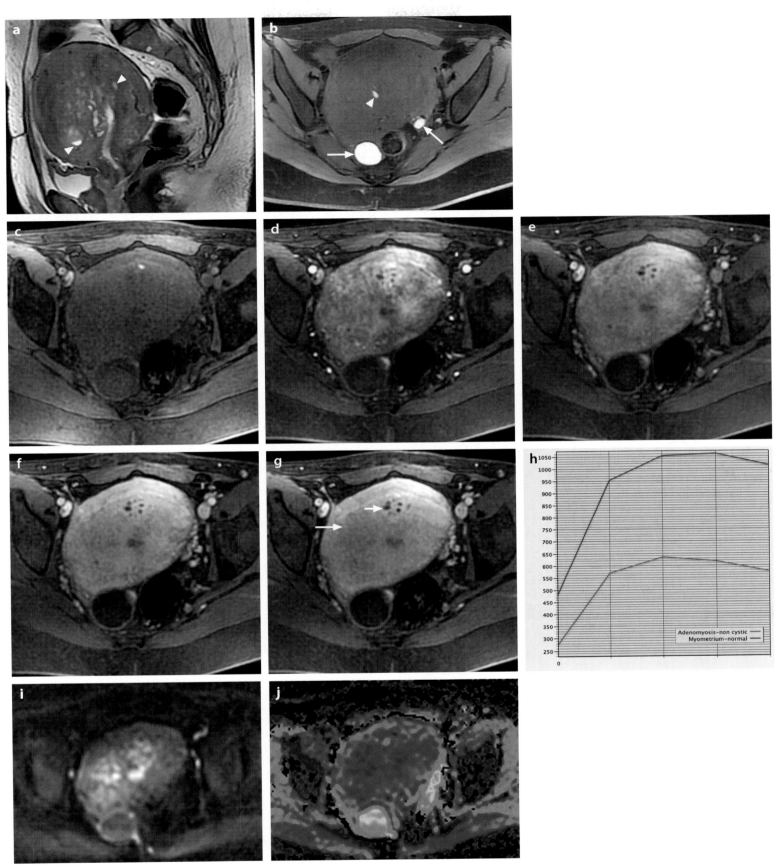

Fig. 24.27 Severe adenomyosis in a 45-year-old woman that necessitated hysterectomy. (**a**) Sagittal T2-weighted images show an enlarged uterus with intramyometrial white areas and spots corresponding to adenomyosis (*arrowheads*). (**b**) Axial T1 fat suppression images show that some of these white spots on T2 are hyperintense related to hemorrhage (*arrowhead*). Ovarian endometriomas are also present (*arrows*). (**c–h**) Dynamic MRI higher than B before (**c**) and 25 (**d**), 70 (**e**), 125 (**f**), and 240 (**g**) seconds after injection with corresponding time-intensity curves shows absence of contrast uptake in some of these white spots on T2 confirming their cystic nature (*short arrow* in **g**). The non-cystic hypointense area of adenomyosis on T2 enhance very progressively (*long arrow* in **g**) less than normal myometrium. (**i**) Diffusion-weighted image at b1000 shows that these cystic areas are often hyperintense due probably to T2 shine-through effect. (**j**) Corresponding ADC map shows a high ADC value (1.6×10^{-3} mm²/s) in some of these cystic spots and a lower ADC value (1×10^{-3} mm²/s) in the less intense solid areas of the myometrium (Mean ADC values at b500 and b1000)

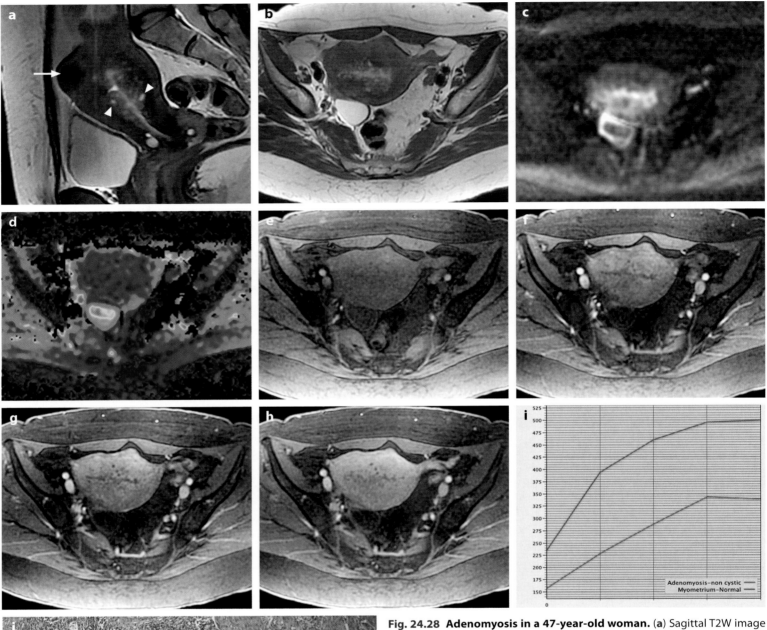

Fig. 24.28 Adenomyosis in a 47-year-old woman. (**a**) Sagittal T2W image shows a hypointense myoma (*arrow*) and multiple hyperintense peri-endometrial spots (*arrowheads*) typical of adenomyosis. In this case, these endometrial spots are essentially located in the peri-endometrial areas with a junctional zone reaching 18 mm in thickness posteriorly. Some Nabothian cysts are present in the cervix. (**b**) Axial T2W image shows small hyperintense endometrial lesions around the endometrium. Cystic simple ovarian structures are seen in the ovaries. (**c**) Diffusion b1000 weighted images at the same levels show a hazy limit of the endometrium due to adenomyosis. (**d**) Corresponding ADC maps show an ADC value of 1.1×10^{-3} mm²/s in the region where adenomyosis is more striking. In the peripheral myometrium where adenomyosis is not evident on imaging, the ADC value is 1.2×10^{-3} mm²/s (mean ADC values computed at b500 and b1000). (**e–i**) Dynamic MRI at the same level as (**c**) before (**e**) and 25 (**f**), 70 (**g**), 125, and 240 (**h**) seconds after injection with corresponding time-intensity curves (**i**) shows absence of contrast uptake in some of these spots confirming their cystic nature. The non-cystic hypointense area of adenomyosis enhances less than normal myometrium. (**j**) Histology of the surgical specimen shows multiple endometrial tissue and glands (*arrow*) inside the myometrium surrounded by muscular hyperplasia (*asterisk*)

Table 24.10 Findings of adenomyosis on MR

1. Topography
- Extends from the deep portion of the endometrium into the myometrium
- Classically most frequent on the posterior wall and the cornua, but can lie anywhere in the myometrium
- May confer a diffuse globulous aspect to the body of the uterus

2. Morphologic findings
(a) **Direct finding: small cysts in the myometrium usually the inner** third; may be more diffuse (characteristic for adenomyosis but only seen in 10–20% of cases).
   - Nonhemorrhagic: hypointense on T1, hyperintense on T2
   - Hemorrhagic: hyperintense on T1 and T1 fat suppression, hyperintense on T2

(b) **Findings of secondary hyperplasia of the myometrium:**
   - On T2, areas of low intensity identical to intensity of the junctional zone extending into the myometrium, with an external irregular and ill-defined border
   - On T1, not clearly depicted because of the same signal as normal myometrium
   - On DMR, at the arterial phase, absence of peripheral vascularization (different from a leiomyoma)

At the venous phase, contrast uptake lower than normal myometrium, and heterogeneous

On the delayed phase, contrast uptake lower than normal myometrium

Exceptionally, contrast uptake superior than myometrium

3. Shape of the area of adenomyosis
- Not round as for a leiomyoma
- Poor limitation between the foci of adenomyosis and the external myometrium

24.6.2 Adenomyoma

It is a circumscribed lesion of adenomyosis, that can mimic a leiomyoma. It can be subserous, interstitial, or pedunculated in the endometrial cavity and can grow as a polyp. About 2% of endometrial polyps are adenomyoma. A rare variant of adenomyomatous polyp, the atypical polypoid adenomyoma, has atypical hyperplastic glands that usually contain foci of squamous metaplasia.

It can be entirely solid or contain cystic cavities. If entirely cystic, the term adenomyotic cyst is used (see below).

24.6.2.1 US

It is hypoechoic. Adenomyoma has usually an ill-defined border unlike leiomyoma or can present a peripheral hyperechoic border (Fig. 24.29). It can contain cystic cavities. Color Doppler does not find vascular rims suggesting leiomyoma but usually depicts irregular vessels in the areas of muscular hyperplasia.

24.6.2.2 MR

On T2W images, the mass is hypointense due to smooth muscle hyperplasia, but can contain cystic hyperintense cavities (Fig. 24.30). On T1W images, it is hypointense except for cavities containing hyperintense blood.

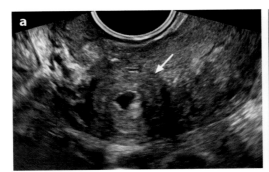
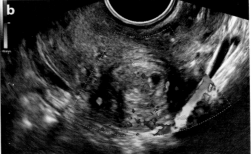

Fig. 24.29 Adenomyoma with intracystic cavity. A 35-year-old woman followed for endometriosis and adenomyosis. Recurrent pain after stopping Decapetyl. (**a**) Transverse transvaginal ultrasound discloses a 1.5-cm well-circumscribed mass (*arrow*) with a small central cavity lined by a hyperechoic wall and surrounded by circular striated muscle hyperplasia. A thin peripheral rim is seen in some places. (**b**) Corresponding color Doppler shows some vessels in the mass but not the characteristic peripheral vascularization of leiomyoma

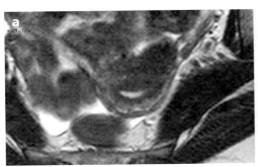
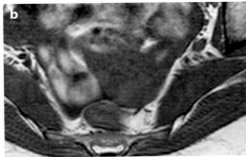
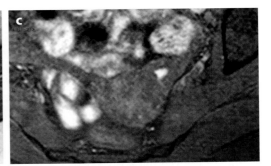
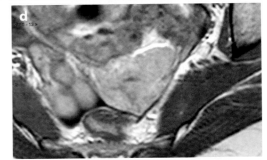

Fig. 24.30 Adenomyoma of the left uterine horn. A 34-year-old woman with cyclic pain. (**a**) Axial T2W image depicts a small hypointense mass of the left uterine horn. (**b**, **c**) T1W images without (**b**) and with (**c**) fat suppression show a hyperintense hemorrhagic focus inside this tumor. (**d**) T1W image after gadolinium injection shows the solid portion of the mass to enhance like the myometrium. The hyperintense hemorrhagic focus is now indistinguishable from the other part of the mass. Surgery and pathology confirmed the presence of a left adenomyoma

On DMR, vascularization is variable. Arterial vascularization and contrast uptake at the venous phase can be more important (Fig. 24.31) or less important than the myometrium or both in case of multiple lesions (Fig. 24.32). The borders are not as well limited as leiomyomas. At the late phase, contrast uptake is very close to contrast uptake of myometrium.

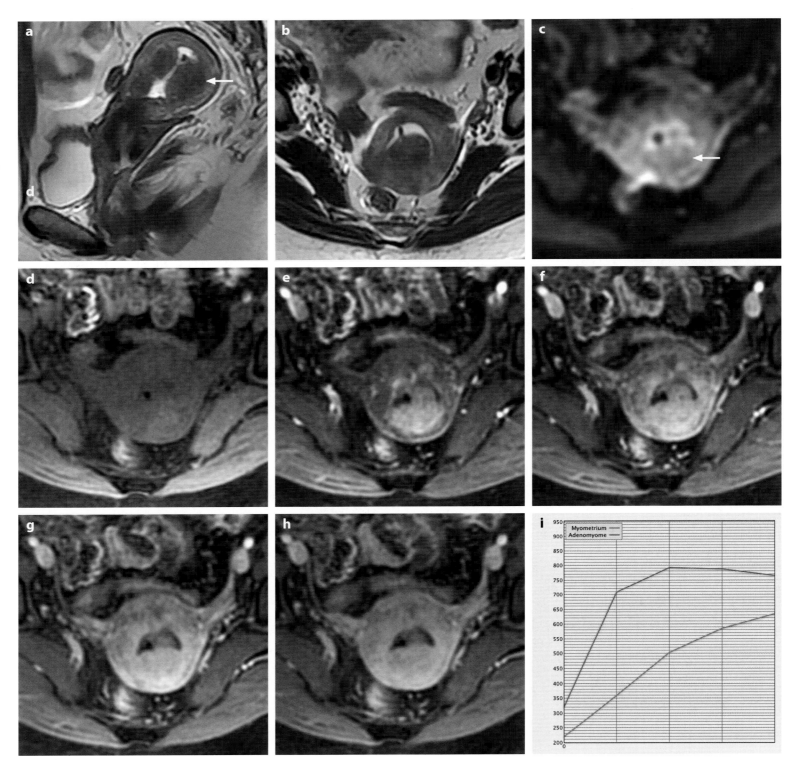

Fig. 24.31 Adenomyomas. Multiple adenomyomas in a 36-year-old woman with metrorrhagia and dysmenorrhea. (**a**) Sagittal T2W image shows three well-circumscribed hypointense myometrial submucosal masses, protruding at different degrees in the uterine cavity, the largest one (*arrow*) being posterior. Part of a uterine device is also seen in the endometrial cavity as a hypointense structure on all sequences. On T1 (not shown), the masses were almost isointense to the myometrium without hyperintense foci suggestive of hemorrhage. Axial T2W (**b**) through the largest mass shows the mass protruding into the endometrial cavity. (**c**) Axial DW image at b500 shows the mass (*arrow*) to be slightly hypointense compared to the myometrium with an ADC value computed at 0.97×10^{-3} mm²/s versus 1.57×10^{-3} mm²/s in the normal adjacent myometrium. DMR before (**d**), at the arterial phase (**e**), at the venous phase (**f**), at the parenchymal phase (**g**), and at the late phase (**h**) with corresponding time-intensity curves (**i**) shows the mass to enhance more rapidly than the myometrium. A preoperative diagnosis of leiomyomas was made. Hysteroscopy was performed and the three masses excised. At pathology, the final diagnosis was adenomyoma.

Fig. 24.31 (*continued*) (**j**) Histologic view showing smooth muscle (*SM*) surrounding endometrial glands (*EG*) and endometrial stroma (*ES*)

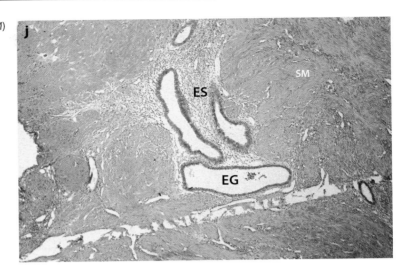

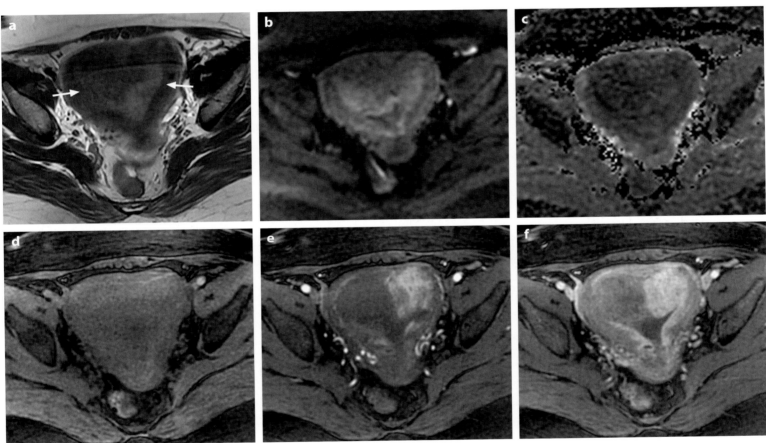

Fig. 24.32 Adenomyosis realizing two pseudomasses (or adenomyomas) protruding into the uterine cavity with different enhancement patterns. Vaginal bleeding in a 51-year-old woman. (**a**) Axial T2W image displays two contiguous ill-defined masses (best defined on the venous phase of the DMR, figure part **f**) or pseudomasses (*arrows*) of the uterine fundus of mixed intermediate and low intensity, protruding into the endometrial cavity. These masses are isointense to myometrium on T1WI and T1-FS-WI (not shown). (**b**, **c**) DWI at b500 (**b**) shows the mass to have high signal intensity in some parts, while on the corresponding ADC map (**c**), it appears uniform with an ADC slightly lower than normal myometrium (0.77×10^{-3} mm^2/s in the right mass and 0.9×10^{-3} mm^2/s in the left mass; mean measurements at b500 and b1000). (**d**–**i**) DMR before (**d**), at the arterial phase (**e**), at the venous phase (**f**), at the parenchymal phase

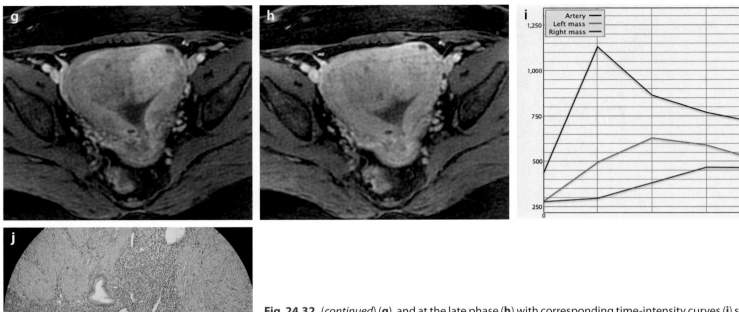

Fig. 24.32 (*continued*) (**g**), and at the late phase (**h**) with corresponding time-intensity curves (**i**) shows that the left part of the mass to enhance more rapidly than the myometrium while the right part of the mass enhances less rapidly than the myometrium. Both became almost isointense to the myometrium on the late phase. Not enhancing blood is seen in the endometrial cavity. The overall impression was that the masses were protruding into the endometrial cavity. At hysteroscopy, two contiguous masses were seen protruding into the endometrial cavity occupying the fundus of the uterus. The masses were excised. (**j**) At histology, the excised tissue was constituted of muscular hyperplasia surrounding benign endometrial glands and stroma. Final diagnosis: benign adenomyosis

24.6.3 Adenomyotic Cyst

Adenomyotic cyst is a rare condition. It may be subserous, within the myometrium, or grow as a polyp originating from the myometrium or endometrium [13] (Fig. 24.33). At pathology, it corresponds to a hemorrhagic cyst surrounded by adenomyotic lesions. On MR and US, the content of the cyst has the same findings as ovarian endometrioma, but its wall is hyperechoic on US and enhances on MR (Figs. 24.34, 24.35, and 24.36).

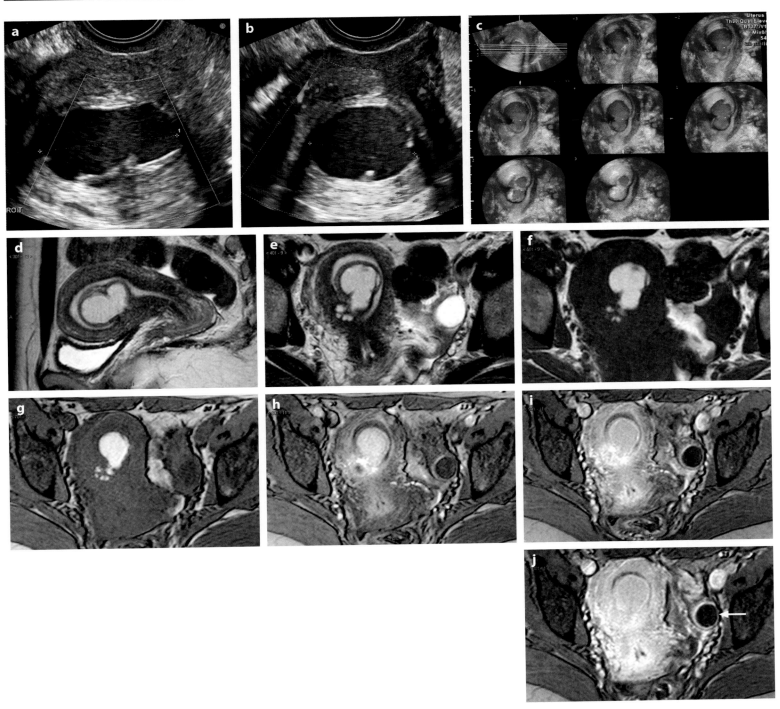

Fig. 24.33 Adenomyotic cyst protruding into the endometrial cavity. A 44-year-old woman with menorrhagia, dysmenorrhea, and history of adenomyosis. (**a**, **b**) Sagittal and transverse transvaginal ultrasound discloses a well-delineated cystic mass within the endometrial cavity. Its content is echoic with small hyperechoic peripheral clots. (**c**) 3D reformations with coronal images show the bilobular shape of the cyst. (**d**, **e**) Sagittal and axial T2W images show the bilocular cystic structure to be surrounded by endometrium. Its content is hyperintense. On the axial view, other small hyperintense cystic structures are seen within the myometrium at the base of implantation of the adenomyotic endocavitary cyst. (**f**) Axial T1W images (**f**) show all the above described endocavitary and intramyometrial cystic structures to have a hyperintense hemorrhagic content persisting after fat suppression and on DMR before injection confirming their hemorrhagic nature. (**g–j**) DMR before injection (**g**), at the arterial phase (**h**), at the venous phase (**i**), and at the late phase (**j**) shows that the wall of the adenomyotic endocavitary cyst enhances roughly like the inner myometrium. A left corpus luteum cyst is also displayed (*arrow* in **j**)

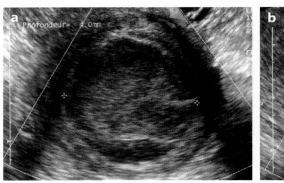

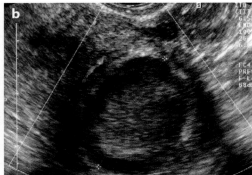

Fig. 24.34 Adenomyotic cyst. Recurrent pelvic pain in a 21-year-old woman followed for adenomyotic cyst proven by MRI. (**a**, **b**), sagittal (**a**) and transverse (**b**) transvaginal ultrasound discloses a 3-cm well-circumscribed mass (*cursors*) with a peripheral hyperechoic rim and a heterogeneous center. No color Doppler could be displayed in the mass

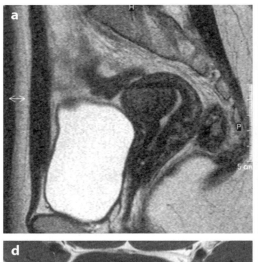

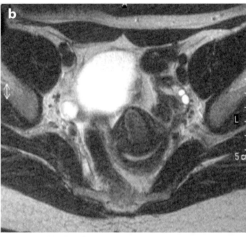

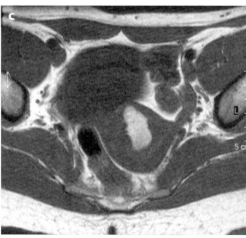

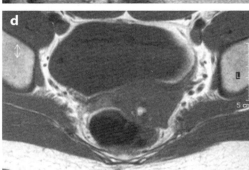

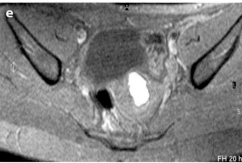

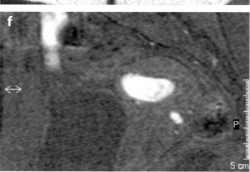

Fig. 24.35 Adenomyotic cyst of the uterus. A 27-year-old woman with postmenarchal pain for several years. Sagittal and axial MR T2-weighted image (**a** and **b**), axial MR T1-weighted images (**c** and **d**), and axial and sagittal MR T1-weighted images with fat suppression (**e** and **f**). (1) A collection with a low signal on T2 (**a**, **b**), a signal equal to adipose tissue on T1 (**c**), and bright on T1 with fat suppression (**e** and **f**) is depicted in the anterior wall of the uterus pushing backward the endometrium (**a**, **b**). These findings are typical for an adenomyotic cyst. (2) Punctiform lesions of adenomyosis are present in the posterior wall (**d** and **f**). *At surgery*, after longitudinal hysterotomy, 15 ml of blood was aspirated from the uterine cyst. Pathologic examination of the wall of the cyst confirms the diagnosis of adenomyosis

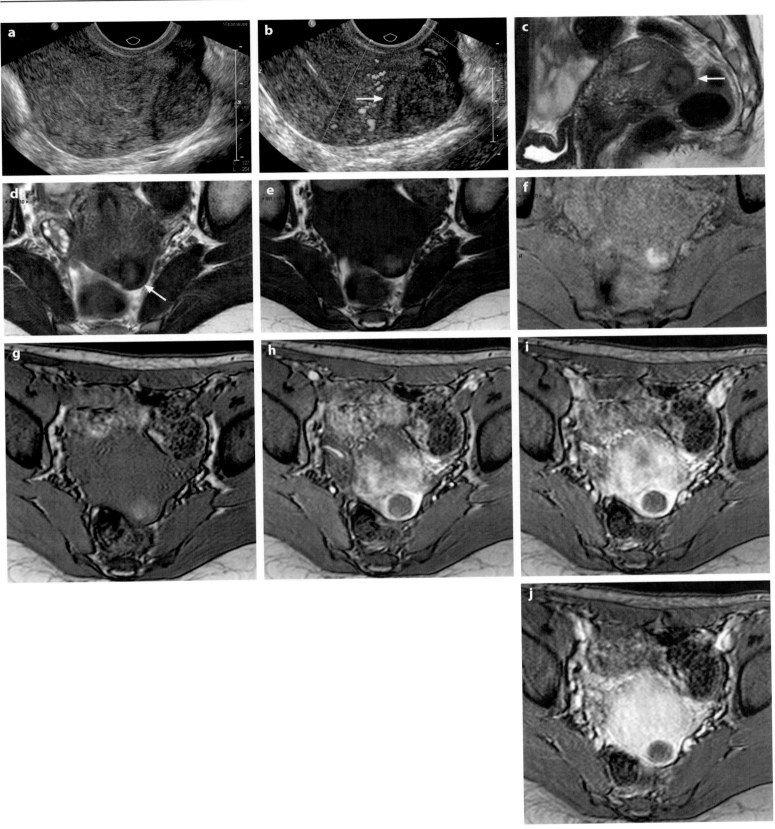

Fig. 24.36 Adenomyotic subserous cyst. A 21-year-old woman with cyclic pain. (**a–b**) Sagittal (**a**, **b**) transvaginal ultrasound with color Doppler shows a subserous mass without color flow, slightly hypoechoic and heterogeneous. A peripheral vascularized echoic rim (*arrow* in **b**) is present. (**c**, **d**) Sagittal and axial T2W images show the subserous posterior mass (*arrows*) to have a center of intermediate intensity and a hypointense periphery. (**e**, **f**) Axial T1W images without (**e**) and with (**f**) fat suppression show the mass to have a hyperintense hemorrhagic center. (**g–j**) DMR before injection (**g**), at the arterial phase (**h**), at the venous phase (**i**), and at the late phase (**j**) shows a cystic lesion with nonenhancing hemorrhagic center and a peripheral enhancing rim

References

1. Andersen J (1998) Factors in fibroid growth. Baillieres Clin Obstet Gynaecol 12(2):225–243
2. Cramer SF, Patel A (1990) The frequency of uterine leiomyomas. Am J Clin Pathol 94(4):435–438
3. Kliewer MA et al (1995) Acoustic shadowing from uterine leiomyomas: sonographic-pathologic correlation. Radiology 196(1):99–102
4. Caoili EM et al (2000) Refractory shadowing from pelvic masses on sonography: a useful diagnostic sign for uterine leiomyomas. AJR Am J Roentgenol 174(1):97–101
5. Wamsteker K, Emanuel MH, de Kruif JH (1993) Transcervical hysteroscopic resection of submucous fibroids for abnormal uterine bleeding: results regarding the degree of intramural extension. Obstet Gynecol 82(5):736–740
6. Salim R et al (2005) A comparative study of three-dimensional saline infusion sonohysterography and diagnostic hysteroscopy for the classification of submucous fibroids. Hum Reprod 20(1):253–257
7. Sahdev A et al (2001) MR imaging of uterine sarcomas. AJR Am J Roentgenol 177(6):1307–1311
8. Torashima M et al (1998) The value of detection of flow voids between the uterus and the leiomyoma with MRI. J Magn Reson Imaging 8(2):427–431
9. Park BK et al (2006) Differentiation of the various lesions causing an abnormality of the endometrial cavity using MR imaging: emphasis on enhancement patterns on dynamic studies and late contrast-enhanced T1-weighted images. Eur Radiol 16(7):1591–1598
10. O'Connor DM, Norris HJ (1990) Mitotically active leiomyomas of the uterus. Hum Pathol 21(2):223–227
11. Yamashita Y et al (1993) Hyperintense uterine leiomyoma at T2-weighted MR imaging: differentiation with dynamic enhanced MR imaging and clinical implications. Radiology 189(3):721–725
12. Oguchi O et al (1995) Prediction of histopathologic features and proliferative activity of uterine leiomyoma by magnetic resonance imaging prior to GnRH analogue therapy: correlation between T2-weighted images and effect of GnRH analogue. J Obstet Gynaecol (Tokyo 1995) 21(2):107–117
13. Zaloudek C (2001) Mesenchymal tumors of the uterus. In: Kurman RJ (ed) Blaustein's pathology of the female genital tract, 5th edn. Springer, New York, pp 561–615
14. Tanaka YO et al (2004) Smooth muscle tumors of uncertain malignant potential and leiomyosarcomas of the uterus: MR findings. J Magn Reson Imaging 20(6):998–1007
15. Parker WH, Fu YS, Berek JS (1994) Uterine sarcoma in patients operated on for presumed leiomyoma and rapidly growing leiomyoma. Obstet Gynecol 83(3):414–418
16. Exacoustos C et al (2007) Can gray-scale and color Doppler sonography differentiate between uterine leiomyosarcoma and leiomyoma? J Clin Ultrasound 35(8):449–457
17. Aviram R et al (2005) Uterine sarcomas versus leiomyomas: gray-scale and Doppler sonographic findings. J Clin Ultrasound 33(1):10–13
18. Goto A et al (2002) Usefulness of Gd-DTPA contrast-enhanced dynamic MRI and serum determination of LDH and its isozymes in the differential diagnosis of leiomyosarcoma from degenerated leiomyoma of the uterus. Int J Gynecol Cancer 12(4):354–361
19. Tamai K et al (2008) The utility of diffusion-weighted MR imaging for differentiating uterine sarcomas from benign leiomyomas. Eur Radiol 18(4):723–730
20. Namimoto T et al (2009) Combined use of T2-weighted and diffusion-weighted 3-T MR imaging for differentiating uterine sarcomas from benign leiomyomas. Eur Radiol 19(11):2756–2764
21. Pecorelli S (2009) Revised FIGO staging for carcinoma of the vulva, cervix, and endometrium. Int J Gynaecol Obstet 105(2):103–104
22. FIGO Committee on Gynecologic Oncology (2009) FIGO staging for uterine sarcomas. Prat J. Int J Gynaecol Obstet 104(3):177–178. Erratum in: Int J Gynaecol Obstet. Sep;106(3):277
23. Scully RE et al (1994) World Health Organization International histological classification of tumours, vol 2, Histological typing of female genital tract tumours. Springer, Berlin
24. Koyama T et al (1999) MR imaging of endometrial stromal sarcoma: correlation with pathologic findings. AJR Am J Roentgenol 173(3):767–772
25. Ueda M et al (2000) Uterine endometrial stromal sarcoma located in uterine myometrium: MRI appearance. Eur Radiol 10(5):780–782
26. Ueda M et al (2001) MR imaging findings of uterine endometrial stromal sarcoma: differentiation from endometrial carcinoma. Eur Radiol 11(1):28–33
27. Gandolfo N et al (2000) Endometrial stromal sarcoma of the uterus: MR and US findings. Eur Radiol 10(5):776–779
28. Silverberg SG, Kurman RJ (1992) Endometrial stromal tumors: tumors of uterine corpus and gestational trophoblastic disease. In: Rosai J (ed) Atlas of tumors pathology, vol 3. AFIP, Washington, pp 91–112
29. Lamboley JL et al (2010) A rare tumor: endometrial stromal nodule. J Radiol 91(11 Pt 1):1161–1163
30. Atri M et al (2000) Adenomyosis: US features with histologic correlation in an in-vitro study. Radiology 215(3):783–790
31. Kilickesmez O et al (2009) Quantitative diffusion-weighted magnetic resonance imaging of normal and diseased uterine zones. Acta Radiol 50(3):340–347

Mixed Epithelial Mesenchymal Tumors

25

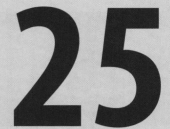

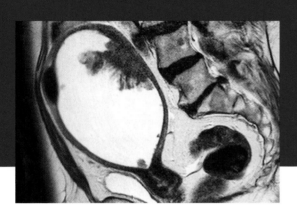

Contents

25.1 Definition

1. Adenofibroma versus adenosarcoma
   - Adenofibroma = adeno (benign epithelial component) + fibroma (benign mesenchymal component)
   - Adenosarcoma = adeno (benign epithelial component) + sarcoma (malignant mesenchymal component, most commonly stromal sarcoma or fibrosarcoma)
2. Malignant Mesodermal Mixed Tumor (MMMT) or carcinosarcoma
   Malignant epithelial and mesenchymal components
   (a) Endometrial origin
      - Malignant epithelium, most often endometrioid carcinoma
      - Malignant sarcoma, most commonly endometrial stromal sarcoma or fibrosarcoma (homologous-type mesenchymal component)
   (b) Endometrial component + homologous type of stromal component (leiomyosarcoma)
   (c) Endometrial component + Heterologous type of stromal component (mainly rhabdomyosarcoma and chondrosarcoma)

25.2 Adenofibroma

25.2.1 US

It appears as a well-defined mass occupying the uterine cavity that can extend into the myometrium. Cystic spaces may be present (Fig. 25.1).

J.N. Buy, M. Ghossain, *Gynecological Imaging*,
DOI 10.1007/978-3-642-31012-6_25, © Springer-Verlag Berlin Heidelberg 2013

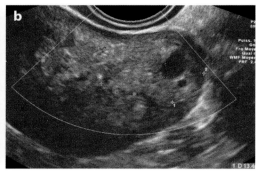

Fig. 25.1 Adenofibroma. Thirty-six-year-old woman with metrorragias for 5 months and previous hysteroscopy for polyp. EVS longitudinal (**a**) and color Doppler (**b**) depict an endometrial mass with an echogenicity close to myometrium extending into the myometrium. The mass contains multiple cystic spaces

25.2.2 CT

It has been described as a well-defined mass expanding the uterine cavity with numerous high-attenuating septum-like strands within it [1].

25.2.3 MR

MR findings have been reported as [1]:
- On T2, a heterogeneous high-intensity mass in the uterine cavity
- On T1, a low signal-intensity mass with multiple septa of higher intensity
- After injection, a latticelike enhancement

25.3 Adenosarcoma

25.3.1 Definition

It is a benign, but occasionally atypical, glandular component and a sarcomatous, usually low-grade, stromal component [2].
In contrast to typical malignant mixed Mullerian tumors, Mullerian adenosarcoma is usually of low malignant potential; only a minority of them are clinically malignant, and many of them pursue an indolent course.

The closely related Mullerian adenofibroma is characterized by epithelial and benign stromal component.

25.3.2 Location

Adenosarcoma most often occurs in the endometrium.

Rare tumors arise in the myometrium presumably from adenomyosis.

In 5–10 % of cases, they arise in the cervix and rarely in extrauterine locations: fallopian tube, ovary, and paraovarian tissues [3].

25.3.3 Clinical Features

Adenosarcoma occurs in women of all ages with a median age of 57–59 years.

Extrauterine adenosarcoma occurs in younger women and is more aggressive than its uterine counterpart.

Patients may have a history of pelvic radiation, tamoxifen therapy for breast cancer, and previous surgery for removal of cervical or endometrial polyp.

Occasional patients are diabetic.

The most common clinical symptom is abnormal vaginal bleeding.

Other findings are vaginal discharge, a palpable pelvic mass, and a tumor protruding from the cervix.

25.3.4 Pathology

25.3.4.1 Macroscopy [3, 4]

Size

One to seventeen centimeters (mean 5 cm).

Aspect

- Typically solitary, sessile, or pedunculated polypoid.
- Variable-sized cysts: the rounded glands vary in size from those of an early proliferative endometrium to cysts with regular wall up to several cm in diameter.
- Or papillary masses grow into the cavity and can enlarge the uterus.
- Tissue protruding from the external cervical os (50 %), in some cases partially filling the vagina.
- Uncommonly
  - Multiple small mucosal polyps
  - Well-circumscribed myometrial masses
- Uncommonly, hemorrhage and focal necrosis
- Extension: invasion of myometrium in 16 % usually the inner third

25.3.4.2 Microscopy

- Epithelium: the most common type resembles inactive or proliferative endometrial epithelium.
- Mesenchymal component generally is a homologous sarcoma such as stromal sarcoma or fibrosarcoma.
- Periglandular stromal hypercellularity is a characteristic feature of adenosarcoma.

25.3.5 Imaging Findings

25.3.5.1 Ultrasound [5]

- A thickened heterogeneous endometrial echo complex mass with cystic spaces
- A polyp-like structure in the uterine cavity with a large feeding extending artery from the myometrium into the stroma of the lesion

25.3.5.2 CT [1]

A large polypoid enhancing mass that had a broad base on the uterine wall with multiple small enhancing polypoid masses expanding the uterine cavity

25.3.5.3 MR

MR findings in the literature are scarce:

(a) A case is reported hereby with solid portion of intermediate intensity on T2 associated to high-intensity cystic pockets, areas of hemorrhage on T1FS, hyperintensity on DWI, and arterial vessels on DMR (Fig. 25.2).

(b) In the case of Chourmouzi [5], the tumor appeared confined to the endometrium:

On T1, multiple well-defined cystic spaces of low signal-intensity area and of high signal intensity presumed to represent hemorrhage.

On T2, well-delineated multiple cystic spaces of high signal intensity.

On T1, after injection, enhancement of the solid component and septa around the cysts creating a latticelike appearance.

(c) In the case of Lee et al. [1], a large polypoid enhancing mass that had a broad base to the uterine wall with multiple small enhancing polypoid masses expanding the uterine cavity.

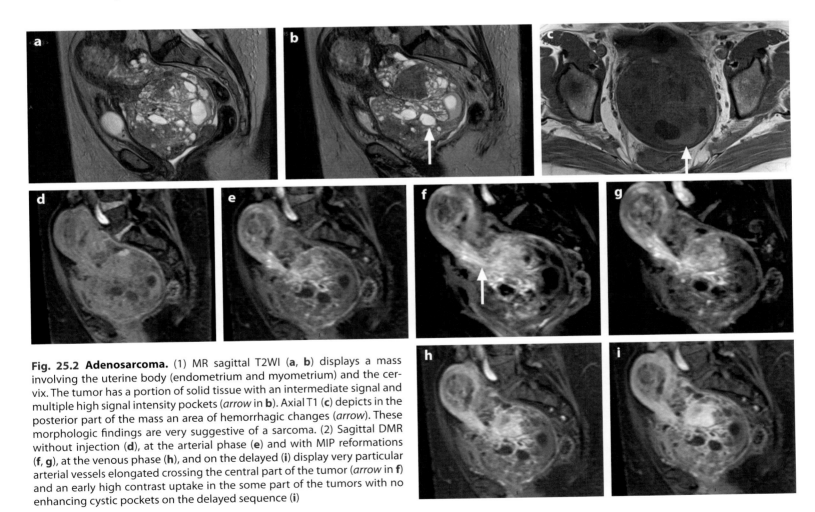

Fig. 25.2 Adenosarcoma. (1) MR sagittal T2WI (**a**, **b**) displays a mass involving the uterine body (endometrium and myometrium) and the cervix. The tumor has a portion of solid tissue with an intermediate signal and multiple high signal intensity pockets (*arrow* in **b**). Axial T1 (**c**) depicts in the posterior part of the mass an area of hemorrhagic changes (*arrow*). These morphologic findings are very suggestive of a sarcoma. (2) Sagittal DMR without injection (**d**), at the arterial phase (**e**) and with MIP reformations (**f**, **g**), at the venous phase (**h**), and on the delayed (**i**) display very particular arterial vessels elongated crossing the central part of the tumor (*arrow* in **f**) and an early high contrast uptake in the some part of the tumors with no enhancing cystic pockets on the delayed sequence (**i**)

25.4 Malignant Mesodermal Mixed Tumor (MMMT) or Carcinosarcoma

They represent about 50 % of uterine sarcoma (Table 25.1).

Table 25.1 Frequency of the different uterine sarcomas [6]

- MMMTs 50 %
- Leiomyosarcomas 30 %
- Endometrial stromal sarcoma 10 %
- Other uterine sarcomas 10 %

25.4.1 Definition

Malignant epithelial and mesenchymal component
(a) Endometrial origin
  - Malignant epithelium, most often endometrioid carcinoma
  - Malignant sarcoma, most commonly stromal sarcoma or fibrosarcoma (homologous-type mesenchymal component)
(b) Endometrial component+homologous type of stromal component (leiomyosarcoma)
(c) Endometrial component+Heterologous type of stromal component (mainly rhabdomyosarcoma and chondrosarcoma)

25.4.2 Pathology

One must distinguish the epithelial and the mesenchymal components [7, 8].

25.4.2.1 Malignant Epithelial Component

- Endometrioid carcinoma isolated (118/203) or accompanied by squamous differentiation (52/203) in most of cases [8].
- Serous, mucinous, clear-cell, and undifferentiated carcinoma can be found (33/203).

25.4.2.2 Malignant Mesenchymal Component

- Homologous (107/203 of cases)
  Homologous=the constituent tissues are encountered in benign uteri.
  In most of the cases, high-grade endometrial stromal sarcoma.
  Less frequently a round cell variant of endometrial stromal sarcoma.
  Even less frequently a leiomyosarcomatous pattern either focally or diffuse.
  Sarcomatous areas resembling malignant fibrous histiocytoma and hemangiopericytoma were also rarely encountered.
- Heterologous (96/203 of cases)
  The most frequent was rhabdomyosarcoma alone (35/96).
  The second most frequent was chondrosarcoma alone (26/96).
  Osteosarcomas alone (7/96), liposarcomas alone (5/96).
  Combinations including rhabdomyosarcomas (16/96) or without rhabdomyosarcomas (7/96).

25.4.3 Macroscopy

- Frequently polypoid, usually fill the entire endometrial cavity
- Areas of necrosis and hemorrhage

- Invasion of the myometrium (3/4 of cases) [8]
- Lymphatic or vascular invasion in half of these cases
- Involves the lower segment (1/2 of cases) and the cervix (1/4 of cases) [8]

25.4.4 MMMT Is a Variant of Endometrial Carcinoma

Since the earliest reports, speculation has centered on whether these tumors represent:
- Collision tumor: a mixture of two histogenetically distinct malignant populations
- Combination tumor: an origin of both elements from a common stem cell
- Composition tumor: pure carcinoma with reactive atypical but benign stromal elements [8]

25.4.5 Risk Factors

Profile: obesity, exogenous estrogen use, nulliparity

Very particular to this type of tumor is *a history of prior radiation in some cases*: in these cases, patients tend to be younger and tend to present with advanced-stage disease.

Microvessel density in the carcinomatous component is higher than in the sarcomatous component, suggesting that the former is responsible for the aggressive biologic behavior of these neoplasms.

Immunohistochemical studies: the mesenchymal components express cytokeratin and epithelial membrane antigens supporting the view that these portions of the tumor arise from carcinomatous component via divergent differentiation.

Molecular genetic studies: identical p53 mutations have been found in the epithelial and mesenchymal components.

25.4.6 Clinical Features

- Most women postmenopausal
- Postmenopausal bleeding (most common)
- Vaginal discharge

25.4.7 Location

(a) Most often, it appears as a large mass growing into the endometrial cavity [9, 10, 13, 14]. It can be pedunculated exophytic or broad based. Uncommonly, it can have a myometrial or cervical epicenter [14].
  - Areas of necrosis and hemorrhage are commonly present
  - Invasion of the myometrium is common but some MMMT are confined to polyps
  - Often, the mass protrudes through the cervical os (protruding part often necrotic)
  - Extension into the endocervix is observed in (1/4 of cases) [8]
(b) Uncommonly, it appears as a large pelvic mass [15].
(c) Extrauterine extension is observed in about 12 % of cases [10] especially ovarian metastases and peritoneal dissemination.

25.4.8 Imaging

25.4.8.1 Ultrasound

Description in the literature is rare.

Teo et al. reported five cases [9]:

- Dilatation of the endometrial cavity (1.6–5.3 cm) was found in three cases. The masses appeared hyperechoic to normal endometrium; myometrial invasion was suspected in two patients.
- A slightly homogeneous echogenic thickening of the endometrium was found in one case.
- A heterogeneous mass replacing the entire uterus was found in one case associated to extrauterine masses
- A case is reported hereby with a particular pattern of an echogenic mass filled with cystic or necrotic spaces (Fig. 25.3).

25.4.8.2 CT

Description in the literature is rare.

Teo et al. reported ten cases [9]:

- Dilatation of the endometrial cavity was present in nine (90 %) cases.
- A mass was present within the endometrial cavity in all ten cases; the largest dimension ranged from 0.9 to 17.0 cm (mean: 4.9 cm).

Six (60 %) of the masses were ill defined, and the remainders were well defined.

- MMMT mostly appeared heterogeneous ($n=9$) except for the smallest mass, which appeared homogeneous.
- All masses appeared hypodense to normal myometrium. Of these, two had areas of hyperdensity that did not constitute 50 % of the mass but affected the measurement of its attenuation; one showed a 0.8-cm calcified nodule, and the other showed a tiny focus of calcification, both within the right lateral aspect of the endometrial cavity.
- In the majority (80 %), enhancement of the mass was about half to almost 70 % of normal myometrium. Interestingly, two masses had almost equal and slightly greater enhancement than normal myometrium, and these were the two masses containing areas of hyperdensity.
- Eight of ten patients were deemed to have myometrial involvement on CT scans.
- Metastatic pelvic and retroperitoneal lymphadenopathy was identified in three patients; omental carcinomatosis and right adnexal involvement in one patient each.

A case is reported hereby with another finding. The mass appears hypodense to myometrium but contains arterial vessel at the arterial phase (Fig. 25.4).

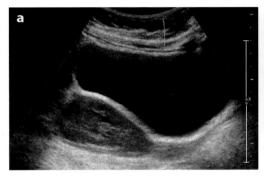 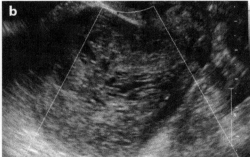 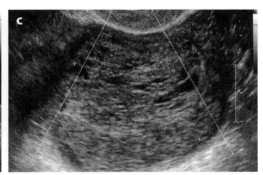

Fig. 25.3 MMMT with poorly differentiated epithelial component and mesenchymal component composed of heterologous sarcoma with predominant rhabdomyosarcoma. Eighty-two-year-old woman with metrorragias. Biopsy of the endometrium: suspicion of endometrial carcinoma. Sagittal TAS (**a**) displays an endometrial mass occupying the endometrial cavity from the fundus to the isthmus. On longitudinal (**b**) and transverse (**c**) EVS with color Doppler, this mass has a very particular echogenicity, containing a lot of cystic or necrotic changes and extending into the myometrium slightly inner to normal external myometrium. Vessels are visualized in the mass. At pathology, extension to the inner part of the myometrium was confirmed, but extension to the endocervical mucosa was missed by ultrasound

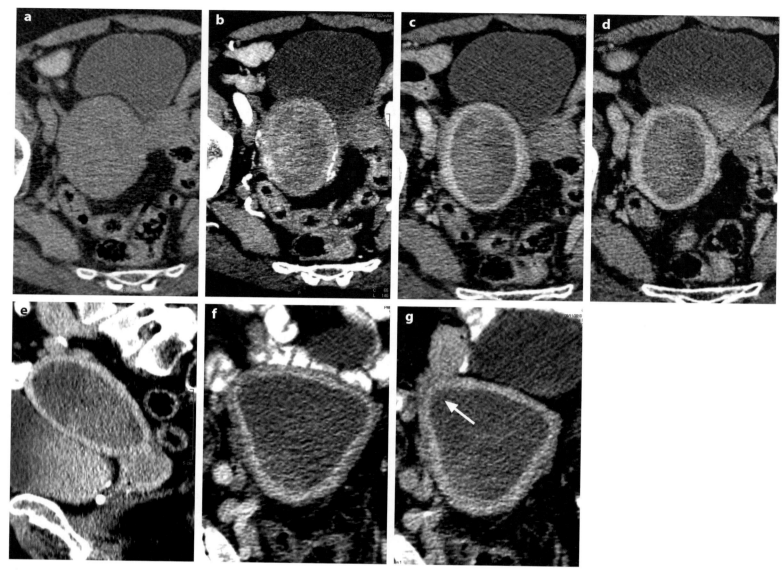

Fig. 25.4 MMMT on CT. (**a**, **d**) Axial DCT before injection (**a**), at the arterial phase (**b**), at the venous phase (**c**), and at the parenchymal phase (**d**), displays a large mass expanding the uterine cavity. At the arterial phase, contrast uptake is seen in the tumor corresponding probably to small arteries.

(**e**–**g**) Sagittal (**e**) and oblique (**f**, **g**) reformations show absence of cervical extension on the sagittal view and invasion of the myometrium on the oblique views especially in the right cornual zone (*arrow*)

25.4.8.3 MR Findings

They are summarized in Table 25.2 (Figs. 25.5, 25.6, and 25.7) [10].

On T2

Signal intensity was compared to myometrium (without making a distinction between inner and outer layers), and to endometrium. In Bharwani's series, the mass was:

- Hyperintense to myometrium (90 %)
- Hypointense (55 %) or isointense (41 %) to endometrium
- Heterogeneous (80 %)

On T1

The mass was [10]:

Predominantly Isointense to myometrium (76 %), with
High T1 signal-intensity foci (27 %)
Heterogeneous (33 %)

Table 25.2 MR findings of MMMT

Location [10]
- Most often (88 %): endometrial growing into the endometrial cavity
- Uncommon
  Myometrial epicenter
  Cervical epicenter

Macroscopic findings [7]
- Frequently polypoid, usually fill the entire endometrial cavity
- Areas of necrosis and hemorrhage
- Invasion of the myometrium common but some confined to polyps
- Often protrudes through the cervical os (protruding part often necrotic)
- Extension into the endocervix (1/4 of cases)

Signal intensity [10]
- On T2, heterogeneous more hyperintense than myometrium
- On T1, isointense to myometrium with possible hyperintense hemorrhagic foci
- Flow voids may be present
- ADC values lower than myometrium
- On DMR, variable enhancement more often heterogeneous and inferior to myometrium but can be superior to myometrium. Arterial vessels at the arterial phase are characteristics

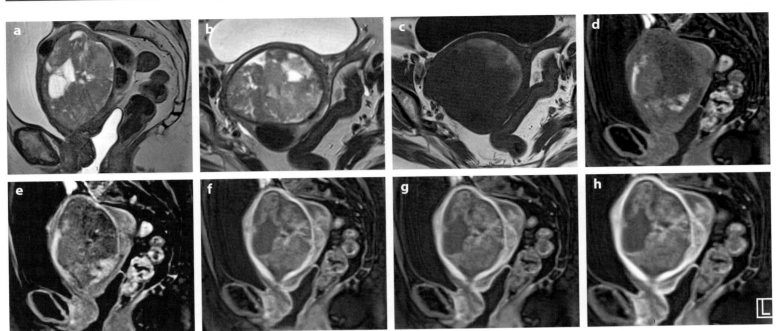

Fig. 25.5 Malignant mesodermal mixed tumor (MMMT) with a heterologous type of stromal component. MR sagittal and axial T2 (**a**, **b**) display an endometrial mass filling the entire endometrial cavity with its lower border at the level of the isthmus without any extension into the cervix. The tumor is composed of solid tissue of intermediate signal and of cystic pockets very suggestive of a sarcoma. Junctional zone is preserved; absence of extension to the myometrium was confirmed at pathology. Axial T1 and sagittal T1 fat suppressions (**c**, **d**) demonstrate hemorrhagic changes in the anterior portion. On sagittal DMR before injection (**d**), at the arterial phase (**e**), at the venous phase (**f**), and at delayed phases (**g**, **h**): At the arterial phase, tumoral vessels are depicted in the posterior and lower part of the tumor allowing diagnosing a malignant tumor. Otherwise, peripheral arterial vessels are seen in the inner myometrium. At the venous phase and on the following phases, contrast uptake is present in the solid portions, while contrast uptake is absent in the hemorrhagic and necrotic degenerative portions. The peripheral enhancing rim, corresponding to the inner myometrium, is now clearly and completely delineated, suggesting absence of myometrial invasion. Surgery: total hysterectomy with bilateral adnexectomy, omentectomy, and bilateral pelvic and lomboaortic lymphadenectomy. Microscopy and immunohistochemical study: MMMT with a heterologous component. Tumor limited to the endometrium without extension outside the uterus

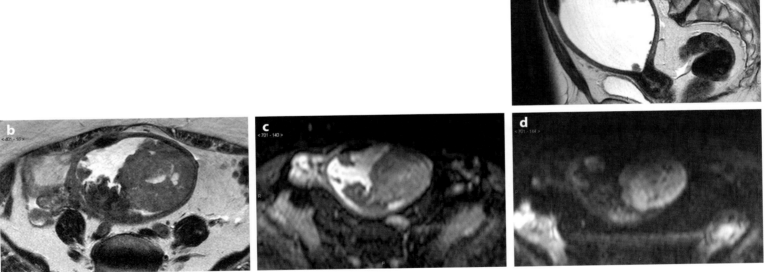

Fig. 25.6 Malignant mixed mesodermal with tubulopapillary epithelial component and rhabdomyosarcoma mesenchymal component. Sixty-nine-year-old woman with metrorragias. MR sagittal T2 (**a**) display an endometrial mass filling the entire endometrial cavity with a solid portion and a large necrotic hyperintense portion. The tissular portion has irregular borders and is associated with multiple small nodules at the periphery. On axial T2 (**b**) passing through the fundus, the right component of the mass extends into the outer part of the myometrium from 6 to 10 h. Right adnexa are invaded by the same proliferation as the primary tumor. At pathology, the tube and the ovary were involved. Diffusion b0 (**c**) and b1000 (**d**) show the solid portion to be hyperintense on b1000

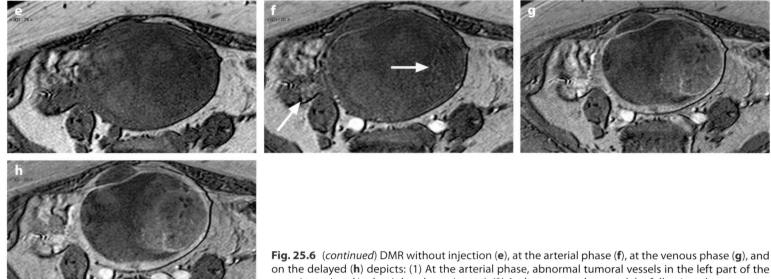

Fig. 25.6 (*continued*) DMR without injection (**e**), at the arterial phase (**f**), at the venous phase (**g**), and on the delayed (**h**) depicts: (1) At the arterial phase, abnormal tumoral vessels in the left part of the mass (*arrow*) and in the right adnexa (*arrow*). (2) At the venous phase and the following phases, extension to the outer part of the myometrium and the right adnexa is depicted. At pathology, the right tube and the right ovary were involved

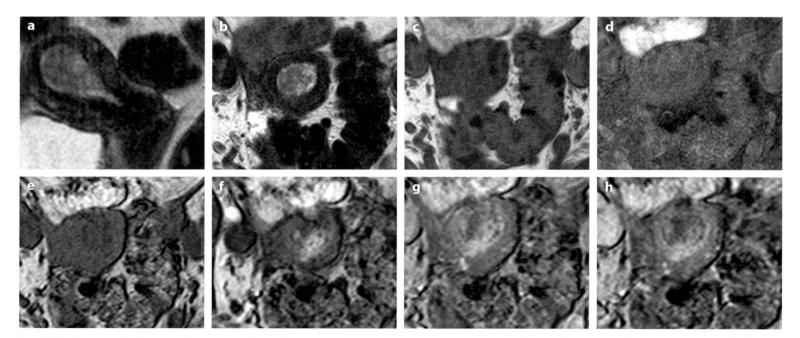

Fig. 25.7 Seventy-eight-year-old woman without hormonal treatment and with metrorragias for 3 months. Hysteroscopy: polypoid mass of the fundus. Biopsy: low-differentiated carcinoma. MR sagittal (**a**) and axial (**b**) T2 images display an endometrial mass with an intermediate signal intensity filling the entire endometrial cavity. Posterior extension to the inner myometrium is visualized. No extension to the cervix is visualized. Axial T1 (**c**) and T1-FS (**d**) do not demonstrate any hemorrhage in the mass. DMR without injection (**e**) and at the arterial phase (**f**) depict large irregular vessels mainly in the left part of the mass. At the venous phase (**g**), a high contrast uptake at the same level is visualized which slightly decreases on the delayed phase (**h**). No pelvic lymph node extension is displayed. Prospective diagnosis: a malignant tumor of the endometrium is diagnosed. Two diagnoses are suggested: (1) a MMMT because of the type of vascularization at the arterial phase and the high contrast uptake at the venous phase and (2) an endometrial carcinoma alone is more unlikely. Surgery: total hysterectomy with bilateral adnexectomy and pelvic lymphadenectomy were performed. Microscopy: MMMT

Flow Voids

Flow voids (sequences not mentioned) were seen inside and/or around the tumor in 2/4 patients [11].

DW

In two cases, ADC values were low with higher intensity than the myometrium on T2 [12].

DMR

Enhancement is more often heterogeneous with arterial vessels often detected at the arterial phase. Overall enhancement may be inferior, equal, or superior to myometrium [10, 11].

25.4.8.4 Extension

• Cervix and vagina
• Pelvic soft tissues
• Peritoneal surfaces of the upper abdomen
• Lymph nodes
• Lungs

25.4.8.5 Differential Diagnosis

While the diagnosis of malignant tumor of the uterus body based on imaging findings particularly MR findings, is usually easily established, differential diagnosis with other types of malignant tumors limited to the endometrium or involving the endometrium and the myometrium (endometrial carcinoma, endometrial stromal sarcoma) is very difficult.

1. Endometrial carcinoma may be focal or diffuse, may appear like MMMT as uniformly exophytic or as polypoid separated masses. Endometrial carcinoma is complicated with necrosis and may be focally hemorrhagic. Some findings can suggest the possibility to differentiate MMMT from endometrial carcinoma Table 25.3 [11].

Table 25.3 Differential MR findings of endometrial carcinoma and MMMT

	Endometrial carcinoma	**MMMT**
Flow voids	Absence	Present in some cases
DMR arterial vessels	Thin and irregular	Larger and usually more regular
Contrast uptake	Usually less than inner myometrium	Areas of early and persistent marked contrast enhancement similar to that of myometrium
Extension	Extension to the lower uterine segment (not as frequent)	The polypoid mass most often protrudes through the cervical os

2. Endometrial stromal sarcoma invades the myometrium, sometimes extensively, and by definition invades the myometrium. Hemorrhage and necrosis are frequently present. In its most frequent pattern of growth, the myometrium is permeated by very particular cords or nodules of tumor.

3. Leiomyosarcoma is usually not a differential diagnosis. Indeed in this case, the mass is roughly round with a focal irregularity of the periphery. The epicenter of the mass is in the myometrium.

References

1. Lee HK et al (1998) Uterine adenofibroma and adenosarcoma: CT and MR findings. J Comput Assist Tomogr 22(2):314–316
2. Clement PB, Scully RE (1974) Mullerian adenosarcoma of the uterus. A clinicopathologic analysis of ten cases of a distinctive type of mullerian mixed tumor. Cancer 34(4):1138–1149
3. Clement PB, Scully RE (1990) Mullerian adenosarcoma of the uterus: a clinicopathologic analysis of 100 cases with a review of the literature. Hum Pathol 21(4):363–381
4. Kaku T et al (1992) Adenosarcoma of the uterus: a Gynecologic Oncology Group clinicopathologic study of 31 cases. Int J Gynecol Pathol 11(2): 75–88
5. Chourmouzi D et al (2003) Sonography and MRI of tamoxifen-associated mullerian adenosarcoma of the uterus. AJR Am J Roentgenol 181(6): 1673–1675
6. Harlow BL, Weiss NS, Lofton S (1986) The epidemiology of sarcomas of the uterus. J Natl Cancer Inst 76(3):399–402
7. Zaloudek C (2002) Mesenchymal tumors of the uterus. In: Blaustein's pathology of the female genital tract. Springer, New York, pp 561–615
8. Silverberg SG et al (1990) Carcinosarcoma (malignant mixed mesodermal tumor) of the uterus. A Gynecologic Oncology Group pathologic study of 203 cases. Int J Gynecol Pathol 9(1):1–19
9. Teo SY et al (2008) Primary malignant mixed mullerian tumor of the uterus: findings on sonography, CT, and gadolinium-enhanced MRI. AJR Am J Roentgenol 191(1):278–283
10. Bharwani N et al (2010) MRI appearances of uterine malignant mixed mullerian tumors. AJR Am J Roentgenol 195(5):1268–1275
11. Ohguri T et al (2002) MRI findings including gadolinium-enhanced dynamic studies of malignant, mixed mesodermal tumors of the uterus: differentiation from endometrial carcinomas. Eur Radiol 12(11): 2737–2742
12. Namimoto T et al (2009) Role of diffusion-weighted imaging in the diagnosis of gynecological diseases. Eur Radiol 19(3):745–760
13. Tanaka YO et al (2008) Carcinosarcoma of the uterus: MR findings. J Magn Reson Imaging 28(2):434–439
14. Shapeero LG, Hricak H (1989) Mixed mullerian sarcoma of the uterus: MR imaging findings. AJR Am J Roentgenol 153(2):317–319
15. Sahdev A et al (2001) MR imaging of uterine sarcomas. AJR Am J Roentgenol 177(6):1307–1311

Embryology, Anatomy, and Histology of the Cervix

26

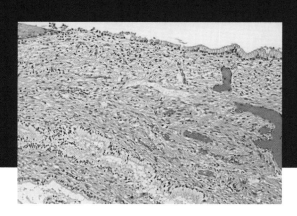

Contents

26.1 Embryology

See Chap. 1

26.2 Anatomy [1, 2]

26.2.1 The Cervix

The cervix is separated from the uterus body by the isthmus. It is about 3.0 cm long and 2.5 cm in diameter.

The cervix is divided into two portions:

(a) A portion that protrudes into the vagina called the portio vaginalis also referred to as the exocervix. This part of the cervix forms with the vaginal wall grooves called vaginal fornices (anterior, lateral, posterior).

(b) A portion above the vagina called the supravaginal portion also referred to as the endocervix.

The portion may be divided into anterior and posterior lips, of which the anterior is shorter and projects lower than the posterior lip.

The upper end communicates with the isthmus by an upper aperture [1]. During pregnancy and childbirth, the part of the cervix closest to the body of the uterus is called by the ob/gyn the internal os. The lower end opens into the vagina by a lower aperture called the external os. The external os is connected to the isthmus by the cervical canal.

There are two longitudinal ridges, one each on its anterior and posterior walls, that give off palmate folds. They ascend laterally like the branches of a tree. The folds interdigitate to close the canal.

J.N. Buy, M. Ghossain, *Gynecological Imaging*,
DOI 10.1007/978-3-642-31012-6_26, © Springer-Verlag Berlin Heidelberg 2013

26.2.2 Relations with the Neighbouring Structures

(a) Anteriorly the cervix is devoid of peritoneum. Its upper limit is in relation with the vesicouterine pouch. The supravaginal part is separated from the bladder by cellular connective tissue, called the vesicouterine septum [1] (Fig. 26.1). This septum is an anterior portion of the parametrium, which is in continuity laterally with the Mackenrodt's ligament.

(b) Posteriorly the peritoneum covers the upper part of the cervix, then the posterior fornix, then reflects on the anterior wall of the rectum to form the Douglas cul-de-sac (Fig. 26.1). On the upper part of the posterior surface of the cervix is a small transverse protrusion, the torus uterinus. On each side of the torus, utero-sacral ligaments go backward on the lateral faces of the rectum to join the anterior face of the sacrum (see Chap. 17). They limit laterally with the rectum the lateral parts of the Douglas (Fig. 26.2).

(c) Laterally the cervix (from its upper part to its inferior part including the vaginal fornices) is separated from the pelvic wall by a portion of the broad ligament the Mackenrodt's ligament or paracervix) (Fig. 26.3) (see Chap. 2).

26.2.3 Vascular Supply and Lymphatic Drainage

26.2.3.1 Arteries

The cervicovaginal artery arises from the uterine artery (its second segment in the Mackenrodt's ligament), immediately medial to the cross of the ureter behind and below the the uterine artery) (see Chap. 2, section broad ligament). It divides into two branches that embrace the anterior and posterior walls of the cervix and the vagina.

26.2.3.2 Veins

Cervical Veins

Cervical veins gather into two groups: mainly an anterior and superior group in front of the ureter, and a posterior and inferior group behind the ureter. These two groups form anastomoses with the vesical veins, the venous vaginal plexus, and end following the uterine artery (in its first extraperitoneal segment) into the hypogastric vein.

26.2.3.3 Lymphatics

The lymphatics of the cervix have a dual origin: coursing beneath the mucosa and deep in the fibrous stroma.

Lymphatics of the cervix drain into four groups:

(a) Forward into nodes near the posterior wall of the urinary bladder.

(b) Laterally in the Mackenrodt's ligament there are two groups of lymphatics. A first group passes in front of the ureter and drains into the middle and superior lymph nodes of the external iliac chain.

A second one passes behind the ureter in the middle and superior lymph nodes of the hypogastric chain and the obturator nodes.

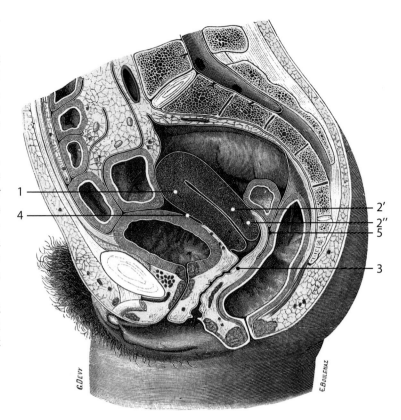

Fig. 26.1 Sagittal section through the pelvis: *1* body of the uterus, *2* cervix: *2'* supravaginalis portion, *2"* infravaginalis portion, *3* vagina, *4* vesicouterine pouch, *5* Douglas (From Testut [1])

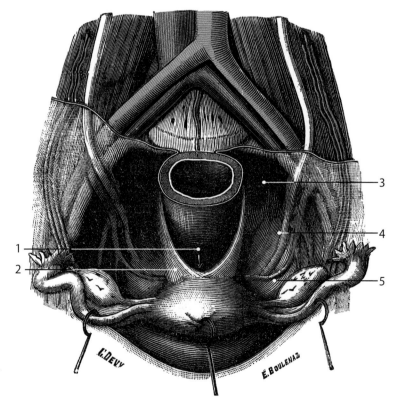

Fig. 26.2 View of the posterior cervix: *1* torus uterinus: small transverse protrusion on the upper part of the posterior cervix (in front of the vertical *arrow*), *2* uterosacral ligaments, *3* posterior parietal peritoneum, *4* ureter, *5* uterine artery (From Testut [1])

In the most extreme example, procidentia, uterus prolapses all the way through the vagina.

26.3 Histology

The cervix is composed of admixture of fibrous, muscular, and elastic tissue. Fibrous tissue is the predominant component. Smooth muscle comprises 15 % of the substance and is located mainly in the endocervix, the portio vaginalis being nearly devoid of smooth muscle fibers. In contrast at the isthmus, 50 % of the supportive connective tissue consists of concentrically arranged smooth muscle that act as a sphincter [2].

26.3.1 Histology of the Exocervix [2]

26.3.1.1 Epithelium

The mature squamous pluristratified nonkeratinized epithelium of the exocervix is similar to the vaginal epithelium but under normal circumstances lacks the rete pegs seen in the vagina. It is divided into three zones:

- The basal/parabasal layer; epithelial regeneration is the major function.
- The midzone occupied by cells undergoing maturation.
- The superficial zone, the most differentiated zone; its function is to protect the underlying epithelial cells and subepithelial vasculature from trauma and infection.

26.3.1.2 Stroma

The squamous epithelium of the exocervix is supported by fibrous connective tissue, devoid (almost entirely) of endocervical glands. There is a well-developed capillary network at the stromal-epithelial junction, with occasional fingerlike extensions into the epithelium, the stroma papillae.

26.3.2 Histology of the Endocervix [2]

26.3.2.1 Epithelium

It is composed of:
- A single layer of mucin-secreting columnar epithelium.
- Endocervical glands representing deep, cleft-like infoldings of the surface epithelium with numerous blind tunnellike collaterals [3].

In multiparous and older women, endocervical glands can appear as distinct tunnel clusters of as many as 50 small glands. These glands are frequently distended by inspissated mucus, so that the epithelium lining is frequently quite flattened.

26.3.2.2 Stroma

The subepithelial stroma with a well-developed capillary network is composed of an admixture of mainly fibrous tissue with some muscular (15 %) and elastic tissue.

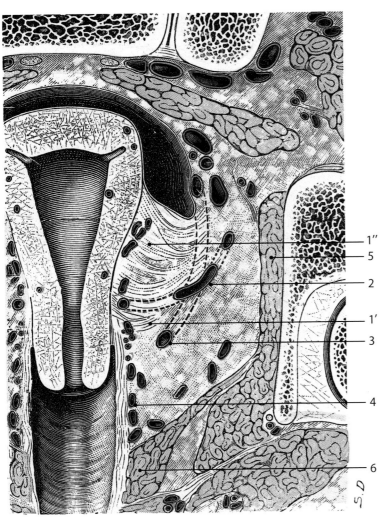

Fig. 26.3 Paracervix or Mackenrodt ligament. Coronal section through the uterus: *1* broad ligament: *1'* Mackenrodt ligament, *1"* mesometrium, *2* uterine artery, *3* ureter, *4* veins, *5* internal obturatis, *6* levator ani (From Testut [1])

Both of these drainages can further involve the common iliac nodes.

(c) Posteriorly lymphatics leave the posterior portion of the cervix, run on both sides of the rectum and go into the presacral lymph nodes and into the lymph nodes situated in front of the promontory.

26.2.4 Nerves

The innervation of the cervix is chiefly limited to the endocervix and the peripheral deep portion of the exocervix. This distribution is responsible for the relative insensitivity of the two-thirds of the portio vaginalis. The cervical nerves are derived from the pelvic autonomic system, the superior, middle, and inferior hypogastric plexuses.

26.2.5 Uterine Support

Uterosacral and Mackenrodt's ligaments may act in varying measure as mechanical supports of the uterus. Failure of these supports may result in prolapse of the uterus through the vagina (see Chap. 37).

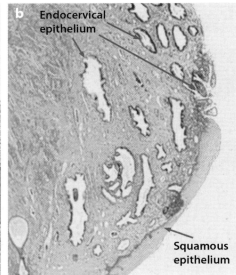

Fig. 26.4 Histology of the squamocolumnar junction. (**a**) This picture illustrates the cervical squamocolumnar junction. The exocervical squamous mucosa is represented on the *left side* of the picture (annotation). The endocervical epithelium is present on the right side, at the surface and lining glandular structures surrounded by stroma (annotated *arrows*). (**b**) In this picture, representing the cervical squamocolumnar junction, the exocervical squamous epithelium (annotated *arrow*) is present at the inferior part, overlying hyperplastic endocervical glands. The endocervical epithelium is present in the upper part (annotated *arrows*). The squamocolumnar junction shows mild chronic cervicitis and squamous metaplasia (From Testut [1])

26.3.3 Definitions of the Original Squamocolumnar Junction, the Physiologic Functional Junction, and the Transformation Zone [2]

Definition of the squamocolumnar junction: The squamocolumnar junction of the cervix is defined as the border between the stratified squamous epithelium of the exocervix and the mucin-secreting columnar epithelium of the endocervix (Fig. 26.4).

Morphogenetically there are two different squamocolumnar junctions:

1) At birth the abrupt original squamocolunar junction.
   - At birth the *original squamocolumnar* junction is at the site at which the native squamous epithelium covering the endocervical canal abuts the columnar epithelium.
   - At 1 year of age, the cervix begins to elongate, which results in migration of the squamocolumnar junction toward the external os.
   - At the time of menarche, both the body and cervix enlarge which results in eversion of endocervical columnar epithelium into the portio vaginalis.
   - Over time, the columnar epithelium that composes cervical ectopy is replaced by metaplastic squamous epithelium. As this occurs, the histologic squamocolumnar junction moves toward the exocervical os. The newly formed squamocolumnar junction is called the *physiologic functional junction*.
2) The post pubertal squamocolumnar junction which is termed the transformation zone.
   - *The transformation zone* is the region between the original squamocolumnar junction and the postpubertal functional squamocolumnar junction.

It is characterized by a metaplastic epithelium which replaces the endocervical mucosa with mature statified squamous epithelium. (Metaplasia is defined as the replacement of one type of mature tissue by another equally mature type of tissue [2]).

At colposcopy, after application of a 5 % solution of acetic acid, the transformation zone appears as a smooth translucent slightly white tissue that corresponds to metaplastic squamous epithelium with circular openings and spherical bumps of 2–4 mm, which correspond to the underlying endocervical glands and nabothian cysts, respectively. Nabothian cysts are formed when the openings of endocervical clefts become obliterated by the proliferating surface metaplastic squamous epithelium. When the flow of mucus is blocked, the secretory products accumulate, leading to cystic glandular dilatations, or Nabothian cysts [2].

The concept of the transformation zone is important for understanding the pathogenesis of squamous cell carcinoma of the cervix and its precursours, because virtually all cervical squamous neoplasia begin at the new squamocolumnar junction and because the extension and limits of cervical cancer precursors coincide with the distribution of the transformation zone [2].

References

1. Testut L (1931) Appareil urogenital, peritoine. In: Latarget A Traité d'anatomie humaine. 8th edn revue par. G Doin et Cie Editeurs, Paris, pp 1–595
2. Wright CT, Ferenczy A (2002) Anatomy and histology of the cervix. In: Kurman RJ (ed) Blaustein's pathology of the female genital tract. Springer, New York, pp 207–224
3. Fluhmann CF (1961) Focal hyperplasia (tunnel clusters) of the cervix uteri. Obstet Gynecol 17:206–214

Benign Diseases of the Cervix

27

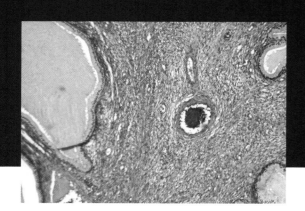

Contents

27.1 Inflammatory Diseases

27.1.1 Cervicitis

Cervicitis can be infectious related to different microorganisms (bacteria, viruses, fungi, protozoa, and parasites) or noninfectious (chemical or mechanical) [1].

Infectious cervicitis can affect either the endocervical-type columnar epithelium producing mucopurulent endocervicitis or the epithelium of the exocervix producing exocervicitis.

In this clinical setting, MR can display retention cysts [2].

27.1.2 Exophytic Condyloma Acuminata [1]

It is one of the common manifestations of human papilloma virus (HPV) infection of the lower anogenital tract. It is caused by HPV types 6 and 11. They are commonly multifocal and may involve the mature squamous epithelium of the exocervix as well as the immature squamous epithelium of the transformation zone.

At colposcopy, they appear white exophytic lesions with papillary projections.

Other aspects include maculopapular, only slightly raised lesions.

27.2 Metaplasia-Hyperplasia

27.2.1 Metaplasia [1]

Metaplasia can be from tubal, tubo-endometrioid, or transitional cell type.

J.N. Buy, M. Ghossain, *Gynecological Imaging*,
DOI 10.1007/978-3-642-31012-6_27, © Springer-Verlag Berlin Heidelberg 2013

In tubal metaplasia, endocervical glands are lined by Müllerian-type epithelium that resembles that of the fallopian tube. It can be quite extensive and can occasionally be mistaken for endocervical glandular neoplasia.

Glands are typically confined to the superficial third of the cervical wall (they extend less than 7 mm into the cervical stroma). It can be typical or atypical.

27.2.2 Hyperplasia

According to its origin (endocervical glands or mesonephric duct remnants), there are two types, microglandular hyperplasia and mesonephric hyperplasia.

27.2.2.1 Microglandular Hyperplasia [1]

Histology

It is a benign proliferation of endocervical glands forming tightly packed glandular or tubular units of varying sizes lined by flattened to cuboidal cells with eosinophilic cytoplasm containing small quantities of mucin. Stroma separating the glands is usually infiltrated with acute and chronic inflammatory cells.

It can be present as a simple focus or as multiple foci. It may involve the surface or deeper portions of endocervical clefts.

Clinical Findings

It is common in women of reproductive age as a result of contraceptive or in pregnant women.

It can result in postcoital bleeding or spotting.

It can form a cervical polyp of 1–2 cm.

MR Findings

They are similar to those of hyperplasia of the endometrium (Fig. 27.1).

Differential Diagnosis

Microglandular hyperplasia with solid areas can be difficult to distinguish from adenocarcinoma on pathology [1].

27.2.2.2 Mesonephric Hyperplasia

Definition

The vestigial elements of the distal ends of the mesonephric ducts are found in 1–22 % of adult cervices. Mesonephric remnants are most commonly present in the lateral aspects of the cervix. They consist of tubules or cysts that are usually located deep in the lateral cervical wall.

Mesonephric remnants may become hyperplastic, resulting in a tubuloglandular proliferation with transmural involvement of the cervix. The most common form is the lobular type that is characterized by clustered mesonephric tubules with or without a centrally mesonephric duct.

Mesonephric hyperplasia is almost always asymptomatic and is detected on cervical biopsy or hysterectomy specimens.

Differential Diagnosis

Minimal-deviation adenocarcinoma of the endocervix can be differentiated by:

1. Lack of complex glandular pattern and periglandular stromal edema
2. Absence of cytologic features: mitosis, intracellular mucin
3. Absent carcinoembryonic antigen (CEA)

27.2.2.3 Imaging Findings

On MR, endocervical hyperplasia appeared as a multicystic mass with thin and regular walls, which can be in some cases partially thickened separating by stroma with contrast uptake. Differential diagnosis can be with Nabothian cysts, tunnel clusters, and adenocarcinoma (Table 27.3).

27.3 Cysts

27.3.1 Nabothian Cyst

27.3.1.1 Definition

They are lined by a single layer of mucin-producing endocervical epithelium, which is flattened. They develop most frequently within the transformation zone secondary to squamous metaplasia.

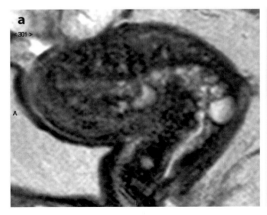 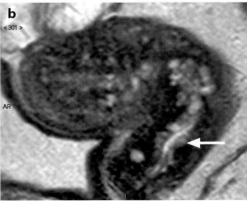

Fig. 27.1 Endometrial hyperplasia with foci of mucinous metaplasia of the endometrium extending into the endocervix (same patient as Fig. 22.20). Seventy-five-year-old woman with metrorrhagia and hydrorrhea. (**a, b**) Sagittal T2W images display thickening of the endometrium and to a lesser extent of the cervical mucosa (*arrow*) with multiple cystic glands. Deeper cystic glands in the myometrium are also present related to adenomyosis

27.3.1.2 Macroscopic and Radiologic Findings

They are very common incidental findings on US and MR. They are frequently multiple and exceptionally large (Fig. 27.2). Their characteristics are reported in Table 27.1.

Table 27.1 Macroscopic and radiologic findings of Nabothian cysts

– Size, usually up to 1.5 cm, exceptionally larger
– Frequently multiple
– Usually in the superficial portion of the cervix, may extend through its wall [3]

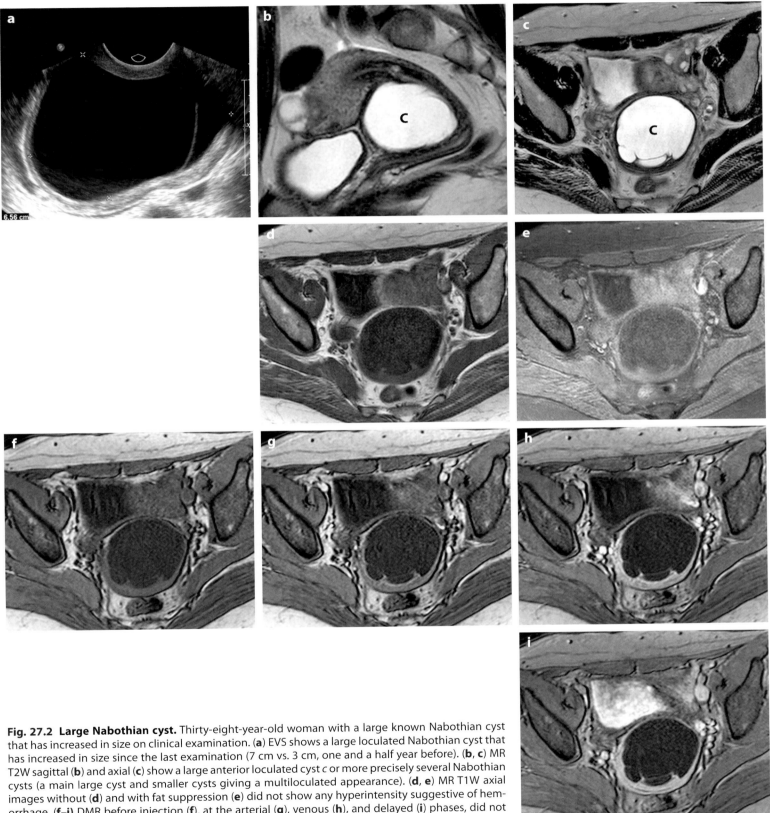

Fig. 27.2 Large Nabothian cyst. Thirty-eight-year-old woman with a large known Nabothian cyst that has increased in size on clinical examination. (**a**) EVS shows a large loculated Nabothian cyst that has increased in size since the last examination (7 cm vs. 3 cm, one and a half year before). (**b**, **c**) MR T2W sagittal (**b**) and axial (**c**) show a large anterior loculated cyst *c* or more precisely several Nabothian cysts (a main large cyst and smaller cysts giving a multiloculated appearance). (**d**, **e**) MR T1W axial images without (**d**) and with fat suppression (**e**) did not show any hyperintensity suggestive of hemorrhage. (**f**–**i**) DMR before injection (**f**), at the arterial (**g**), venous (**h**), and delayed (**i**) phases, did not show any nodular or suspicious contrast uptake in the cysts

27.3.2 Tunnel Clusters

27.3.2.1 Definition

Benign collections of endocervical glands usually located close to the surface epithelium of the cervix

27.3.2.2 Macroscopic and Radiologic Findings

MR findings can mimic adenoma malignum [4]. They are reported in Table 27.2.

Table 27.2 Macroscopic and radiologic findings of tunnel clusters

– Clustered cystic spaces with a round marginated appearance
– Absence of invasion of the deep cervical stroma
– Absence of nodular enhancement in the mass

27.3.2.3 Differential Diagnosis

A minimal-deviation adenocarcinoma of the cervix also designated as adenoma malignum (see Chap. 28); however, this entity often involves more than two-thirds of the thickness of the cervical stroma [3].

All these different cystic entities (hyperplasia, Nabothian cyst, and tunnel clusters) and endocervicosis (see Chap. 17) particularly when they extend beyond several millimeters from the surface look like adenocarcinoma of the cervix, particularly the most well-differentiated mucinous adenocarcinoma usually called adenoma malignum (Table 27.3).

Table 27.3 Differential diagnosis of conditions in which glands extend beyond 7 mm from the surface

– Mesonephric hyperplasia
– Deeply situated Nabothian cysts
– Tunnel clusters
– Endocervicosis of the outer cervical wall (see Chap. 17)
– Adenocarcinoma of the cervix (especially adenoma malignum)

On MR, Okamoto et al. [2] in a series of 22 patients with malignant and benign lesions of the cervix studied if MRI could allow to differentiate these lesions:

1. The main finding of malignancy was the presence of an entirely or mainly solid component (except in one case), while entirely cystic lesions were benign. Mainly cystic with a solid component were benign or malignant.
2. Size and intensity of the fluid did not help in the differential. Lesions composed of cysts smaller than 5 mm tend to be malignant, but some lesions composed of larger cysts can also be malignant. In malignant lesions, signal intensity of fluid on T1W images compared to the cervical stroma could be low, isointense, or high.

27.4 Benign Tumors

27.4.1 Endocervical Polyps

27.4.1.1 Definition

Focal hyperplastic productions of endocervical folds including epithelium and substantia propria

1. Epithelium. It is composed of mucinous epithelium that lines crypts with or without cystic changes. Squamous metaplasia involving the surface or glandular epithelium is frequently observed.
2. Stroma is generally loose with centrally placed feeding vessels, containing almost always a chronic inflammatory infiltrate. It may be fibrous.

Blood vessels may predominate, and the lesion is called a vascular polyp.

27.4.1.2 Clinical Findings

Leukorrhea caused by hypersecretion of the mucus
Abnormal bleeding from ulceration of the surface epithelium

27.4.1.3 Common Macroscopic and Radiologic Findings

They are listed in Table 27.4.

Table 27.4 Common macroscopic and radiologic findings of endocervical polyps

– Round or elongated
– Smooth or lobulated surface
– Most are single
– Size: from a few millimeters to 2–3 cm.
– Vascular pedicle
– Cystic structures may be present

27.4.1.4 Ultrasound Findings

Polyps of the endocervix, because the same echogenicity of the mucosa can be very difficult to identify on transvaginal ultrasound and can be very easily missed. Localized enlargement of the mucosa and overall identification of vascular pedicle can make diagnosis (Fig. 27.3). Cystic spaces may be present (Fig. 27.4). Uncommonly, some fluid in the endocervix allows depicting them clearly (Figs. 27.4 and 27.5).

27.4.1.5 MR Findings

On T2, they are slightly less hypointense than the endometrium and cervical mucosa. On DMR, central arteries are displayed at the arterial phase, and enhancement in the remaining of the polyp is seen on the following phases (Fig. 27.6). This differs from pedunculated submucous leiomyoma where arterial vessels are seen at the periphery at the arterial phase (compare with Figs. 27.7 and 24.1 in Chap. 24). Enhancement is more marked than in the cervical stroma. If cystic structures are numerous, differentiation from tunnel clusters or the lesions cited in Table 27.3 is based on identifying the endocavitary location of the lesion (Fig. 27.8).

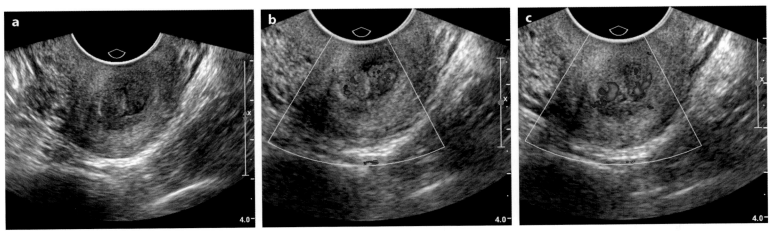

Fig. 27.3 Endocervical polyps. (a) EVS disclose thickening of the cervical mucosa apparently related to two small masses. (b, c) Color Doppler confirms the presence of two vascular pedicles penetrating the masses and confirming the diagnosis of polyps

Fig. 27.4 Mucous fibroglandular polyp of the endocervix. (a) EVS shows an 11×7 mm elongated echogenic structure with a pedicle inserted on the anterior wall of the upper cervix surrounded by a hyperechogenic line and containing a small cystic cavity. (b) Doppler displays a vascular pedicle and vessels inside this echogenic structure. These morphologic and vascular findings are typical for a benign polyp. At microscopy: The surface is covered by a unistratified mucinous epithelium of endocervical type. It lies on a fibrovascular axis containing glandular recesses

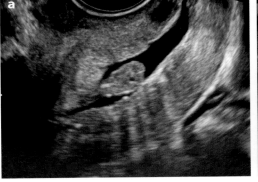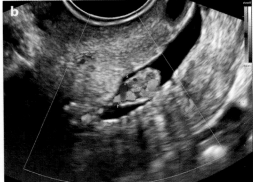

Fig. 27.5 Endocervical polyp associated with endometrial polyp. A 49-year-old woman with menometrorrhagia. (a). Transvaginal sonography discloses a typical corporeal endometrial polyp, hyperechoic compared to the endometrium, partially delineated by liquid. No vascular pedicle could be displayed on color Doppler. (b) In the endocervical canal, a small polyp is seen, well delineated by liquid, with clear vascular pedicle. Hysteroscopy and histology confirmed the presence of endometrial and cervical polyps

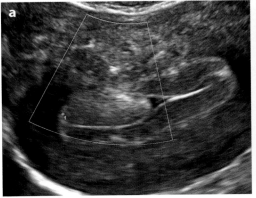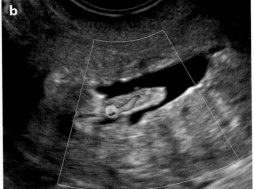

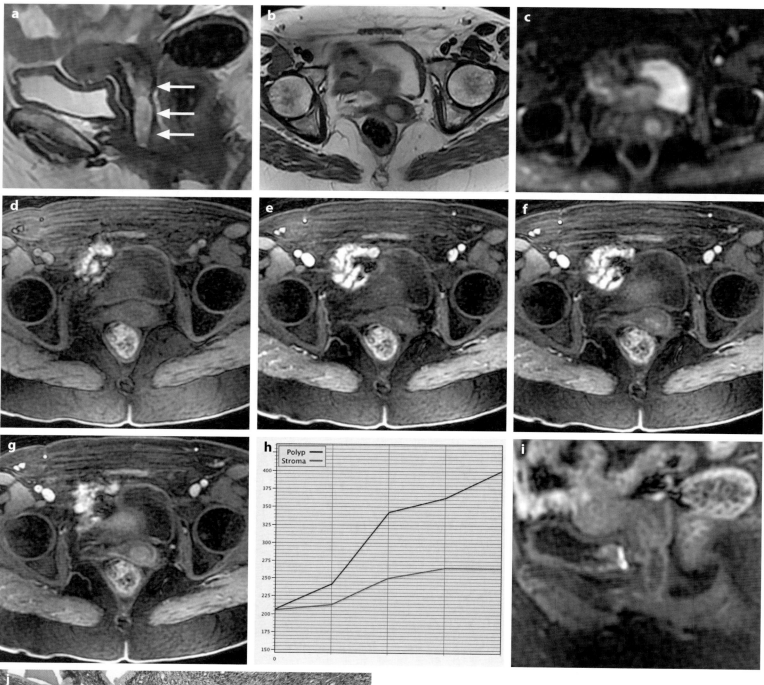

Fig. 27.6 Endocervical polyp protruding in the vagina in a 62-year-old woman. (a, b) Sagittal T2WI (**a**) and axial T2WI at the level of the cervix (**b**) show an elongated polypoid structure (*arrows*) extending from the cervix to the vagina. It has an intermediate intensity higher than that of cervical stroma and slightly lower than fat and normal mucosa. Small barely seen cystic structures are present inside it. Its limits with the inner hypointense cervical stroma and vaginal wall are well delineated except at its insertion on the posterior wall of the cervix. (**c**) DW image at the same level as (**b**) can hardly differentiate the slightly hypointense polyp from the hyperintense mucosa. Both structures are well delineated from the hypointense inner cervical stroma. (**d–h**) DMR at the same level as (**b, c**) before injection (**d**) and 25 (**e**), 70 (**f**), 125, and 240 (**g**) seconds after injection with corresponding time-intensity curves (**h**) shows at the arterial phase central arterial vessels and later on enhancement of the entire polyp; this favors the diagnosis of polyp over leiomyoma. On all phases, the polyp enhances more than the cervical stroma. (**i**) Sagittal T1FS delayed image shows more marked enhancement in the cervical part of the polyp than in the protruding vaginal part where numerous small cystic structures are seen. (**j**) Histology demonstrates a benign polyp with endocervical glands

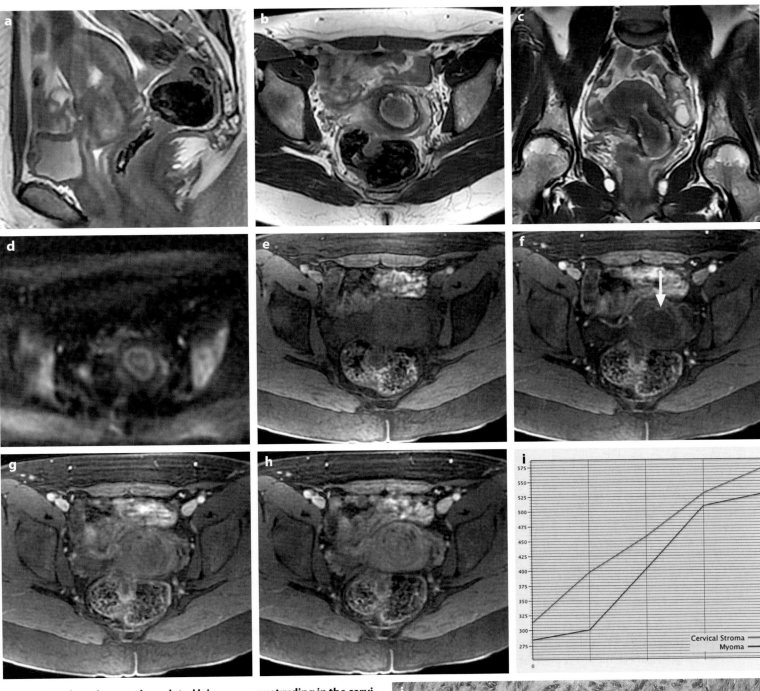

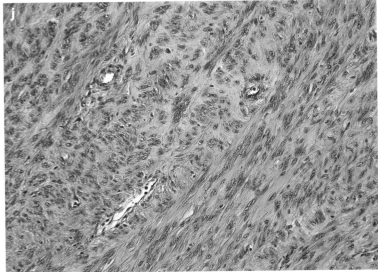

Fig. 27.7 Endocavitary pedunculated leiomyoma protruding in the cervical cavity. Forty-seven-year-old woman with metrorrhagia. (**a–b**) Sagittal and axial T2W images show an intracavitary mass with intermediate signal on T2 (between that of adipose tissue and pelvic muscle). The insertion of the pedicle is well seen on the sagittal view, at the posterior wall of the sus-isthmic portion. Axial view well demonstrates the intracavitary location with the different layers from outside to inside: cervical outer stroma of intermediate signal intensity, hypointense inner cervical stroma, mucosa of high intensity compared to the other structures, and the centrally located myoma of intermediate signal intensity. On (**b**), compressed Nabothian cysts are seen in the anterior and left cervical stroma. (**c**) The pedicle of the cyst is demonstrated at its best on coronal T2W image. (**d**) Axial DWI at the level of (**b**) shows the myoma to be hypointense containing some hyperintense area and surrounded by a hyperintense mucosa. (**e–i**) DMR before (**e**) and 25 (**f**), 75 (**g**), 125 (**h**), and 240 s after injection with corresponding time-intensity curves (**i**) shows a peripheral arterial vessel at the arterial phase (*arrow*) without central vessel favoring the diagnosis of leiomyoma over polyp. Overall, the mass enhances less than the cervical stroma at the arterial phase becoming close to its signal on the late phases. Small nonenhancing structures correspond to Nabothian cysts and some liquid in the cavity. (**j**) A leiomyoma is disclosed at histology

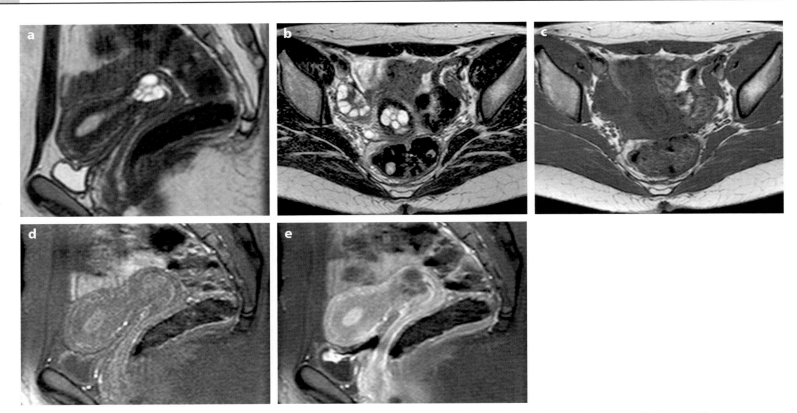

Fig. 27.8 Fibroglandular polyp of the cervix in a 21-year-old woman with metrorrhagia. (a, b) T2W sagittal (**a**) and axial (**b**) disclose an agglomerate of small cystic structures expanding the cervical canal. The inner hypointense band of the cervical stroma that prolongates the junctional zone of the uterus is well delineated and well identified on the sagittal image, confirming the endocavitary location of the lesion. The right ovary is displayed in (**a**). (**c**) Axial T1W image did not show hemorrhagic hyperintense area. (**d, e**) Sagittal T1W image with fat suppression before (**d**) and after injection (**e**) shows nonenhancing cystic structures and tissular portions

27.4.1.6 Differential Diagnosis [1]

- Leiomyoma
- Adenomyoma
- Papillary adenofibroma
- Fibroadenoma
- Papilloma

27.4.2 Mesodermal Stromal Polyps (Pseudosarcoma Botryoides)

It is a benign exophytic proliferation of stroma and epithelium.

They are composed of an edematous stroma covered by a benign-appearing, stratified squamous epithelium [1].

These lesions are seen most frequently in pregnant women and arise more commonly from the vagina than from the cervix [5].

They are more extensively treated in Chap. 30.

27.4.3 Leiomyomas

When intramural or subserous, they produce unilateral enlargement of the cervical portio vaginalis.

When submucosal, they can protrude in the canal resembling an endocervical polyp and in pregnancy may produce dystocia. Submucous leiomyoma of the body of the uterus may protrude in the endocervical canal and mimic a cervical polyp or leiomyoma (Fig. 27.7).

27.4.3.1 US and MR Findings

(a) Morphologic findings are the same as those of the myometrium (see Chap. 24).
(b) Vascular findings: Vascularization of these leiomyomas is in most of the cases much lower than those of the myometrium.

27.4.4 Adenomyoma and Papillary Adenofibroma

Adenomyoma is an admixture of smooth muscles elements with glands lined by predominantly endocervical-type epithelium. They are more frequent in the myometrium where the epithelium is of endometrial type (see Chap. 24).

Adenofibroma is an admixture of fibrous tissue and glands lined by an endocervical-type epithelium or tubal-type epithelium. These neoplasms are rare in the uterus.

27.4.5 Hemangioma and Hemangiofibroma

They can rarely occur in the stroma of the cervix. Hemangiofibroma are less vascularized than hemangioma (Fig. 27.9).

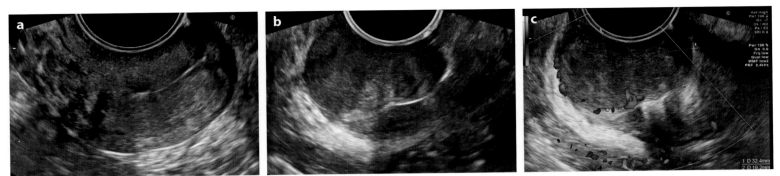

Fig. 27.9 Hemangiofibroma of the cervix. (**a**) Sagittal EVS shows a slightly hyperechoic and heterogeneous ill-defined mass in the anterior wall of the cervix. (**b**, **c**) Transverse EVS through the mass without (**b**) and with color Doppler (**c**) shows large vessels penetrating the mass that measured 32 × 19 mm (*cursors* in **c**)

References

1. Wright CT, Ferenczy A (2002) Benign diseases of the cervix. In: Kurman RJ (ed) Blaustein's pathology of the female genital tract. Springer, New York, pp 225–252
2. Okamoto Y et al (2003) MR imaging of the uterine cervix: imaging-pathologic correlation. Radiographics 23(2):425–445; quiz 534–535
3. Clement PB, Young RH (1989) Deep nabothian cysts of the uterine cervix. A possible source of confusion with minimal-deviation adenocarcinoma (adenoma malignum). Int J Gynecol Pathol 8(4):340–348
4. Sugiyama K, Takehara Y (2007) MR findings of pseudoneoplastic lesions in the uterine cervix mimicking adenoma malignum. Br J Radiol 80(959): 878–883
5. Norris HJ, Taylor HB (1966) Polyps of the vagina. A benign lesion resembling sarcoma botryoides. Cancer 19(2):227–232

Carcinoma and Other Tumors of the Cervix

28

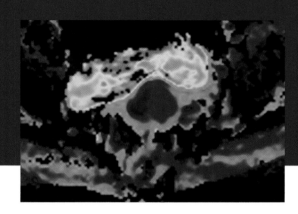

Contents

Carcinoma of the cervix accounts for almost all the malignant tumors of the cervix, with roughly 75–80 % of squamous cell carcinomas and 20–25 % of adenocarcinomas. Other malignant epithelial tumors, mixed epithelial and mesenchymal tumors, mesenchymal tumors, very uncommon miscellaneous tumors and secondary tumors are quite uncommon.

Detection of carcinoma of the cerix is usually made in asymptomatic women on a routine cervical smear or is revealed by clinical findings among the most common one is vaginal bleeding. Vaginal touch and examination with the speculcum can unfortunaly in some cases identify a tumor at a stage already advanced. Colposcopy is essential to visualize small lesions and to guide the biopsy which confirms the carcinoma of the cervix. Imaging modalities in the great majority of cases have no place at all in the detection and in the diagnosis of cervical carcinoma. However they play an important role in the evaluation of the extension of the tumor before surgery or after a neoadjuvant chemotherapy has been performed, and in the followup of the patients in the detection and characterization of recurrences.

28.1 Squamous Cell Carcinoma

28.1.1 Clinical findings [1]

a) Microinvasive squamous cell carcinoma (MICA)

MICA is considered as preclinical stage in the progressive spectrum of squamous intraepithelial lesion (SIL) and frank invasive carcinoma of the cervix uteri.

Definition of MICA:
A tumor that invades to a depth of not more than 5 mm taken from the base of the epithelium, either surface or glandular, from which

J.N. Buy, M. Ghossain, *Gynecological Imaging*,
DOI 10.1007/978-3-642-31012-6_28, © Springer-Verlag Berlin Heidelberg 2013

it originates and a second dimension, the horizontal spread, must not exceed 7 mm according to the FIGO classification [6].

Clinical features:

The majority of MICA occurs in women 35–46 years of age. Most patients are asymptomatic and the tumors are generally discovered on a routine cervical smear. The cervix demostrates a grossly normal appearance or non specific findings, such as chronic cervicitis or true erosion. Colposcopically, detection of MICA requires invasion of more than 1 mm into the cervical stroma. Areas of MICA usually display dense acetowhitening consistent with high grade squamous intraepithelial lesion (SIL). Many colposcopists routinely treat all large biopsy-confirmed, high grade SIL using excisional methods such as loop excision. However a diagnosis of MICA should only be made after a conization has been performed to exclude more advanced disease.

b) Invasive squamous cell carcinoma

There is a considerable body of evidence that invasive squamous cell carcinoma develops from SIL, and consequently, women with invasive squamous cell carcinoma have similar epidemiologic characteristics. Like women with SIL, women with invasive squamous carcinoma began heterosexual activity early in life, married early, are multiparous, and have many sexual partners. These associations suggest a role for a sexually transmitted agent in the etiology of cervical cancer. Multiple types of human papillomavirus (HPV) are resposible for the development of cervical carcinoma, predominantly HPV 16, 18, 45 and 58.

The average age of patients is 51 years (a little older than patients with high-grade SIL or with MICA). Women under the age of 35 years account for 22 % of all patients. The most common and significant feature is bleeding following intercourse or douching. Intermittent spotting, serosanguinous discharge, and frank hemorrhage are also common. Malodorous discharge and pain, often radiating to the sacral region occurs in 10–20 % of patients.

Means for accurate detection and diagnosis of frank invasive carcinoma include cytology, colposcopy, and colpospically directed punch biopsy.

28.1.2 Pathology

28.1.2.1 Macroscopy [1]

Early Lesions

Ninety-eight percent are localized in the transformation zone, with variable degrees of encroachment onto the neighboring native squamous epithelium.

They may be focally indurated or ulcerated or may present as a slightly elevated and granular area.

Advanced Tumors

More advanced tumors have two major types of gross appearance.
(a) Endophytic:
- Are ulcerated or nodular.
- Tend to develop within the endocervical canal.
- This pattern frequently invades deeply into the cervical stroma to produce a large barrel-shaped cervix.
- In some patients, the cervix appears normal.

(b) Exophytic:
- Have a polyploid or papillary appearance

28.1.2.2 Microscopy and Grading

The tumor may be in situ, microinvasive, or invasive.
Grading is reported in Table 28.1.

Table 28.1 Grading of squamous cell carcinoma [1]

Grade 1
– Cells mature with irregular large nuclei and abundant cytoplasm
– Keratin pearls: concentric whorls of abundant keratin in the centers of neoplastic epithelial nests
– Stroma infiltrated by chronic inflammatory cells
Grade 2
– Neoplastic cells are more pleomorphic with large irregular nuclei and scanty cytoplasm
– Cell borders are indistinct
– Keratin pearls are nonexistent
Grade 3
– Neoplastic cells show hyperchromatic oval nuclei with scant indistinct cytoplasm
– Clear-cut squamous differentiation manifested by keratinization may be difficult to find

Variants of Squamous Cell Carcinomas

1. *Verrucous carcinoma*
   At microscopy, they are characterized by frond-like papillae without the central fibroconnective tissue.

2. *Warty carcinoma*
   Unlike verrucous carcinoma, warty carcinomas demonstrate features of a typical squamous cell carcinoma at the deep margin.

Many of the malignant cells have cytoplasmic vacuolization and nuclear changes closely resembling koilocytotic atypia.

3. *Papillary squamous cell carcinoma*

   They are composed of papillary projections that are covered by several layers of atypical epithelial cells.

4. *Lymphoepithelioma-like carcinoma*

28.1.3 MR imaging Findings Before Treatment

28.1.3.1 Tumor

On T2, the lesion has an intermediate signal between cervical stroma and adipose tissue (Figs. 28.1, 28.2, 28.3, and 28.4).

On T1, the lesion is usually difficult to identify because its signal is close to that of stroma.

DMR may be particularly useful in the detection and characterization of tumor.

Signal intensity measurement made in ROIs includes an intratumoral plasma component, an intracellular component, and an intratumoral interstitial component.

1. Typically, cervical carcinoma shows earlier enhancement than that of the myometrium or cervical stroma [2]:
   - Most often homogeneous intense in more than 70 % of the tumor area
   - Less commonly a ringlike peripheral enhancement with poorly enhanced central areas

2. Rarely, poor enhancement

   Tumors with ringlike enhancement and poorly enhanced tumors were significantly larger than those with homogeneous intense enhancement [2].

Vascularization, permeability, and interstitial space in cervical carcinomas are substantially greater than those of normal tissue.

At confrontation with pathology, tumors with homogeneous intense enhancement or peripheral areas in tumors with ringlike enhancement:

(a) Display numerous and leaky capillaries (the basement membrane of the endothelium in malignant tumors is damaged or missing)

(b) Are predominantly composed of abundant tumor cells

(c) Have a thin connective tissue

And conversely at pharmacokinetic analysis, (a) their mean tissue-specific transport parameter k that describes the transfer of contrast medium between the plasma compartment and interstitial space and (b) the ratio of extracellular volume to intravascular volume f were respectively significantly higher and lower than those of the center of large tumor.

Diffusion

In Edwards et al. series [3], ADC values in cervical carcinoma of $757 \times 10^{-6} \, \text{mm}^2/\text{s} \pm 110$ were significantly lower than those in adjacent

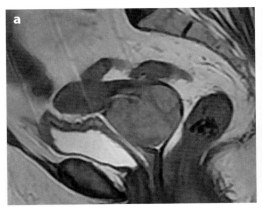 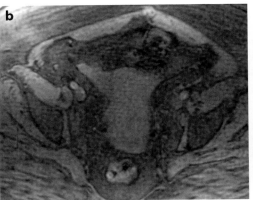 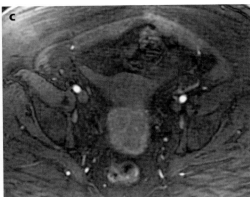

Fig. 28.1 Squamous cell carcinoma with parametrial involvement (stage IIB). (a) Sagittal view 5.2×4.4 cm mass of intermediate signal occupying the entire cervix distending the cervical stroma and vagina. Differentiating distended vagina from cervical thinned stroma is not evident. (**b–f**) DMR before (**b**) and 25 (**c**)

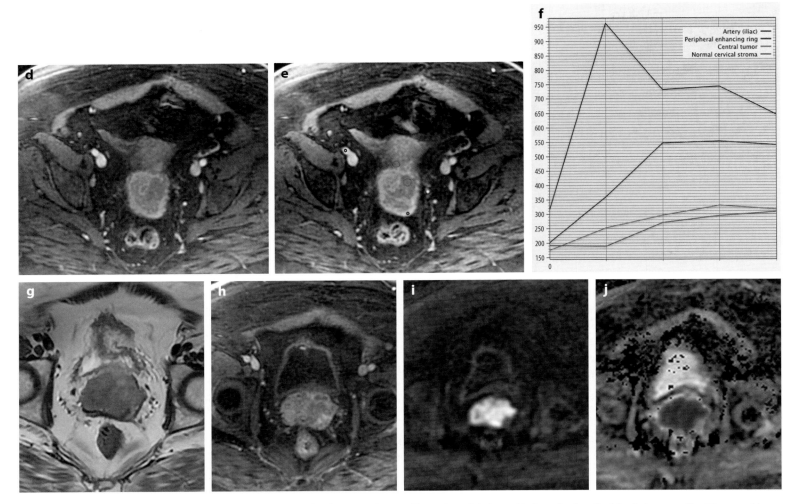

Fig. 28.1 *(continued)* (**d–i**) 70 (**d**), 125, and 240 (**e**) seconds after injection with time-intensity curves (**f**) shows that the central part of the tumor (*red ROI in* **e**) enhances less than a peripheral ring (*blue ROI in* **e**) but more than the normal cervical stroma (*green ROI in* **e**). The peripheral enhancement corresponds probably to a mixture of tumor and adjacent infiltrated stroma. (**g, h**) Axial T2 (**g**) and corresponding DMR at 240 s, (**h**) at low level, show disruption of right and left vaginal wall with obvious cardinal ligament invasion on the left. The anterior wall of the vagina is also disrupted on T2, but there is integrity of the bladder wall on DMR. (**i, j**) DWI at b1000 (**i**) and corresponding ADC map (**j**), at the level of (**g**), show hyperintense tumor with ADC of 0.45×10^{-3} mm²/s. Left lobulation in the cardinal ligament is well seen on both images

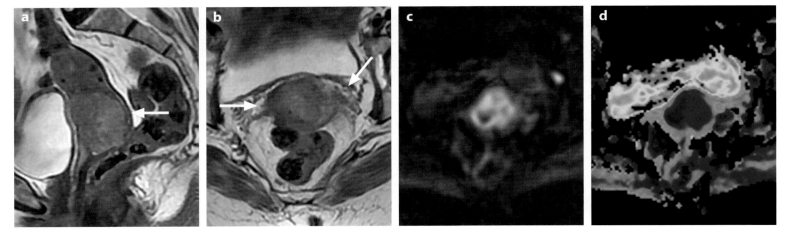

Fig. 28.2 Squamous cell carcinoma of the cervix in a 79-year-old woman (stage IIB). (**a, b**) Sagittal and axial T2W images show a 4.8-cm mass of intermediate signal intensity occupying the endocervical canal, protruding in the external and internal os. On the sagittal image, a thin band of normal hypointense cervical stroma is seen posteriorly (*arrow in* **a**), while it is almost inexistent and disrupted anteriorly. On the axial image, disruption of the stroma is well individualized in several areas with left and right invasion in the cardinal ligament (*arrows in* **b**). (**c, d**) DW image at b1000 (**c**) and corresponding ADC map (**d**) show the tumor to be hyperintense with an ADC of 0.9×10^{-3} mm²/s. However, invasion of the stroma is not evident

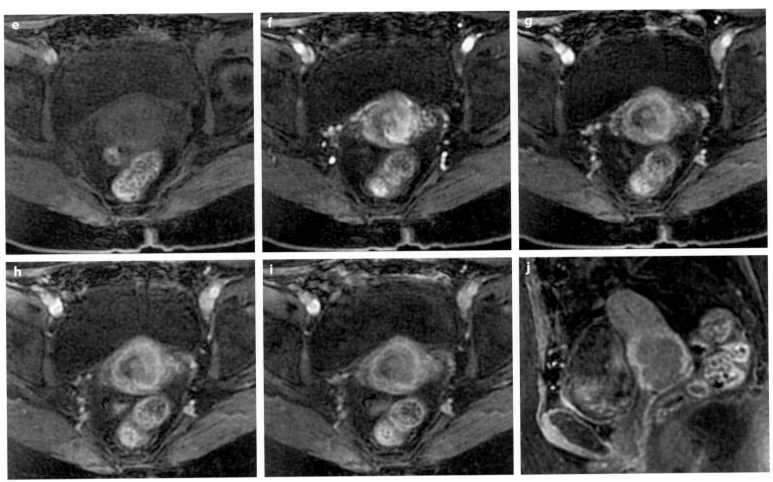

Fig. 28.2 (*continued*) (**e–i**) DMR before (**e**) and 25 (**f**), 70 (**g**), 125 (**h**), and 240 (**i**) seconds after injection shows arterial vessels at 25 s in the mass and the peripheral invaded stroma and cardinal ligaments. On the following phases, a peripheral enhancing incomplete ring is seen that, when compared to T2WI, corresponds probably to the periphery of the main tumor. (**j**) Late sagittal LAVA after injection show the mass surrounded by a highly enhancing ring anteriorly and posteriorly contrary to a normal cervical stroma that enhances less than the myometrium. It is not possible to differentiate the periphery of the tumor and the adjacent invaded stroma from the thin posterior peripheral stroma that appeared preserved on sagittal T2 image. In this case, extension of the tumor was best appreciated on T2WI

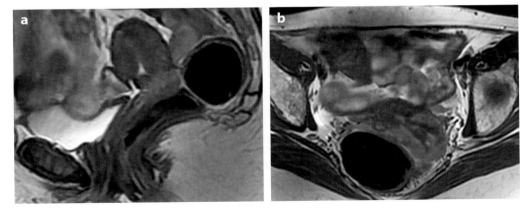

Fig. 28.3 Squamous cell carcinoma of the cervix with vaginal extension. (**a**) Sagittal T2W image shows the tumor of intermediate signal intensity (between adipose tissue and pelvic muscle), higher than that of cervical stroma and myometrium, occupying the cervix and disrupting posteriorly the vaginal wall. (**b**) Axial T2W image at the level of the cervix showing the tumor and adjacent hypointense cervical stroma

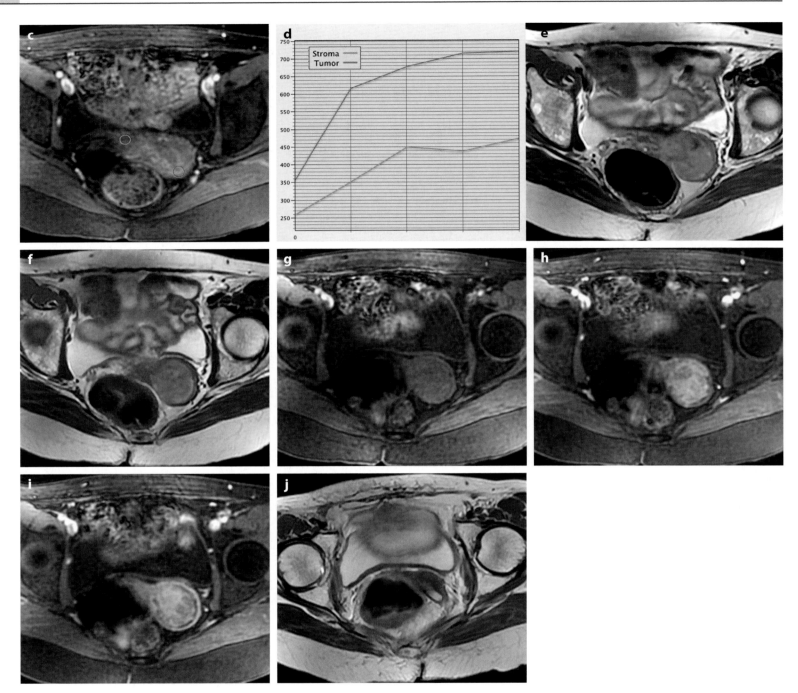

Fig. 28.3 (*continued*) (**c, d**) DMR at the same level as (**b**) at the arterial phase (**c**) and corresponding time-intensity curves (**d**) shows marked higher contrast uptake in the tumor (*red* ROI) compared to normal cervical stroma (*green* ROI). (**e**) Axial T2 image at a lower level shows the tumor extending through the vaginal wall and coming in contact with the rectal wall without disrupting it. (**f**) Axial T2W image at still lower level shows the tumor occupying the entire vaginal lumen. The vagina is left deviated and its wall partially disrupted posteriorly on the right. (**g–i**) DMR at the level of (**f**), before (**g**) and after contrast injection at the arterial (**h**), venous, and late (**i**) phases, shows early contrast uptake in the tumor at the arterial phase, superior to that of the vaginal wall. The uptake in the tumor is slightly heterogeneous. The vaginal wall is ill defined posteriorly on the right. On DWI b1000 (not shown), high-intensity signal was displayed in the tumor with ADC value of 0.64×10^{-3} mm²/s. The tumor was classified FIGO stage IIA. (**j**) Axial T2W image 5 months later, after chemoradiotherapy, shows absence of visible tumor with reappearance of the zonal anatomy and intermediate intensity areas in the surrounding adipose tissue secondary to radiotherapy. These lesions were stable on follow-up confirming their nonneoplastic nature

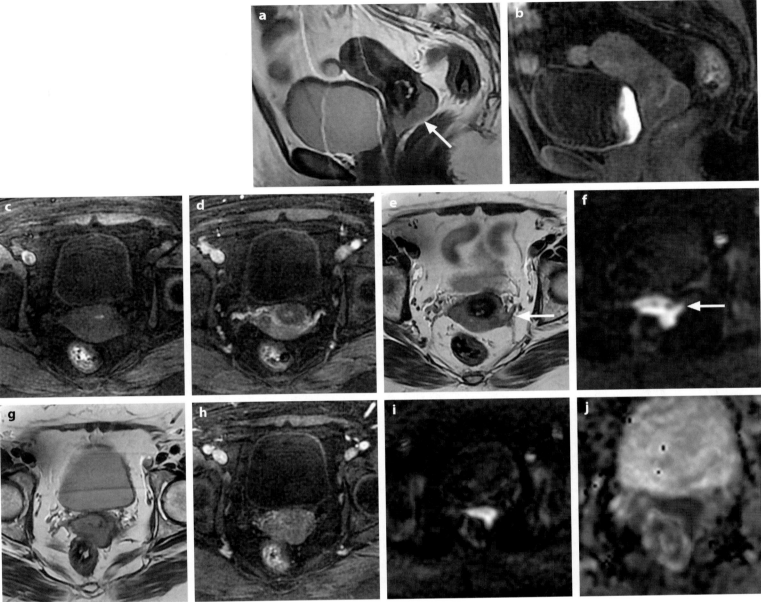

Fig. 28.4 Squamous cell carcinoma of the cervix with vaginal and parametrial involvement in a 55-year-old woman (FIGO stage IIB). (**a**) Sagittal T2W images show a mass of intermediate signal intensity (between signal intensity of adipose tissue and pelvic muscles), measuring 4.3 cm in height and 5 cm in width, eroding the outer cervix, and occupying the upper half of the vagina. The hypointense vaginal wall is clearly disrupted posteriorly (*arrow*). Small Nabothian cysts are present. No endocervical lesion is identified. (**b**) On sagittal acquisition performed after DMR, the vaginal wall that enhances more than the tumor appears disrupted posteriorly, but this finding is better evaluated on T2WI. (**c**, **d**) DMR before (**c**), at the arterial phase 25 (**d**), and on following phases demonstrates that the tumor enhances more than the cervical stroma with a peak at the arterial phase. A small hyperintense spot is seen before injection in the endocervical canal possibly related to hemorrhage. There is suspicious left cardinal ligament involvement. (**e**) Axial T2W images at approximately the same level as (**c**, **d**)

show the tumor surrounding the posterior cervix, disrupting clearly the left vaginal wall and invading the adjacent cardinal ligament (*arrow*). (**f**) DWI at b1000, at approximately the same level as (**e**), shows a hyperintense tumor with an ADC of 0.54×10^{-3} mm^2/s (0.7 at b500). A small lobulation is seen protruding in the left cardinal ligament and confirming its invasion (*arrow*). (**g**) T2WI at a lower level, the tumor is in contact with the rectal wall. (**h**) DMR image at the level of suspicious rectal involvement (arterial phase shown) shows the tumor in contact with the rectal wall but not disrupting it. (**i**, **j**) DWI at b1000 (**i**) and corresponding ADC map (**j**) at the level where the tumor is in contact with the rectum confirms that the rectal wall is well delineated especially on (**j**). Several iliac lymph nodes were seen on the different sequences, the lagest one on the right measuring 18×10 mm. The tumor was classified stage FIGO IIB and treated with chemoradiotherapy. Follow-up MR is shown in Fig. 28.8

epithelium $1,331 \times 10^{-6}$ mm^2/s or cervical intraepithelial neoplasia (CIN) $1,291 \times 10^{-6}$ mm^2/s (Figs. 28.1, 28.2, 28.3 and 28.4). From this study, a threshold of $1,100 \times 10^{-6}$ mm^2/s has been proposed to differentiate invasive cervical carcinoma from nontumoral epithelium. No significant difference was found between ADC of squamous cell, adenocarcinomas, and adenosquamous carcinomas [4].

Extension may be well visualized on DWI or underestimated compared to T2WI (Figs. 28.1, 28.2, and 28.4).

In patients with incompletely excised stage IA or IB1, invasive carcinoma was identified as area of ADC of less than $1,100 \times 10^{-6}$ mm^2/s [3]. Combination of the results obtained with T2 and ADC improves the detection and characterization of invasive cervical carcinoma [3, 5].

When patients had biopsies taken within 2 weeks prior to MR studies, granulation and healing of the cervical epithelium can give a high signal in the adjacent stroma that is indistinguishable from invasive cervical carcinoma on T2 while these lesions could better differentiated with T2 and ADC.

28.1.3.2 Extension

FIGO staging is summarized in Table 28.2.

Table 28.2 FIGO classification [6]

Stage I. The carcinoma is strictly confined to the cervix (extension to the corpus would be disregarded)
IA. Invasive carcinoma which can be diagnosed only by microscopy, with deepest invasion ≤5 mm and largest extension ≤7 mm
IA1. Measured stromal invasion of ≤3 mm in depth and extension of ≤7 mm
IA2. Measured stromal invasion of >3 mm and not >5 mm with an extension of not >7 mm
IB. Clinically visible lesions limited to the cervix or preclinical cancers greater than stage IA[a]
IB1. Clinically visible lesion ≤4.0 cm in greatest dimension
IB2. Clinically visible lesion >4.0 cm in greatest dimension
Stage II. Cervical carcinoma extends beyond the uterus, but not to the pelvic wall or to the lower third of the vagina
IIA. Without parametrial invasion
IIA1. Clinically visible lesion ≤4.0 cm in greatest dimension
IIA2. Clinically visible lesion >4.0 cm in greatest dimension
IIB. With obvious parametrial invasion
Stage III. The tumor extends to the pelvic wall and/or involves the lower third of the vagina and/or causes hydronephrosis or nonfunctioning kidney[b]
IIIA. Tumor involves lower third of the vagina with no extension to the pelvic wall
IIIB. Extension to the pelvic wall and/or hydronephrosis or nonfunctioning kidney
Stage IV. The carcinoma has extended beyond the true pelvis or has involved (biopsy proven) the mucosa of the bladder or rectum. A bullous edema, as such, does not permit a case to be allotted stage IV
IVA. Spread of the growth to adjacent organs
IVB. Spread to distant organs

[a]All macroscopically visible lesions even with superficial invasion are allotted to stage IB carcinomas. Invasion is limited to a measured stromal invasion with a maximal depth of 5.00 mm and a horizontal extension not >7 mm. Depth of invasion should not be >5 mm taken from the base of the epithelium of the original tissue superficial or glandular. The depth of invasion should always be reported in mm, even in those cases with early (minimal) stromal invasion (~1 mm). The involvement of vascular/lymphatic spaces should not change the stage allotment

[b]On rectal examination, there is no cancer-free space between the tumor and the pelvic wall. All cases with hydronephrosis or nonfunctioning kidney are included, unless they are known to be due to another cause

MR findings are summarized in Table 28.3 [7].

Table 28.3 MR findings in cervix carcinoma (all types) correlated to FIGO staging

IA. No evidence of a mass lesion
IB. Tumor completely surrounded by the hypointense stromal ring
IIA. Segmental disruption of the hypointense upper two-thirds of vaginal wall
IIB. Protrusion of the tumor into the cardinal ligament through a disrupted hypointense cervical stromal ring
IIIA. Same finding as for stage IIA in the lower one-third of the vagina
IIIB. Same finding as for stage IIB with obliteration of the entire cardinal ligament directly extending to pelvic muscles or with hydroureter
IVA. Segmental disruption of the hypointense bladder or rectal wall or a segmental thickened rectal wall
IVB. Evidence of mass lesions in distant organs

Extension may involve:

1. *Mackenrodt's ligament and ureter*

   Extension to the proximal part of the Mackenrodt's ligament appears as tissue with irregular limits in continuity with the lateral border of the cervical tumor or as nodules. Signal intensity of this extension is very similar to the signal intensity of the cervical tumor on the different sequences. Extension to the ureter results in dilatation of the pelvic ureter above the obstruction; in some cases, CT can be helpful to precise this extension.

2. *Vagina* (Figs. 28.3, 28.4, 28.5, 28.6, and 28.7)

   Staging in early cervical cancer can be difficult and overestimated, especially if the tumor is slightly extended into the proximal vagina. Vaginal contrast medium better delineates the borders of the tumor; in Akata's series [9], correct staging with vaginal opacification was achieved in 78 % patients.

3. Bladder

   The tumor is classified stage IV only if involvement of the mucosa is present and confirmed at cystoscopy.

   On MR, extension to the bladder wall is diagnosed:
   - On T2, when there is focal interruption of the hypointense signal of the muscle layer or protrusion through the mucosa (Fig. 28.5)
   - After IV contrast injection, when there is a mass protruding into the bladder wall of the same signal intensity as the cervical tumor

   Ultrasound is a good modality to evaluate this extension [10]. A tumor protuberance at the junction of the cervix and the uterine corpus invading the bladder with:
   - Disruption of the echogenic outer wall
   - Thickened bladder wall
   - Irregular mucosa

   CT scan that can be performed to evaluate ureteral extension is also an accurate modality (Fig. 28.5).

4. *Rectum*

   On MR, extension is evaluated with the same findings as for the bladder.

   In questionable case, CT with rectal opacification is very accurate to assess the presence or absence of extension.

5. *Uterus corpus and adnexa* (Fig. 28.7)

   Extension can be evaluated on MR or US.

6. *Pelvic wall*

   Tumor extending to the internal obturator, piriform, or levator ani indicates pelvic wall invasion [11].

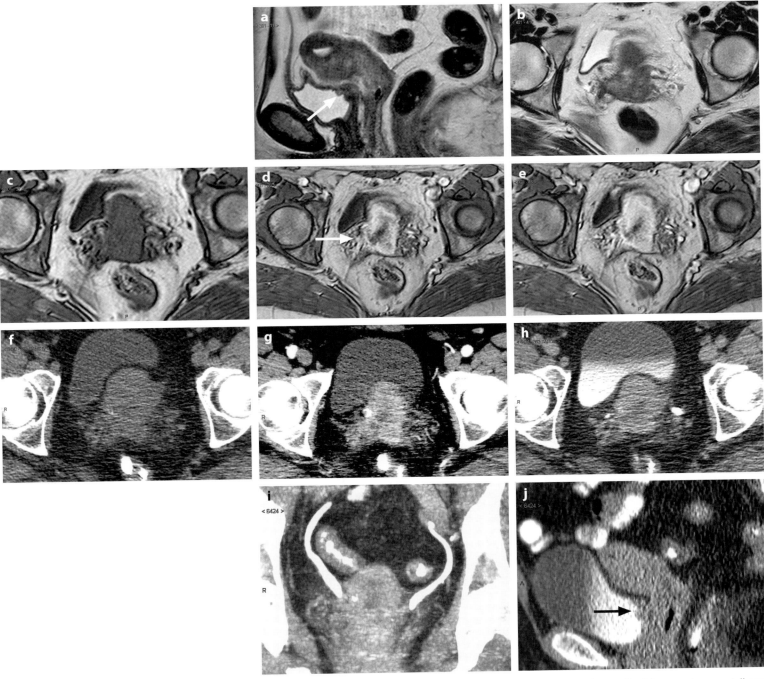

Fig. 28.5 Epidermoid carcinoma stage III. Fifty-year-old woman with metrorrhagia for 2 months. Biopsy of the cervix: epidermoid carcinoma. (1) MR sagittal T2 (**a**) displays a tumor of intermediate signal involving the endometrium, the cervix, and the vagina extending to its lower third. The epicenter of the tumor is in the cervix. Anteriorly, the mass extends into the vesicovaginal septum and the bladder wall protruding under the mucosa (*arrow*). On axial T2 (**b**), the mass extends into the proximal part of the cardinal ligaments especially on the right. DMR without injection (**c**) and at the arterial phase (**d**) displays multiple arterial tumoral vessels in the tumor extending into the proximal right cardinal ligament (*arrow*). At the venous phase and on the delayed (**e**), a high-contrast uptake is visualized in the tumor with a proximal extension into the cardinal ligaments especially on the right. (2) CT scan was performed to precise the urinary extension. DCT without contrast (**f**) and at the arterial phase with MIP reformation (**g**) depicts arterial tumoral vessels in the tumor. At the venous phase and on the delayed (**h**) and coronal reformation (**i**), extension to the right proximal cardinal ligament is confirmed respecting the ureter. On sagittal reformation (**j**), extension to the vesicovaginal septum is clearly shown, with a protrusion into the bladder mucosa (*arrow*). Cystoscopy precised the absence of extension to the mucosa. PET scan confirmed extension to the vesicovaginal septum and to the bladder wall

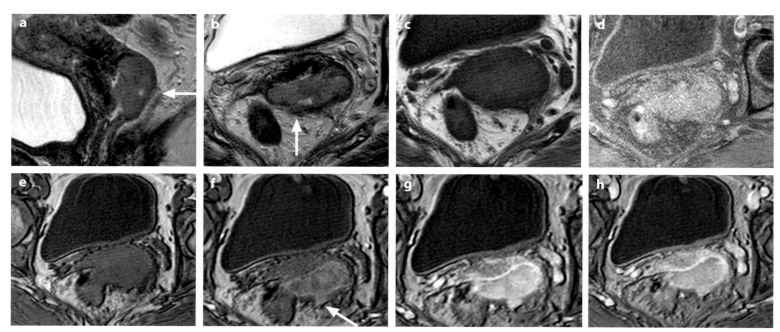

Fig. 28.6 Cervical carcinoma stage IIA. Sixty-year-old woman with metror-rhagia after intercourse. MR Sagittal T2 (**a**) and axial T2 (**b**) display, in the posterior lip of the cervix, a mass of intermediate signal measuring 3.8 cm in height and 5.2 cm of transverse diameter. The posterior wall of the vagina on the middle at the junction of the upper third and the middle third is focally interrupted (*arrows*). Axial T1 (**c**) and fat suppression (**d**) do not demonstrate any hemorrhage in the tumor. DMR without injection (**e**) and at the arterial phase (**f**) confirms invasion of the vagina (*arrow* in **f**), with a contrast uptake that increases at the venous (**g**) and on the delayed (**h**) phases

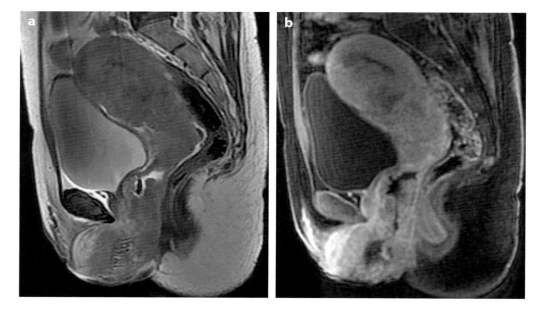

Fig. 28.7 Extensive cervical cancer extending from the vulva to the uterus. Thirty-six-year-old woman with metrorrhagia and vulvar tumor. (**a, b**) Sagittal T2W (**a**) and T1W-FS after gadolinium injection (**b**) show a huge tumor starting in the cervix, extending upward into the uterus body and downward until the vulva

28.1.3.3 Lymph Nodes

Lymphatic spread is initially to the parametrial lymph nodes followed by pelvic and then lomboaortic nodes [12]

Diagnostic criteria have been defined in the different imaging modalities:

- *Size*: Superior to 1 cm (small axis) is considered as a finding of malignancy [13]. However, this finding is not specific, and lymph nodes smaller than 1 cm may contain metastases [14].
- Round shape [15].
- *Structure*: Central necrosis is very suggestive of metastasis. It was present in 27 % on CT and in 17.5 % on MR, and all of these nodes had metastasis at pathology [15].

On US, involved lymph nodes are hypoechoic [16].

However, the accuracy of the different imaging modalities is very low. Indeed, foci of metastasis are commonly overlooked. Moreover, large lymph nodes are not necessarily malignant.

28.1.4 Imaging Findings After Radiation Therapy [17]

Tumors treated with radiation therapy respond with a decrease in size and signal intensity (Fig. 28.8). The response may be immediate (3–6 months) or, in larger tumors, delayed (6–9 months).

The findings of reconstitution of the normal zonal anatomy and the presence of homogeneous low signal intensity stroma are reliable indicators of a tumor-free postirradiation cervix.

28.1.4.1 The First 3 Months

Differentiation between residual tumor and radiation changes cannot be made in the presence of the following findings:

- Widened cervical canal.
- High-intensity stroma on T2.
- Contrast enhancement is seen in postirradiation fibrosis, inflammation, radiation necrosis, and tumor.

Diffusion: It has been reported that between 1 and 3 months, ADC has a potential ability to differentiate normal from persistent disease [5].

28.1.4.2 Later

A significant decrease in size of the uterus and of T2 cervical intensity is common.

Fibrosis of the cardinal ligament is common.
Wall thickening of bladder and rectum.
Symmetric thickening of the uterosacral ligaments.
Presacral space widening.
Inhomogeneous decrease in signal of adipose tissue on T1.
High signal intensity on T2 in skeletal muscles.
High signal intensity on T2 of bone marrow.
At that time, DMR allows to make the differential between tumor and fibrosis.

28.1.4.3 Late Complications

Rectovesical fistula, rectal stricture, sigmoiditis.
Ureteral stricture.
Sacral insufficiency fracture.
Inflammatory lesion of the vagina may occur (Fig. 28.9).

28.1.5 Imaging Findings with Recurrent and Metastatic Disease

28.1.5.1 Location

1. Pelvic and para-aortic adenopathy
2. The most common sites of recurrence:
   - Vaginal cuff (Fig. 28.10)
   - Cervix
   - Parametrium
   - Pelvic side wall
3. Metastases: lung, bone, less frequently peritoneum and GI tract

28.1.5.2 Imaging

Malignant pelvic recurrence and peritoneal implants have usually an intermediate signal on T2, a rapid enhancement, a high intensity on DWI, and a low ADC value (Fig. 28.10).

28.2 Adenocarcinoma

28.2.1 Clinical Findings [1]

28.2.1.1 Macroscopy

The majority arises in the transformation zone.
- Fifty percent has a fungating, polypoid, or papillary mass.
- In 15 % the cervix is diffusely enlarged or nodular.
- In 15 % no gross lesion is visible.

28.2.1.2 Microscopy

Mucinous adenocarcinoma – Endocervical type – Intestinal type – Signet ring cell type	57 %
Endometrioid adenocarcinoma	30 %
Clear cell adenocarcinoma	11 %
Others – Minimal deviation adenocarcinoma – Serous adenocarcinoma – Mesonephric carcinoma – Well-differentiated villoglandular adenocarcinoma	3 %

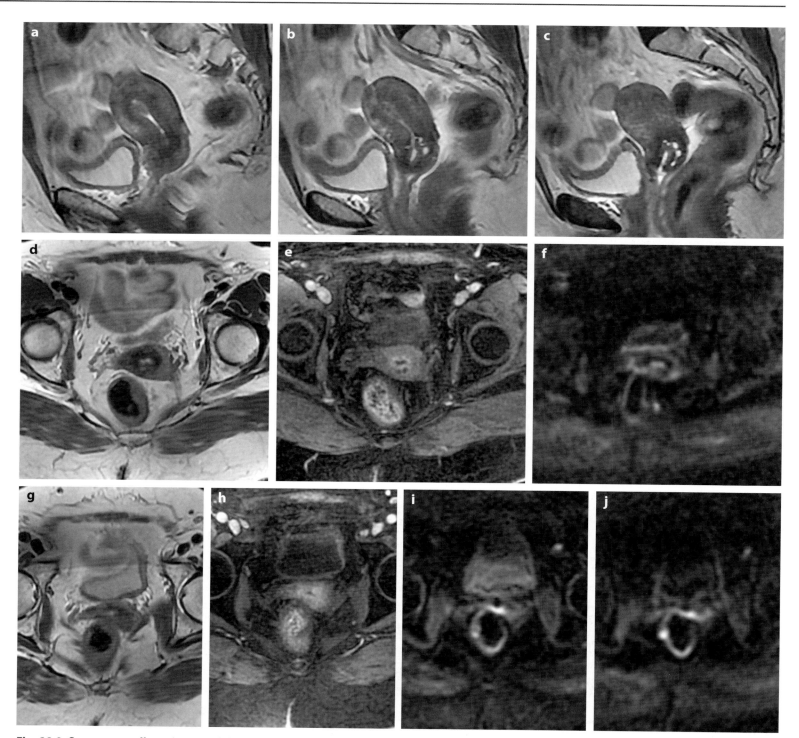

Fig. 28.8 Squamous cell carcinoma of the cervix, 6 months following chemo-radiotherapy, followed by radical surgery (same patient as Fig. 28.4). On Sagittal T2 with contiguous images (**a–c**), a small area of intermediate signal in the cervix and the upper vagina is still visualized in (**a**, **b**) without any abnormality in (**c**). Axial T2 (**d**), DMR at the arterial phase (**e**) and DWI b1000 (**f**) at the same level show a residual intermediate signal on the left border of the cervix on T2 but without abnormality on DMR and DWI. At histology, necrotic tissue with microscopic residual tumor foci was found in the cervix. At a lower level on axial T2 (**g**), the vagina appears still in contact with the rectum. DMR at the arterial phase (**h**) at the same level does not show any abnormality. DWI at b500 (**i**) and b1000 (**j**), at the same level, show on b500 a small hyperintensity between the vagina and the rectal wall that almost disappear on b1000, probably related to T2 through shine effect, with an ADC value of 1.5×10^{-3} mm²/s on b500 and 1.2×10^{-3} mm²/s at b1000. At surgery no significant abnormality was found at this level. Pelvic lymph nodes on MR were of same size as at the initial examination ($\leq 18 \times 10$ mm). At surgery, no lymph node was involved on a total of 20 lymph nodes resected; no rectal or para-rectal involvment was found

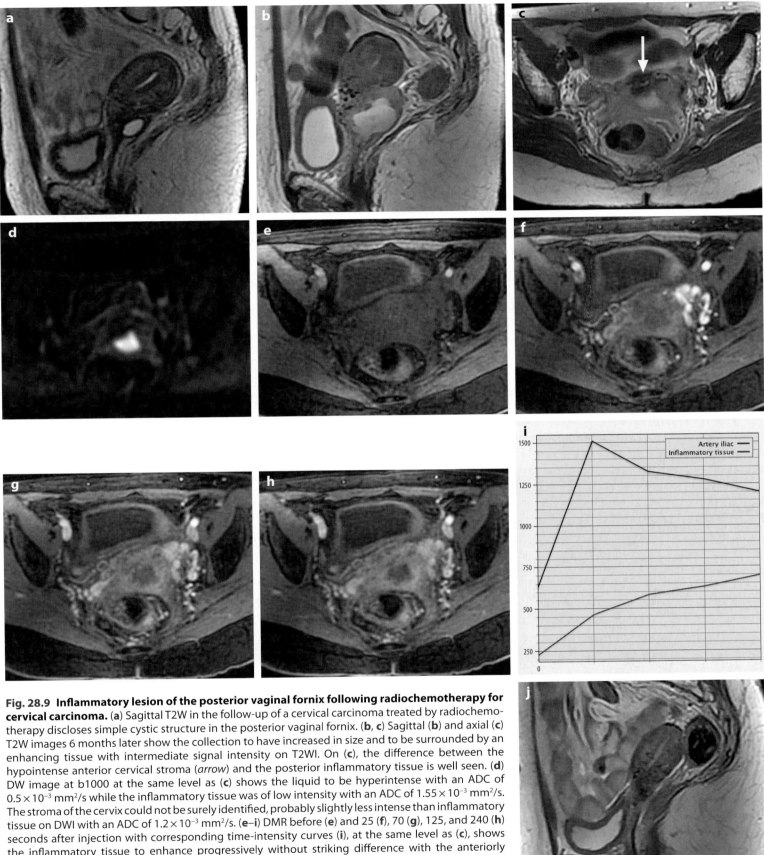

Fig. 28.9 Inflammatory lesion of the posterior vaginal fornix following radiochemotherapy for cervical carcinoma. (a) Sagittal T2W in the follow-up of a cervical carcinoma treated by radiochemotherapy discloses simple cystic structure in the posterior vaginal fornix. **(b, c)** Sagittal **(b)** and axial **(c)** T2W images 6 months later show the collection to have increased in size and to be surrounded by an enhancing tissue with intermediate signal intensity on T2WI. On **(c)**, the difference between the hypointense anterior cervical stroma (*arrow*) and the posterior inflammatory tissue is well seen. **(d)** DW image at b1000 at the same level as **(c)** shows the liquid to be hyperintense with an ADC of 0.5×10^{-3} mm^2/s while the inflammatory tissue was of low intensity with an ADC of 1.55×10^{-3} mm^2/s. The stroma of the cervix could not be surely identified, probably slightly less intense than inflammatory tissue on DWI with an ADC of 1.2×10^{-3} mm^2/s. **(e–i)** DMR before **(e)** and 25 **(f)**, 70 **(g)**, 125, and 240 **(h)** seconds after injection with corresponding time-intensity curves **(i)**, at the same level as **(c)**, shows the inflammatory tissue to enhance progressively without striking difference with the anteriorly located cervical stroma that could not be clearly identified. Colposcopy with biopsy and liquid evacuation revealed inflammatory tissue. **(j)** Follow-up MR at 10 months **(j)** and later on at 17 months shows complete disappearance of the lesion and shrinking of the cervix

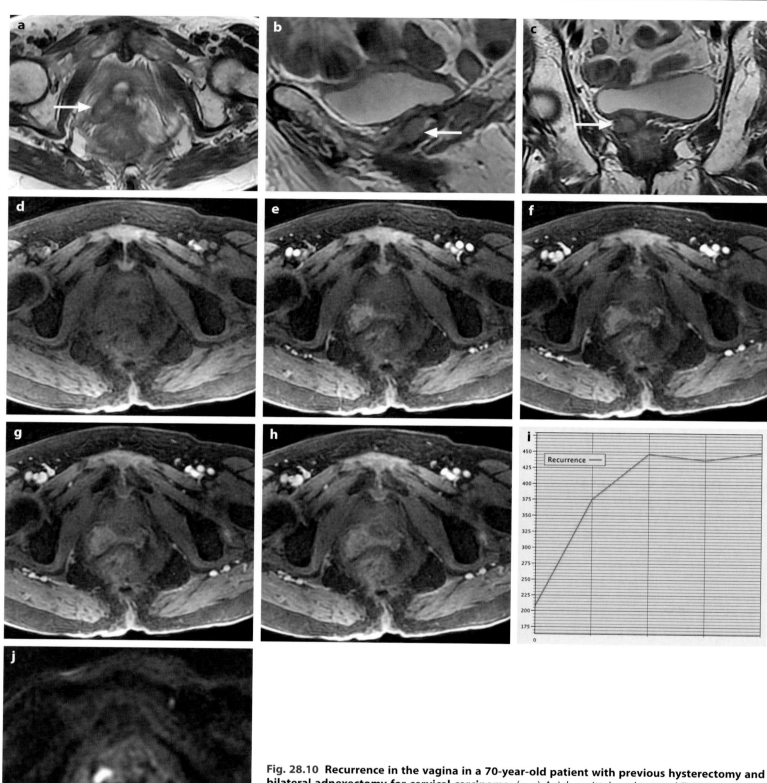

Fig. 28.10 Recurrence in the vagina in a 70-year-old patient with previous hysterectomy and bilateral adnexectomy for cervical carcinoma. (a–c) Axial, sagittal, and coronal T2W images disclose a 2.5×1.5 cm tumor (*arrows*) of intermediate signal intensity (between that of adipose tissue and muscle) in the vagina and right vaginal stump. The hypointense vaginal wall is interrupted in several places. (d–i). DMR before (d) and 25 (e), 75 (f), 125 (g), and 240 (h) seconds after injection with time-intensity curve (i) show a high contrast uptake at the arterial phase with a peak at the venous phase. Contrast enhancement is slightly heterogeneous. (j) DWI at b1000 shows the recurrence to have a high intensity signal with an ADC of 0.85×10⁻³ mm²/s

28.2.2 Pathology

Adenocarcinoma usually arises from the endocervical canal often forming a barrel-shaped mass. But it often presents a false-negative result on a Pap smear due to its high location in the endocervical canal so that punch biopsy, dilatation and curettage, or conization should be required to make a correct diagnosis [18].

28.2.3 MR Findings [19]

Adenocarcinoma (AD) and squamous cell carcinoma (SCC) can be difficult to distinguish on MR because their appearance and the pattern of spread can be similar [20], although in some cases adenocarcinoma (Figs. 28.11 and 28.12) may be suspected because of a particular barrel shape along the endocervical canal and tendency to involve lymph nodes in earlier stages [21].

MR findings of adenocarcinoma versus squamous cell carcinoma are reported in Table 28.4 [19, 21, 22].

Table 28.4 MR findings of adenocarcinoma versus squamous cell carcinoma

	Adenocarcinoma	Squamous cell carcinoma
Location	Endocervical canal (58.8 %)	Exocervical (75 %)
	Downward extension (41.2 %)	Extension endocervix (25 %)
Signal intensity	Higher than myometrium on T2	Higher than myometrium on T2 but not as high as adenocarcinoma
Shape	Barrel shaped	Localized mass or polypoid appearance
Aspect	Intratumoral multiseptations	No multiseptated lesions
Hydrometrocolpos	Yes (17.6 %)	No
Contrast uptake	Low	More intense
	Peripheral enhancement	Global enhancement

The differences in signal intensity between AD and SCC are probably due to cytoplasmic mucin and intraglandular mucinous or serous fluid in the multiple tumorous glands, while in SCC compact cellularity is not associated with mucinous or serous fluid in the cytoplasm or surrounding stroma.

As it has been described by Wright et al. [1], the tumor composed of complex glandular structures may invade the stroma underneath an intact surface of epithelium. In Torashima et al.'s series [22], endocervical superficial mucosa was preserved in 12/13 (92 %) of adenocarcinomas involving the entire cervix.

Pharmacokinetic analysis [2] and perfusion imaging can help predict radiation therapy. There is a wide range of dynamic enhancement values within the tumor. Poor blood supply and hypoxia contribute to radiation therapy failure.

28.2.4 Particular Findings Related to the Histological Type

28.2.4.1 Endocervical Endometrioid Carcinoma

It can be difficult to differentiate mucinous endometrial adenocarcinoma from endocervical adenocarcinoma at histology.

However, primary cervical endometrioid carcinoma tends to expand to the endocervix in the absence of enlargement of the endometrium (Fig. 28.12).

When endometrial carcinoma extends to the endocervix, it usually invades the myometrium and becomes sufficiently bulky to enlarge the uterus.

28.2.4.2 Clear Cell Adenocarcinoma

In case of a history of in utero exposure to diethylstilbestrol (DES), they occur in young women. They develop predominantly on the exocervix.

In the absence of exposure to DES, they occur most commonly in postmenopausal women. They develop in either the exocervix or the endocervix.

Differential Diagnosis

1. Other types of adenocarcinomas
2. Benign processes
   - Arias-Stella reaction during pregnancy (see Chap. 21, Sect. 21.3, for definition).
   - Microglandular hyperplasia. It usually lacks the degree of nuclear atypia of clear cell carcinoma and contains mucin.

28.2.4.3 Minimal Deviation Adenocarcinoma (Adenoma Malignum)

They represent about 3 % of adenocarcinomas [23]. The designation adenoma malignum has been first used because of its deceptively benign histological appearance [24].

Definition

It is an extremely well-differentiated variant of mucinous cervical adenocarcinoma [24]; others also consider endometrioid or clear cell origin [1].

Pathology [24]

Macroscopy

The cervix is typically firm.

It has an intact ectocervical epithelium.

Endocervical mucosa is hemorrhagic, friable, or mucoid.

The wall of the endocervix is thickened with yellow or tan-white tissue. Cysts filled with mucin, measuring up to 2 cm in maximum dimension, can be present.

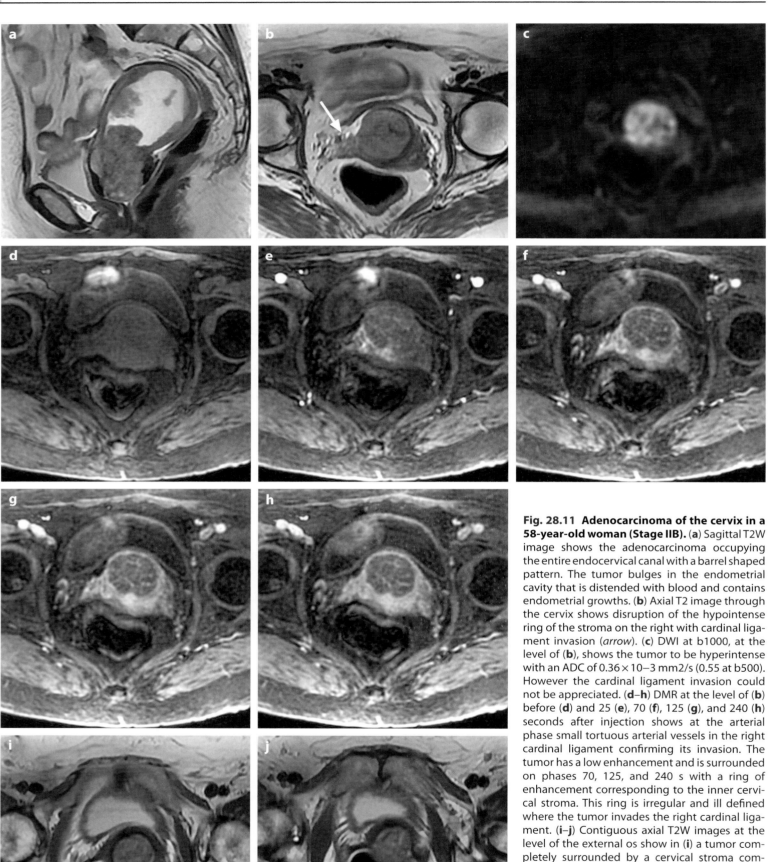

Fig. 28.11 Adenocarcinoma of the cervix in a 58-year-old woman (Stage IIB). (a) Sagittal T2W image shows the adenocarcinoma occupying the entire endocervical canal with a barrel shaped pattern. The tumor bulges in the endometrial cavity that is distended with blood and contains endometrial growths. (b) Axial T2 image through the cervix shows disruption of the hypointense ring of the stroma on the right with cardinal ligament invasion (*arrow*). (c) DWI at b1000, at the level of (b), shows the tumor to be hyperintense with an ADC of 0.36×10^{-3} mm2/s (0.55 at b500). However the cardinal ligament invasion could not be appreciated. (d–h) DMR at the level of (b) before (d) and 25 (e), 70 (f), 125 (g), and 240 (h) seconds after injection shows at the arterial phase small tortuous arterial vessels in the right cardinal ligament confirming its invasion. The tumor has a low enhancement and is surrounded on phases 70, 125, and 240 s with a ring of enhancement corresponding to the inner cervical stroma. This ring is irregular and ill defined where the tumor invades the right cardinal ligament. (i–j) Contiguous axial T2W images at the level of the external os show in (i) a tumor completely surrounded by a cervical stroma composed of two layers: an inner hypointense ring and outer less hypointense ring. However, one cut below (j), the cervical stroma is disrupted especially in its right part with the tumor in contact with the rectal wall but without obvious rectal wall invasion (at rectoscopy, the rectal mucosa was not involved)

Fig. 28.12 Endometrioid adenocarcinoma of the cervix with parametrial and pelvic wall involvement (stage IIIB). (**a**) Sagittal T2W image shows a cervical mass involving the lower uterus body. (**b–d**) Axial T2W images at the level of the isthmus (**b**), the cervix (**c**), and the exocervix (**d**) show right and left cardinal ligaments invasion (*arrows* in **b**) and extension to the pelvic wall (*arrow* in **d**). (**e**) DWI at b1000 shows the mass to be hyperintense with a low ADC value of 0.89×10^{-3} mm²/s (mean of b500 and b1000). Extension is not well appreciated. (**f–j**) DMR at the level of (**b**), before injection (**f**), at 25 (**g**), 70 (**h**), 125 (**i**), and 240 s (**j**) shows arterial vessel in the mass at the arterial phase (*arrow* in **g**), continuous enhancement in the solid part of the mass, and a small central necrotic center with a hyperintense hemorrhagic foci before injection

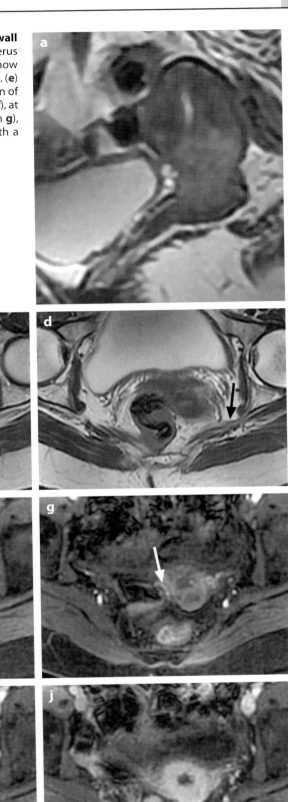

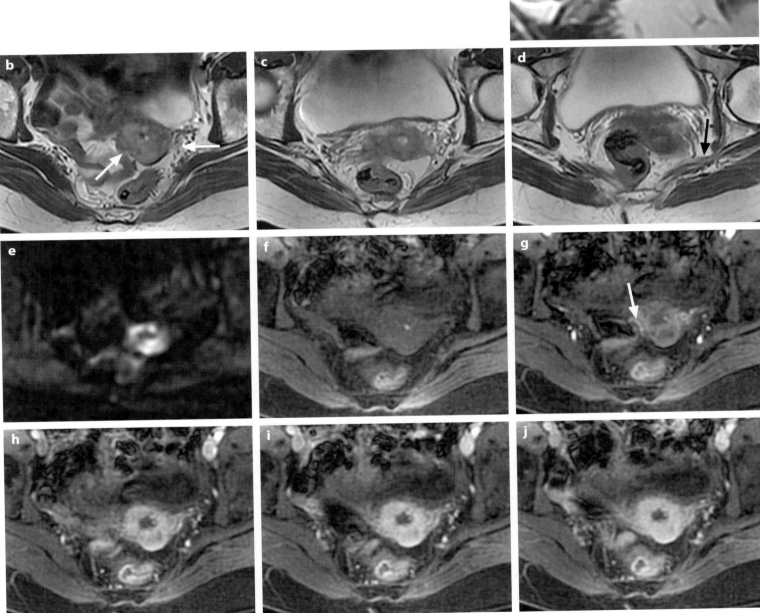

Microscopy

1. Marked irregular, abnormally shaped glands
2. Invasion of the outer half of the cervical wall (>7 mm) while normal crypts rarely extend more than 8 mm from the endocervical surface [25] in premenopausal women and less than 5 mm in postmenopausal women
3. Extension to the serosa or cardinal ligament in almost half of the cases
4. Positive staining for carcinoembryonic antigen

Clinical Features

1. Menometrorrhagia, postmenopausal bleeding
2. Vaginal discharge: mucoid, watery, or purulent
3. Abdominal pain
4. Possible association with Peutz-Jeghers syndrome

Imaging Findings

1. Tumor

US

A multicystic lesion of the cervix consisting of multiple small round anechoic cysts which varied in size and were easily distinguished from cervical stroma [26]

CT

- Without contrast low-density area
- After contrast multiple cysts surrounded by enhanced cervix

MR

MR better than US and CT demonstrates the features of this entity:
1. On T2, an irregular high-intensity image with indistinct margins giving a villous or hazy appearance [26]
2. Multiple small cysts [26] or association of relatively large cysts surrounded by smaller vesicles of various sizes from 1 to 20 mm [26, 27]:
   - On T2 with intensity similar to the signal intensity of urine.
   - After contrast, the walls of the cysts were smooth and thin.
3. Solid parts surround or are adjacent to the cysts [27]:
   - On T2 slightly hyperintense to the uterus
   - After contrast more clearly visualized as enhancing lesions
4. Fluid in the endocervix, vagina [26]
5. Extension to serosa, cardinal ligament, or myometrium.
6. Association with ovarian tumors (17/26 in Gilk et al.'s series) [24]:
   - Mucinous tumor ($n = 13$) with carcinomas more common than borderline than benign. These tumors were synchronous or metachronous.
   - Sex cord tumor with annular tubules ($n = 4$) and particular calcifications (sometimes in the frame of a Peutz-Jeghers syndrome).

Differential Diagnosis

Conditions in which nonneoplastic glands extend beyond 7 mm from the surface:
1. Endocervical tunnel clusters
2. Deeply situated Nabothian cysts
3. Mesonephric hyperplasia
4. Endocervicosis of the cervical wall (see Chap. 17)

On MR, Okamoto et al. [7] in a series of 22 patients with malignant and benign lesions of the cervix studied if MRI could allow to differentiate these lesions:
1. The main finding of malignancy was the presence of an entirely or mainly solid component (except in one case), while entirely cystic lesions were benign. Mainly cystic with a solid component were benign or malignant.
2. Size and intensity of the fluid did not help in the differential. Lesions composed of cysts smaller than 5 mm tend to be malignant, but some lesions composed of larger cysts can also be malignant. In malignant lesions, signal intensity of fluid on T1W images compared to the cervical stroma could be low, isointense, or high.

28.3 Other Epithelial Tumors

Other epithelial tumors include:
- Adenosquamous carcinoma
- Glassy cell carcinoma
- Clear cell adenosquamous carcinoma
- Mucoepidermoid carcinoma
- Adenoid cystic carcinoma
- Adenoid basal carcinoma
- Neuroendocrine tumors (carcinoid tumors)
- Small oat cell carcinoma (2–5 % of all cervical tumors) [1]

28.3.1 Adenoid Cystic Carcinoma

Less than 1 % of all cervical adenocarcinomas

28.3.1.1 Definition

Nests of small basaloid cells of varying sizes with high nuclear-to-cytoplasmic ratios. Cribriform appearance due to cylindrical hyaline bodies or small acini or cysts

28.3.1.2 MR Findings [28]

Low intensity on T1, high intensity on T2

Lobulated contour and multiple septum-like architectures probably representing interglandular fibrous stroma

It contains spots of very high signal intensity that would represent mucin in the glandular lumens.

28.3.2 Small Oat Cell Carcinoma

Small oat cell carcinoma (2–5 % of all cervical tumors) [1]

28.3.2.1 Definition

These tumors are characterized by small anaplastic cells that have scant amounts of cytoplasm, finely stippled chromatin, and inconspicuous nucleoli.

28.3.2.2 Macroscopy

Size ranges from small, clinically inapparent lesions to large ulcerated lesions measuring more than 6 cm in diameter.

Small cell carcinomas are more frequently infiltrative than are squamous or adenocarcinoma, and a barrel-shaped cervix is commonly present [1].

Multiagent chemotherapy and pelvic radiotherapy before surgery produce a better outcome than local treatment alone. However, early accurate diagnosis is limited on routine screening examination because Papanicolaou smear has a very low accuracy, and even microscopic examination is not highly sensitive.

28.3.2.3 MR Findings

1. Although tumor has a tendency toward homogeneous appearance and irregular margins, these findings are not specific.
2. Extension: The high aggressiveness of the tumor is displayed by its degree of extension. Even tumors of 4 cm or smaller have considerable incidence of parametrial invasion (60 %) and lymphadenopathy (80 %).

28.4 Malignant Mesenchymal Tumors

The most common form is leiomyosarcoma. Very uncommonly endocervical stromal sarcoma, embryonal rhabdomyosarcoma, alveolar soft part sarcoma, osteosarcoma, and undifferentiated sarcoma (Fig. 28.13) can occur.

28.5 Mixed Epithelial and Mesenchymatous Tumors (see Chap. 25)

- Malignant mixed Mullerian tumors (MMMT)
- Adenosarcoma

28.6 Miscellaneous

Other rare tumors are:
- Melanoma
- Primary choriocarcinoma
- Lymphoma
- Leukemia
- Primary cervical germ cell tumors
- Primitive neuroectodermal tumors (PNET)

28.6.1 Lymphoma

Primary lymphomas can arise in the cervix. Seventy percent of the tumors are of the diffuse large cell type, and 20 % are lower-grade follicular lymphomas. Most are secondary; they occur in 6 % of generalized disease [1].

28.6.1.1 MR Findings

1. Location
   At histology: True lymphoid follicles, with or without germinal centers, are encountered in the subepithelial stroma of both the exocervix and the endocervix [29]. This is the reason why lack of mucosal involvement as well as sparing of the cervical stroma is the most important findings to differentiate lymphoma from carcinoma [21].
2. Signal [30]
   On T1, they are isointense or hypointense relative to myometrium.
   On T2, signal intensity was high.
   After contrast, there is diffuse enhancement usually homogeneous, but it can be inhomogeneous.
   Diffuse enlargement of the uterus and a relative homogeneous signal intensity in spite of large tumor size are very suggestive of lymphoma [21].

28.6.2 Leukemia

Leukemia are usually secondary (Fig. 28.14) and rarely primary.

28.6.3 PNET

These tumors appear to be identical to PNETs at other sites (see Chap. 24) (Fig. 28.15)

28.7 Secondary Tumors [1]

1. Direct extension from:
   - Endometrium
   - Rectum
   - Bladder
2. Lymphatic or vascular metastases from:
   - Ovarian carcinomas, endometrial carcinomas, and uncommonly transitional cell carcinoma of the bladder
   - Choriocarcinoma
   - Sarcomas of the corpus
3. From distant primary foci:
   - GI tract: colon and stomach
   - Breast

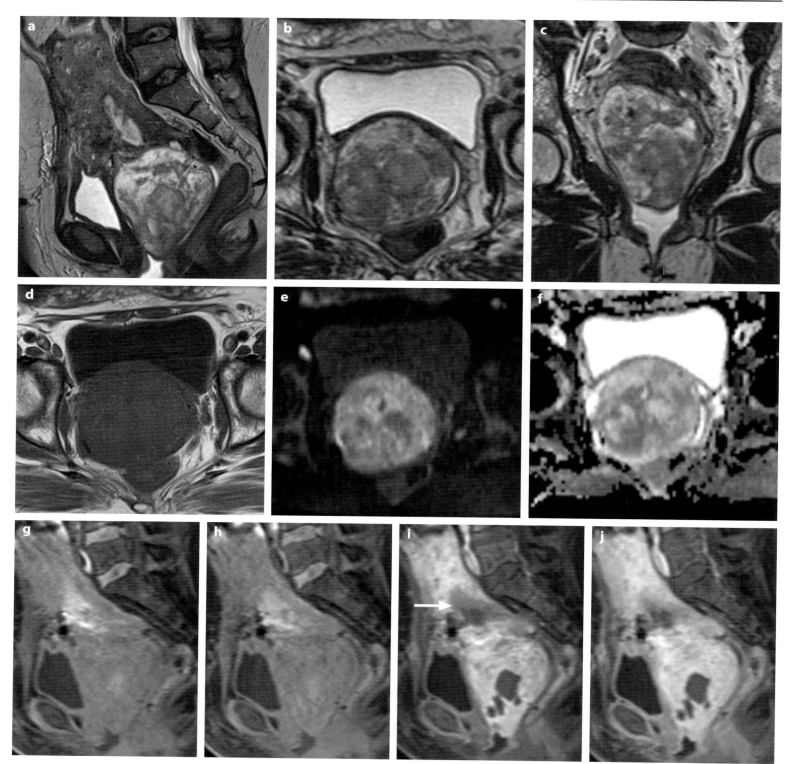

Fig. 28.13 High-grade undifferentiated sarcoma of the cervix. MR in a 41-year-old woman 1 month after cesarian section at 34 weeks of amenorrhea for cervical mass considered as a myoma. Biopsy done 1 week ago was nonconclusive. (**a–c**) Sagittal (**a**), axial (**b**), and coronal T2W (**c**) images show a large mass of heterogeneous intensity occupying almost the entire cervix with persistence of a posterior cervical wall containing Nabothian cysts. An extension to the endometrium is also visualized. (**d**) On axial T1W image, there is no hyperintensity suggestive of hemorrhage. (**e, f**) On axial DWI (**e**), the tumor is overall hyperintense, slightly heterogeneous, with variable ADC values on the corresponding ADC map (**f**). (**g–k**) DMR in the sagittal plane before injection (**g**), at the arterial phase (**h**), the venous phase (**i**), and the late phase (**j**), shows: In the cervical tumor, an enhancement close to that of the myometrium with areas of necrosis. In the endometrial extension, low enhancement (*arrow* in **i**) compared to that of the myometrium. A hysterectomy was performed with at pathology resection in sano of a high-grade undifferentiated sarcoma of the cervix. A bilateral adnexectomy was then performed

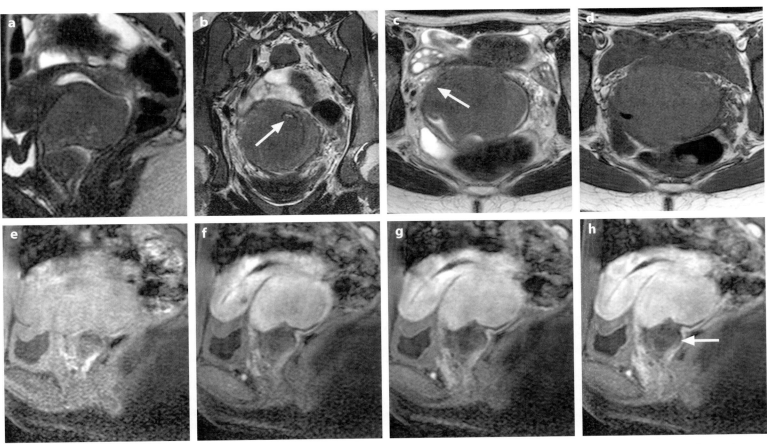

Fig. 28.14 Acute myeloid leukemia with blasts. Seventeen-year-old girl with metrorrhagia. (a–c) Sagittal, coronal, and axial T2W images show a large mass of intermediate intensity surrounding the endocervical canal, more prominent anteriorly and protruding in the vagina. The inner hypointense cervical stroma is disturbed anteriorly (*arrow* in **b**). The vaginal wall is also invaded in some region (*arrow* in **c**). (**d**) Axial T1W image shows absence of hyperintensity suggestive of hemorrhage. (**e–h**) Sagittal DMR before (**e**), at the arterial (**f**), venous (**g**), and delayed (**h**) phases, shows absence of necrosis in the mass and a hypointense vaginal clot (*arrow* in **h**) that was of intermediate intensity on T2

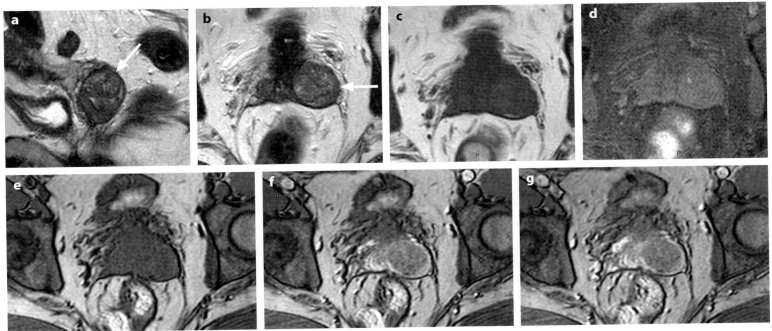

Fig. 28.15 Primitive neuroectodermic tumor of the cervix. A 43-year-old woman with spontaneous metrorrhagia. Left breast carcinoma 10 years ago treated by mastectomy with radiotherapy and chemotherapy. (**a, b**) Sagittal (**a**) and axial (**b**) T2W images show a well-circumscribed 3.5-cm posterior and left intramural mass (*arrows*) abutting against the cervical mucosa and uterine serosa. It has heterogeneous intermediate signal intensity with multiple small hyperintense areas. (**c, d**) Axial T1 (**c**) and T1FS (**d**) images show a hyperintense spot on (**d**) that could be related to hemorrhage. (**e–i**) DMR before injection (**e**), at the arterial (**f**), venous (**g**)

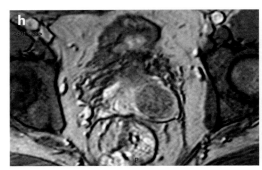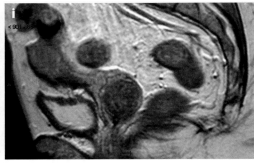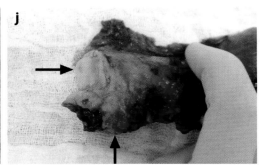

Fig. 28.15 (*continued*) Parenchymal (**h**) phases, followed by delayed T1 sagittal image (**i**) shows a low enhancing tumor compared to cervical stroma and myometrium. (**j**) View of the surgical specimen of hysterectomy showing the cervical tumor (*vertical arrow*) and the exocervix (*horizontal arrow*)

References

1. Wright CT, Ferenczy A, Kurman RJ (2002) Carcinoma and other tumors of the cervix. In: Kurman RJ (ed) Blaustein's pathology of the female genital tract. Springer, New York, pp 325–381
2. Yamashita Y et al (2000) Dynamic contrast-enhanced MR imaging of uterine cervical cancer: pharmacokinetic analysis with histopathologic correlation and its importance in predicting the outcome of radiation therapy. Radiology 216(3):803–809
3. Charles-Edwards EM et al (2008) Diffusion-weighted imaging in cervical cancer with an endovaginal technique: potential value for improving tumor detection in stage Ia and Ib1 disease. Radiology 249(2):541–550
4. McVeigh PZ et al (2008) Diffusion-weighted MRI in cervical cancer. Eur Radiol 18(5):1058–1064
5. Naganawa S et al (2005) Apparent diffusion coefficient in cervical cancer of the uterus: comparison with the normal uterine cervix. Eur Radiol 15(1):71–78
6. Pecorelli S (2009) Revised FIGO staging for carcinoma of the vulva, cervix, and endometrium. Int J Gynaecol Obstet 105(2):103–104, Erratum in: Int J Gynaecol Obstet, 2010; 108(2):176
7. Okamoto Y et al (2003) MR imaging of the uterine cervix: imaging-pathologic correlation. Radiographics 23(2):425–445; quiz 534–535
8. Hricak H et al (2007) Early invasive cervical cancer: CT and MR imaging in preoperative evaluation – ACRIN/GOG comparative study of diagnostic performance and interobserver variability. Radiology 245(2):491–498
9. Akata D et al (2005) Efficacy of transvaginal contrast-enhanced MRI in the early staging of cervical carcinoma. Eur Radiol 15(8):1727–1733
10. Huang WC et al (2006) Ultrasonographic characteristics and cystoscopic correlates of bladder wall invasion by endophytic cervical cancer. Ultrasound Obstet Gynecol 27(6):680–686
11. Nicolet V et al (2000) MR imaging of cervical carcinoma: a practical staging approach. Radiographics 20(6):1539–1549
12. Park JM et al (1994) Pathways of nodal metastasis from pelvic tumors: CT demonstration. Radiographics 14(6):1309–1321
13. Vinnicombe SJ et al (1995) Normal pelvic lymph nodes: evaluation with CT after bipedal lymphangiography. Radiology 194(2):349–355
14. Torabi M, Aquino SL, Harisinghani MG (2004) Current concepts in lymph node imaging. J Nucl Med 45(9):1509–1518
15. Yang WT et al (2000) Comparison of dynamic helical CT and dynamic MR imaging in the evaluation of pelvic lymph nodes in cervical carcinoma. AJR Am J Roentgenol 175(3):759–766
16. Yang WT et al (1999) Comparison of laparoscopic sonography with surgical pathology in the evaluation of pelvic lymph nodes in women with cervical cancer. AJR Am J Roentgenol 172(6):1521–1525
17. Engin G (2006) Cervical cancer: MR imaging findings before, during, and after radiation therapy. Eur Radiol 16(2):313–324
18. Hatch KD, Fu YS (1996) Cervical and vaginal cancer. In: Berek JS, Adashi EY, Hillard PA (eds) Novak's gynecology. Williams & Wilkins, Philadelphia, pp 1111–1153
19. Chung JJ et al (1999) T2-weighted fast spin-echo MR findings of adenocarcinoma of the uterine cervix: comparison with squamous cell carcinoma. Yonsei Med J 40(3):226–231
20. Mezrich R (1994) Magnetic resonance imaging applications in uterine cervical cancer. Magn Reson Imaging Clin N Am 2(2):211–243
21. Kim JC (1998) MR imaging findings of uterine cervical adenocarcinoma. J Korean Soc Magn Reson Med 2(2):113–119
22. Torashima M et al (1997) Invasive adenocarcinoma of the uterine cervix: MR imaging. Comput Med Imaging Graph 21(4):253–260
23. Kaminski PF, Norris HJ (1983) Minimal deviation carcinoma (adenoma malignum) of the cervix. Int J Gynecol Pathol 2(2):141–152
24. Gilks CB et al (1989) Adenoma malignum (minimal deviation adenocarcinoma) of the uterine cervix. A clinicopathological and immunohistochemical analysis of 26 cases. Am J Surg Pathol 13(9):717–729
25. Anderson MC, Hartley RB (1980) Cervical crypt involvement by intraepithelial neoplasia. Obstet Gynecol 55(5):546–550
26. Itoh K et al (2000) A comparative analysis of cross sectional imaging techniques in minimal deviation adenocarcinoma of the uterine cervix. BJOG 107(9):1158–1163
27. Doi T et al (1997) Adenoma malignum: MR imaging and pathologic study. Radiology 204(1):39–42
28. Kaku T et al (1992) Adenosarcoma of the uterus: a Gynecologic Oncology Group clinicopathologic study of 31 cases. Int J Gynecol Pathol 11(2):75–88
29. Wright CT, Ferenczy A (2002) Anatomy and histology of the cervix. In: Kurman RJ (ed) Blaustein's pathology of the female genital tract. Springer, New York, pp 207–224
30. Marin C et al (2002) Magnetic resonance imaging of primary lymphoma of the cervix. Eur Radiol 12(6):1541–1545

Embryology, Anatomy, and Histology of the Vagina

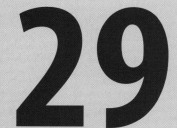

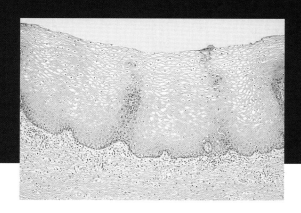

Contents

29.1 Embryology (See Chap. 1) [1, 2]

The vagina originates from two different structures:

The Müller duct which will form the subperitoneal portion from the fornices to the introitus partially obliterated by the hymen (in the virgin woman).

The urogenital sinus which will form the vulvar portion of the vagina, which opens in the vestibule which is a portion of 1.5–2 cm (see Chap. 34).

29.2 Anatomy [3, 4]

Vagina is oblique downward and forward. Its anterior wall is 7.5 cm long, and the posterior wall 9 cm long.

29.2.1 The Upper End

At this level, the muscular wall of the vagina fuses with the homologous wall of the cervix, while its mucosa reflects on the cervix forming a circular vault called the fornix; the annular recess between the cervix and the vagina forms four fornices.

The posterior fornix surrounds the cervix at the junction of the inferior 1/3 and superior 2/3. It measures from 10 to 25 mm.

The anterior fornix is less deep. It is reduced in some cases where the insertion of the vagina is on the lower part of the cervix to a simple gutter.

The lateral fornices are in relation with:
• The ureters.
• The highest part of the vaginal plexus.

J.N. Buy, M. Ghossain, *Gynecological Imaging*,
DOI 10.1007/978-3-642-31012-6_29, © Springer-Verlag Berlin Heidelberg 2013

- Three or four lymphatic canals.

They contain in their wall:
- The Gartner's canal (vestige of the mesonephric duct) that is present in 1/3 of women. It originates at the paroophorum; crosses medially the mesosalpinx, the medial part of the mesometrium; and reaches the superior part of the cervix. At this level, it goes into the wall of the cervix, crossing the entire cervix; goes into the anterolateral wall of the vagina; and goes down until the base of the hymen. At this level, it usually penetrates the thickness of this membrane and ends on its free border, sometimes on its lateral border, more rarely in the nymphohymeneal groove.

During its crossing through the cervix, just immediately above or at the level of the lateral fornices, the Gartner's canal presents a small dilatation, which is the equivalence of the small dilatation of the deferens canal in its retrovesical portion.

29.2.2 The Lower End or Introitus (Fig. 29.1)

It is at the level of the hymen at the junction of the subperitoneal and the perineal portions.

Below it is the vulvar portion of the vagina.

29.2.3 The Anterior Wall (Fig. 29.2)

The inner surface of the vaginal wall has transverse folds (Fig. 29.3). At the inferior part is the vaginal tubercle.

29.2.3.1 The Subperitoneal Segment

The superior half part is in relation with the vesicovaginal septum. Its length is 3 cm, its thickness 8–10 mm. Laterally, the ureters are outside the vesicovaginal septum and penetrate into the bladder at 2 cm below the anterior fornix.

29.2.3.2 The Inferior Half Part

It is in relation with the urethra. The urethra is 4 cm long and 6 mm in diameter.

It begins at the internal urethral orifice of the bladder, approximately opposite the middle of the symphysis pubis, and runs anteroinferiorly behind the symphysis pubis. In its superior 1/3, it is relatively free related to the vagina by a relatively loose tissue, while in its inferior 2/3, it is embedded in the anterior vaginal wall.

It has two segments: (1) a subperitoneal segment and (2) a perineal segment that crosses the perineal membrane and ends at the external urethral orifice as an anteroposterior slit, situated directly anterior to the opening of the vagina and 2.5 cm behind the glans clitoridis.

29.2.3.3 Anatomy and Histology of the Urethra and of the Urethral Sphincter Mechanism

The wall of the urethra consists of:
1. An inner mucosa composed of:
   - An epithelium with: At the upper 1/3, an urothelium with urethral sphincter mechanism.

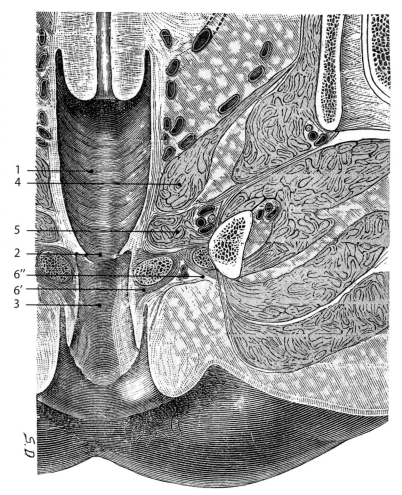

Fig. 29.1 Coronal section through the middle part of the vagina, *1* subperitoneal vagina, *2* vaginal introitus, *3* vestibular vagina, *4* levator ani, *5* deep transverse muscle, *6'* bulbospongiosus muscle, *6"* ischiocavernous muscle

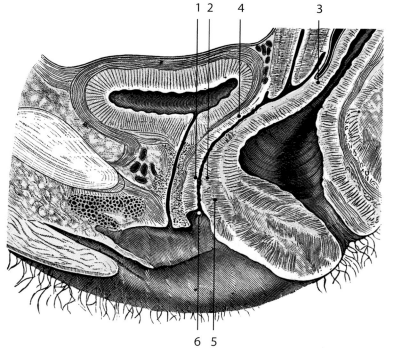

Fig. 29.2 Sagittal section through the vagina. *1* anterior vaginal wall, *2* posterior vaginal wall, *3* bottom of the Douglas, *4* vesicovaginal septum, *5* rectovaginal septum, *6* vaginal introitus

Fig. 29.3 Coronal section with inner view of posterior (a) and anterior (b) wall of the vagina. (**a**) *1* transverse folds, *2* navicular fossa, *3* myrtiform carunculae. (**b**) On this view, the caudal part of the vaginal wall is in continuity with the inferior wall of the bladder and with the urethral orifice and the clitoris which have been drawn backward and downward. *1* transverse folds, *3* carunculae, *4* urethral meat, *5* clitoris, *6* vaginal tubercle

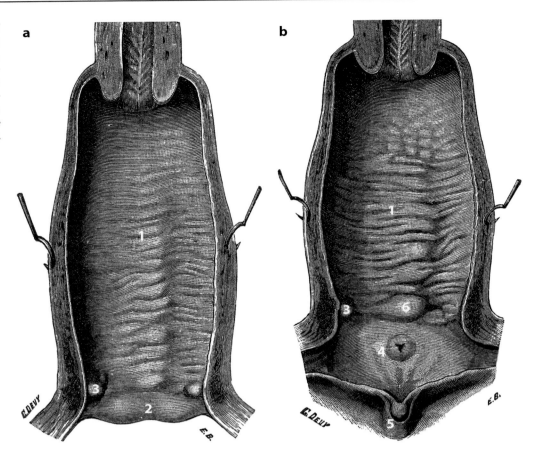

At the lower 2/3, a nonkeratinizing stratified squamous epithelium.

At the urethral meatus, a keratinizing stratified squamous epithelium.

- A lamina propria or loose connective tissue:

    Well vascularized.

    Contains a fine nerve plexus, believed to be derived from sensory branches of the pudendal nerve.

2. An inner coat of smooth muscle fibers that extends throughout the length of the urethra.

3. A sheath of striated muscle: the external urethral sphincter or urethral sphincter mechanism [4]. It forms a sleeve that is thickest anteriorly in the middle 1/3 of the urethra and is relatively deficient posteriorly. It extends in the anterior wall of the upper 1/3 and lower 1/3 but is relatively deficient posteriorly.

It comprises:

- The sphincter urethrae. It consists of intrinsic striated smooth muscle of the urethra and the pubourethralis component of the levator ani that surrounds the urethra. It surrounds the middle and upper thirds of the urethra. It compresses the urethra particularly when the bladder contains fluid. Like the bulbospongiosus, it relaxes during micturition.

- The compressor urethra. It arises from the ischiopubic rami of each side by a small tendon. Fibers pass anteriorly to meet their contralateral counterparts in a flat band that lies anterior to the urethra, below sphincter urethrae.

- The sphincter urethrovaginalis. It arises from the perineal body. Its fibers pass forward on either side of the vagina and urethra to meet their contralateral counterparts in a flat band anterior to the urethra, below compressor urethrae.

- The direction of the fibers of the compressor urethrae and sphincter urethrovaginalis suggests they can produce elongation as well as compression of the membranous urethra and thus aid continence.

29.2.4 The Posterior Wall (Fig. 29.2)

The inner surface of the posterior vaginal wall, as the anterior one, has transverse folds (Fig. 29.3). At the inferior part is the navicular fossa.

29.2.4.1 The Subperitoneal Segment

It is in relation with the Douglas pouch and the rectovaginal septum below.

29.2.4.2 The Perineal Segment

The lower segment of the vagina separates from the rectum forming the rectovaginal triangle. At its top, vagina and rectum are gathered by a rectovaginal muscle, which needs to be cut to separate the vagina from the rectum. The base of the triangle is comprised between the fourchette in front and the anus behind; it measures 25 mm.

It contains the perineal body, a poorly defined aggregation of fibromuscular tissue, located in the midline at the junction of the anal and urogenital triangles.

It is attached to:

Posteriorly with fibers from the middle part of the external anal sphincter and the conjoint longitudinal coat.

Superiorly with the rectovaginal septum.

Anteriorly to the deep transverse perinea, the superficial transverse perinea, and bulbospongiosus.

It is continuous with the perineal membrane and the superficial peritoneal fascia.

It is attached to the posterior commissure of the labia majora and the introitus of the vagina.

29.2.5 Lateral Walls

29.2.5.1 The Subperitoneal Segment

The pelvic upper segment is in relation with the lower part of the mesometrium.

The middle segment is in relation with the levator ani.

29.2.5.2 The Inferior Perineal Segment

It is in relation with the deep transverse perinea, the greater vestibular glands, and the bulbospongiosus muscle.

29.2.5.3 Vascularization

Arteries:

- Superior part: vesicovaginal and cervicovaginal branches of the uterine artery.
- Inferior part: long vaginal artery.

29.3 Histology [5]

The vaginal wall consists of three layers:

29.3.1 Mucosa

It is composed of an epithelium and an underlying layer the lamina propria (Fig. 29.4):

(a) A stratified squamous epithelium nonkeratinizing that is normally glycogenated with:

- A basal/parabasal layer.
- A midzone.
- A superficial layer.

(b) A lamina propria that consists of a loose fibrovascular stroma containing elastic fibers and nerves.

29.3.2 Muscularis

It consists of inner circular and outer longitudinal bundles of smooth muscle.

29.3.3 Adventitia

It contains numerous blood vessels and nerves within adipose tissue.

Anatomy and histology of the urethra are described above.

MR anatomy is displayed in Fig. 29.5.

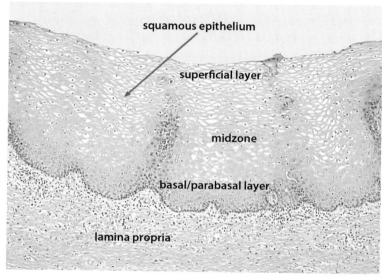

Fig. 29.4 Vaginal mucosa. The figure represents the vaginal mucosa composed of a nonkeratinized squamous epithelium and an underlying lamina propria (see annotations)

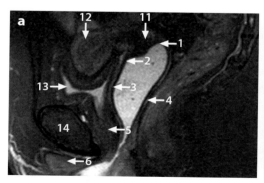 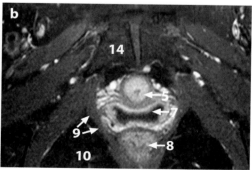

Fig. 29.5 Vaginal anatomy at MRI. (a) Sagittal T2W image of normal vagina distended with ultrasound gel. (**b**) Axial T1W-FS image after gadolinium injection of normal vagina without opacification: Vaginal fornix: posterior (*1*), anterior (*2*), vaginal fibromuscular walls: anterior (*3*), posterior (*4*), urethra (*5*), anterior parts of clitoris and vestibular bulbs (*6*), vaginal inner mucosal layer and mucus secretions (*7*), rectum (*8*), levator ani muscle (*9*), ischiorectal/anal fossa (*10*), uterine cervix (*11*), body of uterus (*12*), urinary bladder (*13*), body of pubis (*14*)

References

1. Moore KL, Persaud TVN, Torchia MG (2008) The developing human. Clinically oriented embryology, 8th edn. Saunders, Philadelphia, pp 243–284
2. Robboy SJ, Bentley RC (2002) Embryology of the female genital tract and disorders of abnormal sexual development. In: Blaustein's pathology of the female genital tract, 5th edn. Springer, New York, pp 3–36
3. Testut L (1931) Appareil urogenital, peritoine. In: Latarget A Traité d'anatomie humaine. 8th edn. revue par. G Doin et Cie Editeurs, Paris, pp 1–595
4. Standring S (ed) (2005) Gray's anatomy. The anatomical basis of clinical practice, 39th edn. Elsevier/Churchill Livingstone, Edinburgh/New York, pp 1331–1338, Chap. 104
5. Zaino RJ, Robboy SJ, Kurman RJ (2002) Diseases of the vagina. In: Kurman RJ (ed) Blaustein's pathology of the female genital tract. Springer, New York, pp 151–206

Diseases of the Vagina

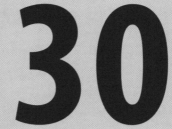

30

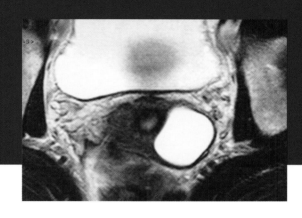

Contents

30.1 Cysts

30.1.1 Clinical Findings

They are often incidental findings on MRI or ultrasound. They are usually asymptomatic but can grow to reach large size, protrude into the vagina, and cause symptoms.

30.1.2 Frequency and Location

Vaginal cysts can be congenital (Müllerian cysts or Gartner's cyst) or acquired (squamous inclusion cysts). The most frequent are Müllerian and squamous inclusion cysts followed by Gartner's cysts [1–3].

Congenital cysts are of paramesonephric origin (Müllerian cysts) or mesonephric origin (Gartner's cyst). Both are located in the anterior-lateral wall of the vagina along the corresponding ducts. When higher situated, they are in the lateral wall of the vagina; at lower level, they are closer to the midline. The same cyst can be seen extending from the anterior midline inferiorly to the lateral wall posteriorly [4]. When large, they can protrude posteriorly in the ischiorectal fossa [5].

Acquired cysts are squamous inclusion cysts (also known as epithelial inclusion cyst, epidermal inclusion cysts). They are secondary to trauma and thus are mostly located at the site of episiotomy posterolaterally.

J.N. Buy, M. Ghossain, *Gynecological Imaging*,
DOI 10.1007/978-3-642-31012-6_30, © Springer-Verlag Berlin Heidelberg 2013

30.1.3 Pathology

30.1.3.1 Müllerian Cysts (Paramesonephric Cysts)

Some may be derived from islands of adenosis. They are usually less than 2 cm. They may be lined by any of the epithelia of the Müllerian duct, including endocervical type (most commonly), endometrial, and ciliated tubal type. Squamous metaplasia may be present.

Their content can be clear mucinous, yellow mucinous, dark brownish mucinous, or hemorrhagic [4–6].

30.1.3.2 Gartner's Duct Cysts (Mesonephric Cysts)
(Figs. 30.1, 30.2, and 30.3)

They are lined by low cuboidal *non-mucin-secreting cells*

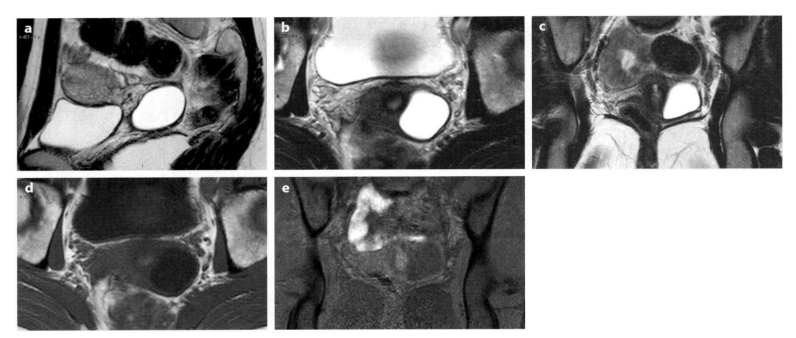

Fig. 30.1 Gartner's cyst. Twenty-three-year-old woman with slight dyspareunia. At speculum examination: swelling on the lateral wall of the vagina. MR sagittal T2 (**a**), coronal T2 (**b**), axial T2 (**c**), axial T1 (**d**), and coronal T1 with fat suppression (**e**). Four centimeter subperitoneal cyst on the left lateral wall of the cervix with a low signal on T1 and T1 with suppression, and a high signal on T2 related to a serous content. Prospective diagnosis based on location: Mullerian or Gartner's cyst. At operation: the cyst is in the wall of the left vaginal cul de sac. At pathology the cyst lies in the stroma. Its lining is a flat or cuboidal non-mucinous epithelium (Gartner's cyst)

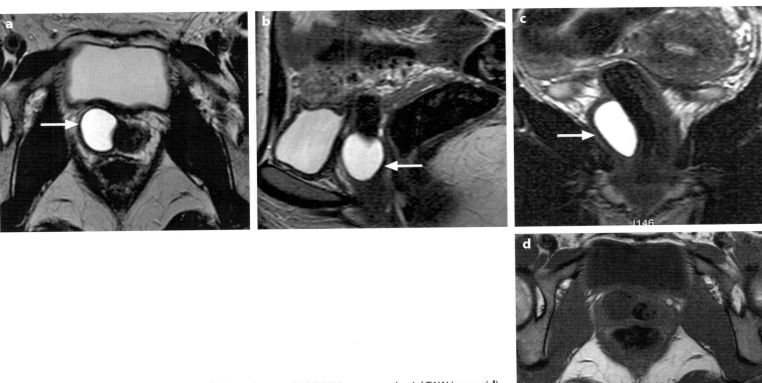

Fig. 30.2 Gartner's cyst. Axial (**a**), sagittal (**b**), and coronal (**c**) T2W images, and axial T1W image (**d**), without vaginal opacification, show a unilocular cyst in the right lateral wall of the midportion of the vagina. Signal intensity is identical to urine on T1 and T2W images (*arrows*)

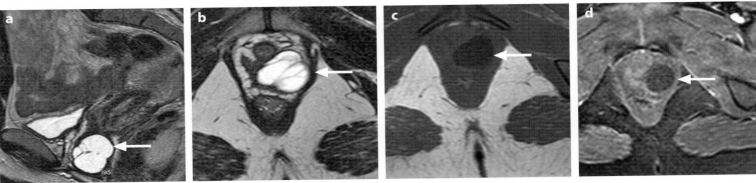

Fig. 30.3 Multilocular Gartner's cyst. (**a**, **b**) Sagittal (**a**) and axial (**b**) T2W images show a hyperintense multilocular cystic mass (*arrows*) with thin regular septa located along the anterolateral wall of the middle third of the vagina. (**c**, **d**) Axial T1W image (**c**) and axial T1W-FS image after gadolinium injection do not show nodular contrast enhancement inside the cyst (*arrows*)

30.1.3.3 Squamous Inclusion Cysts (Also Known as Epithelial Inclusion Cyst, Epidermal Inclusion Cysts)

These cysts arise from entrapment of vaginal mucosa as a result of surgery (episiotomy, obstetrical trauma, or vaginoplasty) or injury.

They are often asymptomatic.

The central content is keratin from desquamated cells. Size ranges from a few millimeters to several centimeters.

30.1.4 Imaging Findings

All these cysts are thin walled with no internal contrast enhancement or internal color Doppler flow. Differentiation between different types could be suggested by their location but not by their internal patterns (see Sect. 30.1.2) (Figs. 30.1, 30.2, and 30.3). As these cysts are usually asymptomatic and not operated, definite histological diagnosis is often missing (Figs. 30.4, 30.5, and 30.6).

On US, they can be anechoic or hypoechoic [4, 6, 7].

Similarly, on MR, they show hyperintense or intermediate signal intensity on T2 [4–6]. On T1, they are most often hypointense but can be of intermediate-to-high signal intensity if proteinaceous or hemorrhagic materials are present [8, 9].

30.2 Benign Neoplasms

Benign solid tumors of vagina arise from vaginal connective tissue such as fibrous muscle, smooth muscle, and skeletal muscle tissues.

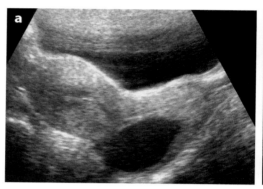
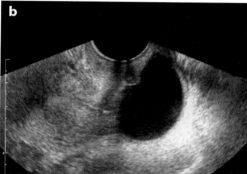

Fig. 30.4 Posterior vaginal cyst in an asymptomatic woman. (**a**, **b**) Transabdominal (**a**) and transvaginal (**b**) ultrasound disclose a posterior vaginal cyst with some internal echos. The cyst was stable on follow-up. As surgery was not performed definite histological diagnosis could not be made but the posterior location of the cyst favors a squamous inclusion cyst

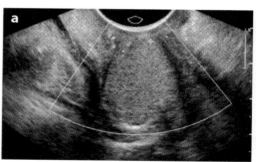
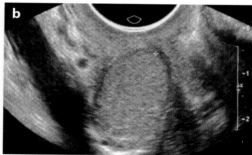

Fig. 30.5 Vaginal cyst. Posterior vaginal mass at clinical examination in an asymptomatic woman. Transvaginal ultrasound (**a**, **b**) discloses a hyperechogenic homogeneous mass of the vagina, avascular on color Doppler study. The mass was stable on follow-up. As surgery was not performed definite histological diagnosis could not be made but the posterior location of the mass and the absence of vascularization on color Doppler favors an inclusion cyst

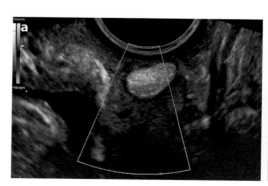
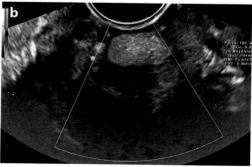

Fig. 30.6 Vaginal cyst. Anterior vaginal cyst in a 42-year-old asymptomatic woman. (**a**, **b**) Transvaginal transverse ultrasound with color Doppler discloses a hyperechogenic homogeneous cystic mass of the anterior wall of the vagina at the junction of the upper third and the middle third of the vagina, measuring 20 mm in diameter. The cyst was stable on follow-up. As surgery was not performed definite histological diagnosis could not be made but the anterior location of the cyst favors a congenital cyst (Mullerian or Gartner's by order of frequency)

30.2.1 Papilloma

Definition: A papillary frond with a central fibrovascular core
Location: Near the hymeneal ring
Aspect: Most commonly clusters
Size: Only a few milliliters

They arise in the wall of the vagina, and the majority occurs early in childhood, before 10 years of age with vaginal bleeding. The clinical findings can mimic those of malignant lesions such as sarcoma botryoides and adenocarcinoma.

30.2.2 Condylomata Acuminata

In order of frequency, they arise in the vulva then the vagina then the cervix, and can be exophytic or less commonly maculopapular almost flat (See Chap. 27, Sect. 27.1.2 and Chap. 35, Sect. 35.2.3).

30.2.3 Fibroepithelial Polyp or Mesodermal Stromal Polyp

Definition: An edematous stroma covered by a stratified squamous epithelium
Mean age: 40 years, 25 % are pregnant at the time of diagnosis
Location: Lateral wall of the lower third of the vagina
Size: 0.5–4 cm
Aspect: A polyp or a cerebriform mass

The most common symptoms are postcoital vaginal spotting or bleeding or a vaginal lump. They most typically present as mobile, rounded submucosal, or polypoid masses.

The distinction from sarcoma is made primarily on the basis of superficial location and small size.

30.2.4 Leiomyoma

The most common mesenchymal neoplasm in the vagina
Location: Anywhere usually submucosal
Size: Most are small

Vaginal leiomyoma usually arises in the midline anterior vaginal wall. But it can be located anywhere within the submucosa of the vaginal wall. Their size ranges from 0.5 to 15 cm. Clinical symptoms include vaginal discomfort, vaginal bleeding, and dyspareunia.

On ultrasound the mass is round or oval, of an echogenicity close to that of myometrium, with characteristic acoustic shadowing (Fig. 30.7).

On MR, they appear as homogeneous low signal intensity on T1 and T2, similar to myometrium. On DMR, on the arterial phase, peripheral arterial vessels are visualized. At the venous phase, there is high and homogeneous contrast uptake identical to myometrium (Fig. 30.7).

While the location to the vagina is clearly established in most cases, in case of low and anterior location, differentiation from urethral leiomyoma may be difficult (Fig. 30.8).

30.2.5 Benign Mixed Tumors

Benign mixed tumors histologically bear some resemblance to salivary gland neoplasm. These tumors occur anywhere in the vagina, but most frequently near the hymenal ring. The mean age at diagnosis is 30 years. They range in size from 1.5 to 5 cm. Microscopically, the neoplasm is characterized by a proliferation of stromal and epithelial cells.

Clinically, they are finger-like protruded polypoid structures, well circumscribed, not encapsulated within the mucosa, and unconnected to the surface of epithelium.

30.3 Malignant Neoplasms

30.3.1 Epidemiology

Primary or secondary malignancies can involve the vaginal walls.
Primary vaginal cancer is relatively rare, accounting for 1–3 % of gynecologic malignant tumors and only approximately 0.1–0.2 % of all cancers [1]. To be considered as primary tumor of the vagina, the neoplasm must be located in the vagina without clinical or histological evidence of involvement of the cervix or vulva.

Bulky tumors located in the upper vagina that have extended on to the portio vaginalis of the cervix are considered as primary cervical carcinoma.

It is predominantly a tumor of elderly women (60–65 years).
Secondary vaginal cancer may represent an extension from a cervical cancer or metastatic disease from a uterine, ovarian, vulvar, bladder, or colon primary tumor.

Squamous cell carcinoma occurring in the vagina within 5 years of therapy for cervical carcinoma is considered to be recurrent cervical carcinoma rather than a new primary carcinoma of the vagina (Fig. 30.9).

30.3.2 The Risk Factors

- HPV infections (human papillomavirus)
- Exposure to diethylstilbestrol (DES) as a fetus (involve young women)
- History of cervical cancer
- History of cervical precancerous conditions
- Vaginal irritation, vaginal adenosis
- Uterine prolapse
- Smoking

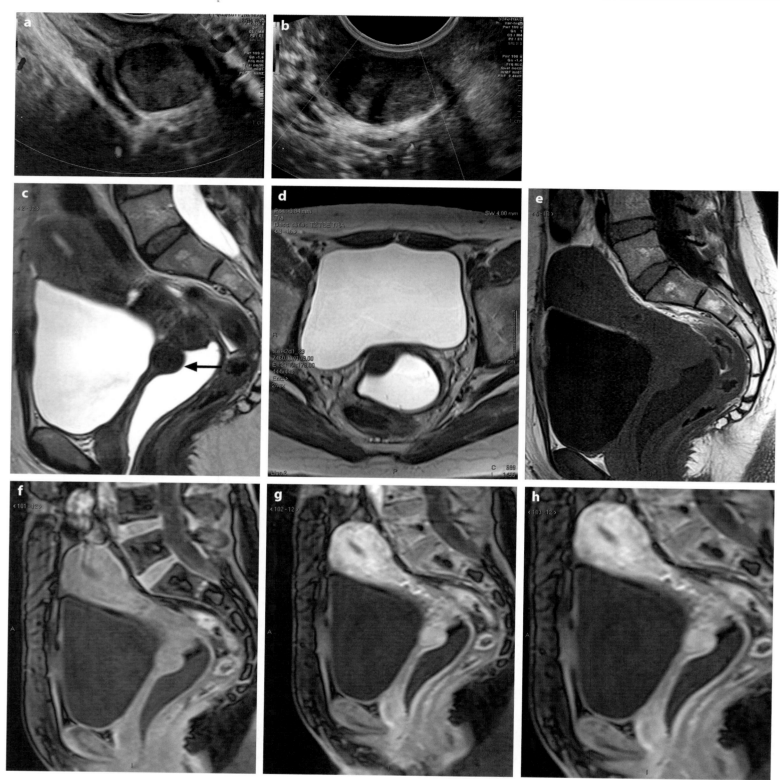

Fig. 30.7 Leiomyoma of the vagina. US Sagittal (**a**) and axial (**b**) view display in the anterior and right upper third of the wall of the vagina a round echogenic mass with foci of ultrasound attenuation very suggestive of a leiomyoma. A hypoechoic rim surrounds the mass. Color Doppler does not display any vessel in the mass. MR sagittal T2 (**c**), axial T2 (**d**), and sagittal T1 (**e**) after vaginal opacification depict that the mass (*arrow* in **c**) arises in the muscular layer of the wall. Signal of the mass is identical to pelvic muscles on T1 and T2. These two findings are very suggestive of a leiomyoma. Sagittal DMR without injection (**f**), at the arterial phase (**g**) and at the venous phase (**h**) demonstrates regular arterial vessels at the periphery of the mass

Fig. 30.7 (*continued*) On the delayed phase (**i**), the contrast uptake is identical to myometrium. These features reinforce the diagnosis of leiomyoma that was confirmed at pathology

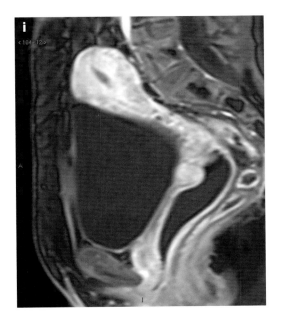

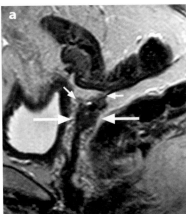
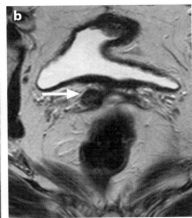
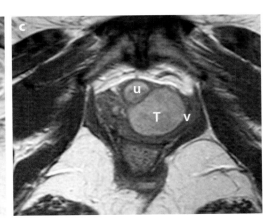

Fig. 30.8 Urethral leiomyoma. Dysuria, dyspareunia, and anterior vaginal wall mass at clinical examination. Axial (**a**) and sagittal (**b**) T2W images display a well-defined mass (letter *T*) of intermediate signal, lying between the urethra and the anterior vaginal wall. The urethral or vaginal origin is impossible to define. On axial T1W image after gadolinium injection (**c**) the mass enhances homogeneously. Urethra *u*, Vagina *v*. The diagnosis of leiomyoma is suggested. Surgery: Leiomyoma of the urethra

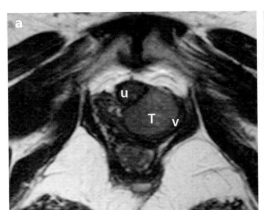
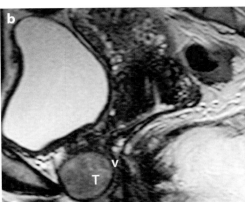
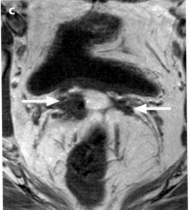
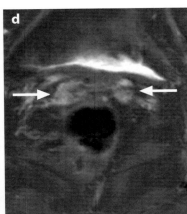

Fig. 30.9 Vaginal squamous cell carcinoma (stage II) after hysterectomy for cervical cancer. A 51-year-old woman with previous hysterectomy for cervical cancer 4 years ago. (**a–d**) Sagittal (**a**) and axial (**b**) T2W images, axial T1W image (**c**), and axial T1W-FS image after gadolinium injection (**d**) show a tumor of the upper vagina and vaginal vault (*arrows*) with subperitoneal nodules (*small arrows* in **a**).

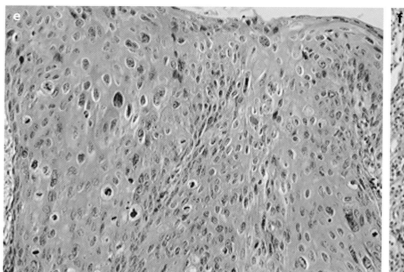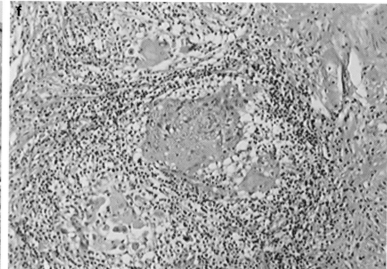

Fig. 30.9 (*continued*) (**e, f**) Microscopic view of the surgical specimen

30.3.3 Histopathology

30.3.3.1 Vaginal Intraepithelial Neoplasia (VAIN)

In contrast to the high prevalence of intraepithelial lesions of the cervix and the vulva, intraepithelial lesions of the vagina are relatively rare.

Gross findings: Most commonly, there is no grossly identifiable lesion. Occasionally, the epithelium appears raised, roughened. More often, the diagnosis is made by a colposcopically directed biopsy.

Microscopic findings are similar to those of the cervix.

MR findings in a case of VAIN 3 are reported (Fig. 30.10).

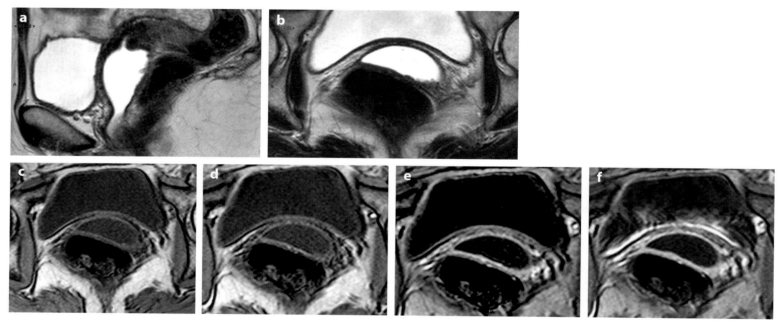

Fig. 30.10 Vaginal intraepithelial neoplasia (VAIN). Sixty-one-year-old woman with dyspareunia and metrorragias following intercourse. Colposcopy: Polypoid fungating hypervascularized lesion extending from the posterior fornix to the upper third of the vagina. Zone of junction of the cervix not visualized, atypical zone of transformation of grade 1. Biopsy: VAIN 3, absence of invasion. MR sagittal (**a**) and axial (**b**) T2W images after vaginal opacification display small polypoid lesions of intermediate signal on the left part of the posterior wall. DMR without injection (**c**) and at the arterial phase (**d**) depicts tiny vessels at the arterial phase in the left portion of the posterior wall with a contrast uptake at the venous phase (**e**) and on the delayed phase (**f**) limited to the wall without extension in the perivaginal tissue

30.3.3.2 Vaginal Squamous Cell Carcinoma

It accounts for 80 % of primary malignant neoplasms [10, 11].

Clinical Findings

The mean age at diagnosis is 64 years.

Painless vaginal bleeding, discharge, dysuria, or frequency.

Up to 10 % of patients have a history of vaginal radiation therapy for cervical carcinoma.

Pathology

Macroscopy

Site: Most arise in the upper third

Fifty-seven percent in the posterior wall

Twenty-seven percent in the anterior wall

Aspect: Variable polypoid, indurated and ulcerated

Microscopy

They resemble those arising in the cervix

30.3.3.3 Clear Cell Adenocarcinoma (9 % of Primary Vaginal Carcinoma)

Clinical Findings

Most cases occur in young women with a past history of DES exposure in utero [12]

• Vaginal bleeding, discharge

Pathology

Macroscopy

• Location: 60 %, vagina.
• The remainder: Cervix or cervix and vagina.

Vaginal tumors are mostly situated in the anterior upper third wall, corresponding to the most frequent site of adenosis.

Tumors are also present on the wall opposite the main tumor, presumably as a result of implantation (kissing lesions).

Aspect: Most are polypoid and nodular.

Some are flat or ulcerated with an indurate surface.

30.3.3.4 Embryonal Rhadomyosarcoma (Rhado-Striated) or Sarcoma Botryoid (Botryo-Brunch of Grapes) [1]

Embryonal rhabdomyosarcoma is the most common malignant neoplasm of the vagina in infants and children, most of which are of the subtype designated sarcoma botryoides.

Ninety percent are diagnosed before 5 years old. The mean age at diagnosis is 2 years, with a range extending from birth to 41 years.

Most children present with a mass or vaginal bleeding.

Location: Anterior wall.

Aspect: Polypoid mass looking like a brunch of grapes, with an intact overlying mucosa.

Microscopy: The distinctions of sarcoma botryoid from the spindle or other variants of embryonal rhabdomyosarcoma are:

• Cambium tumor cell layer (latin cambiare – to change peripheral activity growing layer in tree trunks and branches): A condensed subepithelial layer of rhabdomyoblasts (polyhedral cells with little discernible cytoplasm) in a loose or condensed collagenous stroma
• Focal evidence of rhabdomyogenesis: Eosinophilic cytoplasm containing fibers in which cross striations are seen

Ultrastructural examination can identify both thick and thin fibrils.

Immunohistochemical staining with antibodies directed against actin desmin can be helpful.

30.3.3.5 Leiomyosarcoma

Leiomyosarcoma of the vagina is an uncommon tumor that accounts for less than 3 % of primary vaginal malignancies. It may occur after radiation therapy to the genital tract. Clinically, it originates from the rectovaginal septum, involving vagina, appearing as a bulky submucosal lesion. It may manifest with odorous vaginal discharge, vaginal bleeding, and dyspareunia.

30.3.3.6 Malignant Vaginal Melanoma

Vaginal melanomas arise from vaginal melanophore cells. It is a very rare malignancy that accounts for less than 3 % of all vaginal malignancies. It is a disease of postmenopausal women, with 75 % of women being over 50 years of age. Primary vaginal melanoma may arise anywhere in the vagina, with a predilection for the lower third and for the anterior and lateral walls.

The biological aggressiveness of this tumor results in an extremely poor prognosis, with a 5-year survival rate of 14 %.

Clinically, vaginal melanoma appears as a brownish to black soft mucosal or submucosal nodular lesion; it can also appear as a pedunculated papillary or lobulated mass.

30.3.3.7 Other Sarcomas and Mixed Malignant Tumor

Rhabdomyosarcoma is exceedingly rare, and usually diagnosed in postmenopausal period.

Other forms of vaginal sarcoma are mixed mesodermal tumors, stromal sarcoma, neurofibrosarcoma, and adenosarcoma arising from endometriosis.

30.3.3.8 Secondary Neoplasms

Secondary spread of malignant neoplasms to the vagina by direct extension or lymphatic or hematogenous metastasis is quite common.

Fu et al. [13] found in a series of invasive carcinomas only 16 % of primary tumors.

Among the secondary, the primary sites were:
• Cervix: 32 %
• Endometrium: 28 %
• Colon and rectum: 9 %
• Ovary: 6 %
• Vulva: 6 %
• Urinary tract: 4 %

30.3.4 Symptoms of Vaginal Cancer

Medical history of vaginal cancer can range from the asymptomatic (20 %) to the symptomatic, including:
- Bloodstained vaginal discharge, postcoital vaginal bleeding, postmenopausal (painless) vaginal bleeding, postdouching vaginal bleeding, vaginal hydrorrhea
- Dyspareunia
- Difficult or painful micturition
- Tenesmus or dyschezia or mass

30.3.5 Classical Examination

- Clinical examination
- Colposcopy
- Biopsy

30.3.6 Site and Staging

30.3.6.1 Site of the Tumor

- 53 % in upper vagina
- 22 % in the middle vagina
- 5 % in the lower third
- 20 % all the vagina

30.3.6.2 Staging

Extension of the tumor is established according to the FIGO classification [1].

FIGO staging	
0	Intraepithelial
I	Limited to vaginal wall
II	Extends to subvaginal tissue but not to pelvic side wall
III	Extends to pelvic sidewall
IV	Extends beyond the true pelvis or involves mucosa of the bladder or rectum (bullous edema does not consign the patient to stage IV)
IVA	Tumors invade bladder and/or rectal mucosa and/or direct extension beyond the true pelvis
IVB	Spread to distant organs

Most common distant organs involved are the lung and the liver.

This classification does not take into account lymph node extension. The carcinomas arising in the upper vagina can spread to the pelvic and aortic lymph nodes. Those in the middle vagina spread to the external iliac and hypogastric lymph nodes. Tumors in lower vagina metastasize mainly to inguinal nodes.

30.3.7 MR Imaging of Vaginal Carcinoma

Sagittal T2-weighted allows assessment of vagina tumor extension to the uterus, bladder, urethra, and rectum.

The supplemented oblique axial T2-weighted images allow detailed assessment of the vaginal tumor and their relation to the paravaginal tissues.

Coronal T2-weighted images allow evaluation of the pelvic sidewall in larger tumor.

Dynamic T1-weighted with intravenous contrast agent and fat-saturated sequences may be of value in delineating tumor extent, and can demonstrate small fistulae from the bladder or the rectum.

30.3.7.1 MR Imaging Features

Vaginal Squamous Cell Carcinoma

At T2-weighted imaging: Squamous cell carcinomas appear as a mass of homogeneous intermediate signal intensity different from the low signal intensity of the vaginal wall (Fig. 30.11). At T1-weighted imaging, squamous cell carcinoma appears as isointense to muscle lesion [14, 15]. Stage I tumor: Limited to the vaginal mucosa, as a mass or plaque of tissue of intermediate signal intensity on T2-weighted image, expanding and filling the vagina with preservation of the low signal intensity of the vaginal outer muscularis layer.

Stage II tumor: Extends into the paravaginal tissue and appears on MR as a mass with disappearance of the low signal intensity of the vaginal muscularis layer (Figs. 30.12, 30.13, and 30.14).

Stage III tumor: Extends to the pelvic sidewall laterally, and is well defined on the axial and coronal T2-weighted images (Fig. 30.15).

Stage IVA: The invasion appears as an intermediate signal through the low signal intensity of the bladder or the rectum wall on the T2-weighted images. Bladder or rectal fistulas are also well delineated on the dynamic sagittal T1-weighted, contrast-enhanced fat-saturated sequence. Extension beyond the true pelvis to the perineum can also be well assessed (Fig. 30.16).

Stage IVB: The peritoneal, the small or large bowel involvement are well analyzed by diffusion MR imaging. The most common sites of distant metastasis are the lung, liver, and bone, also well defined on DW MR imaging.

Vaginal Adenocarcinoma

Primary vaginal adenocarcinoma at MR has been described as a mass with homogeneous intermediate signal intensity on T2-weighted sequence and isointense signal to muscle on T1-weighted sequence. Most of these neoplasms are clear cell adenocarcinomas that develop in 1–2 % of women who were exposed in utero to diethylstilbestrol (DES). The uterine abnormalities associated with both DES exposure (hypoplastic, T-shaped uterus) and clear cell adenocarcinoma of the vagina have been depicted with MR imaging.

Vaginal adenocarcinoma secondary to adenocarcinomas of the endometrium (Fig. 30.17), to adenocarcinoma of the rectum (Fig. 30.18) or other organs can be displayed.

Vaginal Malignant Melanoma [15–18]

Typically, they appear hyperintense on T1 and hypointense on T2 because of the paramagnetic effect of melanin and methemoglobin from intratumoral necrosis or hemorrhage.

However, primary vaginal melanoma can also appear as intermediate-to-high signal intensity on T1 and intermediate on T2 (Fig. 30.19). Therefore, the absence of high signal intensity on T1 should not preclude the diagnosis of malignant melanoma.

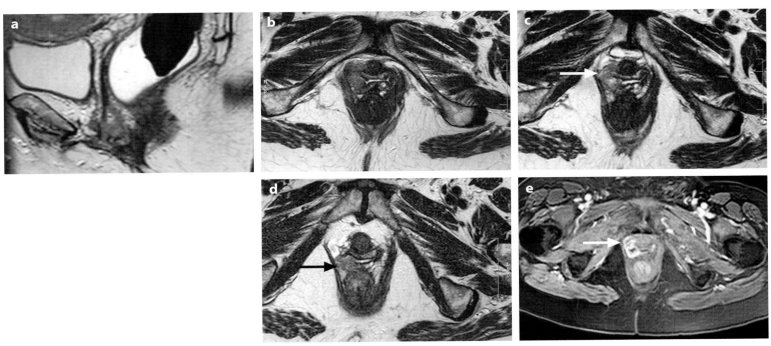

Fig. 30.11 Squamous cell carcinoma (stage II) of lower and mid-vagina. A 69-year-old woman with history of vaginal bleeding. Sagittal (**a**) and axial (**b–d**) T2W images with axial T1W-FS image after gadolinium injection (**e**) show a mass of the lower and mid-vagina arising from the right lateral wall of the vagina and infiltrating the paravaginal tissue (*arrows*). The mass has intermediate signal intensity on T2W images where the vaginal wall appears disrupted. The mass enhances after gadolinium injection

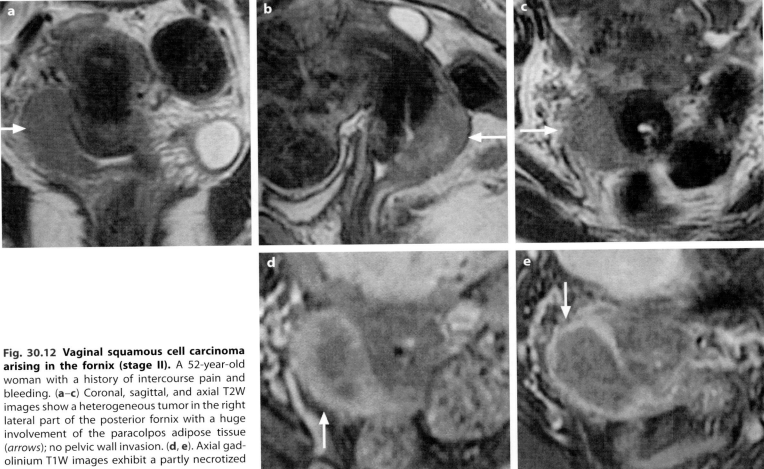

Fig. 30.12 Vaginal squamous cell carcinoma arising in the fornix (stage II). A 52-year-old woman with a history of intercourse pain and bleeding. (**a–c**) Coronal, sagittal, and axial T2W images show a heterogeneous tumor in the right lateral part of the posterior fornix with a huge involvement of the paracolpos adipose tissue (*arrows*); no pelvic wall invasion. (**d, e**). Axial gadolinium T1W images exhibit a partly necrotized mass (*arrows*)

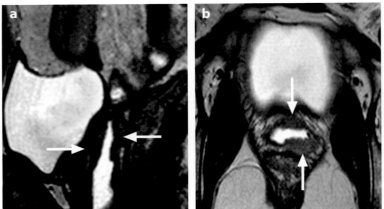

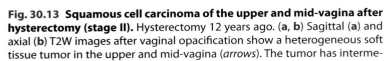

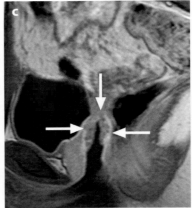

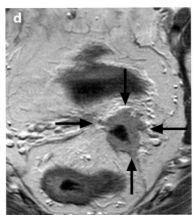

Fig. 30.13 Squamous cell carcinoma of the upper and mid-vagina after hysterectomy (stage II). Hysterectomy 12 years ago. (**a**, **b**) Sagittal (**a**) and axial (**b**) T2W images after vaginal opacification show a heterogeneous soft tissue tumor in the upper and mid-vagina (*arrows*). The tumor has interme- diate signal intensity and reduces the vaginal lumen. (**c**, **d**) Sagittal (**c**) and axial gadolinium T1W images exhibit enhancement of the tumor (*arrows* in **c**) and paracolpos adipose tissue involvement (*arrows* in **d**)

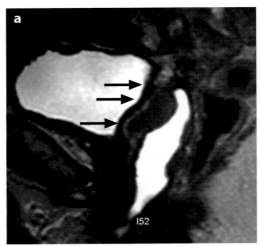

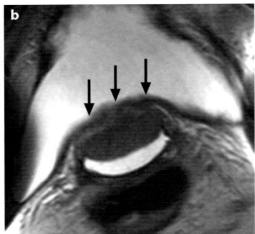

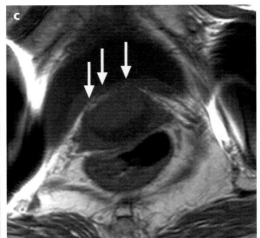

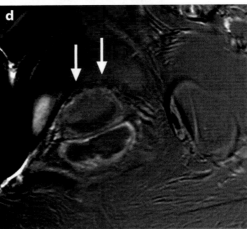

Fig. 30.14 Vaginal squamous cell carcinoma after hysterectomy (stage II). A 79-year-old woman with 40 years previous hysterectomy for leiomyoma. Sagittal (**a**) and axial (**b**) T2W images with vaginal opacification, axial T1W image (**c**), and axial gadolinium T1W-FS image (**d**) show a tumor expanding into the upper anterior vaginal wall and lumen. It involves the paracolpos adipose tissue without bladder involvement (*arrows*). The vaginal wall is clearly disrupted on T2W images. There is also another posterior vaginal wall involvement. Pathology after biopsy: primary vaginal squamous cell carcinoma. Treatment: radiation therapy and brachytherapy

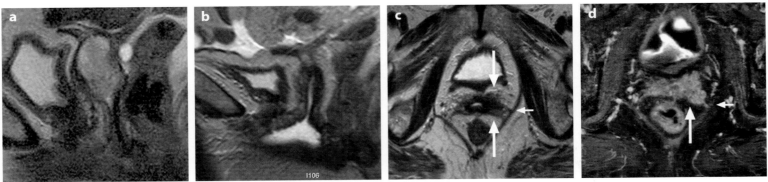

Fig. 30.15 Squamous cell vaginal carcinoma (stage III). (**a**, **b**) Sagittal T2W images show hematocolpos above a narrow vagina. (**c**, **d**) After hematocolpos discharge, axial T2W image, and axial T1W-FS image with gadolinium injections show a vaginal squamous cell carcinoma (*large arrows*) extending through the left lateral vaginal wall to involve the levator ani muscle (*small arrows*)

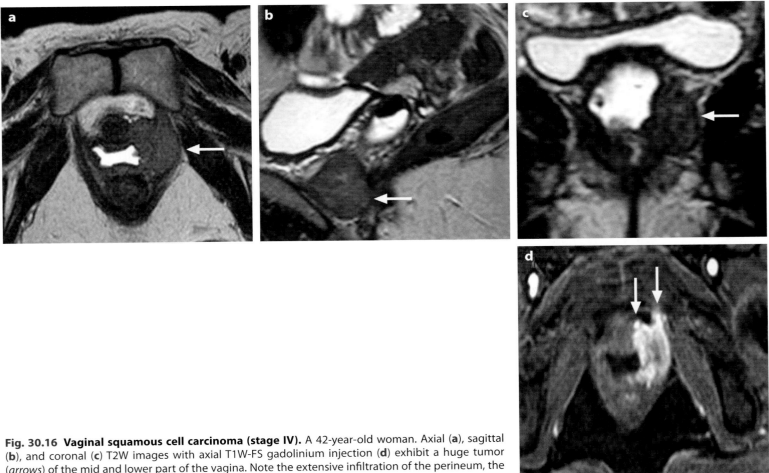

Fig. 30.16 Vaginal squamous cell carcinoma (stage IV). A 42-year-old woman. Axial (**a**), sagittal (**b**), and coronal (**c**) T2W images with axial T1W-FS gadolinium injection (**d**) exhibit a huge tumor (*arrows*) of the mid and lower part of the vagina. Note the extensive infiltration of the perineum, the left puborectalis muscle and the left urethral wall (*arrows* in **d**)

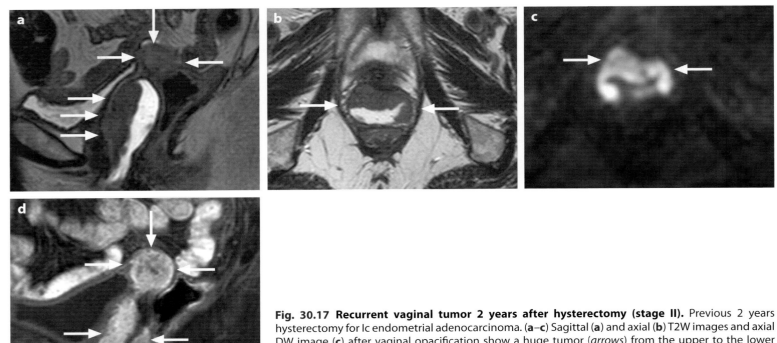

Fig. 30.17 Recurrent vaginal tumor 2 years after hysterectomy (stage II). Previous 2 years hysterectomy for Ic endometrial adenocarcinoma. (**a–c**) Sagittal (**a**) and axial (**b**) T2W images and axial DW image (**c**) after vaginal opacification show a huge tumor (*arrows*) from the upper to the lower vagina, extending through vaginal cuff and vaginal lateral wall without levator ani muscle involvement. (**d**) Sagittal gadolinium T1W-FS image better displays the tumor (*arrows*) extending through vaginal cuff and the subperitoneal space

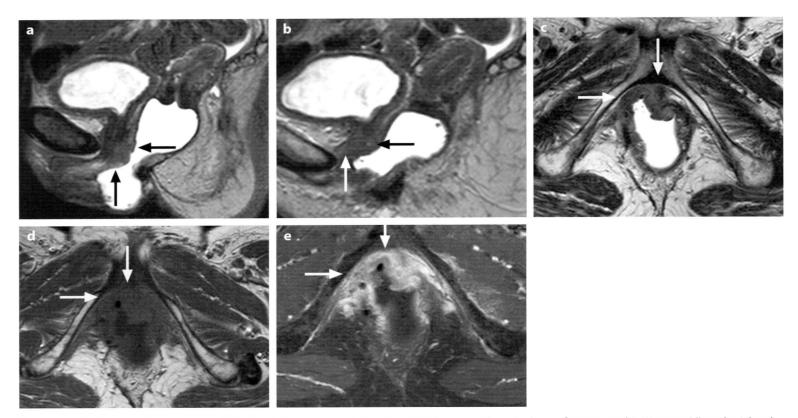

Fig. 30.18 Vaginal carcinoma (stage IV) after total meso-rectal excision. Five years previous abdomino-perineal total meso-rectal excision for a pT3N2M0 rectal cancer in a 43-year-old woman. Sagittal (**a**, **b**) and axial (**c**) T2W images with vaginal opacification, axial T1W image (**d**), and axial gadolinium T1W-FS image (**e**) shows a lower vaginal recurrence (*arrows*) with urethral and right ischiocavernous muscle involvement

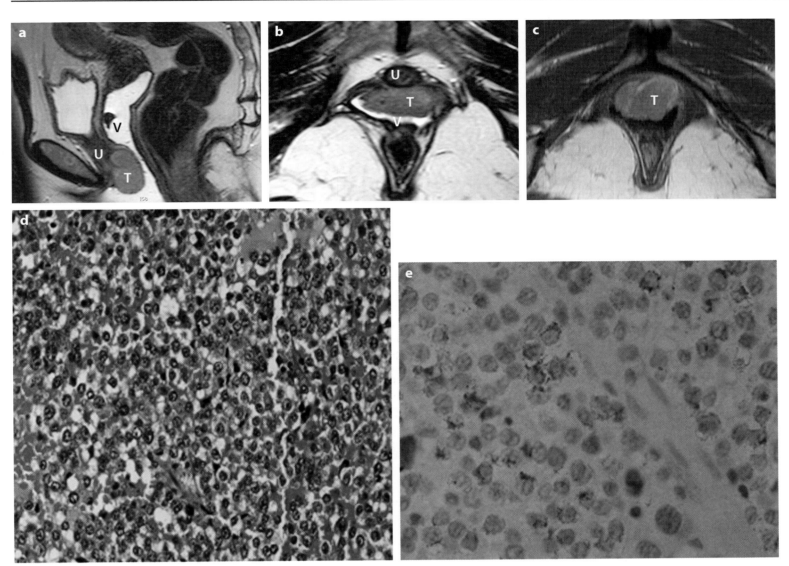

Fig. 30.19 Suburethral melanoma. Sagittal (**a**) and axial (**b**) T2WI with vaginal opacification, and axial T1W image after gadolinium injection (**c**) show a prominent suburethral solid mass (letter *T*) with involvement of the vaginal anterior wall, without invasion of the urethral posterior wall. The mass has intermediate signal intensity on T2W images and protrudes into the anterior vagina. After gadolinium injection, the mass has an intermediate signal with a peripheral more enhancing rim. *U* Urethra, *V* Vagina. (**d**, **e**) At pathology, malignant melanoma with immunohistochemistry positive for HMB 45

Vaginal Sarcomas

- Vaginal rhabdomyosarcoma: The botryoid subtype appears as an intraluminal grape-like mass with a size greater than 5 cm. On MR imaging, the tumor signal intensity is nonspecific: Low signal intensity on T1-weighted imaging and high signal intensity on T2-weighted imaging, with heterogeneity due to hemorrhage and necrosis. There is a pseudocapsule with low signal intensity in both sequences. MR imaging has been recommended as an optimal imaging modality both for initial detection and for post treatment follow-up of these aggressive neoplasm. Signs of poor prognosis that can be ascertained with imaging studies include large size (>5 cm), regional lymphadenopathy, and local organ invasion.
- Vaginal leiomyosarcoma: It appears as a bulky submucosal lesion, involving mainly the upper vagina. MRI shows a bulky mixed cystic solid mass arising from the vagina, of intermediate signal intensity on T1-weighted imaging, and intermediate-to-high signal intensity on T2-weighted imaging. The tumor may be irregular, locally infiltrative mass with high signal intensity on T2-weighted images with areas of necrosis and hemorrhage.
- Vaginal malignant mixed tumor: They include vaginal synovial sarcoma or malignant tumor arising from mesonephric rest.

Vaginal Secondary Neoplasms

- They account for more than 80 % of all vaginal tumor. They arise from direct extension, lymphatic, or hematogenous metastasis. Spread from primary carcinoma of the cervix, the endometrium, colon and rectum, ovaries, vulva, and urinary tract. Eighty percent of vaginal metastasis occurs within the first 3 years after the primary tumor, and 67 % occurs after surgical removal of the primary lesion.
- The most common malignancies to metastasize to the vagina are ovarian, cervical, endometrial, and rectal cancer.
- Seventy-five percent of squamous vaginal metastases arise from the cervix and 14 % from the vulva.

- Cervical advanced cancer involves the vagina. The patterns of involvement of the vagina follow the growth pattern of the primary cervical cancer. The MR imaging features of metastases to the vagina mimic the MR imaging features of the primary tumor: Intermediate-to-high signal intensity on T2-weighted images and low signal intensity on T1-weighted MR images.

Vaginal Lymphoma

- Vaginal secondary lymphoma is more common than the primary vaginal lymphoma. Both of these lymphomas are usually B-cell non-Hodgkin lymphoma. On MR imaging, the mass is infiltrative or lobular with homogeneous low signal intensity on T1-weighted imaging and intermediate-to-high signal intensity on T2-weighted imaging. After contrast injection, the mass demonstrates homogeneous contrast enhancement.

30.4 Other Pathologies

30.4.1 Vaginal Endometriosis

It is not uncommon. Endometriosis may involve the vagina, either superficially, implanted in the squamous mucosa or involving the deep stroma of the rectovaginal septum. Superficial vaginal endometriosis typically involves the vault; but deep vaginal endometriosis is more common, typically associated with pelvic endometriosis and appears as nodular or polypoid masses involving the posterior vaginal fornix.

Endometriotic foci appear as high-intensity lesion on T1-weighted imaging, which are made more conspicuous following fat suppression. They demonstrate intermediate-to-high signal intensity on T2-weighted imaging.

30.4.2 Vaginal Fistulas

The two most common vaginal fistulas are vesicovaginal and rectovaginal.

They are due to complications related to abdominal or vaginal hysterectomy, congenital anomalies, birth trauma, malignancies, inflammatory bowel disease, diverticular disease, and pelvic irradiation.

The majority of *rectovaginal fistulas* [14] occur in the lower third of the vagina (Fig. 30.20) and are the result of incomplete healing of a perineal laceration from obstetric trauma; the other major cause of rectovaginal fistula is radiation therapy for cervical and endometrial carcinoma. The most common cause of *anovaginal fistulas* is inflammatory bowel disease, and most *colovaginal fistulas* are from diverticulitis in elderly women who have undergone a prior hysterectomy. Most *vesicovaginal* fistulas result from hysterectomy and radiation therapy for cervical carcinoma.

Fistulous tracts may be visualized on MRI using T2-weighted imaging or delayed contrast-enhanced T1-weighted sequences with fat suppression.

They can be depicted at best on CT after contrast opacification of one of the cavities (Fig. 30.20).

30.4.3 Hematocolpos

It is usually secondary to imperforated hymen (see Chap. 19).

In menopausal women, it can be secondary to vaginal atresia (Fig. 30.21).

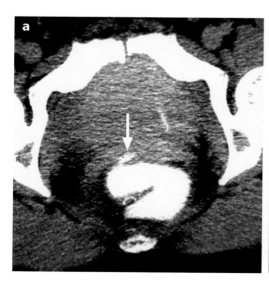 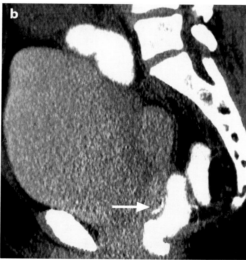

Fig. 30.20 Rectovaginal fistula. Axial CT (**a**) with sagittal 2D reformation (**b**) after rectal opacification discloses the fistula tract (*arrows*)

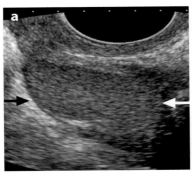
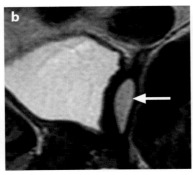
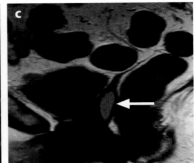
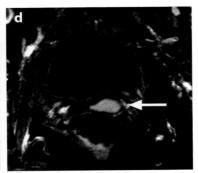

Fig. 30.21 Encysted hematocolpos with vaginal atresia. Vaginal bleeding in a 79-year-old woman previously treated for uterine leiomyoma (total hysterectomy). (**a**) US imaging exhibits a hyperechoic intravaginal mass (*arrows*), homogeneous with no internal Doppler flow. (**b–d**) Sagittal T2 (**b**) shows a homogeneous hyperintense intravaginal collection (*arrow*) with a narrowing of the lumen in the lower part of the vagina. On sagittal T1W (**c**) and on T1W-FS after gadolinium injection (**d**), the collection looks hyperintense related to an hematocolpos (*arrows*). No internal nodule and no mass of the vaginal cuff are seen. On (**d**) the vaginal wall is regular containing normal vessels

30.4.4 Urethral Diverticula

The majority is located in the middle third of the urethra and involves the posterolateral wall. Approximately 1/3 of patients with urethral diverticulum have multiple or compound diverticula. They can be perineal or subperitoneal (Fig. 30.22). See also Chap. 35.

30.5 Recurrence and Follow-Up

After radiotherapy, evaluation of the tumor can be assessed by MRI (Fig. 30.23).

After complete vaginectomy, a neovagina can be performed using bowel (Fig. 30.24) or the surgical cavity left collapsed. In this last case, granulation tissues may be present that must not be confused with recurrence (Fig. 30.25).

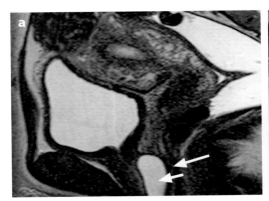
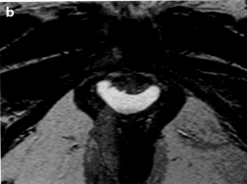
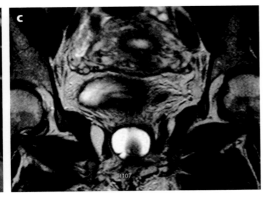

Fig. 30.22 Urethral diverticula. Sagittal (**a**), axial (**b**), and coronal (**c**) T2W images (without vaginal opacification) shows a circumferential urethral diverticulum (*short arrow*), with fluid signal intensity, around the lateral and posterior aspect of the urethra (vaginal wall = *long arrow*)

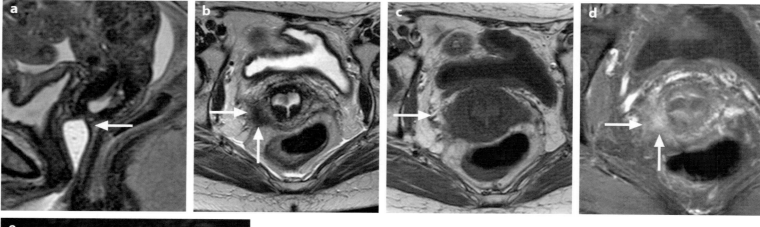

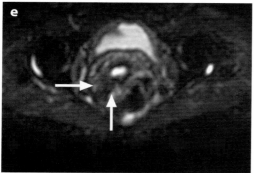

Fig. 30.23 T2 vaginal carcinoma after treatment. Same patient as (Fig. 30.12) following chemora-diation therapy and brachytherapy. Sagittal (**a**) and axial (**b**) T2W images, axial T1W image (**c**) and axial gadolinium T1W-FS image (**d**) shows that the tumor has entirely shrunk (*arrows*). (**e**) No high signal intensity is seen on DWIBS in the previous site of the tumor (*arrows*)

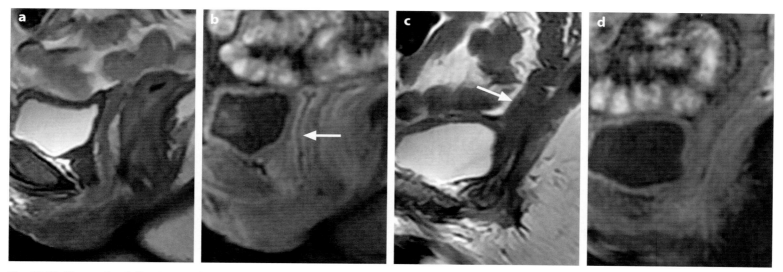

Fig. 30.24 Neovagina following total vaginectomy. A 44 year-old woman with vaginal dysplasia (previous hysterectomy). (**a**, **b**) Sagittal T2W (**a**) and T1W-FS after gadolinium injection (**b**) show no radiographic abnormality of the vagina. The vaginal lumen is well displayed in (**b**) lined by non-enhanc-ing secretions (*arrow*). (**c**, **d**) Sagittal T2W (**c**) and T1W-FS after gadolinium injection (**d**), following total vaginectomy. A neovagina constituted by a sig-moid loop (*arrow* in **c**) is seen in place of the vagina

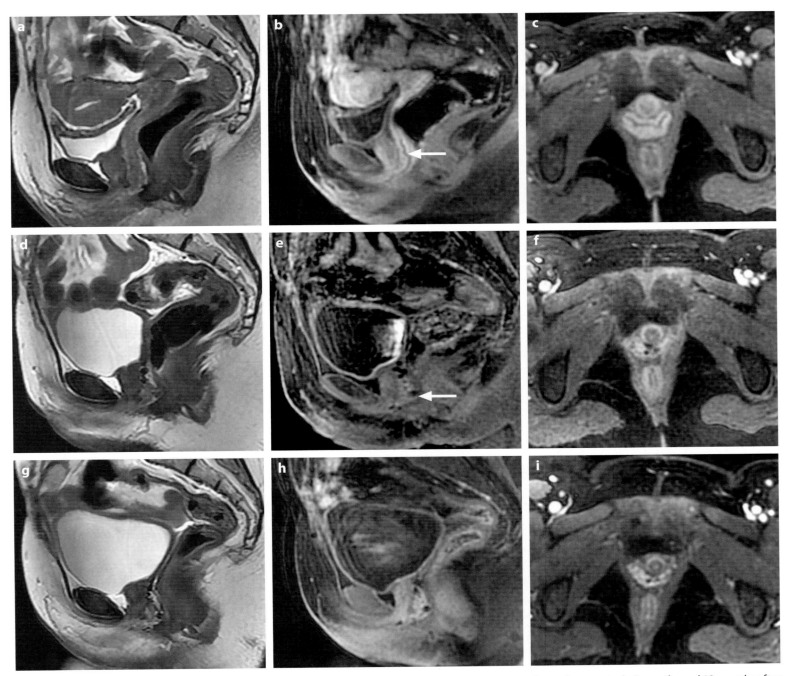

Fig. 30.25 Granulation tissue after total vaginectomy. (a–c) Sagittal T2W image followed by sagittal and axial dynamic MRI images for preoperative evaluation of a patient with vaginal cancer in situ, show no radiological abnormality. The vagina (*arrow*) is well delineated especially after injection where it shows a well-enhanced wall with a hypointense lumen. (d–f) and (g–i) Same sequences performed respectively 6 months and 12 months after surgery show stable granulation tissue (*arrow* in **e**) in the place of the vagina. The granulation tissue appears gray on T2W, enhances after injection, and contains small round, sometimes confluent or serpiginous structures, hypointense on all sequences, corresponding probably to fibrotic tissue

References

1. Zaino RJ, Robboy SJ, Kurman RJ (2002) Diseases of the vagina. In: Kurman RJ (ed) Blaustein's pathology of the female genital tract. Springer, New York, pp 151–206

2. Kondi-Pafiti A et al (2008) Vaginal cysts: a common pathologic entity revisited. Clin Exp Obstet Gynecol 35(1):41–44

3. Pradhan S, Tobon H (1986) Vaginal cysts: a clinicopathological study of 41 cases. Int J Gynecol Pathol 5(1):35–46

4. Cil AP et al (2008) Diagnosis and management of vaginal mullerian cyst in a virgin patient. Int Urogynecol J Pelvic Floor Dysfunct 19(5): 735–737

5. Wai CY et al (2004) Multiple vaginal wall cysts: diagnosis and surgical management. Obstet Gynecol 103(5 Pt 2):1099–1102

6. Hwang JH et al (2009) Multiple vaginal mullerian cysts: a case report and review of literature. Arch Gynecol Obstet 280(1):137–139

7. Lopez-Rasines G et al (1998) Transrectal sonography in the assessment of vaginal pathology: a preliminary study. J Clin Ultrasound 26(7):353–356

8. Grant LA, Sala E, Griffin N (2010) Congenital and acquired conditions of the vulva and vagina on magnetic resonance imaging: a pictorial review. Semin Ultrasound CT MR 31(5):347–362

9. Griffin N, Grant LA, Sala E (2008) Magnetic resonance imaging of vaginal and vulval pathology. Eur Radiol 18(6):1269–1280

10. Creasman WT, Phillips JL, Menck HR (1998) The National Cancer Data Base report on cancer of the vagina. Cancer 83(5):1033–1040

11. Platz CE, Benda JA (1995) Female genital tract cancer. Cancer 75 (1 Suppl):270–294

12. Horwitz RI et al (1988) Clear cell adenocarcinoma of the vagina and cervix: incidence, undetected disease, and diethylstilbestrol. J Clin Epidemiol 41(6):593–597

13. Fu YS, Reagan JW (1989) Pathology of the cervix, vagina, and vulva. Saunders, Philadelphia, pp 336–379

14. Siegelman ES et al (1997) High-resolution MR imaging of the vagina. Radiographics 17(5):1183–1203

15. Parikh JH, Barton DP, Ind TE, Sohaib SA (2008) MRI features of vagina malignancies. Radiographics 28:49–63

16. Chung AF et al (1980) Malignant melanoma of the vagina – report of 19 cases. Obstet Gynecol 55(6):720–727

17. Moon WK, Kim SH, Han MC (1993) MR findings of malignant melanoma of the vagina. Clin Radiol 48(5):326–328

18. Fan SF, Gu WZ, Zhang JM (2001) Cases report/MR finding of malignant melanoma of vagina. Br J Radiol 74:445–447

Broad Ligament

Part 6

Embryology Anatomy, Histology and Diseases of the Broad Ligament

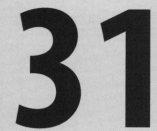

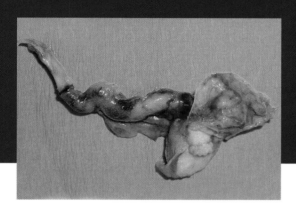

Contents

31.1 Embryology, Anatomy, and Histology

31.1.1 Embryology [1]

See Chap. 1.

31.1.2 Anatomy [2, 3]

See Chap. 2.

31.1.3 Histology

1. In its upper part, the mesovarium and the mesosalpinx are very thin, composed almost exclusively of peritoneum.
2. In the mesometrium, beneath the peritoneum, dense conjunctive fascicles are associated with muscular tissue and adipose tissue.

31.2 WHO Classification of Tumors of the Broad Ligament and Other Uterine Ligaments [4]

There is a broad variety of tumor and tumor-like lesions of the broad ligament (Table 31.1). Simple cysts (often called para-ovarian cysts) are very common and most often correspond to tumor like-lesions (cysts of mullerian, mesonephric or mesothelial origin) rarely to true neoplasms. In the absence of papillary projections or solid components, differentiation of a tumor-like lesion from a true neoplasm can be difficult [4, 5].

J.N. Buy, M. Ghossain, *Gynecological Imaging*,
DOI 10.1007/978-3-642-31012-6_31, © Springer-Verlag Berlin Heidelberg 2013

Table 31.1 WHO classification of tumors of the broad ligament and other uterine ligaments

1. **Epithelial tumors**
   Mullerian
      Serous tumors (cystadenoma, borderline cystadenoma, serous carcinoma)
      Mucinous carcinomas
      Endometrioid tumors
      Clear cell carcinomas
      Brenner tumor
   Wolffian
      Papillary cystadenoma
   Ependymoma
2. **Mesenchymal tumors**
   Benign   leiomyomas, lipomas
   Malignant sarcomas (leiomyosarcomas and other sarcomas)
3. **Mixed epithelial-mesenchymal tumors**
   Adenomyomas
   Adenosarcomas
4. **Miscellaneous tumors**
   Germ cell tumors
   Granulosa cell tumors, thecoma, fibroma, steroid cell tumors
   Adenomatoid tumor
   Pheochromocytoma
5. **Secondary tumors**
   Carcinoma
   Lymphoma and leukemia
6. **Tumor like lesions**
   Cysts
     Mullerian
     Wolffian
     Mesothelial

Table 31.2 Topographic findings of a mass of the broad ligament

1. Location in the mesovarium or the mesosalpinx
   Cystic mass separated from the ovary
      Round shape, different from a hydrosalpinx
2. Location in the mesometrium
   Mass separated from the lateral border of the uterus, moving apart the anterior and posterior leaves of the broad ligament
   Round ligament pushed upward by the mass
   Lateral extension until the pelvic wall
   Inward displacement of the lateral wall of the bladder
   Downward extension until the pubic symphysis
   Mass effect on the pelvic ureter in its parametrial portion

31.3 Imaging Findings

31.3.1 Common Topographic Characters in Favor of the Location to the Broad Ligament

These findings are reported in Table 31.2.

31.3.2 Different Types of Tumors

31.3.2.1 Epithelial Tumors [5]

On US, these tumors are mainly cystic. They can be without any papillary projection or with papillary projection which can be benign, borderline (Fig. 31.1), or carcinomas.

Diagnosis of the extraovarian site is easy when the normal ipsilateral ovary separated from the cyst is clearly depicted (Fig. 31.2). However, the location outside the ovary can be difficult to precise in other cases.

MR can help to localize the cyst, particularly in case of voluminous mass (Fig. 31.3) in displaying the normal ovary.

Uncommonly, these tumors can be complicated with torsion of the adnexa (Fig. 31.4).

Morphologic and vascular findings are identical to ovarian tumors of the same type (see Chap. 9).

These tumors can recur after surgery.

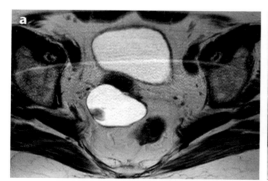 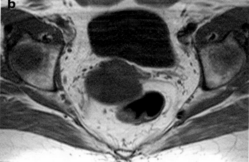 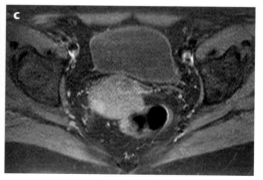

Fig. 31.1 Serous borderline tumor of the broad ligament. MR axial T2 (**a**) depicts a cystic mass with an endocystic papillary projection. Normal ipsilateral ovary was seen separated from the mass. On T1 (**b**) and fat suppression (**c**) the cystic content has a higher signal than urine. Prospective diagnosis: a serous extraovarian tumor was diagnosed; a benign tumor was suggested. At pathology: borderline serous tumor

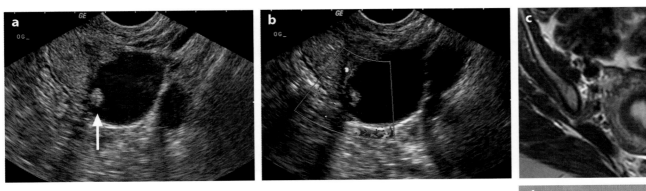

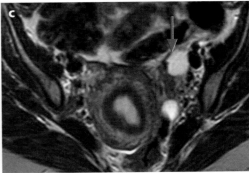

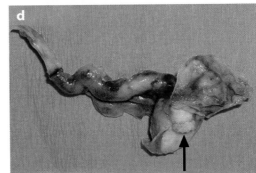

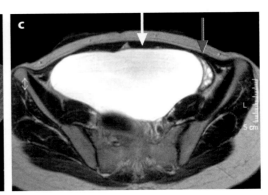

Fig. 31.2 Serous cystadenoma of the mesosalpinx adherent to the left ovary and the tube. (**a**) (EVS): 3-cm left cystic mass containing an endocystic papillary projection (*arrow*), measuring 6 mm with regular border and a short base of implantation, suggestive of a benign tumor. The mass is lying against a normal ovary. Color Doppler (**b**) shows vessels between the cyst and the normal ovary; however, it is difficult to precise its ovarian or extraovarian location. (**c**) MR axial T2. The cyst is clearly separated from the ovary (*arrow*). At laparotomy, the left ovary was normal. The cyst was developed in the mesosalpinx, and a salpingectomy was performed. (**d**) On the pathologic specimen, the benign papillary projection (*arrow*), lying on a fibrous area of the inner wall, is well displayed

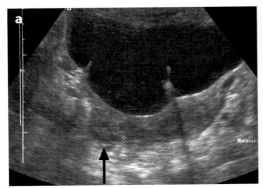

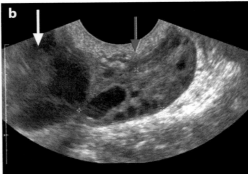

Fig. 31.3 Cyst of the mesosalpinx. Transverse TAS (**a**) displays a unilocular cystic mass with bosselated borders anterior to the uterus; a normal right ovary is depicted (*arrow*). Examination with the endovaginal probe in the lateral portion of left flank (**b**) depicts the left normal ovary (*red arrow*) pushed laterally by the cyst (*white arrow*). (**c**) MR axial T2 confirms the extraovarian location of the cyst (*white arrow*) in contact with the left normal ovary (*red arrow*). Coelioscopy: resection of the cyst. Microscopy: left paraovarian cyst

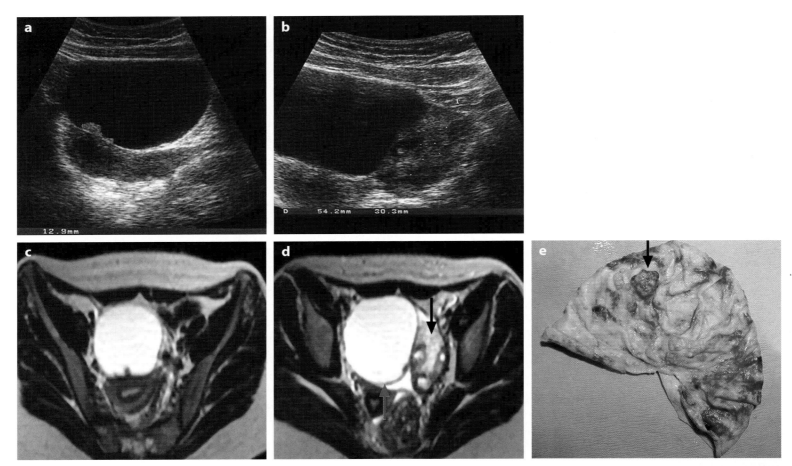

Fig. 31.4 Serous cystadenoma of the mesosalpinx complicated with torsion of the left ovary. Acute pelvic pain in a 16-year-old girl. TAS (**a**, **b**) displays a left enlarged ovary (5.4×3 cm) and an adjacent large anterior cyst containing endocystic vegetations. The largest vegetation measures 13-mm. Axial T2 (**c**, **d**) displays a left extraovarian cystic mass containing vegetations (*red arrow*) and an enlarged left ovary with a hyperintense edematous stroma (*black arrow*), very suggestive of torsion. Surgery confirmed the edematous torsion of a left cystadenoma of the mesosalpinx. Detorsion and cystectomy were performed. Macroscopic specimen (**e**) shows the opened cyst with the papillary projections (*arrow*) (Modified from [5], authors' personal publication)

31.3.2.2 Mesenchymal Tumors

Benign

Leiomyomas (Fig. 31.5). These tumors can arise primarily from the broad ligament. When they are in contact with the uterus, they can be difficult to distinguish from a subserous leiomyomas. In very uncommon cases, they can be discovered total hysterectomy (Fig. 31.6), raising the question of a subserous leiomyoma ignored at the time of hysterectomy or of a primary leiomyoma of the broad ligament discovered one or several years after hysterectomy.

Lipomas are usually small and lie below the tube or in its serosa along the distal portion of the ampulla.

Occasional cases of many other varieties of mesenchymal tumors include fibromas and hemangiopericytoma (Fig. 31.7).

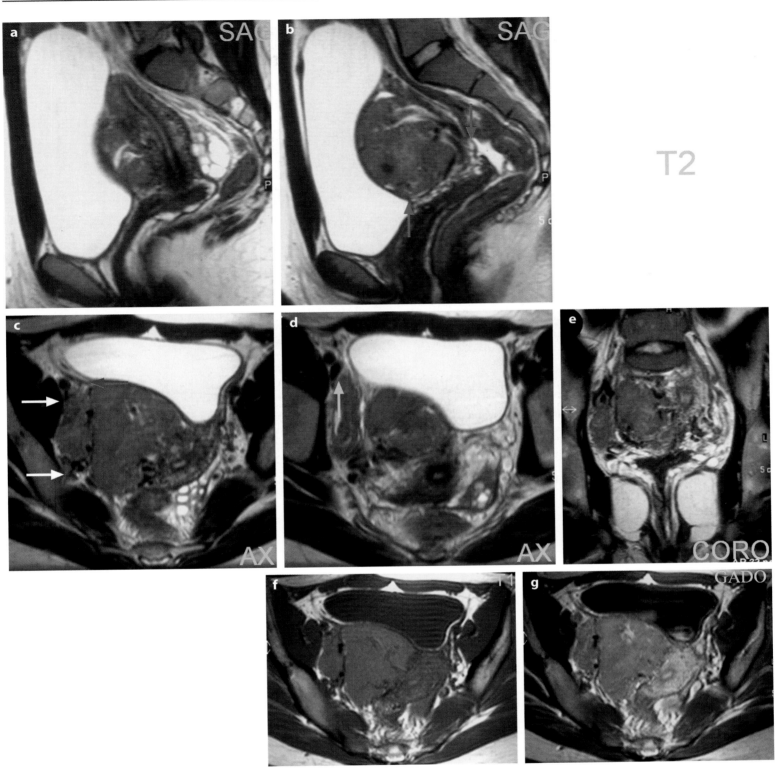

Fig. 31.5 Eighteen-year-old woman. Pelvic pain. MR sagittal T2 (**a**, **b**), axial T2 (**c**, **d**), and coronal T2 (**e**) display a subserous uterine mass of intermediate signal developed from the anterior and right border of the cervix and the uterine body, which: (1) Moves apart the anterior and the posterior leaves of the broad ligament (*red arrows*), (2) Extends laterally until the pelvic wall (*white arrows*), (3) Raises up the round ligament (*blue arrow*), (4) Slightly compresses forward the posterior part of the external iliac vein (*yellow arrow*) and inward the lateral face of the bladder, These different anatomical landmarks allowed to precise the location of the mass in the mesometrium. Large vessels are visualized at the periphery of the mass. Axial T1 without (**f**) and after injection (**g**) displays contrast enhancement less than myometrium. Surgery: the mass is in the broad ligament; resection of the mass was performed. Microscopy: epithelioid leiomyoma

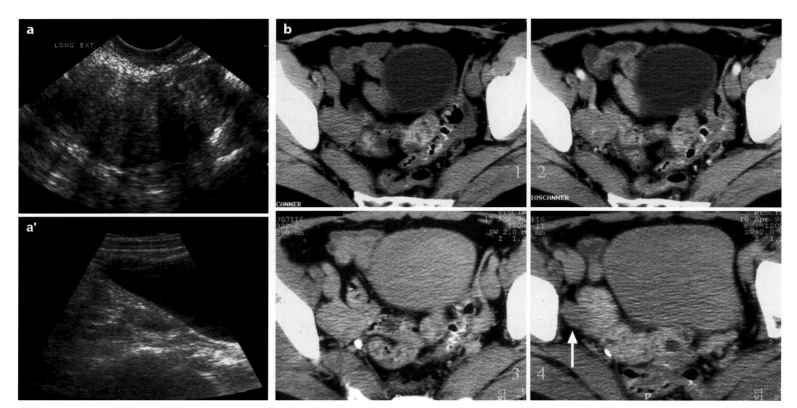

Fig. 31.6 Leiomyoma of the broad ligament after hysterectomy. Fifty-five-year-old woman. Total hysterectomy with preservation of the adnexae 5 years ago. (**a**) EVS (**a**) and TAS (**a′**). EVS displays in the right portion of the pelvis a solid mass with acoustic shadowing suggestive of a fibroma. TAS shows a normal ovary independent from the mass. (**b**) CT performed at the same level without contrast (1), at the arterial phase (2), and on the delayed (3), displays a mass (*red arrow*) with regular peripheral, central vessels and a homogeneous contrast uptake. The mass is in contact anteriorly with the round ligament and extends laterally to the pelvic wall. At a level below (4), the mass is clearly separated from the right ovary (*white arrow*). These criteria are in favor of a location in the broad ligament. Prospective diagnosis: a benign solid mass. Surgery: the mass was developed in the lateral part of the broad ligament. Microscopy: leiomyoma

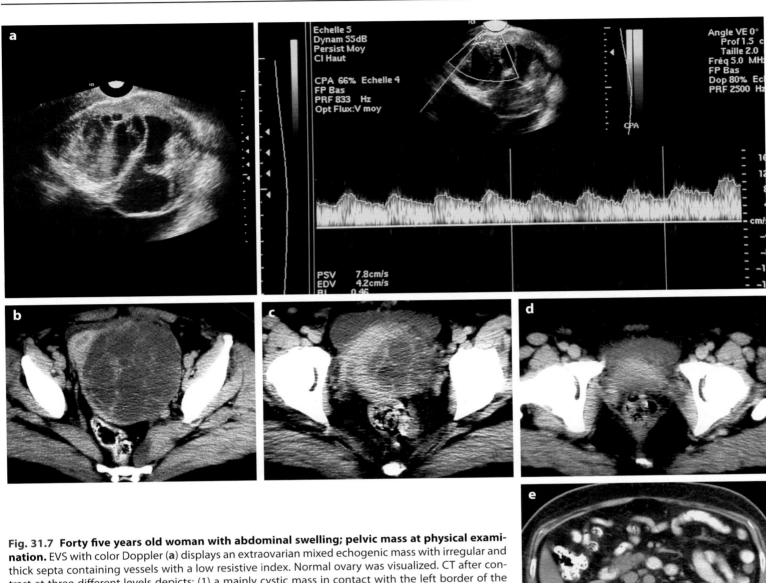

Fig. 31.7 Forty five years old woman with abdominal swelling; pelvic mass at physical examination. EVS with color Doppler (**a**) displays an extraovarian mixed echogenic mass with irregular and thick septa containing vessels with a low resistive index. Normal ovary was visualized. CT after contrast at three different levels depicts: (1) a mainly cystic mass in contact with the left border of the uterus body and the cervix (**b**), with a marked extension downward (**c**, **d**) quite unusual for a subserous leiomyoma. CT performed 4 mn after injection (**e**) visualizes an obstruction of the left urinary tract by the mass; Prospective diagnosis: subperitoneal mass; a subserous leiomyoma is unlikely; a tumor of the broad ligament was discussed because of the pronounced extension downward, the close relationship with the uterus and the obstruction of the ureter. Surgery: Total hysterectomy with resection of the mass. Microscopy: hemangiopericytoma of the broad ligament

Malignant: Sarcomas
(Leiomyosarcomas and Other Sarcomas)

The most common sarcoma is the leiomyosarcoma.

Other sarcomas as synovial sarcoma (Fig. 31.8), embryonal rhabdomyosarcomas, and endometrioid stromal sarcomas have been reported.

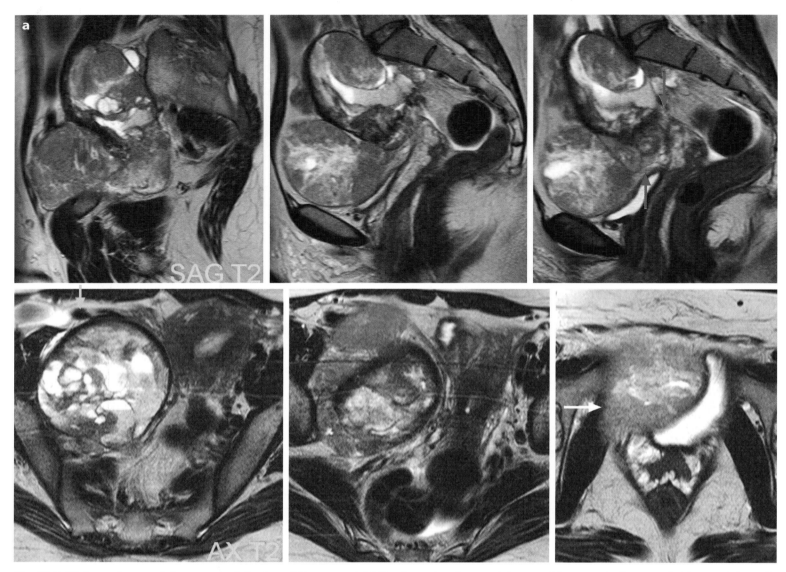

Fig. 31.8 High grade synoviolosacoma of the broad ligament. (a) MR sagittal T2 (in three contiguous planes) (a) displays a round well-delineated mass moving apart the anterior and posterior leaves of the broad ligament (*red arrows*). On axial T2 (a) at three different levels, the mass (1) pushes inward and upward the round ligament (*yellow arrow*), (2) extends laterally until the pelvic wall, and (3) extends downward (*white arrow*) until the pubic symphysis pushing inward the lateral wall of the bladder.

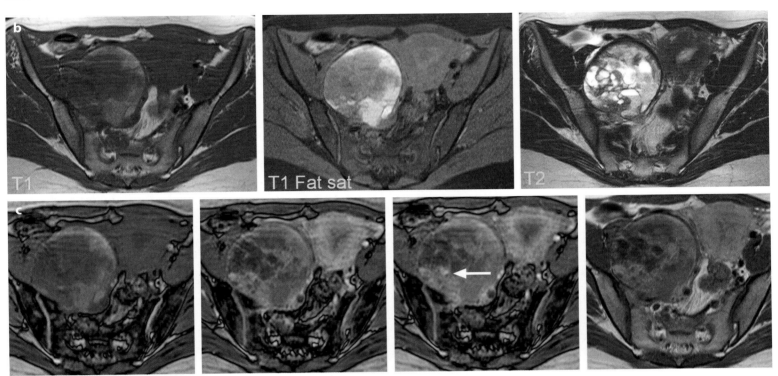

Fig. 31.8 (*continued*) (**b**) On axial T2, the mass contains solid tissue of intermediate signal with multiple cystic spaces. On axial T1 and on T1 with fat suppression, the solid portions contain hemorrhagic areas. (**c**) On DMR without injection, at the arterial phase, at the venous phase, and on the delayed, depict tiny arterial vessels (*arrow*), a contrast uptake in the solid tissue similar to myometrium. Prospective diagnosis: tumor of the broad ligament. Cystic cavities and hemorrhagic changes suggest the possibility of a sarcoma. Definite diagnosis: high-grade synoviolosarcoma of the broad ligament

References

1. Moore KL, Persaud TVN, Torchia MG (2008) The developing human. Clinically oriented embryology, 8th edn. Saunders, Philadelphia, pp 243–284
2. Standring S (2005) Gray's anatomy. The anatomical basis of clinical practice, 39th edn. Elsevier/Churchill Livingstone, London, pp 1331–1338, Chap. 104
3. Testut L (1931) Appareil urogenital, peritoine. In: Latarget A Traité d'anatomie humaine. 8th edn. revue par. G Doin et Cie Editeurs, Paris, pp 1–595
4. Scully RE, Young R, Clement PB (2008) Tumors of the broad ligament and other uterine ligaments. In: Rosai J, Sobin LH (eds) Tumors of the ovary, maldeveloped gonads, fallopian tube, and broad ligament, vol 23. Armed Forces Institute of Pathology, Washington. Chapter 27, pp 499–511
5. Ghossain MA, Braidy CG, Kanso HN et al (2005) Extraovarian cystadenomas: ultrasound and MR findings in 7 cases. J Comput Assist Tomogr 29:74–79

Complications of Adnexal Masses

Part 7

Complications of Adnexal Masses

32

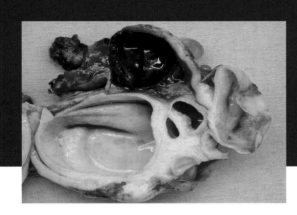

Contents

Ovarian masses are usually asymptomatic and may grow to significant size before they can be palpated and give rise to symptoms. Intracystic hemorrhage, rupture or leakage, and torsion are the most frequent complications; infection, necrosis, fistula, and hernia are rare.

Complication can occur at any age even in utero [1–4].

This chapter will make a rapid recall on hemorrhage in cystic portion, hemorrhage in solid portion, and paraneoplastic syndromes, which are treated extensively in other chapters; it will focus on more severe complications, i.e., leakage (or rupture), torsion, necrosis, infection, fistula, and hernia.

32.1 Intracystic Hemorrhage

Intracystic hemorrhage usually occurs in functional cyst or corpus luteum cyst, and for a lot of authors, "hemorrhagic cyst" is the synonym of "functional hemorrhagic cyst" or "corpus luteum hemorrhagic cyst." However, one must keep in mind that any tumor either benign or malignant can show intracystic hemorrhage (Table 32.1) (Fig. 32.1).

In malignant tumors, hemorrhage in cystic and/or solid portion is frequent, but the features of malignancy usually predominate. Hemorrhage in solid portion of benign tumors is rare.

The patterns of functional hemorrhagic cyst (FHC) and corpus luteum hemorrhagic cyst (CLHC) have been extensively treated in Chap. 7. Intracystic hemorrhage is often asymptomatic, and this chapter will focus on more severe complications.

J.N. Buy, M. Ghossain, *Gynecological Imaging*,
DOI 10.1007/978-3-642-31012-6_32, © Springer-Verlag Berlin Heidelberg 2013

32.2 Hemorrhage in a Solid Portion of a Tumor

It is a common finding in primary and secondary malignant tumors [5, 6]. In the absence of torsion, this finding is rare in benign tumors [7].

This finding can be considered as part of tumor description and will not be treated in this chapter but in each tumor description.

32.3 Rupture or Leakage

Rupture of a cyst is usually spontaneous, sometimes secondary to trauma such as intercourse or blunt trauma like in a motor vehicle accident. Rarely, it could be secondary to infection.

Rupture is usually associated with FHC, but one must be aware that paraovarian cysts, endometrioid cysts, and ovarian tumors may rupture (Table 32.2) (Figs. 32.2 and 32.3).

Table 32.1 Ultrasound pattern of FHC and CLHC

Loculation
– Usually unique and unilocular
– Rarely multilocular, multiple, and/or bilateral (after ovarian stimulation, in newborn, perimenarchal, and perimenopausal age)
Intracystic pattern
  Suggestive
    – Interdigitating fibrin septations
      Thin (fishnet appearance)
      Coarse (like a sponge)
      Spaced (simulating septa or floating membranes)
    – Clot
      Central or eccentric
      Stellate, with digitations, or well circumscribed
    – Fluid level
    – Small echo-free area(s) on diffuse echoic background
  Uncommon
    Diffuse hypoechoic
    Diffuse hyperechoic
  Complex pattern
    Any combination of the above patterns
Wall
– Thick, hyperechoic, and vascular in CLHC
– Thinner, less hyperechoic, and less vascular in FHC
Doppler
– Avascular intracystic content
– Vascularized wall
– Resistivity index may be low (<0.4) in CLHC
Differential diagnosis
– Endometrioma (especially if fluid level or homogeneous isoechoic pattern)
– Dermoid cyst (especially if fluid level or homogeneous hyperechoic pattern)
– Malignant tumor with solid vascularized component if no Doppler study or if Doppler study technically limited (transabdominal approach or bad technical conditions)
– Any cystic tumor with intracystic hemorrhage
– Any solid necrotic tumor
– Abscess
– Ectopic pregnancy

Table 32.2 Ultrasound patterns of ruptured cysts

The cyst
– Partially or totally collapsed
– Well circumscribed
– Nonvisualized
Intracystic pattern
– Same as FHC or CLHC
– May be anechoic
– May depend of the nature of the cyst
Hemoperitoneum
– Anechoic
– Hyperechoic
– Mixed anechoic and hyperechoic
Histology
– Usually FHC or CLHC
– Any benign or malignant cystic tumor
Differential diagnosis
– Differentiating FHC and CLHC from cystic benign or malignant tumor (follow-up or surgery)
– Ectopic pregnancy

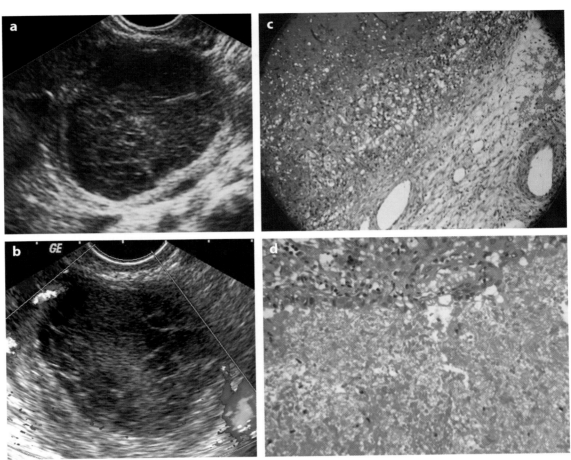

Fig. 32.1 FHC versus hemorrhagic cystadenoma: (a) and (c) correspond to a FHC that has been proved surgically. At histology, the wall of the cyst is lined by granular cells. (b) and (d) correspond to a hemorrhagic cystadenoma without vegetation or solid tissue. At histology, the epithelium of the cyst is abraded but still recognizable. At ultrasound, both cysts contain echoic material avascular on Doppler study, and no criteria can distinguish them

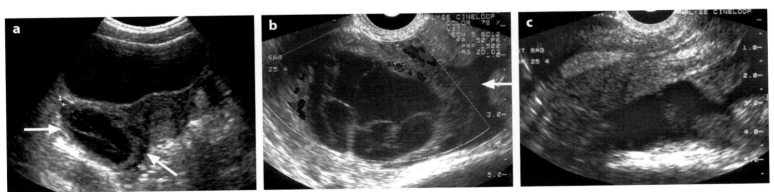

Fig. 32.2 Ruptured FHC with spontaneous regression. (a) Transabdominal ultrasound in a young woman with pelvic pain discloses a right ovarian cyst (*horizontal arrow*) with echoic intracystic materials. A small peritoneal effusion is barely seen (*oblique arrow*). (b) Endovaginal ultrasound with Doppler shows no color flow in the intracystic interlaced fibrin septa. A small peritoneal effusion (*arrow*) is seen abutting the inner side of the cyst, but the site of rupture could not be clearly determined. (c) Sagittal view of the pouch of Douglas better displays the peritoneal effusion that contains echoic materials. Follow-up ultrasound showed complete disappearance of all findings confirming the diagnosis of FHC

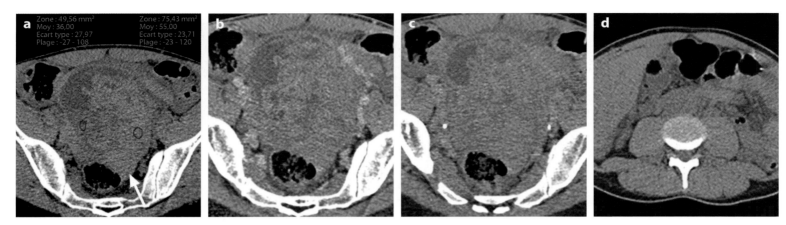

Fig. 32.3 Ruptured granulosa tumor. A 33-year-old woman with sudden pain onset. CT scans before injection (**a**) at the portal phase (**b**) and at 8 min (**c**) show a pelvic mass with low-density liquid, solid portions that enhance after injection (small ROI in a: 36 UH before, 78 UH at portal phase, and 66 UH at 8 min), and high-density liquid that does not enhance (large ROI in a: 55 UH before injection). Only contrast uptake allows to differentiate vascularized tissue from hemorrhage. High-deionsity liquid is also present in the pouch of Douglas which is difficult to differentiate from the mass (*arrow* in **a**). Liquid is also present in the upper abdomen (**d**)

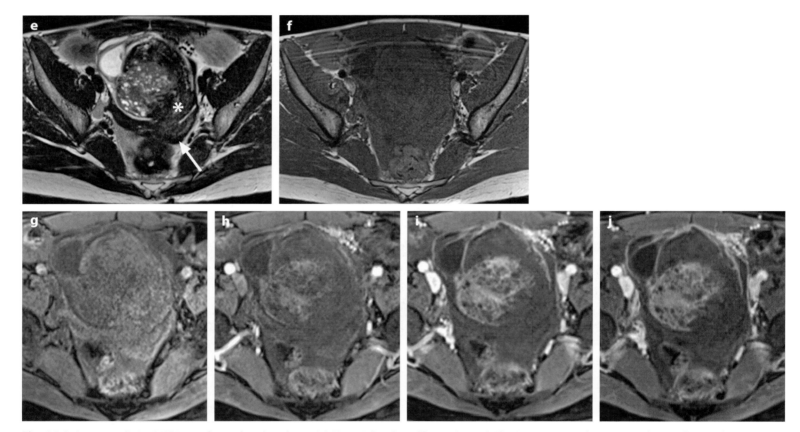

Fig. 32.3 (*continued*) An MRI is performed 2 days later. (**e**) T2-weighted image shows the tumor to contain a solid portion with small cystic components; the ruptured wall is well disclosed between the intracystic hypointense hemorrhagic content (*asterisk*) and the hypointense hemorrhagic effusion (*arrow*). The intracystic and extracystic hemorrhage is hypointense on T1 (**f**) and T1 fat saturation images. Dynamic MRI images before injection (**g**) and at the arterial (**h**), portal (**i**), and late (**j**) phases well disclose the solid component and the ruptured wall

32.3.1 The Cyst

The cyst may conserve a round appearance, and the main finding of rupture is hemoperitoneum (Figs. 32.4 and 32.5). The absence of collapse of the cyst may be due to the presence of an intraluminal clot, the obstruction of the break by a clot, or rupture of a vessel on the external wall of the cyst.

The cyst may appear collapsed with or without visualization of the rupture. Sometimes bowel loops may be seen inside the lumen.

The intracystic pattern is usually that of FHC or CLHC, may be anechoic on ultrasound, or depends of the nature of the cyst (Table 32.2).

In some cases, the ruptured cyst is not visualized at all either because it is entirely collapsed or because adjacent clots in the associated hemoperitoneum prevent visualizing the ovary and/or the cyst.

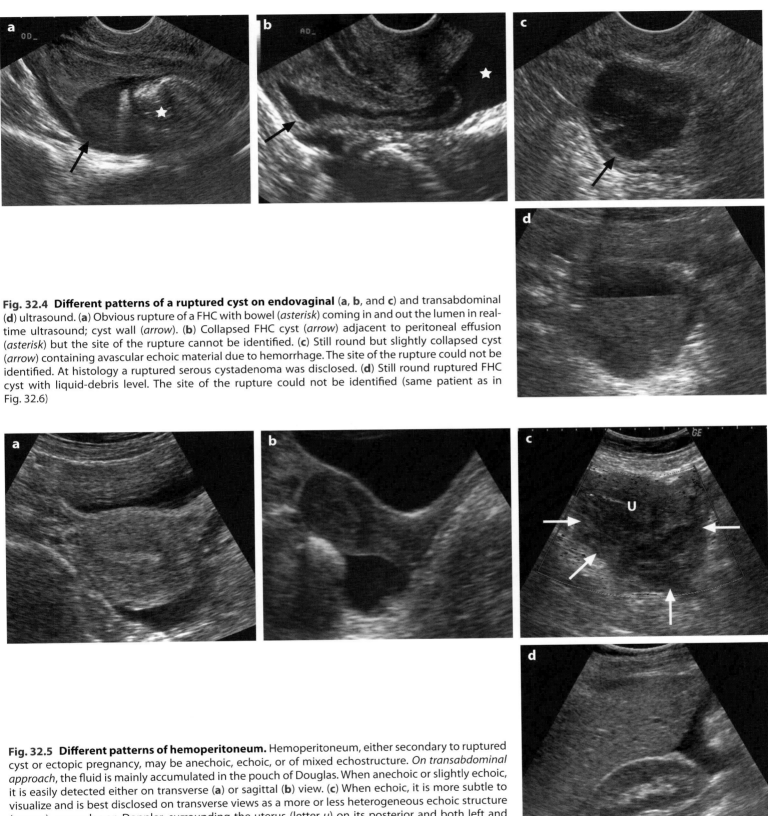

Fig. 32.4 Different patterns of a ruptured cyst on endovaginal (**a**, **b**, and **c**) and transabdominal (**d**) ultrasound. (**a**) Obvious rupture of a FHC with bowel (*asterisk*) coming in and out the lumen in real-time ultrasound; cyst wall (*arrow*). (**b**) Collapsed FHC cyst (*arrow*) adjacent to peritoneal effusion (*asterisk*) but the site of the rupture cannot be identified. (**c**) Still round but slightly collapsed cyst (*arrow*) containing avascular echoic material due to hemorrhage. The site of the rupture could not be identified. At histology a ruptured serous cystadenoma was disclosed. (**d**) Still round ruptured FHC cyst with liquid-debris level. The site of the rupture could not be identified (same patient as in Fig. 32.6)

Fig. 32.5 Different patterns of hemoperitoneum. Hemoperitoneum, either secondary to ruptured cyst or ectopic pregnancy, may be anechoic, echoic, or of mixed echostructure. *On transabdominal approach*, the fluid is mainly accumulated in the pouch of Douglas. When anechoic or slightly echoic, it is easily detected either on transverse (**a**) or sagittal (**b**) view. (**c**) When echoic, it is more subtle to visualize and is best disclosed on transverse views as a more or less heterogeneous echoic structure (*arrows*), avascular on Doppler, surrounding the uterus (letter *u*) on its posterior and both left and right sides. Ovaries are often difficult to visualize in this magma often called hematoma. (**d**) One must always look for fluid in the upper abdomen especially in the Morrison pouch. Fluid in the upper abdomen is indicative of an important hemoperitoneum

32.3.2 The Hemoperitoneum

The main consequence of a ruptured cyst is pain and hemoperitoneum. As the great number of ruptured cysts is functional and the hemoperitoneum moderate, conservative treatment is often possible. Pain usually subsides gradually, and the hemoperitoneum disappears. In rare cases, surgery is necessary to stop bleeding. When performing an ultrasound in patients with ruptured cyst, it is a good habit to have a look at the upper abdomen; presence of liquid in the Morrison pouch is indicative of an important bleeding.

A special case is that of patient with coagulation troubles. In these patients, despite severe bleeding, surgeons favor conservative treatment and correction of coagulation disorders before intervention (Fig. 32.6).

On ultrasound, hemoperitoneum is easily detected when anechoic or slightly echoic. When it is hyperechoic and moderate, it could be missed or underestimated especially by transabdominal ultrasound. When it is hyperechoic and important, it appears as a hyperechoic avascular structure surrounding the uterus on both sides and posteriorly. The two main diagnoses in these cases are ruptured functional cyst and ruptured extrauterine pregnancy. The hyperechoic clotted blood often makes it difficult or impossible to see the normal and/or the diseased ovaries.

On CT scan, the presence of slightly dense ascites in a female patient with sudden pelvic pain should prompt us to look for an ovarian cyst especially a corpus luteum cyst which is the most common cause of rupture (Fig. 32.7).

On MRI, the hemoperitoneum may show a wide range of signal depending of the quantity and age of the blood; sedimentation with level(s) may be present (Figs. 32.6 and 32.8).

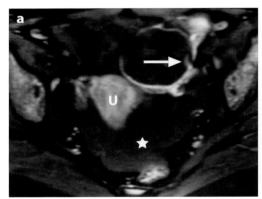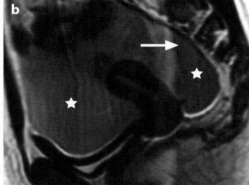

Fig. 32.6 Massive hemorrhage secondary to a ruptured FHC in a 14-year-old girl with myelodysplasia. Ultrasound (Fig. 32.4d) shows a left pelvic cyst with fluid-debris level, but the site of the rupture and the importance of the peritoneal effusion could not be well appreciated. (**a**) T1-weighted image with gadolinium discloses a cyst with a hypointense content and a wall that enhances markedly. The rupture is well seen (*arrow*). (**b**) Sagittal T2-weighted view allows better evaluation of the importance of the hemoperitoneum that contains two fluid levels (*arrow* points to the more dependant part). Uterus (*u*); peritoneal effusion (*asterisks*)

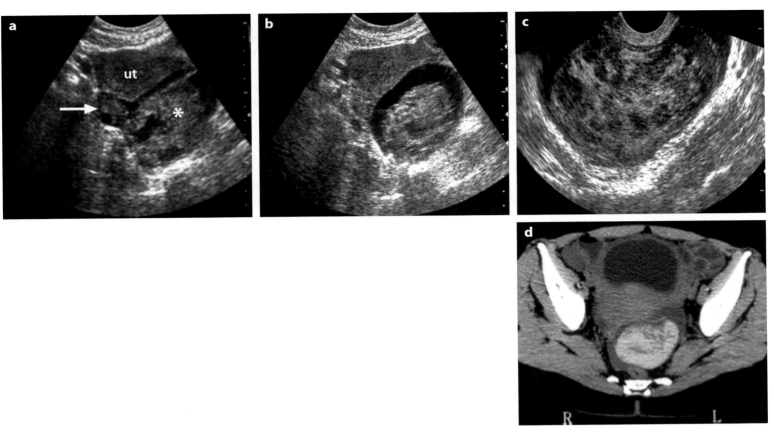

Fig. 32.7 Ruptured FHC on US and CT. (a, b) Transabdominal ultrasound in a young woman with pelvic pain discloses a normal right ovary (*horizontal arrow*) and a hyperechoic left cyst (*asterisk*) surrounded by free liquid. Uterus *ut*. (**c**) Transvaginal ultrasound better demonstrates the echostructure of the cyst grossly resembling a sponge. The site of the rupture could not be determined. No Doppler flow was detected in the cyst. (**d**) CT scan without (not shown) and with injection shows the cyst to be spontaneously hyperdense (without contrast uptake) well delineated by free peritoneal fluid. The site of rupture is probably anterior. Note that the peritoneal effusion is denser than the unopacified urine. Surgery confirmed a ruptured FHC

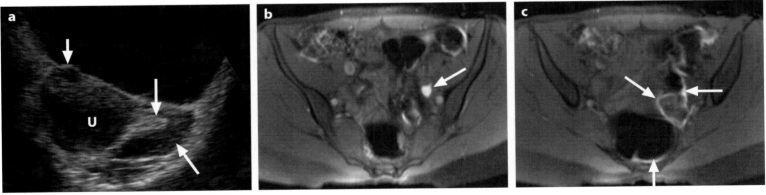

Fig. 32.8 Ruptured corpus luteum with thin T1 hyperintense effusion. (**a**) Ultrasound in a 16-year-old girl with pain during the second part of her menstrual cycle disclosed a small 10-mm hyperechoic structure (*long vertical arrow*) of the left ovary (*oblique arrow*) that merges imperceptibly with adjacent peritoneal fat. The adjacent uterus (*u*) contains a small subserous leiomyoma (*short vertical arrow*). (**b** and **c**) T1-weighted fat saturation MRI images. At MRI, the ovarian lesion appeared hypointense on T2 (not shown), hyperintense on T1 (not shown), and on T1 fat saturation images (*arrow* in **b**). A thin T1 hyperintense effusion related to a small hemoperitoneum is also seen on lower slices (*arrows* in **c**). Coelioscopy confirmed the above findings

32.3.3 The Peritoneum

After spontaneous or surgical resolution of the disease, there is usually no consequence on the peritoneum.

However, spontaneous or surgical rupture of an ovarian cancer may prompt peritoneal carcinomatosis. Pseudomyxoma peritonei may be the consequence of a rupture ovarian mucinous carcinoma although it is believed that it arises more frequently from the appendix.

Granulomatous peritonitis may be secondary to a long-standing hemoperitoneum.

Gliomatosis and melanosis are very rare peritoneal secondary lesions that could be but not necessary associated with rupture of a teratoma [8–10].

32.4 Adnexal Torsion

32.4.1 Physiopathology and Clinical Findings

The clinical and radiological patterns of adnexal torsion are extremely variable. This is due to a complex physiopathology secondary to different factors:
– Usually, the torsion involves the ovary and the tube, but it may involve the ovary alone or rarely the tube alone.
– The torsion may involve normal adnexa but usually is secondary to a preexisting mass in the adnexa.
– The severity of the vascular compression is variable depending on the number of twists and the tightness of the twist(s).
– The dual vascular supply of the ovary from the ovarian and uterine arteries.
– The intermittent severity of the vascular compression due to the alternation of tightness and untightness of the twist(s) that could result sometimes in complete spontaneous detorsion.
  Basically, there are two phases:
(a) Early phase: venous compression with edema
  At this stage, the adnexa are viable. The usual treatment is surgical detorsion either by coelioscopy or laparotomy. If a mass is present, it is removed. Keeping or removing the adnexa will depend on the nature of the associated mass if present and the age of the patient.
(b) Late phase: compression with hemorrhagic necrosis
  The necrosis may be complete or partial. Usually, the surgeon proceeds to detorsion and observes the color of the adnexa. If they are revascularized with only some petechiae, he can keep them. Otherwise, he usually performs adnexectomy or partial resection. The surgical decision will depend also on the nature of the associated mass if present and the age of the patient. Even in case of necrosis, some surgeons advocate keeping the adnexa especially in children or young patients [11–13].
  At both the early and late stage, oophoropexy or shortening of the utero-ovarian ligament is sometimes performed ipsilaterally, contralaterally if the ovary has been removed, or bilaterally especially in children [14].
The evolution of torsion is unpredictable. It can rapidly progress to a stage of hemorrhagic necrosis in a few hours or remain at the stage of edema for several days. The intermittent character of the torsion is translated clinically by intermittent pain that in some cases may evolve into a complete spontaneous detorsion with the patient becoming asymptomatic or to completion of the torsion with hemorrhagic necrosis and loss of the adnexa [15].

Clinically, pain secondary to torsion can be confused with that of renal colic, appendicitis, diverticulitis, ruptured or unruptured hemorrhagic functional cyst, ovulation, or any other pelvic pain.

The complex physiopathology is also reflected by a variable radiological appearance. Multitudes of papers have been published concerning adnexal torsion describing a multitude of findings that may confuse the reader. However, it is easy to understand and remember them if they are separated into two groups: findings due to edema in the early phase and findings due to hemorrhagic necrosis observed later. Combination of these two groups is often found. We can also add a third group, the associated findings (Table 32.3).

32.4.2 Early Phase (Edema)

Edema may involve the ovary and the fallopian tube, the ovary alone or the tube alone, depending on which parts of the adnexa are involved by torsion.

32.4.2.1 Edema of the Ovarian Stroma

Edema of the ovarian stroma is best appreciated when the torsion involves a normal ovary. It results in an increase in size of the ovary that is sometimes spectacular simulating a mass or tumor. We can calculate either the largest cross-sectional area of the ovary or the ovarian volume to appreciate its increase in size. In our practice, we prefer to use the cross-sectional area because it is easier to calculate and more reproducible. To assess the increase in size of an ovary in polycystic ovary syndrome, the threshold of 6 cm^2 is usually used. With regard to adnexal torsion, we set our threshold at 10 cm^2 [16]. A torsion is unlikely if the largest ovarian cross-sectional area is <10 cm^2 and very likely if it is >10 cm^2 in the proper clinical context (Fig. 32.9). Follicles are usually pushed to the periphery by stromal edema.

When a mass is present in the ovary, we must differentiate between an increase in size due to edema and an increase in size due to the mass. To solve this problem, we calculate what we called the corrected cross-sectional area of the ovary corresponding to the entire cross-sectional area of the ovary minus the cross-sectional area of all follicles, cysts, or masses >1 cm [16]. This is done to be in similar conditions to normal ovaries or polycystic ovaries that only contain follicles <1 cm. After choosing on ultrasound the cross section showing the largest area of ovarian parenchyma, we proceed to the calculation of the corrected cross-sectional area. We also use a threshold of 10 cm^2 [16] (Figs. 32.10 and 32.11).

The area(s) needed for computing the cross-sectional or the corrected cross-sectional area can be calculated by drawing it (them) directly on the screen or using the formula: largest diameter (cm) × short diameter (cm) × 0.8 = area (cm^2).

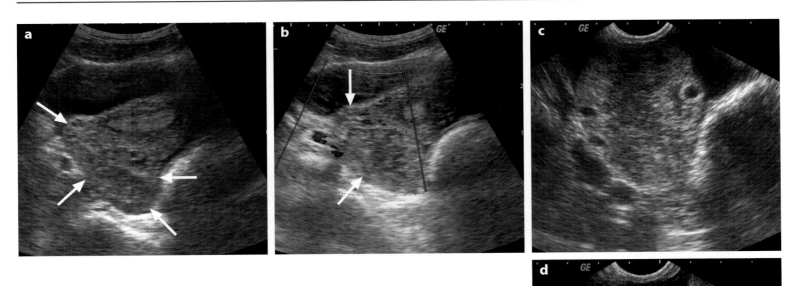

Fig. 32.9 Adnexal torsion without associated mass diagnosed on US. (a) Transabdominal US in a 20-year-old woman complaining of pelvic pain since 36 h displays large right adnexa (*arrows*) next to a uterus with a thickened endometrium. (b) Close US scanning shows that this enlarged adnexa is composed of two parts: a thickened tube (*vertical arrow*) and a large ovary (*oblique arrow*). Some vessels could be detected in the tube by color Doppler. (c) Transrectal ultrasound in this virgin woman clearly identifies a large 5.3×4.2 cm (17.8-cm² cross-sectional area) right ovary with peripheral follicles <1 cm. The ovarian stroma appears partly hyperechoic. (d) Between the ovary (*ov*) and the uterus (*ut*), a thickened tube (*arrow line*), 2.3 cm in width, is seen. A small peritoneal effusion is also present. An arterial flow with a resistivity index of 0.60 could be detected in the ovary. No venous flow could be recorded. Laparoscopy displayed a right adnexal torsion involving the ovary and the tube. The adnexa were viable with some petechiae

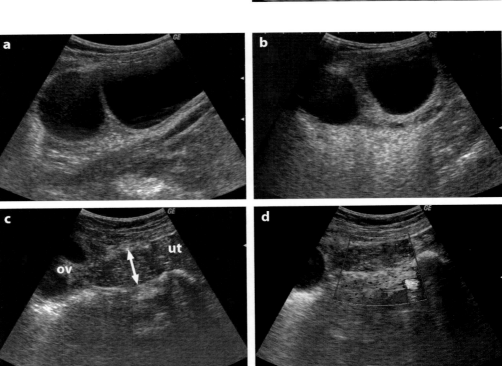

Fig. 32.10 US before and after adnexal torsion in a pregnant patient with follicular cysts. (a) Routine US at 9 weeks and 4 days of amenorrhea shows two right ovarian follicular cysts. The patient was asymptomatic. Notice that the ovarian stroma separating the cysts is not enlarged. (b) At 13 weeks and 1 day of amenorrhea, the patient developed right pelvic pain. Repeated US shows increase in stroma thickness with a corrected cross-sectional area of 13.9 cm². (c and d) A 19–27-mm thickened tube (*arrow line*) is seen joining the right ovary (*ov*) to the uterus (*ut*). Venous and arterial flow could be recorded in the tube and the ovary. Laparoscopy with detorsion and aspiration of the cysts was performed. The patient completed her pregnancy normally

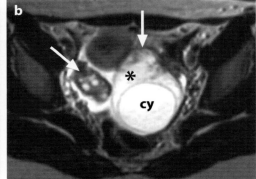

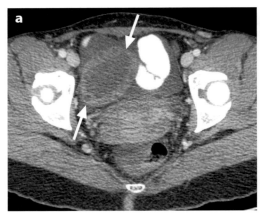

Fig. 32.11 Isolated ovarian torsion with high intensity T2-weighted ovarian edema. A 20-year-old woman with pelvic pain since 24 h. (**a**) Power Doppler shows a vascularized enlarged ovary containing a 45-mm anechoic cyst (largest ovarian cross-sectional area, 34.11 cm²; largest corrected ovarian cross-sectional area, 17.79 cm²). (**b**) Axial T2-weighted image (4500/96) shows both ovaries in the same plane. The right ovary (*oblique arrow*) has a normal-intensity stroma and is surrounded by ascites. On the left, large areas of the ovarian stroma

(*asterisk*) have signal intensity equal to that of the content of the cyst (*cy*) and to that of ascites. Some areas of the stroma (*vertical arrow*), the wall of the cyst, and the most external layer of the cortical parenchyma (tunica albuginea) remain hypointense. Laparoscopy confirmed the presence of a left ovarian torsion with a follicular cyst; the left tube was not involved by torsion. The ovary was edematous and viable. Conservative surgery, cystectomy and detorsion, was performed (Figures from Authors' personal publication: Ghossain et al. [16])

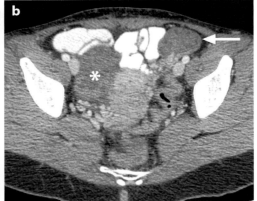

Fig. 32.12 Ovarian torsion without tubal involvement at a viable stage. (**a**, **b**) CT scan after contrast injection shows a large right ovary (*arrows* in **a**) with 24-cm² cross section and only small follicles <1 cm without any large mass. The left ovary (*arrow* in **b**) is also enlarged due to polycystic disease but not exceeding a cross section of 8.9 cm². The right ovary is hypodense due to edema with a density in its central portion of 25 HU versus 47 HU for

the opposite side. The difference of density is less obvious in the periphery of the ovaries where small follicles are present. *Asterisk* in **b** = upper part of the right ovary. No tubal thickening is seen. At surgery, the ovary was twisted but not the tube. It was cyanotic but recovered its normal color after detorsion. No hemorrhagic areas were seen

Ultrasound

We do not rely on the echogenicity of ovarian parenchyma because it is very subjective and difficult to assess. We compute the cross-sectional area or the corrected cross-sectional area as defined above.

The main difficulty is to differentiate between ovarian parenchyma and an echoic cyst as a hemorrhagic functional cyst, a dermoid cyst, or an endometrioma. This can be particularly difficult by suprapubic ultrasound even for experienced sonographers. Another difficulty is to differentiate between the ovarian parenchyma and an adjacent edematous fallopian tube (Fig. 32.9). At this stage, color flow is usually detected in the ovary and tube (Figs. 32.10 and 32.11). Because of technical limitations, absence of color flow does

not mean necessarily that the adnexa are not vascularized especially by transabdominal approach.

CT Scan

On CT scan, the ovary is increased in size and appears hypodense relative to the opposite side (Fig. 32.12). The stromal edema is more difficult to assess than in MRI but can be detected easily if the increase in size is important and if one is aware of this finding (Fig. 32.13). Comparison of pre- and postcontrast images allows differentiating edema from liquid and vascularized from nonvascularized areas and detection of spontaneous hyperdense hemorrhagic necrosis if present (Fig. 32.14).

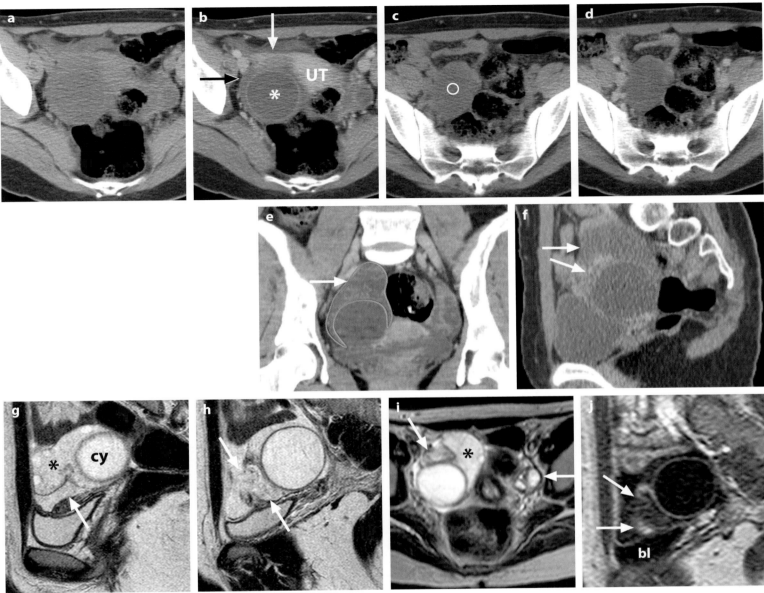

Fig. 32.13 Adnexal torsion at the edematous stage in a 23-year-old woman. CT scans (**a**) before and (**b**) after contrast injection display a cyst (*asterisk*) with an enhancing wall, an enhancing 17-mm thickened tube (*vertical arrow*) and a slightly enhancing peripheral ovarian parenchyma (*horizontal arrow*). Uterus = *ut*. CT scans (**c**) before and (**d**) after contrast injection, at a higher level, show more ovarian parenchyma (*circle*), allowing better density measurement with an enhancement from 23 to 38 HU. (**e**) Coronal and (**f**) sagittal reformatting allows to better measure the corrected cross-sectional surface of the ovary (*horizontal arrows*) that reached (19.3 cm²). In (**e**) is shown an example of computing the cross-sectional sur-face of the ovary using direct surface measurement. The thickened tube is also seen in (**f**) (*oblique arrow*). (**g, h**) Sagittal MR T2-weighted images show that the ovarian parenchyma is hyperintense due to edema (*asterisk*), slightly less than the cystic content of the cyst (*cy*). The tube is also displayed (*arrows*) and hyperintense, reaching 32 mm in thickness. (**i**) Axial T2-weighted image allows comparison between the enlarged right hyperintense ovarian stroma (*asterisk*) and the small hypointense stroma of the left ovary (*horizontal arrow*) that can be barely seen between follicles. Right thickened tube = *oblique arrow*. (**j**) Dynamic sagittal MRI at a late phase shows serpigi-nous vessels in the thickened tube (*arrows*). Bladder *bl*

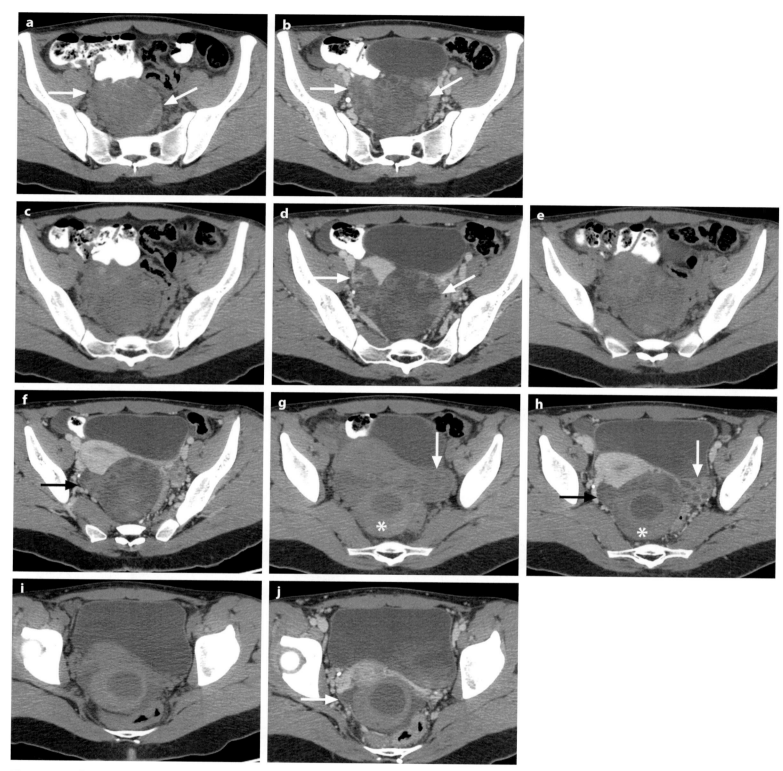

Fig. 32.14 Adnexal torsion with partial necrosis. Serial CT scans before injection (a,c,e,g,i) and after injection (b,d,f,h,j), at the same levels. (**a, b**) At high level, it is difficult to differentiate between the thickened tube (*horizontal arrow*) and the ovary (*oblique arrow*). (**c–j**) At lower levels, the uterus is well visualized after contrast injection, allowing to better distinguish the thickened tube (*horizontal white* and *black arrows*) from the right ovary (*oblique arrow* in **d**). Left ovary = *vertical arrow* in **g** and **h**. The tube could be followed on serial section from cornua utera to cervix on the right side of the ovary. Contrast enhancement could be demonstrated in the tube but not in the entire ovary. Part of the ovary (*asterisk*) appeared hyperdense before injection, not enhancing, corresponding to hemorrhagic necrosis. At surgery, the tube was edematous and the ovary partially necrotic. Detorsion and partial ovariectomy were performed

MRI

MRI has two major advantages over ultrasound and/or CT:

(a) It allows to distinguish clearly between the ovary and adjacent tube and occasionally between the ovarian parenchyma and intraovarian masses, allowing accurately computing the corrected cross-sectional area of the ovary and the thickness of the tube (Figs. 32.13 and 32.15).

(b) While the echogenicity of the ovarian parenchyma on ultrasound or its density on CT is difficult to appreciate, ovarian parenchyma appears hyperintense on T2 considerably higher than the contralateral side, sometimes confused with liquid (Figs. 32.11 and 32.13). Several clinical cases have been pub-

lished in the literature where a large edematous ovary has been confused with a cystic mass [17, 18]. The clue to the diagnosis is to demonstrate vascularization in the pseudo-liquid zones either by Doppler or contrast enhancement [16]. Follicular and cyst walls, as well as the most external layer of the cortical parenchyma (tunica albuginea), tended to remain hypointense provided that adequate window settings are used (Fig. 32.11) [16]. It seems also that fibrous tissue is less involved by edema than the normal ovarian parenchyma (Fig. 32.16). In some cases, not all the stroma appears hyperintense on T2. This can be due to areas spared by edema or areas with hemorrhagic necrosis (Figs. 32.11 and 32.15).

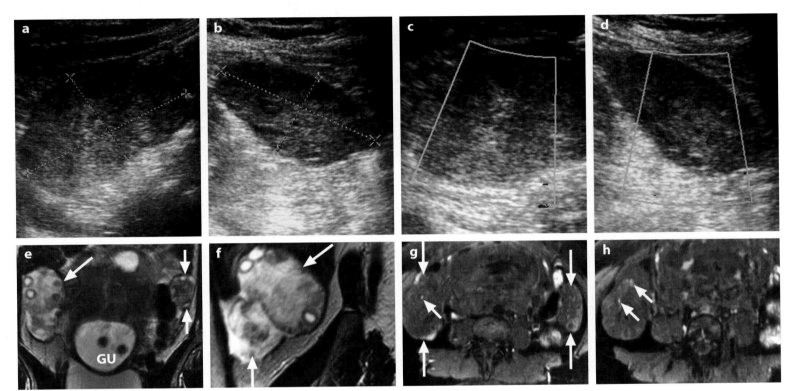

Fig. 32.15 Right adnexal torsion in an 18-week pregnant woman with previous ovarian stimulation. Transabdominal ultrasound in an 18-week pregnant woman complaining of right pelvic pain 1 week after losing one of two fetuses shows both ovaries to be enlarged due to previous ovarian stimulation. However, the right ovary (**a**) is larger with a 27-cm² cross-sectional area against 16 cm² for the left ovary (**b**). Moreover, color Doppler could not be detected in the right ovary (**c**), while it was present in the left ovary (**d**). The diagnosis of right ovarian torsion was made, but the surgeon asked to have more proofs before undergoing surgery in this patient with precious and high-risk pregnancy. MRI without gadolinium injection was performed. (**e**) The right ovary was enlarged and its stroma hyperintense on T2 (*oblique arrow*); note some hypointense areas that can be related to normal stroma not still involved by edema or areas where edematous stroma was replaced by necrotic hemorrhage. The left ovary is of smaller size with a normal hypointense stroma on T2 (*short vertical arrows*). Gravid uterus = GU. (**f**) Sagittal T2 MRI of the right ovary disclosed not only the large ovary (*oblique arrow*) but a thickened hyperintense fallopian tube (*vertical arrow*). (**g** and **h**) T1-weighted fat saturation images show both enlarged ovaries (*long vertical arrows*) and some punctiform hyperintensity hemorrhagic spots of the right ovary (*short oblique arrows*). At surgery, the right adnexa were twisted twice and appeared blue. After detorsion, the adnexa recovered their normal color and were kept in place after ovarian fixation. Follow-up was uneventful with no recurrent torsion and delivery by cesarean section at 31 weeks and 3 days

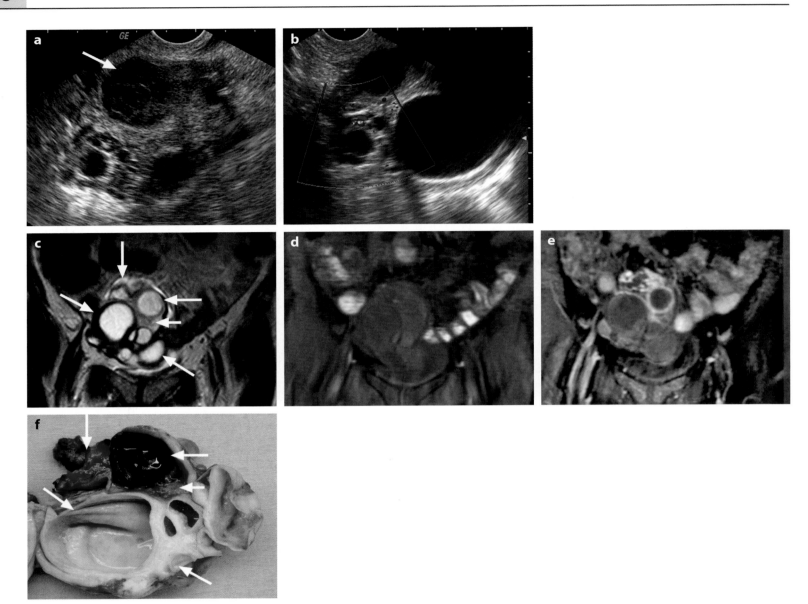

Fig. 32.16 Adnexal torsion with cystadenofibroma and FHC. (a and **b)** Transabdominal and endovaginal ultrasound in a 40-year-old woman with right pelvic pain discloses a large multicystic right ovary with an echoic structure suggesting an FHC (*arrow*). The ovary was vascularized on Doppler. (**c**) T2-, (**d**) T1- fat saturation, (**e**) T1-weighted fat saturation gadolinium images, and (**f**) photography of the surgical specimen disclose: A *cystadenofibroma* (*oblique arrows*) with hypointense solid tissue on T2, slightly enhancing after gadolinium injection, corresponding to fibrous white tissue at pathology. An *FHC* (*long horizontal arrow*) hyperintense on T2 and hypointense on T1 with a wall that enhances markedly, frankly hemorrhagic on pathology corresponding to the FHC described on ultrasound. An *edematous ovarian stroma* (*short horizontal arrow*) hyperintense on T2, enhancing more than the fibrous tissue of the cystadenofibroma. A *thickened tube* (*vertical arrow*) hyperintense on T2, enhancing heterogeneously. At surgery, a right adnexal torsion involving the tube and the ovary was present. The right adnexa were edematous and viable. However, because of the presence of a tumor, a right adnexectomy was performed

32.4.2.2 Edema of the Fallopian Tube

Edema of the tube results in tubal thickening that can also be detected on ultrasound, CT, and MRI. A threshold of 15 mm can be proposed [19]. When only the tube is twisted and not the ovary, findings of torsion are only present in the tube and not in the ovary; the leading cause in this condition is a paraovarian cyst or a hydrosalpinx (Figs. 32.17 and 32.18).

Exceptionally, the fallopian tube is not twisted, but an edematous twisted lombo-ovarian ligament can be confused with an edematous tube; clue to the diagnosis is to follow the tubular structures that instead of joining the uterine, cornua joins the pelvic wall (Fig. 32.19).

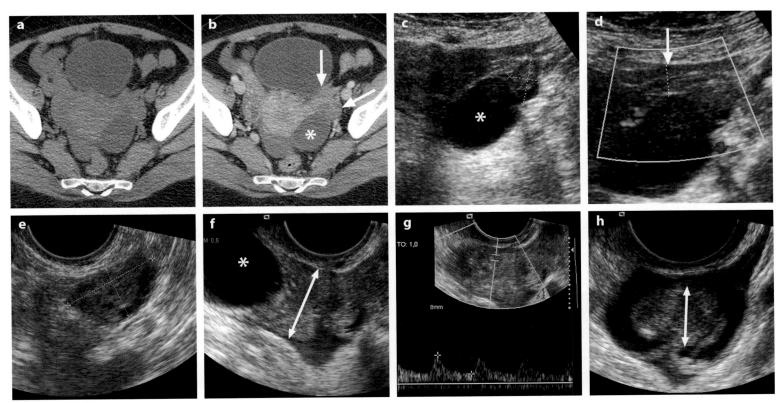

Fig. 32.17 Isolated tubal torsion secondary to paraovarian cyst. (a, b) CT scan before (**a**) and after (**b**) contrast injection shows an enlarged vascularized left adnexa but with difficulty to differentiate between a cyst (*asterisk*), the left ovary (*oblique arrow*), and the left tube (*vertical arrow*). (**c, d**) Transabdominal ultrasound showed a cyst (*asterisk*) adjacent to a normal-sized ovary (*cursors* in **c**) and a vascularized tube 12 mm in thickness (*vertical arrow* in **d**). (**e–h**) Transvaginal US shows a normal left ovary (*cursors* in **e**) distant from the cyst (*asterisk* in **f**) from which arises a 22 mm thickened tube (*arrow line*), vascularized on Doppler, that could be followed away from the cyst surrounded in some places by peritoneal effusion. At surgery, only the tube was twisted and edematous. Detorsion with ablation of the paraovarian cyst was performed. The adnexa were viable

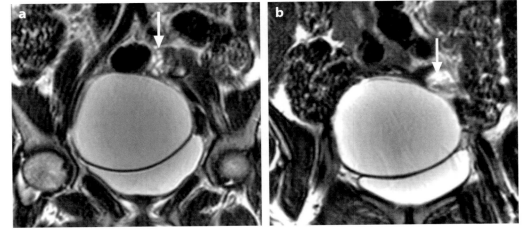

Fig. 32.18 Left isolated tubal torsion associated to a paraovarian cyst. Transabdominal ultrasound in a 27-year-old woman with left pelvic pain disclosed a normal right ovary and an 11-cm cyst. The left ovary was not visualized. (**a** and **b**) Coronal T2-weighted images displayed a normal left ovary (*vertical arrow* in **a**) and an edematous thickened hyperintense left fallopian tube (*vertical arrow* in **b**). At surgery, a tubal torsion was present with a mesosalpinx cyst as a leading factor. Detorsion with cystectomy was performed. The tube was edematous and viable. The ovary was not involved by torsion

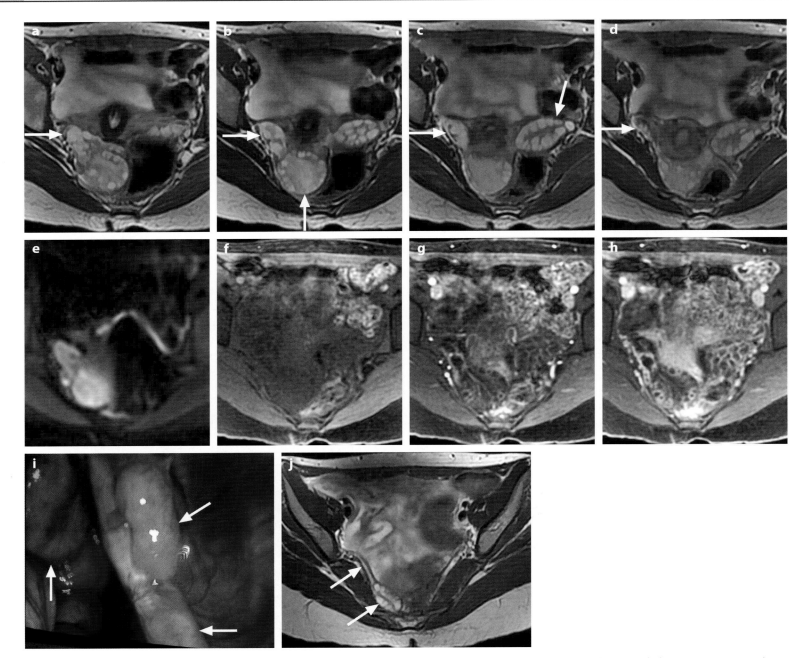

Fig. 32.19 Ovarian torsion involving the lombo-ovarian ligament sparing the fallopian tube. (a–d) Axial T2WI from down to up shows an enlarged right ovary (*vertical arrow* in **b**) with a cross section of 13 cm², peripheral small follicles, and hyperintense edematous stroma. Note the difference with the left ovary that is smaller with hypointense stroma (*oblique arrow* in **c**). A hyperintense tubular structure (*horizontal arrows* from **a** to **d**), 16 mm in thickness, is seen extending from the ovary to the pelvic wall corresponding to a thickened lombo-ovarian ligament. Axial TWI without and with fat suppression (not shown) shows no hyperintense area suggestive of hemorrhage. (**e**) Axial DWI easily detects the ovary and the lombo-ovarian ligament that are hyperintense. ADC measurements show high ADC value in the ovarian stroma ($1.8-2 \times 10^{-3}$ mm²/s) and in the tube (2.4×10^{-3} mm²/s) confirming that high intensity on DWI is due to edema (T2-shine-through effect) rather than necrosis. (**f–h**) DMR before injection (**f**), at the arterial (**g**) and delayed (**h**) phases, shows at the arterial phase tortuous arterial vessels in the tubular structure and straight arterial vessels in the ovarian parenchyma. On following phases, contrast uptake is well seen in the entire ovarian parenchyma, but serpiginous nonenhancing structures are seen in the tubular structures probably related to engorged nonopacified veins. The diagnosis of ovarian torsion was made. (**i**) After MR, the patient presented an acute pain, and urgent coelioscopy was performed. It showed an edematous right ovary (*vertical arrow*) and an edematous very thick lombo-ovarian ligament (*horizontal arrow*). The right fallopian tube (*oblique arrow*) was normal. Torsion was no more present probably due to spontaneous detorsion while inflating the abdominal cavity at the beginning of coelioscopy. (**j**) Six months later, the 18-year-old girl is still asymptomatic with on control MR (axial T2WI shown) normal right ovary and lombo-ovarian ligament (*arrows*)

Ultrasound

The thickened fallopian tube appears as a tubular structure extending from the uterine horn to the ovary often partially enrobing it. This tubal thickening is not always fully detectable. Often only a part of it will be visible. Upon contact with the ovary, we must be careful not to confuse it with the ovarian parenchyma (Figs. 32.9 and 32.10). Although, one can observe a whirled pattern in the tube, the diagnosis is made on the increase in size of the tube diameter.

CT Scan

Tubal thickness can also be assessed on CT [19, 20] (Figs. 32.13 and 32.17). It is usually better assessed than on ultrasound, especially if a mass is present. However, one must be aware of this finding and look to it on serial slices. Serpigeneous vessels are often observed in the thickened tube.

MRI

MRI can assess not only the tubal thickening but also the high signal intensity on T2 of the edematous tube [16]. As on CT, one must be aware of this finding and look to it in the different planes, sometimes detecting it on only one plane (Figs. 32.13 and 32.15). A serpigeneous pattern can be seen on T2 and after injection.

32.4.2.3 Vascularization at the Early Stage

At the early stage of edema, the adnexa are still vascularized.

On Doppler study, venous and/or arterial flow may be detected in the tube and ovary (Figs. 32.9 and 32.10). Some authors suggested that an increase in size of the diameter of the vessels is indicative of torsion [21], but we do not rely on this finding considering the large number of asymmetrical para-uterine vessels. Theoretically, venous flow is supposed to disappear before arterial flow, but considering the difficulty to detect flow either arterial or venous in normal ovaries, one must be cautious with this finding [22]. Because of technical limitations, absence of color flow does not mean necessarily that the adnexa are not vascularized especially by transabdominal approach.

On CT and MRI, contrast uptake is often more important in the tube than in the ovarian parenchyma allowing better differentiating the tube from adjacent structures (Fig. 32.13). The uptake in the wall of follicles and functional cysts is often more easy to detect than in ovarian parenchyma. The uptake in the edematous parenchyma is often less marked than the normal side because of vascular perfusion impairment and edema that reduce the ratio of vessels to extracellular fluid (Figs. 32.12 and 32.20).

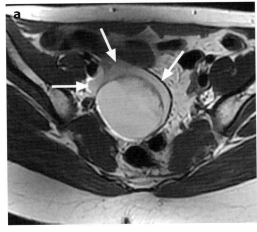
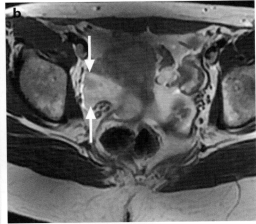
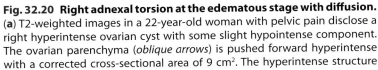

Fig. 32.20 Right adnexal torsion at the edematous stage with diffusion. (**a**) T2-weighted images in a 22-year-old woman with pelvic pain disclose a right hyperintense ovarian cyst with some slight hypointense component. The ovarian parenchyma (*oblique arrows*) is pushed forward hyperintense with a corrected cross-sectional area of 9 cm². The hyperintense structure (*horizontal arrow*) at the right of the ovary is a hyperintense edematous thickened tube that can be followed on lower sections wrapping the cyst and (**b**) reaching 25-mm thickness on the lower slices (*vertical arrows*). Axial dynamic MRI before injection

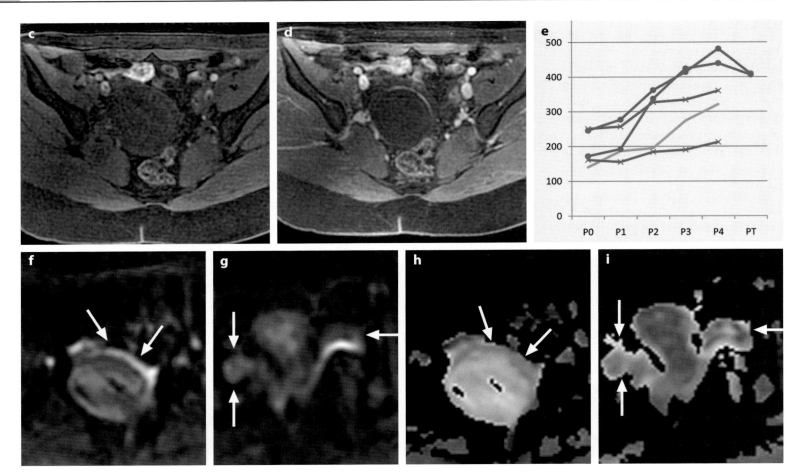

Fig. 32.20 (*continued*) (**c**) and at the late phase (**d**) shows contrast uptake in the tube, the wall of the cyst, and the parenchyma. No uptake is seen inside the cyst that corresponded to a functional hemorrhagic cyst on surgery. (**e**) Time intensity curves in the torsed right ovary (*blue x line* for stroma and *blue point line* for wall of cyst) and the normal left ovary (*red x line* for stroma and red point line for wall of follicles) show less marked uptake in the right edematous stroma compared to the normal left stroma. Concerning the wall of the follicles and cyst, the difference is no significant. Uptake in the torsed tube (*green line*) is more marked than in the edematous right stroma but less than in the follicular walls. (**f** and **g**) B-1000 DWI and (**h** and **i**) the corresponding ADC maps, at the same levels as the preceding T2-weighted images, show the ovarian parenchyma (*oblique arrows*) and the tube (*vertical arrows*) to be hyperintense on DWI with high ADC values (2.75×10^{-3} mm^2/s and 2.47×10^{-3} mm^2/s) compatible with edema and T2-shine-through effect. The left ovary (*horizontal arrows*) is slightly less hyperintense on DWI than the right one with an ADC value of 2.24×10^{-3} mm^2/s, 24% lower than the right one. ADC values were calculated as mean of b500 and b1000

32.4.2.4 Stromal Edema (Pitfalls)

The hyperintense ovarian parenchyma on T2 is a very good finding, but one must be aware that a normal hyperintensity can be seen close to a corpus luteum (Fig. 32.21). Computing the corrected cross-sectional area of the ovary helps differentiating this hyperintensity from hyperintensity secondary to torsion; the corrected cross-sectional area is normal or in the upper limit of normal with uncomplicated corpus luteum while it is usually increased (>10 cm^2) in torsion. Often, the clinical findings can be useful, the patient being asymptomatic or having pain on the opposite side. If

ambiguity persists and the ovary is well vascularized after contrast injection, follow-up is sufficient.

A second difficulty is ovarian hyperstimulation syndrome where the ovaries and ovarian parenchyma are enlarged. The ovaries are normally increased in size, and thus, it is difficult to use this finding to diagnose torsion. However, an increase in size of an ovary superior to the opposite side (>5 cm^2) [16], associated with pain on the same side, and in some cases the presence of a thick adjacent tube help in making the diagnosis (Figs. 32.15 and 32.22).

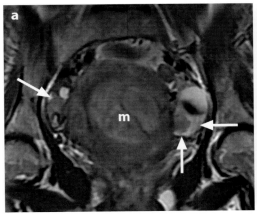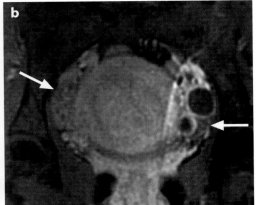

Fig. 32.21 Pitfall in the diagnosis of torsion on T2-weighted images: hyperintensity of the stroma next to a corpus luteum. (**a**) MRI in an asymptomatic 45-year-old woman for evaluation of a uterus leiomyoma (letter *m*) shows on coronal T2-weighted image a normal right ovary (*oblique arrow*). The left ovary contains a hypointense corpus luteum (*vertical arrow*), a functional hemorrhagic cyst of mixed intensity, and a hyperintense stroma (*horizontal arrow*). The corrected cross-sectional ovarian area is 7.5 cm^2 (5.25 cm^2 for the right ovary). (**b**) On coronal LAVA after injection, the corpus luteum is well identified with its hypervascular peripheral rim. No contrast uptake is seen inside the FHC. The left ovarian stroma (*horizontal arrow*) enhances slightly less than the right one (*oblique arrow*) probably related to edematous reaction around the corpus luteum

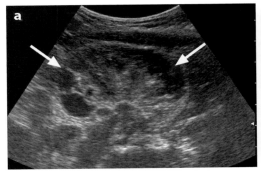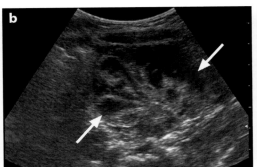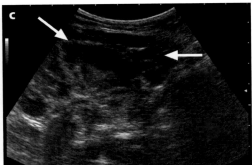

Fig. 32.22 Ovarian torsion in a 4-month-old newborn. A 4-month-old female newborn complained of sudden and severe abdominal pain since 24 h. A transabdominal ultrasound disclosed two large ovaries. The right ovary was larger and more heterogeneous than the left, measuring 6 cm in length and containing multiple follicles of different sizes (*oblique arrows* in **a**, **b**, and **c**). The left ovary was seen next to the right (*horizontal arrow* in **c**), measuring 4 cm in length and also containing several follicles. Doppler study was not conclusive in this restless patient because of too many artifacts. Coelioscopy disclosed a right ovarian torsion without tubal torsion. The ovary was necrotic. The left ovary was enlarged with multiple follicles but not torsed. Detorsion, partial right ovariectomy, and bilateral ovarian fixation were performed

32.4.3 Hemorrhagic Necrosis

At the stage of hemorrhagic necrosis, increased size of the ovary and the tube persists, but the blood supply is no longer present. Findings of edema are gradually replaced by those of hemorrhagic necrosis.

32.4.3.1 Ultrasound

The ovarian parenchyma or the tubes are increased in size and the echo pattern often slightly hyperechoic without detectable Doppler flow (Fig. 32.23).

If a cyst is associated, we can observe intracystic bleeding, but this finding can also be observed at the early stage of edema.

32.4.3.2 CT Scan

The ovarian parenchyma and the tube are increased in size, not enhancing after contrast injection. Hyperdensity may be present before injection due to hemorrhage, making it necessary to perform CT before and after contrast injection to confirm the absence of contrast uptake (Figs. 32.24 and 32.25).

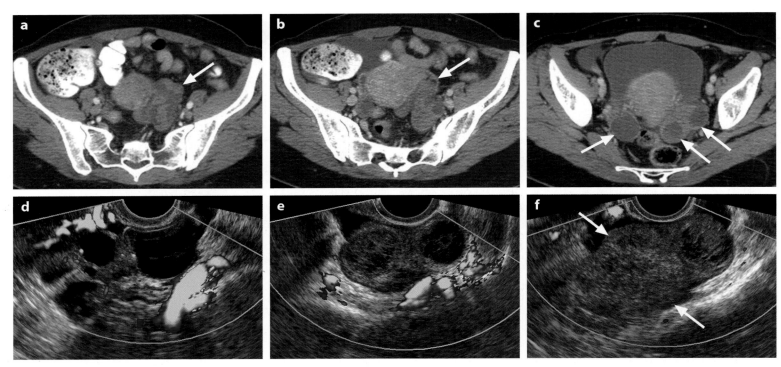

Fig. 32.23 Necrotic left adnexal torsion detected on contrast enhanced CT scan and confirmed by Doppler US. (a–c) Contrast enhanced abdominopelvic CT scan in a 43-year-old woman with nonspecific pelvic pain since 3 days shows two large ovaries containing cystic structures of follicular type (*arrows* in **c**) and a thickened tubular structure joining the left uterine cornua to the ovary, corresponding to a thickened fallopian tube (*arrows* in **a** and **b**). The diagnosis of left adnexal torsion was made. Contrast uptake in the adnexa could not be evaluated because precontrast images were not obtained. (d–f) Immediate Doppler US was performed to evaluate the vascularization of the left adnexa. (**d**) The right ovary was well vascularized with two large follicles and a corrected ovarian cross-sectional area of 4.5 cm². (**e**) The left ovary was enlarged with two large follicules, one of which echogenic hemorrhagic, and a corrected ovarian cross-sectional area of 7.5 cm². No color flow was detected in the left ovary. (**f**) A large slightly hyperechoic and heterogeneous thickened tube (*arrows*), 4.3 cm in thickness, avascular on Doppler, was seen joining the ovary to the left uterine cornua. At surgery, the left adnexa were torsed and necrotic; left adnexectomy was performed

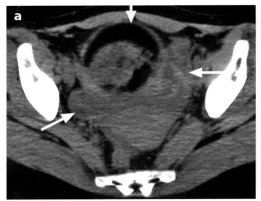
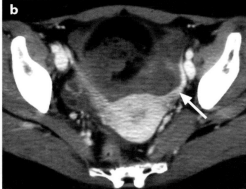

Fig. 32.24 CT scan before and after contrast injection of a left adnexal torsion with necrosis. (**a**) CT scan before injection shows a normal-sized right ovary (*oblique arrow*), a dermoid cyst containing fat (*vertical arrow*), and a left thickened fallopian tube (*horizontal arrow*) containing spontaneous high-density small areas corresponding to hemorrhage. (**b**) CT scan after injection at approximately the same level shows normal contrast uptake in a normal right ovary containing a corpus luteum, in the uterus and round ligaments (*oblique arrow* for left round ligament), but no contrast uptake in the wall of the dermoid cyst and in the thickened fallopian tube

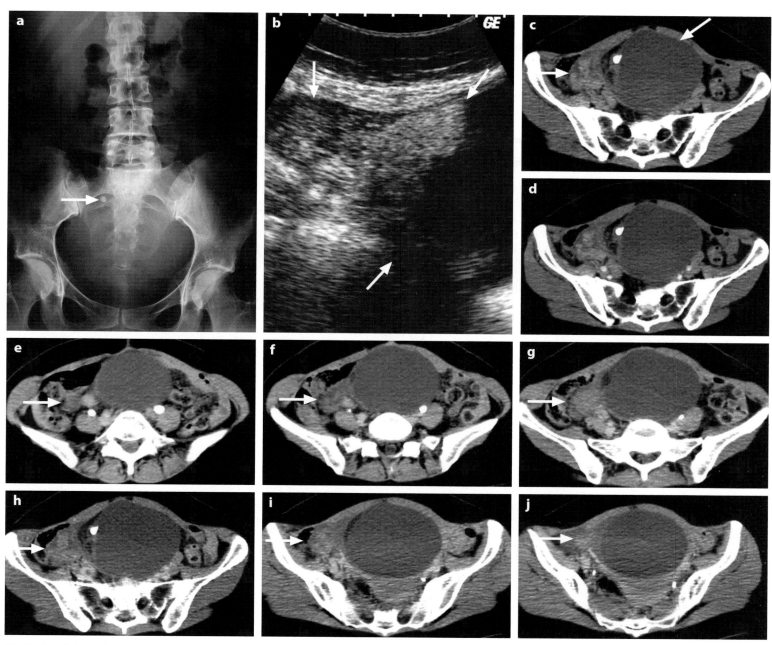

Fig. 32.25 Adnexal torsion with necrosis first treated as a renal colic. (**a**) Plain film of the abdomen in a 40-year-old woman treated for right renal colic since 3 days showed a pelvic calcification (*right arrow*). (**b**) Ultrasound showed a complex pelvic mass (*oblique arrows*) with a possible thickened tube (*vertical arrow*). CT scan at the same level before (**c**) and after (**d**) contrast injection shows a dermoid cyst (*oblique arrow*) containing a large loculation without fat density, a calcification, and a smaller loculation with fat density. A thickened right tube (*horizontal arrow*) with high-density areas before injection, due to hemorrhage, is seen. No contrast uptake is detected in the dermoid cyst and the tube (**d**). (**e–j**) Selected CT slices after contrast injection show how the thickened tube (*arrows*) can be followed from the level of the upper cyst to the level of the uterine cornua. At surgery, the right adnexa were torsed and necrotic. Adnexectomy was performed

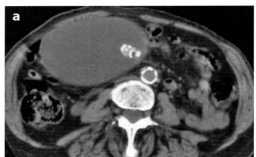 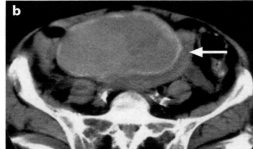 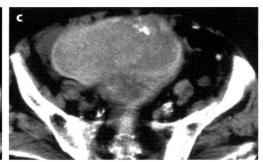

Fig. 32.28 Right ovarian cystadenofibroma with adnexal torsion in an 84-year-old woman. (**a**) CT scan obtained 8 months before the onset of torsion shows 12-cm thin-walled right ovarian cyst. Note calcified vegetation lying on posterior wall. (**b**) Unenhanced CT scan obtained 8 months later shows wall of the cyst to be thickened and hyperdense, indicating hemorrhage. Note enlarged structure (*arrow*) covering posterior and left side of the ovary, corresponding to thickened hemorrhagic fallopian tube at surgery. (**c**) CT scan at level of vegetation shows it is now lying on the anterior wall of the cyst (From Authors' personal publication: Ghossain et al. [26])

Table 32.3 Imaging patterns of adnexal torsion

	Size	Threshold	T2-images signal intensity	Vascularization
Early phase (edema)				
Tube	Thickened	>15 mm	High	Usually present
Ovarian stroma	Thickened	Corrected cross-sectional area >10 cm²	High	Usually present
Adnexal mass	Findings are usually more obvious in the tube and/or the stroma. Intracystic hemorrhage is frequent but not specific			
Location	Findings may present in the tube alone, in the ovary alone or may predominate in one structure. Exceptionally an edematous thickened lombo-ovarian ligament can mimic a tube			
Late phase (hemorrhagic necrosis)				
Tube	Thickened	>15 mm	Low	Usually absent
Ovarian stroma	Thickened	Corrected cross-sectional area >10 cm²	Low	Usually absent
Adnexal mass	Findings of necrosis such a thickened wall, hemorrhage, air in the cyst, etc.			
Location	Findings may present in the tube alone, in the ovary alone, or may predominate in one structure			
Intermediate phase				
	Often there is a mixture of early and late findings of torsion			
Associated findings				
	Beak sign			
	Rotation of a focal element			
	Peritoneal effusion			
	Peritoneal fat infiltration			
	Deviation of the uterus (not reliable)			

In some cases, only edema findings are present; in others, only findings of hemorrhagic necrosis are present, and sometimes, at the transition stage, there is a mixture of these two groups of findings.

These findings may be seen in the ovary alone if only the ovary is twisted (Fig. 32.12) and in the tube alone if only the tube is twisted (Fig. 32.18) and most often involve both structures but may predominate or be detectable in one structure.

As for associated findings, they are useful to make us think of the diagnosis or to make our diagnosis more confident, but the diagnosis is made mainly on direct findings of thickening of the tube and/or enlarged ovarian stroma and the findings related to edema or necrosis.

In some cases, despite tremendous advances in the diagnosis of torsion, specific findings of torsion could not be detected, and diagnosis is suspected on the association of pain and enlarged adnexa (Fig. 32.29).

Table 32.4 summarizes the main differential diagnosis of acute pelvic pain.

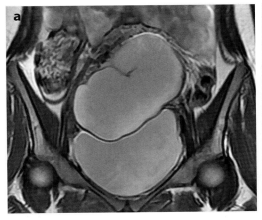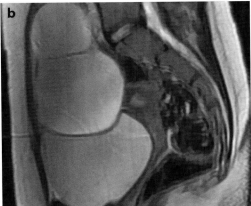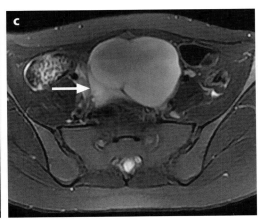

Fig. 32.29 Ovarian torsion on an atypical dermoid cyst, without tubal torsion. (a) Coronal and **(b)** sagittal MR T2-weighted images in a 14-year-old girl with severe pelvic pain show a large indented cystic structure, hyperintense on T2 and hypointense on T1 (not shown) without identifiable enlarged ovarian parenchyma or thickened tube. **(c)** On axial T2-weighted fat suppression image, a small hyperintense area (*arrow*) was suspected to be edematous ovarian parenchyma and/or tube but this was doubtful. On dynamic MR imaging (not shown), the wall of the cystic structure was enhancing. The diagnosis of torsion was suggested mainly based on the combination of pain and pelvic mass. At surgery, an ovarian torsion with a dermoid cyst containing some hair was demonstrated. Detorsion and cystectomy were performed. The tube was not involved by torsion. The ovary was viable and corresponded to the small hyperintense area on T2

Table 32.4 Differential diagnosis of adnexal torsion and other main causes related to acute pelvic pain

	Tube thickening	Corrected ovarian cross-sectional area	Vascularization	T2 signal	Others
Adnexal torsion (early stage of edema)	>15 mm	>10 cm²	Usually present	High	Findings may predominate in the tube or ovary Intermittent pain
Adnexal torsion (late stage of necrosis)	>15 mm	>10 cm²	Usually absent	Low	Continuous severe pain Previously intermittent
Spontaneous adnexal detorsion	>15 mm	>10 cm²	Present and even high if study performed after pain disappearance	High	Disappearance of pain before or after the imaging study (preferably MRI)
Renal colic or gastrointestinal disease	<15 mm	<10 cm²	Present	Normal	Usually no adnexal mass and clinical and radiological findings related to urinary or gastrointestinal disease
FHC and CLHC	<15 mm	<10 cm²	Present	High if close to CL	Pain may be contralateral to the cyst
Ruptured FHC or CLHC	<15 mm	<10 cm² If hematoma allow correct computing	Present	High if close to CL	Echoic peritoneal effusion and sometimes collapsed cyst
Ectopic pregnancy	May be enlarged due to hematosalpinx	<10 cm² If hematoma allow correct computing	Present	MRI usually not performed	Hemoperitoneum if ruptured Typical adnexal mass if present β-HCG+
Salpingitis and/or ovarian abscess	Present but rarely >15 mm	Increased but rarely >10 cm²	Increased+++	High but not as in torsion	Typical biological and clinical findings of pelvic inflammatory disease

FHC functional hemorrhagic cyst, *CLHC* corpus luteum hemorrhagic cyst, *CL* corpus luteum

32.4.6 Spontaneous Detorsion

The concept of intermittent pain in adnexal torsion is well known. Spontaneous complete detorsion is less known and more difficult to prove. Indeed, even if clinically suspected, diagnosis can be confirmed only if imaging shows clear findings of torsion [15] (Fig. 32.30). Although few cases have been published in the old literature [28, 29], it is only through better knowledge of torsion findings especially with MRI that the diagnosis became possible in some well-documented cases [15]. Several conditions must be present:

– Pain compatible with adnexal torsion that disappears spontaneously.
– Imaging findings very suggestive of torsion at the edematous phase especially hyperintensity on T2 of an enlarged ovarian parenchyma or tube. These findings can be observed before or after the untwisting because the edema does not disappear immediately.
– The return to normal of the adnexa on follow-up ultrasound or MRI.

The evolution of this spontaneous detorsion is little known in view of the limited number of cases published in the literature. If the surgeon operates, he will find untwisted adnexa with sometimes findings of edema and congestion of the tube and/or ovary. Stabilizing ovarian procedures such as oophoropexy or shortening of the utero-ovarian ligament can be performed.

Based on what we published [15] and several other cases that we observed, surgical abstention without recurrence was the most frequent outcome, but we also observed several recurrences in the same patients until stabilizing procedure of the ovary was performed and in one case loss of the ovary because the patient could not be operated on time.

In case of abstention, it is important for the radiologist to confirm the good vascularization of the adnexa and to make the patient aware of the possibility and danger of recurrence (Figs. 32.27 and 32.30).

32.4.7 Massive Ovarian Edema

In the cases of spontaneous detorsion we followed, the ovarian parenchyma returned to normal size or to the upper limit of normal. However, it is possible that in certain chronic conditions, the increased size of the ovary persists and becomes irreversible. In the entity known as massive ovarian edema (MOE), the ovary is enlarged and edematous. Adnexal torsion was present at surgery in approximately half number of cases, and intermittent torsion was incriminated in the other cases [30, 31]. The T2 hyperintensity of MOE was described relatively early; it was only later that the use of T2 hyperintensity in the context of an acute or subacute torsion has been highlighted [16–18, 32, 33]. Some cases of MOE have been reported in association with ovarian lymphatic obstruction secondary to metastatic disease [31].

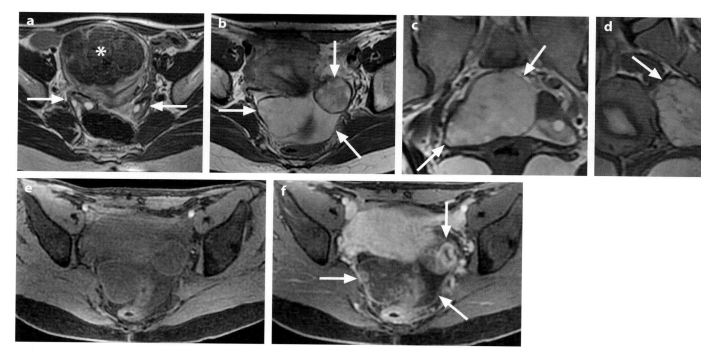

Fig. 32.30 Spontaneous detorsion with recurrence. (a) T2-weighted axial MR image in a 35-year-old woman showed normal ovaries (*arrows*) and a large uterine leiomyoma (*asterisk*); myomectomy was performed. Two years later, she complained of intermittent pelvic pain. **(b)** Axial T2-weighted image shows a slightly enlarged and hyperintense left ovary (*vertical arrow*), an enlarged hyperintense right ovary (*horizontal arrow*), and peritoneal effusion (*oblique arrow*). **(c, d)** Coronal and sagittal T2-weighted images better display the enlargement of the right ovary (*arrows*) that contains only small follicles with a cross-sectional area of 18.2 cm². **(e, f)** Dynamic MR before (**e**) and at the late 240-s phase (**f**) shows that the slight enlargement of the left ovary and its slight hyperintensity on T2-weighted images were due to a typical corpus luteum with hypervascular ring (*vertical arrow*); the corrected cross-sectional area of the left ovary was inferior to 10 cm². The right ovary (*horizontal arrow*) also shows contrast uptake with well-delineated follicular walls, medullar vessels, and a stroma enhancing slightly less than on the opposite side (*oblique arrow*) peritoneal effusion. The diagnosis of torsion was made, but the pain disappeared the same day. The patient refused surgery, and an ultrasound follow-up 3 months later showed normal-sized ovaries. Three months later, torsion recurred, and this time she was operated and ovarian fixation performed

Some authors consider ovarian fibromatosis, a rare lesion characterized by diffuse ovarian fibrosis, to be closely related to MOE. Young and Scully consider MOE as simply ovarian fibromatosis following torsion and accumulation of edema fluid, while Russel and Farnsworth consider ovarian fibromatosis the "burned-out" stage of a reactive fibroblastic proliferation that at one end of the spectrum is represented by MOE and at the other end by a variety of highly cellular fibroblastic tumorlike lesions [31, 34, 35]. The imaging pattern of ovarian fibromatosis is described in the Chap. 7.

32.4.8 Diffusion Sequences

The sequences with diffusion are increasingly used in pelvic MRI although their exact usefulness is not clearly established. Two papers have already been published on adnexal torsions [36, 37]: one case report with a necrotic adnexa that showed high signal of necrotic tissue on DWI and low ADC values [36] and a series of 11 cases that suggested that high signal intensity on DWI is indicator of a twisted adnexa but without evaluating ADC values and without correlation with surgical and pathologic findings [37]. However, with regard to adnexal torsion, it is always useful to distinguish between the early phase where findings of edema predominate and the late phase where findings of hemorrhagic necrosis predominate.

Our experience is based on 11 cases (under publication) and shows:

1. DW images are not necessary to make the diagnosis of torsion. In the only case where the diagnosis could not be made on the main findings of thickened tube and/or enlarged ovarian stroma, DW images were not useful to the diagnosis. In this case, the tube was not involved by torsion, and there was a large ovarian mass with a small ovarian parenchyma difficult to detect on all classical and DW sequences.

2. With viable adnexa, the signal of the ovarian stroma compared to the contralateral size was either comparable or higher. This is probably due to T2-shine-through effect secondary to edema as proved by a high ADC value always superior to the opposite nontorsed side. In about half the case, the tube was also hyperintense on DW images (Fig. 32.20).

3. With ovary containing hemorrhagic necrosis, the signal on DW images was either high due to necrosis or T2-shine-through effect secondary to persistent areas of edema, or low due to artifacts secondary to the presence of hemorrhagic necrosis, i.e., hemoglobin degradation products. In some cases, due to these artifacts, the entire ovary appears hypointense on DWI, while on ADC map and T2-weighted images, detection of the less suffering areas was possible (Figs. 32.26 and 32.31). Spin-echo diffusion-weighted sequences may be more accurate but are too long in a context of emergency, and their usefulness is doubtful because the diagnosis is already made on usual sequences. The ADC was always lower than the opposite side.

4. A low ADC value was a good indicator of hemorrhagic necrosis as the hypointensity on T2.

In summary, DWI are not necessary to make the diagnosis of torsion and even sometimes cannot do it, but a high intensity signal on DWI may alert the radiologist to the presence of a thickened tube and/or enlarged ovarian stroma if he did not already notice them on T2-weighted images. A low ADC value is indicative of hemorrhagic necrosis but T2 images also (Table 32.5).

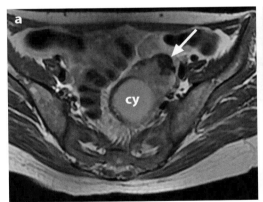
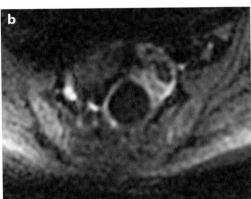
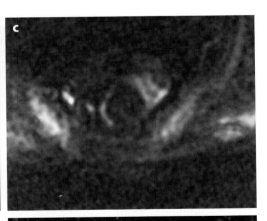
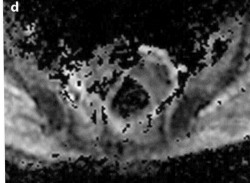

Fig. 32.31 Neglected ovarian torsion with necrosis at surgery. (**a**) T2-weighted ovarian torsion shows a left ovary with a cyst (*cy*) that proved to be a dermoid on other sections and a necrotic ovarian parenchyma that contains a very dark area (*arrow*) and a gray area. (**b**) On b-500 and (**c**) b-1000 DWI, the *dark area* on T2 appeared mainly hypointense and the *gray area* hyperintense. (**d**) On b-1000 ADC map, the *darkest area* has an ADC of 0.62×10^{-3} mm²/s and the *lighter areas* 1.15×10^{-3} mm²/s. Darkest area corresponds to the most severe lesions of hemorrhagic necrosis

Table 32.5 T2-weighted images versus diffusion-weighted images in adnexal torsion

	T2-images intensity	DWI intensity	ADC values	Vascularization
Early phase (edema)	High	Normal or high	Normal or high	Usually present
Late phase (hemorrhagic necrosis)	Low	High or low	Low	Usually absent

32.5 Necrosis

In the absence of torsion, this finding is rare.

Rarely, a subserous leiomyoma or an ovarian solid benign tumor may undergo massive necrosis and hemorrhage without clear relation to torsion (Fig. 32.32).

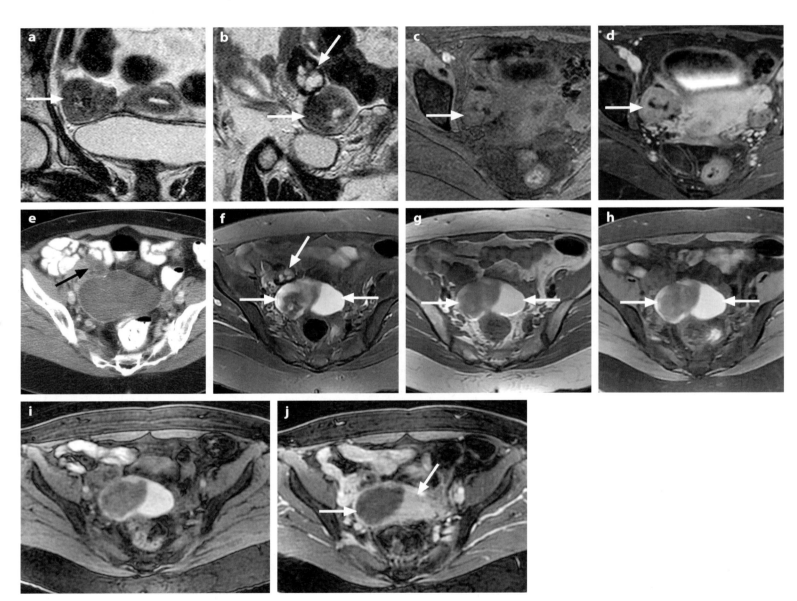

Fig. 32.32 Necrotic solid adnexal mass of imprecise origin. (a) Coronal and **(b)** sagittal T2-weighted images show a right adnexal mass (*horizontal arrow*) in close contact to the uterus and right ovary (*oblique arrow*). The mass is mainly hypointense in comparison to myometrium and contains small cystic hyperintense areas. The ovary also contains small agglomerated cystic structures. T1-weighted image with fat suppression before **(c)** and after **(d)** gadolinium injection shows the adnexal mass (*arrows*) to enhance except for small cystic areas. The mass was considered as a pedunculated leiomyoma and the ovarian cystic structures as follicles. *One year and a half later*, the patient complained of pelvic pain and mild inflammatory syndrome. **(e)** A CT scan with contrast injection showed the right ovary still con-taining the agglomerate of small cystic structures that corresponded in fact to a small cystadenofibroma on histology and the adnexal mass that seems cystic with a density of 50 HU surrounded by edematous peritoneal fat threads. **(f)** Axial T2-weighted fat saturation, **(g)** T1-, and **(h)** T1-weighted fat suppression images show the adnexal mass (*horizontal arrows*) to have a heterogeneous signal with hyperintense hemorrhagic areas on T1 images. Right ovary = *oblique arrow*. **(i, j)** Dynamic MR before **(i)** and at the late venous phase **(j)** show absence of enhancement in the mass except for a thin peripheral rim (*arrows*). Right adnexectomy and histology showed a small right intraovarian cystadenofibroma and a necrotic mass with imprecise histology probably ovarian fibroma (Courtesy of Dr Georges Nawfal)

32.6 Infection

Infection with eventual abscess formation is a rare but recognized complication of ovarian tumor. It could be found in the absence of fistula. It was described in dermoid cyst, mucinous cystadenoma, cystadenocarcinoma, and even in nonneoplastic mass such as endometrioma [38–45]. Subsequent abscess rupture and fistula may follow [38, 42]. Imaging features may be absent or correspond to usual findings of infections such as wall thickening, peritoneal fat infiltration, and air in the cyst [46] (Table 32.6) (Figs. 32.33 and 32.34). Distinction between a true ovarian abscess and infected or not infected cyst is not always possible (Fig. 32.35).

Table 32.6 Infected cystic mass

Intracystic pattern
– Dependant of the nature of the cyst and not related to infection
– Echoic or dense content due to pus
– Rarely air due to infection or fistula
The cyst wall
– Dependant of the nature of the cyst and not related to infection
– Thickened due to inflammation
Peritoneum
– Normal
– Peritoneal fat threads due to inflammation
Rupture or fistula
– Absent
– Present and visible
– Present and not visible

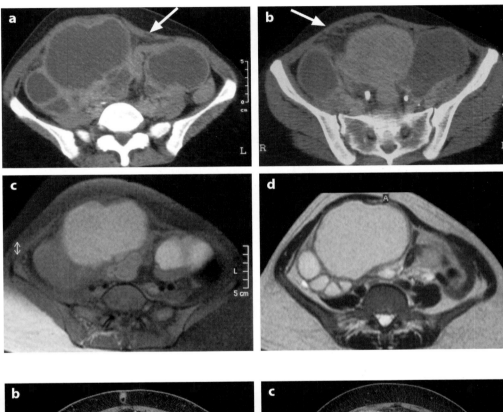

Fig. 32.33 Pyosalpinx and infected endometriomas in a 40-year-old woman who complained of fever and pelvic pain. (**a, b**) CT scan shows multilocular cystic masses with peritoneal fat infiltration (*arrows*). (**c**) T1 and (**d**) T2 MRI show part of the mass to be hyperintense on T1 corresponding to infected endometriomas at surgery and a posterior part multilocular hypointense on T1 and hyperintense on T2 corresponding to a pyosalpinx at surgery. No communication between the pyosalpinx and the cysts was seen either at surgery or at pathology. The culture grew in *Escherichia coli*

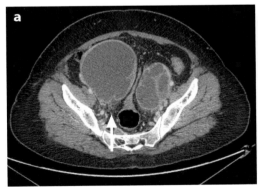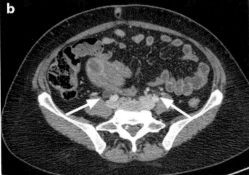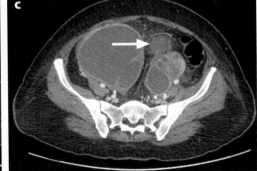

Fig. 32.34 Infected endometriomas with secondary rupture in a 45-year-old woman who complained of fever and pelvic pain during menstruations: (**a**) CT scan shows multilocular cystic mass with slightly dense content (18–25 HU). Slight peritoneal fat infiltration is seen against some area of the cyst (*arrow*). (**b**) The ureters are slightly dilated (*arrows*) abutting against the masses. Despite antibiotic treatment, she developed lumbar pain, and a double J was installed bilaterally. (**c**) Repeated CT scan shows rupture of the cyst and extravasation of dense material (*arrow*). Peritoneal fat infiltration is also more prominent. Surgery disclosed infected endometriomas with a frozen pelvis and ureter infiltration. Hysterectomy and bilateral annexectomy were performed. Salpingitis was present, but no communication between the tubes and the cysts was seen either at surgery or at pathology. The culture grew in *Escherichia coli* (Courtesy of Dr Lina Menassa-Moussa)

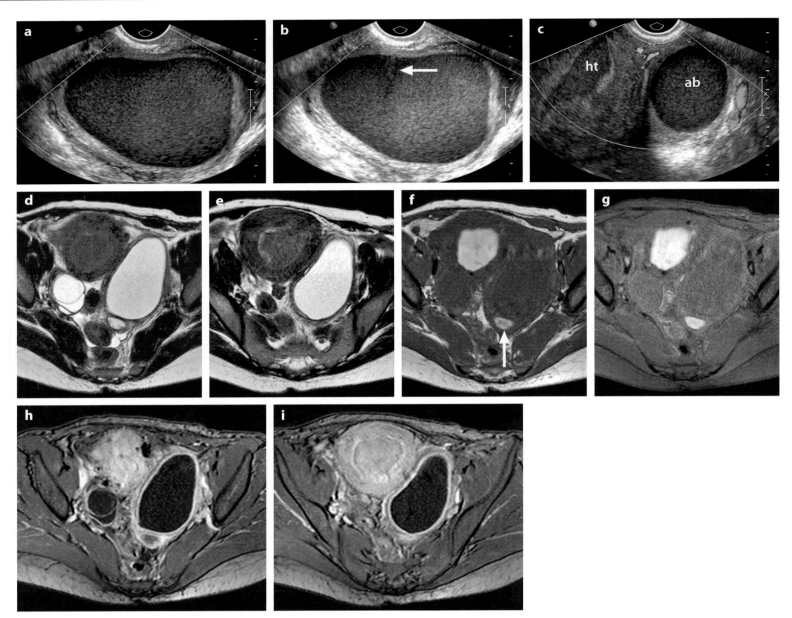

Fig. 32.35 Ovarian abscess in a 39-year-old woman with history of several genital infection and hematometra secondary to cervical stenosis. (**a**) Transvaginal US discloses a 7.3 cm homogeneously echoic cyst with avascular content on Doppler US. (**b**) Care must be taken not to confuse Doppler flow artifact (*arrow*) with true vascular flow. (**c**) Hematometra (*ht*) is also seen; abscess (*ab*). (**d** and **e**) T2-weighted axial images show a right ovary containing several large follicles and the left ovarian abscess that is hyperintense. A small peritoneal effusion is also present. (**f** and **g**) T1-weighted axial images with and without fat suppression at the same level show the hematometra (*ht*) to be hyperintense as well as a left corpus luteum (*arrow*) also seen on T2. (**h** and **i**) T1-weighted fat suppression images with contrast uptake confirm absence of enhancement in the abscess and the right follicles. The wall of the corpus luteum is convoluted. Surgery confirmed the above findings

Most primary infections are bacterial, and the most incriminated organisms were Salmonella and Escherichia coli, but other types of infection may be present. A special case is echinococcosis. The ovary is a rare localization of this parasitic infection that involves mostly the liver, but primary or secondary hydatid cysts have occasionally been described in endemic areas [47, 48]. The diagnosis may be suspected in case of previous ruptured hydatid cyst and another localization or in the presence of daughter cysts or floating membrane [47]. However, even in case of high clinical suspicion of echinococcosis, one must be careful not to confuse on ultrasound daughter cysts and floating membranes with intracystic material in dermoid cyst; CT scan or MRI by showing fat can easily make the diagnosis of mature cystic teratoma that is much more frequent even in endemic areas [49, 50].

32.7 Fistula

Although rare, a fistula between a primary ovarian mass and adjacent structure can be present as a consequence of abscess rupture, benign or malignant tumor growth, endometriosis, or an extraovarian process such as diverticulitis. The fistula is usually between the cyst and the intestine or the cyst and the bladder, but involvement of the uterus or the vagina has also been described [38, 51–54].

Radiological description of this complication is even rarer. Most authors had emphasized on the role of contrast enema in entero-cystic fistula [52, 55]. Radiological findings may be absent (Figs. 32.33 and 32.34).

Fistula, not involving the primary tumor, can be seen in ovarian cancer as a complication of surgery, radiotherapy, or intraperitoneal catheter for chemotherapy [56–58].

32.8 Hernia

Metastatic lesions of an ovarian tumor may be found in inguinal hernia, but herniation of an ovarian tumor is rare [59–62]. An umbilical hernia may also harbor these lesions [63, 64]. Incarceration of such lesions has been occasionally described [65, 66]. Rare cases of internal herniation through the broad ligament have been reported [67].

Radiological descriptions are rare. In female children, differential diagnosis by ultrasound is possible between an inguinal hernia containing normal ovary and tube and a hydrocele of the canal of Nuck [68].

References

1. Abolmakarem H, Tharmaratnum S, Thilaganathan B (2001) Fetal anemia as a consequence of hemorrhage into an ovarian cyst. Ultrasound Obstet Gynecol 17(6):527–528
2. Adamsbaum C, Metsdagh P, Andre C, Rocourt N, Robert Y (2000) Cystic ovarian pathology excepting genital activity. J Radiol 81(12 Suppl):1789–1797
3. Kirkinen P, Jouppila P (1985) Perinatal aspects of pregnancy complicated by fetal ovarian cyst. J Perinat Med 13(5):245–251
4. Suita S, Handa N, Nakano H (1992) Antenatally detected ovarian cysts – a therapeutic dilemma. Early Hum Dev 29(1–3):363–367
5. Hann LE, Lui DM, Shi W, Bach AM, Selland DL, Castiel M (2000) Adnexal masses in women with breast cancer: US findings with clinical and histopathologic correlation. Radiology 216(1):242–247
6. Lee KR, Young RH (2003) The distinction between primary and metastatic mucinous carcinomas of the ovary: gross and histologic findings in 50 cases. Am J Surg Pathol 27(3):281–292
7. Hayes MC, Scully RE (1987) Ovarian steroid cell tumors (not otherwise specified). A clinicopathological analysis of 63 cases. Am J Surg Pathol 11(11):835–845
8. Jaworski RC, Boadle R, Greg J, Cocks P (2001) Peritoneal "melanosis" associated with a ruptured ovarian dermoid cyst: report of a case with electron-probe energy dispersive X-ray analysis. Int J Gynecol Pathol 20(4):386–389
9. Muller AM, Sondgen D, Strunz R, Muller KM (2002) Gliomatosis peritonei: a report of two cases and review of the literature. Eur J Obstet Gynecol Reprod Biol 100(2):213–222
10. Levy AD, Shaw JC, Sobin LH (2009) Secondary tumors and tumorlike lesions of the peritoneal cavity: imaging features with pathologic correlation. Radiographics 29(2):347–373
11. Bider D, Ben-Rafael Z, Goldenberg M, Shalev J, Mashiach S (1989) Pregnancy outcome after unwinding of twisted ischaemic-haemorrhagic adnexa. Br J Obstet Gynaecol 96(4):428–430
12. Shalev J, Goldenberg M, Oelsner G, Ben-Rafael Z, Bider D, Blankstein J, Mashiach S (1989) Treatment of twisted ischemic adnexa by simple detorsion. N Engl J Med 321(8):546
13. Aziz D, Davis V, Allen L, Langer JC (2004) Ovarian torsion in children: is oophorectomy necessary? J Pediatr Surg 39(5):750–753
14. Abes M, Sarihan H (2004) Oophoropexy in children with ovarian torsion. Eur J Pediatr Surg 14(3):168–171
15. Ghossain MA, Hachem K, Aoun NJ, Haddad-Zebouni S, Mansour F, Suidan JS, Abboud J (2006) Spontaneous detorsion of the ovary: can it be diagnosed by MRI? J Magn Reson Imaging 24(4):880–885
16. Ghossain MA, Hachem K, Buy JN, Hourany-Rizk RG, Aoun NJ, Haddad-Zebouni S, Mansour F, Attieh E, Abboud J (2004) Adnexal torsion: magnetic resonance findings in the viable adnexa with emphasis on stromal ovarian appearance. J Magn Reson Imaging 20(3):451–462
17. Hall BP, Printz DA, Roth J (1993) Massive ovarian edema: ultrasound and MR characteristics. J Comput Assist Tomogr 17(3):477–479
18. Umesaki N, Tanaka T, Miyama M, Nishimura S, Kawamura N, Ogita S (2000) Successful preoperative diagnosis of massive ovarian edema aided by comparative imaging study using magnetic resonance and ultrasound. Eur J Obstet Gynecol Reprod Biol 89(1):97–99
19. Ghossain MA, Buy JN, Bazot M, Haddad S, Guinet C, Malbec L, Hugol D, Truc JB, Poitout P, Vadrot D (1994) CT in adnexal torsion with emphasis on tubal findings: correlation with US. J Comput Assist Tomogr 18(4):619–625
20. Kim YH, Cho KS, Ha HK, Byun JY, Auh YH, Rhim HC, Shim JC, Cha SJ, Hur G (1999) CT features of torsion of benign cystic teratoma of the ovary. J Comput Assist Tomogr 23(6):923–928
21. Shalev J, Mashiach R, Bar-Hava I, Girtler O, Bar J, Dicker D, Meizner I (2001) Subtorsion of the ovary: sonographic features and clinical management. J Ultrasound Med 20(8):849–854; quiz 856
22. Kupesic S, Plavsic BM (2010) Adnexal torsion: color Doppler and three-dimensional ultrasound. Abdom Imaging 35(5):602–606
23. Jain KA (1995) Magnetic resonance imaging findings in ovarian torsion. Magn Reson Imaging 13(1):111–113
24. Bader T, Ranner G, Haberlik A (1996) Torsion of a normal adnexa in a premenarcheal girl: MRI findings. Eur Radiol 6(5):704–706
25. Kawahara Y, Fukuda T, Futagawa S, Sakamoto I, Takao M, Kinoshita Y, Hayashi K (1996) Intravascular gas within an ovarian tumor: a CT sign of ovarian torsion. J Comput Assist Tomogr 20(1):154–156
26. Ghossain MA, Buy JN, Sciot C, Jacob D, Hugol D, Vadrot D (1997) CT findings before and after adnexal torsion: rotation of a focal solid element of a cystic adjunctive sign in diagnosis. AJR Am J Roentgenol 169(5):1343–1346
27. Kimura I, Togashi K, Kawakami S, Takakura K, Mori T, Konishi J (1994) Ovarian torsion: CT and MR imaging appearances. Radiology 190(2):337–341
28. Warnock NG, Brown BP, Barloon TJ, Hemann LS (1994) Spontaneous detorsion of the ovary demonstrated by ultrasonography. J Ultrasound Med 13(1):57–59
29. Guerriero S, Ajossa S, Caffiero A, Mais V (1995) Relationship between abnormally high levels of plasma CA 125 and resolution of acute pelvic pain in two women with endometrioma. Gynecol Obstet Invest 40(1):61–63
30. Scully RE, Young RH, Clement PB (1998) Tumor-like lesions. In: Rosai J, Sobin LH (eds) Tumors of the ovary, maldeveloped gonads, fallopian tube, and broad ligament, vol 23. Armed Forces Institute of Pathology, Washington, pp 409–450
31. Clement PB (2002) Nonneoplastic lesions of the ovary. In: Kurman RJ (ed) Blaustein's pathology of the female genital tract, 5th edn. Springer, New-York, pp 675–727
32. Kramer LA, Lalani T, Kawashima A (1997) Massive edema of the ovary: high resolution MR findings using a phased-array pelvic coil. J Magn Reson Imaging 7(4):758–760
33. Haque TL, Togashi K, Kobayashi H, Fujii S, Konishi J (2000) Adnexal torsion: MR imaging findings of viable ovary. Eur Radiol 10(12):1954–1957
34. Young RH, Scully RE (1984) Fibromatosis and massive edema of the ovary, possibly related entities: a report of 14 cases of fibromatosis and 11 cases of massive edema. Int J Gynecol Pathol 3(2):153–178
35. Russell P, Farnsworth A (1997) Massive edema and fibromatosis. In: Russell P, Farnsworth A et al (eds) Surgical pathology of the ovaries. Churchill Livingstone, New York, pp 147–154
36. Kilickesmez O, Tasdelen N, Yetimoglu B, Kayhan A, Cihangiroglu M, Gurmen N (2009) Diffusion-weighted imaging of adnexal torsion. Emerg Radiol 16(5):399–401
37. Fujii S, Kaneda S, Kakite S, Kanasaki Y, Matsusue E, Harada T, Kaminou T, Ogawa T (2011) Diffusion-weighted imaging findings of adnexal torsion: initial results. Eur J Radiol 77(2):330–334
38. Zarain Garcia F (1974) Cystic teratoma of the ovary associated with abscess and vaginal fistula. Ginecol Obstet Mex 36(213):49–53
39. Reina J, Borrell N (1991) Infection of a neoplastic ovarian cyst caused by Salmonella enterica subspecies enterica, serotype Enteritidis. Enferm Infecc Microbiol Clin 9(3):185–186
40. Hsueh PR, Hwang CC, Yen KP, Lin M, Young C (1992) Abscess formation complicated in ovarian mucinous cystadenoma: a case report. Kansenshogaku Zasshi 66(3):416–420
41. Wan YL, Chen WJ, Chien CC, Lee TY, Tsai CC (1993) Ovarian dermoid cyst associated with tuberculosis, cystadenoma and torsion. J Formos Med Assoc 92(9):851–853

42. Yoshida M, Katsuragawa H, Miyamoto U, Ohnishi S, Katsura Y (1993) Estrogen-producing ovarian adenocarcinoma with large abscess formation. Gynecol Obstet Invest 35(4):245–248

43. Burgmans JP, van Erp EJ, Brimicombe RW, Kazzaz BA (1997) Salmonella enteritidis in an endometriotic ovarian cyst. Eur J Obstet Gynecol Reprod Biol 72(2):207–211

44. Liu Z, Lang J, Huang R, Li B, Zhang L (1998) Secondary infection of the ovarian endometriotic cysts. Zhongguo Yi Xue Ke Xue Yuan Xue Bao 20(1):49–53

45. Matsubayashi T, Hamajima T, Asano K, Mizukami A, Seguchi M, Kohno C, Inukai K, Tobayama S (2001) Salmonella infection of an ovarian dermoid cyst. Pediatr Int 43(2):164–165

46. Le Bouedec G, Raynaud F, Glowaczower E, Quibant A, Dauplat J (1993) Ovarian abscess. A case of a dermoid cyst with a secondary infection. Rev Fr Gynecol Obstet 88(1):23–26

47. Hiller N, Zagal I, Hadas-Halpern I (2000) Echinococcal ovarian cyst. A case report. J Reprod Med 45(3):224–226

48. Konar K, Ghosh S, Konar S, Bhattacharya S, Sarkar S (2001) Bilateral ovarian hydatid disease – an unusual case. Indian J Pathol Microbiol 44(4):495–496

49. El Fortia M, Elhajaji E, Elmadani B, Khalil M, Eldergash O, Elhamroush H (2006) Are they spherules of ovarian cystic teratoma or daughter cysts of echinococcosis? Ultraschall Med 27(6):582–584

50. Gurel H, Gurel SA (2008) Ovarian cystic teratoma with a pathognomonic appearance of multiple floating balls: a case report and investigation of common characteristics of the cases in the literature. Fertil Steril 90(5):2008.e17–2009.e17

51. Floberg J, Backdahl M, Silfersward C, Thomassen PA (1984) Postpartum perforation of the colon due to endometriosis. Acta Obstet Gynecol Scand 63(2):183–184

52. Shiels WE, Dueno F, Hernandez E (1986) Ovarian dermoid cyst complicated by an entero-ovarian fistula. Radiology 160(2):443–444

53. Allimant P, Bietiger M, Attipou L, Rosburger C, Babini E, Zeyer B, Dalcher G (1990) Sigmoid perforation in an ovarian cyst. J Chir (Paris) 127(11):559–560

54. Skipper D, Moran B, Dormandy JA, Heald RJ (1995) Two cases of colo-ovarian cyst fistula. Int J Colorectal Dis 10(2):70–72

55. Landmann DD, Lewis RW (1988) Benign cystic ovarian teratoma with colorectal involvement. Report of a case and review of the literature. Dis Colon Rectum 31(10):808–813

56. Chamberlain RS, Kaufman HL, Danforth DN (1998) Enterocutaneous fistula in cancer patients: etiology, management, outcome, and impact on further treatment. Am Surg 64(12):1204–1211

57. Takai N, Utsunomiya H, Kawano Y, Nasu K, Narahara H, Miyakawa I (2002) Complete response to radiation therapy in a patient with chemotherapy-resistant ovarian clear cell adenocarcinoma. Arch Gynecol Obstet 267(2):98–100

58. Milczek T, Emerich J, Klasa-Mazurkiewicz D (2003) Surgical complications connected with intraperitoneal chemotherapy in ovarian cancer. Ginekol Pol 74(9):817–823

59. Nicholson CP, Donohue JH, Thompson GB, Lewis JE (1992) A study of metastatic cancer found during inguinal hernia repair. Cancer 69(12):3008–3011

60. van Heesewijk HP, Smit FW, Heitbrink MA, Kok FP (1990) Herniation of an ovarian cyst through the inguinal canal: diagnosis with CT. AJR Am J Roentgenol 154(1):202–203

61. Prasad KR, Aruna C, Saheb DA (1993) Primary leiomyoma of ovary. Indian J Med Sci 47(2):39–41

62. Takeuchi K, Tsuzuki Y, Ando T, Sekihara M, Hara T, Kori T, Kawakami T, Ohno Y, Kuwano H (2003) Malignant mixed Mullerian tumor of the ovary growing into an inguinal hernia sac: report of a case. Surg Today 33(10):797–800

63. Millar RC, Geelhoed GW, Ketcham AS (1975) Ovarian cancer presenting as umbilical hernia. J Surg Oncol 7(6):493–496

64. Wolfson N, Graves K, Pastorek JG 2nd, Suleman M (1991) Benign cystic teratoma manifested as an umbilical hernia. South Med J 84(3):405

65. Slizovskii GV, Sigailo ZS (1990) Ovarian polycystosis in a strangulated inguinal hernia in a newborn infant. Vestn Khir Im I I Grek 145(11):99–100

66. Poenaru D, Jacobs DA, Kamal I (1999) Unusual findings in the inguinal canal: a report of four cases. Pediatr Surg Int 15(7):515–516

67. Demir H, Scoccia B (2010) Internal herniation of adnexa through a defect of the broad ligament: case report and literature review. J Minim Invasive Gynecol 17(1):110–112

68. Huang CS, Luo CC, Chao HC, Chu SM, Yu YJ, Yen JB (2003) The presentation of asymptomatic palpable movable mass in female inguinal hernia. Eur J Pediatr 162(7–8):493–495

Pelvic Inflammatory Disease (PID)

Part 8

33.3.3 Ovarian Involvement

33.3.3.1 Tubo-Ovarian Abscess (TOA)

Ovarian involvement by PID is almost always secondary to salpingitis and typically takes the form of a tubo-ovarian abscess [18]. Inadequately treated PID may lead to unilateral or bilateral TOA [4]. Unfortunately, clinical symptoms secondary to uncomplicated salpingitis and TOA are often similar and up to 20% of patients with TOA lack clinical signs of infection [19].

Macroscopic and Radiologic Findings

They are summarized in Table 33.4.

Table 33.4 Macroscopic and radiologic findings of TOA

– Uni- or bilateral
– Tubular or round shape
– Most commonly cystic
– Uni- or multilocular or multicystic
– 7–12 cm
– Thickened wall, irregular margins
– Complete or incomplete septa
– Rarely, mostly solid

Vascular Findings

Two types of findings: angiogenesis and increase of the vascular permeability are responsible for characteristic findings on DCT or DMR.

US Findings

Morphologic Findings

The most common appearance is an adnexal mass including the tube and the ovary. The shape may be roughly round or oval or tubular. It looks hypoechoic and homogeneous sometimes with a ground-glass pattern resembling an endometrioma (Figs. 33.1, 33.9, 33.10, and 33.12) or complex. The margins are regular or irregular. Posterior acoustic enhancement can be present.

Ultrasound Patterns

Internal echoes (with or without septations), fluid-debris levels [4] can be present. Prominent echogenic foci related to gas can be displayed.

Color Doppler

It usually allows distinction of complex fluid component from tissular masses.

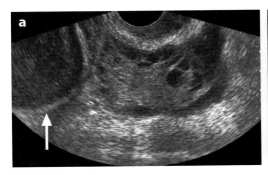
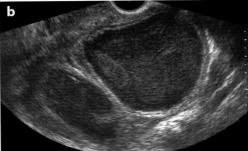
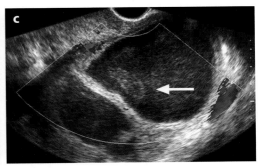

Fig. 33.9 Right TOA resembling endometriosis on US. A 26-year-old woman with asthenia and inflammatory syndrome. Longitudinal EVS (**a**) displays a right tubal collection (*arrow*) in front of a normal left ovary. EVS (**b**) with color Doppler (**c**): multiple collections of fluid of diffuse homogeneous low echogenicity associated with hyperechogenic foci (*arrow*) resembling clots highly suggest an endometrioma (**c**). However, hypervascularization in the wall of the collection is unusual in endometriosis (**c**)

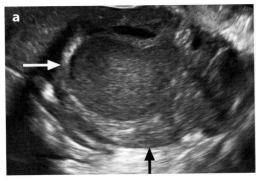
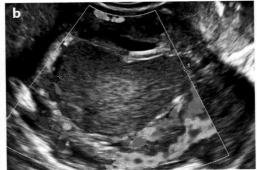
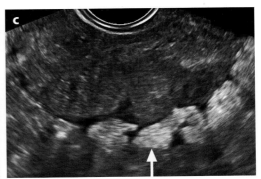

Fig. 33.10 Tubo-ovarian abscess. Thirty-two year-old woman. After a hysteroscopy for suspicion of hyperplasia of the endometrium, left pelvic pain, fever, RCP 106, increase white cell count 11,000/ml. (**a, b**) Transversal EVS of the left adnexa without (**a**) and with Doppler (**b**) display: (1) in the ovary a collection with a ground-glass pattern (*white arrow*), containing however a more echogenic central portion; (2) next to its superior and medial border a tubal collection is visualized (*black arrow*). A hypervascularization in the wall of the ovarian and the tubal collection is depicted. Association of these findings is typical for a TOA. (**c**) On a transverse view of the uterus and adnexa, the mesosigmoid looks thickened and echogenic (*arrow*), with some peritoneal fluid due to peritoneal reaction. Prospective diagnosis: TOA with peritonitis. Coelioscopy: left TOA with an inflammatory tube wrapping around the ovarian abscess. Adhesion to the sigmoid. Inflammatory adhesions in the Douglas

Associated Findings

There is often purulent complex fluid within the cul-de-sac of Douglas or the peritoneal cavity [4].

However, TOA can be difficult to distinguish from other adnexal masses:

- Ovarian carcinoma.
- A benign epithelial tumor.
- Endometrioma; hemorrhagic cyst.

Drainage

US is not only valuable in the diagnosis of TOA but also has a therapeutic role in the management. US-guided abscess drainage, either aspiration alone or catheter placement, has been shown to speed recovery in conjunction with antibiotic therapy [4, 20].

CT Findings (Figs. 33.11 and 33.12)

1. On the noncontrast CT: The density of the cystic content is usually higher than urine. The most specific sign of abscess is the presence of gas [21], but this sign is unusual in TOA. It was absent in all cases of Wilbur's series [22] and was present in only 1/9 cases of Ellis' series [23].

2. On the dynamic CT:
   - At the arterial phase (20 s after the beginning of IV injection), thin regular vessels are displayed in the wall and the septa.
   - 30 s after injection, contrast uptake is already visualized in the wall and septa.
   - At the parenchymal phase (40 s after injection), a significant contrast uptake more than double compared to the noncontrast CT is visualized in the wall and septa.
   - On the following phases, a plateau curve of contrast uptake is displayed.

3. On the delayed CT, accumulation of contrast is visualized in the wall and septa. Diffusion of contrast in the area of ovarian parenchyma surrounding the abscess is very likely related to inflammation surrounding the abscess.

   CT is particularly useful to evaluate complications:
   - In case of bladder fistula (Fig. 33.13).
   - In case of perforation with peritonitis (Fig. 33.14).

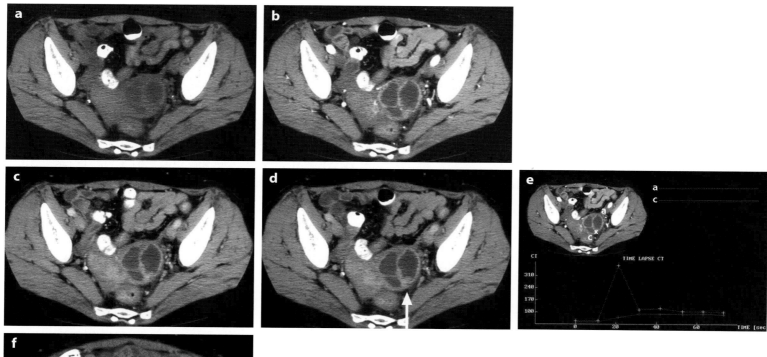

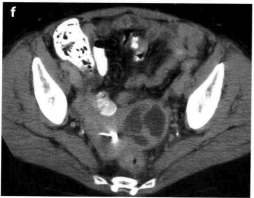

Fig. 33.11 Typical TOA on the dynamic CT with IUD. CT without injection (**a**) and at the arterial phase (**b**) depict three contiguous collections in the right ovary with regular vessels in the walls. Thirty second after injection (**c**) and moreover 60 s after injection (**d**), a significant contrast uptake with diffusion of contrast is visualized in the walls of the abscesses (*arrow*). Evolution of contrast uptake is shown on the ROC curve (**e**). Presence of an IUD in the uterus (**f**)

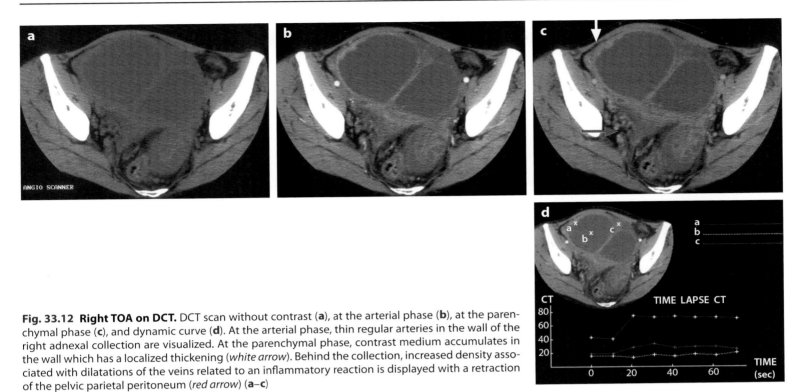

Fig. 33.12 Right TOA on DCT. DCT scan without contrast (**a**), at the arterial phase (**b**), at the parenchymal phase (**c**), and dynamic curve (**d**). At the arterial phase, thin regular arteries in the wall of the right adnexal collection are visualized. At the parenchymal phase, contrast medium accumulates in the wall which has a localized thickening (*white arrow*). Behind the collection, increased density associated with dilatations of the veins related to an inflammatory reaction is displayed with a retraction of the pelvic parietal peritoneum (*red arrow*) (**a–c**)

Fig. 33.13 Bilateral tuboovarian abscess with bladder fistula. TAS (**a**) displays a bilateral echogenic adnexal mass. On EVS of the right (**b**) and of the left (**c**) masses multiple hyperechogenic dots are seen at the periphery of the right mass and in the middle of the left mass suggesting the presence of air. Color Doppler of the left mass (**d**) confirms its cystic nature, associated with a peripheral rim of vascularization very suggestive of an abscess. DCT without injection

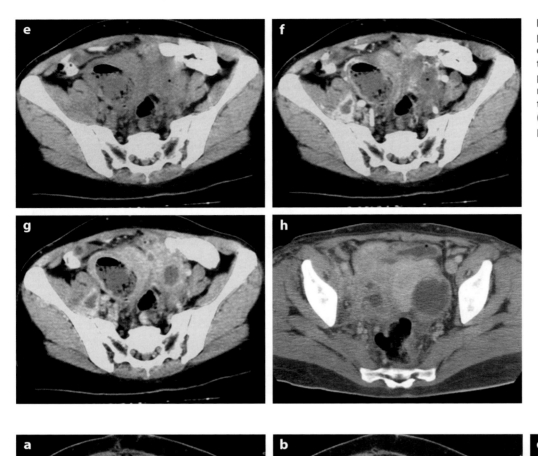

Fig. 33.13 (*continued*) (**e**) definitely confirms the presence of air in both masses and therefore the diagnosis of abscess. At the arterial phase (**f**) a typical peripheral arterial vascularization is displayed with a progressive diffusion of contrast medium in the wall at the venous phase (**g**).On the delayed CT performed at a little lower level (**h**) air is visualized in the bladder indicating the presence of a bladder fistula

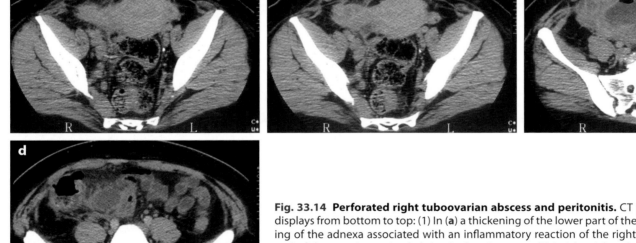

Fig. 33.14 Perforated right tuboovarian abscess and peritonitis. CT performed after IV contrast displays from bottom to top: (1) In (**a**) a thickening of the lower part of the adnexa. (2) In (**b**) a thickening of the adnexa associated with an inflammatory reaction of the right parietal pelvic peritoneum and of the anterior parietal abdominal peritoneum. (3) In (**c**) a right adnexal mass with a thickened wall containing an air fluid level related to an abscess, with an inflammatory reaction of the peritoneum in front of the mass. (4) In (**d**) a marked inflammatory reaction of the anterior and of the posterior parietal peritoneum and a thickening of the medial wall of the caecum are displayed. Preoperative diagnosis: tuboovarian abscess complicated with peritonitis. Coelioscopy confirmed the diagnosis and displayed a tiny rupture of the collection

MR Findings (Figs. 33.15 and 33.16)

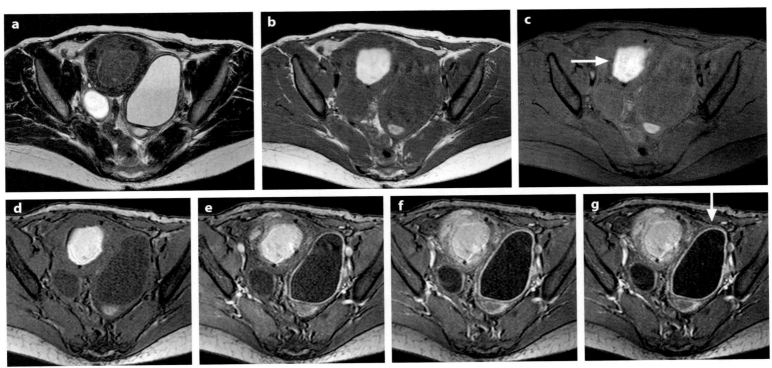

Fig. 33.15 Left tuboovarian abscess with pyometria. Axial T2W (**a**), axial T1W (**b**), T1W fat suppression (**c**) display (1) in the left ovary a cystic mass with a high signal on T2, a signal identical to pelvic muscle on T1 and low signal on fat suppression, (2) at the posterior part of the left ovary a corpus luteum with a hyperintense signal on T2, T1, and T1 fat suppression; (3) in the endometrial cavity a collection with a high signal on T1 and T1 fat sup-pression (*arrow* in **c**) and a low signal on T2 related to a retention of pus. DMR without injection (**d**), at the arterial phase (**e**) depict a regular rim of enhance-ment in the wall, with a slight diffusion of contrast at the venous phase (**f**) and on the delayed phase (**g**) (*arrows* in **g**); these findings are typical for an ovarian abscess. In the right ovary, functional hemorrhagic cyst

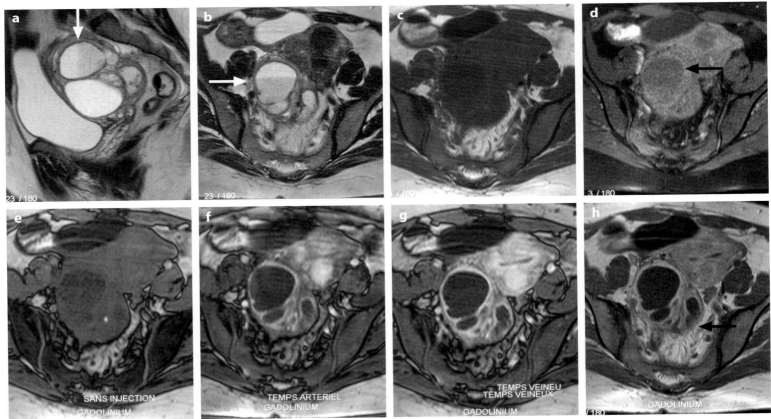

Fig. 33.16 Right tubo-ovarian abscess. (**a, b**) MR sagittal (**a**) and axial (**b**) T2W images: right multicystic adnexal mass with fluid level (*arrow*) in one of the collections. (**c, d**) Axial T1W (**c**) and fat suppression (**d**) images: intensity of the cystic content is like pelvic muscle; in one collection the wall is slightly hyperintense (*arrow*). (**e–h**) Dynamic axial MR before injection (**e**), at the arterial (**f**), parenchymal (**g**), and late (**h**) phases. A significant contrast uptake is displayed at the arterial phase in the wall of the fluid collections. Contrast uptake increases at the parenchymal phase. It persists on the delayed MR and contrast diffuses in the stroma (*arrow*)

The Abscess

The Cystic Content

The signal intensity of the fluid is variable according to its viscosity or protein concentration [16].

On T1W images: the cystic components most commonly have signal characteristics equal close to pelvic muscle. Rarely signal intensity is similar to blood [24].

On fat suppression, signal intensity can be very high like in endometriosis (Fig. 33.17).

On T2W images: signal intensity is hyperintense equal or superior to urine, homogeneous or heterogeneous [19]. Shading of a hypointense area mostly in the peripheral portion of the abscess is commonly present [19].

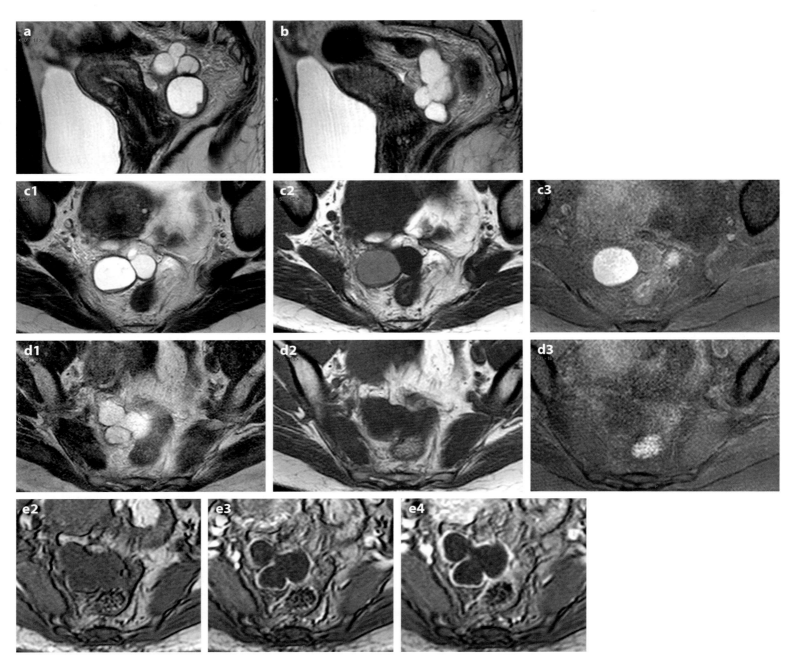

Fig. 33.17 TOA. Fifty-year-old woman. Menopause without hormonal replacement. Right pelvic pain for 2 months. MR sagittal T2 (**a**, **b**) display in (**a**) a right adnexal mass with two different components : a tubular structure related to a dilatation of the tube and a round cystic mass with a fluid level (**a**). Both collections seem to communicate on (**b**). Axial T2 (**c1**), T1 (**c2**) and fat suppression (**c3**) of the round cystic mass display a high signal intensity on T2 (**c1**), an intermediate signal on T1 (between muscle and adipose tissue), and a high signal on fat suppression. Axial T2 (**d1**), T1 (**d2**), and fat suppression (**d3**) of the tubular collection display a high signal on T2, and low signal on T1 and on fat suppression. On DMR, at the arterial phase (**e2**), depict regular arterial vessels in the wall of the collections, at the venous phase (**e3**) a high contrast uptake which increases significantly on the delayed (**e4**) with an ill defined outer border. This type of contrast enhancement is typical for a TOA. Prospective diagnosis: right TOA. Definite diagnosis: coelioscopy confirmed the diagnosis

The Wall

On microscopy, the wall consists of two layers:

- An outer layer of fibrosis.
- An inner layer of granulation tissue massively infiltrated by lymphocytes, histiocytes, and plasma cells [19].

The inner layer appears as a thin rim from 1 to 3 mm in thickness in the innermost portion, hyperintense or of intermediate signal on T1 (Fig. 33.18), hypointense on T2, with contrast uptake [19]. This finding has been observed in 8/9 cases in Ha's series. The hyperintensity within the layer on T1W may be attributed to focal areas of fresh hemorrhage. This finding is different from a thin inner rim in endometrial cyst caused by hemosiderin-laden macrophages; in this case, the rim is hypointense on T1 and T2W images [19]; it slightly enhances after contrast.

A capsule surrounding the abscess of low intensity, mainly visualized on T2W images, was seen in 4/10 cases in Wall's series. Although this finding did not have any pathologic correlation, it could be related to fibrosis in the outer wall.

DMR at the arterial phase displays regular arterial vessels in the wall. At the venous phase, a significant contrast uptake is visualized in the wall. On the delayed phases, accumulation of contrast medium in the wall and the surrounding parenchyma is visualized. These findings are very typical for an abscess (Fig. 33.17).

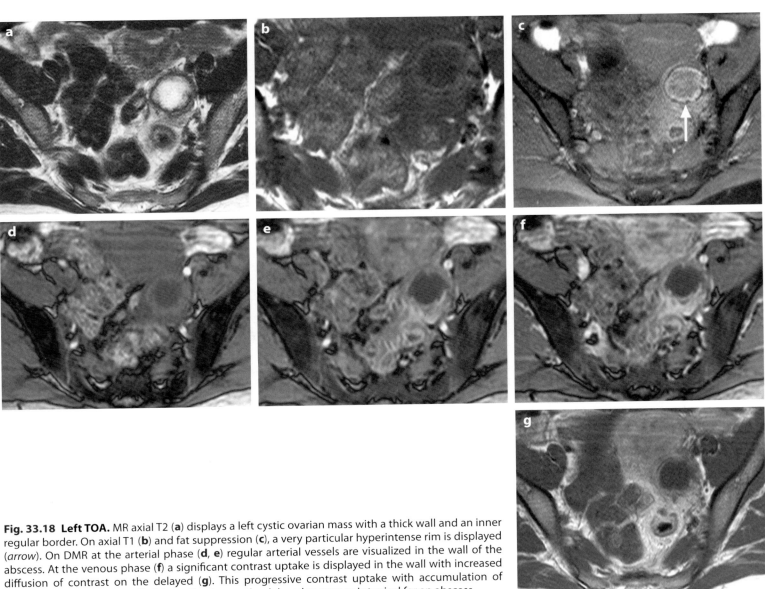

Fig. 33.18 Left TOA. MR axial T2 (**a**) displays a left cystic ovarian mass with a thick wall and an inner regular border. On axial T1 (**b**) and fat suppression (**c**), a very particular hyperintense rim is displayed (*arrow*). On DMR at the arterial phase (**d**, **e**) regular arterial vessels are visualized in the wall of the abscess. At the venous phase (**f**) a significant contrast uptake is displayed in the wall with increased diffusion of contrast on the delayed (**g**). This progressive contrast uptake with accumulation of contrast medium in the wall of the collection on the delayed sequence is typical for an abscess

Secondary Changes in the Adjacent Pelvic Structures

Mesh-like networks or strands in the pelvic fat planes or along the US ligaments related to dense adhesions at surgery were seen in all cases in Ha's series [19]. They appear as isointense on T1W, hypointense on T2W and densely enhance after IV injection.

Solid Forms

In some cases, the lesion is mainly solid (Fig. 33.19).

A pseudotumoral form can be seen in actinomycosis (Fig. 33.20).

Rarely a chronic ovarian abscess may result in a solid tumor-like mass, variably designated ovarian xanthogranuloma or inflammatory pseudotumor [25]. The involved ovary in such cases is replaced by a solid yellow lobulated mass.

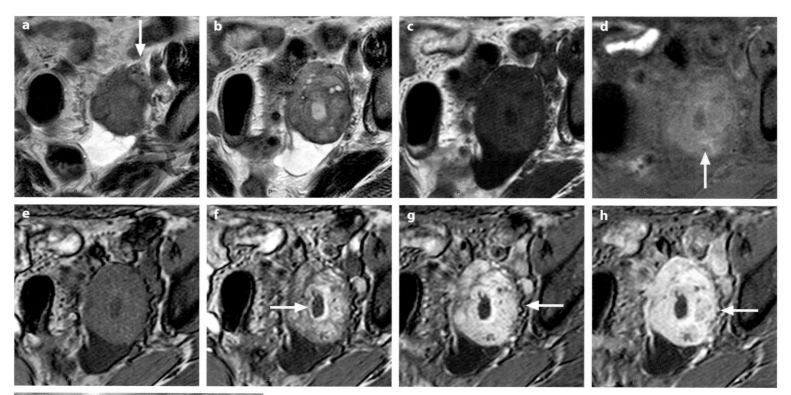

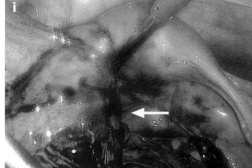

Fig. 33.19 Solid pattern of tubo-ovarian abscess. Forty-two-year-old woman; left pelvic pain, fever, white discharge for a month, and increased white cell count. (**a, b**) MR axial T2 (**a, b**) display a left mainly tissular ovarian mass containing small cystic areas, pushing normal ovarian parenchyma forward (**a**) (*arrow*) with adhesion on its medial border with the sigmoid (**b**). (**c, d**) On axial T1 (**c**), signal intensity of the mass is close to pelvic muscle. On T1 fat suppression (**d**), slight hyperintensity and especially a focal hyperintense area in the posterior part of the mass are visualized (*arrow*). (**e–h**) On DMR without injection (**e**) and at the arterial phase (**f**) depict regular arterial vessels in the central part of the mass around the cystic cavities (*arrow*) and at the periphery. At the venous phase (**g**), a marked contrast enhancement is visualized in the parenchyma (*arrow*), which involves the entire mass and is even more pronounced on the delayed phase (**h**) (*arrow*). Such diffusion of contrast enhancement highly suggests the diagnosis of an abscess. (**i**) At coelioscopy, a left tubo-ovarian abscess was excised (*arrow*)

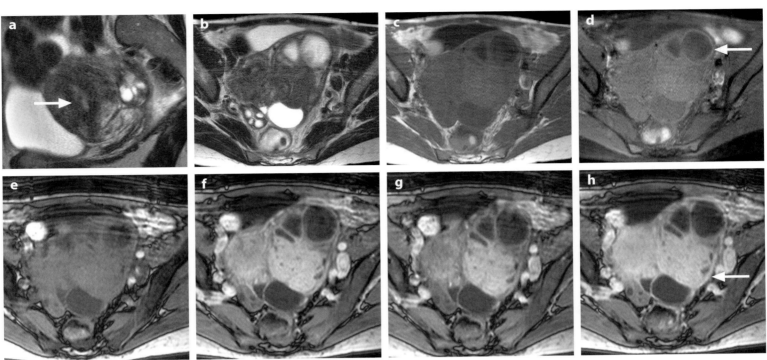

Fig. 33.20 Pseudotumoral form of abscess in actinomycosis. A 41-year-old woman with an IUD. A pelvic mass is discovered during a routine examination. CA 125 is 18 IU/ml. On US, a mixed ovarian mass with a hypervascularized solid portion is displayed. (**a–d**) Sagittal (**a**) and axial (**b**) T2W images, axial T1W (**c**), and T1 fast suppression (**d**). Some debris are present in the uterine cavity very likely related to endometritis in **a** (*arrow*). In the left adnexal mass the ovarian mass is not separated from the tube. The mass is mainly tissular. It contains cystic portions that are outlined by a thin hyperintense layer on the inner wall better visualized on the fat suppression (*arrow*). However, differential diagnosis with an ovarian carcinoma is discussed. Right ovary looks normal. (**e–h**) DMR on the noncontrast (**e**) and at the arterial phase (**f**) does not display tumoral arterial vessels. At the parenchymal phase (**g**), an intense contrast uptake is depicted in the solid tissue and in the walls of the cystic portions. On the delayed MR (**h**), accumulation of contrast persists in these previous areas and contrast diffuses in the neighboring areas (*arrow*)

Mild Forms

Pathology

In inactive PID, histologic and functional consequences of periovarian adhesions have been reported by Quan [26]. Some similarities with PCOD are described:

1. Periovarian fibrosis.
2. Follicular development and ovulation: ovaries have over three times as many developing and atretic follicles as normal subjects and less than one-fifth as many corpora albicantia.

However:

1. The ovary is not conspicuously enlarged.
2. The fibrous covering of the ovary is irregular and formed from extrinsic and newly laid down connective tissue and has a sharp transition with the underlying ovarian stroma. In PCOD, the cortical fibrosis is regular, arises from the ovarian stroma, and blends smoothly with the underlying stroma.
   Thecomatosis of the ovarian stroma is not present.
3. Luteinization of the theca interna in cystic follicles is less frequent than in normal subjects while it is prominent in PCOD.

Ultrasound

In acute PID, inflamed ovaries demonstrate enlargement, indistinct contours, and periovarian thickening or fluid collections [4]. At laparoscopy, sonographic contour indistinctness and periovarian findings corresponded to periovarian exudates and adhesions [4].

Follow-Up

During the healing process, the metabolic demand decreases. The network of the capillaries regress and the scar shrinks. The resistance to flow grows. However, if the infection results in the formation of a chronically infected pyosalpinx, the low-resistance flow remains detectable.

33.3.4 Peritonitis

33.3.4.1 Definitions

Peritoneal Reaction

Serous peritoneal fluid can be present.
Macroscopy: congestion and edema of the peritoneum.
Microscopy: deposits of fibrin on the peritoneum.

Peritonitis

Purulent peritoneal fluid can be present.
Macroscopy: gray white false membranes on the peritoneum.
Microscopy: deposits of fibrin and leukocytes on the peritoneum.

33.3.4.2 US Findings

1. Pelvic fluid
   On US pelvic fluid with internal echoes can be displayed [27].

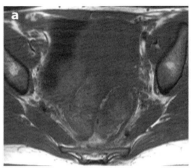
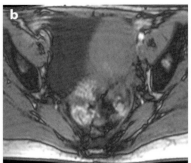
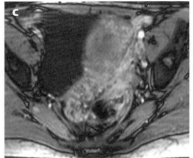
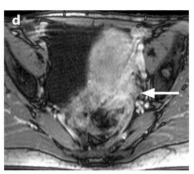

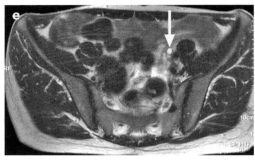

Fig. 33.21 Inflammatory parietal pelvic peritoneum with ureteral obstruction. DMR with non contrast (**a**), at the arterial phase (**b**), at the parenchymal phase (**c**), on the delayed (**d**): thickening of the left USL associated with infiltration of the parietal peritoneum with a significant contrast uptake (*arrow* in **d**). Axial T2W (**e**): Left ureteral dilatation (*arrow*) was very likely related to parietal pelvic peritoneum inflammation

2. Modifications of the peritoneum
   - Fat planes are obliterated between the mass, adjacent bowel loops, and rectosigmoid bladder [23].
   - Echogenicity of the mesos.
   - Anterior displacement and thickening of the mesosalpinx. Because the mesosalpinx normally arches anteriorly and superiorly to the mesovarium, expansion of the ovary or of the mesovarium by inflammatory or neoplastic process displaces the mesosalpinx anteriorly [22]. Although suggestive of adnexal disease, it is not specific for TOA (Fig. 33.2).

33.3.4.3 CT Findings

Three different findings may suggest the presence of peritonitis: (1) a higher density than urine related to the purulent content, (2) debris, and (3) a significant contrast uptake of the peritoneum surrounding the fluid (Figs. 33.2 and 33.14).

33.3.4.4 MR Findings

According to Togashi, MR is more sensitive than US and CT in the diagnosis of peritonitis secondary to PID.
- Peritoneal fluid
  Inflammatory exudates along the uterine and adnexal surfaces and in the CDS display signal intensity equal to or greater than simple fluid on T1 and T2W images.
- Peritoneal thickening
  Inflammatory changes within the pelvic fat, indistinct borders of the pelvic organs, and thickening of the fascial planes are identified on T1W images.
  Sequence of diffusion displays thickening and high signal intensity of the peritoneum.
- Subperitoneal posterior spread of inflammation.
- Uterosacral ligaments
  The uterosacral ligaments are two subperitoneal muscular cords extending from the posterior and superior parts of the cervix to the posterior peritoneum. Posterior extension of PID may cause

thickening of the USL and increase density of the presacral and perirectal fat [22] (Fig. 33.21). USL thickening in conjunction with anterior displacement of the mesosalpinx provides additional evidence for adnexal disease.
- Rectosigmoid involvement
  Because the inflammation and fibrosis associated with TOA tend to spread posteriorly into the perirectal and presacral fat, barium enema frequently shows extrinsic rectosigmoid involvement. The mucosa appears intact with serrated spiculated margins. Phillips [28] found constriction of the sigmoid colon in 28/32 (88%) patients with TOA who had barium enema.
  On CT luminal narrowing, infiltration of perirectal fat and indistinct borders between the pelvic mass and bowel suggest rectosigmoid involvement.
  Fistulous communication between the TOA and sigmoid colon is a rare complication [28].
- Indistinct borders with the uterus [22].
- Ureteral involvement
  The pelvic ureters form the posterior boundary of the ovarian fossa and as such may be compressed in patients with TOA or by the inflammation of the peritoneum. Phillips [28] observed proximal ureter dilatation in 17 (39%) of 44 patients with TOA who had excretory urography (Fig. 33.21).

33.3.5 Vascular Thrombosis

Ovarian vein thrombosis is an uncommon but potentially fatal disorder that most often occurs postpartum but may follow pelvic operations or pelvic trauma or complicate other pelvic disorders such as pelvic inflammatory disease.

The clinical picture may simulate acute appendicitis or pyelonephritis.

The ovarian vein is markedly enlarged, and associated with marked inflammation of the surrounding retroperitoneal tissues.

On color doppler the thrombus is echogenic with absence of color flow. On DCT or DMR, at the venous phase, the ovarian vein is enlarged with an intraluminal defect and a significant contrast enhacement of the wall. The ovary is congested but not infarcted because of the compensation by the arterial vascularization provided by the uterine artery. The thrombus may extend to the inferior vena cava on the right or to the renal vein on the left.

33.3.6 Lomboaortic Lymphadenopathy

The lymphatic drainage of the ovaries and fallopian tubes parallels the gonadal veins. As a result, inflammatory para-aortic lymphadenopathy occurs in the lymph nodes below the renal hila.

33.4 Chronic Manifestations of PID

33.4.1 Chronic Salpingitis (CS) (Fig. 33.22)

The mucosa plicae, secondary to surface fibrin deposition, agglutinate and adhere to one other. Healing and organization then lead to permanent bridging between folds. In the classical case, this results in follicular salpingitis. Often, the height of the plicae is reduced, or their intricate pattern, so prominent in the ampulla and infundibulum, is subtly altered.

The mucosa may become hyperplastic, forming cribriform pseudoglands and invaginations of epithelium into the muscularis.

Agglutination of the fimbriae may coalesce, blocking the lumen and causing a hydrosalpinx. The proximity of the ovary to the fimbriae allows multiple tubo-ovarian adhesions. Fibrinous adhesions develop between the serosa and surrounding peritoneal surfaces.

Psammoma bodies are an occasional finding in CS associated with IgG antibodies to Chlamydia [29] (Fig. 33.23) but may be seen in otherwise normal-appearing epithelium. Accumulation of lipofuscin accompanied by scanty iron pigment in macrophages in the mucosa has been reported in pigmentosis tubae and in endometriosis.

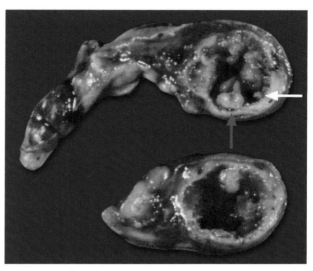

Fig. 33.22 Persistent plicae appear as focal thickening of the mucosa, some resembling papillary projections (*red arrow*) while others are more elongated (*white arrow*)

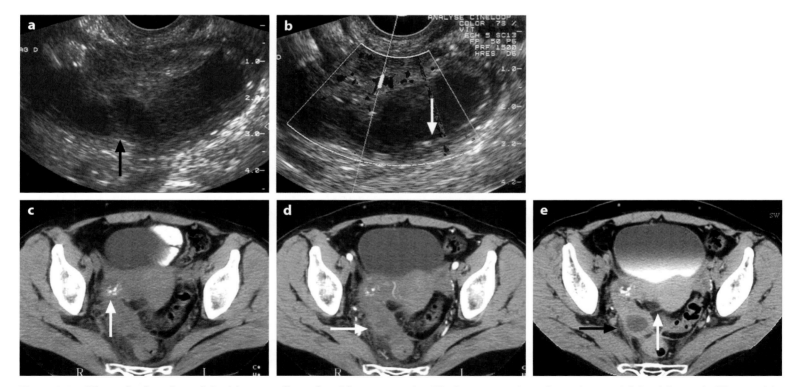

Fig. 33.23 Bilateral chronic salpingitis complicated with acute inflammatory reaction. Right acute salpingitis superimposed on chronic salpingitis with inflammatory reaction in the mesosalpinx. A 59-year-old woman with replaced hormonal treatment. Right pelvic mass at physical examination. CA 125: 254 IU/ml. CA 19–9:57 IU/ml. (**a**, **b**) EVS without (**a**) and with color Doppler (**b**): Right dilated tube with thickened hypervascularized wall containing hyperechogenic foci (*white arrow*) very likely related to fibrin deposits at pathology. On the inner wall, most of the plicae are obliterated (*black arrow*) while others are thickened owing to the inflammatory reaction. The lumen contains echogenic material. (**c–e**) Dynamic CT scan without IV injection (**c**), at the arterial phase (**d**), and on the delayed CT (**e**): (**c**) Right ovary containing small calcifications related to psammoma bodies (*arrow*). (**d**) Right thickened tube with absence of abnormal vessel at the arterial phase; tiny regular vessels (*arrow*) in the wall were only visualized 40 s after injection. (**e**) On the delayed CT, a collection of fluid was displayed. Adhesions between uterus and tube are present (*white arrow*). Increased density on the right side of the tube related to the inflammatory reaction of the mesosalpinx (*black arrow*)

33.4.2 Hydrosalpinx

Hydrosalpinx is one of the complications of salpingitis.

Definition: Obliteration of the fimbriated end and dilatation of the tube, usually the ampullary and infundibular portions.

The tube contains clear serous fluid with low protein content.

33.4.2.1 Pathology

Because a luminal communication usually can be demonstrated between dilated and nondilated portions of the tube, the etiology of dilatation is obscure but may result from a sphincter-like action of the isthmic muscularis.

1. Most of the epithelial lining consists of low cuboidal cells. The selective damage of the tubal folds leads to:
   (a) Occasional plicae may remain with intact columnar epithelium.
   (b) Marked blunting of the plicae (related to chronic salpingitis) (Fig. 33.22).
   (c) Plical disappearance (Fig. 33.24).
   If the ovary is first involved in tubo-ovarian adhesions, the dilated tube may compress the ovary.
2. The muscle wall is both thin and atrophic or replaced by collagenous connective tissue.
3. Occasional fibrous adhesions on its surface are present.

33.4.2.2 Ultrasound

One of the most common difficulties in the diagnosis of the origin of an adnexal mass is to make the differential between an

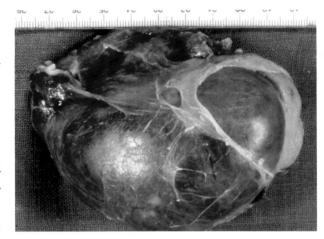

Fig. 33.24 Hydrosalpinx. The isthmic portion is only slightly enlarged, while the ampulla and the infundibulum are significantly distended

hydrosalpinx and a cystic ovarian mass [4]. Identification of the ipsilateral ovary separated from the cystic adnexal mass is very suggestive but is not always possible (Fig. 33.25).

The tubular shape, the foldings, and the plicae lead to a correct diagnosis [4, 13]. However, these plicae can be mistaken for papillary projections (Figs. 33.22 and 33.26) in a cystic ovarian mass [5]. Scanning in multiple planes and 3D reformation are useful to make the differential diagnosis (Fig. 33.27).

Color Doppler allows distinguishing a hydrosalpinx from prominent parametrial veins. Hydrosalpinx can be distinguished from bowel loops by visible peristaltism during real-time imaging.

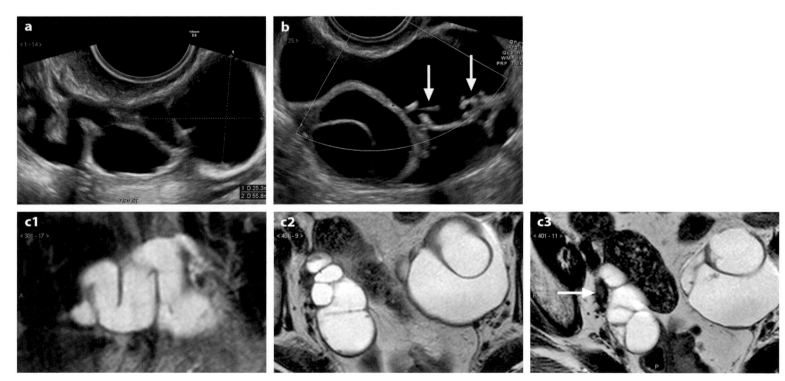

Fig. 33.25 Bilateral cystic adnexal mass: left hydrosalpinx resembling an ovarian cystadenoma. Fifty-eight-year-old woman. Operated from appendicular peritonitis 5 years ago. EVS of the right adnexa (**a**) depicts a tubular collection with thickened plicae typical for a hydrosalpinx. Normal right ovary was clearly identified. EVS of the left adnexa with color Doppler (**b**) depicts a cystic round collection which looks multilocular while normal left ovary is not identified; on the inner wall of the loculi, echogenic round and elongated echogenic structures (*arrows*) could be related either to papillary projections of a surface epithelial ovarian tumor or to thickened plicae in a hydrosalpinx. Because of the impossibility to definitely conclude, MR is performed. MR of the right adnexa on sagittal (**c1**) and axialT2 (**c2**) displays a typical right hydrosalpinx with some thickened plicae. Normal right ovary (**c3**) is clearly shown (*arrow*)

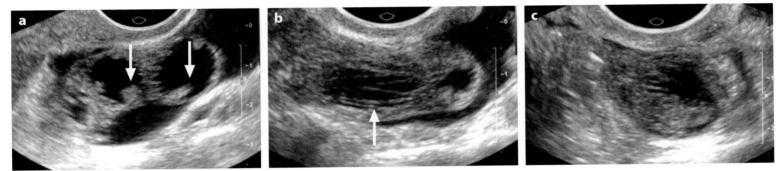

Fig. 33.25 (*continued*) MR of the left adnexa on sagittal T2 (**d1**) shows that the mass has a tubular shape; on coronal T2 (**d2**) low-intensity round and elongated structures are seen against the inner wall, but not as well as on EVS. However, on axial T2 (**d3**) a normal left ovary of small size (*arrow*) is well visualized against the medial part of the cystic collection, which can be diagnosed as a hydrosalpinx

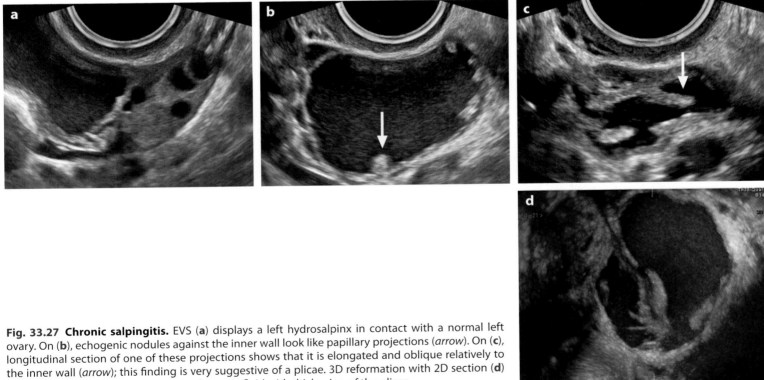

Fig. 33.26 Chronic salpingitis with hydrosalpinx. EVS (**a**) depicts a hydrosalpinx with a thickened wall and thickened plicae, some of them resembling papillary projections (*arrows*). Longitudinal (**b**) and transverse section (**c**) of the ampulla display thickened plicae of the mucosa (*arrow*)

Fig. 33.27 Chronic salpingitis. EVS (**a**) displays a left hydrosalpinx in contact with a normal left ovary. On (**b**), echogenic nodules against the inner wall look like papillary projections (*arrow*). On (**c**), longitudinal section of one of these projections shows that it is elongated and oblique relatively to the inner wall (*arrow*); this finding is very suggestive of a plicae. 3D reformation with 2D section (**d**) displays the dilated tube containing echogenic fluid with thickening of the plicae

33.4.2.3 MR

In case of voluminous adnexal collection, MR can be helpful to identify the tubal origin of the mass in identifying the normal ovary (Fig. 33.25).

A hydrosalpinx usually has thinner walls than a pyosalpinx (Figs. 33.28 and 33.29). The dilatation can involve all the tube or be limited to the ampulla and the infundibulum (Fig. 33.7) because of the mechanism of sphincter of the isthmic muscularis described above.

Hydrosalpinx may be complicated by torsion.

33.4.2.4 CT

The wall is usually thin with a mild wall enhancement.

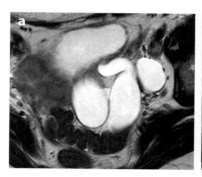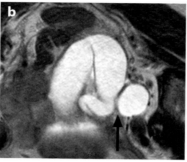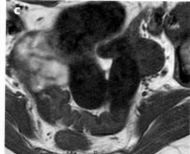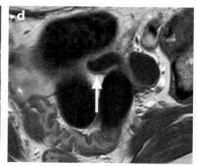

Fig. 33.28 Left hydrosalpinx. A 53-year-old woman. Interannexial total hysterectomy 10 years ago. Pelvic pain. US examination demonstrates a left hydrosalpinx, but is enable to know if it is uni- or bilateral. MR axial T2 supine (**a**) displays a left tubular adnexal extraovarian collection typical for a hydrosalpinx. Axial T2 on prone position (**b**) demonstrates that the fluid is slightly moving in the tube; this sequence can be helpful in the differential of other cystic adnexal masses. Medial face of the left ovary lies against the isthmic ampullary junction; ovary contains a functional cyst (which has slightly increased in size 2 weeks after the US). Axial T1 without injection (**c**) shows that the content of the dilated tube is a watery hypointense; after injection (**d**), a slight contrast uptake is visualized in the wall of the hydrosalpinx (*arrow*)

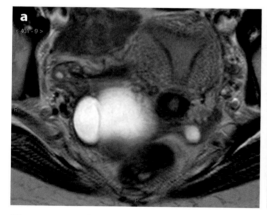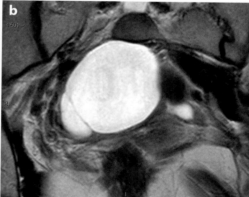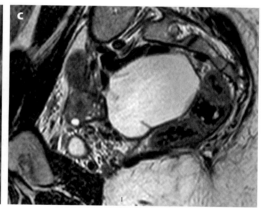

Fig. 33.29 Hydrosalpinx. MR axial T2 (**a**) depicts a right cystic collection with a folding, independent from the ovary. Coronal T2 (**b**) shows the collection is not round like it is the case in a hydrosalpinx. Sagittal oblique in the longitudinal axis of the collection (**c**) using 2 mm thick section, depicts clearly the hydrosalpinx lying against the posterior wall of the ovary

33.4.3 Adhesions

Tuboovarian or peritoneal adhesions may occur after PID. These adhesios may appear as cords between two neighbouring structures or as an obliteration of plane between two contiguous organs. These adhesions may be complicated with peritoneal pseudocyst or induce particularly with some infectious agents a Fitz Hugh Curtis syndrome.

33.4.3.1 Peritoneal pseudocyst (see Chap. 16.2.1)

33.4.3.2 Fitz-Hugh-Curtis Syndrome

Definition: adhesions between the visceral peritoneum covering the liver and the parietal peritoneum covering the right hemidiaphragm, which have a typical stringy look, called "violin-string" adhesions.

It occurs mainly after mycoplasma and chlamydia infection, more uncommonly after gonorrhea.

In some individuals, these adhesions cause no symptoms. Others have pain in the upper right upper quadrant of the abdomen wih sometimes irradiation to the right shoulder.

Radiologic diagnosis is made uncommonly. On CT, strings or perihepatic peritoneal thickening (Fig. 33.30) may be displayed.

Fitz Hugh Curtis may be an incidental finding at laparoscopy, or laparoscopy can confirm the diagnosis.

33.4.4 The Two Main Complications

33.4.4.1 Infertility

Tubal factors for infertility are multiple. Distortion of the tube, immotile cilia (like in the Kartagener's syndrome), obliteraive fibrosis which can be complicated with obstruction at the uterotubal junction, peritubal adhesions can be isolated or associated.

Hysterosalpingography allows to identify the level of the obstruction, the chronic lesions of the mucosa, the rigidity of the tube, the absence of diffusion of contrast medium in the peritoneal cavity, and eventually with a selective catheter to correct the obstuction.

33.4.4.2 Ectopic Pregnancy

Most often ectopic pregnancy is secondary to PID. It is usually discovered in a woman with 5 to 6 weeks of amenorrhea, associated with metrorrhagia and unilateral pelvic pain, and sympathetic findings of pregnancy.

Diagnosis is made by ultrasound with color doppler. Absence of a gestational sac in the endometrial cavity, and visualization of a small hematoma or a sac close to the ovary (containg usually the corpus luteum) with a ring finding on color doppler allow to make the diagnosis. Ectopic pregnancy can be associated with an acute hemoperitoneum secondary to a rupture of the tube, or an hemoperitoneum

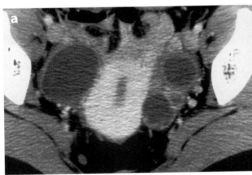
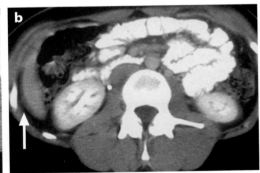
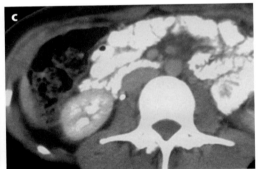

Fig. 33.30 Fitz-Hugh–Curtis syndrome. (a) CT after contrast displays a bilateral adnexal collection. (**b**, **c**) in the subhepatic space, thickening of the peritoneum is displayed (*arrow*). AT coelioscopy peritoneal strings were visualized

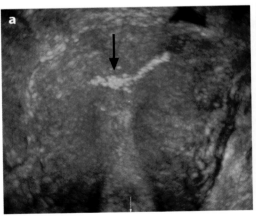
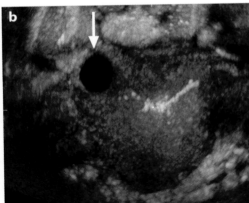
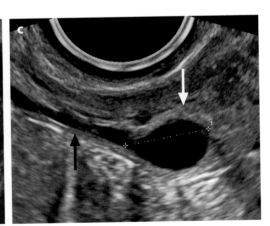

Fig. 33.31 Tuberculosis. Thirty-two-year-old woman, nulligeste. Primary infertility, secondary amenorrhea. EVS with 3D reformation: 2D coronal view (**a**) and 2D transverse view (**b**) of the uterus display a hyperechogenic band that corresponds to a fibrous adhesion at hysteroscopy (*arrow in a*). On (**b**) and on 2D transverse (**c**) view of the right adnexa, a cystic formation in the right horn (**b**, **c**) (*white arrows*) is related to the proximal portion of the dilatation of the tube with a particular racket aspect and a rigid aspect of the tubal wall (**c**) (*black arrow*). Prospective diagnosis: association of these lesions suggested the possibility of tuberculosis. Biopsy made through hysteroscopy confirmed the diagnosis

without clinical findings of state of shock related to a slow diffusion of blood through the infundiulum.

Diagnosis of pregnancy is confirmed by elevated betaHCG.

33.5 Chronic with Acute Inflammatory Response

Acute salpingitis may complicate a chronic salpingitis (Fig. 33.23).

Subacute salpingitis may persist after insufficient antibiotherapy.

33.6 PID Related to Uncommon Infections

33.6.1 Genital Tuberculosis (Figs. 33.31 and 16.5)

Involvement of the female genital tract by mycobacterium tuberculosis can resemble a nontuberculosis PID. However, the predominant involvement of the tubes, the common location to the peritoneum, and particular morphologic findings may suggest the possibility of TB. However, in case of extensive involvement to the peritoneum, the pattern can wrongly suggest a carcinoma of the adnexae with peritoneal metastases.

Typically, the lesions are bilateral:
1. Calcifications in the adnexa and in nodes.
2. Endometrium (involvement in 60% of cases)
   Diffuse endometrial thickening.
   Fluid in the endometrial cavity.

Particular to TB synechiae, which can be associated with a deformity of the endometrial cavity.
3. Tubes (involvement in 95% of cases)
   Obstruction of the fallopian tube at the junction of the isthmus and the ampulla.
   More suggestive of TB: multiple constrictions with a beaded appearance, multiple diverticules surrounding the ampulla, rigid pipe stem appearance.
4. Ovary (involvement in 15% of cases)
   Mixed ovarian masses.
5. Peritoneal involvement (involvement in 50% of cases)
   Ascites: free or more suggestive loculated peritoneal fluid, uncommonly of dry type. Density of the liquid can be high on CT.
   Nodules and thickening of the peritoneum, omental cake, and mesenteric mass with stellate appearance can mimic peritoneal metastases.
6. Lymphadenopathy typically with caseation necrosis
   US: hypoechoic with central necrosis.
   CT and MR: peripheral enhancement with absence of enhancement in the center.

33.6.2 Parasitic Infections (Echinococcus Granulosus)

Very uncommonly, echinococcus granulosus may involve the adnexae. An exceptional case is reported (Fig. 33.32).

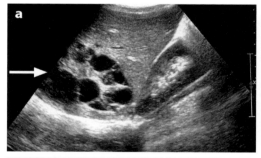
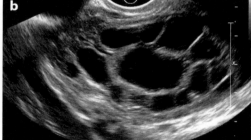
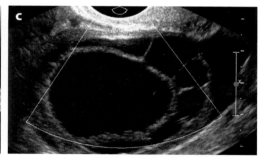
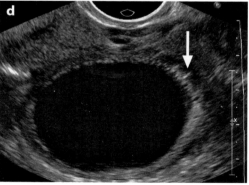

Fig. 33.32 Ovarian hydatid cyst associated with hydatidose of the liver. A 24-year-old woman, epigastric pain. CT discovered two multicystic lesions with calcifications in the liver, and a left ovarian mass of 6 cm in diameter. TAS longitudinal of the right lobe of the liver (**a**) depicts a multicystic round lesion in the segment VII near the capsule (*arrow*). EVS without (**b**) and with Doppler (**c**) depicts a multilocular cystic mass of the left ovary of the same echostructure as the liver without vascularization, pushing the normal ovarian parenchyma to the periphery. The cystic portions are anechoic with thin septa. On EVS with magnification (**d**), we can see tiny calcifications (*arrow*) and the irregularity of the inner wall of the largest cyst, which is probably related to the presence of daughter vesicles. Prospective diagnosis: the similarity of the echostructure of the liver and ovarian lesion, the presence of fine calcifications at the periphery of these cysts is in favor of the diagnosis of several localization of hydatidose. Surgery: left ovariectomy and resection of two cysts of the liver. Presence of scolex after excision of the ovarian cyst

References

1. Molander P et al (2000) Laparoscopic management of suspected acute pelvic inflammatory disease. J Am Assoc Gynecol Laparosc 7(1):107–110
2. Paavonen J et al (1985) Comparison of endometrial biopsy and peritoneal fluid cytologic testing with laparoscopy in the diagnosis of acute pelvic inflammatory disease. Am J Obstet Gynecol 151(5):645–650
3. Sellors J et al (1991) The accuracy of clinical findings and laparoscopy in pelvic inflammatory disease. Am J Obstet Gynecol 164(1 Pt 1):113–120
4. Patten RM et al (1990) Pelvic inflammatory disease. Endovaginal sonography with laparoscopic correlation. J Ultrasound Med 9(12):681–689
5. Rowling SE, Ramchandani P (1996) Imaging of the fallopian tubes. Semin Roentgenol 31(4):299–311
6. Terry J, Forrest T (1989) Sonographic demonstration of salpingitis. Potential confusion with appendicitis. J Ultrasound Med 8(1):39–41
7. Puylaert JB (1986) Acute appendicitis: US evaluation using graded compression. Radiology 158(2):355–360
8. Jeffrey RB Jr, Laing FC, Lewis FR (1987) Acute appendicitis: high-resolution real-time US findings. Radiology 163(1):11–14
9. Deutsch A, Leopold GR (1981) Ultrasonic demonstration of the inflamed appendix: case report. Radiology 140(1):163–164
10. Molander P et al (2001) Transvaginal power Doppler findings in laparoscopically proven acute pelvic inflammatory disease. Ultrasound Obstet Gynecol 17(3):233–238
11. Tinkanen H, Kujansuu E (1993) Doppler ultrasound findings in tubo-ovarian infectious complex. J Clin Ultrasound 21(3):175–178
12. Orlandi C, Dunn CJ, Cutshaw LG (1988) Evaluation of angiogenesis in chronic inflammation by laser-Doppler flowmetry. Clin Sci (Lond) 74(2):119–121
13. Tessler FN et al (1989) Endovaginal sonographic diagnosis of dilated fallopian tubes. AJR Am J Roentgenol 153(3):523–525
14. Timor-Tritsch IE, Rottem S (1987) Transvaginal ultrasonographic study of the fallopian tube. Obstet Gynecol 70(3 Pt 1):424–428
15. Timor-Tritsch IE et al (1998) Transvaginal sonographic markers of tubal inflammatory disease. Ultrasound Obstet Gynecol 12(1):56–66
16. Sam JW, Jacobs JE, Birnbaum BA (2002) Spectrum of CT findings in acute pyogenic pelvic inflammatory disease. Radiographics 22(6):1327–1334
17. Outwater EK et al (1998) Dilated fallopian tubes: MR imaging characteristics. Radiology 208(2):463–469
18. Clement PB (2002) Nonneoplastic lesions of the ovary. In: Kurman RJ (ed) Blaustein's pathology of the female genital tract. Springer, New-York, pp 675–727
19. Ha HK et al (1995) MR imaging of tubo-ovarian abscess. Acta Radiol 36(5):510–514
20. Teisala K, Heinonen PK, Punnonen R (1990) Transvaginal ultrasound in the diagnosis and treatment of tubo-ovarian abscess. Br J Obstet Gynaecol 97(2):178–180
21. Callen PW (1979) Computed tomographic evaluation of abdominal and pelvic abscesses. Radiology 131(1):171–175
22. Wilbur AC, Aizenstein RI, Napp TE (1992) CT findings in tuboovarian abscess. AJR Am J Roentgenol 158(3):575–579
23. Ellis JH et al (1991) CT findings in tuboovarian abscess. J Comput Assist Tomogr 15(4):589–592
24. Mitchell DG et al (1987) Adnexal masses: MR imaging observations at 1.5T, with US and CT correlation. Radiology 162(2):319–324
25. Pace EH, Voet RL, Melancon JT (1984) Xanthogranulomatous oophoritis: an inflammatory pseudotumor of the ovary. Int J Gynecol Pathol 3(4):398–402
26. Quan A, Charles D, Craig JM (1963) Histologic and functional consequences of periovarian adhesions. Obstet Gynecol 22:96–101
27. Bulas DI et al (1992) Pelvic inflammatory disease in the adolescent: comparison of transabdominal and transvaginal sonographic evaluation. Radiology 183(2):435–439
28. Phillips JC (1974) A spectrum of radiologic abnormalities due to tubo-ovarian abscess. Radiology 110(2):307–311
29. Martin DC, Khare VK, Miller BE (1995) Association of Chlamydia trachomatis immunoglobulin gamma titers with dystrophic peritoneal calcification, psammoma bodies, adhesions, and hydrosalpinges. Fertil Steril 63(1):39–44

Vulva

Part 9

Vulva or Pudendum Embryology, Anatomy, and Histology

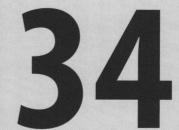

34

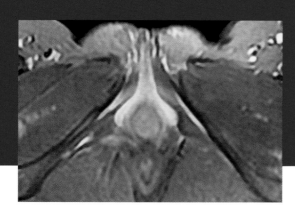

Contents

34.1 Definitions

Pelvic diaphragm: Levator ani and ischiococcygeus (also called coccygeus) form the pelvic diaphragm and delineate the lower limit of the true pelvis.

Perineum

(a) Limits

The deep limit: the inferior surface of the pelvic diaphragm
The superficial limit: the skin which is continuous with that over the medial aspect of the thighs and the lower abdominal wall.

(b) Comprises

Anal triangle
Urogenital triangle

Urogenital triangle comprises from deep to the superficial:

Deep perineal space (between deeply the endopelvic fascia of the pelvic floor and superficially the perineal membrane)
Superficial perineal space (between deeply the perineal membrane and superficially the superficial perineal fascia)
Vulva or pudendum or external female genitalia compartment (between the superficial fascia and the skin)

Anatomical definition of vulva or pudendum or external female genitalia comprises the following anatomical structures:

Labial formations: Mons pubis, pubis, labia major, labia minora
Erectile organs (clitoris and bulbs of the vestibule)
Glands and their ducts (Bartholin's and Skene's glands)
Vestibule containing vaginal orifice (introitus), hymen vaginae
External urethral orifice also called external urethral meatus.

Although most of these anatomical structures belong to the most superficial anatomical compartment of the anterior urogenital triangle (female external genitalia compartment), in fact some of them

J.N. Buy, M. Ghossain, *Gynecological Imaging*,
DOI 10.1007/978-3-642-31012-6_34, © Springer-Verlag Berlin Heidelberg 2013

Table 34.1 Components of the vulva

Anatomical Compartment		
Anatomical structures	**Vulva**	**Superficial perineal space**
1. Labial formations		
Mons pubis	Mons pubis	
Labia majora	Labia majora	
Labia minora	Labia minora	
2. Erectile organs		
Clitoris		
Corpora cavernosa		Corpora cavernosa
Corpus clitoridis	Corpus clitoridis (1/2 anterior)	Corpus clitoridis (1/2 posterior)
Glans	Glans	
Bulbs of the vestibule	Bulbs of the vestibule (anterior part: joins to the posterior part of corpus clitoridis)	Bulbs of the vestibule (posterior and middle part)
3. Glands		
Greater vestibular glands	Greater vestibular glands (anterior part)	Greater vestibular glands (posterior and middlepart)
Ducts	Ducts	
Skene's glands	Skene's glands	Skene's glands
Skene's ducts	Skene's ducts	Skene's ducts
4. Vestibule (between labia minora)		
Urethra	Urethral meatus (in vestibule)	Urethra (part of perineal portion)
Vagina	Vaginal orifice (in vestibule)	Vagina (part of perineal portion)
	Hymen	

are located or arise in the superficial perineal space (Table 34.1) (Figs. 34.1 and 34.2)

Vulva or pudendum or female external genitalia compartment is limited by:

Deeply

The superficial perineal fascia also called Colles' fascia which is attached to:

Posteriorly, the fascia over the superficial transverse perinei and the posterior limit of the perineal membrane.

Laterally, the margins of the ischiopubic rami and the ischial tuberosities; from here it runs more superficially to the skin of the urogenital triangle, lining the external genitalia, where it ends in the labia majora.

Superficially

The skin.

Superficial perineal space

(a) Is limited by

Deeply

The perineal membrane, which is triangular and is attached

Laterally to the periosteum of the ischiopubic rami

The posterior border is fused with the deep part of the perineal body and is continuous with the fascia over the deep transverse perinei. The upper sheet is continuous posteriorly with the lower part of the rectovaginal septum

Anteriorly at the apex fascia over transverse perinei and the perineal membrane join to form very tight aponeurotic fibres, the transverse ligament of Henlé also called the pubourethral ligament. Its apex is attached to the arcuate ligament of the pubis

Superficially

The superficial perineal fascia also called Colles' fascia.

(b) It contains

Superficial transverse perinei (mainly posteriorly)

Bulbospongiosus (medially)

Attaches to the perineal body

On each side is separate

Covers the superficial part of the vestibular bulbs and greater vestibular glands; the vestibular bulbs run anteriorly on each side of the vagina to attach to the corpora cavernosa clitoridis

Ischiocavernosus (laterally)

Attaches on the ischiopubic ramus on both sides of the corpus clitoridis

Covers the corpora cavernosa of the clitoridis, ends in an aponeurosis attached to the sides and under surface of the of the crus; anteriorly corpora cavernosa of the clitoridis join to form the corpus clitoridis (hidden part)

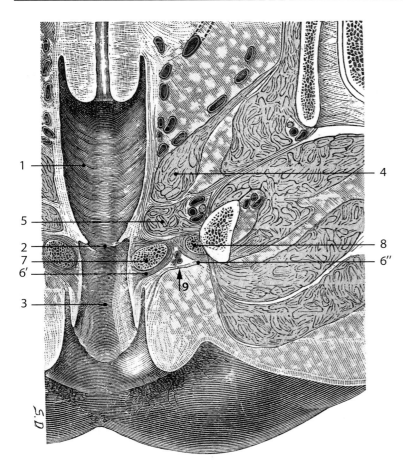

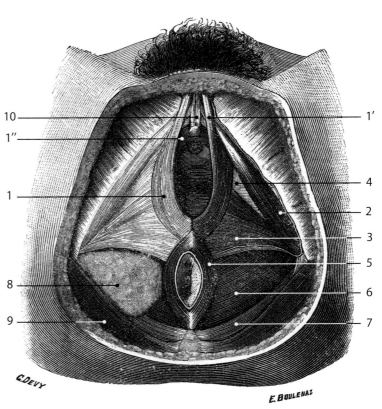

Fig. 34.1 Coronal section through the middle part of the vagina. *1* subperitoneal vagina, *2* vaginal introitus, *3* vestibular vagina, *4* levator ani, *5* deep transverse perinei with the perineal membrane superficial to this muscle, *6′* bulbospongiosus muscle, *6″* ischiocavernosus muscle, *7* bulb of vestibule, *8* crus of clitoris, *9* superficial perineal fascia (From Testut [2])

Fig. 34.2 Muscles of the perineum. On the right side superficial perineal fascia or Colles' fascia is present while on the left side this fascia has been removed. *1* Bulbospongiosus muscle (covered with superficial perineal fascia), *1′* internal fascicle, *1″* external fascicle, *2* ischiocavernosus muscle covering the root of the clitoris, *3* superficial transverse perinei, *4* perineal membrane, *5* external anal sphincter, *6* levator ani, *7* ischiococcygeus muscle, *8* adipose tissue of the ischiorectal fossa, *9* gluteus maximus, *10* clitoris (From Testut [2])

34.2 Embryology [1] (See Fig. 1.4)

34.2.1 Common Development in Female and Male

Up to the seventh week, the external genitalia are similar in both sexes. Distinguishing sexual characteristics begin to appear during the ninth week, but the external genitalia are not fully differentiated until the 12th week.

In the fourth week, proliferating mesenchyme produces a *genital tubercle at the cranial end* of the cloacal membrane.

Labioscrotal swellings and urogenital folds soon develop on each side of the cloacal membrane. The genital tubercle elongates to form a primordial phallus.

When the urorectal septum fuses with the cloacal membrane at the end of the sixth week, it divides the cloacal membrane in a dorsal anal membrane and a ventral urogenital membrane.

The urogenital membrane lies in the floor of a median cleft, the urethral groove, which is bound by the urogenital folds. The anal and urogenital membranes rupture a week later, forming the anus and urogenital orifices. The urethra and the vagina open in a common cavity, the vestibule.

34.2.2 Development of Male External Genitalia

Masculinization of the indifferent external genitalia is induced by testosterone produced by the interstitial cells of the fetal testes.

As the phallus enlarges and elongates to become the penis, the urethral folds form the lateral walls of the urethral groove on the ventral surface of the penis.

34.2.3 Development of Female External Genitalia

(a) The primordial phallus gradually becomes the clitoris.
(b) The urogenital folds fuse posteriorly to form the frenulum of the labia minora or nymphae. The unfused parts form the labia minora.
(c) The labioscrotal folds fuse posteriorly to form the posterior labial commissure and anteriorly to form the anterior labial commissure and the mons pubis. The unfused parts form the labia majora.

34.2.4 Auxiliary Genital Glands

Buds grow from the urethra into the surrounding mesenchyme and form the bilateral mucus-secreting urethral glands and paraurethral glands. These glands correspond to the prostate in the male.

Outgrowths from the urogenital sinus form the greater vestibular glands in the lower third of the labia majora. These tubuloalveolar glands also secrete mucus and are homologous to the bulbourethral glands in male.

34.2.5 Development of the Inguinal Canals

(a) The Gubernaculum. As the mesonephros degenerates, a ligament, the gubernaculum, develops on each side of the abdomen from the caudal pole of the gonad.

The gubernaculum passes obliquely through the developing anterior abdominal wall at the site of the future inguinal canal and attaches caudally to the internal surface of the labioscrotal swellings (future labia majora).

The gubernaculum is also attached to the uterus near the attachment of the uterine tube. The cranial part becomes the ovarian ligament, the caudal part the round ligament of the uterus.

(b) The Processus Vaginalis. The processus vaginalis is an evagination of peritoneum, which develops ventral to the gubernaculum, and herniates through the abdominal wall along the path formed by the gubernaculum. The vaginal process carries along extensions of the layers of the abdominal wall with it, which forms the walls of the inguinal canal. This relatively small processus vaginalis obliterates and disappears before birth. A processus vaginalis that persists after birth is called a *canal of Nuck*.

34.3 Anatomy [2, 3]

34.3.1 Labial Formations (Fig. 34.3)

(a) The mons pubis or the mons veneris lies over the anterior superior part of the symphysis pubis and is composed of skin, hair, and subcutaneous adipose tissue.

(b) The labia majora are two symmetrical cutaneous folds, which measure from 7 to 8 cm in length, 2–3 cm width, and 1.5–2 cm in thickness [2]:
– The lateral face of each labium is separated from the medial aspect of the thigh by a marked groove the genito-crural groove.
– The medial face is separated from the labia minora by a labial groove.
– The superior border is adherent to the ischiopubic ramus.
– The inferior border demarcates with the inferior border of the other labia majora the pudendal cleft.
– The anterior extremities join on the midline and form the anterior commissure, thick and arciform, which is in continuity with the posterior part of the mons pubis.
– The posterior extremities merge into the neighbouring skin, ending near to each other. The connecting skin between them forms a ridge called the fourchette. This overlies the perineal

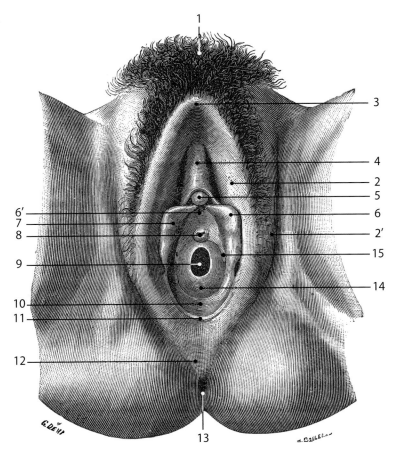

Fig. 34.3 External view of the vulva in a virgin woman: *1* mons veneris, *2* medial part of the labia majora, *2'* lateral part of the labia majora, *3* anterior commissure of the vulva, *4* junction of the anterior roots of the labia minora forming the clitoral hood, *5* glans of the clitoris, *6* labia minora, *6'* junction of the posterior roots of the labia minora forming the frenulum of the clitoris, *7* vestibule (medially to the point indicated on the figure), *8* urethral meatus, *9* vaginal orifice, *10* navicular fossa, *11* fourchette, *12* perineal body, *13* anus, *14* hymen, *15* external orifice of the Bartholin's gland (From Testut [2])

body and is the posterior limit of the vulva. Between the fourchette and the vaginal orifice is a small depression called the navicular fossa.

The uterine round ligament may end in the adipose tissue and skin in front of labium. A congenital inguinal hernia or a persistent processus vaginalis may also reach a labium.

(c) The labia minora or nymphae lie between the labia majora and are two symmetrical thin skin folds that measure 3–3.5 cm in length, 1–1.5 cm in width, and 5 mm in thickness [2].

Lateral face is related to the medial face of the labium majorum.

Medial face is related to the pudendal cleft.

Superior border is adherent and leans against the bulb of the vestibule.

Inferior border is floating in the pudendal cleft.

Anterior extremity a little before reaching the clitoris bifurcates in two layers:
– The posterior, short, runs to the posterior face of the clitoris and inserts on it, forming with its fellow the frenulum of the clitoris.
– The anterior, longer than the previous one, passes in front of the clitoris, meets with its fellow to form the prepuce or hood of the clitoris.

Posterior extremity ends on the medial face of the corresponding labium majorum most often at the junction of its middle part and the third posterior part.

Labia minora are formed by a double layer of cutaneous tissue, containing in their center a thin layer of conjonctive tissue, rich in elastic fibres, but devoid of adipose tissue.

34.3.2 Vestibule (Figs. 34.3 and 34.4)

The vestibule is bounded by:
- Anteriorly: the frenulum of the clitoris
- Laterally: the medial faces of the labia minora
- Posteriorly: the posterior part of the vaginal orifice

It includes:
(a) The external urethral orifice also called the external urethral meatus and the openings of the Skene ducts.
(b) The vaginal orifice or introitus at the level of the hymen.
(c) Opening of the greater vestibular glands of Bartholin (situated in the superficial perineum) by a duct of 2 cm in the groove between the hymen and a labium minus.

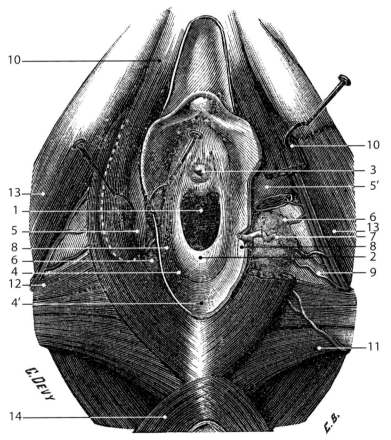

Fig. 34.4 Vulva and superficial perineal space. *1* Introitus, *2* hymen, *3* urethral meatus, *4* labio-hymeneal groove, *4'* navicular fossa, *5 right* bulb of the vestibule, *5' partly* resected bulb on the left side, *6* greater vestibular gland with its duct (*7*) and its orifice (*8*) and its artery (artery to the bulb arising from the pudendal artery) (*9*), *10* bulbospongiosus partly resected on the left side, *11* superficial transverse perinei, *12* ischiobulbous (inconstant muscle), *13* ischiocavernosus, *14* external anal sphincter (From Testut [2])

34.3.3 Erectile Apparatus

34.3.3.1 The Clitoris

The clitoris has two portions in the superficial perineal space and in the vulva.
1. In the superficial perineal space
   The roots of the corpora cavernosa are connected by their superior border with the crus which inserts on the inferior border of the ischiopubic ramus; the corpora cavernosa go then into the lateral part of the superficial perineal space covered deeply by the perineal membrane and superficially by the ischiocavernosus muscles.
   The roots join anteriorly on the midline in front of the urethra to form the posterior part of the corpus clitoridis. Corpus clitoridis has two corpora cavernosa, which are composed of erectile tissue and enclosed in dense fibrous tissue, the albugine, separated medially by an incomplete fibrous pectiniform septum. Below the pubic symphysis is the pubourethral ligament. At this level, the corpus of the clitoris passes below the ligament into the vulva, the dorsal vein of the clitoris through the ligament.
2. In the vulva
   A little in front of the symphysis, is the elbow of the corpus [2]. The corpus clitoridis bends backward and downward. The suspensory ligament inserts on the lower part of the anterior face of the pubic symphysis and wraps around the elbow of the clitoris; the dorsal artery of the clitoris, terminal branch of the pudendal artery goes through this ligament. Then the short visible portion of the clitoris is covered with the hood (anterior layer of the anterior extremity of the labia minora) with the frenulum (posterior layer of the anterior extremity of the labia minora) (see Sect. 34.3.1). The glans of the clitoris is a small round tubercle of spongy erectile tissue.
   The clitoris measures 6–7 cm in length: 3 cm for the crura, 3 cm for the body, and 7 mm for the glans.

34.3.3.2 Bulbs of the Vestibule

They are mainly located in the medial part of the superficial perineal space, while the anterior extremity is located in the vestibular area. They have:
- A superior face which is in contact deeply and is attached to the perineal membrane.
- An inferior face covered superficially with the bulbospongious muscle.
- A posterior round extremity, covering the Bartholin's gland.
- An anterior extremity which is thin and tapered and is situated in the vestibular area between the urethral meatus and the clitoris. At this level, the bulb communicates with its fellow by venous channels. At this site the bulbs communicate with the posterior part of corpus clitoridis through a rich network of veins, called Intermediate network by Kobelt in Testut [2] where bulbous veins and clitoris veins participate.
- A lateral border surrounded by the bulbospongious muscle.
- A medial border surrounding the lateral border of the vagina and the urethra.

There are two elongated erectile masses, flanking the vaginal orifice, below the middle perineal aponeurosis. Each mass is 3 cm length.

Benign Diseases of the Vulva

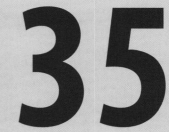

35

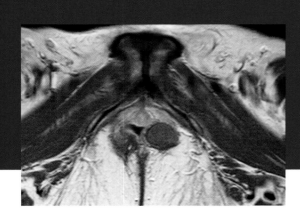

Contents

35.1 Cysts [1]

35.1.1 Bartholin Gland Cyst

35.1.1.1 Anatomy and Histology of the Glands

The major vestibular (Bartholin) glands are bilaterally adjacent to the posterior vestibular bulb with acini composed of simple columnar mucus-secreting epithelium.

Each gland is drained just external to the hymen ring of the vestibule posterolaterally. The Bartholin duct 2.5 cm length is lined:
- Proximally by mucus-secreting epithelium
- Then transitional epithelium
- At its exit squamous epithelium

35.1.1.2 Pathology of the Cyst

Duct obstruction occurs at their vestibular orifice, situated at the 5 and 7 o'clock positions between the hymen and labia minora, with subsequent accumulation of secretion and cystic dilatation. The cyst can appear posterolaterally or laterally in the vestibule. The cyst lining varies from mucin secreting to squamous or transitional. The content of an uninfected Bartholin cyst is either clear or mucoid highly viscous and thick.

35.1.1.3 MR Imaging

When the content is clear fluid, the signal intensity on T1 and T2 is like urine (Fig. 35.1). When mucoid, their signal intensity is intermediate on T1 and intermediate or high on T2 (Fig. 35.2).
Complications
- Infection (see below)
- Association of Bartholin adenocarcinoma

J.N. Buy, M. Ghossain, *Gynecological Imaging*,
DOI 10.1007/978-3-642-31012-6_35, © Springer-Verlag Berlin Heidelberg 2013

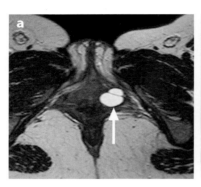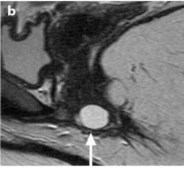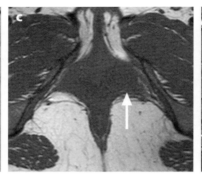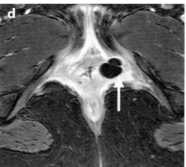

Fig. 35.1 MRI of an uninfected Bartholin gland cyst with translucent liquid. Axial (**a**) and sagittal (**b**) T2W images, axial T1W image (**c**), axial T1W-FS image after gadolinium injection (**d**). Biloculated cystic lesion (*arrows*) developed lateral to the introitus. This topography is typical for a Bartholin cyst. Signal intensity identical to urine is related to its aqueous uninfected content as confirmed at excision

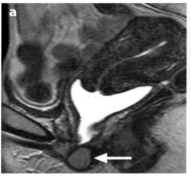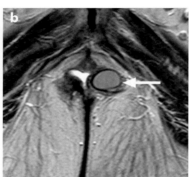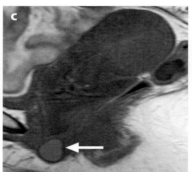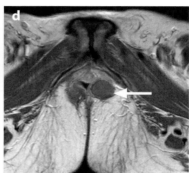

Fig. 35.2 Mucoid uninfected Bartholin cyst. Sagittal (**a**) and axial (**b**) T2W images with vaginal opacification, Sagittal T1W image (**c**), and axial T1W images (**d**). Two centimeters cyst (*arrows*) located posterolaterally to the introitus at 5 o'clock, compressing the wall of the vagina. This topography is typical for a Bartholin cyst. The cyst has an intermediate signal on T1 and on T2 related to its mucoid content confirmed at excision

35.1.2 Epithelial Inclusion Cysts

Definition: Lined by a stratified squamous epithelium
　　Location: The labia majora and clitoris
　　Size: 2–5 mm
　　Content: Keratinous

35.1.3 Mucinous Cysts

Definition: Lined by mucus-secreting columnar epithelium
　　Location: Minor vestibular gland
　　Content: Mucinous

35.1.4 Mesonephric-Like Cysts

Definition: The epithelium is cuboidal to columnar
　　Location: Lateral aspects of the vulva
　　Content: Clear fluid

35.1.5 Cyst of the Canal of Nuck

Location:
– The superior aspect of the labia majora
– Inguinal canal

They must be distinguished from an inguinal hernia with which they are associated in one-third of cases [2].

There are comma-shaped cysts with their tails directed cranially toward the inguinal canal.

35.1.6 Urothelial Cysts (Skene Duct Cysts)

Skene ducts run parallel to the urethra and are located lateral and posterior to the external urethral meatus.

The majority of the ducts of the paraurethral glands lie in the middle to distal urethra, near the 3 and 9 o'clock positions, and terminates in the paraurethral ducts of Skene. Skene duct cysts appear as round or oval masses that show hyperintense signal on T2-weighted imaging.

35.1.7 Suburethral Diverticulum

Location: The majority is located in the middle third of the urethra and involves the posterolateral wall.

They are horseshoe-shaped [3].

35.1.8 Differential Diagnosis According to Location

Differential diagnosis of vulvar cysts is mainly based on their location (Table 35.1).

Table 35.1 Differential location of vulvar cysts according to their location

Bartholin cyst	Posterolateral to lower vagina
Epithelial inclusion cysts	Labia majora
	Clitoris
Mucinous cysts	Vestibule
Mesonephric-like cysts	Lateral aspects of vulva
Cyst of the canal of Nuck	The superior aspect of the labia majora
	Inguinal canal
Skene duct cysts	Posterolateral to urethra
Suburethral diverticulum	Posterolateral to urethra (Horseshoe-shaped)

35.2 Inflammatory Diseases [1]

35.2.1 Bartholinitis

(a) The Bartholin cysts may be recurrent and occasionally are associated with primary infection of the Bartholin gland.

(b) Bartholin abscess results from acquired infection of the Bartholin gland duct or from secondary infection of a Bartholin cyst. Polymicrobial organism (Staphylococcus or other anaerobic bacteria) frequently causes the infection.

It is an acute process. The patient presents with tenderness and swelling in the Bartholin gland area.

MRI can be used if there is doubt about the diagnosis or to assess complications.

Abscess appears as a thick-walled cystic mass of variable signal intensity on T1-weighted imaging, high or intermediate signal intensity on T2-weighted. High signal intensity in surrounding tissues due to edema can be seen, but more constant is enhancement of surrounding tissue due to inflammation (Fig. 35.3).

35.2.2 Labial Cellulitis (Fig. 35.4)

This infection can be secondary to infection of a follicle hair.

On US, the process can be echogenic and eventually associated with a low echogenic cavity. Color Doppler can display hypervascularization at the periphery of the cyst.

On MR, the process can appear with a low intensity on T1 and a high intensity on T2. A high contrast enhancement with ill-defined limits of the process is highly suggestive of an inflammatory process.

35.2.3 HPV Infection

HPV is responsible for benign tumors termed *condyloma acuminata* (see Chap. 27) and precursor lesions of certain types of vulvar carcinomas.

35.3 Benign Tumors [1]

35.3.1 Epithelial

They can be:
- Squamous epithelial
- Fibroepithelial polyp
- Papilloma (see Chap. 30)
- Glandular

35.3.2 Mesenchymal Tumors

35.3.2.1 Leiomyoma

Leiomyomas are the most common soft tissue tumors of the vulva. They may arise from the smooth muscle elements surrounding the crura of the clitoris. They also may be seen along the labia majora. The lesion may enlarge during pregnancy.

MR findings are the same as elsewhere (see Chap. 24.3.1).

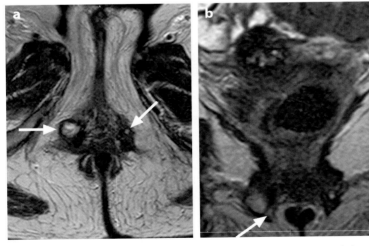 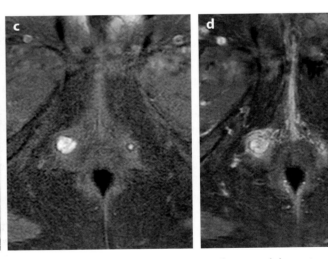

Fig. 35.3 Bartholinitis. Axial (**a**) and coronal (**b**) T2WI shows bilateral Bartholin cysts (*arrow*). Their signal is intermediate on T2 with a thick hypointense wall. The right one is larger. On (**b**), the right vestibular bulb is seen (*arrow*) in contact with the cyst. Axial T1WI before (**c**) and after (**d**) gadolinium injection shows marked contrast uptake around the cysts especially on the right. Clinical and radiological diagnosis: Bilateral bartholinitis confirmed at marsupialization

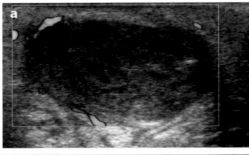
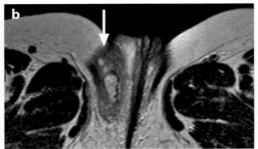
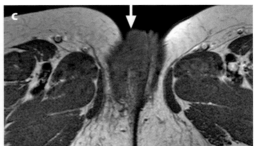
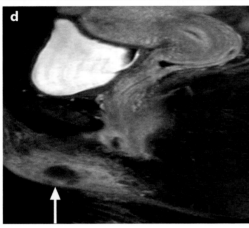

Fig. 35.4 Labial cellulitis. (**a**) Ultrasound of the anterior part of the right labia majora shows an overall hypoechoic area, slightly heterogeneous, containing some anechoic zones. Association with a peripheral color flow is very suggestive of an inflammatory process. (**b**) Axial T2W image shows this area (*arrow*) to contain an ovoid hyperintense center and some hyperintense spots; all of them surrounded by tissue of intermediate signal intensity. (**c**) On T1W image, the entire area is hypointense (*arrow*). (**d**) Sagittal T1W-FS image after gadolinium injection shows an ovoid non-enhancing area corresponding to pus surrounded by enhancing inflammatory peripheral tissue (*arrow*)

Myxoid change may occur, associated with pregnancy. Epithelioid leiomyoma during pregnancy has also been reported.

35.3.2.2 Lipoma

Vulvar lipoma is the second most common solid tumor found in the vulva area.

They arise from the vulvar subcuticular fat pads located on the mons pubis and the labia majora. It is a slow-growing tumor and may reach excessive size.

On CT and MRI, their fatty content is characteristic.

35.3.2.3 Hemangioma

Acquired Hemangiomas: They are far more common than other hemangiomas of the vulva. They are typically multiple, from 1 to 3 mm.

Cavernous Hemangiomas: They are rare in the vulva. Cavernous hemangioma results from dilated blood vessels, with resultant formation of the vascular tumor deep within the dermis or subcutaneous tissues.

It is usually discovered incidentally. Histologically, randomly arranged thin-walled capillaries separated by thin connective tissue septa are seen. The diagnosis is made by visual inspection.

For large hemangiomas, MRI is useful to define the depth, the extension into the pelvic sidewalls, and the perirectal spaces. This observation is of significance clinically for those patients who require therapy and for those patients who plan to conceive.

A deep-seated cavernous hemangioma in the perivaginal wall and the perirectal spaces may bleed significantly when exposed to the trauma of vaginal delivery.

35.4 Endometriosis of the Vulva (Fig. 35.5)

They are uncommon lesions.

Most of them occur secondary to obstetrical and surgical trauma. Furthermore, a large proportion of them are observed on episiotomy scars in the posterior part of the labia majora.

Symptoms are cyclic and synchronized with the menstrual cycle.

Their aspect is like endometriosis elsewhere, mainly in the abdominal wall (see Chap. 17):
- High intensity foci on T1 and T1 with fat suppression and low or high intensity on T2
- A fibromuscular component of low signal on T1 and T2 with a contrast uptake after injection

35.5 Congenital Abnormalities

Different congenital disorders have been reported, like congenital clitoris hypertrophy, hypertrophy or hypoplasia of the labia minora, and low transverse vaginal septum (Fig. 35.6).

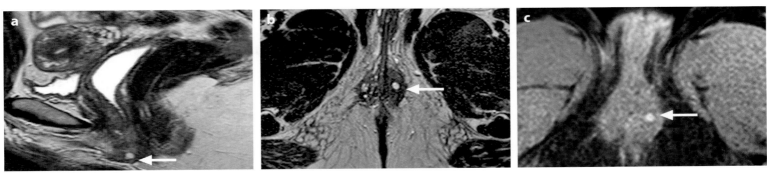

Fig. 35.5 Vulvar endometriosis. Sagittal (**a**) and axial (**b**) T2W images with vaginal opacification and axial T1W image (**c**) show a left vulvar mass (*arrows*) with a central hemorrhagic focus of intermediate signal on T2 that is hyperintense on T1 and T1 fat suppression (not shown). This focus is surrounded by fibrous tissue hypointense on T2. This pattern is typical for endometriosis

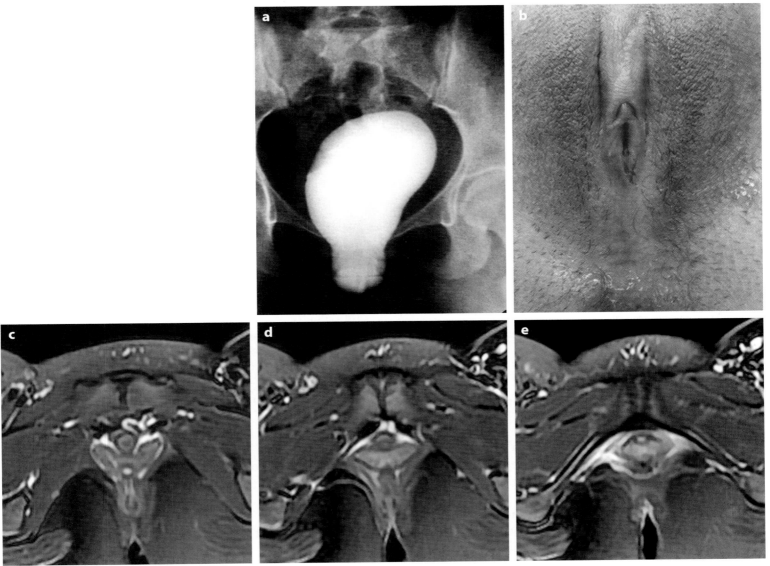

Fig. 35.6 Congenital anomaly of the vestibule in a 16-year-old girl. Since birth, she had a thick membrane covering the vaginal and urethral outlets with a tiny hole allowing passage of urine and later of menses. However, she had continuous leak. (**a**) An attempt to make a retrograde cystography opacified a structure that obviously was not the bladder. As it will be shown later on, the upper ovoid part corresponds to the distended vagina above the hymen and the lower part to a pouch constituted by the lower vagina (below the hymen) where the urethra opened. (**b**) View of the vulva before surgical repair shows a normal labia majora easily recognizable due to the pigmented skin of their outer borders. The clitoris is also easily identified. Behind it, there are two tiny labia minora bordering a membrane containing a tiny hole (not seen in this picture). The anus is posterior, normally situated. (**c–g**) Serial T2 FS from upper to lower shows: In (**c**), a normal H-shaped vagina, above the hymen, with in front of it a normal urethra. In (**d** and **e**), below the hymen, the vestibule has a non-shaped form, which is normal, but appears slightly ovoid and enlarged with no liquid. The urethra is still well delineated in front of it.

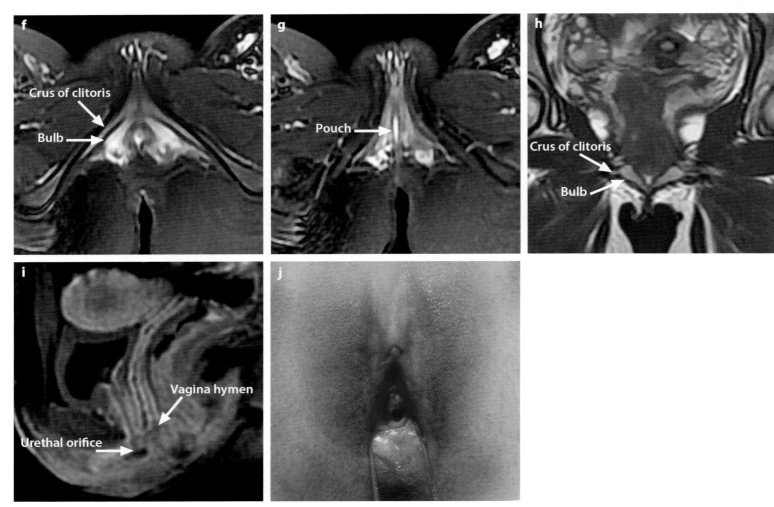

Fig. 35.6 *(continued)* In (**f**), the urethra is seen opening in the lower part of the pouch formed by the enlarged vestibule; at this level, the enlarged vestibule contains a small quantity of hyperintense liquid. The erectile organs are best delineated at this level. The paired bulbs of the vestibule (*labeled arrow*) are seen laterally. More laterally, the paired crus of the clitoris (*labeled arrow*) are seen converging to form anteriorly the corpus of the clitoris. In (**g**), the bottom end of the vestibular pouch (*labeled arrow*) is seen containing some hyperintense liquid. The glans of the clitoris is seen anteriorly. (**h**) Coronal T2 FS at the level of the opening of the urethra in the vestibular pouch shows in the midline the narrow bottom of the pouch containing some hyperintense fluid and laterally the erectile organs: bulbs (*labeled arrow*) and crus of the clitoris (*labeled arrow*). (**i**) Delayed midline sagittal T1 FS after injection shows the urethra and its lower orifice (*labeled arrow*) situated at the level of (**f**), and the vagina that is well delineated until the hymen (*labeled arrow*) that is situated between the levels of (**c** and **d**). (**j**) View of the vulva after surgical repair. During surgery, the membrane that was about 1 cm thick was cut and the incision enlarged posteriorly through the perineal body. The vestibular pouch contained a small quantity of thick mucinous material. The vestibule is now well seen, bounded superiorly by the hymen and its orifice; in front of the hymen, the urethral meatus is visible

References

1. Wilkinson EJ, Xie DL (2002) Benign diseases of the vulva. In: Kurman RJ (ed) Blaustein's pathology of the female genital tract, 5th edn. Springer, New York, pp 37–98
2. Schneider CA, Festa S, Spillert CR, Bruce CJ, Lazaro EJ (1994) Hydrocele of the canal of Nuck. N J Med 91(1):37–38
3. Chou CP, Levenson RB, Elsayes KM, Lin YH, Fu TY, Chiu YS, Huang JS, Pan HB (2008) Imaging of female urethral diverticulum: an update. Radiographics 28(7):1917–1930

Premalignant and Malignant Tumors of the Vulva

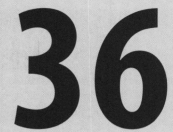

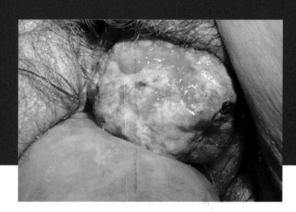

Contents

36.1 Introduction

Vulvar carcinoma is rare, accounting for 3–5 % of female tract cancers. Sixty-six percent of cases occur over the age of 70 years.

Over 85 % of malignant tumors are squamous cell carcinomas (SCC), followed by melanoma that accounts for 5–10 %.

Vulvar cancer is a visible and palpable disease and should be diagnosed early, but unfortunately 39 % of patients are diagnosed with advanced stages (III or IV).

36.2 Squamous Tumors

36.2.1 Vulvar Intraepithelial Neoplasia (VIN) (Dysplasia, Carcinoma In Situ)

Fifty percent of these women have other neoplasia involving the genital tract, most often cervical intraepithelial neoplasia.

Fifty percent have a history of a preexisting or concomitant sexually transmitted disease, of which condylomata acuminata is the most frequent.

Most patients are symptomatic with pruritus.

J.N. Buy, M. Ghossain, *Gynecological Imaging*,
DOI 10.1007/978-3-642-31012-6_36, © Springer-Verlag Berlin Heidelberg 2013

36.2.2 Invasive Squamous Cell Carcinoma

36.2.2.1 Etiology

There are three main groups of patients:

1. Women (mean age, 55 years) who have VIN associated with squamous cell carcinoma. They have a high rate of cervical and vaginal neoplasia. They tend to be heavy cigarette smokers. The tumors are predominantly of the warty or basaloid types. HPV is detected in 75 % of cases.
2. Older women (mean age 77 years) who do not have associated VIN, but often have vulvar dermatoses especially lichen sclerosus. They do not have a history of heavy cigarette smoking. The tumors are well-differentiated keratinizing squamous cell carcinomas. They rarely contain HPV.
3. Women with chronic granulomatous disease, mainlygranuloma inguinale.

Diabetes mellitus, immunosuppression, and achlorhydria may be associated with vulvar squamous cell carcinoma.

36.2.2.2 Special Histological Subtypes

Different subtypes of SCC exist; among them is verrucous carcinoma [1].

Verrucous carcinoma is a well-differentiated squamous cell hyperkeratotic epithelial tumor.

It is predominantly locally invasive neoplasia. The condition may occur in young women.

The prevalence is estimated to be 6.5 % among malignant lesions of the vulva.

The diagnosis is based on extensive vulvar pruritus, similar to squamous cell carcinoma.

Warty carcinoma (condylomatous carcinoma) is frequently associated to HPV type 16.

36.2.2.3 Clinical Features

Women presenting with vulvar carcinoma may have a wide variety of presenting complaints relevant to the vulvar tumor, especially if the tumor is at an advanced stage.

- No symptoms in 20 % of cases
- Long history of pruritus: ++++
- Itching, burning, and soreness
- A lump or mass on the vulva: +++, or a wite hyperkeratotic plaque
- Painful urination
- Bleeding or bloodstained vaginal discharge

36.2.2.4 Site of the Tumor

- Most often in the labia majora and the labia minora
- But can be found anywhere on the vulva: clitoris, fourchette

36.2.2.5 Diagnosis

Classical procedure:
- Pelvic clinical examination under anesthetic
- Colposcopy
- Biopsy (punch or excisional)

36.2.2.6 MR Imaging [2–4]

Primary Tumor

The tumor is best seen on T2-weighted sequences as intermediate signal intensity mass or thickening of the vulvar skin (Figs. 36.1 and 36.2). The relationship of the tumor to the clitoris, urethra, vagina, and anus is important prognostically. If deep invasion is suspected, T2-weighted images in the sagittal or coronal planes can be helpful to assess the cranial extent of tumor.

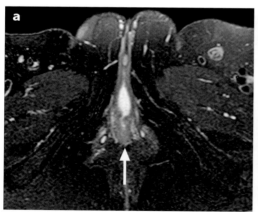 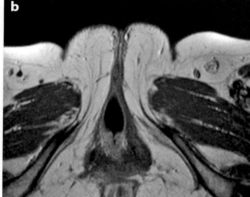 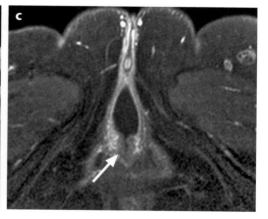

Fig. 36.1 Squamous cell carcinoma of the posterior fourchette (stage IA). Forty five year-old woman with a clinical ulcerated mass of the vulva. Vulvovaginal opacification. On Axial T2W-FS (**a**), a "horseshoe" tumor of the fourchette (*arrow*), of intermediate signal, less than 2 cm in diameter, regular, and well confined is displayed (**c**). On axial T1 (**b**), and after injection of gadolinium (**c**), the tumor slightly enhances (*arrow* in **c**), and does not extend to the adjacent perineal structures. A normal left inguinal lymphnode is depicted on the different sequences. At pathology resection of the tumor was stage 1A; sentinel ymph nodes were negative

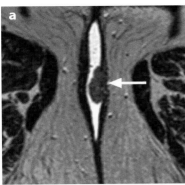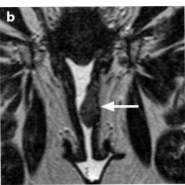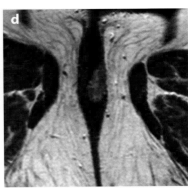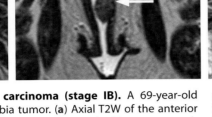

Fig. 36.2 Squamous cell vulvar carcinoma (stage IB). A 69-year-old woman with clinically left minor labia tumor. (**a**) Axial T2W of the anterior vulva, (**b**) coronal T2W in front of the vagina and uretral orifice, corresponding, (**c**) axial T1W, and (**d**) axial gado-T1W images, after vulvo-vaginal opacification, show a left minor labia tumor (*arrows*) partially surrounded by gel, 2.5 cm in largest diameter. It has intermediate signal intensity on T2W images and a hypointense signal on T1 image and enhances after gadolinium injection. Radical vulvectomy was performed. At pathology, left sentinel lymph nodes were negative; the tumor was 2.5 cm in size and corresponded to an infiltrative squamous cell carcinoma

Invasion is indicated by replacement of the relatively hypointense muscular coast of the urethra, vagina, or anorectum by intermediate signal intensity tumor, contiguous with the vulvar primary tumor.

Pitfalls of MRI

Stage I cancer may be too small to be detected on MRI.

Huge stage I or II tumors that are "en plaque" may be difficult to identify.

Superficial invasion can be difficult to exclude in tumors confined to the labia but lying adjacent to the urethral meatus, introitus, or anal margins.

36.2.2.7 Extension

Carcinoma of the vulva is commonly staged using the FIGO staging classification, which is based on the surgical-pathological findings (Table 36.1) [5].

Imaging procedures, especially MRI, help to assess:

(a) The depth of invasion of the tumor

(b) Local extension:
- Urethral meatus (Fig. 36.3)
- Vagina (Fig. 36.4)
- Perineal muscles
- Anal canal (Fig. 36.5)

(c) Lymphatic and hematogenous spread:
Vulvar cancer spreads by direct extension, followed by lymphatic embolization to inguino-femoral then pelvic lymph nodes

Table 36.1 FIGO staging of vulvar carcinoma

Stage I: Tumor confined to the vulva
IA: Lesions ≤2 cm in size, confined to the vulva or perineum and with stromal invasion ≤10 mm[a], no nodal metastasis
IB: Lesion >2 cm in size or with stromal invasion >10 mm[a], confined to the vulva or perineum, with negative nodes
Stage II: Tumor of any size with extension to adjacent perineal structures (1/3 lower urethra, 1/3 lower vagina, anus) with negative nodes
Stage III: Tumor of any size with or without extension to adjacent perineal structures (1/3 lower urethra, 1/3 lower vagina, anus) with positive inguino-femoral lymph nodes
IIIA: With 1 lymph node metastasis (≥5 mm), or 1–2 lymph nodes metastases (≤5 mm)
IIIB: With 2 or more lymph node metastases (≥5 mm), or 3 or more lymph node metastases (<5 mm)
IIIC: With positive nodes with extracapsular spread
Stage IV: Tumor invades other regional (2/3 upper urethra, 2/3 upper vagina) or distant structures
IVA: Tumor invades any of the following:
Upper urethral and/or vaginal mucosa, bladder mucosa, rectal mucosa, or fixed to pelvic bone
Fixed or ulcerated inguino-femoral lymph nodes
IVB: Any distant metastases including pelvic lymph nodes

[a]The depth of invasion is defined as the measurement of the tumor from the epithelial-stromal junction of the adjacent most superficial dermal papilla to the deepest point of invasion

(Figs. 36.5, 36.6, and 36.7) and finally by hematogenous spread to distant sites. MRI and CT scan often help in performing a sentinel node biopsy.

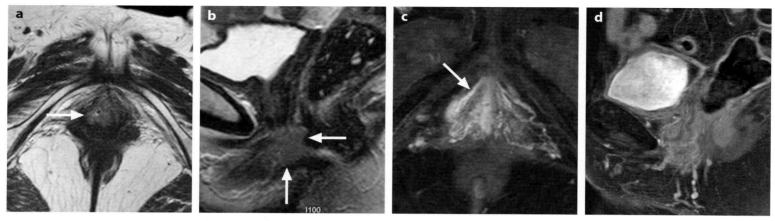

Fig. 36.3 Squamous cell vulvar carcinoma (stage II). Primary basal squamous cell carcinoma of the vulva in a 50-year-old woman primarily treated for cervical squamous cell cancer 10 years ago. Axial (**a**) and sagittal (**b**) T2W images and axial (**c**) and sagittal (**d**) T1W-FS images after gadolinium injection show (*arrows in* **a** *and* **b**) a mass with intermediate signal intensity on T2W images and gadolinium enhancement after injection that corresponds to a tumor of the junction of right labia minora and majora. In (**a**), the tumor (*arrow*) is seen invading and surrounding the lower urethra. Right crus of the clitoris is well seen in **c** (*oblique arrow*). The tumor size was underestimated between 1.7 and 2 cm with MRI, while pathology showed a 3-cm basal squamous tumor

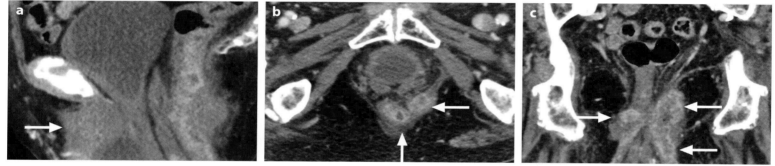

Fig. 36.4 Squamous cell vulvar carcinoma (stage IVB). An 87-year-old woman with prolapse of the three compartments. (**a–c**) CT scan with multi-planar reconstruction in sagittal (**a**), axial (**b**), and coronal (**c**) views shows a vulvar carcinoma (*arrows*) involving upper lateral wall of the vagina, the left ischiocavernosus, and the levator ani muscles. Pelvic lymph nodes were present

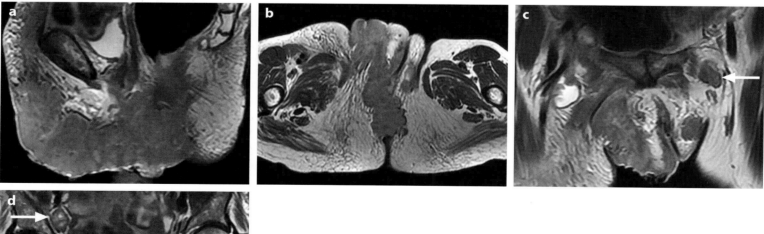

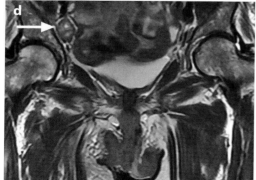

Fig. 36.5 Squamous cell carcinoma (stage IVB) under chemotherapy. MRI in a 75-year-old woman for follow-up of a T4B squamous cell carcinoma under chemotherapy. (**a–d**). Sagittal (**a**), axial (**b**), and coronal (**c**, **d**) T2W images show a huge tumor invading the perineum from the pubis to the anus. Inguinal and pelvic lymph nodes are present, well displayed on coronal images (*arrows*). Pubic bone involvement is also present, well seen in **c**.

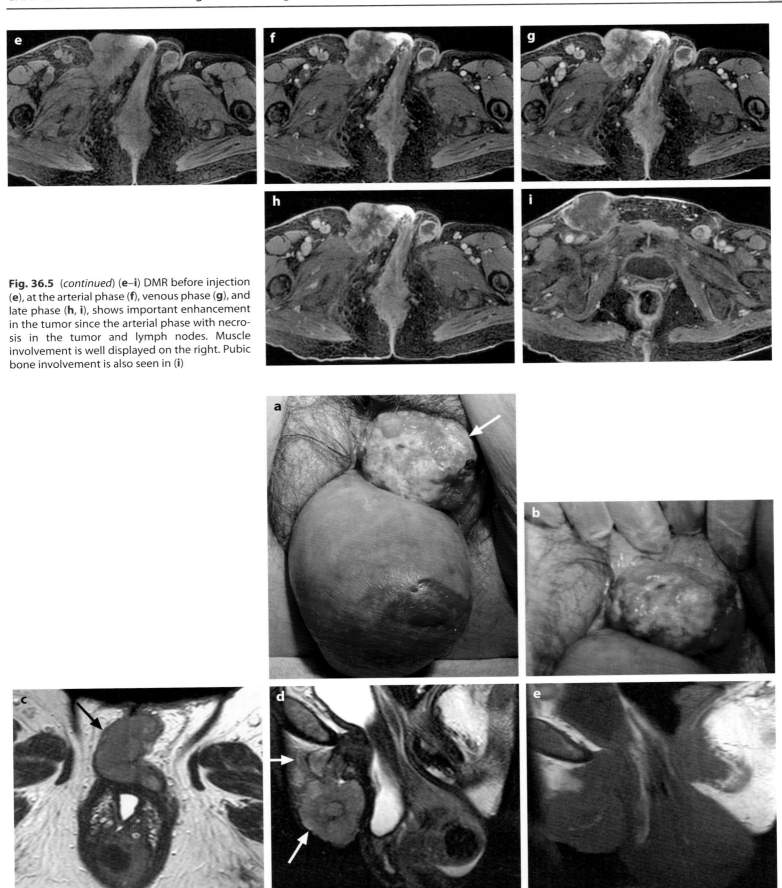

Fig. 36.5 (*continued*) (**e–i**) DMR before injection (**e**), at the arterial phase (**f**), venous phase (**g**), and late phase (**h**, **i**), shows important enhancement in the tumor since the arterial phase with necrosis in the tumor and lymph nodes. Muscle involvement is well displayed on the right. Pubic bone involvement is also seen in (**i**)

Fig. 36.6 Squamous cell vulvar carcinoma (stage IIIA). (**a**, **b**) Squamous cell carcinoma of the left labia majora (*arrow*) in a 79-year-old woman with a 3-compartment prolapse. (**c–e**) Axial T2W (**c**), sagittal T2W (**d**), and sagittal (**e**) T1W images well disclose the vulvar tumor (*oblique arrows* in **c** and **d**) mainly of intermediate intensity on T2W image and low intensity on T1W image and the 3-compartment prolapse (*horizontal arrow* in **d** = glans of clitoris)

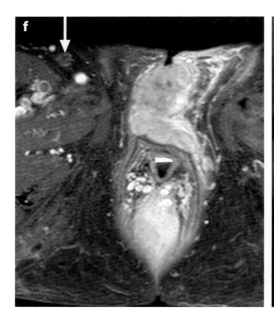

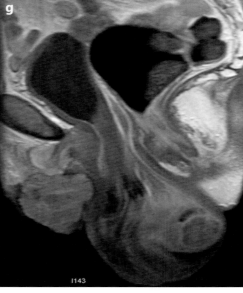

Fig. 36.6 (*continued*) (**f**, **g**) Axial T1W-FS (**f**) and sagittal (**g**) T1W images after gadolinium injection show the mass to infiltrate the left labia majora without involvement of the clitoris, urethra, vagina, and anus. The inguinal small lymph nodes nonclinically palpable are well defined on MRI, but only one right inguinal node was positive at pathology (*vertical arrow* in **f**). Radical vulvectomy and colpectomy were performed

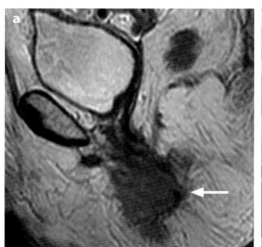

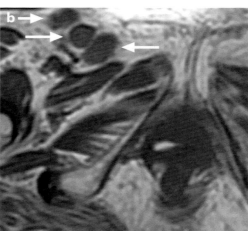

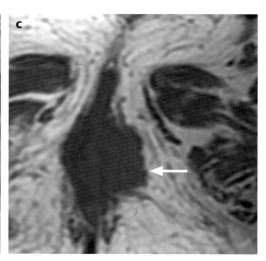

Fig. 36.7 Squamous cell carcinoma of the vulva associated to positive lymph nodes with extracapsular spread (stage IIIC). Sagittal (**a**) and axial (**b**) T2W images and axial T1W image (**c**) exhibit a vulvar mass (*arrows* in **a** and **c**) involving adjacent perineal structures with positive enlarged inguinal lymph nodes showing some irregular borders (*arrows* in **b**). Palliative chemoradiation therapy was performed

36.2.2.8 Treatment

Treatment is closely related to the stage, type, and location of the tumor.

Surgery is the most common treatment of the vulvar cancer:
- Wide local excision taking out the cancer with a safety margin of at least 1 cm.
- Radical local excision taking out the cancer and a larger area of normal tissue all around the tumor with lymph node dissection.
- Partial or hemi-vulvectomy removes part of the vulva.
- Simple vulvectomy: multiple lesions or lesion crossing the median line without lymph nodes.
- Radical vulvectomy takes out the entire vulva with surrounding lymph nodes.
- Pelvic exenteration: if the cancer has spread beyond the vulva.

Chemoradiation therapy
Palliative radiotherapy

36.2.2.9 Prognosis

The prognosis of patient with vulvar cancer is generally good when appropriate treatment is initiated. The number of positive groin nodes is the most important prognostic factor. Other factors are tumor size and ploidy.

36.3 Glandular Tumors

Adenocarcinomas of the vulva are relatively rare. Most arise as primary malignant tumors of the Bartholin glands; however, they may arise from other glands (sweat glands or other skin appendages, Skene glands) or from Paget disease [1].

36.3.1 Bartholin Gland Carcinoma [1, 6]

Several primary malignancies may arise from Bartholin gland; the estimated prevalence of adenocarcinoma is 40 %, squamous cell carcinoma 40 %, adenoid cystic carcinoma 15 %, and other tumors less than 5 %.

The tumor affects women 40–70 years of age.

The criteria for the diagnosis are that the neoplasm must arise at the site of Bartholin gland, be consistent histologically with primary neoplasm of Bartholin gland, and not be metastatic.

At clinical examination, carcinoma of Bartholin gland usually presents as an enlargement in the gland area and may be confused with a Bartholin cyst.

Macroscopically, Bartholin gland tumors are typically solid, deeply infiltrative. They range from 1 to 7 cm and may clinically be mistaken for inflammatory process.

36.3.2 Paget Disease

Adenocarcinoma may be associated with Paget disease.

Paget disease can present as either an erythematous lesion, often involving the vestibule and adjacent areas, or an eczematous lesion that appears as a red to pink area with white islands of hyperkeratosis and usually involving hair-bearing skin [1].

36.4 Mesenchymal Tumors

36.4.1 Vulvar Sarcomas

It arises from a connective component of the vulva. It may occur at any age.

Leiomyosarcomas of the vulva are the most commonly occurring lesions among sarcomas and can affect women from 18 to 66 years of age.

They may be present on the labia majora, clitoris, or Bartholin gland.

Rhabdomyosarcoma is the most common soft tissue sarcoma in children and adolescents; it is thought to originate from primitive mesenchymal tissue that has the capacity to form rhabdomyoblasts.

MRI is the optimal imaging modality for initial diagnosis and for posttreatment follow-up.

36.5 Other Malignant Vulvar Tumors

- Melanoma
- Primary malignant lymphoma
- Yolk sac tumor
- Metastatic tumors

36.5.1 Primary Vulvar Malignant Melanoma [7]

Vulvar malignant melanoma constitutes 5–10 % of all malignant lesions of the vulva.

These entities are the second most common vulvar malignancy after squamous cell carcinoma. The cause is unknown. They may evolve from benign preexisting pigmented lesions. Vulvar bleeding is the most common symptom; pruritus, irritation, and burning are the other symptoms. The lesion is most frequently located on thea clitoris, labia minora, or labia majora. Macroscopically, primary vulvar melanoma appears as a slightly elevated pigmented or non-pigmented lesions or nodular tumor or like a nevi.

On MR, some primary vulvar melanomas appear as typical high signal intensity lesion on T1-weighted images with low signal intensity on T2-weighted or as intermediate to high signal intensity on T1-weighted images and intermediate to high signal intensity on T2-weighted images. They are much more clearly demonstrated on fat-suppressed images with brighter signal.

References

1. Wilkinson EJ (2002) Premalignant and malignant tumors of the vulva. In: Kurman RJ (ed) Blaustein's pathology of the female genital tract, 5th edn. Springer, New-York, pp 99–149
2. Siegelman ES, Outwater EK, Banner MP, Ramchandani P, Anderson TL, Schnall MD (1997) High-resolution MR imaging of the vagina. Radiographics 17(5):1183–1203
3. Griffin N, Grant LA, Sala E (2008) Magnetic resonance imaging of vaginal and vulval pathology. Eur Radiol 18(6):1269–1280
4. Lee SI, Oliva E, Hahn PF, Russell AH (2011) Malignant tumors of the female pelvic floor: imaging features that determine therapy: pictorial review. AJR Am J Roentgenol 196(3 Suppl):S15–S23, Quis S24–S27
5. Pecorelli S (2009) Revised FIGO staging for carcinoma of the vulva, cervix, and endometrium. Int J Gynaecol Obstet 105(2):103–104
6. Ray K, Rocconi RP, Novak L, Straughn JM Jr (2006) Recurrence of endometrial adenocarcinoma in a prior Bartholin's cyst marsupialization incision. Gynecol Oncol 103(2):749–751
7. Piura B, Rabinovich A, Yanai-Inbar I (2002) Primary malignant melanoma of the vagina: case report and review of literature. Eur J Gynaecol Oncol 23(3):195–198

Pathology of the Pelvic Floor

Part 10

Pelvic Floor Dysfunction

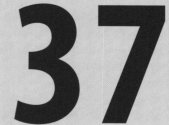

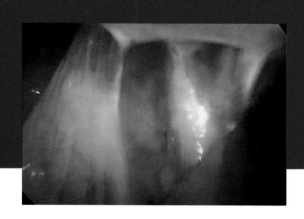

Contents

37.1 Introduction

The pelvic floor is a complex system, with passive and active components that provide pelvic support, maintain continence, and coordinate relaxation during urination and defecation [1].

Whereas exact mechanisms of pelvic floor weakness are subject to debate, established risk factors [2–4] include vaginal childbirth, advancing age as pelvic floor weakness progresses with age, and increasing body mass index. Potential risk factors include ethnicity (most common among Caucasian women, followed by Hispanic, Asian, and Afro-Caribbean women), genetics (higher incidence in some families), collagen-related disorders [5], hysterectomy, and repetitive straining (such as chronic constipation or chronic cough) [6].

Pelvic floor dysfunction is an umbrella term for a heterogeneous group of disorders affecting up to 50 % of middle-aged and older women presenting with stress incontinence, pelvic organ prolapse (POP), and defecatory dysfunction (incomplete defecation or fecal incontinence). In addition, over the next 30 years, the population of women over the age of 60 years is expected to increase at a higher rate than the general population, resulting in a projected 45 % increase in the demand for all services related to treating patients with pelvic floor disorders [7].

Most patients with incontinence and minimal pelvic floor weakness can be treated on physical examination and basic urodynamic findings. But around 15 % of the patients are more symptomatic, and by the age of 70 years, an estimated one in ten undergoes pelvic floor surgical repair. Moreover, despite surgeons' best efforts, symptoms recur in 10–30 % of patients [8]. Although the factors that lead to failure of surgical repair are not well understood, it appears likely that an incomplete physical examination, along with the failure to recognize defects in other compartments that are asymptomatic at the initial evaluation, is contributory for this failure.

J.N. Buy, M. Ghossain, *Gynecological Imaging*,
DOI 10.1007/978-3-642-31012-6_37, © Springer-Verlag Berlin Heidelberg 2013

Consequently, the treatment of pelvic floor dysfunction is becoming increasingly dependent on accurate preoperative imaging to elucidate the presence and extent of pelvic floor abnormalities.

37.2 Definitions

Pelvic organ prolapse and pelvic floor relaxation are two related and often coexistent but separate pathologic entities, which need to be defined and differentiated.

37.2.1 Pelvic Floor Relaxation

There are two components of pelvic floor relaxation: one antero-posterior with a widening of the puborectal hiatus and one vertical with pelvic floor descent.

37.2.2 Prolapse

Pelvic organ prolapse (POP), also called urogenital prolapse, is downward descent of the pelvic organs that results in a protrusion through the urogenital hiatus.

Colpocele is bulging of this organ in the vagina.

POP is distinct from rectal prolapse that is protrusion of the rectum through the anus as a rectal intussusception.

- Different types of POP

  Surgeons view the female pelvis as three functional compartments: anterior compartment (bladder and urethra), middle compartment (vagina, cervix, uterus, *and adnexa*), and posterior compartment (peritoneum and content, rectum *and anus*).

Prolapse can affect the anterior vaginal wall (anterior colpocele), posterior vaginal wall (posterior colpocele), and uterus or apex of the vagina (apical prolapse), usually in some combination.

- Anterior compartment
  - (a) *Urethrocele or urethral hypermobility* is defined as horizontal translation of the urethra away from the normal vertical axis. The angle of the urethral axis is abnormal when it is greater than 30° from the vertical.
  - (b) *Cystocele* results in an anterior colpocele with herniation of the posterior bladder wall through the anterior vaginal wall.
- Middle compartment
  Apical prolapse is protrusion of the uterus or the vaginal cuff in case of hysterectomy in the vagina or beyond it.
- Posterior compartment
  - Posterior Colpocele (Fig. 37.1)
    - (a) *Peritoneocele/enterocele/sigmoidocele*
      These are a herniation of the pelvic peritoneal sac and contents (fat = peritoneocele, small bowel = enterocele/mesenterocele, and less frequently sigmoid = sigmoidocele) beyond the normal confines of the cul-de-sac, through rectovaginal septum, protruding into the posterior vaginal wall.
    - (b) *Rectocele* is herniation of the anterior wall of the rectum above the anal canal through the posterior vaginal wall. Less frequently in context of prior surgery, rectocele can involve the posterior or lateral wall of the rectum.
  - Rectal prolapse
    Rectal prolapse is the protrusion of either the rectal mucosa or the entire wall of the rectum. Partial prolapse involves only the inner lining of the rectum (rectal mucosa) and is usually anterior and protrudes by a few centimeters. Complete prolapse involves all layers of the rectal wall with both the mucosa and muscular layer and is usually circumferential.

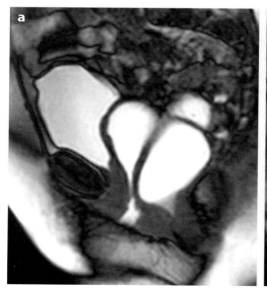
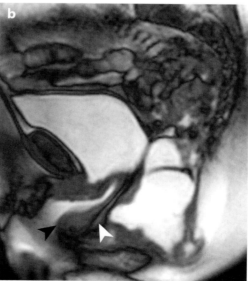

Fig. 37.1 Posterior colpocele in a 78 years old woman with prior hysterectomy. (**a**) resting midsagittal T2 weighted image and (**b**) corresponding midsagittal T2 weighted image at maximal straining image show a peritoneocele with peritoneum in rectovaginal space (*white arrowhead*) bulging to the posterior vaginal wall (*black arrowhead*). Note the presence of a small rectocele

37.3 Clinical Findings

37.3.1 Pelvic Organ Prolapse (POP)

37.3.1.1 Physical Examination

Women presenting with symptoms suggestive of POP undergo pelvic examination. Assessment of POP should be done with the patient resting and straining while supine and standing to define the extent of the prolapse and establish the segments of the vagina affected (anterior, posterior, or apical) (Fig. 37.2).

POP can involve any combination of the following:

- Anterior compartment
  - Urethrocele (also called urethral hypermobility)
  In cases where there is loss of fascial support, an increase of abdominal pressure with coughing or sneezing allows the urethrovesical junction descent and rotation of the urethral axis into the horizontal plane. Bladder pressure rises above urethral pressure, resulting in urine leakage. Thus, patients with urethral hypermobility can have urinary incontinence, and urine leakage may be seen when the patient is asked to perform a Valsalva maneuver. The diagnosis of urethral hypermobility is made at physical examination and cystourethroscopy. Direct observation of urethral mobility is made by placing a Q-tip at the urethrovesical junction and asking the patient to strain.
  - Cystocele: anterior colpocele
  As the bladder neck and proximal urethra are mobile, descent of the bladder neck during strain may result in clockwise rotational descent of the bladder neck and proximal urethra and can cause kinking of the proximal urethra that may mask stress urinary incontinence and may be a potential cause of urinary retention leading to urinary stasis and infection.
  Other signs include a vaginal mass with symptoms of heaviness and bulging of tissues in the vagina that are exacerbated by physical exertion or standing for prolonged periods of time

and back pain if the bladder prolapse is severe enough as the muscular pelvic floor may entrap the ureters and create ureteral obstruction (hydronephrosis).

- Middle compartment
  - Apical prolapse entails either the uterus or post-hysterectomy vaginal cuff
  In severe cases of complete eversion, cervical and uterine prolapses (procidentia) are seen as a bulging mass outside the external genitalia as the vaginal walls form a sac containing the prolapsing organs. If this prolapse is long standing, the mucosa can become thick. Patients with vaginal eversion have difficulty walking or sitting as well as pelvic pressure and protrusion of tissue through the vagina.
- Posterior compartment: posterior colpocele
  Posterior vaginal wall prolapse (or a posterior colpocele) involves the rectum, peritoneum with or without bowel, or both.
  - Peritoneocele/enterocele/sigmoidocele
  On physical examination, enlargement of the enterocele may produce a bulge at the introitus and the presence of a bulge in the superoposterior vaginal wall. The examiner places one finger in the vagina and another one in the rectum. The presence of small bowel in the rectovaginal space is suggested by loops of small bowel palpated between an examiner's fingers or by observation of peristalsis behind the posterior vaginal wall. Peristalsis of small bowel may also be appreciated if the vaginal wall is thin. The incidence of enterocele has markedly increased as a result of the widespread performance of both hysterectomy and cystourethropexy because both of these procedures open up the posterior cul-de-sac.
  Patients may have a dragging sensation in the pelvis as well as pelvic pressure. Stretching of the mesentery with straining can cause pain in the lower abdomen or back. An enterocele may result in compression of the distal part of the anorectum and finally in incomplete evacuation due to outlet obstruction.

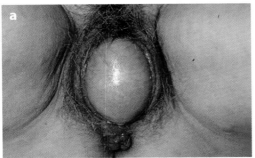
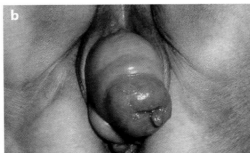
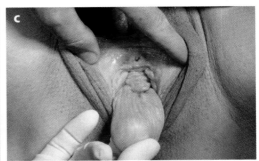
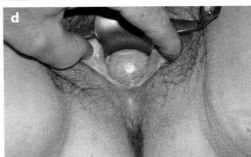

Fig. 37.2 Photographs in lithotomy position. Pelvic organ prolapse might include (**a**) bladder (cystocele), (**b**) uterus (hysterocele), (**c**) peritoneum (peritoneocele), (**d**) rectum (rectocele)

Peritoneocele/enterocele may not always be detected clinically or can also be confused with high rectoceles. Exceptionally peritoneocele can occur between the bladder and the vagina through the vesicovaginal septum (only in the context of hysterectomy).

– Rectocele

A rectocele is diagnosed when a coincident anterior and inferior rectal wall bulge occurs during evacuation. Most are not apparent at rest. Rectoceles are common in women because the rectovaginal septum is relatively weak, and rectoceles are likely to be a normal variant [9] but only become clinically significant when symptoms develop. Patients may present with obstructed defecation or incomplete evacuation as the association between a large rectocele and difficult evacuation is well recognized. Many need to assist defecation by applying digital pressure to the perineal body or posterior vaginal wall. Asymptomatic rectoceles are present in up to 80 % of patients with multicompartment disease.

Other symptoms include a bulge along the superoposterior wall of vagina, perineal fullness, dyspareunia, and low back pain.

Very uncommonly, posterolateral herniation of the rectum may result from levator ani damage during childbirth or prior to surgery in the rectal region.

37.3.1.2 Clinical Classification

Although several prolapse grading systems exist, the only system with international acceptance is the pelvic organ prolapse quantification (POP-Q) system [10].

The amount of prolapse is systematically defined during a pelvic examination by measuring anterior, posterior, and apical segments of the vaginal wall in centimeters relative to a fixed anatomical structure (the vaginal hymen). Six points are measured with reference to the plane of the hymen. Points above or proximal to the hymen are described by the distance from the hymenal plane in centimeters preceded by a minus sign, while points below or distal to the hymen are described by the distance in centimeters preceded by a positive sign. Three other measurements include total vaginal length, genital hiatus, and perineal body, for a total of nine points, which can be documented on the 3×3 grid (Fig. 37.3). Enterocele is not a part of the POP-Q system and should be noted by the examiner.

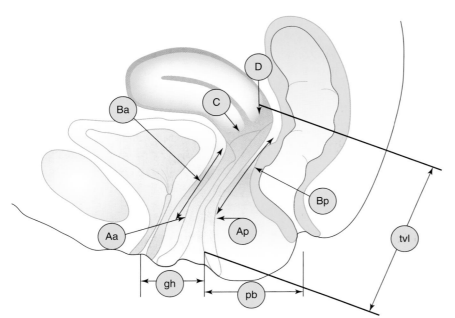

anterior wall		anterior wall		cervix or cuff	
	Aa		Ba		C
genital hiatus		perineal body		total vaginal length	
	gh		pb		tvl
posterior wall		posterior wall		posterior fornix	
	Ap		Bp		D

Fig. 37.3 Graphic of the different points and measurements of POP Q system and the 3x3 grid. *Anterior Vaginal Wall: Point Aa* corresponds approximately to the urethrovesical junction. *Point Ba:* Represents the most distal position of any part of the upper anterior vaginal wall from the vaginal cuff or anterior vaginal fornix to *point Aa. Posterior Vaginal Wall:* Posterior vaginal wall points are measured with the woman straining after single speculum blade is turned to retract the anterior vaginal wall. *Point Ap:* Located in the midline of the posterior vaginal wall, 3 cm proximal to the hymen. *Point Bp:* The most distal position of any part of the upper posterior vaginal wall from the vaginal cuff or posterior vaginal fornix to *point Ap. Superior Vagina:* Points located on the superior vagina represent the most proximal location of the normally positioned pelvic organs. These points are assessed with the woman straining with an assembled speculum in place. *Point C:* The most distal (most dependent) edge of the cervix or the leading edge of the vaginal cuff after hysterectomy. *Point D:* Marks the location of the posterior fornix in a woman who still has a cervix. *Additional Measurements: Total Vaginal Length (TVL):* With an assembled speculum in place and point C or D reduced completely to its normal position, the total vaginal length is measured as the greatest depth of the vagina in centimeters. *Genital Hiatus (GH):* Measured from the middle of the external urethral meatus to the posterior midline hymen while the patient is straining. *Perineal Body (PB):* Measured from the posterior margin of the GH to the midanal opening

Table 37.1 Quantification of stages of prolapse

Stage	Definition
Stage 0	Points Aa, Ap, Ba, and Bp are assigned value of −3 cm. Value for point D or C is less or equal to TVL (cm) −2 cm and has a negative sign. This stage represents no prolapse
Stage I	The most distal portion of the prolapse is more than 1 cm above the level of the hymen
Stage II	The most distal portion of the prolapse is 1 cm or less above the level of the hymen or within one centimeter below the hymen
Stage III	The most distal portion of the prolapse is more than 1 cm below the hymen, but no further than 2 cm less than the total vaginal length in centimeters
Stage IV	Almost complete eversion of the total length of the vagina is present. The protrusion minimally extends beyond hymen further than TVL-2 cm

Prolapse is quantified by stages, which are assigned according to the most severe portion of the prolapse when the maximum protrusion has been demonstrated (Table 37.1).

37.3.2 Rectal Prolapse

It is important to understand that POP is distinct from rectal prolapse, in which the rectum protrudes through the anus as a rectal intussusception.

Although mucosa alone may prolapse (anterior mucosal prolapse), invagination or intussusception is defined as a full-thickness rectal wall prolapse involving both the mucosa and muscular layer. Both can be associated with a rectocele during straining. Infolding of the rectal wall may be intrarectal, intra-anal, or complete rectal prolapse. Extra-anal invagination is currently clinically termed rectal prolapse [11]. This causes a mechanical obstruction to the passage of stool. Similar to a rectocele, small degrees of rectal intussusception can also be seen in asymptomatic individuals (50 % in volunteers [9]). Rectoanal or extra-anal intussusceptions can be associated with rectal ulcer.

37.3.3 Spastic Pelvic Floor Syndrome

Spastic pelvic floor syndrome (also known as anismus, pelvic floor dyssynergy, or paradoxical puborectalis contraction) is a functional abnormality that affects some constipated patients who experience evacuation failure associated with involuntary, inappropriate, and paradoxical contraction of striated pelvic floor musculature (mainly the puborectalis muscle) [12]. The etiology of this condition is unclear and can include both abnormal muscle activity and psychological or cognitive factors [1]. Increased pressure at rest and during defecation is shown with anorectal manometry, while pathological signals are evident at electromyography.

37.3.4 Incontinence

37.3.4.1 Urinary Incontinence

Urinary incontinence has been defined as "a condition in which involuntary loss of urine is a social or a hygienic problem and is objectively demonstrable" [13].

Urinary incontinence in women is divided into stress urinary incontinence, urge urinary incontinence, and overflow urinary incontinence. Stress urinary incontinence is defined as uncontrolled urine leakage during stress or activity such as sneezing, coughing, or exercise. Two types of stress urinary incontinence are identified: genuine stress incontinence, caused by hypermobility of the bladder neck, and the less frequent intrinsic sphincter deficiency, caused by a sphincter defect. Urge incontinence and overflow urinary incontinence are related to bladder abnormalities. In urge incontinence, there is detrusor overactivity due to damage to the nervous system supplying the urinary bladder, such as in multiple sclerosis, stroke, or pelvic injury, and a large amount of urine leaks when the patient experiences a sudden urge to urinate. In overflow incontinence, a small amount of urine leaks when the urinary bladder is overdistended because of weakness of the bladder muscles in a neurogenic bladder or in chronic bladder outlet obstruction.

37.3.4.2 Anal Incontinence

Anal incontinence is common, especially in women, with a prevalence increasing with age, and has a considerable economic impact [14]. Patients can present with either fecal leakage suggesting an internal sphincter abnormality or with urge incontinence, indicating external sphincter damage. The most common cause of incontinence is vaginal delivery that causes direct sphincter laceration or indirect damage to sphincter innervation. Other causes include iatrogenic damage (as a complication of anal surgery) or neuropathy.

37.4 Anatomy of Pelvic Floor Structures and Physiopathology

The pelvic floor is a complex, integrated, multilayered anatomic and functional unit that provides active and passive support. Endopelvic fascia and ligaments to the bony pelvis provide passive support, while the muscles of the pelvic floor, mainly the levator ani, provide active support.

Support of the pelvic structures depends on the interplay between the fascia and ligaments and the levator ani muscle. Disruption with tears or dysfunction (weakness) of both or one of the structures may be compensated for by the others but will predispose to eventual pelvic floor disorders leading to various degrees and combinations of pelvic organ prolapse and pelvic floor relaxation.

37.4.1 Active Support: Levator Ani

37.4.1.1 Anatomy

In many mammal quadruped species, the levator ani is composed of different muscles which are distinct, the ones of the cloacae sphincter and the ones of the caudo-pelvic muscle. But in primates, the levator ani is a broad muscular sheet which is subdivided into named portions according to their attachments and the pelvic viscera to which they are related. These parts are often referred to as separate muscles, but it must be kept in mind that the boundaries between each part cannot be easily distinguished. Considering the Terminologia Anatomica (international anatomical terminology), the levator ani complex comprises five distinct origin-insertion pairs or subdivisions [15], each with its own unique mechanical effect. The puboanalis, puboperinealis, and pubovaginalis muscles form a single mass in some regions and are separately classified because of their different insertion points. They are, therefore, displayed together as a single structure for visual clarity referred to the term pubovisceralis (pubococcygeus). The two other parts are the puborectalis and iliococcygeus muscles (Fig. 37.4).

To simplify, two perpendicular components can be described [16]: an inferomedial part (composed of the pubovisceralis and the puborectalis) which is central, vertical, thick, and has sphincter function and the superoposterolateral part (composed of the iliococcygeus) which is lateral, horizontal, thin, and has a function of elevating.

The inferomedial part of the levator ani is attached to the back of the body of the pubis and passes back almost vertically. It can be divided in two parts: the pubovisceralis and the puborectalis. The pubovisceralis lies medial to the puborectalis, arises high on the pubis near the superior pubic ramus where it forms a single mass, and is then divided into separate parts according to the pelvic viscera to which they relate: the pubovaginalis, puboperinealis, and puboanalis muscles which are separately classified because of their different insertion points, the vagina, perineal body, and anus, respectively. The puborectalis arises near the inferior pubic ramus and passes, as a thick muscular sling, behind the rectum around the anorectal junction just cephalad to the anal sphincter.

The superoposterolateral part (iliococcygeus part) is a wide, thin, and horizontal sheetlike structure attached to the inner surface of the ischial spine below and anterior to the attachment of the ischiococcygeus and to the obturator fascia as far forward as the obturator canal. The most posterior fibers are attached to the tip of the sacrum and coccyx, but most join with fibers from the opposite side to form the raphe (anococcygeal ligament).

The innervations of the levator ani consist of fibers originating mainly in the second, third, and fourth sacral spinal segments to reach the muscle from below and above in a variety of routes.

The levator ani is supplied by branches of the inferior gluteal artery, the inferior vesical artery, and the pudendal artery.

Unlike other skeletal muscles in the body, in healthy women, the LA remains in constant tone even during rest. It is well recognized

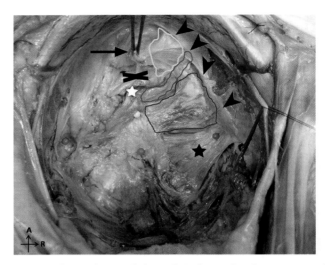

Fig. 37.4 View from above of the pelvic floor. The three major subdivisions of the right part of the levator ani are contoured: the pubovisceralis (*pink*), the puborectalis (*brown*), and the iliococcygeus (*purple*). Urethra cut (*black arrow*), vagina cut (*black cross*), rectum cut (*white star*), arcus tendineus of levator ani (*arrow heads*), ischiococcygeus ligament (*black star*), *red mark* (right ischial spine), *blue mark* (left ischial spine), *green mark* (sacrococcygeus junction), *yellow mark* (tip of the coccyx)

that the levator ani must relax appropriately to permit expulsion of urine and particularly feces. This striated muscle has slow-twitch (type I) muscle fibers [17] that continuously contract at rest and provide tone to the pelvic floor, against the stress that comes from gravity and intra-abdominal pressure. Its activity automatically adjusts to variations in posture and abdominal pressure to provide upward support to the pelvic viscera. Its action minimizes the load on connective tissues that attach the organs to the pelvis.

Tonic contraction closes the urogenital hiatus and provides a supportive platform during normal activity and standing. At rest, by forming a U-shaped sling between the pubis and the anus, the puborectalis particularly acts as an anterior sling keeping the rectum, vagina, and urethra elevated and closed by pressing them anteriorly toward the pubic symphysis, resulting in an acute angle between the bladder neck and the urethra as between the anus and the rectum.

37.4.1.2 MRI

The subdivisions of the levator ani muscle are clearly seen in MRI scans on T2-weighted MR images, each with distinct morphology and characteristic features [18].

- The inferomedial part (pubovisceralis and puborectalis) (Figs. 37.5, 37.6, and 37.7)
  The axial plane provides a clear view of the pubovisceralis and its subdivisions. Near the pubic origin, the pubovisceralis subdivisions cannot be distinguished. However, the different insertion points of the pubovaginalis, puboperinealis, and puboanalis muscles can be seen. The pubovaginalis attachment is identified as medial fusion of the muscle with the vaginal wall. The puboperinealis muscle can be seen entering into the perineal body.

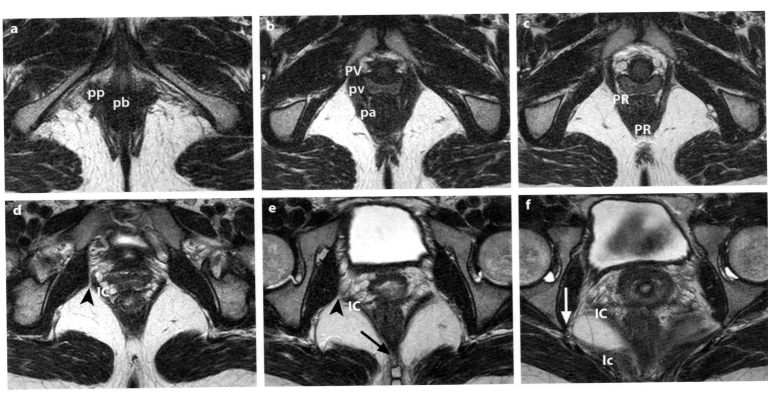

Fig. 37.5 Axial T2-weighted scan of a 22-year-old nullipara volunteer showing subdivisions of the levator ani from bottom to top. (a) axial image shows the puboperinealis (*pp*) entering the perineal body (*pb*). (b) axial image shows the anterior retropubic part of the pubovisceralis (*PV*) and distal insertions with attachment to the vaginal wall (the pubovaginalis (*pv*)) and with attachment to the anal canal wall (the puboanalis (*pa*)). (c) axial image shows the puborectalis (*PR*) appearing as a sling dorsal to the rectum. (d–f) axial images show the iliococcygeus (*IC*) arising from the arcus tendineus levator ani (*arrow head*) and passing around the rectum above the fibers of the puborectalis to form the anococcygeal raphe (*black arrow*). Note that the iliococcygeus is up to the ischial spine (*white arrow*) behind the ischiococcygeus (*Ic*)

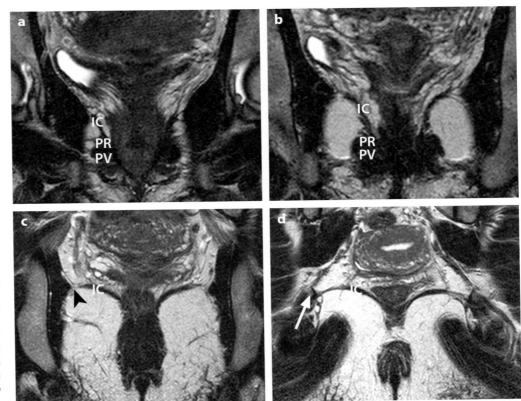

Fig. 37.6 Coronal T2-weighted scan of a 22-year-old nullipara volunteer showing subdivisions of the levator ani from back to forth. (a, b) coronal images show well the two perpendicular components of the levator ani with its inferomedial part composed of the pubovisceralis and the puborectalis (*PV + PR*) and its superoposterolateral part composed of the iliococcygeus (*IC*). (c, d) coronal images show the iliococcygeus (*IC*) with its winglike configuration arising from the arcus tendineus levator ani (*arrow head*) up to the ischial spine (*white arrow*)

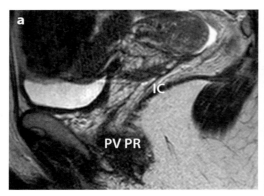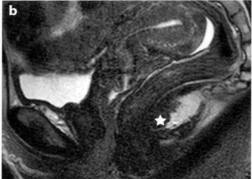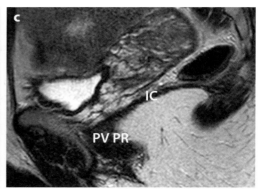

Fig. 37.7 Sagittal T2-weighted scan of a 22-year-old nullipara volunteer showing subdivisions of the levator ani from right to left. (a, c) sagittal images show the shelflike orientation of the iliococcygeus (*IC*) which is dorsal and above the pubovisceralis and puborectalis (*PV + PR*). (**b**) median sagittal image shows the puborectalis that passes dorsal to the rectum with decussating fibers forming a "bump" (*star*)

The puboanalis portion can be seen passing into the intersphincteric space.

The puborectalis is a subdivision that can be distinguished from the three elements of the pubovisceralis. It originates lateral to the pubovisceralis and appears as a sling dorsal to the rectum. The aspect of the right puborectalis may appear slightly thinner than the left, a finding that is caused by chemical shift artifact in most cases.

The coronal view is perpendicular to the fiber direction of the puborectalis and pubovisceralis and shows them as "clusters" of muscle on either side of the vagina because their fibers are contiguous and without visible separation; the two together are seen as a single body of muscle lateral to the vagina. Similarly, the subdivisions composing the pubovisceralis cannot be separated in the coronal MRI cross sections.

The sagittal plane offers the distinct advantage of being parallel to the pubovisceralis and puborectalis fiber directions, allowing the fibers of the puborectalis to be seen as they pass dorsal to the rectum forming a "bump" that is consistently visible.

• The superoposterolateral part/iliococcygeus (Figs. 37.5, 37.6, and 37.7)

The coronal plane is optimal for viewing the iliococcygeus in the dorsal parts of the pelvis. This winglike configuration is visible as it arises from its lateral attachments to the arcus tendineus levator ani over the obturator internus muscle. On coronal images, the iliococcygeal muscle should be intact and upwardly convex. As women age, some thinning of the levator ani muscle occurs normally; however, no tears should be identified. In axial images, it can be seen passing around the rectum above the fibers of the puborectal muscle. The sagittal images show the shelf like orientation of the iliococcygeus muscle, which has been referred, with the addition of the anococcygeal raphe, as the "levator plate" by various authors.

37.4.1.3 Pathology

The injury to the levator ani plays a significant role in prolapse [19, 20], and different studies add to a growing body of data concerning connective-tissue abnormalities [21] and smooth muscle [22, 23]

in the development of prolapse. For instance, it is plausible that failure in one element (levator ani muscle) could lead to increased demands on other components (connective tissue and smooth muscle) which may eventually fail as well. The fact that 30 % of the women with prolapse had no evidence of a muscle defect on MRI supports the fact that the disease process involves other factors as well. This fact does not diminish the importance of levator ani injury but is a reminder that multiple aspects of the system underlie failure. Decline of normal levator ani tone – by denervation or direct muscle trauma – results in an open urogenital hiatus, weakening of the horizontal orientation of the iliococcygeus, and a bowl-like configuration [24].

Each component of the levator ani muscle has a unique origin-insertion pair and, thus, a unique line of action. An injury to each individual subdivision of the levator ani would be expected to have a specific functional effect resulting in a unique deficit. But there are no clear-cut boundaries between normal and abnormal morphologic condition of the pelvic floor considering the morphologic variants of the levator ani muscle [19, 25]. For example, the absence of a visible insertion of the LA inside the pubic bone on both sides in 10 % of all women can be a surprising result, because all anatomy books describe this connection. If some of anatomic variants that may favor prolapse after vaginal birth may be questioned, for now, findings on MRI can be regarded as pathological only if the corresponding clinical symptoms are present.

In addition to direct muscle trauma, neuropathic injury of the levator ani muscles can result from vaginal delivery [26]. Chronic straining to achieve defecation has also been associated with pelvic muscle denervation [27]. The excess straining and associated perineal descent are thought to cause stretch injury to nerve and result in neuropathy.

37.4.2 Passive Support

37.4.2.1 Bone

The bony pelvis and lumbar osseous system plays a role in the orientation of the forces to the pelvic structures. Variations in orientation and shape of the bony pelvis have been associated with development of pelvic organ prolapse. Specifically, a loss of lumbar lordosis and a pelvic inlet that is less vertically oriented is more usual in women who develop genital prolapse than in those who do not [28, 29]. A less vertical orientation of the pelvic inlet is thought to result in alteration of intra-abdominal vector forces that are usually directed anteriorly to the pubic symphysis such that a greater proportion is directed toward the pelvic viscera and their connective-tissue and muscular supports.

37.4.2.2 Fascia

Anatomy

- The endopelvic fascia is the connective-tissue network that envelops all organs of the pelvis and connects them loosely to the supportive musculature and bones of the pelvis. The endopelvic fascia and the ligaments formed from fascia are not seen on MRI.
  - Anteriorly, the endopelvic fascia forms a supportive layer called the pubocervical fascia between the pubis, the urinary bladder, and the anterior vaginal wall. It attaches to the arcus tendineus fasciae pelvis anterolaterally and to the cervix posteriorly and attaches the lateral part of the vagina to the pelvic sidewalls.
  - In the middle compartment, the endopelvic fascia also attaches the uterus-cervix and vagina to the pelvic sidewall via the elastic condensations known as the parametrium and paracolpium, respectively. The parametrium is made up of the cardinal and uterosacral ligaments (which suspend the uterus and upper vagina from the presacral fascia) and provides support to the body of the uterus. The uterosacral ligaments suspend the cervix and upper vagina from the presacral fascia. This attachment pulls these structures superiorly and posteriorly over the levator ani toward the sacrum. This mechanism is protective because the vagina moves into the hollow of the sacrum and forms a horizontal supporting shelf when abdominal pressure increases. The paracolpium stretches the vagina transversely between the bladder and the rectum. Vaginal support in the pelvis has been described by DeLancey [30] as having three levels of support. The cephalic 2–3-cm portion of the vagina, described as level 1, is suspended from the pelvic sidewall by the parametrium and paracolpium, which are condensations of the endopelvic fascia. Level 3 is described as the level that starts at the hymen ring and extends 2–3 cm cephalad to it, and level 2 is between levels 1 and 3. Level 2 of the vagina is attached to the arcus tendineus, although level 3 is directly attached to its surrounding structures: anteriorly to the urethra, posteriorly to the perineal body, and laterally with the levator ani muscles, rather than being attached to or suspended from the pelvic walls.
  - Posteriorly the endopelvic fascia forms a supportive layer, the rectovaginal fascia, between the posterior vaginal wall and the rectum, which attaches the posterior part of the vagina to perineal body and prevents the rectum from protruding

forward and the bowel from herniating inferiorly. One of the muscles of the levator ani, the iliococcygeus muscle, is a horizontally oriented sheet of muscle that, together with the rectovaginal fascia, forms a diaphragm that provides support to the pelvic organs, especially those in the posterior compartment.

- Two dense aggregations of obturator and levator ani fascia, the arcus tendineus fasciae pelvis and arcus tendineus levator ani, provide important passive lateral support. The arcus tendineus fasciae pelvis provides lateral anchoring for the anterior vaginal wall where it underlies and supports the urethra, while the arcus tendineus levator ani provides anchoring for the levator ani muscles. While the arcus tendineus levator ani can be identified on MRI images as the origin of the iliococcygeus at the internal obturator fascia, the arcus tendineus fasciae pelvis cannot be visualized on MRI.

Pathology

Disruption or stretching of these connective-tissue attachments happens during vaginal delivery or hysterectomy, with chronic straining, or with normal aging [8].

In the anterior compartment, defects in the pubocervical fascia with loss of support to the urethra and bladder can allow urethral hypermobility and ultimately a cystocele. Four types of defects can occur in the pubocervical fascia: lateral or paravaginal defects when the pubocervical fascia detaches from the arcus tendineus fasciae pelvis, transverse defects when the pubocervical fascia detaches from its central attachment at the pericervical ring of fibrous tissue, central defects when the pubocervical fascia is disrupted in the midline under the bladder base, and distal defects when the fascia detaches from the urogenital diaphragm. The most common type of defect is the paravaginal defect, which may be unilateral or bilateral and is often seen in patients with urethral hypermobility. More important stretching or tearing of the pubocervical fascia and levator ani muscle allows the posterior aspect of the bladder to bulge into the anterior vaginal wall.

In the middle compartment, abnormalities of the pubocervical fascia, parametrium, paracolpium, or uterosacral ligaments allow mobility and descent of the uterus, cervix, or vaginal cuff. In patients who have undergone a hysterectomy, prolapse of the vaginal apex can arise because of weakness of the paracolpium, resulting in apical prolapse.

In the posterior compartment, prolapse of peritoneal contents is due to deficiency of the supporting ligaments, the rectovaginal fascia and iliococcygeus muscle, resulting in widening of the rectovaginal space. There are two types of enterocele: the one with a mechanism of traction (follows vaginal/uterine prolapse) and the one with a mechanism of pulsion (occurs with chronic pressure on vaginal vault). In normal individuals, the rectovaginal space caudal to the upper third of the vagina is closely apposed [31]. Widening of this space will allow inferior herniation of the peritoneal fat, small bowel, sigmoid colon, and fluid into the pouch of Douglas. Prior hysterectomy may cause disruption of the rectovaginal fascia

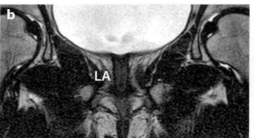
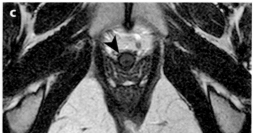

Fig. 37.8 Normal urethra of a 24-year-old nullipara volunteer. (**a**) sagittal T2-weighted image shows the normal position of the urethra (*arrow heads*). (**b**) coronal T2-weighted image shows the relationships of the urethra with the levator ani (*LA*). (**c**) axial T2-weighted image shows the midportion of the urethra well delineated by the outer striated muscle layer which appears hypointense

and is a risk factor for peritoneocele as a vaginal vault descent causes a traction effect on the cul-de-sac, displacing it inferiorly, and creates a wider potential space for the peritoneal cul-de-sac to descend through or can cause a traction effect on it [1], resulting in a peritoneocele.

A rectocele results from defects in the prerectal and pararectal fascia as well as the rectovaginal septum.

In addition, the smooth muscle of the posterior [22] and anterior [23] vaginal walls, which normally reinforce the rectovaginal and the pubocervical fascia respectively, is altered in women with POP.

37.4.3 Sphincters

The female urethra is approximately 4.5 cm long, with two-thirds of the urethra above the levator ani. The urethral sphincter is composed of involuntary inner smooth muscle that is continuous with the bladder as well as the voluntary external sphincter, which is composed of striated muscle. The amount of striated muscle decreases with aging, and this may play a role in incontinence. The urethra can be appreciated on MRI (Fig. 37.8), but its different layers and its supporting ligaments are readily visible at high-resolution MR imaging with an endovaginal or endourethral coil on T2-weighted images [1, 32].

The anorectal junction is defined as the point of angulation between rectum and anal canal, corresponding to the posterior impression of the puborectal muscle (Fig. 37.9). In healthy patients, the anorectal angle closes during squeezing, and the anorectal junction can rise 1–2 cm from the rest position. During straining and defecation, the anorectal angle becomes more obtuse, the anal canal opens and shortens, and the rectum is rapidly evacuated. Finally, the anal canal closes, and the anorectal junction and anorectal angle return to their pre-evacuation positions.

The anal sphincters form two cylindrical layers, between which lies the longitudinal muscle. The internal sphincter forms the innermost muscular layer and is the terminal condensation of the circular rectal smooth muscle. The internal sphincter extends from the anorectal junction to approximately 1 cm below the dentate line. It is composed of smooth muscle fibers with autonomous innervation from sympathetic presacral nerves. The longitudinal muscle is the continuation of the longitudinal muscle of the rectal wall [1]. The deep part of the external anal sphincter is fused with or intimately related to the puborectalis muscle. Anteriorly, it is closely related to the superficial transverse muscle of the perineum and the perineal body. Posteriorly, the muscle is continuous with the anococcygeal raphe. The anal sphincter muscles are well visualized on MRI (Fig. 37.10), but their study is usually not performed during a dynamic study of the pelvis. It can be performed with an endoanal coil after the dynamic evaluation if desired or is usually a separate study [1].

37.4.4 Urogenital Diaphragm

The most caudal part of the pelvic floor, the urogenital diaphragm, is composed mainly of connective tissue and the deep transverse perineal muscle, oriented transversely just deep to the pelvic diaphragm and anterior to the anorectal junction. It is a diamond-shaped combination of two contiguous triangles (anterior and posterior), whose common base is the transverse perineal muscle. The apex of the anterior triangle is the symphysis pubis, and the sides are the pubic bones. The apex of the posterior triangle is the tip of the coccyx. The anterior triangle is penetrated by the urethra and vagina, whereas the posterior triangle is penetrated by the anus.

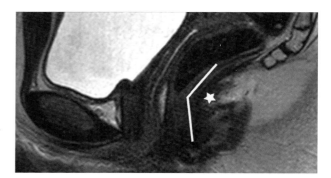

Fig. 37.9 Normal anorectal junction of a 24-year-old nullipara volunteer. Sagittal T2-weighted image shows the anorectal junction at the point of the angulation of the rectum and the anal canal. Note the posterior impression of the puborectal muscle (*star*)

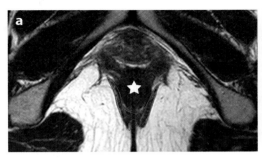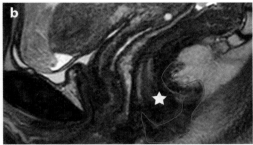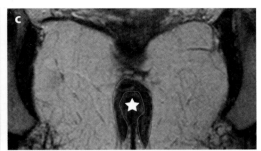

Fig. 37.10 Normal canal anal sphincters of a 22-year-old nullipara volunteer. (**a**) axial, (**b**) paramedian sagittal, and (**c**) coronal T2-weighted images show the external sphincter (*red line*) wrapped behind the internal sphincter (*star*)

Directly anterior to the anal sphincter is the perineal body (central tendon of the perineum) which can be considered as a passive support structure. In women, it lies between vaginal introitus and anal canal. Many structures insert fibers into the perineal body, including the external anal sphincter, the deep and superficial transverse muscles of the perineum, and the bulbocavernosus and puborectalis muscles. The perineal body prevents expansion of the urogenital hiatus, which is the orifice through which pelvic organ prolapse occurs. The perineal body may be damaged during vaginal delivery via an episiotomy. Although the urogenital diaphragm is variably visualized in routine clinical MR imaging applications, it has been imaged with high resolution with the use of endoluminal coils [1].

37.5 Imaging

37.5.1 Indication

Treatment for the most patients with incontinence and minimal pelvic floor weakness can be based on physical examination and basic urodynamic findings. In patients with moderate to severe symptoms, imaging will be useful. Imaging is complementary to physical examination and assists urogynecologists in localizing and grading pelvic floor dysfunction for surgical triage and planning to avoid recurrence.

Although the factors that lead to failure of surgical repair are not well understood, it appears likely that the limitations of physical examination and the failure to recognize asymptomatic defects are contributory. It is advisable to identify all of the areas of prolapse preoperatively as coexisting asymptomatic defects may become symptomatic within a relatively short time and all may require correction; ideally, this is done at one surgical setting. For example, experience with dynamic imaging has shown that peritoneoceles (enteroceles and sigmoidoceles) are difficult to diagnose on physical examination [33] and only 50 % of enteroceles are diagnosed on physical examination.

Imaging is indicated under the following circumstances:
- Preoperative planning tool:
  - Multicompartmental involvement with a planned complex repair. For some, imaging is indicated every time a surgery is planned to avoid failure.
  - Prior pelvic surgery or prior hysterectomy.
  - Recurrence after previous repair of pelvic floor dysfunction.
- To characterize a posterior colpocele (rectocele, peritoneocele, and its contents): Peritoneocele/enteroceles may not always be detected clinically or can also be confused with high rectoceles. Imaging allows direct visualization of the content and easily differentiates a rectocele from an enterocele, which can alter clinical management.
- In case of suboptimal physical examination (obesity, clinical discordance between physical examination and symptoms).
- In case of suspicion of associated pelvic disease.

37.5.2 MRI

37.5.2.1 Protocol (Table 37.2)

Table 37.2 Protocol

Patient preparation		
The patient is asked to void before the exam and perform a rectal evacuating enema few hours before the exam		
Explanations of the modality of the exam are given to the patient to achieve complete cooperation		
No oral or intravenous contrast agents nor bowel preparation		
Opacification	Vaginal opacification with 15–50 cc of sonographic gel	
	Rectal opacification with 120 cc of sonographic gel	
Patient installation: supine position with legs somewhat apart, with headphones attached		
MRI technique		
Morphologic sequences	Dynamic sequences	
Three planes in T2 ponderation sequences with 5-mm-thick images	6- to 10-mm-thick sagittal images of the midline obtained with a steady-state T2-weighted imaging sequence obtained at rest, during squeezing, and during Valsalva maneuver with straining and defecation	
	Repeat sequence at least two or three times up to satisfactory results	

Patient Preparation

Classic contraindications are a patient with a pace maker or a metallic foreign body. Claustrophobia may be prevented by medication.

1. Explanations to the patient:

   The more extensive abnormalities detected with imaging compared with physical examination are likely, at least partly, due to the ability to image the patient during defecation compared with only the Valsalva maneuver with physical examination. Complete relaxation of pelvic floor muscles occurs only during defecation (and micturition), thereby permitting maximal pelvic organ prolapse.

   Thus, because the patient's cooperation is of major importance in achieving a satisfactory examination, explanation with clear and simple instructions is crucial during the preparatory phase, since defecating in the supine position could be difficult for some patients. Comprehension and cooperation of the patient are essential, and the importance of defecating is explained to the patient. It is important to review the concept of the Valsalva maneuver with the technologists so as to coach the patient on how to perform it properly without lifting the pelvis.

   Lack of comprehension or poor cooperation may be a cause of underestimation of the pelvic floor dysfunction.

2. The patient is asked to void immediately before the study. The bladder should be empty because of modification of anatomy, and straining is better if the bladder is empty as patients are afraid to void on the table. Moreover, overdistention of the bladder can mask prolapse in other compartments. Because of their pelvic dysfunction, patients always maintain a small amount of urine in the bladder which permits its visualization.

3. The MRI protocol requires no oral or intravenous contrast agents, and bowel preparation is not necessary either.

4. Patient installation:

   The patient should be dressed in a light cotton gown and without any undergarments, continence garments, and vaginal pessaries to maximize relative movement of pelvic organs. She is placed in a supine position, over protection, with the legs slightly flexed and apart, and knees bent over a pillow so as not to interfere with organ prolapse, especially during the straining phase of the study. A multicoil array is wrapped around the inferior portion of the pelvis and is positioned slightly lower than usual to cover the proximal thighs to ensure complete coverage of pelvic organ descent.

   The patient keeps in contact by headphones (volume should be adjusted in case of deafness): training and coaching the patient is performed during the examination to achieve optimal straining.

5. *Opacification*: The contrast material takes a few minutes to administer:

   - *Vaginal opacification*: While it is not systematic for some radiologists, the opacification of the vagina with 15–50 cc of sonographic gel (introduced with a Foley catheter) seems better in practice. It improves detection of prolapse (especially vaginal vault and peritoneocele by defining the fornix). A tampon is not recommended as it disturbs anatomy and does not always stay in the medial position.

   - *Rectal opacification*: It improves rectal evacuation which is necessary to allow good straining [34] and improves detection of rectocele and rectal prolapse. First, a rectal evacuating enema is prescribed few hours before the exam. Then using 60-cc syringes, 120 cc of sonographic gel is placed into the rectum. Gel is introduced into the rectum via a short flexible tube while the patient lies in the lateral decubitus position on the MRI table before being moved into the gantry.

   - Owing to the high intrinsic soft-tissue contrast of MR imaging, it is not necessary to opacify bowel loops or bladder.

MRI Technique

There is no standardized protocol for MRI of patients with pelvic floor disorders. However, the key element of any protocol is to image the patient during maximal strain or rectal evacuation. The examination can be completed in 15 min.

- Morphologic/static sequences: Three planes in T2 ponderation sequences with a small field of view (20–24 cm, approximately from 3 cm above the pubic bone up to S1) and 5-mm-thick images are acquired to obtain high-resolution images of the muscles and fascia of the pelvic floor. T1 sequence is not necessary for exploration of pelvic floor disorder.

- Dynamic sequences:

  - 6- to 15-mm-thick sagittal images of the midline are obtained with a steady-state T2-weighted imaging sequence and a 30–40-cm field of view acquiring with one section per second. These images are obtained at rest, during squeezing, and during Valsalva maneuver with straining and defecation. The patient is instructed to progressively strain to a maximum. Many patients require coaching to achieve maximal pelvic strain. Patients are asked to defecate on the table, and their ability to do so is taken as evidence of adequate straining. The variation between resting and straining images helps define the severity of the support defects. This procedure is repeated several times at the same level up to satisfactory results.

  - Images are analyzed on a workstation, then placed in a cine loop and videotaped mode.

37.5.2.2 Advantages of MRI Compared to Other Techniques and Limits

Dynamic cystocolpoproctography (DCP) is also a valuable tool to evaluate patients with pelvic floor abnormalities [35, 36] as its is able to image patients in more physiologic standing or seated positions. Indeed, fluoroscopic studies are often considered the gold standard for the diagnosis of pelvic floor abnormalities when newer techniques are introduced because fluoroscopic studies have been widely used for the past 20 years. But, there is really no true gold standard to which fluoroscopy can be compared with.

Unlike MR imaging, DCP does not always allow simultaneous assessment of all of the pelvic compartments in one examination nor assessment of the pelvic organs and the pelvic floor itself and requires multiple examinations and radiation exposure to the patient even with a low dose program. On the contrary, MRI is simple, with no radiation exposure and less invasive since bladder catheterization and bowel opacification are not necessary, and allows multiplanar imaging capability with a comprehensive, high-resolution, high-contrast evaluation of the entire pelvis.

The disadvantage of MRI is the supine position necessary with most magnets. This can result in suboptimal straining or defecation, which can lead to false-negative diagnoses regarding the presence and severity of prolapse and also suboptimal evaluation of evacuation disorders. The primary advantage of DCP is the ability of the patient to defecate on a commode. This approximates normal conditions and can be used to assess evacuation disorders. However, there have been no large studies comparing the two techniques. And the results may be partly dependent on the technique of the MRI study, especially whether rectal contrast was given. In a study of ten patients who underwent both dynamic MRI and fluoroscopic cystocolpoproctography [37], the MRI and fluoroscopic results were similar. Ten rectoceles and nine cystoceles were shown on both studies. Seven enteroceles were diagnosed on fluoroscopy, one of which was not initially seen on MRI, and two sigmoidoceles were diagnosed on MRI, one of which was not identified fluoroscopically [37].

When comparing MRI defecography in a vertical configuration magnet with fluoroscopy, the tests were comparable for anorectal pathology [38].

On the other hand, MRI is an accurate modality for evaluating peritoneocele because of its ability to help identify the content of the peritoneal sac (fat or bowel loops), to assess the role of the content in the dynamics of evacuation obstruction, and to survey the entire pelvis simultaneously. Moreover, unlike with DCP, bowel loops are easily identified on MR images without the need for selective opacification as the small bowel needs to be opacified with an oral contrast preparation 1–2 h before the study on DCP. MRI has been shown to be superior to DCP, which fails to demonstrate up to 20 % of enteroceles [31]. Another advantage is that because of its multiplanar imaging capability, MRI can depict a lateral rectocele or enterocele [39].

By contrast, intussusceptions can be difficult to detect on MRI, and fluoroscopy has been shown to reveal more intussusceptions than MRI. The sensitivity for diagnosing rectal intussusceptions on MRI has been reported to be 70 % relative to evacuation proctography. But these findings are of no clinical importance nor change the treatment because of the low grade of these findings.

Another limit with the MRI examination is the competition between the different compartments. A large enterocele may mask a coexisting cystocele or rectocele because of the tight space in the pelvic floor. Reduction of the enterocele may be required before assessment of the other compartments of the pelvic floor can be performed. Conversely, a persistently large rectocele or incomplete evacuation of the rectal contents in a large rectocele may also underestimate or even mask an enterocele or a cystocele [40]. Thus, compartment competition can be a cause of underestimation of some prolapse with MR defecography, and that is why a physical examination with a speculum is always needed and performed. The MRI examination with valves of a speculum improves detection or severity of prolapse [41], but its realization is difficult in practice.

Transabdominal, transvaginal, endoanal, transperineal, and 3D techniques can be used to evaluate the pelvic floor sonographically. But the role of ultrasound in evaluating pelvic organ prolapse is still under investigation [42].

Finally, although there is no consensus as to which technique is superior in the evaluation of pelvic organ prolapse, in our practice, MRI is the first choice modality to explore the pelvic floor dysfunction, and DCP can be used in a complementary fashion when assessing patients with complex defecatory disorders.

37.5.2.3 MRI Interpretation

Morphologic/Static Sequences

Pelvic Organ

Organ Lesions

MRI allows study of the pelvic organs. This is almost important when patients are treated by perineal access.

The management of pelvic floor dysfunction is delayed when a malignant neoplasm of cervix, endometrium (Fig. 37.11), ovary, bladder, or rectum or ascites is found.

The presence of a benign neoplasm is important as it may explain symptoms, and the management will be different, e.g., a huge uterine leiomyoma with a mass effect on the bladder (Fig. 37.12) or the presence of a urethral diverticulum (Fig. 37.13).

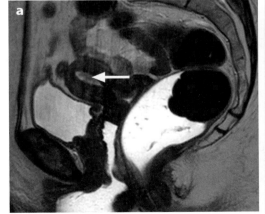 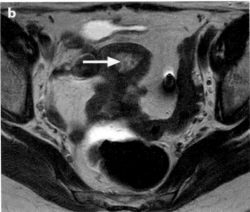

Fig. 37.11 Stress incontinence and cystocele in a 67-year-old woman. (**a**) sagittal and (**b**) axial T2-weighted images show an endometrial thickening (*arrow*) which recommended further gynecologic studies

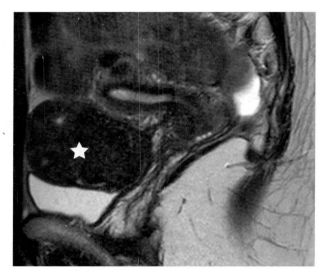

Fig. 37.12 Symptoms of heaviness and involuntary loss of urine in a 45-year-old woman. Sagittal T2-weighted image depicts a huge subserous leiomyoma (*star*) in the vesicouterine space with a mass effect on the bladder. The symptoms resolved after the leiomyoma removal

MRI also has the advantage of exploring the lower lumbar segment to depict spina bifida occulta or meningocele which may explain some symptoms.

- Organ lesions associated with prolapse
  - Hypertrophic elongation of the cervix (Fig. 37.14). The normal length of the cervix is around 3 cm. In case of hypertrophic elongation, the most distal part of the anterior lip of the cervix is clearly lower compared to posterior vaginal fornix, and the anterior lip measures much more than 3 cm. Even if it can be associated with uterine prolapse, it should be differentiated as it can be caused by chronic cystocele.
  - Hydronephrosis when the bladder prolapse is severe enough. The muscular pelvic floor may entrap the ureters and create ureteral obstruction (Fig. 37.15).
  - Hernia of the posterior wall of the bladder in case of a cystocele (Fig. 37.16) or enlargement of the inferior rectovaginal space just anterior to the rectal wall, in the case of a rectocele (Fig. 37.17), in case of long-standing prolapse.

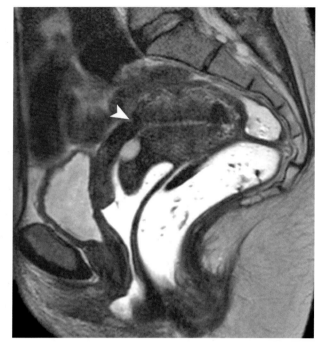

Fig. 37.14 Urinary incontinence and vaginal mass in a 50 year-old-woman. Sagittal T2-weighted image shows a hypertrophic elongation of the cervix. Note the well-defined upper limit of the anterior lip by the cesarean scar (*arrowhead*)

  - Urethral funneling at rest is an abnormality in which there is dilatation of the proximal urethral lumen and apparent shortening of the urethra can also be observed. This finding may indicate intrinsic urethral sphincter incompetence in incontinent women [34]. However funneling is a nonspecific sign of incontinence, since it can be observed in continent women as well.
- Pelvic adhesions
  In the case of prior pelvic surgery, MRI is an interesting tool to depict pelvic adhesions, particularly in case of adhesions of the fundus of the uterus to the pelvic wall, within the uterorectal space or between bowel and the abdominal wall (Fig. 37.18). Sometimes the diagnosis of these adhesions may be overlooked or underestimated.

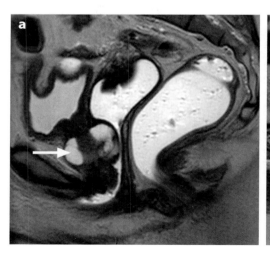
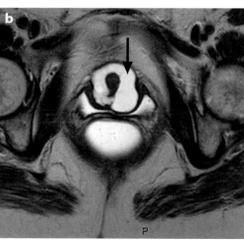

Fig. 37.13 Urine incontinence in a 45-year-old woman. (**a**) sagittal and (**b**) axial T2-weighted images show a circumferential urethral diverticulum (*arrow*). Symptoms resolved after surgical treatment

Fig. 37.15 Exteriorized prolapse in an 81-year-old woman. (**a**) sagittal T2-weighted image at rest shows a cystocele (*arrow*) associated with a uterine procidentia (*star*). Note also the fecal incontinence with spontaneous loss of rectal sonographic gel. (**b**) coronal T2-weighted image at rest shows bilateral ureteral dilatation (*arrows*)

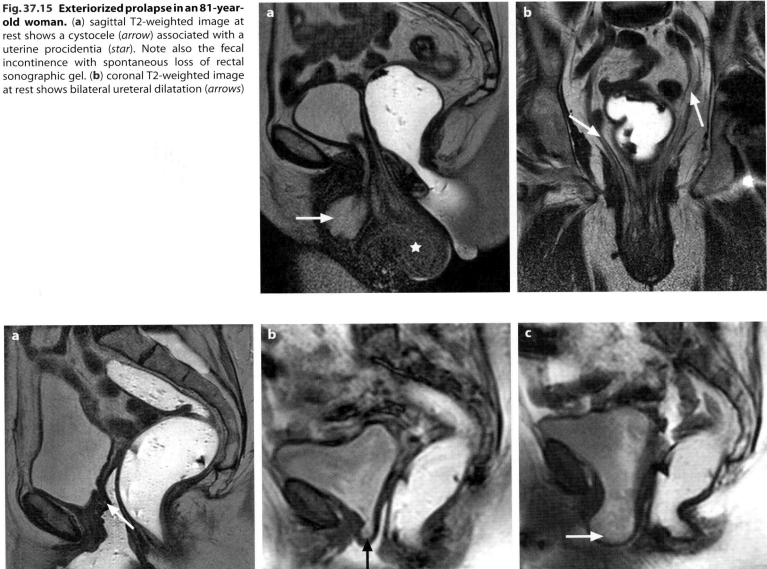

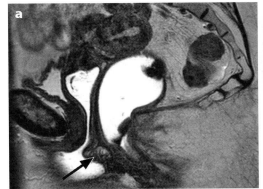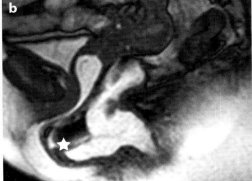

Fig. 37.16 Cystocele in a 70-year-old woman. (**a**) resting, (**b**) at mild, and (**c**) at maximum straining sagittal T2-weighted images show a small parietal hernia of the posterior wall of the bladder (*arrow*) which increases during straining consisting with a cystocele

Fig. 37.17 Symptoms of perineal mass and incomplete evacuation in a 51-year-old woman. (**a**) resting sagittal T2-weighted image shows an enlargement of the inferior rectovaginal space (*arrow*) probably due to the chronic distension by the rectocele (*star*) depicted on the (**b**) straining T2-weighted midsagittal image

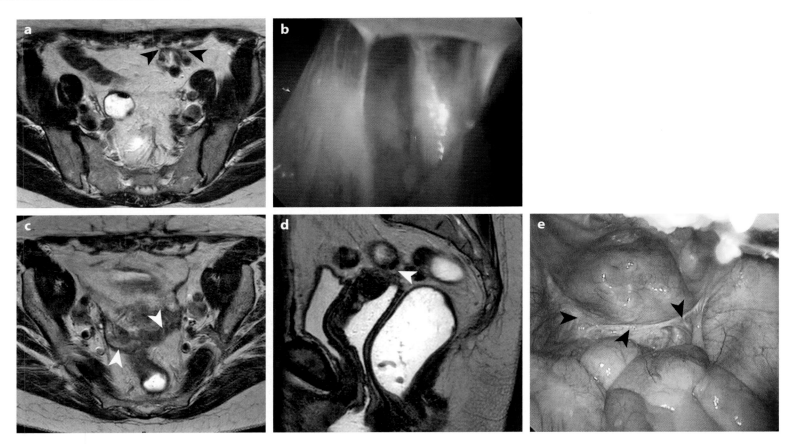

Fig. 37.18 Cystocele in a 56-year-old woman with prior subtotal hysterectomy. (**a**) axial T2 image and (**b**) laparoscopic photograph show adhesions (*arrowheads*) between the anterior abdominal wall and bowels. (**c**) axial image, (**d**) sagittal T2-weighted image, and (**e**) laparoscopic photograph show pelvic adhesion with complete peritonization (*arrowheads*)

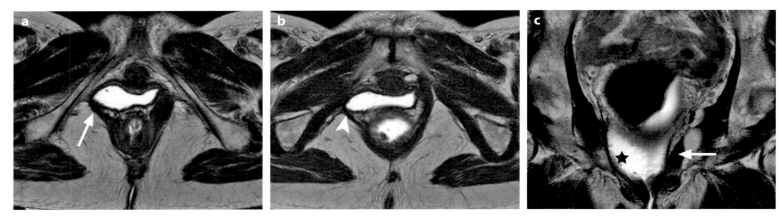

Fig. 37.19 Cystocele in a 61-year-old woman. (**a**, **b**) axial T2-weighted images show thin right pubovisceralis (*arrow*) and puborectalis (*arrowhead*) with anterior retropubic desinsertion and homolateral vaginal deformation. (**c**) coronal T2-weighted image shows the muscle defect with the muscle bulk loss compared to the right (*arrow*) and the homolateral deformation of the vagina (*star*) in place of the muscle loss

These results help surgeons to select appropriate access for the intervention (perineal or pelvic access) and to prevent any difficulties when passing instruments through the abdominal wall during a coelioscopy.

Levator Ani

Pubovisceralis and puborectalis defects are defined as thinning (half or more than a half of the muscle is missing up to the complete muscle bulk lost [20, 43]) or tears with anterior retropubic desinsertion (Figs. 37.19, 37.20, and 37.21).

Weakness of the iliococcygeus is based on its aspect: loss of superior convexity to an inverse shape on coronal plane, a posterior widening (bowl-like configuration) on axial plane, and lateral tears with desinsertion and/or atrophy (Figs. 37.22 and 37.23).

Fig. 37.20 Stress urinary incontinence and vaginal mass sensation in a 65-year-old woman. (a) axial T2- and (b) axial T1-weighted images show a bilateral fatty involution of pubovisceralis with linear hypersignal within the muscle (*arrows*)

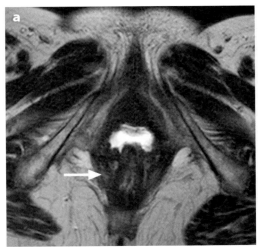
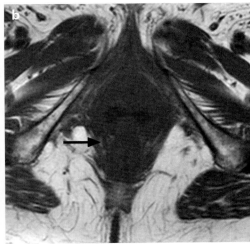

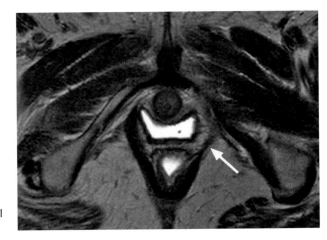

Fig. 37.21 Urinary incontinence and hysterocele in a 48-year-old woman. Axial T2-weighted image shows a thin left puborectalis (*arrow*) with anterior tear

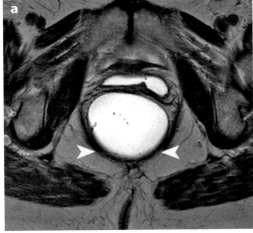
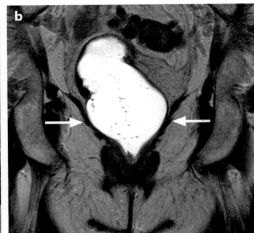

Fig. 37.22 Hysterocele and posterior colpocele in a 77-year-old woman. (a) axial and (b) coronal T2-weighted images show bilateral weakness of the iliococcygeus with a bowl-like posterior widening (*arrowheads*) and a plate shape (*arrows*)

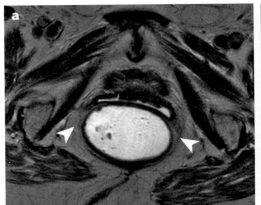
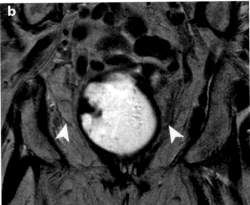

Fig. 37.23 Cystocele in a 74-year-old woman. (a) axial and (b) coronal passing through the rectum T2-weighted images show bilateral weakness of the iliococcygeus with a bowl-like posterior widening and posterior muscle atrophy (*arrowheads*)

Fascia

Pelvic fascias are delicate structures which are below imaging resolution, but their defects may be inferred indirectly through secondary findings.

Because of attachment of the uterosacral ligaments to the presacral fascia, the normal proximal two-thirds of the vagina extends posteriorly over the levator ani. On the sagittal images, its normal configuration is often lost in cases of prolapse, as the vagina appears straightened (Fig. 37.24).

A defect in the fascia of level I and II of DeLancey can be visualized, in the axial plane, as sagging of the fluid-filled posterior urinary bladder wall due to the detachment of the vaginal supporting fascia from the lateral pelvic wall, known as the "saddlebags sign" (Fig. 37.25).

A defect in the fascia of level III of DeLancey can be suspected when the vagina loses its "H" shape and has a flattened appearance. On axial images, the shape of the distal thirds of the vagina is assessed. Normally, the vagina has an "H" shape (or butterfly shape) with anterior extension of the left and right lateral walls because of insertions of the overlying endopelvic fascia which indicates adequate lateral fascial support. The disruption to the paravaginal ligaments will weaken support to the urethra because the middle and distal thirds of the urethra are closely related to and supported by the anterior vaginal wall. But, loss of the normal shape of the vagina on MRI can also be seen in nulliparous asymptomatic women and in the absence of relevant clinical symptoms; therefore, the diagnosis of weakening of vaginal support should not be made based on vaginal shape alone [44]. A paravaginal fascia defect of level III of DeLancey is more obvious when recognized by the "drooping mustache sign," which is formed by fat in the prevesical space against the bilateral sagging of the detached lower third of the anterior vaginal wall from the arcus tendineus fasciae pelvis [45] (Fig. 37.26).

Sphincter

Sphincter lesions are almost seen with specific endovaginal, endourethral, or endoanal coil or with thin images, but even on a routine MR defecography, lesions can be seen.

On axial images, the anterior external urethral sphincter and thin fascial condensations that support the upper portion of the urethra can be seen. In a study by Kim et al. [46], distortion of the periurethral and paraurethral ligaments was frequently noted in patients with stress urinary incontinence. Urethral ligament abnormalities can be classified as distorted when internal architectural changes with waviness of the ligaments were seen and as a defect when there was discontinuity of the ligament with visualization of the torn parts [47].

Anal sphincter lesions are reported according to the muscle injured (the internal or the external sphincter) and according to the lesion type (defect and/or scarring). A sphincteric defect is defined as a discontinuity of the muscle ring and a scarring as a low signal intensity deformation of the normal pattern of the muscle layer [48].

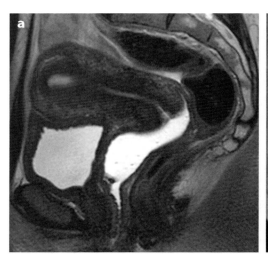
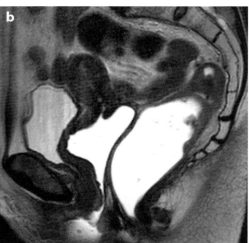

Fig. 37.24 Vaginal configuration in prolapse. (**a**) sagittal T2-weighted image in a 23-year-old woman suspected of endometriosis shows the normal "banana-shaped" configuration of the vaginal axis with a slightly anteroposterior horizontal configuration. (**b**) sagittal T2-weighted image in a 65-year-old woman with prolapse shows that the vagina assumes a more vertical orientation than on (**a**) and with an anterior convexity of its anterior wall

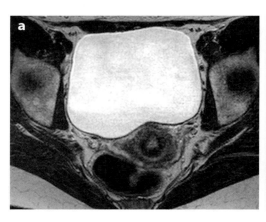
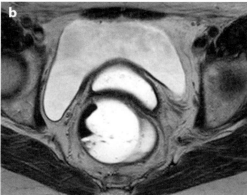

Fig. 37.25 Fascial defect of level I and II of DeLancey. (**a**) axial T2-weighted image in a 21-year-old volunteer shows normal posterior convexity of the posterior bladder wall. (**b**) axial T2-weighted image in a 70-year-old woman with prolapse shows bilateral asymmetric sagging of the fluid-filled posterior urinary bladder wall

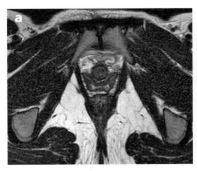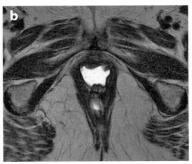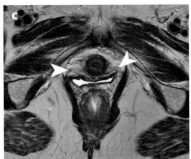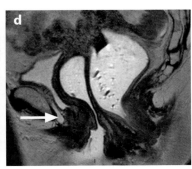

Fig. 37.26 Fascial defect of level III of DeLancey. (a) axial T2-weighted image in a 19-year-old volunteer shows the normal "H" shape of the distal third of the vagina. (b) axial T2-weighted image in a 72-year-old woman with prolapse shows loss of the normal shape of the vagina with a flattened appearance. (c) axial T2-weighted and (d) sagittal T2-weighted images in a 79-year-old woman with prolapse show fat in the prevesical space of Retzius (*arrow*) with a "drooping mustache sign" on (a) (*arrowheads*), consisting of paravaginal fascia defects

Dynamic Sequences

Pelvic Floor Relaxation

Pelvic floor relaxation develops over time as the fascia and the muscular levator ani become weakened. As the pelvic floor is pathologically descending, so do the organs above that it is supposed to support. Consequently, pelvic floor relaxation and organ prolapse are not synonymous and should be differentiated [49]. In fact, many combinations of pelvic floor relaxation and pelvic organ prolapse can occur in a given patient.

To help standardize interpretation and grading of pelvic floor dysfunction with MR imaging, the HMO (H line, M line, organ prolapse) system was developed, which is applied to a midsagittal T2-weighted image obtained during maximal patient strain [34, 49, 50]. This system clearly defines and differentiates between the pelvic floor relaxation and pelvic organ prolapse. There are two components of pelvic floor relaxation: one anteroposterior with a widening of the hiatus and one vertical with pelvic floor descent.

On the midsagittal image obtained during maximal strain, three points of reference are first defined: *A*, the inferior margin of the symphysis pubis; *B*, the convex posterior margin of the puborectalis muscle sling; and, *C*, the last joint of the coccyx. The two anatomic references in the HMO system are the pubococcygeal line (PCL), which is drawn between points *A* and C and the point *B*.

The first component of pelvic floor relaxation is the H line (puborectal hiatus line) which represents the puborectal. The H line allows grading of the maximal widening of the pelvic sling in the anteroposterior dimension during straining and is the linear distance between points *A* and *B*. The second component of pelvic floor relaxation is the M line, which is the measure of the vertical descent of the puborectal hiatus. The M line extends perpendicularly from the PCL to the posterior end of the H line (point *B*) (Fig. 37.27).

The H and M lines tend to elongate with pelvic floor relaxation, representing puborectal hiatus widening and pelvic floor descent, respectively [50]. In asymptomatic patients, the H line is less than 6 cm, and the M line is no more than 2 cm in length. The abnormal widening of the pelvic floor, measured with the H line, is graded progressively when it exceeds 6 cm in length. Abnormal descent (M line) is progressively graded when its length exceeds 2 cm (Fig. 37.27) (Table 37.3) [49, 50].

Taking into account the importance of the pelvic floor relaxation may help the surgeon to choose the route and the planning repair of POP that also best limit levator ani descent and hiatal widening.

Fig. 37.27 Landmarks and lines of the HMO system for grading pelvic floor relaxation. (a) resting midsagittal T2-weighted image and (b) corresponding midsagittal T2-weighted image at maximal straining show the three-point landmarks: *A* the inferior margin of the symphysis pubis; *B* the convex posterior margin of the puborectalis muscle sling; and, *C* the last joint of the coccyx. The pubococcygeal line (between points *A* and *C*, *white line PCL*), the H line (distance between points *A* and *B*, *blue line HL*), and M line (perpendicular line from the PCL to the point *B*, *green line ML*) are drawn on figure (b) which show grade 1 pelvic floor widening with an anteroposterior puborectal hiatus length of 7.5 cm and grade 1 pelvic floor descent of 3.7 cm

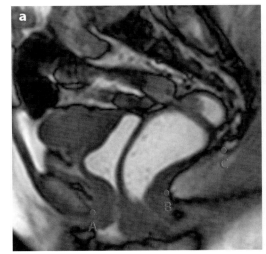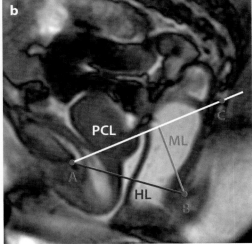

Table 37.3 Grading of pelvic floor relaxation at maximal strain

Grade	Hiatal enlargement (cm)	Pelvic floor descent (cm)
0 (normal)	<6	0–2
1 (mild)	6–8	2–4
2 (moderate)	8–10	4–6
3 (severe)	≥10	≥6

Table from: Boyadzhyan et al. [49]

Table 37.4 Grading of pelvic organ prolapse at maximal strain

Grade	Organ location relative to the H line
0 (no prolapse)	Above
1 (mild or small)	0–2 cm below
2 (moderate)	2–4 cm below
3 (severe or large)	≥4 cm below

Table from: Boyadzhyan et al. [49]

Pelvic Organ Prolapse
References Lines
Clinical pelvic organ prolapse quantification systems use the plane of the hymen as the reference line [10] (see Sect. 37.3.1.2). But, over the years, radiologists have been proposed several reference lines for rest and stress measurements in order to stage pelvic organ prolapse on MRI.

The three most commonly used lines are the H line of the HMO system [49], the PCL line [51, 52] that represents for some authors the level of the pelvic floor, and the midpubic line (MPL) extending caudally along the long axis of the symphysis pubis that has been shown to correspond to the level of the vaginal hymen on cadaveric dissection [53]. The choice of reference line for MRI interpretation may be dependent on radiologist experience and referring physician preference. Once the MR reference line is chosen, staging of pelvic organ prolapse in all three compartments can be performed by measuring the perpendicular distance from the anatomic reference point in each compartment to the reference line.

On the contrary to the PCL and MPL, the HMO system, with the H line which is moving, allows consistent definition, differentiation, and grading of pelvic organ prolapse and pelvic floor relaxation. There seems for authors [49] to be more clinical correlation by using the H line because it is closer to the hymen. Considering this line, pelvic organ prolapse is any protrusion of a given organ (urethra, bladder, uterus or apex of the vagina, peritoneum and content, or rectum) through the puborectal hiatus or the H line. This constitutes the final *O* component of the HMO classification system (Table 37.4). It is measured as the shortest distance between the most caudal aspect of a given organ (considered as the reference point) and the H line on the midsagittal MR image obtained at maximal straining (Fig. 37.28).

Posterior Compartment: The Particular Case of the Rectocele
In case of a rectocele, the radiologic definition and grading are more commonly based on different criteria than the HMO system (i.e., the shortest distance between the most caudal aspect of the rectum during Valsalva maneuver and the H line). Indeed, the size of a rectocele is usually based on its maximal depth measured at right angles to a line extended upward through the anterior wall of the anal canal (Fig. 37.29). A rectal bulge into the vaginal lumen of greater than 2–3 cm anterior to this line is described as a rectocele [50, 54]. For some, a rectocele has been considered small if it is less than 2 cm in depth, moderate if it is 2–4 cm in depth, and large if it is more than 4 cm in depth [33]. According to this definition, most asymptomatic women harbor a rectocele [9]. Thus, this definition has been questioned and has led others to restrict the diagnosis of rectocele to those anterior rectal bulges that are greater than 3 cm in depth [54]. In general, a rectocele less than 2 cm in depth should be dismissed as a normal finding.

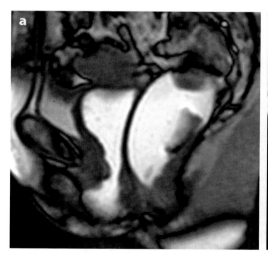 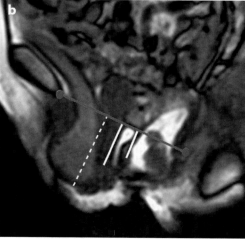

Fig. 37.28 HMO system for grading organ prolapse. (a) resting midsagittal T-weighted image and **(b)** corresponding midsagittal T2-weighted image at maximal straining show a grade 3 cystocele with the bladder 5.1 cm below H line (*dot line*), a grade 2 hysterocele with the cervix 3.8 cm below H line (*long white line*), and a grade 1 rectocele with anterior rectum wall 2.2 cm below the H line (*short white line*). Note that the rectocele can be underestimated because of the potential competition with the hysterocele and cystocele

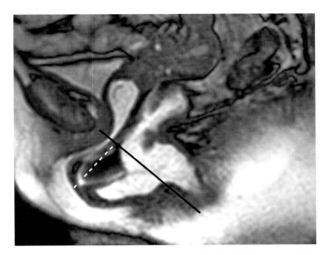

Fig. 37.29 Rectocele measurement. A midsagittal T2-weighted image at maximal straining shows a 5-cm-depth anterior rectocele measured at right angles (*white dot line*) to a line extended upward through the anterior wall of the anal canal (*black line*)

Description

On the midsagittal T2-weighted image, prolapse of the urethra, bladder, vagina, and rectum is each assessed and graded separately along with any associated pelvic floor relaxation to help determine their relative clinical relevance.

1. Anterior Compartment
   - Urethrocele and urethral hypermobility
   A change in the urethral axis can be observed with straining in patients with urethral hypermobility [34], but it is not always clearly visualized. Sagittal MR images obtained with the patient at rest usually show the urethra to be vertical in orientation. With increased abdominal pressure, the proximal urethra moves inferiorly, and the axis of the urethra becomes more horizontal. The angle of the urethral axis is abnormal when it is greater than 30° from the vertical (Fig. 37.30).
   - Cystocele
   In case of a cystocele, the posterior wall of the bladder descends along an arc, initially moving posteriorly and inferiorly to deform the anterior wall of the vagina and then bulging forward as it exits the introitus. The anterior wall of the bladder is fixed by the median umbilical ligament to the anterior abdominal wall and remains relatively stationary, giving the bladder an elongated appearance (Fig. 37.31). The bladder may prolapse completely to lie outside the pelvic cavity (Fig. 37.32).
   Because the bladder neck and proximal urethra are mobile, descent of the bladder neck during strain may result in clockwise rotational descent of the bladder neck and proximal urethra. In this condition, cystocele can be associated with or

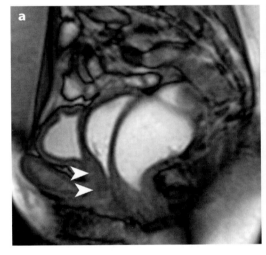

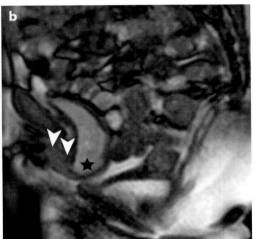

Fig. 37.30 Stress urinary incontinence in a 54-year-old woman. (**a**) resting midsagittal T2-weighted image and (**b**) corresponding midsagittal T2-weighted image at maximal straining show a hypermobility of the urethra (*arrowheads*) which assumes a clockwise rotation during straining and a small cystocele (*star*)

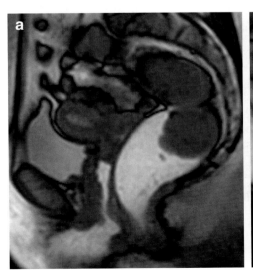

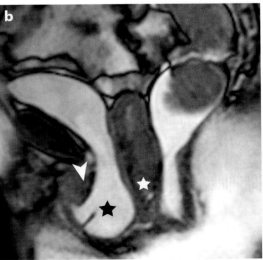

Fig. 37.31 Vaginal mass with feeling of incomplete bladder voiding and without stress urinary incontinence in a 66-year-old woman. (**a**) resting midsagittal T2-weighted image shows no organ prolapse, and (**b**) corresponding midsagittal T2-weighted image at maximal straining shows a large cystocele (*black star*) with kinking of the urethra (*arrowhead*) which caused urinary retention and masked stress urinary incontinence, as it appeared after pelvic floor surgery. Note the small hysterocele (*white star*)

mask symptoms of stress urinary incontinence (urethral hypermobility) and may lead to urinary retention with urinary stasis and infection (Fig. 37.31).

2. Middle compartment: uterine and vaginal vault prolapse
   The vagina may appear shortened due to partial eversion of the vault and is pathologically displaced inferiorly on dynamic MR images (Fig. 37.33).

   In severe cases of complete eversion, cervical and uterine prolapses are seen as a bulging mass outside the external genitalia (called uterine procidentia) (Fig. 37.15) as the vaginal walls form a sac containing the prolapsing organs. This makes diagnosis of any concomitant pelvic organ prolapse very difficult [5, 50].

   A fibroma in the uterus may prevent descent of the uterus and cause underestimation of the true degree of pelvic floor dysfunction and supporting fascial damage.

   In cases of hysterectomy, superior defects in the vaginal supports can cause vaginal descent, infolding of the vaginal apex, or complete eversion of the mucosa.

Because vaginal vault prolapse is usually associated with prolapse of other organs, comprehensive assessment of the entire pelvis with MR imaging is particularly important [5].

3. Posterior Compartment
   Posterior colpocele: hernia through the posterior vaginal wall
   • Peritoneocele/enterocele/sigmoidocele
   On MR dynamic images, weakness in the cul-de-sac results in the formation between the rectum and vagina of peritoneoceles (Fig. 37.34), enteroceles (Fig. 37.35), and sigmoidoceles (Fig. 37.36), which contain peritoneal fat, small bowel, and sigmoid colon, respectively.

   This usually occurs at the end of evacuation as a consequence of increased intra-abdominal pressure and when both the bladder and rectum are empty because a filled rectum or bladder frequently pushes the small bowel out of the pelvis and does not allow sufficient space for small bowel to descend into the pelvis [55]. Repeated straining after evacuation may be essential and needed for the depiction and quantification (into the rectovaginal

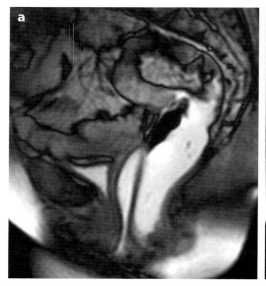
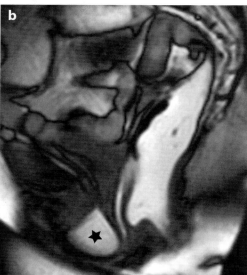

Fig. 37.32 **Vaginal mass and difficulty to urinate in a 56-year-old woman.** (**a**) resting midsagittal T2-weighted image shows no organ prolapse, and (**b**) midsagittal T2-weighted image at maximal straining shows a large cystocele lying outside the pelvic cavity (*star*)

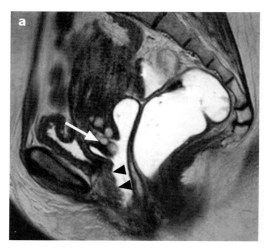
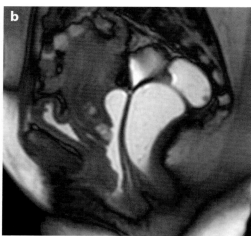
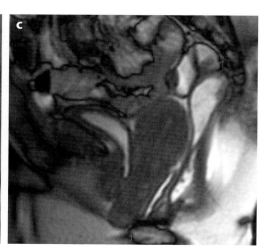

Fig. 37.33 **Urinary incontinence, cystocele, and hysterocele in a 48-year-old woman.** (**a**) sagittal T2-weighted image shows the partial shortening of the vagina (*arrowheads*). Note the hypertrophic elongation of the cervix (*arrow*). (**b**) resting midsagittal T2-image shows no organ prolapse, and (**c**) corresponding midsagittal image at maximal straining shows a mild hysterocele with a small accompanying cystocele. Note that because of the competition between the middle and the anterior compartments, the cystocele described at the physical examination is mask by the major hysterocele

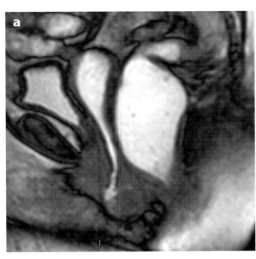 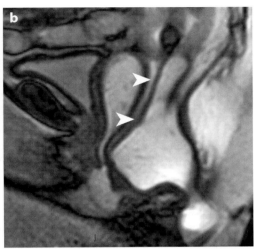 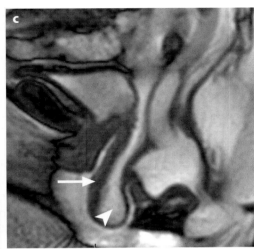

Fig. 37.34 Posterior colpocele in a 72-year-old woman prior hysterectomy. (**a**) resting midsagittal T2-weighted image, (**b**) midsagittal T2-weighted image at the beginning of the strain, and (**c**) midsagittal T2-weighted image at maximal straining show a progressive peritoneocele with peritoneum in rectovaginal space (*arrowheads*) bulging to the posterior vaginal wall (*arrow*). Note the association with a rectocele

Fig. 37.35 Pelvic heaviness sensation during defection in an 85-year-old woman. (**a**) resting midsagittal T2-weighted image and (**b**) corresponding midsagittal T2-weighted image at maximal straining show an enterocele with small bowels filling the rectovaginal space (*star*) and bulging to the posterior vaginal wall (*arrowhead*)

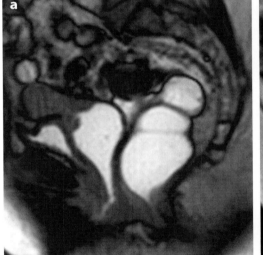 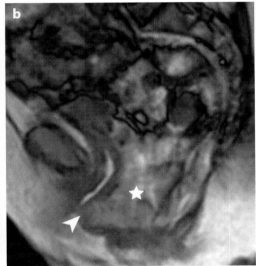

space and/or with intravaginal extension) of peritoneocele (Fig. 37.37).

It must be remembered that compared with all other forms of organ prolapse, these herniation defects present the biggest diagnostic challenge at physical examination, especially when multiple organs are involved. Undiagnosed peritoneocele or enterocele may change the surgical approach from a transvaginal to a transabdominal route of entry. Preoperative recognition of a sigmoidocele is important so that colorectal surgery and repair of associated pelvic floor defects can be accomplished at one surgical setting. Dynamic MRI is ideally suited and far better than physical examination to preoperative characterization of these bulges [34].

- Rectocele
  MR defecography provides information about the size and dynamics of rectocele emptying, retention of gel within the rectocele, and coexistent abnormalities. Retention of gel in the rectocele during rectal voiding is a supporting evidence for this abnormality and explains the symptoms of incomplete evacuation (Fig. 37.38).

For the rare condition in which a lateral or posterior rectocele is suspected (suspected in case of levator ani damage on static images or prior surgery in the rectal region), coronal, sagittal, and/or axial dynamic sequences should be performed.

Rectal Prolapse

Analysis of defecation with luminal contrast allows detection of rectal prolapse. It starts approximately 6–8 cm from inside the rectum and has varying degrees of severity with intrarectal, intra-anal, and extra-anal involvement.

MR defecography has the potential advantage of clearly distinguishing between partial rectal prolapse (usually anterior mucosal prolapse) (Fig. 37.39) and complete rectal prolapse (full-thickness wall prolapse), a difference which is relevant in that the treatment for the two conditions is different. Complete rectal prolapse is with a circular infolding of the rectal wall (folds are greater than 3 mm thick) that narrows the lumen (Fig. 37.40) [56].

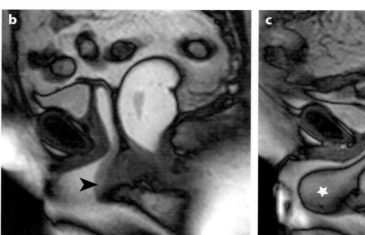

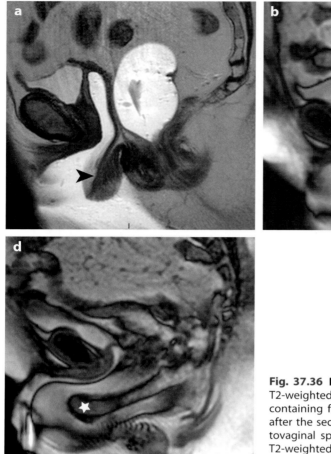

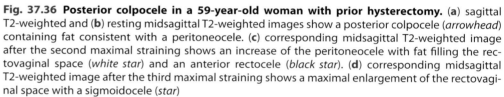

Fig. 37.36 Posterior colpocele in a 59-year-old woman with prior hysterectomy. (a) sagittal T2-weighted and (b) resting midsagittal T2-weighted images show a posterior colpocele (*arrowhead*) containing fat consistent with a peritoneocele. (c) corresponding midsagittal T2-weighted image after the second maximal straining shows an increase of the peritoneocele with fat filling the rectovaginal space (*white star*) and an anterior rectocele (*black star*). (d) corresponding midsagittal T2-weighted image after the third maximal straining shows a maximal enlargement of the rectovaginal space with a sigmoidocele (*star*)

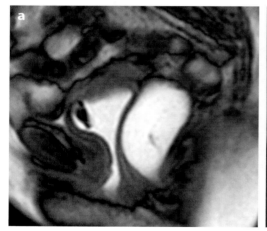

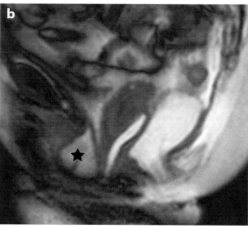

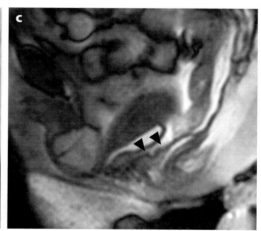

Fig. 37.37 Sensation of vaginal mass at the end of the day in a 58-year-old woman. (a) resting midsagittal T2-weighted image shows no prolapse. (b) corresponding midsagittal T2-weighted image after the first maximal straining shows a large cystocele (*star*). (c) corresponding midsagittal T2-weighted image after the third maximal straining, when the rectum is empty, shows a small peritoneocele (*arrowheads*)

Fig. 37.38 Feeling of incomplete evacuation and posterior vaginal mass during defecation in a 48-year-old woman. (**a**) resting midsagittal T2-weighted image shows an enlargement of the inferior rectovaginal space (*arrow*) probably due to the chronic mild rectocele (*star*) bulging into the vagina which is depicted on (**b**) corresponding midsagittal T2-weighted image at maximal straining. During defecation, the rectocele is filled with intrarectal sonographic gel and is unable to empty

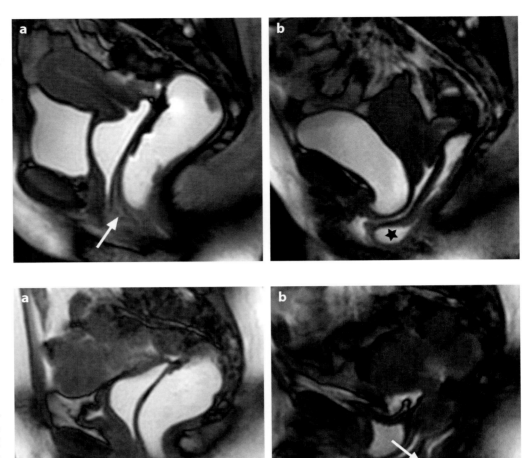

Fig. 37.39 Feeling of incomplete rectal voiding in a 56-year-old woman. (**a**) resting and (**b**) at maximal straining midsagittal T2-weighted images show a small anterior rectocele associated with an intra-anal anterior mucosal prolapse (*arrow*) that may be obstructive to stool passage during rectal voiding. Note also the small cystocele

Defecatory Function

Four criteria can be retained for a normal evacuation proctographic study on MRI: increase in anorectal angulation, obliteration of the puborectal impression, wide anal canal opening, and evacuation of at least some of the rectal contrast material to a total evacuation [57].

Spastic Pelvic Floor Syndrome

The major findings are the failure of the anorectal angle to open, prolonged (more than 30 s of straining) and incomplete evacuation as on DCP [58, 59], and a long interval between opening of the anal canal and start of defecation [1] (Fig. 37.41). Because puborectal dysfunction has been the main focus of the syndrome, MR imaging clearly shows lack of physiologic relaxation and descent of the pelvic floor during defecation and paradoxical contraction of the puborectalis muscle (frequently hypertrophic) with visualization of a prominent puborectal impression during voiding.

If the patient is unable to evacuate the rectal contrast material on the first attempt, the sequence is repeated at least twice to ensure that the inability to evacuate contrast material is not due to a lack of communication or effort.

Assessment of the anorectal angle during attempted defecation may help differentiate between patients with true paradoxical contraction of the puborectalis muscle and patients who have difficulty

defecating due to supine positioning. No change in the anorectal angle or a more acute change in the anorectal angle with attempted defecation may suggest pelvic dyssynergia [58], whereas a more obtuse change in the anorectal angle may suggest difficulty defecating in a supine position [60].

Anal Incontinence

Clinical findings remain essential for the diagnosis. Anal canal manometry is also important for determining whether sphincter function is normal, although it is unable to help differentiate traumatic damage from atrophy.

Imaging of fecal incontinence relies on endoanal MR imaging or ultrasonography of the anal sphincter, with the aim of detecting sphincter tear or atrophy and thus selecting patients likely to benefit from surgical repair [14].

However, MR defecography findings such as inability to hold an enema, anorectal angle changes of less than 10°, pelvic floor descent, intussusception, and rectocele may change the surgical approach for surgery candidates for treatment of incontinence [52]. A recent study reported that MR defecography findings led to changes in surgical approach in 67 % of patients who were candidates for treatment of fecal incontinence with some form of surgery [52]. In particular, if a simple sphincter repair was planned, the evidence of a rectocele or enterocele modified the treatment to

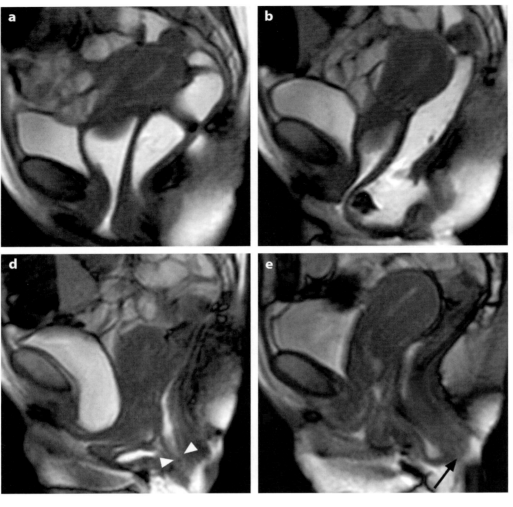

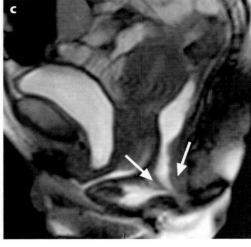

Fig. 37.40 Rectal prolapse during defecation in a 36 years old woman. (**a**) resting, (**b**) at the beginning of the straining and (**c**) at the end of the first maximal straining midsagittal T2 weighted images show an anterior rectocele and a intrarectal intussusceptions (*white arrows*). (**d**) at the mid part of the straining and (**e**) at the end of the second maximal straining midsagittal T2 weighted images show the rectal intussusception progressing to intra anal position (*arrowheads*) up to exteriorization (*black arrow*)

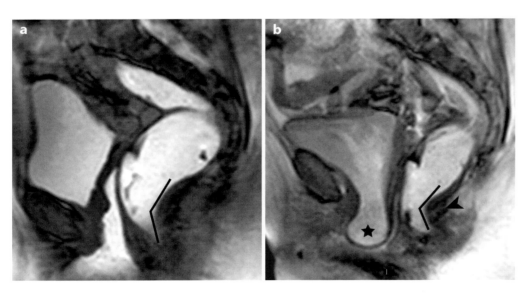

Fig. 37.41 Chronic history of outlet obstruction syndrome symptoms with recent onset of a cystocele in a 60-year-old woman. (**a**) resting midsagittal T2-weighted image and (**b**) midsagittal T2-weighted images at maximal straining (fourth attempt) show paradoxical closure of the anorectal angle (*black angles*) and shortening of the puborectal hiatus with visualization of a prominent puborectal impression (*arrowhead*) associated with failure to open of the anal sphincter. Note that the cystocele is still displayed (*star*)

Table 37.5 Reporting MR imaging findings

	Morphologic sequences	
Pelvic organs	Organ lesion	
	Organs lesion associated to the prolapse	
Levator ani	Pubovisceralis and puborectalis: thickness, tears	
	Iliococcygeus: shape, trophicity, tears	
Fascia	Level I and II: "saddlebags sign"	
	Level III: loss of the "H" shape of the vagina, vaginal deformation, and "drooping mustache sign"	
	Dynamic sequences	
Pelvic floor relaxation	Puborectal hiatus widening: H line > 6 cm	
	Pelvic floor descent: M line > 2 cm	
Pelvic organ prolapse (compared to H line)	Anterior compartment	Urethrocele
		Cystocele
	Middle compartment	Hysterocele or vaginal vault prolapse
	Posterior compartment	Peritoneocele, enterocele, sigmoidocele
		Rectocele
		Rectal prolapse

sphincteroplasty and anterior levatorplasty. Even patients with constipation may complain of fecal incontinence (e.g., overflow incontinence or post defecation leakage). In these patients, MR defecography is helpful for demonstrating the causes of associated outlet obstruction.

37.5.2.4 Reporting MR Imaging Findings

Findings reported at dynamic MR imaging of the pelvic floor are valuable for selecting patients who are candidates for surgical treatment and for choosing the appropriate surgical approach.

Radiology report of a pelvic floor MR examination can be broken down into the assessment of five components: pelvic organs, pelvic floor support structures (the location of muscle tears and inferred fascial tears), pelvic floor relaxation, pelvic organ prolapse (location and number of compartments), and rectal evacuation (Table 37.5).

37.6 Conclusion

Dynamic MRI is a functional method of evaluating the global pelvic floor for pelvic organ prolapse and defecatory disorders. Clinicians find it a useful diagnostic tool that can alter management decisions from surgical to medical and vice versa in many cases. It has become clear that pelvic floor disorders rarely occur in isolation and that global pelvic floor assessment is necessary. It should be understood that the imaging POP examination is not intended to compete with the clinical POP-Q examination. The clinical POP-Q examination looks at different vaginal points, whereas the imaging POP examination is organ specific. Imaging is meant to complement the deficiencies of clinical examination as the clinical treatment of patients with anorectal and pelvic floor dysfunction is often difficult.

To conclude, pelvic floor disorders are a common and complex problem in which imaging plays a key role in effective diagnosis and treatment.

References

1. Stoker J, Halligan S, Bartram CI (2001) Pelvic floor imaging. Radiology 218:621–641
2. Bump RC, Norton PA (1998) Epidemiology and natural history of pelvic floor dysfunction. Obstet Gynecol Clin North Am 25:723–746
3. DeLancey JO (1993) Anatomy and biomechanics of genital prolapse. Clin Obstet Gynecol 36:897–909
4. Jelovsek JE, Maher C, Barber MD (2007) Pelvic organ prolapse. Lancet 369:1027–1038
5. Deval B, Haab F (2003) What's new in prolapse surgery? Curr Opin Urol 13:315–323
6. Fielding JR (2002) Practical MR imaging of female pelvic floor weakness. Radiographics 22:295–304
7. Luber KM, Boero S, Choe JY (2001) The demographics of pelvic floor disorders: current observations and future projections. Am J Obstet Gynecol 184:1496–1501; discussion 1501–1503
8. DeLancey JO (2005) The hidden epidemic of pelvic floor dysfunction: achievable goals for improved prevention and treatment. Am J Obstet Gynecol 192:1488–1495
9. Shorvon PJ, McHugh S, Diamant NE, Somers S, Stevenson GW (1989) Defecography in normal volunteers: results and implications. Gut 30:1737–1749
10. Bump RC, Mattiasson A, Bo K et al (1996) The standardization of terminology of female pelvic organ prolapse and pelvic floor dysfunction. Am J Obstet Gynecol 175:10–17
11. Roos JE, Weishaupt D, Wildermuth S, Willmann JK, Marincek B, Hilfiker PR (2002) Experience of 4 years with open MR defecography: pictorial review of anorectal anatomy and disease. Radiographics 22:817–832
12. Preston DM, Lennard-Jones JE (1985) Anismus in chronic constipation. Dig Dis Sci 30:413–418
13. Bates P, Bradley WE, Glen E et al (1979) The standardization of terminology of lower urinary tract function. J Urol 121:551–554
14. Terra MP, Stoker J (2006) The current role of imaging techniques in faecal incontinence. Eur Radiol 16:1727–1736
15. Kearney R, Sawhney R, DeLancey JO (2004) Levator ani muscle anatomy evaluated by origin-insertion pairs. Obstet Gynecol 104:168–173
16. Singh K, Reid WM, Berger LA (2002) Magnetic resonance imaging of normal levator ani anatomy and function. Obstet Gynecol 99:433–438
17. Critchley HO, Dixon JS, Gosling JA (1980) Comparative study of the periurethral and perianal parts of the human levator ani muscle. Urol Int 35:226–232
18. Margulies RU, Hsu Y, Kearney R, Stein T, Umek WH, DeLancey JO (2006) Appearance of the levator ani muscle subdivisions in magnetic resonance images. Obstet Gynecol 107:1064–1069
19. Tunn R, Delancey JO, Howard D, Ashton-Miller JA, Quint LE (2003) Anatomic variations in the levator ani muscle, endopelvic fascia, and urethra in nulliparas evaluated by magnetic resonance imaging. Am J Obstet Gynecol 188:116–121
20. DeLancey JO, Morgan DM, Fenner DE et al (2007) Comparison of levator ani muscle defects and function in women with and without pelvic organ prolapse. Obstet Gynecol 109:295–302
21. Jackson SR, Avery NC, Tarlton JF, Eckford SD, Abrams P, Bailey AJ (1996) Changes in metabolism of collagen in genitourinary prolapse. Lancet 347:1658–1661
22. Boreham MK, Wai CY, Miller RT, Schaffer JI, Word RA (2002) Morphometric properties of the posterior vaginal wall in women with pelvic organ prolapse. Am J Obstet Gynecol 187:1501–1508; discussion 1508–1509
23. Boreham MK, Wai CY, Miller RT, Schaffer JI, Word RA (2002) Morphometric analysis of smooth muscle in the anterior vaginal wall of women with pelvic organ prolapse. Am J Obstet Gynecol 187:56–63
24. Singh K, Jakab M, Reid WM, Berger LA, Hoyte L (2003) Three-dimensional magnetic resonance imaging assessment of levator ani morphologic features in different grades of prolapse. Am J Obstet Gynecol 188:910–915
25. Loubeyre P, Copercini M, Petignat P, Dubuisson JB (2012) Levator ani muscle complex: anatomic findings in nulliparous patients at thin-section MR imaging with double opacification. Radiology 262:538–543
26. Weidner AC, Jamison MG, Branham V, South MM, Borawski KM, Romero AA (2006) Neuropathic injury to the levator ani occurs in 1 in 4 primiparous women. Am J Obstet Gynecol 195:1851–1856
27. Snooks SJ, Barnes PR, Swash M (1984) Damage to the innervation of the voluntary anal and periurethral sphincter musculature in incontinence: an electrophysiological study. J Neurol Neurosurg Psychiatry 47:1269–1273
28. Mattox TF, Lucente V, McIntyre P, Miklos JR, Tomezsko J (2000) Abnormal spinal curvature and its relationship to pelvic organ prolapse. Am J Obstet Gynecol 183:1381–1384; discussion 1384
29. Nguyen JK, Lind LR, Choe JY, McKindsey F, Sinow R, Bhatia NN (2000) Lumbosacral spine and pelvic inlet changes associated with pelvic organ prolapse. Obstet Gynecol 95:332–336
30. DeLancey JO (1986) Correlative study of paraurethral anatomy. Obstet Gynecol 68:91–97
31. Lienemann A, Anthuber C, Baron A, Reiser M (2000) Diagnosing enteroceles using dynamic magnetic resonance imaging. Dis Colon Rectum 43:205–212; discussion 212–213
32. Macura KJ, Genadry RR, Bluemke DA (2006) MR imaging of the female urethra and supporting ligaments in assessment of urinary incontinence: spectrum of abnormalities. Radiographics 26:1135–1149
33. Kelvin FM, Maglinte DD, Hornback JA, Benson JT (1992) Pelvic prolapse: assessment with evacuation proctography (defecography). Radiology 184:547–551
34. Pannu HK, Kaufman HS, Cundiff GW, Genadry R, Bluemke DA, Fishman EK (2000) Dynamic MR imaging of pelvic organ prolapse: spectrum of abnormalities. Radiographics 20:1567–1582
35. Maglinte DD, Bartram CI, Hale DA et al (2011) Functional imaging of the pelvic floor. Radiology 258:23–39
36. Kelvin FM, Hale DS, Maglinte DD, Patten BJ, Benson JT (1999) Female pelvic organ prolapse: diagnostic contribution of dynamic cystoproctography and comparison with physical examination. AJR Am J Roentgenol 173:31–37
37. Kelvin FM, Maglinte DD, Hale DS, Benson JT (2000) Female pelvic organ prolapse: a comparison of triphasic dynamic MR imaging and triphasic fluoroscopic cystocolpoproctography. AJR Am J Roentgenol 174:81–88
38. Schoenenberger AW, Debatin JF, Guldenschuh I, Hany TF, Steiner P, Krestin GP (1998) Dynamic MR defecography with a superconducting, open-configuration MR system. Radiology 206:641–646
39. Etlik O, Arslan H, Odabasi O et al (2005) The role of the MR-fluoroscopy in the diagnosis and staging of the pelvic organ prolapse. Eur J Radiol 53:136–141
40. Mellgren A, Johansson C, Dolk A et al (1994) Enterocele demonstrated by defaecography is associated with other pelvic floor disorders. Int J Colorectal Dis 9:121–124
41. Maubon A, Martel-Boncoeur MP, Juhan V et al (2000) Static and dynamic magnetic resonance imaging of the pelvic floor. J Radiol 81:1875–1886
42. Woodfield CA, Krishnamoorthy S, Hampton BS, Brody JM (2010) Imaging pelvic floor disorders: trend toward comprehensive MRI. AJR Am J Roentgenol 194:1640–1649
43. Margulies RU, Huebner M, DeLancey JO (2007) Origin and insertion points involved in levator ani muscle defects. Am J Obstet Gynecol 196:251.e1–255.e1
44. Law YM, Fielding JR (2008) MRI of pelvic floor dysfunction: review. AJR Am J Roentgenol 191:S45–S53
45. Huddleston HT, Dunnihoo DR, Huddleston PM 3rd, Meyers PC Sr (1995) Magnetic resonance imaging of defects in DeLancey's vaginal support levels I, II, and III. Am J Obstet Gynecol 172:1778–1782; discussion 1782–1784
46. Kim JK, Kim YJ, Choo MS, Cho KS (2003) The urethra and its supporting structures in women with stress urinary incontinence: MR imaging using an endovaginal coil. AJR Am J Roentgenol 180:1037–1044
47. El Sayed RF, El Mashed S, Farag A, Morsy MM, Abdel Azim MS (2008) Pelvic floor dysfunction: assessment with combined analysis of static and dynamic MR imaging findings. Radiology 248:518–530

48. Rociu E, Stoker J, Zwamborn AW, Lameris JS (1999) Endoanal MR imaging of the anal sphincter in fecal incontinence. Radiographics 19 Spec No:S171–S177

49. Boyadzhyan L, Raman SS, Raz S (2008) Role of static and dynamic MR imaging in surgical pelvic floor dysfunction. Radiographics 28:949–967

50. Comiter CV, Vasavada SP, Barbaric ZL, Gousse AE, Raz S (1999) Grading pelvic prolapse and pelvic floor relaxation using dynamic magnetic resonance imaging. Urology 54:454–457

51. Yang A, Mostwin JL, Rosenshein NB, Zerhouni EA (1991) Pelvic floor descent in women: dynamic evaluation with fast MR imaging and cinematic display. Radiology 179:25–33

52. Hetzer FH, Andreisek G, Tsagari C, Sahrbacher U, Weishaupt D (2006) MR defecography in patients with fecal incontinence: imaging findings and their effect on surgical management. Radiology 240:449–457

53. Singh K, Reid WM, Berger LA (2001) Assessment and grading of pelvic organ prolapse by use of dynamic magnetic resonance imaging. Am J Obstet Gynecol 185:71–77

54. Lienemann A, Anthuber C, Baron A, Kohz P, Reiser M (1997) Dynamic MR colpocystorectography assessing pelvic-floor descent. Eur Radiol 7:1309–1317

55. Kelvin FM, Maglinte DD, Benson JT, Brubaker LP, Smith C (1994) Dynamic cystoproctography: a technique for assessing disorders of the pelvic floor in women. AJR Am J Roentgenol 163:368–370

56. Felt-Bersma RJ, Cuesta MA (2001) Rectal prolapse, rectal intussusception, rectocele, and solitary rectal ulcer syndrome. Gastroenterol Clin North Am 30:199–222

57. Mahieu P, Pringot J, Bodart P (1984) Defecography: I. Description of a new procedure and results in normal patients. Gastrointest Radiol 9:247–251

58. Kelvin FM, Maglinte DD, Benson JT (1994) Evacuation proctography (defecography): an aid to the investigation of pelvic floor disorders. Obstet Gynecol 83:307–314

59. Halligan S, Bartram CI, Park HJ, Kamm MA (1995) Proctographic features of anismus. Radiology 197:679–682

60. Mortele KJ, Fairhurst J (2007) Dynamic MR defecography of the posterior compartment: indications, techniques and MRI features. Eur J Radiol 61:462–472

Index

J.N. Buy, M. Ghossain, *Gynecological Imaging*,
DOI 10.1007/978-3-642-31012-6, © Springer-Verlag Berlin Heidelberg 2013